Designed for the maintenance of good nutrition of practically all health people in the United States

Water-Soluble Vitamins							Minerals						
Vitamin C (mg)	Thiamin (mg)	Riboflavin (mg)	Niacin (mg NE)	Vitamin B6 (mg)	Folate (µg)	Vitamin B12 (µg)	Calcium (mg)	Phosphorus (mg)	Magnesium (mg)	Iron (mg)	Zinc (mg)	Iodine (µg)	Selenium (µg)
30	0.3	0.4	5	0.3	25	0.3	400	300	40	6	5	40	10
35	0.4	0.5	6	0.6	35	0.5	600	500	60	10	5	50	15
40	0.7	0.8	9	1.0	50	0.7	800	800	80	10	10	70	20
45	0.9	1.1	12	1.1	75	1.0	800	800	120	10	10	90	20
45	1.0	1.2	13	1.4	100	1.4	800	800	170	10	10	120	30
50	1.3	1.5	17	1.7	150	2.0	1,200	1,200	270	12	15	150	40
60	1.5	1.8	20	2.0	200	2.0	1,200	1,200	400	12	15	150	50
60	1.5	1.7	19	2.0	200	2.0	1,200	1,200	350	10	15	150	70
60	1.5	1.7	19	2.0	200	2.0	800	800	350	10	15	150	70
60	1.2	1.4	15	2.0	200	2.0	800	800	350	10	15	150	70
50	1.1	1.3	15	1.4	150	2.0	1,200	1,200	280	15	12	150	45
60	1.1	1.3	15	1.5	180	2.0	1,200	1,200	300	15	12	150	50
60	1.1	1.3	15	1.6	180	2.0	1,200	1,200	280	15	12	150	55
60	1.1	1.3	15	1.6	180	2.0	800	800	280	15	12	150	55
60	1.0	1.2	13	1.6	180	2.0	800	800	280	10	12	150	55
70	1.5	1.6	17	2.2	400	2.2	1,200	1,200	320	30	15	175	65
95	1.6	1.8	20	2.1	280	2.6	1,200	1,200	355	15	19	200	75
90	1.6	1.7	20	2.1	260	2.6	1,200	1,200	340	15	16	200	75

Retinol equivalents. 1 retinol equivalent = 1 µg retinol or 6 µg β-carotene.

[d] As cholecalciferol. 10 µg cholecalciferol = 400 IU of vitamin D.

[c] α-Tocopherol equivalents. 1 mg d-α tocopherol = 1 α-TE.

[f] 1 NE (niacin equivalent) is equal to 1 mg of niacin or 60 mg of dietary tryptophan.

Estimated Safe and Adequate Daily Dietary Intakes of Selected Vitamins and Minerals[a]

Category	Age (years)	Vitamins	
		Biotin (µg)	Pantothenic Acid (mg)
Infants	0-0.5	10	2
	0.5-1	15	3
Children and adolescents	1-3	20	3
	4-6	25	3-1
	7-10	30	4-5
	11+	30-100	4-7
Adults		30-100	4-7

Category	Age (years)	Trace Elements[b]				
		Copper (mg)	Manganese (mg)	Fluoride (µg)	Chromium (µg)	Molybdenum (mg)
Infants	0-0.5	0.4-0.6	0.3-0.6	0.1-0.5	10-40	15-30
	0.5-1	0.6-0.7	0.6-1.0	0.2-1.0	20-60	20-40
Children and adolescents	1-3	0.7-1.0	1.0-1.5	0.5-1.5	20-80	25-50
	4-6	1.0-1.5	1.5-2.0	1.0-2.5	30-120	30-75
	7-10	1.0-2.0	2.0-3.0	1.5-2.5	50-200	50-150
	11+	1.5-2.5	2.0-5.0	1.5-2.5	50-200	75-250
Adults		1.5-3.0	2.0-5.0	1.5-4.0	50-200	75-250

*Because there is less information on which to base allowances, these figures are not given in the main table of RDA and are provided here in the form of ranges of recommended intakes.

*Since the toxic levels for many trace elements may be only several times usual intakes, the upper levels for the trace elements given in this table should not be habitually exceeded.

CONTEMPORARY NUTRITION

ISSUES AND INSIGHTS

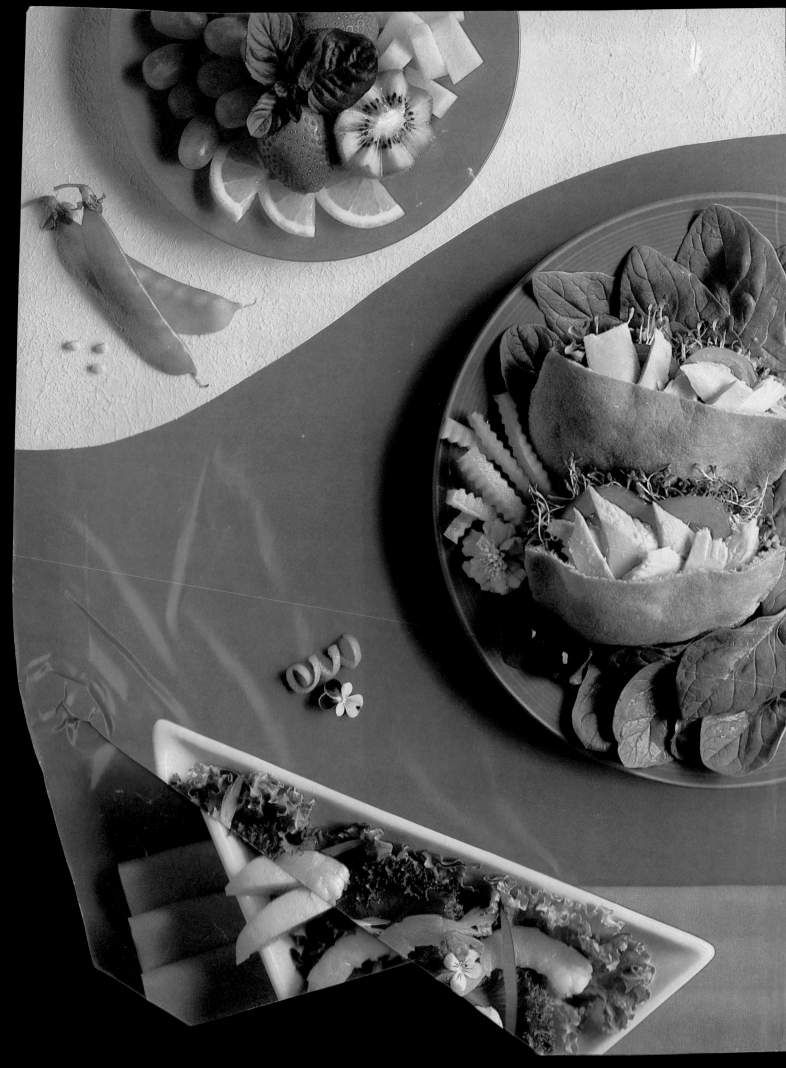

CONTEMPORARY NUTRITION

ISSUES AND INSIGHTS

GORDON M. WARDLAW, Ph.D., R.D., L.D.
The Ohio State University

PAUL M. INSEL, Ph.D.
Stanford University School of Medicine

MARCIA F. SEYLER, M.Phil.

with 309 illustrations

Illustrations by
Medical and Scientific Illustration:
William C. Ober, M.D.
Claire Garrison, R.N., B.A.

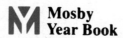

Mosby
Year Book

St. Louis   Baltimore   Boston   Chicago   London   Philadelphia   Sydney   Toronto

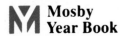

Mosby
Year Book

Dedicated to Publishing Excellence

Publisher: Edward F. Murphy
Acquisitions Editor: Vicki Van Ry-Malinee
Developmental Editor: Loren Stevenson
Project Manager: Karen Edwards
Production Editor: Cindy Miller
Production: Cindy Miller, Jeanne Genz,
            Ginny Douglas, and Jeanne Wolfgeher
Photographic Researcher: Kathy Sedovic
Text Design: WRK, Inc.
Design Coordinator: Jeanne Wolfgeher
Cover Design: Jeanne Wolfgeher
Cover Photography: WANS STUDIO, INC.
Cover Food Stylist: Irene Bertolucci

Printed in the United States of America

Mosby–Year Book, Inc.
11830 Westline Industrial Drive
St. Louis, MO 63146

Library of Congress Cataloging-in-Publication Data

Wardlaw, Gordon M.
    Contemporary nutrition: issues and insights / Gordon M. Wardlaw,
Paul M. Insel, Marcia F. Seyler.
      p.   cm.
    Includes bibliographical references (p.   ) and index.
    ISBN 0-8016-2348-0
    1. Nutrition.   I. Insel, Paul M.   II. Seyler, Marcia F.
III. Title.
QP141.W378   1991
613.2—dc20
                                      91-29473
                                          CIP

92 93 94 95 96 CL/CLD/VH 9 8 7 6 5 4 3 2

CONTEMPORARY NUTRITION

ISSUES AND INSIGHTS

GORDON M. WARDLAW, Ph.D., R.D., L.D.

The Ohio State University

PAUL M. INSEL, Ph.D.

Stanford University School of Medicine

MARCIA F. SEYLER, M.Phil.

with 309 illustrations

Illustrations by
Medical and Scientific Illustration:
William C. Ober, M.D.
Claire Garrison, R.N., B.A.

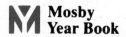 **Mosby**
Year Book

St. Louis   Baltimore   Boston   Chicago   London   Philadelphia   Sydney   Toronto

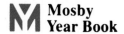
Mosby
Year Book
Dedicated to Publishing Excellence

Publisher: Edward F. Murphy
Acquisitions Editor: Vicki Van Ry-Malinee
Developmental Editor: Loren Stevenson
Project Manager: Karen Edwards
Production Editor: Cindy Miller
Production: Cindy Miller, Jeanne Genz,
         Ginny Douglas, and Jeanne Wolfgeher
Photographic Researcher: Kathy Sedovic
Text Design: WRK, Inc.
Design Coordinator: Jeanne Wolfgeher
Cover Design: Jeanne Wolfgeher
Cover Photography: WANS STUDIO, INC.
Cover Food Stylist: Irene Bertolucci

Printed in the United States of America

Mosby–Year Book, Inc.
11830 Westline Industrial Drive
St. Louis, MO 63146

Library of Congress Cataloging-in-Publication Data

Wardlaw, Gordon M.
    Contemporary nutrition: issues and insights / Gordon M. Wardlaw,
  Paul M. Insel, Marcia F. Seyler.
      p.   cm.
    Includes bibliographical references (p.   ) and index.
    ISBN 0-8016-2348-0
    1. Nutrition. I. Insel, Paul M. II. Seyler, Marcia F.
  III. Title.
  QP141.W378   1991
  613.2—dc20   91-29473
                                            CIP

92 93 94 95 96 CL/CLD/VH 9 8 7 6 5 4 3 2

ABOUT THE AUTHORS

GORDON M. WARDLAW, Ph.D., R.D., L.D., teaches nutrition to a variety of students at The Ohio State University. Dr. Wardlaw is the author of numerous articles in prominent nutrition, biology, physiology, and biochemistry journals and was the 1985 recipient of the Mary P. Huddleson Award from the American Dietetic Association. In 1991 Dr. Wardlaw was voted into the prestigious American Institute of Nutrition as a full member based on meritorious nutrition research.

PAUL M. INSEL, Ph.D., is currently Clinical Associate Professor of Psychiatry and Behavioral Sciences at Stanford University. He has been the principle investigator of numerous NIH studies, is the senior author of the leading introductory health text, and is Editor-in-Chief of *Healthline* magazine.

MARCIA F. SEYLER, M.Phil., is a freelance science writer and editor. She has been involved in the development of many college textbooks, specifically *Perspectives in Nutrition* by Gordon M. Wardlaw and Paul M. Insel. She has written numerous articles for *Healthline* magazine and other publications.

CONTENTS IN BRIEF

CONTENTS

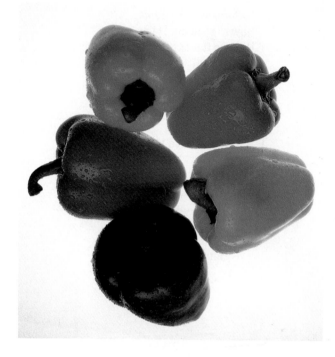

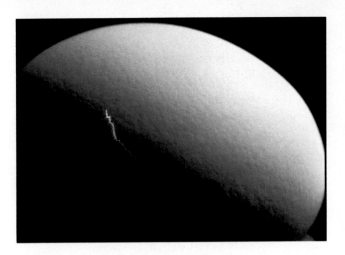

8 PROTEINS, 218

9 VITAMINS, 246

10 WATER AND MINERALS, 290

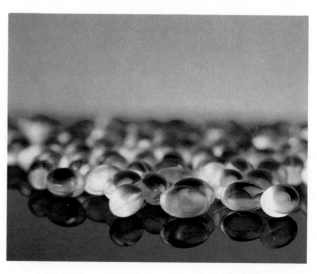

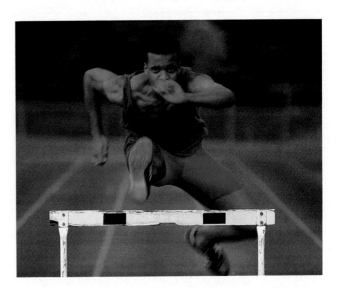

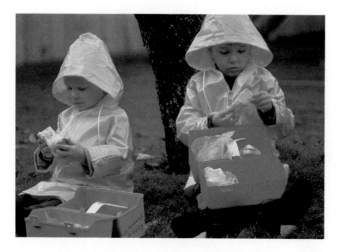

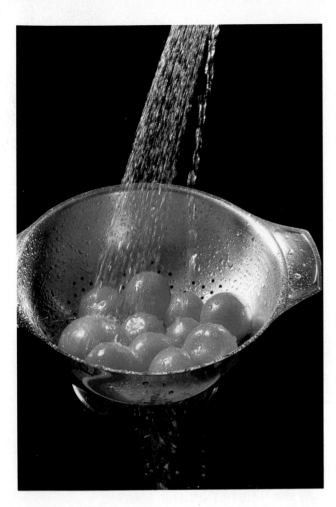

PART 5 • NUTRITION: BEYOND THE NUTRIENTS THEMSELVES

APPENDICES

PREFACE FOR THE INSTRUCTOR

As a professor, you undoubtedly already find nutrition a fascinating topic. However, it can also be quite frustrating to teach. There are countless claims and counterclaims about the need for certain constituents in our diet, such as dietary cholesterol. One group of researchers promotes a reduction in dietary cholesterol intake by all Americans over 2 years of age, while other researchers show that many people can eat a few eggs every day without significantly increasing their fasting blood cholesterol levels.

We, too, are frustrated by conflicting data in our field, and so have attempted to draw on as many sources as possible in writing this textbook. Many new major publications have guided us, such as the Surgeon General's Report on Nutrition and Health, the latest National Academy of Sciences Reports on Diet and Health and Nutrition During Pregnancy, and the tenth edition of the RDA. We have incorporated much of the material from these sources, especially the new RDA values, as well as information from many current review articles and basic scientific reports. We also have consulted with a number of experts who have provided their opinions of the current state of nutrition research as applicable to each chapter.

This textbook makes a break from all others in the field. Like other textbooks, it focuses on the latest research in nutrition. But it goes further to document important recent research studies and list those references at the back of the chapters. Nutrition Issues in each chapter then reexamine the most controversial nutrition topics of our day. In all, we provide students with a well-rounded view of current nutrition research so that they can more clearly understand and take part in the debate over current nutrition issues.

PERSONALIZING NUTRITION

One overriding theme in nutrition research today is *individuality*. Not all of us find that salt intake raises our blood pressure levels over recommended standards. Sugar does not raise everyone's blood glucose levels above accepted guidelines. We often respond in an idiosyncratic manner to nutrients, a fact that is constantly pointed out in this textbook.

Even at this basic level we do not try to put every nutrition student through the same square hole. We constantly ask students to learn more about themselves and their health status and suggest they apply the information given in a manner appropriate to improving their health. After reading this textbook, students will have a much clearer understanding of how the nutrition information given on the evening news, on cereal box labels, in popular magazines, and by government agencies applies to them. Most importantly, they will become knowledgeable consumers of nutrients and nutrition information. They will come to understand that nutrition knowledge allows them to personalize their diet, rather than following every guideline issued to a population—which by definition actually consists of separate individuals with separate genetic backgrounds and responses to diet.

In addition, we cover important questions that students often raise concerning vegetarianism, diets for athletes, the safety of our food supply, and fad diets. We emphasize the importance of behavior in terms of understanding one's food choices and changing one's diet. We discuss food behaviors in Chapter 1, behavior modification in Chapter 3, and behaviors that lead to obesity in Chapter 11.

AUDIENCE

This book has been designed for a nonmajors audience. The chemistry has been kept to a bare minimum. This book will be most suitable as a beginning textbook for any student interested either in an introduction to nutrition or in fulfilling a general science requirement. Health majors, Home Economics majors, Nursing students, Physical Education students, and students in other health-related areas will also find this text quite appropriate. Because of the flexibility of chapter organization and content, this book can be adapted to students of diverse backgrounds.

While the book is most suitable for a semester-length course, it can also be used in a quarter-length course by omitting chapters. A unique feature of this text is that it is presented in five segments:

Part 1: NUTRITION: A Foundation for Health
Part 2: NUTRIENTS: The Heart of Nutrition
Part 3: ENERGY: Balance and Imbalance
Part 4: NUTRITION: A Focus on Life Stages
Part 5: NUTRITION: Beyond the Nutrients Themselves

This organization facilitates tailoring the text to your specific course needs.

FEATURES
Content

We have organized this text to make up for weaknesses seen in many current textbooks:

Emphasis on changing behaviors. Chapter 3 encourages the student to plan his or her own diet to enhance health maintenance and then outlines how to do so. This chapter allows the student to take the foundations of a healthy food plan and apply it to daily life, allowing him or her to set nutritional goals and then change his or her own diet accordingly.

Detailed discussion of consumerism. In chapter 2 the student will learn how to decipher a food label. Chapter 4 discusses nutrition fads and fallacies in detail. These topics are often poorly covered by nutrition textbooks.

Separate chapters on weight control and eating disorders. The student receives a thorough discussion on these very controversial and current topics.

Early introduction of digestion and absorption. These topics are discussed before the energy-yielding nutrients. This enables students to obtain a good background in the basic entry of nutrients into the body before they learn how nutrients function in the body.

Review boxes. Some chapters contain large detailed review boxes that include the major points made in the chapter. These tables provide convenient capsules for reference.

Content and controversial topics are well referenced. Approximately 90% of the referenced material is from sources published since 1987; 60% is from sources published since 1988. As professors, we demand the latest information to present to our students. Providing this up-to-date research will not only give students the most accurate picture of nutrition today, but will also point them to current materials for further study.

DESIGN

Organizing the illustration program for this textbook has been quite exciting. We have drawn heavily from the nutrition expertise of Mosby–Year Book, and especially from the illustrators under the direction of William Ober, M.D. This textbook is far ahead of any in the field in depicting important nutrition-related phenomenons, such as cholesterol metabolism, emulsification, vitamin D. metabolism, digestion and absorption, the progression of cancer, and fetal development, in a nonthreatening way. The extensive, three-dimensional graphic presentations in this book will make nutrition come alive for students.

In addition, we have drawn on many sources to provide what we consider the best photographic program in any nutrition text. The numerous four-color photos for this text were researched and selected to reflect a modern view of food consumption and food presentation. This visually provides the student with the most outstanding and up-to-date view of the nutrition arena today.

Humor has been sprinkled throughout the text to aid the learning process. We have combed recent newspapers for the best work of our nation's leading cartoonists. The cartoons make important nutrition points in a way students will remember, such as Gary Larson's wolves hesitating to eat raw pork in Chapter 17.

PEDAGOGY

The following extensive pedagogical features were designed not only to interest the student but also to constantly reinforce the learning process.

Assess Yourself. This exercise at the beginning of each chapter helps students explore their food habits and ideally peaks their interest in the nutritional information in the chapter. For example, the assessment in Chapter 6 is on fiber intake, which is a key discussion point in the chapter.

Another Bite. These are short paragraphs spaced throughout the book that examine the application of the material or provide another vantage point from which to view, and possibly better appreciate, the text material.

Margin Definitions. Important key terms are boldfaced at first mention. More difficult terms include a definition in the text's margin. All boldfaced terms are included in the glossary at the back of the text.

Margin Notes. A liberal use of margin notes appear throughout the book. These notes provide extra examples, references to other chapters, clarification of ideas, and further details for important concepts.

Concept Checks. This material summarizes chapter content every few pages, providing the student with the opportunity to monitor his or her understanding of the material presented.

Rate Your Plate. This activity at the end of each chapter provides the student with an opportunity to put theory into practice. The suggested assignments generally have the student carefully analyze part of their current diet or nutrition-related lifestyle.

Nutrition Insights. Each chapter contains two to three short boxed essays on often controversial topics in nutrition, such as bottled water and fat replacements.

Summary Points. Chapter content is summarized by highlighting up to ten major points. This feature, together with the Concept Checks, should help students study for examinations.

Up-to-date References. Each chapter contains approximately 20 current references, most published since 1988.

How Much Have I Learned? This set of 15 true/false questions at the end of each chapter with answers at the end of the text serve to heighten awareness of chapter content. This feature also provides students with an opportunity to gauge how much they learned by repeating the quiz and comparing their scores in preparation for examinations.

Nutrition Issues. These essays at the end of each chapter extend the chapter content by adding more detailed and often controversial material. Topics include reading labels, conducting nutrition research, food allergies, and the safety of pesticides in foods.

Glossary. A comprehensive glossary is included for the student's reference. The glossary contains a list of common medical terms and their root definitions, as well as pronunciation inclusions for many unfamiliar terms.

SUPPLEMENTARY MATERIALS

Both the student and the instructor are provided with the latest materials to make better use of the text and the concepts of the course.

Instructor's manual and test bank. Prepared by Jeff Harris, D.H.Sc., R.D., this comprehensive teaching aid includes chapter summaries with suggestions for teaching difficult material; activities; suggested readings; nutrition assessments; conversion notes; source lists of supplementary materials; and a unique chapter on survival that discusses class organization, scheduling, and problem areas such as cheating. This chapter is addressed to the novice instructor.

Extensively reviewed for clarity and accuracy, the test bank features more than 1400 test items (multiple-choice, short-answer, and matching) coded for level of difficulty, the kind of knowledge being tested, and topic reference. Test items in each chapter follow the sequence of chapter discussions to make selection easy. The resource manual also includes 75 transparency masters of key illustrations selected from the text.

Diploma II computerized test bank. Qualified adopters of the text receive a computerized test bank package compatible with the IBM, Macintosh, Apple IIc, or Apple IIe microcomputers. This test bank provides a unique combination of user-friendly aids and enables the instructor to select, edit, delete, or add questions, and construct and print tests and answer keys. The Gradebook segment features computerized record-keeping, and class, test, or individual grade analysis displayed as bar charts. The Proctor segment allows instructors to set up student tutorials, using items from the Test Bank or specially written tests.

Study guide. Prepared by the primary author of the textbook Gordon M. Wardlaw, this student aid has been thoroughly reviewed by experienced instructors. This comprehensive guide reinforces concepts presented in the text and integrates them with study activities, such as the use of flash cards to reinforce key concepts. It features vocabulary review and sample examinations structured to reflect the actual examinations students will face in the classroom. An application of chapter material to the student's current lifestyle highlights each chapter.

Mosby Diet Simple nutrient analysis software. This interactive software includes a unique food list with more than 1900 items, selected activities, and food exchange lists. The disk allows students to input food intake and physical activities to determine total kcalories consumed and expended in a 24-hour period.

Transparency acetates. 72 full-color transparency acetates feature key illustrations from the text with large, easy-to-read labels.

ACKNOWLEDGMENTS

Text development

Barbara Freden, M.S. aided the authors in the difficult task of tailoring the content for a nonmajors audience. A scientist herself, she has extensive experience editing biology and general science textbooks.

Reviewers

As our goal throughout this project has been to provide the most accurate, up-to-date, and useful introductory nutrition text available, we have constantly called on the expert assistance of many noted colleagues in nutrition research and instruction:

Stephen Barrett, M.D.
Psychiatrist and Consumer Advocate
Index and Chapter 4

Linda Boyne, M.S., R.D.
The Ohio State University
Chapter 15

Sarah Burroughs, Ph.D.
California Polytechnic Institute
Chapter 14

Robert DiSilvestro, Ph.D.
The Ohio State University
Chapter 10

Murray Kaplan, Ph.D.
Iowa State University
Chapter 11

Alice Kubernick, M.S., R.D.
Cypress Community College
Chapter 18

Rose Ann Kutschke, Ph.D.
University of Texas-Austin
Chapter 7

Donald McCormick, Ph.D.
Emory University
Chapter 9

Robert Moffatt, Ph.D.
Florida State University
Chapter 12

Marla Reicks, Ph.D.
University of Minnesota
Chapter 17

Daphene Roe, M.D.
Cornell University
Chapter 16

Karla Roehring, Ph.D.
The Ohio State University
Chapter 6

Special gratitude must go to those people who reviewed the entire text. They will find their "fingerprints" throughout the text, because their valuable reviews shaped its outcome:

Sara Anderson, Ph.D., R.D.
Southern Illinois University-Carbondale

Joan Benson, M.S., R.D.
University of Utah

Effie Creamer, Ph.D.
Eastern Kentucky University

Julie Ray Friedman, Ph.D.
State University of New York-Farmingdale

Deloy Hendricks, Ph.D.
Utah State University

Michael Hudecki, Ph.D.
State University of New York-Buffalo

Wendy Hunt, M.S., R.D.
American River College

Gladys Jennings, M.S., R.D.
Washington State University

Nelda Loper, M.S., R.D.
Seminole Community College

Margaret Ann McCarthy, M.P.H., R.D.
Eastern Kentucky University

Marsha Read, Ph.D.
University of Nevada

Joanne Spaide, Ph.D.
University of Northern Iowa

Diana Spillman, Ph.D., R.D.
Miami University

Kay Stanek, Ph.D., R.D.
University of Nebraska

Ann Stasch, Ph.D.
California State University-Northridge

We would like to thank those people whose insight and direction guided us in the proposal stages, especially Richard Ahrens, University of Maryland, and Nelda Loper, Seminole Community College.

Special thanks also goes to Jeffrey Harris D.H.S.C. R.D., West Chester University, for his creative ideas and suggestions for the pedagogy.

SPECIAL ACKNOWLEDGMENTS

We would like to thank our developmental editors, first Vicki Van Ry, and later Loren Stevenson, who nurtured and assisted us every step of the tortuous journey. Vicki Van Ry, eventual Acquisitions Editor, and Ed Murphy, Vice President and Publisher, facilitated the difficult decisions that frequently arose. Kathy Sedovic researched most of the outstanding photographs, Cindy Miller provided excellent and careful copyediting and production work, and Karen Edwards managed the text through the production schedule.

This book would never have been completed without the help of Lorie Wardlaw. Many times the daily task of reforming the manuscript through numerous drafts fell on her shoulders. While this book was taking much of our free time for the last 2 years, our children William and Elizabeth Wardlaw and Claire and Philip Insel had to sometimes wait for their parents to finish the book in order to have their bedtime stories, go to the swimming pool, or walk the dog.

The book began with a commitment to simplify nutrition science for the nonmajor student, was fostered by the sense of accomplishment that finishing each element brought, and has ended in the establishment of an innovative and exciting textbook that we feel sets a new standard for nonmajors nutrition textbooks.

GORDON M. WARDLAW
PAUL M. INSEL
MARCIA F. SEYLER

STUDENT PREFACE

Oat bran, saturated fat, vegetarianism, high-fiber diets, cholesterol, anorexia nervosa, and *Salmonella* food poisoning—we suspect you have heard these terms. Which of these are important enough to be a consideration in your life?

Americans pride themselves on being individuals. Nutritional advice should be given in that manner. Not all of us have high cholesterol levels, and so don't face a high risk for heart disease. The need to tailor dietary advice to our individual nature is the basic philosophy behind this book. First, we give you a brief introduction to the study of nutrition and give you information on how to be a good consumer. With so much information floating around—both accurate and inaccurate—you will need to know how to make informed decisions about your nutritional well-being. Then, we encourage you to discover the basics of nutrition and how to apply the concepts in this book that specifically pertain to you.

We think you will find the study of nutrition fascinating. The text combines some of the most interesting and important elements of nutrition and food consumption to help you understand both how your body works and how what you eat affects your health.

FEATURES

We have included some features in this book that you should find especially interesting and valuable:

Planning a new way of eating. Chapter 3 begins by giving you useful advice on how to improve your dietary patterns. You will follow Alan, a typical college student, as he attempts to improve his diet. We'll show you how to set nutritional goals and design a diet plan to help you attain those goals.

Becoming an informed consumer. In Chapter 4, we discuss the critical information you will need to sort nutritional advice. With so much misleading information being published today, this chapter gives you, the consumer, the tools you will need to separate nutrition fact from fiction.

Understanding the world around us. In a college environment, it is often difficult to envision how real the problem of world hunger is. Chapter 18 examines the problem of undernutrition and the conditions that create it. The chapter allows you to examine possible solutions and visualize hope for the future of our planet.

PEDAGOGY

Contemporary Nutrition: Issues and Insights incorporates some important tools (called pedagogy) to help you learn nutrition. The next few pages graphically point out how to use these study aids to your best advantage.

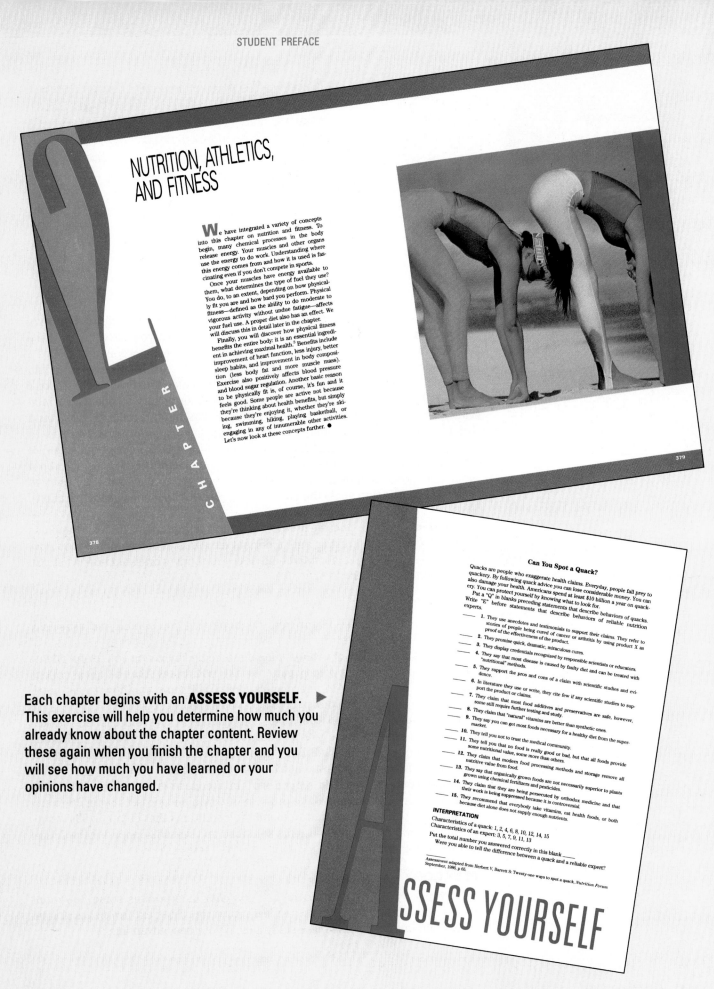

NUTRITION, ATHLETICS, AND FITNESS

We have integrated a variety of concepts into this chapter on nutrition and fitness. To begin, many chemical processes in the body release energy. Your muscles and other organs use the energy to do work. Understanding where this energy comes from and how it is used is fascinating even if you don't compete in sports.

Once your muscles have energy available to them, what determines the type of fuel they use? You do, to an extent, depending on how physically fit you are and how hard you perform. Physical fitness—defined as the ability to do moderate to vigorous activity without undue fatigue—affects your fuel use. A proper diet also has an effect. We will discuss this in detail later in the chapter.

Finally, you will discover how physical fitness benefits the entire body; it is an essential ingredient in achieving maximal health.[3] Benefits include improvement of heart function, less injury, better sleep habits, and improvement in body composition (less body fat and more muscle mass). Exercise also positively affects blood pressure and blood sugar regulation. Another basic reason to be physically fit is, of course, it's fun and it feels good. Some people are active not because they're thinking about health benefits, but simply because they're enjoying it, whether they're skiing, swimming, hiking, playing basketball, or engaging in any of innumerable other activities. Let's now look at these concepts further. ●

379

378

Each chapter begins with an ASSESS YOURSELF. ▶ This exercise will help you determine how much you already know about the chapter content. Review these again when you finish the chapter and you will see how much you have learned or your opinions have changed.

Can You Spot a Quack?

Quacks are people who exaggerate health claims. Everyday, people fall prey to quackery. By following quack advice you can lose considerable money. You can also damage your health. Americans spend at least $10 billion a year on quackery. You can protect yourself by knowing what to look for.

Put a "Q" in blanks preceding statements that describe behaviors of quacks. Write "E" before statements that describe behaviors of reliable nutrition experts.

_____ 1. They use anecdotes and testimonials to support their claims. They refer to stories of people being cured of cancer or arthritis by using product X as proof of the effectiveness of the product.

_____ 2. They promise quick, dramatic, miraculous cures.

_____ 3. They display credentials recognized by responsible scientists or educators.

_____ 4. They say that most disease is caused by faulty diet and can be treated with "nutritional" methods.

_____ 5. They support the pros and cons of a claim with scientific studies and evidence.

_____ 6. In literature they use or write, they cite few if any scientific studies to support the product or claims.

_____ 7. They claim that most food additives and preservatives are safe, however, some still require further testing and study.

_____ 8. They claim that "natural" vitamins are better than synthetic ones.

_____ 9. They say you can get most foods necessary for a healthy diet from the supermarket.

_____ 10. They tell you not to trust the medical community.

_____ 11. They tell you that no food is really good or bad, but that all foods provide some nutritional value, some more than others.

_____ 12. They claim that modern food processing methods and storage remove all nutritive value from food.

_____ 13. They say that organically grown foods are not necessarily superior to plants grown using chemical fertilizers and pesticides.

_____ 14. They claim that they are being persecuted by orthodox medicine and that their work is being suppressed because it is controversial.

_____ 15. They recommend that everybody take vitamins, eat health foods, or both because diet alone does not supply enough nutrients.

INTERPRETATION

Characteristics of a quack: 1, 2, 4, 6, 8, 10, 12, 14, 15
Characteristics of an expert: 3, 5, 7, 9, 11, 13

Put the total number you answered correctly in this blank _____
Were you able to tell the difference between a quack and a reliable expert?

Assessment adapted from Herbert V, Barrett S: Twenty-one ways to spot a quack, *Nutrition Forum* September, 1986, p 65.

SSESS YOURSELF

◀ At the end of each chapter is a **RATE YOUR PLATE** section that will help you put a major concept in each chapter into focus for your own life. The activity encourages you to look more carefully at your diet, examine your family history, or apply information learned to help others.

RATE YOUR
P L A T E

DOES YOUR DIET MEET THE RDA?

Instructions: Perform either part I or part II. Then perform part III. (For assistance in following the instructions for this activity, see the sample Assessment in Appendix D.)

Part I.

A. Take the information from the 1-day food intake record you completed in Chapter 1 and record it on the blank form provided in Appendix D. Make sure to record the food or drink ingested and the amount (weight) consumed. NOTE: Your professor may require you to keep the food record for more than 1 day.

B. Review the 1989 RDA on the inside cover of the book and choose the appropriate recommendations for your gender and age. Write the appropriate value for each nutrient on the line labeled "Your RDA."
NOTE: The values for sodium and potassium from the table on the inside cover of the book are labeled, "Estimated Sodium, Chloride, and Potassium Minimum Requirements of Healthy Persons."

C. Look up the foods and drinks you've listed on the form in the food composition table, Appendix A. Record on the form the amounts of each nutrient and kcalories present in them.

D. For each food and drink, add the amounts in each column and record the results on the line labeled "Totals."

E. Compare the totals to your RDA's. Divide the total for each nutrient by the specific RDA or minimum requirement and multiply that by 100. Record the result on the line labeled, "% of your RDA."

F. Hold on to this assessment for use in subsequent activities for other chapters.

Part II.

A. Obtain copies of the computer software, Mosby Diet Simple, from your instructor, as well as directions for using it. Follow the instructions and load the software into the computer.

B. Choose your RDA based on your age and gender.

C. Enter the information from the 1-day food intake record you completed in Chapter 1. Make sure to enter each food and drink and the appropriate serving size.

D. This software program will give you the following results:
   a. Your 1989 RDA value for each nutrient.
   b. The total amount of each nutrient and kcalories consumed for the day.
   c. The percentage of the RDA 1989 values you consumed for each nutrient.

E. Hold on to this assessment for use in subsequent activities in other chapters.

The numerous **tables** throughout the text provide convenient capsules of information for your reference. ▶

TABLE 2-1

The Guide to Daily Food Choices—a summary

Food Group	Serving	Major Contributions	Foods and Serving Sizes*
Milk, yogurt, and cheese	2 (adult‖) 3 (children, teens, young adults, and pregnant or lactating women)	Calcium Riboflavin Protein Potassium Zinc	1 cup milk 1½ oz cheese 2 oz processed cheese 1 cup yogurt 2 cups cottage cheese 1 cup custard/pudding 1½ cups ice cream
Meat, poultry, fish, dry beans, eggs, and nuts	2-3	Protein Niacin Iron Vitamin B-6 Zinc Thiamin Vitamin B-12†	2-3 oz cooked meat, poultry, fish 1-1½ cups cooked dry beans 4 T peanut butter 2 eggs ½-1 cup nuts
Fruits	2-4	Vitamin C Fiber	¼ cup dried fruit ½ cup cooked fruit ¾ cup juice 1 whole piece of fruit 1 melon wedge
Vegetables	3-5	Vitamin A Vitamin C Folate Magnesium Fiber	½ cup raw or cooked vegetables 1 cup raw leafy vegetables
Bread, cereals, rice, and pasta	6-11	Starch Thiamin Riboflavin§ Iron Niacin Folate Magnesium‡ Fiber‡ Zinc‡	1 slice of bread 1 oz ready-to-eat cereal ½-¾ cup cooked cereal, rice, or pasta
Fats, oils, and sweets		Foods from this group should not replace any from the other groups. Amounts consumed should be determined by individual energy needs.	

This is a practical way to turn the RDA into food choices. You can get all essential nutrients by eating a balanced variety of foods each day from the food groups listed here. Eat a variety of foods in each food group and adjust serving sizes appropriately to reach and maintain desirable weight.

*May be reduced for child servings.
†Only in animal food choices.
‡Whole grains especially.
§If enriched.
‖≥ 25 years of age.

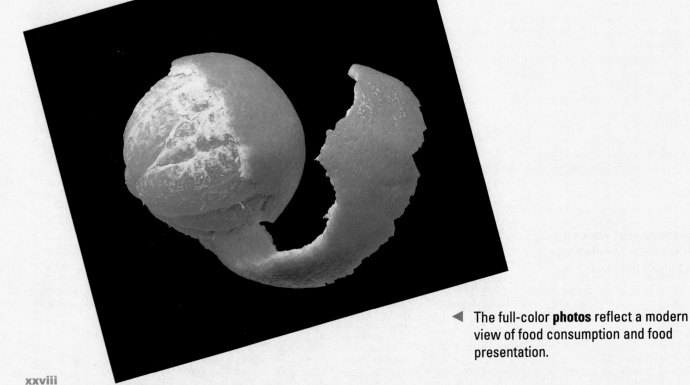

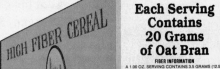

Nutritional information is required on all products that make a nutritional claim or add a nutrient.

Making Sense of the U.S. RDA

U.S. RDA are recommended daily nutrient standards developed for use in the nutrition labeling of food products. Because nutrient needs vary among individuals, the U.S. RDA are set high enough to cover the needs of nearly everyone.

To calculate the amount of iron in one serving, multiply 0.30 times the U.S. RDA of 18 milligrams (see Appendix E): $0.3 \times 18 = 5.4$ milligrams of iron per serving.

You'll find that the numerous full-color, 3-dimensional **illustrations** almost jump off the page. No other nutrition textbook provides you with effective, detailed anatomical drawings that virtually "come alive."

Oat Bran Per Serving

Label lists the grams of oat bran per serving. The serving size of ready-to-eat Oat Bran cereal is 28 grams (1 ounce or ¾ cup). Serving size, which is arbitrary, affects per serving amounts of everything else.

Fat

There are 9 kcalories in each gram of fat. The percentage of kcalories from fat is determined by multiplying the number of fat grams by nine, dividing that by the number of kcalories, and then multiplying by 100. This cereal derives 18% of its kcalories from fat.

Sodium

Sodium is frequently listed on food product labels. Sodium occurs naturally in some foods and is sometimes added for taste or in production.

Ingredients

For most foods, the ingredients must be listed on the label. The ingredient present in the largest amount, by weight, must be listed first, followed by other ingredients in descending order. However, an ingredient label doesn't tell you how much of an ingredient is actually in the product. For example, although sugar is listed as the second ingredient, it is actually a relatively small portion of the ingredients.

Manufacturer's Name and Address

The manufacturer's name and address is included on the package.

◀ The full-color **photos** reflect a modern view of food consumption and food presentation.

How Much Have I Learned? questions at the end of each chapter help you determine how well you have retained chapter material. These questions will help you prepare and study for examinations. ▶

HOW MUCH HAVE I LEARNED?

9 VITAMINS

What have you learned from Chapter 9? Here are 15 statements about vitamins. Read them to test your current knowledge. If you think the answer is true or mostly true, circle T. If you think the answer is false or mostly false, circle F. Use the scoring key at the end of the book to compute your total score. To review, take this test again later, and especially before tests.

1. T F If a vitamin is missing from your diet for 1 week, you are risking a vitamin deficiency.
2. T F People who use mineral oil as a laxative at mealtimes are susceptible to fat-soluble vitamin deficiencies.
3. T F Vitamin D improves calcium absorption.
4. T F Vitamin A is important for night vision.
5. T F Vitamin D is synthesized by sunlight.
6. T F Vitamin K is important for blood clotting.
7. T F Vitamin B-6 can prevent premenstrual syndrome by influencing neurotransmitter levels.
8. T F Thiamin needs are related to the amount of fat one eats.
9. T F Milk is a good source of riboflavin.
10. T F Using an amino acid, the body can make niacin.
11. T F A niacin deficiency causes severe skin inflammation.
12. T F The term folate comes from the word foliage.
13. T F Vitamin B-12 is concentrated only in animal foods.
14. T F Vitamin C enhances iron absorption.
15. T F High doses of vitamin C can prevent the common cold.

289

Throughout each chapter are **boldfaced key terms.** These are terms you will need to be familiar with throughout your study. The more difficult terms will include a definition in the text's margins. All boldfaced terms will appear with their definitions and pronunciations in the **glossary** at the end of the text.
▼

2 THE RIGHT DIET FOR YOU

RDA for all recommended nutrients rather than run the risk of developing health problems from poor nutrition.[8]

Estimated Safe and Adequate Daily Dietary Intakes

The Food and Nutrition Board sets **estimated safe and adequate daily dietary intakes (ESADDI)** for several nutrients that have no true RDA, including copper, biotin, and chromium (see the inside cover for values). The board feels that information on these nutrients is too incomplete to set an RDA but detailed enough to set a range for a reasonable group intake.[8] By providing a range, the ESADDI not only recommend intake to meet nutritional needs, but also discourage people from eating too much of these nutrients. The Board also sets **minimum requirements for health** for sodium, potassium, and chloride. Note that these nutrients do not have RDA or ESADDI.[8]

Some nutrients—carbohydrates and fats, for example—still have no RDA, ESADDI, or minimum requirement for health. Still, our needs for these nutrients can easily be met by eating a diet that meets our established nutrient needs. Chapters 6 and 7 will discuss this issue in more detail.

RDA for energy needs

The RDA for energy estimates average energy needs for physically active people of various age groups and then suggests a wide range for the allowance (see inside cover for recommendations). Note that no extra amount is added for variabilities, as is done for nutrient RDA. Energy intake really are only rough estimates. For most adults, weight maintenance is the best gauge of whether energy intake matching kcalorie output.

Estimated Safe and Adequate Daily Dietary Intake (ESADDI) • Nutrient intake recommendations made by the Food and Nutrition Board where a range for intake of some nutrients is given because not enough information is available to set an RDA.

U.S. Recommended Daily Allowances (U.S. RDA) • Nutrient standards established by the FDA for use on nutrition labels. Generally the four existing versions use the highest nutrient recommendation in the appropriate age and gender category from the 1968 publication of the RDA. The version that includes children over 4 years and adults is most commonly used on nutrition labels.

Nutrition Insights are boxed essays that allow you to explore timely topics that are of interest to you.

Another Bite boxes are short paragraphs within the text designed to provide you with a different perspective on chapter material. You'll discover new and different ways to apply information.

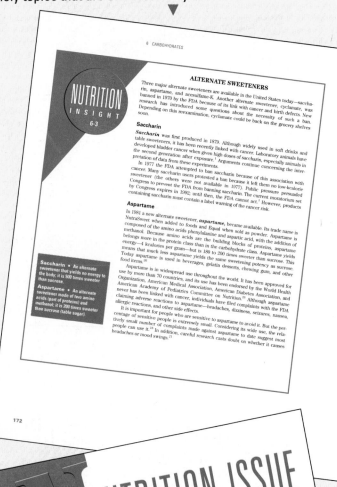

6 CARBOHYDRATES

NUTRITION INSIGHT 6-3

ALTERNATE SWEETENERS

Three major alternate sweeteners are available in the United States today—saccharin, aspartame, and acesulfame-K. Another alternate sweetener, cyclamate, was banned in 1970 by the FDA because of its link with cancer and birth defects. New research has introduced some questions about the necessity of such a ban. Depending on this reexamination, cyclamate could be back on the grocery shelves soon.

Saccharin

Saccharin was first produced in 1879. Although widely used in soft drinks and table sweeteners, it has been recently linked with cancer. Laboratory animals have developed bladder cancer when given high doses of saccharin. Arguments concerning the interpretation of data from these experiments.[1]

In 1977 the FDA attempted to ban saccharin because of this association with cancer. Many saccharin users protested a ban because it left them no low-kcalorie sweetener (the others were not available in 1977). Public pressure persuaded Congress to prevent the FDA from banning saccharin. The current moratorium set by Congress expires in 1992; until then, the FDA cannot act.[1] However, products containing saccharin must contain a label warning of the cancer risk.

Aspartame

In 1981 a new alternate sweetener, *aspartame*, became available. Its trade name is NutraSweet when added to foods and Equal when sold as powder. Aspartame is composed of the amino acids phenylalanine and aspartic acid, with the addition of methanol. Because amino acids are the building blocks of proteins, aspartame belongs more in the protein class than in the carbohydrate class. Aspartame yields energy—4 kcalories per gram—but is 180 to 200 times sweeter than sucrose. This means that much less aspartame yields the same sweetening potency as sucrose. Today aspartame is used in beverages, gelatin desserts, chewing gum, and other food items.[20]

Aspartame is in widespread use throughout the world. It has been approved for use by more than 70 countries, and its use has been endorsed by the World Health Organization, American Medical Association, American Diabetes Association, and American Academy of Pediatrics Committee on Nutrition.[20] Although aspartame never has been linked with cancer, individuals have filed complaints with the FDA claiming adverse reactions to aspartame—headaches, dizziness, seizures, nausea, allergic reactions, and other side effects.

It is important for people who are sensitive to aspartame to avoid it. But the percentage of sensitive people is extremely small. Considering its wide use, the relatively small number of complaints made against aspartame to date suggest most people can use it.[18] In addition, careful research casts doubt on whether it causes headaches or mood swings.[21]

Saccharin • An alternate sweetener that yields no energy to the body; it is 500 times sweeter than sucrose.

Aspartame • An alternate sweetener made of two amino acids (part of proteins) and methanol; it is 200 times sweeter than sucrose (table sugar).

172

6 CARBOHYDRATES

ANOTHER BITE

You may be left still feeling hungry after consuming an aspartame-sweetened beverage on an empty stomach.[19] This is because you essentially tried to quell hunger with carbonated water. Your usual sugared soft drink would have led to a rise in blood glucose levels and in turn reduced hunger (see Chapter 11 for a look at the glucose-hunger link). A possible solution is to combine these diet beverages with a small meal. This way you can save the kcalories that you would have consumed from the simple sugar-laden beverage and provide energy to quell your hunger from healthier foods.

Aspartame's high phenylalanine content concerns some people. They feel the blood levels of this amino acid may increase too much because aspartame is not balanced by the other amino acids normally found in protein foods. This situation can be easily avoided by consuming aspartame with protein foods. Some people also are concerned about aspartame's methanol content. However, the amount of methanol in a soft drink sweetened with aspartame is not more than is found in a cup of many fruit or vegetable juices.

Overall, the scientific community agrees that aspartame itself is safe; as we said numerous scientific and medical groups support its use. An acceptable daily intake set by FDA is equivalent to about 14 cans of diet soft drinks a day for an adult, or about 80 packets of Equal. Aspartame is safe for children and pregnant women to consume, but some scientists suggest cautious use by these groups.[15,20]

One final note about aspartame. A rare disease called *phenylketonuria* (PKU) prevents a person from metabolizing phenylalanine. We discuss PKU in Chapter 8. For now, note that you were tested for this disease as an infant, usually before leaving the hospital. Labels on products containing aspartame warn people with PKU against using the product. Individuals carrying only one PKU gene do not have the disease and can consume aspartame.[26] Only a person with two PKU genes has inherited the disease and should not use aspartame.

Acesulfame-K

The newest alternate sweetener in the United States, *acesulfame-K* (Sunette), was approved by the FDA in July 1988. Acesulfame-K is 200 times sweeter than sucrose. Presently, it can be used in chewing gum, powdered drink mixes, gelatins, puddings, and nondairy creamers. It contributes no kcalories to the diet because it is not broken down by the body.

Some studies show that laboratory animals develop cancer after exposure to acesulfame-K. However, the FDA's analysis of these studies suggests that the tumors were not caused by acesulfame-K consumption. They were routinely seen in the untreated animal species studied. Therefore acesulfame-K has FDA approval. It is already used as a sweetener in foods and beverages in at least 20 countries. Acesulfame-K can be used in baking, whereas the current form of aspartame cannot because it breaks down when heated. So acesulfame-K may see wider uses. Currently, little information has been published about acesulfame-K. ●

Phenylketonuria (PKU) • A disease in which the liver cannot readily metabolize the amino acid phenylalanine. Toxic byproducts of phenylalanine can then build up in the body and lead to mental retardation.

Acesulfame-K • An alternate sweetener that yields no energy to the body; it is 200 times sweeter than sucrose.

A few other alternate sugars—single-sugar alcohols—appear in foods. Today the major one used is sorbitol. This is found in sugarless gum. It yields kcalories but is not readily metabolized in the mouth. Thus sorbitol does not promote dental caries (cavities).

173

To briefly clarify and expand concepts presented, **margin notes** are provided for you. These help reinforce concepts you'll learn in every chapter.

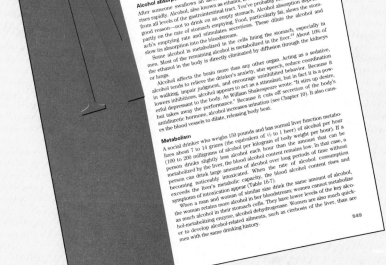

NUTRITION ISSUE

ETHANOL—ITS METABOLISM AND POTENTIAL TO INFLUENCE HEALTH

Alcoholism is an important issue for all adults to carefully examine. From early adulthood through elderly years, alcohol's ability to tear away at nutritional and overall health is enormous.

Alcohol absorption and action

After someone swallows an alcoholic beverage, their blood level of alcohol rises rapidly. Alcohol, also known as ethanol, is readily absorbed into the blood from all levels of the gastrointestinal tract. You've probably been warned—with good reason—not to drink on an empty stomach. Food, particularly fat, slows the stomach's emptying rate and stimulates secretions. These dilute the alcohol and slow its absorption into the bloodstream.

Some alcohol is metabolized in the cells lining the stomach, especially in men. Most of the remaining alcohol is metabolized in the liver.[24] About 10% of the ethanol in the body is directly eliminated by diffusion through the kidneys or lungs.

Alcohol affects the brain more than any other organ. Acting as a sedative, alcohol tends to relieve the drinker's anxiety, slur speech, reduce coordination in walking, impair judgment, and encourage uninhibited behavior. Because it lowers inhibitions, alcohol appears to act as a stimulant, but in fact it is a powerful depressant to the body. As William Shakespeare wrote: "It stirs up desire, but takes away the performance." Because it cuts off secretion of the body's antidiuretic hormone, alcohol increases urination (see Chapter 10). It also causes the blood vessels to dilate, releasing body heat.

Metabolism

A social drinker who weighs 150 pounds has normal liver function metabolizes about 7 to 14 grams (the equivalent of ½ to 1 beer) of alcohol per hour (100 to 200 milligrams of alcohol per kilogram of body weight per hour). If a person drinks slightly less alcohol each hour than the amount that can be metabolized by the liver, the blood alcohol content remains low. In that case, a person can drink large amounts of alcohol over long periods of time without becoming noticeably intoxicated. When the rate of alcohol consumption exceeds the liver's metabolic capacity, the blood alcohol content rises and symptoms of intoxication appear (Table 16-7).

When a man and woman of similar size drink the same amount of alcohol, the woman retains more alcohol in her bloodstream; women cannot metabolize as much alcohol in their stomach cells. They have lower levels of the key alcohol-metabolizing enzyme, alcohol dehydrogenase. Women are also much quicker to develop alcohol-related ailments, such as cirrhosis of the liver, than are men with the same drinking history.

549

Nutrition Issues are essays at the end of chapters that develop current topics in nutrition in greater detail than the chapter can. Topics include nutrition and alcohol, heart disease, cancer, fad diets, and nutrition labeling.

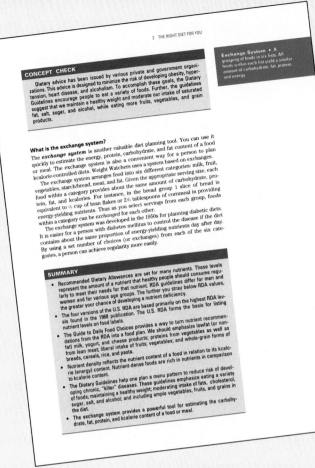

CONCEPT CHECK

Dietary advice has been issued by various private and government organizations. This advice is designed to minimize the risk of developing obesity, hypertension, heart disease, and alcoholism. To accomplish these goals, the Dietary Guidelines encourage people to eat a variety of foods. Further, the guidelines suggest that we maintain a healthy weight and moderate our intake of saturated fat, salt, sugar, and alcohol, while eating more fruits, vegetables, and grain products.

Exchange System • A grouping of foods in six lists. All foods within each list yield a similar amount of carbohydrate, fat, protein, and energy.

What is the exchange system?

The *exchange system* is another valuable diet planning tool. You can use it quickly to estimate the energy, protein, carbohydrate, and fat content of a food or meal. The exchange system is also a convenient way for a person to plan kcalorie-controlled diets. Weight Watchers uses a system based on exchanges.

The exchange system arranges food into six different categories: milk, fruit, vegetables, starch/bread, meat, and fat. Given the appropriate serving size, each food within a category provides about the same amount of carbohydrate, protein, fat, and kcalories. For instance, in the bread group 1 slice of bread is equivalent to ½ cup of bran flakes or 2½ tablespoons of cornmeal in providing energy-yielding nutrients. Thus as you select servings from each group, foods within a category can be *exchanged* for each other.

The exchange system was developed in the 1950s for planning diabetic diets. It is easier for a person with diabetes mellitus to control the disease if the diet contains about the same proportion of energy-yielding nutrients day after day. By using a set number of choices (or exchanges) from each of the six categories, a person can achieve regularity more easily.

SUMMARY

- Recommended Dietary Allowances are set for many nutrients. These levels represent the amount of a nutrient that healthy people should consume regularly to meet their needs for that nutrient. RDA guidelines differ for men and women and for various age groups. The further you stray below RDA values, the greater your chance of developing a nutrient deficiency.
- The four versions of the U.S. RDA are based primarily on the highest RDA levels found in the 1968 publication. The U.S. RDA forms the basis for listing nutrient levels on food labels.
- The Guide to Daily Food Choices provides a way to turn nutrient recommendations from the RDA into a food plan. We should emphasize lowfat (or nonfat) milk, yogurt, and cheese products; proteins from vegetables as well as from lean meat; liberal intake of fruits; vegetables; and whole-grain forms of breads, cereals, rice, and pasta.
- Nutrient density reflects the nutrient content of a food in relation to its kcalorie (energy) content. Nutrient-dense foods are rich in nutrients in comparison to kcalorie content.
- The Dietary Guidelines help one plan a menu pattern to reduce risk of developing chronic, "killer" diseases. These guidelines emphasize eating a variety of foods; maintaining a healthy weight; moderating intake of fats, cholesterol, sugar, salt, and alcohol; and including ample vegetables, fruits, and grains in the diet.
- The exchange system provides a powerful tool for estimating the carbohydrate, fat, protein, and kcalorie content of a food or meal.

The **Concept Checks** list the major points made in a chapter section. If you don't understand what the Concept Check says, you should reread the preceding section in the textbook.

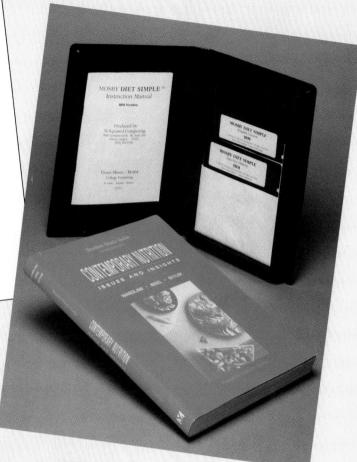

A Student Study Guide and Mosby Diet Simple software are available to you with *Contemporary Nutrition: Issues and Insights.* These instructional aids are designed to help you practice the major concepts developed in each chapter and prepare for classroom examinations.

Student Study Guide

Reviewed by instructors and developed in consultation with a learning theory expert, this valuable Study Guide by Gordon Wardlaw reinforces concepts presented in the text and integrates them with activities to facilitate learning.

- Sample examinations reflect the actual tests you will face in the classroom.
- Vocabulary review exercises increase your knowledge of terminology.
- Flash cards help you practice explaining the major concepts in the chapter to yourself, and in turn test your understanding of these important concepts.
- Activities include fill-in tables, labeling, and matching terms. These activities follow the text discussion and are anchored with quotations and page citations from the text. An ongoing dietary analysis highlights the content of many chapters.

Mosby Diet Simple nutrient analysis software

Created by N-Squared Computing, the nutrient analysis computer software is designed to help you quickly calculate the nutrient content of your diet, learn more about the exchange system, and calculate how many kcalories you use each day. You will find that learning to use this software will help you analyze your diet more efficiently.

1

NUTRITION

A
FOUNDATION
FOR
HEALTH

WHAT YOU EAT AND WHY

Do you need vitamin and mineral supplements? Are you getting too much cholesterol? Is much of what you eat unsafe? Are *junk foods* really that bad? Should you become a vegetarian? If you're confused about what you should eat, welcome to what is probably the fastest-growing club in the country.

Why should a daily activity that is necessary and usually enjoyable pose so many problems? For some time the media have been blasting us with information about nutrition and health. Headlines trumpet *breakthroughs* that frequently break down after further study.[12] Bookstores display row after row of nutrition books—some excellent, some so-so, some ridiculous—that presumably are the last word on what to eat and what to avoid. Some food manufacturers gleefully cash in on the latest nutritional marvel (whose wonders often turn out to be based on limited research).

But both the overrated claims and the sensible information spring from the same root. As the 1988 *Surgeon General's Report on Nutrition and Health* put it: "For the two out of three adult Americans who do not smoke and do not drink excessively, one personal choice seems to influence long-term health prospects more than any other: what we eat."[20] What some of us eat isn't in tune with our personal health risks. So, sooner or later, we're in trouble. Because we live longer than our ancestors did, we must focus more on preventing nutrition-related diseases.[7,10] ●

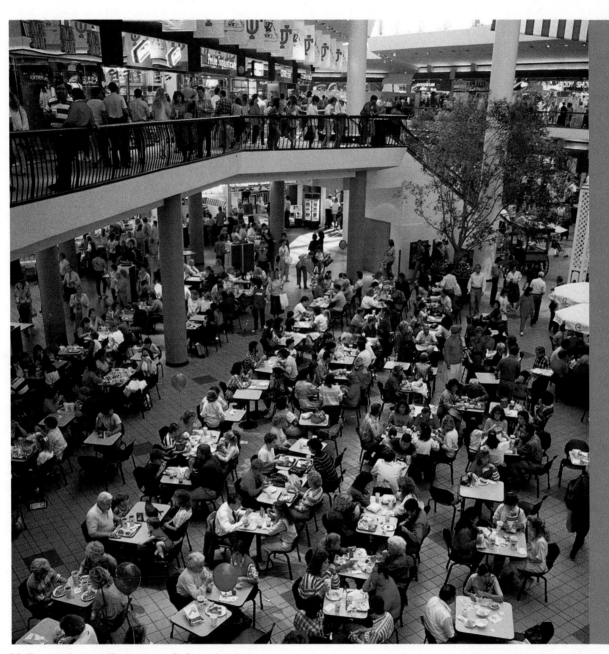

Mall munchers roll eating and shopping into one.

What Factors Determine Your Food Choices?

What are your favorite foods? Why do you like them? If only the taste buds determine food preferences, you probably wouldn't try strong tasting or spicy foods. Which foods do most of the members of your family enjoy together? Which foods are consistently excluded, if any? Use the following survey to discover how significantly the factors listed determine why you eat the way you do? Circle the number reflecting the most appropriate answer.

	Not significant at all					Very significant
1. Weight Control	(0)	1	2	3	4	5
2. Health	(0)	1	2	3	4	5
3. Food Costs	0	1	(2)	3	4	5
4. Convenience/Time	0	1	(2)	3	4	5
5. Family Background	(0)	1	2	3	4	5
6. Advertisements (TV or Radio)	0	(1)	2	3	4	5
7. Emotions	(0)	1	2	3	4	5
8. Peers (Friends, Coworkers)	(0)	1	2	3	4	5
9. Customs/Ethnic Background	0	(1)	2	3	4	5
10. Physical Activity Level	(0)	1	2	3	4	5

INTERPRETATION

Take note of the factors that scored 4 or 5. These are your most significant influences. Next to these put a PLUS (+) or MINUS (−) sign to indicate whether you feel they have been a positive or negative influence in terms of health.

In this chapter we want you to examine what you eat and why so you understand the origins of your eating habits. We begin with a general discussion of why we eat what we do. Then we ask you to complete an activity that focuses on your reasons for choosing certain foods in a day's menu.

ASSESS YOURSELF

HOW DO YOUR OWN FOOD HABITS MEASURE UP?

Although the science of **nutrition** is relatively young, we already know what nutrients are needed for an adequate diet and the foods that provide them. In a lifetime you will eat about 70,000 meals and 60 tons of food. In this opening chapter we encourage you to take a close look at your eating habits and discover the underlying reasons for them. This is an important first step. If you make even small changes in your behavior toward food, you can increase your chances for enjoying a long and vigorous life.[20] The more you know about nutrition and your health risks, the better you can plan diets to meet your nutritional needs.

Recent evidence points to poor diet as a **risk factor** for **chronic** diseases that are the leading causes of death: **heart disease, stroke, hypertension, diabetes mellitus,** and some types of **cancer.**[20] Together, these disorders account for two thirds of all deaths in North America (Table 1-1).[16] Not getting enough **nutrients** also makes us more likely to suffer later bone fractures (from the disease **osteoporosis**) and iron-deficiency **anemia.** At the same time, taking too much of a nutrient supplement, such as vitamin A, vitamin B-6, or copper, can be harmful. Another dietary problem, drinking too much alcohol, is associated with **cirrhosis** of the liver, some forms of cancer, accidents, and suicides.[20] As you gain understanding about your nutritional habits and increase your knowledge about nutrition, you can dramatically cut your risk for these problems.

As you begin your study of nutrition in this chapter, you will learn the names of the nutrients you need. Then you will discover what those nutrients do in your body. Later you will learn how to evaluate a person's nutritional health, as well as evaluate how healthy the current North American diet is. Finally, you will discover why people eat the things they do and how to apply the scientific method to nutritional concepts.

Nutrition • The Council on Food and Nutrition of the American Medical Association defines nutrition as "the science of food, the nutrients and the substances therein, their action, interaction, and balance in relation to health and disease, and the process by which the organism (i.e., body) ingests, digests, absorbs, transports, utilizes, and excretes food substances."

TABLE 1-1

Ten leading causes of death in the United States (1989)

Rank Order	Cause of Death	Percent of Total Deaths
. . .	All causes	100.0
1	Diseases of heart	34
2	Malignant neoplasms, including neoplasms of lymphatic and hematopoietic tissues (cancer)	23
3	Cerebrovascular diseases (stroke)	7
4	Accidents and adverse effects	4
. . .	Motor vehicle accidents	2
. . .	All other accidents and adverse effects	2
5	Chronic obstructive pulmonary diseases and allied conditions (lung diseases)	4
6	Pneumonia and influenza	4
7	Diabetes mellitus	2
8	Suicide	1
9	Chronic liver disease and cirrhosis	1
10	Homicide and law enforcement	1

NOTE: Acquired immune deficiency syndrome (AIDS) is ranked no. 11.
Modified from National Center for Health Statistics: Monthly Vital Statistics Report, August 30, 1990.

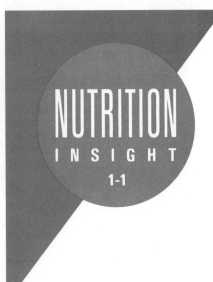

MATH TOOLS FOR NUTRITION

You will use a few mathematical concepts in studying nutrition. Besides performing addition, subtraction, multiplication, and division, you need to know how to calculate percentages and convert English units of measurement to metric units.

PERCENTAGES

The term **percent** (%) refers to a part of the total when the total represents 100 parts. For example, if you earn 80% on your first nutrition examination, you will have answered the equivalent of 80 out of 100 questions correctly. This equivalent could be 8 correct answers out of 10; 80% also describes 16 of 20 ($^{16}/_{20}$ = 0.8% or 80%. The best way to master this concept is to calculate some percentages. Some examples are given below:

Question	Answer
What is 6% of 45?	$0.06 \times 45 = 2.7$
What is 32% of 8?	$0.32 \times 8 = 2.6$
What percent of 16 is 6?	$^{6}/_{16} = 0.375$ or 37.5%
What percent of 99 is 3?	$^{3}/_{99} = 0.03$ or 3%

Joe ate 15% of the adult recommended dietary allowance (RDA) for vitamin C at lunch. How many milligrams did he eat? (RDA = 60 milligrams)

$$0.15 \times 60 \text{ milligrams} = 9 \text{ milligrams}$$

It is difficult to succeed in a nutrition course unless you know what a percentage means and how to calculate one. Percentages are used frequently when referring to menus and nutrient composition.

THE METRIC SYSTEM

The basic units of the metric system are the meter, which indicates length, the gram, which indicates weight, and the liter, which indicates volume. The inside cover of this textbook lists conversions from the metric system to the English system (pounds, feet, cups) and vice versa. Here is a brief summary:

One **meter** is 39.4 inches long, or about 3 inches longer than 1 yard (3 feet).

A meter can be divided into 100 units of **centi**meters, or into 1000 units of **milli**meters.

NUTRIENTS COME FROM FOOD

What is the difference between food, nutrients, and nutrition? Food provides both the energy and the materials needed to build and maintain all body cells. **Nutrients** are the nourishing substances found in food. These essential substances are vital for growth from infancy to adulthood and maintenance of body functions throughout life.[16] Nutrition is the study of nutrients: what they consist of, how the body **metabolizes** them, and what they finally do in the body to keep us healthy.

Classes of nutrients

You have probably heard the terms **carbohydrates, proteins, lipids** (fats and oils), **vitamins,** and **minerals.** These, plus water, make up the six classes of nutrients found in food (Table 1-2). Today we know that the minimum diet for human growth and development must contain about 45 essential nutrients. They are *essential* for a diet because we must get these substances from food. With few exceptions, our bodies cannot manufacture them.

Nutrients • Chemical substances in food that nourish us by providing energy, materials for building body parts, and factors to regulate needed chemical processes in the body. The body either can't make these nutrients or can't make them fast enough for its needs.

Metabolism • Chemical processes in the body that allow for life.

Kcalorie • A kcalorie is actually a measure of the energy content in foods. It is the heat needed to raise 1000 grams (1 liter) of water 1° C. This is the same as raising about 4 cups of water 2° F.

A millimeter is about the thickness of a dime.

There are 2.54 centimeters in 1 inch and about 30 centimeters in 1 foot.

A person 6 feet tall is equivalent to 183 centimeters tall.

A *gram* is about 1/30 of an ounce (28 grams to the ounce).

Five grams of sugar or salt is about 1 teaspoon.

A *kilo*gram is 1000 grams, equivalent to 2.2 pounds.

A pound weighs 454 grams.

A 154-pound man weighs 70 kilograms (154/2.2 = 70).

A gram can be divided into 1000 milligrams or 1,000,000 *micro*grams.

15 micrograms of zinc (approximately the adult RDA)
would be a small speck of zinc oxide.

Liters are divided into 1000 units called milliliters.

One teaspoon equals about 5 milliliters, 1 cup is about 240 milliliters,
and 1 quart (4 cups) equals almost 1 liter (0.946 liters to be exact).

If you plan to work in any scientific field, you will need to learn the metric system. For now, remember that a kilogram equals 2.2 pounds, an ounce weighs 28 grams, 2.54 centimeters equals 1 inch, and a liter is almost the same as a quart. In addition, know what the prefixes micro (1/1,000,000), milli (1/1,000), centi (1/100), and kilo (1,000) represent.

For your review, key units in the English system are:

- 3 teaspoons per tablespoon
- 16 tablespoons per cup
- 2 cups to a pint
- 2 pints or 4 cups to a quart
- 4 quarts to a gallon
- 12 inches to a foot
- 3 feet to a yard
- 16 ounces to a pound

Nutrients can be divided into three groups: (1) those that primarily provide us with *kcalories* (energy); (2) those that are important for growth and maintenance; and (3) those that act to keep body functions running smoothly. Some overlap exists between these groupings. The energy-yielding nutrients, which make up a major portion of most foods, are introduced first.

Carbohydrates. Carbohydrates provide a major source of fuel for your body. Small carbohydrate forms are called sugars or simple sugars. Table sugar is an example. Simple sugars, such as glucose, can chemically link together to form large storage carbohydrates called complex carbohydrates. One example is *starch* in potatoes.

Sugars impart sweetness to many foods we eat. Aside from enjoying this taste,[15] we need sugars or other carbohydrates in our diets primarily to satisfy the energy needs of certain body *cells,* like red blood cells. When you do not eat enough carbohydrates to supply one particular sugar (glucose) to cells, your body will be forced to make this sugar from proteins. However, because we eat two to four times more carbohydrates than our bodies need, this rarely happens.

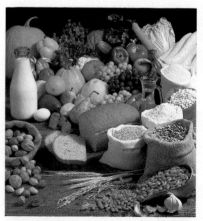

Carbohydrates nourish us by providing energy.

TABLE 1-2

Essential nutrients[*] in the human diet and their categories

| Energy Nutrients | | | | | |
Carbohydrate	Lipids (Fat)[†]	Proteins (Amino Acid)	Vitamins	Minerals	Water
Glucose[‡] (or a carbohydrate that yields glucose)	Linoleic acid α-Linolenic acid	Histidine Isoleucine Leucine Lysine Methionine Phenylalanine Threonine Tryptophan Valine	A D[§] E K Thiamin Riboflavin Niacin Pantothenic acid Biotin B-6 B-12 Folate C	Arsenic[¶] Boron[¶] Calcium Chloride Chromium Copper Cobalt Fluoride[‖] Iodide Iron Magnesium Manganese Molybdenum Nickel[¶] Phosphorus Potassium Selenium Silicon[¶] Sodium Sulfur Tin[#] Vanadium[#] Zinc	Water

This table includes nutrients the current RDA publication lists for humans. Some debate over other minerals not listed does exist.

[*]Dietary fiber could be added to the list of essential substances, but it is not a nutrient (see Chapter 6).

[†]The fats (lipids) listed are needed in only slight amounts, about 2% of total kcalorie needs (see Chapter 5).

[‡]In order to prevent ketosis and thus the muscle loss that would occur as protein was used to synthesize carbohydrate (see Chapter 6).

[§]Sunshine on the skin also allows the body to make vitamin D for itself (see Chapter 9).

[‖]Primarily for dental health.

[¶]Based only on animal studies. True roles in humans need more investigation.

[#]Evidence for these as an essential part of a diet is weak.

Modified from Wardlaw GM, Insel PM: Perspectives in nutrition, St Louis, 1990, Mosby–Year Book.

Molecule • A group of like or unlike atoms chemically linked together. It is similar to a compound, which is a group of different types of atoms bonded together in definite proportion.

We begin digesting some of the starches in our diets as soon as we put them into our mouths. The process continues until starches and large sugars break down into single sugar molecules (like *glucose*) for absorption into the bloodstream. The links between the sugar *molecules* in certain complex carbohydrates cannot be broken down by human digestive processes. These carbohydrates are part of what is called *dietary fiber*.[20] These fibers then pass down the intestinal tract to provide bulk for the stool (feces) formed in the large intestine (colon).[7] Chapter 6 focuses on the family of carbohydrates.

Lipids. Lipids are a second general class of nutrients that contain the familiar fats and oils. These supply another major fuel for the body. By definition fats are solid at room temperature and oils are liquid. There are two basic types of fat found in food: *saturated* and *unsaturated.* (We will discuss these chemical definitions in detail in Chapter 7.) Fats in food are a combination of both saturated and unsaturated fatty acids. The dominant type of fatty acid determines the fat's characteristics, such as whether it is solid or liquid at room temperature. Plant oils tend to be unsaturated. This makes them liquid. Animal fats are often quite saturated, and this makes them solid.

Certain unsaturated fats are essential parts of the diet. Their components help regulate some important body functions, such as blood pressure. They are also needed for the synthesis and repair of vital cell parts. You only need about 1 tablespoon of a common vegetable oil (like those found in supermarkets) per day to supply your body with essential fats. The average American diet supplies about 3 times the amount needed. Chapter 7 focuses on fats, especially their connection to heart disease.

Proteins.   Proteins are a third class of nutrients. These form a major part of the body structure. Muscles contain much protein. A major part of bones is also protein. Important parts of blood, *enzymes,* some *hormones, cell membranes,* and components of the immune system come from proteins. The basic unit of protein structure is the *amino acid.* Amino acids join together to form proteins. Twenty common amino acids are found in food; nine of these are essential parts of an adult's diet.

Most of us eat about one and a half to two times more protein than the body needs to maintain health. In a healthy person this extra protein in the diet is not harmful—it simply reflects the standard of living and the dietary habits that most Americans enjoy. The excess is used for fuel or made into fat or carbohydrate. Chapter 8 focuses on proteins.

Again, aside from water, food is mostly a mixture of carbohydrates, fats, and proteins (Figure 1-1).

Enzyme • A compound that speeds the rate of a chemical process but is not altered by the process. Almost all enzymes are proteins (see Chapters 5 and 8).

Hormone • A compound secreted into the bloodstream that acts to control the function of distant cells.

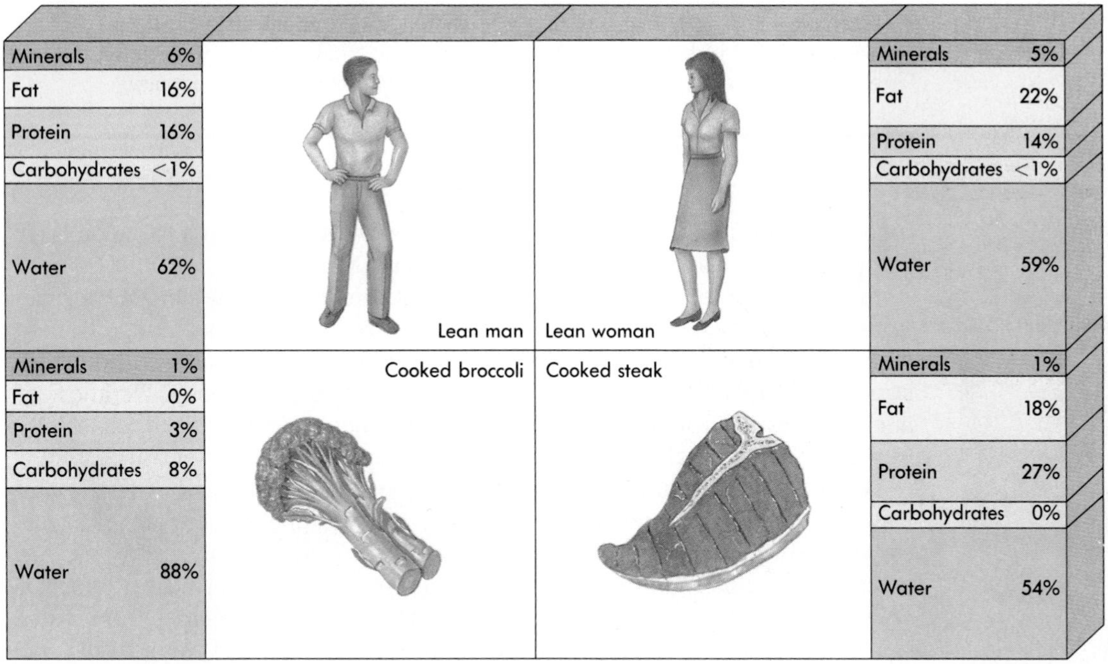

FIGURE 1-1
You aren't what you eat! The proportions of nutrients in the human body do not match those found in typical foods—animal or vegetable.

The fourth and fifth classes of nutrients are vitamins and minerals. These nutrients form the bulk of the regulators and structural parts in the body. While vitamins and minerals are vital to good health, they are needed only in small amounts in our diet.

Vitamins.   Vitamins are compounds that enable many chemical reactions to occur in the body, some of which release the energy stored in carbohydrates, fats, and proteins. The vitamins themselves provide no kcalories to the body. We need 13 different vitamins; four are fat soluble (they dissolve in fat) and

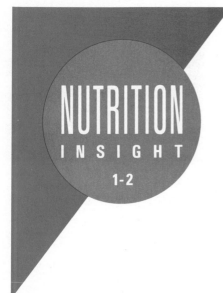

NUTRITION
I N S I G H T
1-2

A FOUNTAIN OF YOUTH?

While most of us wish for long life, we do not like to think of ourselves as suffering poor health when we are old. And rightfully so! We can only truly enjoy long life if we are productive and free of illness. Rather than suffer the ravages of heart disease, stroke, diabetes mellitus, osteoporosis, and other chronic diseases from age 50 or 60 years until death, we should strive to be as free of disease as possible and to enjoy vitality even in the last several years of life.[10] If we can reach this state, we will have achieved a state of physical, mental, and social well-being.

Aging is a natural process: your body cells age no matter what health practices you follow. But to a considerable extent you can choose how fast you age throughout your adult years. Genetic background has a great effect, but you also have some control in the matter (Table 1-3). How you act now is important to your later health. *Successful* aging is the goal. *Age fast or age slow—you choose.*

A BASIC PLAN FOR HEALTH PROMOTION AND DISEASE PREVENTION

Adults can best promote health and prevent disease by doing the following things:

- Eat a healthful diet—A varied diet that maintains a desirable weight should be a priority. The Guide to Daily Food Choices, discussed in Chapter 2, is a great place to start. Especially emphasize lowfat dairy products, lean meats, plant proteins, whole grains, plant oils, fruits, and dark green or leafy vegetables.[16,20]
- Exercise—Research suggests that you should spend about 2000 kcalories per week in brisk walking, jogging, swimming, stair climbing, and other activities that stimulate the cardiovascular system. See Chapter 12 for more details.

Organic • Anything that contains carbon linked to hydrogen in the chemical structure.

Inorganic • Anything that is free of carbon linked to hydrogen in the chemical structure.

Alcohol • Ethyl alcohol or ethanol. An energy-yielding substance found in beer, wine, and distilled spirits.

Bond • A sharing of electrons, charges, or attractions used to link two atoms.

---

nine are water soluble (they dissolve in water). Vitamins, with a focus on their role in the fight against cancer, are discussed in Chapter 9.

Minerals. Minerals also play an important role in the body's chemical reactions, such as magnesium for carbohydrate use. In addition, minerals help make up the body's structure and form key components of parts of the bloodstream. Minerals by themselves provide no kcalories to the body. We know of about 17 essential minerals. Minerals are the focus of Chapter 10, especially how they relate to bone health and high blood pressure (hypertension).

Water. Water is the sixth and last class of nutrients. It nourishes us in many ways. It is vital in the body because it dissolves substances, lubricates processes, and provides a way to transport nutrients and waste. Our body cells are composed of mostly water. The body can even make water as a by-product of ***chemical reactions*** in cells. The bulk of our dietary needs comes from water (about 10 cups a day from a combination of foods, fluids, and water itself) and kcalories. Compare this to our daily needs of 9 tablespoons of protein, one-fourth teaspoon of calcium, and one-thousandth teaspoon (a 2-microgram speck) of vitamin B-12 each day. Water is examined in detail in Chapter 10.

ANOTHER BITE

Nutrients such as carbohydrates, fats, and proteins contain carbons attached to hydrogens. This attachment by definition makes these nutrients *organic* compounds in strict chemical terms. Because minerals and water do not contain carbons attached to hydrogens, they are called *inorganic* compounds. These terms are part of the language of nutrition and based on simple chemistry concepts. Note that they have little to do with organic gardening (see Chapter 4).

- Don't smoke—Lung cancer, primarily caused by smoking cigarettes, is the only form of cancer where yearly rates still increase.
- Limit alcohol intake—Don't drink more than 1 to 2 ounces of alcohol per day.[16,20] One 12-ounce beer, a 4 ounce glass of wine, or a mixed drink supplies about 1/2 ounce (15 grams) of alcohol. Furthermore, women should avoid alcohol during pregnancy as this can harm the baby (Chapter 14 discusses the disease that can result—fetal alcohol syndrome).
- Limit stress, or adjust to the causes of stress—Practice better time management, relax, listen to music, have a massage, and exercise regularly. Do your favorite things to reduce stress.
- Consult health care professionals when necessary—Early diagnosis is especially important for controlling the damaging effects of many diseases.

Your key to optimal health is to discover how to maintain your best physical, mental, psychological, and social states. There is no general formula for achieving this ideal. Each of us must juggle and balance personal goals with opportunities and obstacles we encounter. Proper diet is not the only thing to consider. As we have discussed, other lifestyle choices are also critical. Taking responsibility for yourself is central to achieving long-lasting health. As individuals we can do a lot to improve our health by establishing good health behaviors. Focusing on disease prevention may not allow you to live longer—because of heredity, accidents, or other things outside your control—but you'll probably live a healthier life.[10]

We can begin our journey to better nutrition by looking at what influences our food choices and deciding to take responsibility for making changes in our eating habits that will promote our health. This is the goal of Chapters 1 to 3. ●

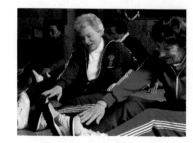

Regular physical activity is one component of a healthy lifestyle.

CONCEPT CHECK

The food you eat contains six vital classes of nutrients: carbohydrates, lipids (fats and oils), proteins, vitamins, minerals, and water. The kcalories (energy) you need for activity come mainly from carbohydrates and lipids. Growth and replacement of body cells require proteins and lipids. Vitamins and minerals have many functions, including aiding in the chemical processes of energy production. Water is the medium of life—a liquid that transports the substances in the body.

We need energy for body functions

We get the energy (again, expressed as kcalories) to perform body functions and to do work from carbohydrates, fats, and proteins (Table 1-3). *Alcohol* is also an energy source for some of us. It is not considered a nutrient, however, because it has no required function. Still, alcoholic beverages are the third leading contributor of kcalories to the diet of people living in the United States.[5]

Energy is held in the chemical *bonds* of carbohydrates, fats, proteins, and alcohol. In Chapter 12 we discuss how energy is released and used by cells.

Kcalories—a closer look

To figure out how many kcalories are in a particular food portion, we would need to use an instrument called a *bomb calorimeter* (Figure 1-2). Information from the bomb calorimeter is used to calculate the energy available to us from 1 gram of carbohydrate, fat, protein, and alcohol. Specifically, carbohydrates yield 4 kcalories per gram, proteins yield 4 kcalories per gram, fats yield 9 kcalories per gram, and alcohol yields 7 kcalories per gram. From

TABLE 1-3

What can we expect from good nutrition and health habits?

Diet

Meeting our needs for protein, kcalories, and other essential nutrients helps prevent:
  Birth defects and low birth weight in pregnancy
  Poor growth and poor resistance to disease in infancy and childhood
  Poor resistance to disease in adult years
  Deficiency diseases, such as cretinism (lack of the mineral iodide), scurvy (lack of vitamin C), and anemia (lack of the mineral iron, the vitamin folate, or other nutrients)
Meeting our needs for the mineral calcium helps prevent:
  Some adult bone loss
Obtaining adequate intake of the mineral fluoride and minimizing sugar intake helps prevent:
  Dental caries (decay)
Eating enough dietary fiber helps prevent:
  Digestive problems, such as constipation, and possibly some forms of cancer
Eating enough vitamin A and beta-carotene (plant form of vitamin A) may help reduce:
  Susceptibility to some cancers, especially in smokers
Moderation in kcalorie intake helps prevent:
  Obesity and related diseases, such as diabetes mellitus, hypertension, cancer, and premature heart disease
Limiting intake of the mineral sodium helps prevent:
  Hypertension and related disease of the heart and kidney in susceptible people
Avoiding intake of saturated fat helps prevent:
  Premature heart disease
Moderation in intake of essential nutrients by using vitamin and mineral supplements wisely, if at all, prevents:
  Most chances for nutrient toxicities

Exercise

Adequate, regular exercise helps prevent:
  Obesity
  Noninsulin-dependent (adult-onset) diabetes mellitus
  Premature heart disease
  Some adult bone loss
  Loss of muscle tone

Lifestyle

Minimizing alcohol intake helps prevent:
  Liver disease
  Fetal alcohol syndrome
  Accidents

In addition, not smoking, minimal use of medications, no illicit drug use, adequate sleep, and limiting stress provides a more complete approach to good nutrition and health.

Because a calorie is such a tiny unit of heat measurement—like a penny in relation to a ten dollar bill—we can more efficiently express food energy in terms of kilocalories, which are 1000-calorie units. The abbreviation kcalorie (or kcal) is used throughout this book.

this you can see that fat yields much more energy per gram than carbohydrates and proteins. Once you know the gram quantities of these substances in a food, it is easy to estimate the total kcalories in that food using the kcalorie values. For example, if a banana-rum drink has 10 grams of carbohydrate, 1 gram of protein, 1 gram of fat, and 15 grams of alcohol, it contains $(10 \times 4) + (1 \times 4) + (1 \times 9) + (15 \times 7) = 158$ kcalories.

Are you what you eat?

The amounts of nutrients that your body needs vary widely from one nutrient to another. Nutrient quantities found in food also vary. Each day we need about

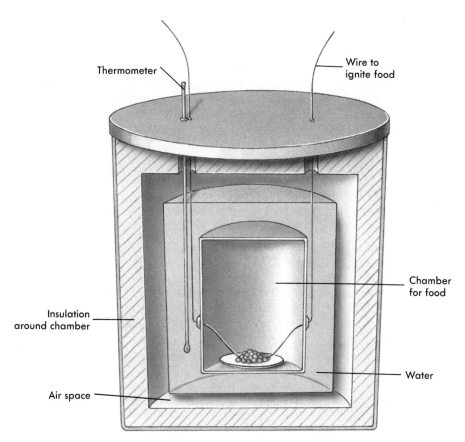

FIGURE 1-2

Cross section of a bomb calorimeter. First, a dried portion of food is burned inside a chamber that is surrounded by water. As the food is burned, it gives off heat. This raises the temperature of the water surrounding the chamber. The increase in water temperature indicates the amount of kcalories contained in the food. Recall 1 kcalorie equals the amount of heat needed to raise 1 kilogram of water 1° C.

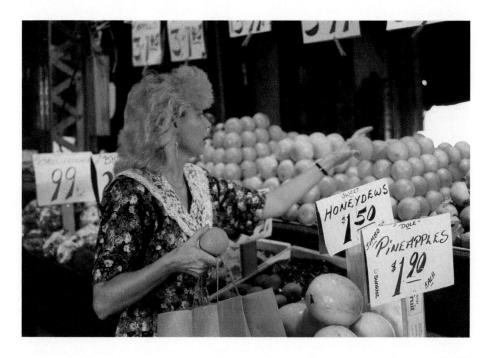

Choose fruits each day as part of your plan for a healthy diet.

a pound (500 grams) of energy-yielding substances in the food we eat. Add to this about 5 pounds of water. We need to take in vitamins regularly, but in very small amounts, 100 milligrams or less. Although we should eat nearly a gram of some minerals like calcium and phosphorus each day, many minerals are needed in quantities of only milligrams or less. For example, you need about 15 milligrams of zinc each day, which is just a few grains of zinc oxide. Figure 1-1 shows the proportion of nutrients in a human body compared with the proportions of the same nutrients in cooked steak and a cooked stalk of broccoli. Note how different your body's nutrient makeup is from that of the foods you eat!

STATES OF NUTRITIONAL HEALTH
Desirable nutritional state

Theoretically, your body needs a certain amount of each nutrient.[3] You reach a desirable amount of a particular nutrient when the body tissues have enough of that nutrient for (1) routine chemical processes and (2) surplus stores of it for use during times of increased need (Table 1-4).

Undernutrition

If you don't take in enough nutrients to meet the nutrient needs for cell activities and body maintenance, surplus stores of nutrients soon become used up, resulting in *undernutrition.* Although body stores of nutrients can make up for a poor diet over a short period of time, the stores will not last indefinitely. Once nutrient stores are depleted, a continuing nutritional deficit drains body tissues. Eventually some of the body's chemical processes slow down, or even stop. *Biochemical changes* in cells then occur.[3]

TABLE 1-4

States of nutritional health with respect to iron

General Conditions	Conditions with Respect to Iron
Desirable nutritional state	
Sufficient amount of nutrients to support body functions, and stores of nutrients for times of increased need	Body has desirable liver stores of iron and normal values for iron-related compounds
Undernutrition	
Stores depleted; tissue levels fall	Serum ferritin,* an iron-containing protein in the blood, drops below normal levels
Body deficiency	
Reduced biochemical function	Hemoglobin, an iron-containing pigment in red blood cells, drops below normal levels
Clinical symptoms	Pale complexion, greatly increased heart rate during activity, and poor body temperature regulation
Overnutrition	
Nutrients consumed in excess of body needs (degree of toxicity varies for each nutrient)	Results in toxic damage to liver cells

*Serum is the liquid portion of blood present after blood clots.
This general scheme can apply to all nutrients. We have chosen iron because you are likely to be familiar with this nutrient.

When the body does not have enough iron, the level of the red blood cell protein **hemoglobin** falls, because iron is needed to make hemoglobin. Serious problems, such as iron deficiency anemia, then can arise. Some women in North America develop anemia because they do not consume enough iron and eventually deplete their iron stores (see Chapter 10 for details).[20]

Body deficiency

If a biochemical change that results from depleted nutrients becomes severe, *clinical symptoms* eventually develop. Changes can be seen in the body, skin, hair, nails, tongue, and eyes (see Appendix B for common clinical symptoms of nutritional deficiencies). Perhaps you have noticed people who appear unhealthy; they lack the vigorous glow that comes with good health. In the case of iron deficiency, the person may appear very pale and may have a much faster heart rate during even moderate activity.

Overnutrition

One nutritional state that is reaching epidemic proportions in North America today is *overnutrition*.[20] Many of us simply overeat. This overloads the body mostly with too many kcalories, but excesses of certain nutrients can build up as well. Overnutrition over a 1- or 2-week period generally causes no symptoms. But keep it up, and blood levels of some nutrients can increase, along with body weight. The average adult gains 15 to 20 pounds from ages 18 to 54 years.[16] Can you afford that extra weight? In the long run, an overweight condition can lead to serious diseases, such as adult onset diabetes mellitus and hypertension.

In recent times taking too many vitamin and mineral supplements (another type of overnutrition) has become a concern.[14] For most nutrients there is a wide gap between the right amount and too much. Therefore a typical multiple vitamin and mineral supplement taken daily probably won't supply a harmful amount of any nutrient. Some possible exceptions are vitamin A, vitamin D, and iron (see Chapters 9 and 10). However, recent studies indicate that very high doses of vitamin B-6 and niacin can also cause health problems. Usually toxic levels build up in the body if supplements are taken in high doses on a regular basis. Therefore high doses of some vitamins and minerals can cause problems. Chapter 3 reviews some potential problems with supplement use in greater detail.

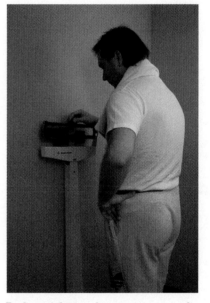

Body weight is a key component of a nutrition assessment.

> **Overnutrition •** A state where nutritional intake exceeds the body's needs.

CONCEPT CHECK

Foods are better sources for nutrients than supplements primarily because each food contains a wide variety, and rarely a potentially toxic amount, of nutrients. Getting a balanced nutrient intake from foods is unlikely to lead to an excessive intake of nutrients as long as good nutritional habits have been developed. A good nutrient intake can prevent the development of biochemical and clinical deficiency symptoms.

In the past people didn't get enough of the right nutrients in their diets. Undernutrition was the nutritional battle cry at the beginning of the twentieth century. Today problems also arise from overnutrition.[20] In fact, the major nutritional problems in America today result from overnutrition combined with too little physical activity. Many of us end up taking in more kcalories than we need. Others of us eat too much sodium and saturated (mostly animal) fats.[16] Both of these habits can reduce heart health.

Some of us should monitor what we eat more carefully because our biological makeup is more susceptible to some diseases. Otherwise, the result can be health problems. This is an issue we will help you focus on throughout the book.

Cholesterol • A waxy fat found in all body cells; it has a structure containing multiple chemical rings (see Chapter 7).

Heart Attack • Rapid fall in heart function caused by reduced blood flow through the heart's blood vessels. Often part of the heart dies in the process (see Chapter 7).

Anthropometry • The measurement of weight, lengths, circumferences, and thicknesses of the body.

Anthropometry, biochemical, clinical, and dietary evaluations make up the ABCD of nutrition assessment.

A warning

Often you can go a long time with poor nutritional habits before you see the first outward (clinical) sign of a problem. For example, a person can eat a diet high in saturated fat, which often leads to a higher blood **cholesterol** level, but not notice any symptoms for years. Eventually, as blood vessels build up deposits of cholesterol and other materials, the person may begin to notice shortness of breath and then chest pain during physical activity. This buildup of fatty substances can one day lead to a **heart attack** (see Chapter 7). Thus a person may be on the road to developing a serious disease, but because it progresses slowly, the effects won't be obvious until quite late—perhaps too late.

Furthermore, symptoms of nutritional deficiencies are often not very specific. Typical effects to look for—diarrhea, an irregular walk, facial sores—can be caused by many different problems. It's often hard to decide if the problem is caused by poor nutrition or by some other medical disorder. Long lag times and vague symptoms often make it difficult to establish a link between an individual's current diet and his or her overall nutritional state.

How could you measure your nutritional state?

The measurements of your height, weight, and body circumferences—called **anthropometry**—reveal something about your nutritional state (Table 1-5). This type of evaluation is simple, but less informative than a full biochemical evaluation, which measures blood levels of some nutrients and their by-products.[3] While useful, a biochemical evaluation is an expensive procedure, and most of the tests can only be done in specialized laboratories. Another way to find out about your nutritional state is to get a thorough physical (clinical) examination and make a detailed evaluation of what you eat.[2]

TABLE 1-5

Components of a nutritional assessment

Component	Example
Anthropometry	Assessment of height, weight, body fat composition, etc.
Biochemical evaluation	Assessment of blood, urine, etc.
Clinical examination	Medical history, physical examination, etc.
Dietary evaluation	Detailed assessment of what you eat

Does what you eat make any difference?

You may wonder why some people show no outward symptoms of poor health even though they have very poor diets. We don't always know the answer to this. Given more time, though, problems may become apparent. We can usually distinguish between undernutrition and good nutrition, but the gray area—the gradual slide from a good to a poor nutritional state—is hard to detect. A lot of research is being done in the field of nutrition that may lead to better methods for early detection of nutritional problems. It is important to strive to regularly meet your nutrient needs; otherwise, a subtle decline in health and performance may occur and you probably will not know why.

THE AMERICAN DIET

For most of us living in America, our main dietary sources of energy are carbohydrates, fats, and proteins. Adults consume about 14% to 16% of their kcalories as proteins, 44% to 47% as carbohydrates, and 35% to 38% as fats. These percentages are estimates and change slightly from year to year. Individual diets also vary widely.[13]

In the American diet most protein comes from animal sources; vegetable sources supply only about one third of our protein. In many other parts of the world vegetable proteins, like those found in rice, beans, and corn, supply most of the protein intake. About half of the carbohydrates in the diets of Americans comes from simple sugars, such as table sugar; the other half comes from starches, such as found in pasta, bread, other grain products, and potatoes. About 60% of our fats come from animal sources and 40% from vegetable sources.[5]

Salt • Generally refers to a mixture of sodium and chloride in a 40:60 ratio.

An American nutrition profile

Our information about the American diet comes from large surveys[19,22] designed to find out what and when people eat. Results from these surveys and other studies show that we eat a wide variety of foods. Many people are meeting their nutrient needs; others are not. The studies show that some of us should choose more foods that are rich in iron, calcium, vitamin A, vitamin B-6, vitamin C, magnesium, zinc, and dietary fiber. Many experts recommend we eat less fat. Chapter 2 gives specific suggestions on how to do just that. In addition, we should match kcalorie intake with need. Overnutrition usually stems from overindulgence in fat and alcoholic beverages.[16] Blacks may need to pay special attention to the amount of sodium (**salt** is a mixture of sodium and chloride) and alcohol in their diets because they have a greater chance of developing hypertension than do whites.[20] Actually, a careful look at sodium and alcohol intake—along with fat—is worth the effort for all of us.

CONCEPT CHECK

Surveys in the United States show that we generally have a variety of food available to us. However, some of us could improve our diets by focusing on good food sources of iron, calcium, vitamin A, vitamin B-6, vitamin C, magnesium, zinc, and dietary fiber. In addition, some of us should use more moderation when consuming kcalories, fat, sodium, and alcoholic beverages.

How aware are we of our nutritional health?

Judging from the responses of over half of the people in several large surveys, Americans are concerned about good nutrition and have a general awareness of possible health hazards from overeating, especially the dangers of too much fat, sodium, and kcalories.[17] But many individuals just aren't willing to critically examine their own food habits. While they may be concerned, they don't necessarily make changes to improve their diets (Figure 1-3). Most people enjoy eating and cooking, but they don't think of or use the principles of nutritional science. We hope you will.

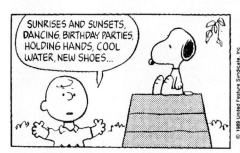
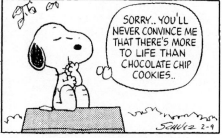

FIGURE 1-3
Peanuts.

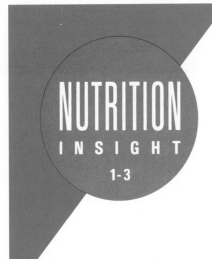

NUTRITION INSIGHT

1-3

ON A TYPICAL DAY IN THE UNITED STATES . . .

- 34 new restaurants open and eight go out of business.
- 134 million people eat out, 16 million eat at McDonald's. Note that McDonald's spends $500 thousand per day to encourage this.
- Each person eats about 4 pounds of food. This includes 16 teaspoons of fat and 32 teaspoons of sugar.
- 11 thousand girls ages 12 to 19 go on a diet, joining the 101 million people already on diets.
- 100 million M&Ms are sold. 2 million Hershey's kisses and 17 million Tootsie Rolls are produced.
- 25 million hot dogs are eaten.
- 524 million Coca-Colas are consumed. To encourage this, Coca-Cola spends $500 thousand per day on advertising.
- $3.5 million are spent on both tortilla chips and vitamin supplements, while $10.4 million are spent on potato chips.
- In total, $22 million are spent on snack foods, while $203 million are spent on low-calorie foods. $1.4 million are spent on laxatives.
- Children see approximately five beer and wine commercials on television. $3 million a day is spent to advertise beer, wine, and other liquors.
- $2 million are spent on baby food.

The United States has about 250 million people.

———

Modified from Heyman T: *On An Average Day*, New York, 1989, Fawcett Columbine.

WHERE DO OUR FOOD CHOICES COME FROM?

Does what you eat say something about you? Your daily food choices have a lot to do with your age, gender, genetic makeup, occupation, where you live, lifestyle, and your family and cultural background.[6] We eat primarily for nourishment, but food means far more to us than that.[1] Food symbolizes much of what we think about ourselves. We can use it to project a desired image.

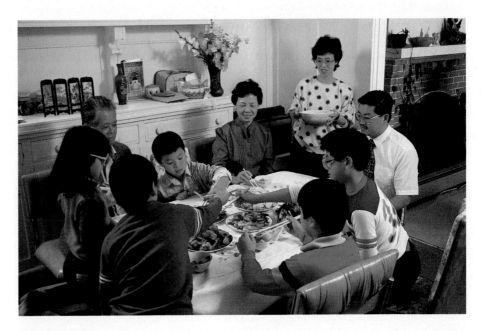

FIGURE 1-4
Meals bring families together. This habit helps create bonds that last a lifetime.

We bond relationships and express friendships around the dinner table (Figure 1-4). We show our creativity and sensitivity by what we serve to others in our homes.[15] The common use of food as a gift is evidence that food signifies friendliness. We cope with stress and tension by eating or not eating. Food can be used as a reward—a dinner out to celebrate a new job or an ice cream cone for an A on a test. Some of us make special foods and elaborate preparations to observe national holidays and religious feast days.

Throughout our lives, we spend 13 to 15 years of our waking hours eating. Taste and texture are two of the most important things that influence our choice of food. After that we consider the cost of food. What we eat ends up revealing much about who we are—politically, religiously, and socially. Behavior, perception, and environment influence food habits (Figure 1-5).[18] While some people have no concern for nutrition, others will agonize endlessly over the taste, kcalories, fat content, and general nutritional value of everything they eat. Where do you fit into the food and nutrition picture?

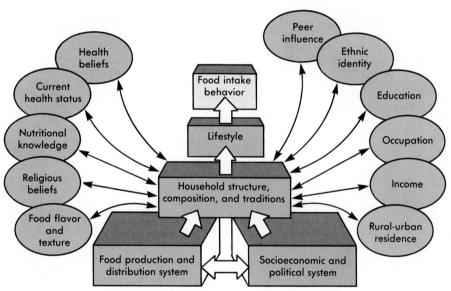

FIGURE 1-5
Food behavior can be influenced by many sources. Which are important in your life?

Our early experiences with food

Our food preferences begin early in life and then change as we interact with parents, friends, and peers (Figure 1-6).[4] Exposure to people, places, and situations often leads us to expand and change our food patterns. Our earliest food memories may include pancakes on Saturday mornings or hot cocoa on cold winter days. Unfortunately, as young children our food experiences may have been severely limited by our parents or other adults responsible for us. Adults may have introduced us to only a small subset of foods available because some excellent foods are often considered inappropriate for children. For example, at what age did you discover lentils, spinach salad, or salmon?

Just being exposed to a variety of foods can help make us less resistant to try new foods. Young children prefer foods that are sweet or familiar.[4] Preschoolers are usually quite willing to try new things. During school years, children are often strongly influenced by their peers. Adults need to give children under their care a variety of foods to try. It may take time, but children usually come to accept new foods (see Chapter 15).

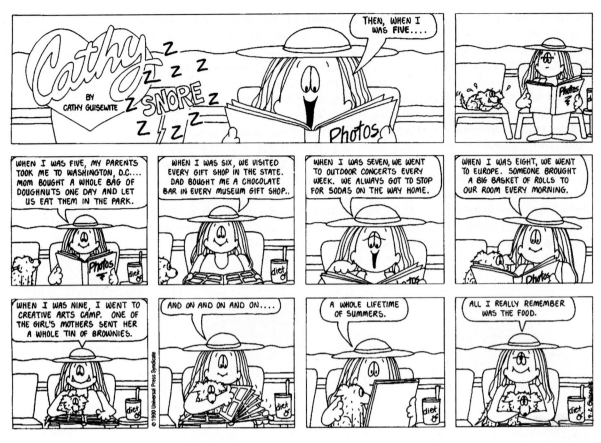

FIGURE 1-6

Our inborn reactions to foods are important, including universal enjoyment of sweet and salty foods and dislike of bitter and sometimes spicy, burning ones.[15] Sweet foods are usually safe to eat. We need to eat *salt* (both the sodium and chloride in table salt are essential nutrients) in foods even though the recommended amount is only about ¼ teaspoon a day. Things that are bitter tasting are often poisonous.

However, our inborn responses to some foods can change once we know a food is safe, allowing us to enjoy foods of different cultures, such as jalapeno peppers and fiery curries.

Habit

Our food choices are tied to our routines and habits. The ease with which we can obtain certain foods influences our choices. Most of us eat from a core group of foods. Only about 100 basic items account for 75% of an individual's total food intake. Narrowing our food choices provides us with security. In this context eating fast food at McDonald's provides common expectations, experiences, and behaviors and can be compared with a *security blanket*.[18]

People often agree that their cooking habits are very similar to those of their mothers. How much do your habits reflect what your mother taught you? Have you considered taking a cooking class to expand your food choices?

Culture

Religious rules about foods can further influence our diet:[1] Hindus would no more eat beef than they would eat a cat. Some Jewish people do not eat pork or serve milk products and meat at the same meal. There are also ethnic taboos. For example, Swedish people, who regard corn as food for hogs, would not enjoy an ear of sweet corn. In the United States insects are rejected almost entirely as foodstuff, whereas in other cultures insects are choice foods. We even have fixed ideas about what time of day we eat certain foods. When was the last time you had vegetable noodle soup for breakfast? Many Japanese people prefer it at that time of day. Even where you live can affect food choices. Different foods are available in different areas. For example, it is sometimes difficult to find a wide variety of fresh vegetables in the winter in some areas or ethnic foods in an isolated town.

Health

About half of us consider nutrition, or what we think are good food habits, an important factor in influencing our food purchases. Americans who focus on better nutrition are mainly well-educated, middle-class professionals.[9] These are the same people who often are health oriented and who have an active lifestyle. Still all of us should pay attention to nutritional health. In fact, increased health awareness among minority people is a major goal of current federal government health strategies.

Sugar used to be the main kcalorie monster; now fat has the limelight.[21] As a result, manufacturers are racing to the market with reduced-fat or nonfat items (many also are lower in cholesterol and sodium), including mayonnaise, salad dressings, cheese, dairy spreads, frozen desserts, luncheon meats, sausage, and butter sprinkles.

Some of us are concerned enough about our health that we want to change our diets. Even so, our food tastes and habits still strongly influence us. When people are asked why they don't include foods they know to be healthy in their diets—for instance, yellow vegetables, lowfat milk, margarine, and whole wheat bread—they say they don't like them. Similarly, people don't want to give up foods such as whole milk, rich cheeses, and fatty meat because they like them too much. This is even the case if they think they should and lower-fat varieties are available.

The modern supermarket is responding to our health concerns by providing fresh, frozen, ready-to-eat, international, gourmet, ethnic, *vegetarian,* and even not-so-healthy foods.[17] Salad bars in supermarkets have become a big hit, especially for single people. Stores are stocking more foods lower in fat, salt,

Vegetarian • A person who avoids eating animal products to a varying degree, ranging from no animal products consumed to simply not consuming four-footed animal products (see Chapter 8).

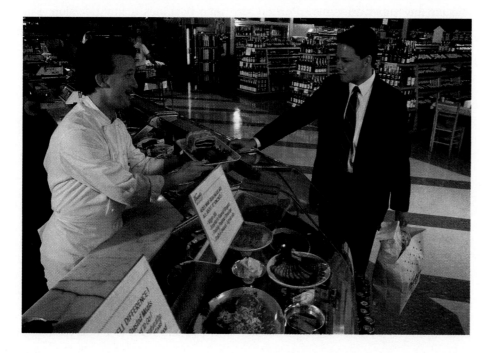

Our options for food choices and sites to purchase food on-the-go expand each decade.

and sugar. They are carrying low-fat varieties of cheeses, yogurts, and peanuts, pure fruit juices, high-fiber cereals, whole-grain breads, fruits canned in natural juices, low-sodium soups and sauces, low-fat turkey and chicken franks, and many kinds of fish. We can select from a variety of bulk foods sold in bins, including beans, rice, flours, dried fruits, nuts, and grains. Often market shelves have tags that provide information on the nutritional content of foods, such as kcalories, vitamins, and minerals. There are many options for us on the road to good nutrition. We just have to follow the right directions.[16]

Advertising

In recent years some of the most successful food products introduced in the United States are advertised as being healthful.[9] However, many of these new products fail to live up to the claims. Popular products of the 1980s have included fruit rolls and bars, bottled mineral water, granola bars, fruit juices, bulk frozen vegetables without sauce, frozen pasta, soft cookies, microwave popcorn, kiwifruit, and Equal (**aspartame**). Ice cream lovers have been able to choose frozen yogurt and new fat-free ice creams as alternatives. Are all these good food choices? Chapter 2 will help you decide.

To capture the interest of consumers, food producers spend well over $32 billion annually on advertising and packaging. Some of this advertising is helpful—when it promotes the importance of calcium and dietary fiber in our diets and encourages us to consume more lowfat milk products, fruits, vegetables, and lean meats. On the other hand, the current hype of cholesterol-free foods is meaningless for many of us, as we describe in Chapter 7. Over half of all food references during prime-time television programs are for low-nutrient beverages and sweets. In the supermarket some poor food choices are placed for higher visibility. Highly sweetened cereals, cookies, cakes, pastries, and alcoholic beverages are given choice spots for display. Food manufacturers often pay for the best place in the supermarkets—at the end of the aisle and, depending on the product, at a child's or adult's eye level.

Fast-food restaurants make especially appealing overtures to consumers. Many now offer healthy alternatives to their high-kcalorie and fat-laden foods.[9] Cutting fat has become a major preoccupation. Still, careful choices must be made. Even a salad bar is not always as healthy as it sounds. Many of the items are loaded with fat and kcalories, such as potato salad, macaroni salad, nachos, and creamy salad dressings. Portion size then becomes a key decision. For some people, such as traveling sales representatives, students, and truck drivers, it is convenient to stop for fast food on a regular basis. For regular consumers of fast food, what they choose to eat is crucial if they want to have a nutritious diet (see Chapter 3 for a look at Eating on the Run).

Social factors

Social changes in recent years have had a strong impact on the food industry. Growing numbers of working mothers and single parents, both young and old, find less time to prepare meals.[9] A general *time-famine* is emerging. Most people still turn to fast-food emporiums for quick meals, but supermarket food counters are stealing restaurant customers. Microwave ovens and frozen food—often complete meals—have come to the rescue, resulting in a whole new array of products.[9] Even products geared for young children are available. Shopping malls have created a new generation of "mall munchers," who eat everything from ethnic foods to high-priced cookies. Drive-through restaurants are now a large part of our culture, whereas 30 years ago they were much less common. It is convenient to drive through, wolf down 1200 kcalories (about half your daily needs) *via* a burger, fries, and shake, and you're on your way.

While people have become more educated about nutrition, and families are starting to eat more meals together than in the recent past, it is still relatively

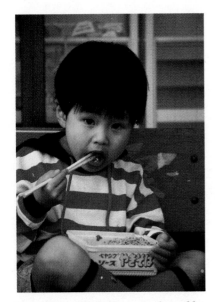

Food likes and dislikes are shaped by early experiences, among other factors.

You eat because you see it, you hear it cooking, you smell it, or it's time to eat. All those stimuli are concentrated in a mall; the food is there, it smells good, and there's so much to choose from. In addition, food may be the most affordable temptation at the mall. After a few hours of trekking through a mall, you would swear you had walked miles. But you would have to walk almost twice around the average mall to chalk up a mile—and that's only 100 kcalories worth of exercise.

The source of shopper's fatigue is psychological—styles, prices, lines, crowds . . .

Tired and frustrated,
the next step is hungry!

Think about that the next time you go shopping. Eat before you go, take a healthful snack, or be on your guard as you sample the smells.

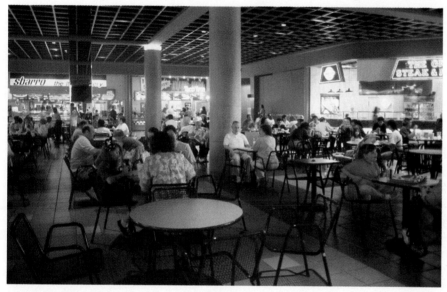

Mall munching can be convenient but costly.

common to eat out and to skip meals. Over one-half of college students report that they eat only two meals a day with many snacks in between. Approximately 30% of adults skip breakfast, a habit that can interfere with proper nutrition. Breakfast is your chance to replace carbohydrate stores used during the night's sleep.

Economics

Food costs affect what we eat. As we make more money, we tend to eat out more often. Two-paycheck households purchase more precooked and prepackaged foods and devote a much larger share of the food budget to eating away from home.[9] However, the relationship between income and overall food consumption is not as strong as you might expect. This is probably because food is relatively inexpensive in the United States compared to other parts of the world.[1] Nevertheless, high beef prices have led people to choose chicken and turkey as alternatives. The high cost of restaurant meals has made fast food a quick and economical choice for families, even though the fare is sometimes limited and of mediocre quality.

CONCEPT CHECK

Our food choices are influenced mainly by taste preferences and habit. Social factors, health concerns, and advertising also enter into the equation. Good food habits, developed and strengthened now, will benefit you in years to come.

Who are you?

Researchers have grouped adults into roughly four categories based on food habits. The factors that have been discussed influence what pigeon hole you fit into.[17]

- **Harried households** (32% of adults). As the name implies, people who live in harried households never feel they have enough time. Convenience is the driving force behind their daily food purchases and consumption decisions.
- **Traditional households** (29% of adults). Traditional households are those in which at least one adult is not employed outside the home. These families have a little more time but a little less money to devote to shopping, preparing foods, and eating.
- **Financially restricted households** (22% of adults). Financially restricted households choose food primarily on the basis of available resources. Time and convenience are not primary concerns.
- **Working singles** (17% of adults). Students often fall into this category. Working singles, like those in harried households, tend to eat on the run. They simply want eating to be convenient.

GIVEN OUR FOOD CHOICES, WE CAN DO BETTER

Americans can take pride in their cultural diversity, varied diets, and overall adequate nutritional health. The 1990s promise a tremendous variety of food choices.[17] Though many recent diet changes are advantageous, some are not. We are eating more fresh and frozen fruits and vegetables than in previous years, but we also drink less milk and more soft drinks. We live longer than ever before and enjoy better general health.[11] Some of us also have more money and time to relax and enjoy life. This can leave us overwhelmed with food and lifestyle choices.

Soft drinks are today more popular than milk, although not as beneficial to the diet.

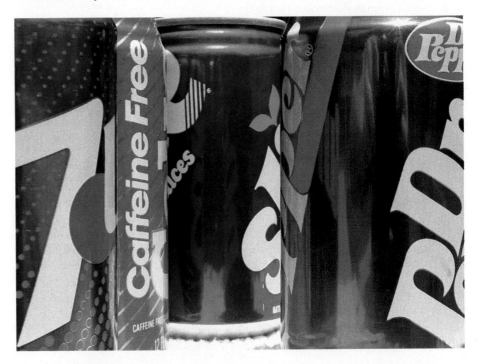

The final outcome of these trends is not fully known, but deaths from heart disease and stroke have dropped dramatically since the late 1960s.[16] This is partly the result of better medical care and more nutritious diets. On the other hand, affluence can lead us into a sedentary and unhealthy lifestyle and lull us into alcoholism and/or *obesity*.[20] Even though greater variety and food availability makes it easier for us to eat a more nutritious diet than ever before, we must also make the best choices.

Overall the American diet has improved, but many of us can do better. The goal of this book is to help you find the best path to good nutrition. There are no junk foods or bad foods, only junk or bad diets. A diet full of nutrient-rich foods can balance a few empty kcalorie foods—foods that have many kcalories but few other nutrients. One's overall diet is the proper focus in a nutritional evaluation. Chapter 2 will emphasize this point and show you how to *balance* a diet.

As you move toward your nutritional goals, remember your health is partly your responsibility.[20] Your body has a natural ability to heal itself. Offer it what it needs, and it will serve you well.[8]

> **Obesity** • A condition characterized by excess body fat, usually defined as 20% above desirable body weight (see Chapter 11).

SUMMARY

- Nutrition is the study of what foods are vital for health and how your body uses nutrients to promote and support growth, maintenance, and reproduction of cells.

- The metric system is used throughout science. Lengths are expressed in meters, weights are expressed in grams, and volumes are expressed in liters. A meter equals about 39 inches, a kilogram is about 2.2 pounds, and a liter is about 1 quart.

- There are six classes of nutrients found in foods: (1) carbohydrates, (2) lipids (fats and oils), (3) proteins, (4) vitamins, (5) minerals, and (6) water. Carbohydrates, lipids, and proteins provide kcalories (energy) for the body to use.

- A basic plan for health promotion and disease prevention includes eating a proper diet, exercising regularly, not smoking, limiting alcohol intake, and limiting or coping with stress.

- As nutritional health diminishes, nutrient stores in the body are depleted. Biochemical reactions in the body then slow down. Finally, outward clinical symptoms appear.

- Overnutrition is a problem in the United States today. This is a condition in which too many kcalories, too much fat, or too much of certain vitamins and minerals are consumed.

- Good nutrition should be based on eating the right foods and not on taking supplements. Getting necessary nutrients from foods prevents severe nutrient imbalances.

- Results from large nutrition surveys suggest that some Americans need to consume foods that supply more vitamin A, vitamin C, vitamin B-6, calcium, magnesium, iron, zinc, and dietary fiber.

- Our food choices are greatly affected by our taste preferences, food habits, culture, upbringing, self-image, and the image we want to present to others. There are no true *junk foods*. The focus should be on balancing a total diet.

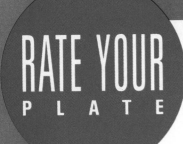

RATE YOUR
P L A T E

FACTORS AFFECTING EATING

Choose one or more days of the week, as your professor directs, that are typical of your eating pattern. In the table below write down all the foods and drinks you consumed for each day. In addition, write down the approximate amounts you ate in units like CUPS, OUNCES, TEASPOONS, AND TABLE-SPOONS. Figure 3-2 in Chapter 3 provides an example of how to record your intake. A blank form is provided on p. 29 and in Appendix D for your use. Copy either form if you are to record more than 1 day. Check the food composition table in Appendix A for examples of appropriate serving units for different types of food, such as meat, vegetables, etc. After completing this activity you will use this list of foods for future activities.

After you record each food/drink and serving size in the table, indicate why you chose to consume it. Draw the symbols given in parentheses below to indicate your reasons. Place the symbols in the space provided to indicate why you picked that particular food or drink.

Taste/Texture (tongue)   Hunger (stomach)
Convenience/Time (clock)   Family and Cultural Background (house)
Emotions (violin)   Peers (stick figures)
Availability (refrigerator)   Cost (dollar sign)
Advertisement (television)   Health (apple)
Weight Control (bathroom scale)

Remember that there can be more than one reason for choosing a particular food or drink.

APPLICATION

Now ask yourself what is your most frequent reason for eating or drinking. To what degree is health a reason for your food choices? Should it be made a greater priority?

Time	Minutes Spent Eating	M or S[*]	H[+]	Activity While Eating	Place of Eating	Food ✓ and Quantity	Others Present	Reason for Food Choice

[*]M or S; meal or snack
[+]Hunger (0 none; 3 maximum)

REFERENCES

1. Axelson ML: The impact of culture on food-related behavior, *Annual Reviews of Nutrition* 6:345, 1986.

2. Bastiotis PP and others: Number of days of food intake records required to estimate individual and group nutrient intakes with defined confidence, *Journal of Nutrition* 117:1638, 1987.

3. Beaton GH: Towards harmonization of dietary, biochemical, and clinical assessments: the meaning of nutritional status and requirements, *Nutrition Reviews* 44:349, 1986.

4. Birch LL: The acquisition of food acceptance patterns in children. In Boakes RA and others, editors: *Eating habits: food, physiology, and learned behavior*, New York, 1987, John Wiley & Sons.

5. Block G and others: Nutrient sources in the American diet, *American Journal of Epidemiology* 122:13, 1985.

6. Boakes RA, Piopplewell D, Burton M: *Eating habits: food, physiology, and learned behavior*, New York, 1987, John Wiley & Sons.

7. Burkitt DP, Eaton SB: Putting the wrong fuel in the tank, *Nutrition* 5:189, 1989.

8. Burton RR and others: NCI dietary guidelines: rationale, *American Journal of Clinical Nutrition* 48:88, 1988.

9. Cassell JA: Commentary: American food habits in the 1980s, *Topics in Clinical Nutrition* 4(2):47, 1989.

10. Fries JF and others: Health promotion and compression of morbidity, *Lancet*, March 4, 1989, p 481.

11. Garn SM, Leonard WR: What did our ancestors eat? *Nutrition Reviews* 47:337, 1989.

12. Harper AE: Nutrition: from myth and magic to science, *Nutrition Today*, January/February, 1988, p 8.

13. Kim WW et al: Evaluation of long-term dietary intakes of adults consuming self-selected diets. *American Journal of Clinical Nutrition* 40:1327, 1984.

14. Koplan JP and others: Nutrient intake and supplementation in the United States (NHANES II), *American Journal of Public Health* 76:287, 1986.

15. McKee LM, Harden ML: Genetic and environmental origins of food patterns, *Nutrition Today*, September/October, 1990, p 26.

16. National Research Council, National Academy of Sciences: *Diet and health*, Washington DC, 1989, National Academy Press.

17. Owen AL: Healthy foods for the future, *Topics in Clinical Nutrition* 5(2):72, 1990.

18. Parraga IM: Determinants of food consumption, *Journal of The American Dietetic Association* 90:661, 1990.

19. Peterkin BB and others: Nationwide food consumption survey, 1986, *Nutrition Today*, January/February, 1988, p 18.

20. Surgeon General's report on nutrition and health, *Nutrition Today*, September/October, 1988, p 22.

21. Webb L: Changing dietary habits of consumers, *Topics in Clinical Nutrition* 5(3):34, 1990.

22. Wotecki CE and others: National health and nutrition examination survey—NHANES, *Nutrition Today*, January/February, 1988, p 25.

HOW MUCH HAVE I LEARNED?

How much have you learned from reading Chapter 1? Here are 15 statements about Chapter 1 designed to help you test your current knowledge. If you think the statement is true or mostly true, circle T; if you think the statement is false or mostly false, circle F. Use the scoring key at the end of the book to compute your total score. You will find this test helpful as a periodic review now and before other tests.

1. (T) F   Your body's cells are mostly water. *lean body 60% water*

2. T (F)   Minerals can be broken down into vitamins.

3. T (F)   The terms kcalories and calories can be used interchangeably. *Kcalories: 1000-cal. units*

4. (T) F   Fats yield more energy per gram than do carbohydrates. *1g fat 9 Kcal. 1g carbohydrate 4 Kcal*

5. (T) F   Vitamins yield no energy.

6. (T) F   Nutrient stores refer to nutrients your body can call upon when needed.

7. T (F)   The body requires greater amounts of vitamins than minerals. *some minerals are req. in greater amt. than vitamins (i.e., calcium)*

8. T (F)   The term organic is similar to the term organic gardening.

9. T (F)   A hypothesis is about the same as a theory. *a hypothesis leads to a theory after it has been verified numerous times)*

10. (T) F   Fatigue and poor temperature control can be signs of an advanced iron deficiency.

11. (T) F   Increased weight can be a sign of overnutrition. *can lead to long term consequences: diabetes, high blood pressure*

12. T (F)   It is necessary to use vitamin and mineral supplements to maintain your nutritional health. *should get nutrients from foods* *Vit. A & D can be harmful if taken in lrg. amts. for a long time*

13. (T) F   Alcohol provides a large source of energy for some people. *3rd leading contributor in U.S.*

14. (T) F   Many people who have poor diets are aware of it, but find themselves unable to change their eating behavior. *often resist changing diets even tho concerned about their nutritional health*

15. (T) F   There is no such thing as junk food. *no food is totally worthless*

NUTRITION ISSUE

APPLYING LOGIC TO NUTRITION

Like other sciences the study of nutrition has developed by using the scientific method, a procedure for testing that is designed to detect and eliminate error. Scientists begin by observing life. They speculate about the causes of the phenomena and suggest possible explanations called *hypotheses* for what they observe. Hypotheses must then be tested in controlled, scientific *experiments.* The data gathered from these experiments may either support or refute each hypothesis. If data or evidence from many experiments support a hypothesis, it becomes generally accepted by scientists and can be called a *theory* (such as the theory of gravity). Very often, the results from one experiment suggest a new set of questions to be answered.

A scientist must be skeptical of hypotheses and theories by not accepting them immediately when there is little evidence and then rejecting those that fail to pass critical analyses (Figure 1-7). In nutrition science we must keep a healthy skepticism and be very critical of many current ideas about nutrition.[12]

WHERE DO HYPOTHESES COME FROM?

By studying the history of diseases and specific health disasters, such as the large outbreaks of scurvy during the fifteenth through nineteenth centuries, scientists reveal clues to causes of poor health. Other clues come from observing more general patterns of diseases and diet habits in whole populations of people in various parts of the world. The study of disease patterns in populations is called *epidemiology.*

When European explorers left Europe to come to the Americas in the fifteenth and sixteenth centuries, they developed *scurvy* while at sea. The sailors developed scurvy but their land-dwelling counterparts didn't. This was an epidemiological observation. Only after many years was scurvy proven to be a vitamin deficiency. The sailors weren't getting enough vitamin C from the few fruits and vegetables available aboard the ship.

In the 1920s epidemiological studies helped Dr. Joseph Goldberger determine that the disease pellagra was caused by a dietary deficiency rather than by an infection. He noticed that prisoners in jail—but not their jailers—suffered from *pellagra.* If pellagra were an *infectious disease,* the prisoners would pass the infection to their jailers and the disease would be seen in both populations.

During World War II, the German army blockaded the Russian city of Leningrad and the people began to suffer from undernutrition. Along with widespread undernutrition there was an increase in infant deaths at childbirth, an occurrence which had been much rarer when the population was able to eat a nutritious diet. Scientists in North America later speculated that pregnant women might benefit from food supplements in terms of survival for their infants.

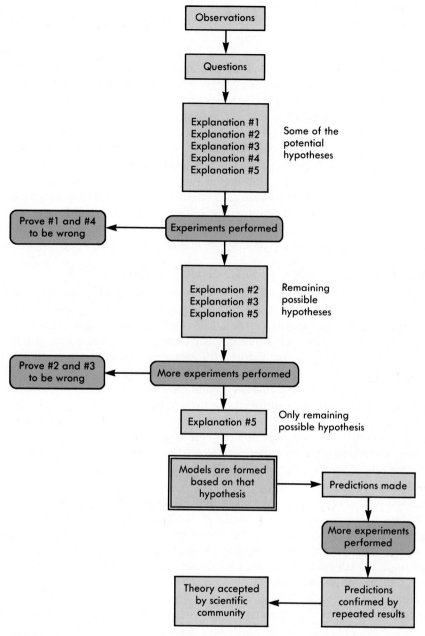

Epidemiology • The study of how disease rates vary between different population groups, for example, a comparison of the rates of stomach cancer in Japan and in Germany.

Scurvy • The deficiency disease that results after a few months of not consuming enough vitamin C (see Chapter 9).

Infectious Disease • Any disease caused by an invasion of the body by microorganisms, such as bacteria, fungi, or viruses.

FIGURE 1-7
From question to theory—the process of science applied to nutrition. Only after careful and thorough analysis does a research finding deserve to have influence over our food choices.

In the 1970s Dr. Denis Burkitt noted that Africans have a low rate of intestinal problems compared to North Americans and Europeans. Burkitt speculated that the large amount of dietary fiber eaten by Africans led to greater intestinal health, while the little amount of dietary fiber eaten by North Americans and Europeans caused problems.

TESTING THE ASSUMPTIONS OF EPIDEMIOLOGY
Epidemiological observations by themselves do not establish that a dietary problem causes a certain disease. We need better evidence. This requires experimental testing. In the case of scurvy, British scientists eventually discov-

ered that lime juice cured the scurvy. But it wasn't until about 300 years later that vitamin C, the crucial substance in citrus fruit that prevents scurvy, was discovered.

As science grew more sophisticated, so did experimental tests. In the 1920s various foods were fed to people in mental asylums who suffered from pellagra. The experiment showed that yeast and high-protein foods could cure pellagra. In another experiment food supplements were given to poor women in Boston and Toronto at risk for nutrient deficiencies to see what effect supplements had on their pregnancies. Results of this experiment showed that food supplements did increase the chances of having a healthy baby.

Experiments in these cases have shown without doubt that dietary deficiencies can cause scurvy, pellagra, and impair pregnancy outcome. However, it is not always as easy to prove a cause and effect relationship. For example, the importance of dietary fiber is still being established. So far, experiments have shown that adding fiber to your diet will often improve the health of your intestines,[7] but more testing is needed. This is discussed in Chapter 6.

USING ANIMAL EXPERIMENTS TO STUDY EPIDEMIOLOGY

When scientists cannot test their hypotheses on humans, they often use animals. Much of what we know about human nutritional needs and functions has come from animal experiments. In the 1930s scientists showed that a pellagra-like disease seen in dogs, called blacktongue, was cured by nicotinic acid. But only when nicotinic acid actually cured the disease in humans were scientists convinced that nicotinic acid, later called niacin (a vitamin), was the critical dietary factor. Thus when a disease found in animals mimics a particular human disease, the *animal model* can be used to test the human hypothesis.

Today we know that low doses of the mineral fluoride in the diet can strengthen teeth (see Chapter 10). It can also stimulate growth in rats. However, we still don't have experimental evidence for its effect on growth in humans. While some speculate that fluoride might stimulate growth in humans, there is no real proof.

In addition, there are ethical considerations in animal and human experiments. Some people think it is reasonable to feed rats a low copper diet to study copper's importance in the formation of blood vessels, while others argue that animal experiments are unethical. Almost universally, however, people would find it unethical to study how a copper deficiency, which is potentially deadly, influences the formation of blood vessels in infants.

Ethical considerations, lack of animal models for specific human diseases, and insufficient funds are all reasons why scientists are often unable to test hypotheses that are suggested by epidemiological evidence.

ANOTHER BITE

Throughout this book we will point out areas where more research is needed to answer important nutritional questions. Some of these questions come from epidemiological studies or observations of scientists, which await testing in an experimental setting (either in an animal model or, even better, in the human clinical laboratory). Until overwhelming evidence supports a hypothesis, it should not be considered a nutrition "fact."

CONDUCTING EXPERIMENTS—THE DOUBLE-BLIND STUDY

An important type of experimental approach used to test hypotheses is the *double-blind study*. This starts with a group of *subjects* that follow specific instructions, such as eating certain foods. In addition, the experiment must balance this experimental group against a **control group** of subjects who do not change their normal pattern of living. Scientists then observe the experimental group over time to see if there are changes in this group that are not found in the control group. Sometimes subjects are used as their own control: first, they are observed for a period of time, and then they are observed after being treated to see what changes occur.

The bias (prejudice) of the subject or the experimenter can easily affect the outcome of an experiment. Either may have a stake in the outcome. Thus researchers need to limit the amount of bias they and their subjects bring to the experiment. The best way to do that is to *blind* the subjects and the scientific investigators so that neither knows which subjects are in the experimental group and which are in the control group. In addition, the outcome of the experiment is not disclosed until the entire study has been completed. Now we have all parts of a double blind study: experimental group, control group, and "blinding" of all parties. This approach avoids the chance that the subjects may begin to feel better, for example, simply because they know they are part of an experimental group rather than a control group. Also, it avoids the possibility that researchers may see the change they want to see in the subjects in order to prove a certain hypothesis, even though the change did not actually occur.

In a double-blind experiment, a **placebo** (fake medicine) is often given to the control group in order to camouflage who is in what group. Until the experiment is complete, only a third party knows which group is which. For some experiments, only a single-blind setup is possible. In single-blind experiments, either the subjects or the researchers are kept in the dark, but not both.

Vitamin experiments are often double-blind because it is easy to develop a placebo that looks like a vitamin pill. However, food studies often cannot be placebo-controlled. It is hard to disguise a diet high in fruits and vegetables from one that has none. In such cases the experimenters should try to keep the results from the blood studies or other samples a secret until the end of the study. This way much of the bias in the subjects can be eliminated. The less bias in an experiment, the more confidence we can have in the results.

> **Double-blind Study •** An experiment where the subjects and researchers are unaware of their actual subject assignment until the study is completed.
>
> **Control Group •** Participants in an experiment whose habits are not altered.

SHARING EXPERIMENTAL RESULTS WITH OTHER SCIENTISTS

Once scientists complete an experiment, they summarize the findings and publish the results in a scientific journal. At the end of each chapter in this book you'll find a list of references for important experiments that have been published in scientific journals. Most of these journals are **peer-reviewed.** This means other scientists have been asked to review and judge the quality of the research; this ensures that only high-quality research findings are published. Because of peer review, research results published in the *American Journal of Clinical Nutrition*, the *New England Journal of Medicine*, or the *Journal of The American Dietetic Association* are much more reliable than those found in popular magazines, newspapers and health newsletters, or promoted on television talk shows.

THE NEED FOR FOLLOW-UP STUDIES

Even if a study follows all the rules and is accepted by the scientific community, one set of experimental results is not enough. Results from one laboratory must be confirmed by other laboratories. Only then can we really trust and use the results. We don't advise accepting new nutritional ideas as fact or applying them in your life until they are proven by several lines of evidence. Instead of drastically changing your diet in response to new scientific evidence, your best approach, in general, is to eat a variety of foods in moderate amounts.[12] See the discussions on olive oil and oat bran in Chapter 7 for further elaboration of this point. ●

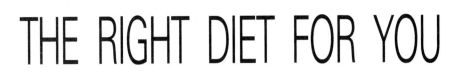

THE RIGHT DIET FOR YOU

How many times have you been bombarded with wild claims about how healthful certain foods are for you? As consumers focus more and more on diet and disease, food manufacturers are responding with products that claim all sorts of health benefits. Supermarket shelves have begun to look like an 1800s medicine show: "Take fish oil capsules to avoid a heart attack." "Eat more olive oil and oat bran to lower your blood cholesterol level." "Strengthen your bones with calcium-fortified orange juice." What's behind these claims? Hearing them, you would think that food manufacturers have solutions to all our health problems. They see today's consumers searching for a cure-all tonic and are happy to use this advertising *hook*.

Advertising aside, nutrition *is* linked to many leading causes of death in America—hypertension, coronary heart disease, cancer, liver disease, and adult-onset diabetes mellitus.[18] How should we respond? In this chapter we will explore the healthy diet that many nutritionists recommend—a diet that minimizes the risks for developing these diseases. How well will your diet stand up to this standard? ●

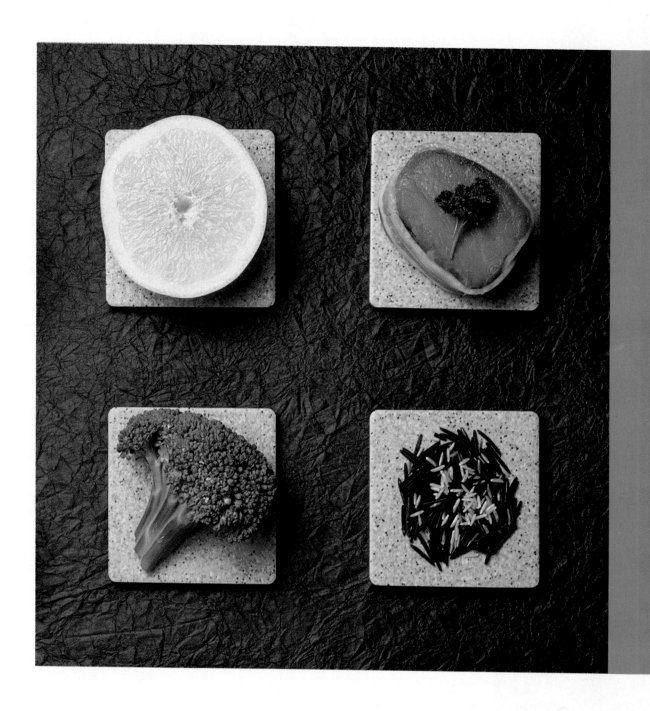

How Does Your Diet Rate for Variety?

Directions: Check the box that best describes your eating habits.

How often do you eat:	Seldom or never	1 or 2 times a week	3 to 4 times a week	Almost daily
1. At least six servings of bread, cereals, rice, crackers, pasta, or other foods made from grains (a serving is one slice of bread or ½ cup cereal, rice, etc.) per day?..........................	☑	☐	☑	☐
2. Foods made from whole grains?......................	☑	☐	☐	☐
3. Three different kinds of vegetables per day?...	☑	☐	☐	☐
4. Two servings of lean meat, poultry, fish, eggs, dry beans, or nuts per day?..............................	☐	☐	☐	☑
5. A dark green leafy vegetable, such as spinach or broccoli?...	☐	☑	☐	☐
6. Two kinds of fruit or fruit juice per day?........	☑	☐	☐	☐
7. Two servings (three if teenager, pregnant, or breastfeeding) of milk, cheese, or yogurt per day?...	☐	☐	☑	☐

Scoring: Compare your answers to the best answers.

Question 1: Almost Daily

Eating breads and cereals will not make you fat. Extra kcalories often come from the fat and/or sugar you may eat with them. Both whole-grained and enriched breads and cereals provide starch and essential nutrients.

Question 2: Almost Daily

Whole-grained breads and cereals contain vitamins, minerals, and dietary fiber that are low in the diets of many Americans. Select whole-grain cereals and bakery products, or make your own and use whole-wheat flour.

Question 3: Almost Daily

Vegetables vary in the amounts of vitamins and minerals they contain. So, it's important to include several kinds every day.

Question 4: Almost Daily

Most Americans include some meat, poultry, or fish in their diets regularly. Dry beans and peas, peanuts (including peanut butter), nuts and seeds, and eggs can be used as alternatives.

Question 5: 3 to 4 Times a Week

Spinach and other dark green leafy vegetables are excellent sources of some nutrients that are low in many diets.

Question 6: Almost Daily

Fruits taste good and are good for you. Choose several different kinds each day.

Question 7: Almost Daily

Adults as well as children need the calcium and other nutrients found in milk, cheese, and yogurt.

ASSESS YOURSELF

WHAT SHOULD I EAT?

You may be surprised to learn that what you should eat is exactly what you've heard many times before—a great variety of foods balanced by moderation with each food.[18] A variety of foods is best because no natural food meets all your nutrient needs. Human milk comes close to meeting the needs of an infant, except it provides only low amounts of iron and vitamin D. Cow's milk also contains very little iron. Meat provides protein but little calcium. Eggs have no vitamin C, and the calcium is mostly in the shell. This is why you need a variety of foods—the nutrients you need are scattered among many foods.

A food plan that works

One way to balance a variety of foods is to select foods from the five major food groups everyday. These groups are: (1) vegetables; (2) fruits; (3) breads, cereals, and other grain-based foods; (4) milk, cheese, and other dairy products, such as yogurt; and (5) meats, fish, poultry, and dry beans and peas. The foods are grouped based on having similar nutrient contents. A bean burrito with tomatoes, accompanied by a glass of milk and an apple takes care of all groups. Fats, oils, and sweets also can be added to one's diet to increase it's desirability. An easy way to further help achieve *balance* in your total diet is to vary the foods within each group so you don't eat only a small group of foods.

Eating *moderately* requires planning. By reviewing your entire day's diet, you can plan ahead on how to juggle nutrient sources. For example, when you plan to eat something relatively high in fat, sugars, salt, or kcalories, such as a bacon cheeseburger at a fast-food restaurant, you should eat other foods that are lower in the same nutrients, like fruits and salad greens, that same day. If you choose salty ham for dinner, opt for fresh or frozen vegetables prepared without salt to accompany it. If you prefer whole milk to lowfat or skim milk, cut the fat elsewhere in your meals. Try lowfat salad dressings or use jam instead of butter or margarine on toast.

Most important, eat foods that appeal to you. There are no *good* or *bad* foods.[12] Focus on your total day's intake when you make a "health" evaluation. Fortunately we live in a time when the food supply is abundant and safe. For most of us a good diet is affordable, and we have a huge variety of food choices. A well-balanced and healthful diet can be planned to match your family and cultural traditions, lifestyle, and budget. Even so, white bread, whole milk, doughnuts, cookies, French fries, hot dogs, hamburgers, and meat loaf—all high in fat—along with sugared soft drinks make up a major part of the American diet.[3] As a nation, we have our work cut out for us to improve our nutrition and health habits.[11,18]

Many people would like to live on pizza alone. What are pizza's nutrient strengths and inadequacies? Check the food composition table, Appendix A, for the vitamin C content of pizza. How many slices would you need to eat to yield the RDA of 60 milligrams?

These foods make up a major part of the American diet.

Health professionals have recommended the same basic diet plan for the last 10 years: watch how much you eat, focus on the major food groups, and stay physically active.[6] Let's now fine-tune this advice.

RECOMMENDED DIETARY ALLOWANCES (RDA)

Before designing a diet, we need to know how frequently we need each nutrient and how much is enough (or too much). People have puzzled over this question for centuries. During World War II, when many men were rejected from military service because of the effects of poor nutrition on their health, the need for official dietary recommendations was recognized. In 1941 a group of 25 scientists formed the first Food and Nutrition Board. They established dietary standards for evaluating the nutritional intakes of large populations and for planning agricultural production. This board developed the first *Recommended Dietary Allowances (RDA)*. They left open the option to revise RDA as better scientific evidence became available. Every four or five years the RDA are revised using the following guidelines:[8]

1. Estimate how much of each essential nutrient the average person requires to be healthy and how much those requirements vary among people.

2. Increase the average requirement by about 30% to 50% in order to cover the needs of most members of the population. For example, if the average requirement for a vitamin is found to be 20 milligrams per day, the RDA may be approximately 28 milligrams per day (40% higher).

3. Increase the RDA again to make up for inefficient use, such as poor absorption of a nutrient by the body.

4. Use scientific judgment to interpret and establish allowances when specific scientific data is limited.

Using this process the Food and Nutrition Board determines RDA for healthy males and females of different age groups.[8] See the inside cover of this book for the specific recommendations.

The RDA is your guide for estimating your nutritional needs. However, make sure these nutrients come from foods rather than mainly from vitamin and mineral supplements. Using foods is important because they contain all essential nutrients. Only 19 of approximately 45 necessary nutrients—not counting certain essential amino acids that make up food protein—have an RDA. Not enough is known about many nutrients for the Food and Nutrition Board to establish an RDA. However, all essential nutrients should be part of your diet.

The RDA are not for amateurs

One common misconception about the abbreviation RDA is that the "D" stands for "daily." It stands instead for "dietary." We don't need to eat the RDA for each nutrient every day because our bodies store nutrients for later use. Think instead of averaging the RDA for vitamins and minerals over a week's time: some days you eat more, and some days you eat less, but the average for 3 to 7 days should meet the RDA. That can be extended to months for vitamin A and vitamin B-12 because they are readily stored by the body.

Notice also that the "R" does not stand for "required," but "recommended." Because the RDA actually apply to groups rather than to individuals, RDA should be used primarily to plan and evaluate diets for groups of people.[8] Because the allowances are set quite high, healthy people should not expect their health to improve if they eat more than RDA levels of various nutrients.[13] The Food and Nutrition Board's goal in establishing RDA is to protect Americans from getting either too much or too little of the needed nutrients. Too often people think that if a little of something is good, a lot must be better.[16] This can lead to trouble with some nutrients, as you will see in Chapter 3.

Recommended Dietary Allowances (RDA) • Recommended nutrient intakes that meet the needs of essentially all people of similar age and gender. These are established by the Food and Nutrition Board of the National Academy of Sciences.

The RDA assumes we eat a wide variety of foods (mixed diet), experience no temperature extremes, and do not participate in long, strenuous physical activity.

While the original purpose of the RDA was to plan and evaluate soldiers' diets, its scope now includes all healthy groups of Americans, such as college students eating in a campus dormitory cafeteria.

POSITIVE BALANCE	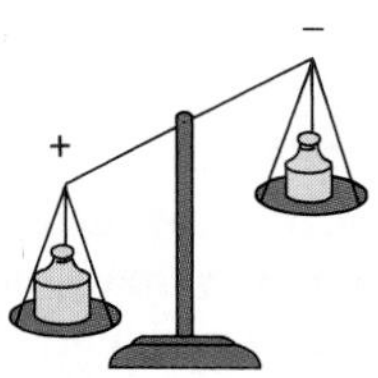	The body absorbs more protein than it loses	• Growing children • Pregnant women • Adults recovering from disease
EQUI-LIBRIUM	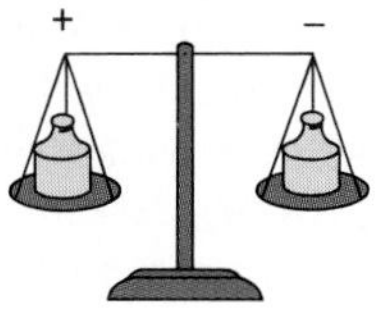	Protein intake equals losses	• Healthy adults
NEGATIVE BALANCE	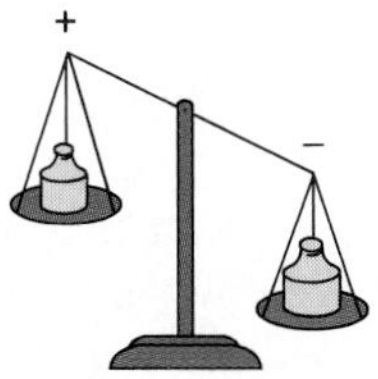	The body loses more protein than it takes in	• Adult with disease (as in cancer) • Fasting person

FIGURE 2-1

Nutrient balance using protein as an example. This balance concept can be applied to all nutrients. Practice your knowledge by substituting calcium for protein in the example, focusing on bone health.

Equilibrium • In nutritional terms, a state where nutrient intake equals nutrient losses. This allows the body to maintain a stable condition.

A close look at one RDA: Protein

A regular intake of protein is critical to maintain health. The RDA for protein is 0.8 grams per kilogram of desirable body weight for an adult.[8] That amount allows daily protein intake to balance the body's protein losses from hair, skin, stool, etc., and allows the body to maintain protein *equilibrium* (Figure 2-1). (Chapter 8 contains more details on proteins in the body.) The recommendation also allows for some extra protein to keep the body's protein stores full. In this way protein status of the body should stay about the same each day.

When setting the RDA for children, scientists must add extra protein to accommodate daily growth needs in new cells. For children it is not enough to balance daily protein losses and store a little extra: to provide for growth, children regularly must take in more protein than they lose. The RDA is adjusted to account for this.

If you total the amount of protein you eat in 1 week and divide by seven, you will have your average daily protein consumption. If that value is close to the RDA, you are most likely eating enough protein. Even if you eat less protein than the RDA, you might not suffer ill effects as your needs are most likely less than the RDA.[8] As a general rule, however, the further you stray below the RDA—particularly as you approach less than half the recommendation—the greater your risk of a nutritional deficiency.

Symptoms of nutritional deficiencies may be subtle and develop slowly. Problems such as a weakened immune system, reduced chemical processing in body cells, or an impaired ability to carry oxygen in the blood may not become apparent for a long period of time. If you suspect that you have an inadequate diet, don't wait for warning signs to develop. Start eating a diet that meets your

RDA for all recommended nutrients rather than run the risk of developing health problems from poor nutrition.[8]

Estimated Safe and Adequate Daily Dietary Intakes

The Food and Nutrition Board sets *estimated safe and adequate daily dietary intakes (ESADDI)* for several nutrients that have no true RDA, including copper, biotin, and chromium (see the inside cover for values). The board feels that information on these nutrients is too incomplete to set an RDA but detailed enough to set a range for a reasonable group intake.[8] By providing a range, the ESADDI not only recommend intake to meet nutritional needs, but also discourage people from eating too much of these nutrients. The board also sets *minimum requirements for health* for sodium, potassium, and chloride. Note that these nutrients do not have RDA or ESADDI.[8]

Some nutrients—carbohydrates and fats, for example—still have no RDA, ESADDI, or minimum requirement for health. Still, our needs for these nutrients can easily be met by eating a diet that meets our established nutrient needs. Chapters 6 and 7 will discuss this issue in more detail.

RDA for energy needs

The RDA for energy estimates average energy needs for physically active people of various age groups and then suggests a wide range for the allowance (see the inside cover for recommendations). Note that no extra amount is added for human variabilities, as is done for nutrient RDA.

The energy RDA are only rough estimates. Energy intake really should depend on energy use.[8] For most adults, weight maintenance is the best indicator of energy balance—kcalorie intake matching kcalorie output.

U.S. RDA

One practical application of the RDA is the *U.S. Recommended Daily Allowances (U.S. RDA).* Note the "D" stands for "daily," not "dietary" as in RDA. This standard was first set in 1974 by the U.S. Food and Drug Administration (FDA) to be used on nutrition labels on foods and vitamin/mineral supplements (Figure 2-2). It replaced the minimum daily requirements (MDR). The U.S. RDA for adults are primarily based on the highest RDA values determined in 1968 for this specific age group. For example, the 1968 RDA for iron for adult men was 10 milligrams per day; for adult women it was 18 milligrams per day. The U.S. RDA for adults uses the higher value of 18 milligrams per day. Appendix E lists U.S. RDA values. The values set for children over 4 years of age and adults are commonly listed on food products.

Mainly for economic reasons, the U.S. RDA have not been updated since they were first set, but new food labeling laws will soon lead to changes.[4,7] The new name will be *Reference Daily Intakes (RDI).* Values will be based on the 1989 RDA and represent an average value of the RDA for that nutrient over the age range that the RDI is applied to (Appendix E). Current U.S. RDA values are in general slightly higher than the RDA. An example is the above mentioned U.S. RDA for iron for adults. Even though the highest RDA value for iron for adult women has been lowered from 18 to 15 milligrams per day in 1989, the U.S. RDA still uses the earlier value of 18 milligrams of iron per day for adults. Therefore when you read a cereal label that claims a serving provides 25% of the U.S. RDA for a nutrient, you can be almost sure that it will provide at least 25% of the RDA for your age and gender. Your need, if it is different from the U.S. RDA, will probably be lower. An exception is calcium for the age group 11 to 24 years; the U.S. RDA is 200 milligrams lower than the RDA.

Figure 2-2 shows a typical *nutrition label* that lists the U.S. RDA for the adult category in terms of percentages. New labeling regulations will likely change this format within the next few years. The label in Figure 2-2 states that

Estimated Safe and Adequate Daily Dietary Intake (ESADDI) • Nutrient intake recommendations made by the Food and Nutrition Board where a range for intake of some nutrients is given because not enough information is available to set an RDA.

Minimum Requirements for Health • Nutrient intake recommendations set by the Food and Nutrition Board for sodium, potassium, and chloride.

U.S. Recommended Daily Allowances (U.S. RDA) • Nutrient standards established by the FDA for use on nutrition labels. Generally the four existing versions use the highest nutrient recommendation in the appropriate age and gender category from the 1968 publication of the RDA. The version that includes children over 4 years of age and adults is most commonly seen on nutrition labels.

Reference Daily Intakes (RDI) • Standards for expressing nutrient content on nutrition labels. RDI are based on average 1989 RDA values set for a nutrient that span a particular age range, such as from children over 4 years through adults. RDI will replace the U.S. RDA by November, 1992.

FIGURE 2-2
A nutrition label. This label is a source of detailed nutrient information on about half of all foods. See the Nutrition Issue on p. 60 for the details about the parts of this label.

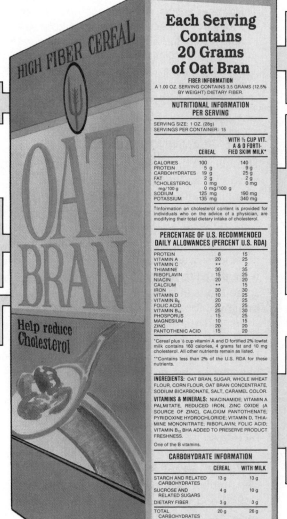

Nutritional information is required on all products that make a nutritional claim or add a nutrient.

Making Sense of the U.S. RDA
U.S. RDA are recommended daily nutrient standards developed for use in the nutrition labeling of food products. Because nutrient needs vary among individuals, the U.S. RDA are set high enough to cover the needs of nearly everyone.

To calculate the amount of iron in one serving, multiply 0.30 times the U.S. RDA of 18 milligrams (see Appendix E): $0.3 \times 18 = 5.4$ milligrams of iron per serving.

Oat Bran Per Serving
Label lists the grams of oat bran per serving. The serving size of ready-to-eat Oat Bran cereal is 28 grams (1 ounce or ¾ cup). Serving size, which is arbitrary, affects per serving amounts of everything else.

Fat
There are 9 kcalories in each gram of fat. The percentage of kcalories from fat is determined by multiplying the number of fat grams by nine, dividing that by the number of kcalories, and then multiplying by 100. This cereal derives 18% of its kcalories from fat.

Sodium
Sodium is frequently listed on food product labels. Sodium occurs naturally in some foods and is sometimes added for taste or in production.

Ingredients
For most foods, the ingredients must be listed on the label. The ingredient present in the largest amount, by weight, must be listed first, followed by other ingredients in descending order. However, an ingredient label doesn't tell you how much of an ingredient is actually in the product. For example, although sugar is listed as the second ingredient, it is actually a relatively small portion of the ingredients.

Manufacturer's Name and Address
The manufacturer's name and address is included on the package.

Label Text

Each Serving Contains 20 Grams of Oat Bran

FIBER INFORMATION
A 1.00 OZ. SERVING CONTAINS 3.5 GRAMS (12.5% BY WEIGHT) DIETARY FIBER.

NUTRITIONAL INFORMATION PER SERVING

SERVING SIZE: 1 OZ. (28g)
SERVINGS PER CONTAINER: 15

	CEREAL	WITH ½ CUP VIT. A & D FORTI-FIED SKIM MILK*
CALORIES	100	140
PROTEIN	5 g	9 g
CARBOHYDRATES	19 g	25 g
FAT	2 g	2 g
†CHOLESTEROL mg/100 g	0 mg	0 mg/100 g
SODIUM	125 mg	190 mg
POTASSIUM	135 mg	340 mg

†Information on cholesterol content is provided for individuals who on the advice of a physician, are modifying their total dietary intake of cholesterol.

PERCENTAGE OF U.S. RECOMMENDED DAILY ALLOWANCES (PERCENT U.S. RDA)

PROTEIN	8	15
VITAMIN A	20	25
VITAMIN C	**	2
THIAMINE	30	35
RIBOFLAVIN	15	25
NIACIN	20	20
CALCIUM	**	15
IRON	30	30
VITAMIN D	10	25
VITAMIN B₆	20	25
FOLIC ACID	20	25
VITAMIN B₁₂	25	30
PHOSPORUS	15	25
MAGNESIUM	10	15
ZINC	20	20
PANTOTHENIC ACID	15	20

*Cereal plus ½ cup vitamin A and D fortified 2% lowfat milk contains 160 calories, 4 grams fat and 10 mg cholesterol. All other nutrients remain as listed.

**Contains less than 2% of the U.S. RDA for these nutrients.

INGREDIENTS: OAT BRAN, SUGAR, WHOLE WHEAT FLOUR, CORN FLOUR, OAT BRAN CONCENTRATE, SODIUM BICARBONATE, SALT, CARAMEL COLOR.

VITAMINS & MINERALS: NIACINAMIDE; VITAMIN A PALMITATE, REDUCED IRON, ZINC OXIDE (A SOURCE OF ZINC); CALCIUM PANTOTHENATE; PYRIDOXINE HYDROCHLORIDE; VITAMIN D, THIAMINE MONONITRATE; RIBOFLAVIN; FOLIC ACID; VITAMIN B₁₂ BHA ADDED TO PRESERVE PRODUCT FRESHNESS.

One of the B vitamins.

CARBOHYDRATE INFORMATION

	CEREAL	WITH MILK
STARCH AND RELATED CARBOHYDRATES	13 g	13 g
SUCROSE AND RELATED SUGARS	4 g	10 g
DIETARY FIBER	3 g	3 g
TOTAL CARBOHYDRATES	20 g	26 g

AVENA OAT CO
PO BOX 1760
ST. LOUIS MO 63148

HIGH FIBER CEREAL

OAT BRAN

Help reduce Cholesterol

NET WT 7 OZ. (198 G)

one serving of this food contains 30% of the U.S. RDA for iron. Since the U.S. RDA for iron is 18 milligrams, this product contains about 5.4 milligrams of iron per serving ($0.3 \times 18 = 5.4$). The label also states that one serving contains 20% of the U.S. RDA for the vitamin niacin. Because the U.S. RDA for niacin is 20 milligrams, the niacin content is 0.20×20 or 4 milligrams. See the Nutrition Issue on p. 60 to learn more about regulations that apply to nutrition labels on foods.

CONCEPT CHECK

Recommended Dietary Allowances represent the nutrient needs of groups—not of individuals. RDA are established for specific age and gender categories. No one knows personal nutritional requirements unless they have been scientifically measured in a laboratory. The best general rule is the further you stray below the RDA for your age and gender, the greater the chance of experiencing a nutritional deficiency. The U.S. RDA was designed in 1974 by FDA as a means of expressing nutrient content of foods on nutrition labels. Nutrient content is listed as a percentage of the U.S. RDA. Soon RDI will replace the U.S. RDA. RDI values will reflect the 1989 RDA.

MEAL PLANNING TOOLS

Throughout the twentieth century nutritionists have worked to clarify nutrition concepts so that people can estimate whether their food selections supply enough of all essential nutrients. By the mid-1950s various food plans evolved into a plan that consisted of four food groups: (1) milk, (2) meat, (3) fruits and vegetables, and (4) breads and cereals. In 1979 the names of the groups were revised by the USDA, and a fifth group that contains fats, sweets, and alcoholic beverages was added as part of the "Hassle-Free Daily Food Guide." People were urged to use caution in consuming items from the fifth group, even though some foods in it supply needed vitamin E. This plan was designed to provide a minimum foundation for a diet, representing about 1200 to 1400 kcalories.

In 1991 the USDA revised the Hassle-Free Daily Food Guide to represent a total diet, rather than simply a foundation for a diet. This latest plan is called USDA's Food Guide—A Pattern for Daily Food Choices (Figure 2-3). The major changes in this guide for daily food choices are an increase in fruit and vegetable servings from four per day to five to nine per day, and bread and cereal servings from four per day to six to eleven per day. The goal of these changes is to provide the bulk of dietary energy intake from carbohydrate while limiting fat intake.

Using the Guide to Daily Food Choices

The number of servings and portion sizes from each food group in the Guide to Daily Food Choices depend on a person's age and kcalorie needs (Table 2-1). Basically, the plan for adults over the age of 25 consists of two servings from the milk, yogurt, and cheese group; two to three servings from the meat, poultry, fish, dry beans, eggs, and nuts group (5 to 7 ounces total); three to five servings from the vegetable group; two to four servings from the fruit group; and six to eleven servings from the bread, cereals, rice, and pasta group. A final group that requires cautious use includes fats, oils, and sweets. Some population groups—children, teenagers, adults under age 25, and pregnant or lactating women—need three servings of the milk, yogurt, and cheese group. Table 2-1 lists the major nutrients each food group supplies. Note the similarities and differences between the groups.

Here are several important points to keep in mind when you use this plan:

1. The guide does not apply to infants.

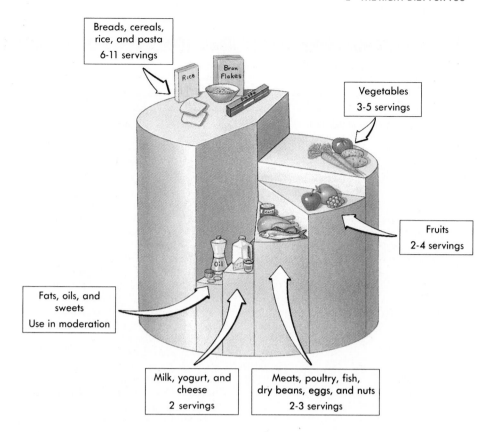

FIGURE 2-3

USDA's Food Guide—A Pattern for Daily Food Choices. This plan forms the basis for a healthy diet if one follows the average American food pattern.

2. No one food is absolutely essential to good nutrition. Each food is low in at least one essential nutrient.

3. No one food group provides all essential nutrients adequately. Each food group offers some important nutrients.

4. Variety is the key to the plan. Variety is guaranteed by choosing foods from all groups and selecting different foods from within each group.

Again, the foundations of nutrition are variety, balance, and moderation. Choosing from every group and varying choices within groups allows a healthy variety of foods.

By following the Guide to Daily Food Choices you can easily create daily diets that contain as little as 1400 to 1600 kcalories and still meet the adult RDA for protein, thiamin, niacin, riboflavin, calcium, and other important nutrients. To ensure enough vitamin E, vitamin B-6, magnesium, iron, and zinc we recommend the following advice:

1. Choose lowfat and nonfat items from the milk, yogurt, and cheese group.

2. Make sure to regularly include servings of vegetable protein sources.

3. For vegetables and fruits, include a vitamin C source and a dark green vegetable each day.

4. Choose whole-grain varieties of breads, cereals, rice, and pasta often.

By following these suggestions, you would still consume only about 1600 kcalories. While 1600 kcalories is not enough for an active adult, it is probably sufficient for a sedentary adult or an elderly person.

If an energy intake of 1600 kcalories is too much for you, the first step in offsetting the excess is to increase your level of physical activity. It is difficult to get enough nutrients from a daily diet containing fewer kcalories. It isn't usual-

TABLE 2-1

The Guide to Daily Food Choices—a summary

Food Group	Serving	Major Contributions	Foods and Serving Sizes[*]
Milk, yogurt, and cheese	2 (adult[‖]) 3 (children, teens, young adults, and pregnant or lactating women)	Calcium Riboflavin Protein Potassium Zinc	1 cup milk 1½ oz cheese 2 oz processed cheese 1 cup yogurt 2 cups cottage cheese 1 cup custard/pudding 1½ cups ice cream
Meat, poultry, fish, dry beans, eggs, and nuts	2-3	Protein Niacin Iron Vitamin B-6 Zinc Thiamin Vitamin B-12[†]	2-3 oz cooked meat, poultry, fish 1-1½ cups cooked dry beans 4 T peanut butter 2 eggs ½-1 cup nuts
Fruits	2-4	Vitamin C Fiber	¼ cup dried fruit ½ cup cooked fruit ¾ cup juice 1 whole piece of fruit 1 melon wedge
Vegetables	3-5	Vitamin A Vitamin C Folate Magnesium Fiber	½ cup raw or cooked vegetables 1 cup raw leafy vegetables
Bread, cereals, rice, and pasta	6-11	Starch Thiamin Riboflavin[§] Iron Niacin Folate Magnesium[‡] Fiber[‡] Zinc[‡]	1 slice of bread 1 oz ready-to-eat cereal ½-¾ cup cooked cereal, rice, or pasta
Fats, oils, and sweets		Foods from this group should not replace any from the other groups. Amounts consumed should be determined by individual energy needs.	

This is a practical way to turn the RDA into food choices. You can get all essential nutrients by eating a balanced variety of foods each day from the food groups listed here. Eat a variety of foods in each food group and adjust serving sizes appropriately to reach and maintain desirable weight.

[*]May be reduced for child servings.
[†]Only in animal food choices.
[‡]Whole grains especially.
[§]If enriched.
[‖]≥ 25 years of age.

ly necessary to meet the RDA for all nutrients, but you may not know what nutrients you can eat less of and still remain healthy. If you can't increase your energy output, you should consider including some nutrient-fortified foods in your diet, such as ready-to-eat breakfast cereals. Chapter 3 discusses whether nutrient supplements are a wise choice; they are usually not needed. In addition, if your diet does not include meat or other animal products, see the Nutrition Issue on vegetarianism in Chapter 8.

Using nutrient density as a diet planning tool

Today kcalories are often a great concern for many of us. How can we evaluate foods so that we choose those that have the most nutrients and the fewest kcalories? The concept of *nutrient density* is one way. This is a measure that compares the vitamin or mineral content of a food to its number of kcalories. The higher the nutrient density in the food, the more nutrient there is per kcalorie and the better the food source is for that particular nutrient. Still, the focus on menu planning is the total diet, not whether one food is the key to an adequate diet.[10,12] Nonetheless, nutrient-dense foods help balance less nutrient-dense choices we often make, like cookies and chips. The latter are often called empty-calorie foods because they supply energy and little else.

> **Nutrient Density** • The ratio formed by dividing a food's contribution to nutrient needs by its contribution to kcalorie needs. When the contribution to nutrient needs exceeds that of kcalorie needs, the food is considered to have a favorable nutrient density.
>
> **Goiter** • An enlargement of the thyroid gland (located in the neck area) often caused by a lack of iodine in the diet.

CONCEPT CHECK

The Guide to Daily Food Choices translates nutrient needs into a food plan. This guide recommends adults over age 24 consume:

1. Two servings from the milk, yogurt, and cheese group (three if age 24 or younger, pregnant, or lactating).
2. Two to three servings from the meat, poultry, fish, dry beans, eggs, and nuts group.
3. Three to five servings from the vegetable group.
4. Two to four servings from the fruit group.
5. Six to eleven servings from the bread, cereals, rice, and pasta group.
6. Cautious use of fats, oils, and sweets.

The concept of nutrient density provides another diet planning tool. Thus evaluate nutrient contributions of a food by comparing its kcalorie value for a specific nutrient to its contribution to total kcalorie needs. Nutrient-dense foods provide ample nutrients in comparison to kcalorie content.

Further guidelines to help you plan your meals

The Guide to Daily Food Choices primarily focuses on supplying enough essential nutrients to keep our body systems functioning well. Yet, many deficiency diseases that were common in years past, such as *goiter* (iodide deficiency) and pellagra (niacin deficiency), are no longer a big problem. In fact most chronic, "killer" diseases prevalent in America, such as heart disease, cancer, diabetes mellitus, and cirrhosis of the liver, are not associated with nutrient deficiencies or general poor body function. The real problems in the American diet are excess kcalories, saturated fat, cholesterol, alcohol, and sodium (salt)[15,18] (Figure 2-4). For some people, too little calcium, iron, zinc, or dietary fiber in the diet also is a problem.

FIGURE 2-4

Is our current diet in our best interests? Many scientists evaluating the relationship between diet and health have concluded we should eat more carbohydrate-rich foods and less fat-rich foods.

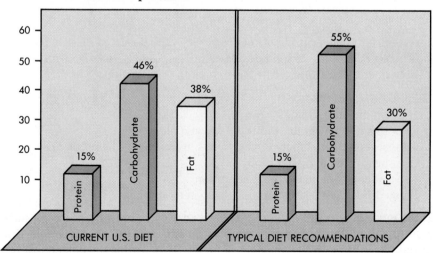

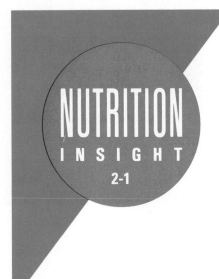

NUTRITION
I N S I G H T
2-1

A shortcut method estimates 100 pounds for the first 60 inches for women and adds an extra 5 pounds for every inch thereafter. The corresponding values for males are 106 pounds for the first 60 inches and 6 additional pounds per inch thereafter.

A DIET FOR LIFE

Recently the Surgeon General,[18] the American Heart Association (AHA), the National Cancer Institute (NCI), and the National Academy of Sciences (NAS)[15] have added recommendations to the framework of the Dietary Guidelines.[6,15,18] Following is a summary of the advice provided by the Dietary Guidelines with additional comments from various health-related organizations.

1. **Eat a variety of foods.** Most groups specifically suggest variety and moderation in food choice. An NAS report entitled *Diet and Health*, suggests limiting protein intake to no more than twice the RDA and not taking nutrient supplements in quantities greater than the RDA in any 1 day. Both the NAS report and the Surgeon General encourage everyone to meet the RDA for calcium, especially adolescent girls and women.

2. **Maintain healthy weight.** You can use the middle ranges of the Metropolitan Life Insurance Table as a standard (see Chapter 11). Both the NAS report and the Surgeon General emphasize balancing food intake with regular physical activity to avoid gradual weight increases that can lead to obesity.

For those who are trying to lose weight, the recommended rate of weight loss is 1 or 2 pounds a week. To do this, the Surgeon General suggests increasing physical activity and eating low-kcalorie, nutrient-rich foods: more fruits, vegetables, and grains; less fat and fatty foods, sugar and sweets, and alcoholic beverages.

3. **Choose a diet low in fat, saturated fat, and cholesterol.** The Dietary Guidelines, NAS report, AHA, and NCI suggest limiting fat intake to 30% of total kcalories. The Dietary Guidelines, NAS report, and AHA recommend limiting saturated fat to at least one-third of total fat intake (10% of total kcalories). A common dietary cholesterol limit is 300 milligrams per day. (The average American consumes 13% to 15% of total kcalories as saturated fat and about 400 to 500 milligrams of dietary cholesterol per day.) The NAS report recommends choosing lean meat, fish, poultry, and dry beans and peas as protein sources; using nonfat or lowfat milk and milk products; limiting intake of fats and oils high in saturated fat; trimming fat off meats; broiling, baking, or boiling instead of frying; and moderating consumption of fat-containing foods, such as breaded or deep-fried foods.

4. **Choose a diet with plenty of vegetables, fruits, and grain products.** The NAS report suggests you have five or more servings of vegetables plus fruits daily and six or more servings of a combination of breads, cereals, and legumes (beans) daily. The NCI recommends 20 to 30 grams of dietary fiber per day. These food choices should meet that goal. The current U.S. average for dietary fiber intake is closer to 15 grams per day.

Dietary Guidelines • General goals for nutrient intakes and diet composition set by the USDA and DHHS.

In response to concerns about the frequency of diet-related disease patterns in the United States, the federal government has issued *Dietary Guidelines* for people over 2 years of age. The latest version (1990) states:[17]

1. Eat a variety of foods.
2. Maintain healthy weight.
3. Choose a diet low in fat, saturated fat, and cholesterol.
4. Choose a diet with plenty of vegetables, fruits, and grain products.
5. Use sugars only in moderation.
6. Use salt and sodium only in moderation.
7. If you drink alcoholic beverages, do so in moderation.

These guidelines refer to your total day's or week's intake, not to one meal or a certain food choice. Overall, the plan aims to ensure you get ample vitamins and minerals by eating a variety of foods. By following the guidelines, you

As mentioned in Chapter 1, dietary fiber is a term used to describe parts of plant foods that human digestive processes can't break down. There are several kinds of fiber, each with different chemical structures and biological effects (see Chapter 6 for details). Since foods differ in the kinds of fiber they contain, it's best to include a variety of fiber-rich foods.

5. **Use sugars only in moderation.** The Surgeon General suggests that those people who are prone to *dental caries* (cavities), especially children, should limit the amount of sugary food they eat. Some authorities recommend that we eat no more than 10% of our total kcalories as sugars. This would amount to about 40 pounds per year, as opposed to the average American's current intake of approximately 145 pounds per year. On a daily basis, this amounts to a limit of 10 teaspoons (50 grams) of sugar on a 2000 kcalorie diet.

6. **Use salt and sodium only in moderation.** The NAS report suggests limiting sodium intake to 2.4 grams per day. This is the amount of sodium contained in 6 grams of salt (40% of salt is sodium). The average person currently eats 4 to 7 grams of sodium per day. The NAS report and Surgeon General suggest we use a limited amount of salt in cooking and avoid adding it to food at the table. In addition, only very small amounts of salty, highly processed, salt-preserved, and salt-pickled foods should be eaten.

A sodium restriction to 2.4 grams a day would require a great change in food habits for many of us. It would mean not eating processed (lunch) meats, salted snack foods, most canned and prepared soups, most types of cheese, and many tomato-based products.

7. **If you drink alcoholic beverages, do so in moderation.** Both the NAS report and Surgeon General recommend no more than two drinks daily—the equivalent of 8 ounces of wine, 24 ounces of beer, or 3 ounces of distilled spirits. Pregnant women should completely avoid alcohol. If you are concerned about excess kcalories and want a nutritious diet, keep in mind that alcoholic beverages are high in kcalories and low or devoid in essential nutrients.

Beyond these overall recommendations, the NCI suggests eating moderate amounts of salt-cured, smoked, and *nitrate*-cured foods because they are thought to increase the risk of certain forms of cancer. The NAS report and Surgeon General also recommend obtaining adequate fluoride, particularly during the growing years. By strengthening tooth structure, fluoride in the diet allows for fewer dental caries. Finally, the Surgeon General recommends that children, adolescents, and women of childbearing age eat iron-rich foods, primarily to avoid developing iron-deficiency anemia. ●

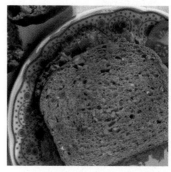

A diet that contains fiber-rich foods is beneficial.

Nitrate ● A nitrogen-containing compound used to cure meats. Its use contributes a pink color to meats, and confers some resistance to bacterial growth.

can reduce your risk for obesity, hypertension, heart disease, diabetes mellitus, and alcoholism (Table 2-2). If you eat the typical American high-meat diet, you will need to make a few changes to follow this plan by increasing your consumption of vegetables, fruits, and grain products (Table 2-3).[15] This plan is easily incorporated into the Guide to Daily Food Choices. In fact, incorporation of the Dietary Guidelines was a key consideration in the guide's development.

Putting dietary guidelines into perspective

The Dietary Guidelines suggested for Americans have disturbed some nutritionists. They think many of the guidelines are too general to meet specific individual nutrition needs. As individuals, we vary in our tendencies toward developing high blood cholesterol levels, hypertension, obesity, cancer, and other health problems that the guidelines are designed to prevent.[10] Genetic background is one key reason for the variation.

Do you know your blood cholesterol level? Blood pressure values? Although you may feel you are not susceptible to the problems listed above, it is still a good idea to have your blood cholesterol levels and blood pressure measured every few years to verify you are right.

An example of how nutrition advice must accommodate individual differences can be seen with sugar intake. People who don't expend much energy should eat a nutrient-dense diet—supplying many nutrients per kcalorie. A high sugar intake, which contributes many kcalories and few nutrients, would not fit in with such a goal. However, someone with a very active lifestyle who practices good dental hygiene can add some sugar to his or her diet with no negative health effects. The same is true of sodium. There are no scientific data that

TABLE 2-2

Putting dietary guidelines into practice

For variety:
- Include foods from all of these groups on a daily basis: breads, cereals, and other grain products; fruits; vegetables; meat, poultry, fish, and alternates; milk, cheese, and yogurt.

For balance:
- If you eat foods high in fat, sugars, or sodium, during the day include other foods that are lower in these components.

To maintain healthy weight:
- Choose a variety of foods that provide needed nutrients.
- Go easy on foods that supply mainly calories—sugars, sweets, fats and oils, foods high in sugars and fats, and alcoholic beverages.

To lose weight:
- Eat a variety of foods that are low in calories and high in nutrients:
  Eat more fruits, vegetables, and whole grains.
  Eat less fat and fatty foods.
  Eat less sugar and sweets.
  Drink less alcoholic beverages.
- Increase your physical activity.

To help control overeating:
- Eat slowly.
- Take smaller portions.
- Avoid "seconds."

To choose a diet low in fat, saturated fat, and cholesterol:
- Choose lean meat, fish, poultry, and dry beans and peas as protein sources.
- Use skim or lowfat milk and milk products.
- Use egg yolks and organ meats in moderation.
- Use fats and oils, especially those high in saturated fat, such as cream, lard, and butter, in moderation.
- Use foods high in fat, such as deep-fried or breaded foods, in moderation.
- Trim fat off meats; remove skin from poultry.
- Broil, bake, boil, steam, or microwave, rather than fry.

- Read labels carefully to determine both amount and type of fat present in foods.

To choose a diet with plenty of vegetables, fruits, and grain products:
- Choose foods that are good sources of starch—breads, cereals, pasta, rice, dry beans and peas, and starchy vegetables, such as potatoes, corn, and lima beans.
- Choose foods that are good sources of fiber, such as whole-grain breads, cereals, and pasta; vegetables and fruits with edible skins; dry beans and peas.

To use sugars only in moderation:
- Use less of all sugars and foods containing large amounts of sugars, including white sugar, brown sugar, raw sugar, honey, and syrups. Examples include soft drinks, candies, cakes, and cookies.
- Remember, how often you eat sugar and sugar-containing food is as important to the health of your teeth as how much sugar you eat. It will help to avoid eating sweets between meals.
- Read food labels for clues on sugar content. If the name sugar, sucrose, glucose, maltose, dextrose, lactose, fructose, or syrups appears first, then there is a large amount of sugar.
- Select fresh fruits or fruits processed without syrup or with light, rather than heavy, syrup.

To use salt and sodium only in moderation:
- Learn to enjoy the flavors of unsalted foods.
- Cook without salt or with only small amounts of added salt.
- Try flavoring foods with herbs, spices, and lemon juice.
- Add little or no salt to food at the table.
- Limit your intake of salty foods, such as potato chips, pretzels, salted nuts and popcorn, condiments (soy sauce, steak sauce, garlic salt), pickled foods, cured meats, some cheeses, and some canned vegetables and soups.
- Read food labels carefully to determine the amounts of sodium.
- Use lower sodium products, when available, to replace those you use that have higher sodium content.

TABLE 2-3

Advice for applying the Dietary Guidelines to practical situations

You usually eat this:	Reconsider and eat this:
White bread	Whole-wheat bread—not as many nutrients have been lost in refinement/processing
Sugared breakfast cereal	Low sugar cereal; use the kcalories you save for a side dish of fruit
Cheeseburger and French fries	Hamburger (hold the mayonnaise) and baked beans (for less fat and the benefits of plant proteins)
Potato salad at the salad bar	Three-bean salad
Doughnut	Bran muffin or bagel (no cream cheese)
Soft drinks	Water, diet soft drinks, or iced tea (save the kcalories for more nutritious foods)
Boiled vegetables	Steamed vegetables (more nutrient retention)
Canned vegetables	Frozen vegetables (less nutrients lost in processing)
Fried meats	Broiled meats (watch the fat drain away)
Fatty meats, like ribs	Lean meats, like ground round; also, eat chicken and fish often
Whole milk and ice cream	1% Milk and sherbet or frozen yogurt (to reduce saturated fat intake)
Mayonnaise or sour cream salad dressing	Oil and vinegar dressings or diet varieties (to save kcalories)
Cookies	Popcorn (air popped with minimal margarine)

support the contention that people who currently have normal blood pressure values will later develop hypertension if they consume excess amounts of sodium. In addition, of the 15% or so of Americans who develop hypertension, only about half are sensitive to the amount of salt in their diets.

You could argue that since causes of hypertension can't be identified until a problem arises, everyone, especially blacks (who have an unusually high rate of hypertension) and people who have a family history of hypertension, should go easy on the salt.[15] However, a more relaxed posture that advises changing your diet when your blood pressure increases also has scientific credibility.

It is best to consider your own state of health when using these guidelines.[10] Make specific changes and see if they are effective. However, results are sometimes disappointing, even when you are following a diet change very closely.[9] Some people can eat a lot of saturated fats and still keep desirable blood cholesterol levels. Other people, unfortunately, have high blood cholesterol levels even if they eat low fat, low-cholesterol diets. Such people don't benefit from the same diet that helps other people.[9,10] Again, differences in genetic background are a likely reason.

Still, most nutrition and health researchers agree with at least some of the guidelines set by our major health and science institutions. The need for varying food choices; controlling body weight; reducing total fat intake for adults; eating many fruits, vegetables, and cereal grains; and moderating alcohol intake is well-accepted advice.[15,18] These recommendations should guide a total day's intake. However, many scientists do not agree on general recommendations for sugar, starches, dietary fiber, salt, specific vitamins, and cholesterol. Rather, they believe that these recommendations must be based both on a person's family history for the major chronic diseases and on the person's current health status. Later in this chapter we offer advice on finding a nutrition expert to help you decide how to change your diet to meet your specific health needs.

Whether or not you need to change your diet to improve your health, you should try to understand the goals embodied in the Dietary Guidelines. The emphasis on lowfat dairy products, lean meats and plant proteins, fruits and vegetables, and breads and cereals is consistent with the suggestions of the

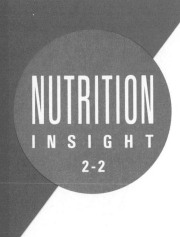

NUTRITION
I N S I G H T
2-2

WHERE TO GET RELIABLE NUTRITION ADVICE

If you have a question about nutrition, the most convenient person to ask is probably your professor or another nutrition faculty member on your campus. Local *registered dietitians (RDs)* or your family physician are also good resources. Most large communities have a service called "Dial a Dietitian" where you can get free nutrition information from a registered dietitian by telephone.

When you are seeking nutrition counseling, it is important to find a registered dietitian. They are specially trained to help you meet your nutritional needs through healthful, tasty diets. Hospitals and health departments are good places to begin your search. A person obtains an RD certification by earning a bachelor's degree in nutrition, completing extensive professional practice under expert supervision, and successfully passing a comprehensive examination.

People who do not have the appropriate training and education sometimes claim to be nutrition professionals. They may have a doctorate degree in a non-nutrition field or a mail order diploma, but they are not qualified to give nutritional advice. Although some of these people may give sound advice, others may promise results that sound too good to be true. They may encourage the use of bogus tests, such as inappropriate allergy tests or hair analyses. They may promote pills, gimmicks, and gadgets and boast success with numerous testimonials from other clients. They may refuse to consult with your physician and try to convince you that no medical doctor has the answer for your ailment. The consumer must be wary of such claims.

Currently 23 states license the right to use the title *dietitian*. In other states, however, people can legally call themselves dietitians or nutritionists even though they have no training in those fields. An RD credential guarantees that the person has a good background in nutrition.

When you meet with a nutrition professional, you should expect that he or she:

- asks questions about your medical history, lifestyle, and current eating habits. The professional may ask you to keep a detailed diet diary in order to establish a baseline before making major diet changes or recommendations.
- formulates a diet plan tailored to your needs, as opposed to simply tearing a form from a tablet that could apply to almost anyone.
- schedules follow-up visits to track your progress, answers any questions, and helps keep you motivated.
- involves family members in the diet plan, when appropriate.
- consults directly with your physician, and readily refers you back to the physician for health problems a nutritionist is not trained to treat.

Usually you need to see a physician for conditions calling for detailed nutrition advice. An exception to this might be losing weight when you are otherwise healthy. If you have high blood cholesterol levels, hypertension, diabetes mellitus, suffer from food *allergies* (sensitivities) or digestive problems, or are beginning to develop osteoporosis, you should have a careful evaluation by a physician. You could have a condition that actually results from another disease. A physician needs to evaluate your total health in order to properly diagnose problems. The next step is to consult a registered dietitian to help you design an appropriate diet.

Steer clear of nutritionists who say that everyone needs vitamin supplements to be sure they're getting enough essential nutrients. Likewise, avoid the advice of anyone who suggests that most diseases are caused by faulty nutrition or that large doses of vitamins and minerals will cure many diseases. Anyone who uses a computer-scored nutrition deficiency test as the basis for prescribing vitamins should not be trusted. And, above all, beware of any practitioner—licensed or not—who sells vitamins in his or her office. We will discuss nutrition fraud further in Chapter 4. Chapter 11 gives tips for separating facts from fiction regarding weight loss diets. ●

Guide to Daily Food Choices. This is the best overall way for you to maintain optimal nutritional health based on current scientific knowledge. Diets of many different cultures already meet these guidelines. Does your diet?

If what you are currently eating is very different from what Figure 2-3 recommends, try to make some changes. To learn more about what you eat, read food labels. The Nutrition Issue on p. 60 will give you some help. Chapter 3 will help you with methods to use to make needed changes in your diet.

Exchange System • A grouping of foods in six lists such that all foods within each list yield a similar amount of carbohydrate, fat, protein, and energy.

CONCEPT CHECK

Dietary advice has been issued by various private and government organizations. This advice is designed to minimize the risk of developing obesity, hypertension, heart disease, and alcoholism. To accomplish these goals, the Dietary Guidelines encourage people to eat a variety of foods. Further, the guidelines suggest that we maintain a healthy weight and moderate our intake of saturated fat, salt, sugar, and alcohol, while eating more fruits, vegetables, and grain products.

What is the exchange system?

The *exchange system* is another valuable diet planning tool. You can use it quickly to estimate the energy, protein, carbohydrate, and fat content of a food or meal. The exchange system is also a convenient way for a person to plan kcalorie-controlled diets. Weight Watchers uses a system based on exchanges.

The exchange system arranges food into six different categories: milk, fruit, vegetables, starch/bread, meat, and fat. Given the appropriate serving size, each food within a category provides about the same amount of carbohydrate, protein, fat, and kcalories. For instance, in the bread group 1 slice of bread is equivalent to ½ cup of bran flakes or 2½ tablespoons of cornmeal in providing energy-yielding nutrients. Thus as you select servings from each group, foods within a category can be *exchanged* for each other.

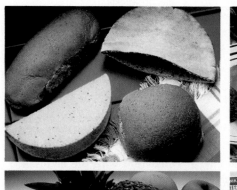 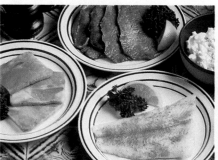 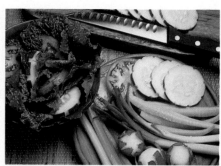

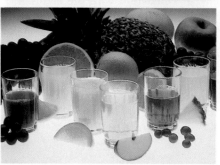 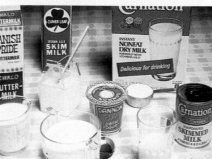 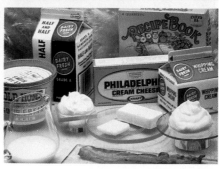

Above left, the starch/bread exchange group; *above center*, the meat exchange group; *above right*, the vegetable exchange group; *below left*, the fruit exchange group; *below center*, the milk exchange group; *below right*, the fat exchange group.

DIETARY ADVICE FOR CANADIANS

Canada has its own version of RDA, called Recommended Nutrient Intakes (RNI), published by the Minister of National Health and Welfare.[5] These are listed in Appendix C. A separate Canadian food guide provides a plan to meet these nutrient needs (Figure 2-5).

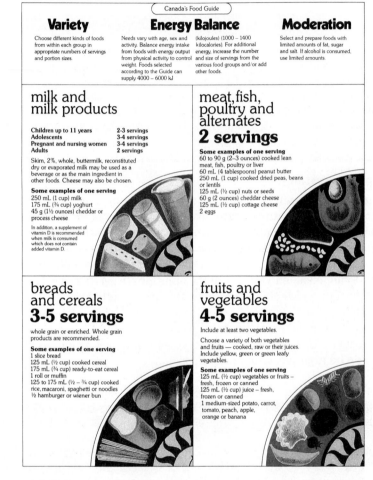

FIGURE 2-5
The Canadian food guide.

A summary of the desired characteristics of the Canadian diet is given below:

1. **The Canadian diet should provide energy consistent with the maintenance of body weight within the recommended range.** Physical activity should be appropriate to circumstances and capabilities. While the importance of maintain-

ing some activity throughout life can be stressed, it is not possible to specify a level of physical activity appropriate for the whole population. As a general guideline it is desirable that adults, for as long as possible, maintain an activity level that permits an energy intake of at least 1800 kcalories while keeping weight within the recommended range.

2. **The Canadian diet should include essential nutrients in amounts recommended in this report.** While it is important that the diet provide the recommended amounts of nutrients, it should be understood that no evidence was found that intakes in excess of the RNI confer any health benefit. There is no general need for supplements except for vitamin D for infants and folate during pregnancy. Vitamin D supplementation might be required for elderly persons not exposed to the sun, and iron for pregnant women with low iron stores.

3. **The Canadian diet should include no more than 30% of energy as fat (33g/1000 kcalories) and no more than 10% as saturated fat (11g/1000 kcalories).** Dietary cholesterol, though not as influential in affecting levels of blood cholesterol, is not without importance. A reduction in cholesterol intake normally will accompany a reduction in total fat and saturated fat. The recommendation to reduce total fat intake does not apply to children under the age of 2 years.

4. **The Canadian diet should provide 55% of energy as carbohydrate (138g/1000 kcalories) from a variety of sources.** Sources should be selected that provide complex carbohydrates, a variety of dietary fiber, and ***beta-carotene.***

5. **The sodium content of the Canadian diet should be reduced.** The present food supply provides sodium in an amount greatly exceeding requirements. While there is insufficient evidence to support a precise recommendation, potential benefit would be expected from a reduction in current sodium intake.

6. **The Canadian diet should include no more than 5% of total energy as alcohol, or two drinks daily, whichever is less.** The harmful influence of alcohol on blood pressure provides a more urgent reason for moderation. During pregnancy it is prudent to abstain from alcoholic beverages because a safe intake is not known with certainty.

7. **The Canadian diet should contain no more caffeine than the equivalent of four regular cups of coffee per day.** This is a prudent measure in view of the increased risk for cardiovascular disease associated with high intakes of caffeine.

8. **Community water supplies containing less than 1 mg/liter should be fluoridated to that level.** Fluoridation of community water supplies has proven to be a safe, effective, and economical method of improving dental health.

More details are available on RNI and diet recommendations in the 1990 publication entitled Nutrition Recommendations: The Report of the Scientific Review Committee. ●

From Canadian nutrient and dietary recommendations, *Nutrition Today*, November/ December, 1990, p 4.

The exchange system was developed in the 1950s for planning diabetic diets. It is easier for a person with diabetes mellitus to control the disease if the diet contains about the same proportion of energy-yielding nutrients day after day. By using a set number of choices (or exchanges) from each of the six categories, a person can achieve regularity more easily.

In addition, because the exchange system also provides a quick way to estimate the content of energy and carbohydrate, protein, and fat in a food or meal, it has a more general use. You can use it to design meal patterns containing specified amounts of protein, carbohydrate, fat, and kcalories. As in learning a foreign language, you will need some practice before you feel comfortable with the exchange system. Appendix F describes the system fully and demonstrates how to use it.

SUMMARY

- Recommended Dietary Allowances are set for many nutrients. These levels represent the amount of a nutrient that healthy people should consume regularly to meet their needs for that nutrient. RDA guidelines differ for men and women and for various age groups. The further you stray below RDA values, the greater your chance of developing a nutrient deficiency.

- The four versions of the U.S. RDA are based primarily on the highest RDA levels found in the 1968 publication. The U.S. RDA forms the basis for listing nutrient levels on food labels.

- The Guide to Daily Food Choices provides a way to turn nutrient recommendations from the RDA into a food plan. We should emphasize lowfat (or nonfat) milk, yogurt, and cheese products; proteins from vegetables as well as from lean meat; liberal intake of fruits; vegetables; and whole-grain forms of breads, cereals, rice, and pasta.

- Nutrient density reflects the nutrient content of a food in relation to its kcalorie (energy) content. Nutrient-dense foods are rich in nutrients in comparison to kcalorie content.

- The Dietary Guidelines help one plan a menu pattern to reduce risk of developing chronic, "killer" diseases. These guidelines emphasize eating a variety of foods; maintaining a healthy weight; moderating intake of fats, cholesterol, sugar, salt, and alcohol; and including ample vegetables, fruits, and grains in the diet.

- The exchange system provides a powerful tool for estimating the carbohydrate, fat, protein, and kcalorie content of a food or meal.

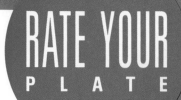

DOES YOUR DIET MEET THE RDA?

Instructions: Perform either part I or part II. Then perform part III. (For assistance in following the instructions for this activity, see the sample Assessment in Appendix D.)

Part I.

A. Take the information from the 1-day food intake record you completed in Chapter 1 and record it on the blank form provided in Appendix D. Make sure to record the food or drink ingested and the amount (weight) consumed. NOTE: Your professor may require you to keep the food record for more than 1 day.

B. Review the 1989 RDA on the inside cover of the book and choose the appropriate recommendations for your gender and age. Write the appropriate value for each nutrient on the line labeled "Your RDA."
NOTE: The values for sodium and potassium from the table on the inside cover of the book are labeled, "Estimated Sodium, Chloride, and Potassium Minimum Requirements of Healthy Persons."

C. Look up the foods and drinks you've listed on the form in the food composition table, Appendix A. Record on the form the amounts of each nutrient and kcalories present in them.

D. For each food and drink, add the amounts in each column and record the results on the line labeled "Totals."

E. Compare the totals to your RDA's. Divide the total for each nutrient by the specific RDA or minimum requirement and multiply that by 100. Record the result on the line labeled, "% of your RDA."

F. Hold on to this assessment for use in subsequent activities for other chapters.

Part II.

A. Obtain copies of the computer software, Mosby Diet Simple, from your instructor, as well as directions for using it. Follow the instructions and load the software into the computer.

B. Choose your RDA based on your age and gender.

C. Enter the information from the 1-day food intake record you completed in Chapter 1. Make sure to enter each food and drink and the appropriate serving size.

D. This software program will give you the following results:
   a. Your 1989 RDA value for each nutrient.
   b. The total amount of each nutrient and kcalories consumed for the day.
   c. The percentage of the RDA 1989 values you consumed for each nutrient.

E. Hold on to this assessment for use in subsequent activities in other chapters.

Part III. Evaluation

Remember that you don't necessarily need to consume 100% of the 1989 RDA values. A safe standard is to consume at least 70%. It would be best not to exceed 500% to avoid potential toxic effects. There is no advantage in exceeding 100%.

A. For which nutrients do you fall below 70%?
B. Did you exceed the minimum requirements for sodium? To what degree?
C. For which nutrients did you exceed the RDA by greater than 500% (5 times greater)?
D. What dietary changes could you make to correct or improve your dietary profile? If unsure, future chapters will help guide your decisions.

REFERENCES

1. ADA testifies on nutrition labeling and education act of 1989, *Journal of the American Dietetic Association* 90:12, 1990.
2. American Dietetic Association: Nutrition and health information on food labels. *Journal of the American Dietetic Association* 90:583, 1990.
3. Block G and others: Nutrient sources in the American diet, *American Journal of Epidemiology* 122:13, 1985.
4. Blumenthal D: A new look at food labeling, *FDA Consumer*, November, 1989, p 15.
5. Canadian nutrient and dietary recommendations, *Nutrition Today*, November/December, 1990, p 4.
6. Cronin FJ, Shaw AM: Summary of dietary recommendations for healthy Americans, *Nutrition Today*, November/December, 1988, p 26.
7. FDA announces examination of food labeling issues, *Journal of the American Dietetic Association* 89:1594, 1989.
8. Food and Nutrition Board, National Academy of Sciences-National Research Council: *Recommended dietary allowances, revised*, Washington DC, 1989, the Board.
9. Harper AE: Scientific substantiation of health claims: how much is enough, *Nutrition Today*, March/April, 1989, p17.
10. Harper AE: Nutrition: from myth and magic to science, *Nutrition Today*, January/February, 1988, p 8.
11. Harris SH, Welch S: How well are our food choices meeting our nutrition needs? *Nutrition Today*, November/December, 1989, p 20.
12. Herbert V: Health claims in food labeling and advertising. *Nutrition Today*, May/June, 1987, p 25.
13. Monsen ER: The 10th edition of the recommended dietary allowances: what's new in the 1989 RDAs, *Journal of the American Dietetic Association* 89:1748, 1989.
14. Mullis RM and others: Developing nutrient criteria for food-specific dietary guidelines for the general public, *Journal of the American Dietetic Association* 90:847, 1990.
15. National Research Council: *Diet and Health*, Washington DC, 1989, National Academy Press.
16. Olson JA: Recommended nutrient intakes: guidelines for the prevention of deficiency or prescription for total health, *Journal of Nutrition* 116:1581, 1986.
17. Perkin BB: Dietary guidelines for Americans, 1990 edition, *Journal of the American Dietetic Association* 90:1725, 1990.
18. Surgeon General's report on nutrition and health, *Nutrition Today*, September/October, 1988, p 22.

HOW MUCH HAVE I LEARNED?

What have you learned from Chapter 2? Here are 15 statements about The Right Diet for You. Read them to test your current knowledge. If you think the statement is true or mostly true, circle T. If you think the statement is false or mostly false, circle F. Use the scoring key at the end of the book to compute your total score. To review, take this test again later, especially before tests.

1. T (F) Scientific data clearly demonstrate that typical sodium intakes for North Americans can produce hypertension in people presently having normal values.

2. (T) F When comparing nutrition labels on different food products, it is important to note the serving size.

3. T (F) The term *sodium free* means that the product contains no sodium. *contains less than 5 milligrams sodium per serving*

4. T (F) Sugar is harmful to include in a diet. *moderate sugar intake not harmful if good dental hygiene is practiced*

5. T (F) Meat should make up the bulk of a diet. *veg., grains, fruit should make up bulk of diet*

6. T (F) RDA is the abbreviation for recommended daily allowance. *→ dietary*

7. T (F) Vitamins are needed daily to maintain good health. *no nutrient is required daily. can maintain health 4 days w/o water 10 days w/o thiamin*

8. (T) F Recommended nutrient needs differ from country to country.

9. T (F) Establishing personal nutritional needs is the main purpose of the RDA. *recommendation for group needs*

10. T (F) An intake of 1500 kcalories per day is considered adequate for most people. *active people require 2200-2800 or more to meet energy needs*

11. T (F) It is sufficient for children to just have protein intake meet daily losses. *need positive protein balance, eat more than they lose*

12. (T) F The exchange system works on the premise that foods with similar fat, protein, and carbohydrate composition can be substituted for each other. *don't need to memorize nutrients found in foods. quick way to est. fat, protein etc. content in food*

13. (T) F Nutrient density is one way to evaluate a food's nutrient composition. *important tool for people on low-kcalorie diet*

14. T (F) In addition to eating a balanced diet, it is important to take vitamin supplements to be certain you are getting enough nutrients. *by practicing good nutrition; variety, balance, moderation, a healthy person can obtain all necessary vitamins from foods.*

15. (T) F There is no perfect food. *all foods are low in one or more nutrients that we need*

NUTRITION ISSUE

WHAT'S ON THE LABEL?

In the United States the Food and Drug Administration (FDA) is responsible for most food labeling.[7] Exceptions are meat and poultry products, which are regulated by the USDA, and alcoholic beverages, which are regulated by the Bureau of Alcohol, Tobacco and Firearms. The Federal Trade Commission (FTC) regulates the advertising of food products and has authority to take action against unsubstantiated claims with enforcement by the FDA.

Most foods packaged and sold in the United States must be labeled with the product name, the manufacturer's name and address, the amount of product in the package, and the ingredients.[4] Note the ingredients are listed in order of amount from most to least by weight. So, when you buy a breakfast cereal, for example, choose one that has a whole grain listed first (such as whole wheat or oatmeal). Exceptions to current labeling laws are fresh fruits, vegetables, and meats—they require no label.

Another exception to required labeling is foods with a set list of ingredients or **standard of identity.** Such products must follow a specific, *standard* recipe on file with the FDA. Examples of these foods are ketchup, ice cream, mustard, mayonnaise, and margarine. In these cases the manufacturer does not have to list ingredients. However, many manufacturers now list ingredients anyway—even though they are not legally required to—because consumers want to know what ingredients are in foods.

Since 1973, if a manufacturer (1) adds a nutrient to a food product or (2) makes a nutritional claim about the product, a *nutrition label* must be provided. The next time you see a food package that announces the product is "low in sodium" or "high in fiber," check the nutrition label for more specific information. Today 60% of the foods under FDA control carry a nutrition label. Of those, about half are voluntary—no nutrition label is legally required. Many foods, however, give us no nutrient information aside from contents. This will change soon because of a new law passed in 1990 that requires most foods to be labeled.

An example of a nutrition label is shown in Figure 2-2. The label lists serving size of the product, servings per package, kcalories, protein, carbohydrate, fat, and sodium content. If the product contains more than 2% of the U.S. RDA for certain nutrients, the percentages of the U.S. RDA must be listed. These nutrients include protein, vitamin A, vitamin C, thiamin, riboflavin, niacin, calcium, and iron. Additional information may be provided on other vitamins and minerals, dietary fiber, and the amount of sugar, types of fats, and cholesterol.

Always check serving sizes when comparing nutrition labels because currently manufacturers determine their own serving sizes, and these vary from product to product. A product may be lower in kcalories than another similar one because the manufacturer simply listed a smaller serving size. Don't be fooled (Figure 2-6).

FRANK & ERNEST® by Bob Thaves

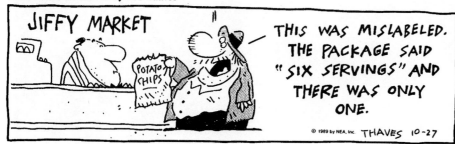

FIGURE 2-6

As we mentioned, FDA is in the midst of changing labeling regulations.[4,7] Proposed regulations will require changes in nutrition labels. The new nutrition labels will have four additional components, including a listing of:

- saturated fat content
- cholesterol content
- total dietary fiber content
- total kcalories from fat in the product

In addition, the U.S. RDA will be updated to more closely conform to the current RDA and undergo a name change to RDI, as we noted earlier. Serving size will follow more uniform patterns. ***Daily reference values (DRV)*** will also be set by FDA for certain parts of a diet not covered by the 1989 RDA, such as carbohydrate, fat, and dietary fiber. The DRV are intended to help us further evaluate food choices as we compare food values to desirable intakes. Final changes in food labeling regulations will be in place by November, 1992.

Labeling pitfalls

Food marketers are happy to satisfy our cravings for *healthy* foods with healthy-sounding food choices labeled "no cholesterol," "low fat," "organic," and "sugar free." How trustworthy are these claims? Though technically true, many of the claims are irrelevant; others are misleading or only paint part of the picture.[12] Below is a list of today's most-used labeling buzzwords. Note that some of these definitions will change in the near future as food labeling regulations change:

Diet or *dietetic:* Usually the product contains no more than 40 kcalories per serving (also called low calorie) or has at least one-third fewer kcalories than the regular product (also called reduced calorie).

Low calorie: The product contains no more than 40 kcalories per serving and no more than 0.4 kcalories per gram. Still, serving size is up to the manufacturer!

Reduced calorie: The product contains at least one-third fewer kcalories than the regular product.

Light (lite): This is labeling language that usually suggests a food is lower in kcalories. A *lite* product intended for reducing body weight or kcalorie intake must satisfy FDA requirements for low- or reduced-calorie foods (as described above) and provide full nutrition labeling information. Still, lite can simply refer to the color of the product.

For meats the terms "light," "lite," "leaner," or "lower fat" mean 25% or greater reduction in fat from a comparable product; "extra lean" means no more than 5% fat by weight; and "lean" or "low fat" mean no more than 10% fat by weight.

Imitation: The product does not follow the usual recipe for that type of product. For instance, more water may have been added to margarine to make it lower in kcalories. Note that such products may also be lower in nutrients, such as protein, vitamins, or minerals.

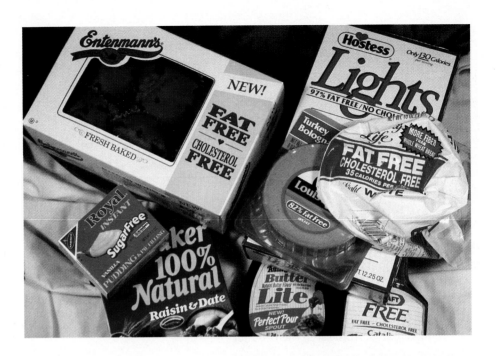

Natural: This term is usually meaningless. It simply states that the product occurs in nature. When applied to meats, it means the meat contains no added artificial flavors, colors, preservatives, or synthetic ingredients.

Organic: This term currently has no legal meaning as far as the U.S. federal law is concerned, but the U.S. Congress has recently passed a law that mandates standards be set. Again, chemists use this term to refer to chemicals with carbon-hydrogen links in them.

Sugar free: The product cannot contain sucrose (table sugar), honey, fruit juice, molasses, or other simple sugars.

Sodium free: The product contains less than 5 milligrams of sodium per serving.

Very low sodium: The product contains no more than 35 milligrams of sodium per serving.

Low sodium: The product contains no more than 140 milligrams of sodium per serving.

Reduced sodium: The product contains 75% less sodium than the product it replaces.

No cholesterol: The product contains no cholesterol.

Cholesterol free: The product contains less than 2 milligrams of cholesterol per serving. Under proposed rules, *cholesterol free* could be used only if a product has less than 2 milligrams of cholesterol per serving and less than 5 grams of fat—no more than 2 grams of which can be saturated fat.[4]

Low cholesterol: The product contains 20 milligrams or less of cholesterol per serving.

Reduced cholesterol: The product contains 75% less cholesterol than the product it replaces.

Low fat: Milk described as such can contain by weight 0.5% to 2% milk fat. Lowfat meat can contain no more than 10% fat by weight (also called lean meat).

No artificial flavors: The product contains no flavors other than those from naturally occurring products.

No artificial coloring: The product contains only colors from naturally occurring products, such as beet juice, grape skin, or carrot oil.

May contain one or more of the following: The product can contain any of the ingredients listed after this phrase. Usually the ingredient(s) will be the one(s) found to be least expensive at the time of production. This is especially true for added fats.

New: The product is either brand new or has been substantially changed within the last 6 months.

Wheat: The product contains wheat but not necessarily whole wheat. The label will say whole wheat if the product uses only whole-wheat flour.

There are other fine points to labeling laws. These definitions represent the most important ones to keep in mind.

Health claims on labels

Authorities are still debating how far a manufacturer should be able to go in claiming health benefits on a food product label. Today manufacturers are allowed to state that a food contains certain nutrients as long as a nutrition label backs up the claim. The actual debate is about whether a manufacturer can state that these nutrients provide specific health benefits, such as saying that dietary fiber in food helps prevent some types of cancer. Manufacturers want to make health claims to sell their products. Since 1984 the Kellogg Company has marketed its high-fiber cereals as a possible preventive measure against some forms of cancer. Whether this should be allowed is far from settled.

The FDA traditionally has viewed health-related messages as drug claims, meaning that foods making these claims should be regulated as drugs. This status would require manufacturers to prove that the food does what it is advertised to do and is safe to use at advertised dosages. However, manufacturers simply want to promote products that are healthful and feel consumers want such information to help them select healthy foods. After relaxing rules to allow for this in 1987, government agencies are now not sure how far they should let manufacturers go. Labeling regulations currently under development will set standards for some of the more common claims, such as "no cholesterol" and "high fiber."

A major problem that likely will continue is that a *good food/bad food* comparison is promoted by many claims on labels,[12] and the emphasis on total diet is ignored. As we have discussed, one's total meal plan and nutrient intake should be the focus because nutrients work together to maintain health—not as separate entities existing in a vacuum. Protein metabolism needs vitamin B-6, iron metabolism needs vitamin C, and vitamin A metabolism needs zinc.

Again, health claims for specific foods or food supplements ignore the importance of the entire diet and are irresponsible because they do not warn of the dangers of excess intakes of specific foods or supplements.[12] Thus the idea of promoting health claims on labels may not be a good one.

The American Dietetic Association (ADA) feels health claims are permissible as part of a labeling or marketing system as long as the claims are presented in the context of total diet recommendations and are generally supported by the scientific community.[1,2] But, too often, these claims deceive us by leaving out information (e.g., not pointing out missing nutrients or high amounts of ingredients that can be harmful). The consumer can't choose wisely if information is missing. The ADA endorses claims that support the recommendations of the Dietary Guidelines. The association also supports listing both positive and negative health claims on food labels so that the public will not be misled.[2] For example, a label that claims a food is high in fiber should also state whether the food is high in fat. In this way important information about the food is not hidden from the consumer.

The bottom line for health claims on food packages is honesty. The whole story needs to be told.[12] How federal agencies in the United States intend to make sure this happens is not known. Your best tactic is to shop defensively: read the small print and question what it says. ●

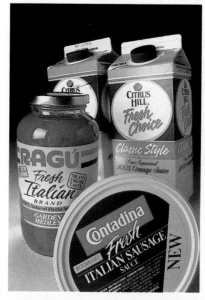

FDA currently is enforcing labeling regulations more strictly. This includes foods that use the term "fresh" but are obviously not since they are packaged.

HOW TO IMPROVE YOUR DIET

When you think of an ideal diet, what do you see? In your mind imagine the shapes and colors of the foods chosen. Smell the aromas of a nutritious hot meal. Savor the sweetness of foods fresh from a garden. These *mind pictures* help us visualize the appeal of our ideal foods. The senses of sight, smell, and taste are strategic guides to our nutrition goals.

Imagery, such as mind pictures, is a useful technique in changing eating behaviors.[7] This chapter presents such strategies to help you make choices about your eating habits. You will learn how to set goals about food choices and weight changes. Although behavior strategies emphasized in this discussion mostly deal with weight control, these same techniques are powerful tools for changing other eating behaviors important to you.

Any diet or nutrition book can give the basics. But how many of those books speak to you as an individual? Do they consider the fact that you are pressed for time and eat most meals on the run? Is the author aware that you eat when you are "stressed out?" Does the standard dose of diet advice take into consideration your family history, health status, or how work affects your eating habits? An important goal of this chapter is to offer you a way to tailor good nutrition advice to your needs. Overall, the behavior change process involves making choices—choosing to do or to stop doing something. You are in control. Is it time to become more involved? ●

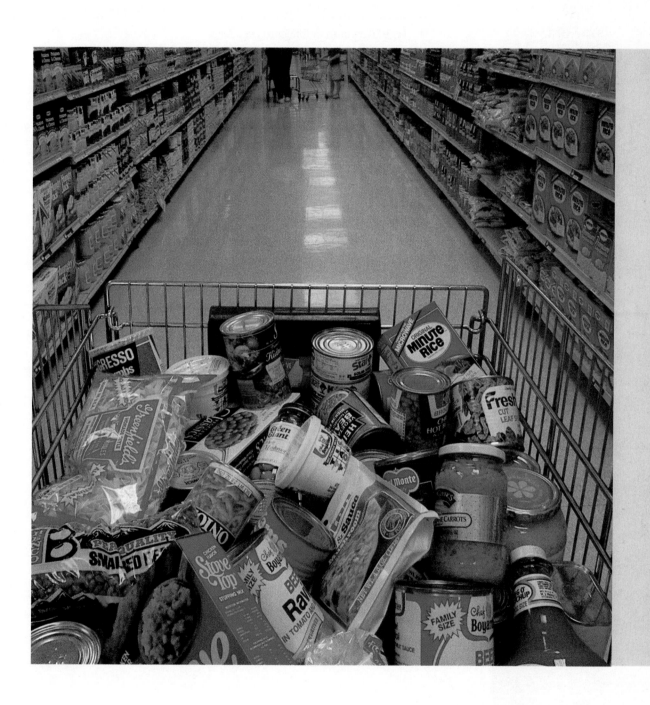

Do Your Eating Habits Encourage Weight Maintenance?

How often do you do the following (circle the appropriate number):

	Rarely	Sometimes	Often
1. Take 20 minutes or longer to eat a meal.	1	2	(3)
2. Eat foods that are baked, boiled, or broiled rather than fried.	1	2	(3)
3. Eat in one main place in your residence.	1	2	3
4. Drink plenty of water.	(1)	2	3
5. Eat breakfast.	1	(2)	3
6. Store foods out of sight in your house or room.	1	2	(3)
7. Plan ahead of time the food you will eat.	1	2	(3)
8. Avoid skipping meals.	1	2	(3)
9. At a restaurant request salad dressing on the side or bring your own.	(1)	2	3
10. Eat until you are comfortably full rather than overeat.	1	2	(3)
11. Exercise regularly.	(1)	2	3
12. Choose lowfat foods.	(1)	2	3
13. Avoid the influence of friends and peers on your eating habits.	1	2	(3)
14. Leave food on your plate.	1	(2)	3
15. Do nothing else while eating (e.g., reading, watching television).	1	2	(3)

ADD TOGETHER THE NUMBERS YOU CIRCLED
AND ENTER THE TOTAL HERE ___36___

INTERPRETATION

Interpret your total score this way:

15-25	*Dietary Doldrums:*	your eating habits need some attention
26-35	*Munching Mediocrity:*	you are doing well for going to college, but it may not get you through to the "golden years"
36-45	*Nutritional Stardom:*	this score gets you into the nutrition hall of fame (however, don't reward yourself by overeating)

ASSESS YOURSELF

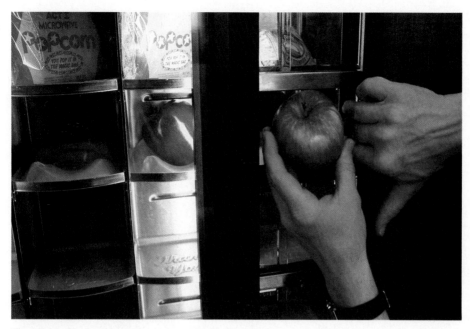

Receptive Framework for Learning • The process by which a person opens and responds to learning more about a problem—it usually involves seeking more information about an issue from books and people.

Healthy food choices pop up everywhere. We just have to look a little harder sometimes.

THE BEHAVIOR CHANGE PROCESS

Behavior patterns that have evolved throughout a lifetime do not change or disappear overnight. Planned behavior changes occur gradually and with some effort. First, a person must perceive that a problem exists.[7] For someone who is overweight, this might mean becoming more aware of health risks, recognizing a lack of physical stamina, or balking at the need to expand one's wardrobe.

After recognizing that a problem indeed exists, an interested person then develops a *receptive framework for learning* more about the problem. This might involve weighing the costs and benefits of changing behaviors: for example, balancing the time and effort required for exercising and sacrificing some favorite foods against the benefits of lowering weight, decreasing health risks, and feeling and looking better (Figure 3-1).

Having decided that the change is sufficiently beneficial, the person then must ask "Can I do it?" We know ourselves best. Is the change feasible? Can one's lifestyle accommodate the new goal? Can the person continue the new behaviors for years? Long-term commitment is a key part of any behavior change plan.[1] It may help a person to speak with others who have worked on similar health problems and to read about others' experiences. The changes then may seem less threatening and more possible. A health professional can often provide the information and encouragement necessary to start the change process.[7]

Are there parts of your health lifestyle that need improvement?

Starting on a new path

Having decided to attempt a change, the person begins a trial run. Ideally, unwanted patterns are changed one step at a time, beginning with the easiest habit to discard. Changing too many habits too soon can be overwhelming, making it hard to adhere to a plan.[1] As we try new behaviors, we experience both difficulties and rewards: some hunger and discomfort versus compliments and greater self-esteem. Some experiences may be perceived as positive, but some will be perceived as negative—otherwise, the old practices would not

Reinforcement • A reaction by others in response to a person's behavior. Positive reinforcement entails encouragement; negative reinforcement entails criticism or penalty.

BENEFITS AND COSTS ANALYSIS

1 Benefits of losing weight?
What do you expect to get, now or later, that you want? What do you get to avoid that would be unpleasant?

- better job possibilities
- Feel better physically and psychologically
- look better
- people pay more attention to me

3 Costs involved in losing weight?
What do you have to do that you don't want to do? What do you have to stop doing that you would rather continue doing?

- cut down on fast food
- cut down on alcohol
- take time to exercise

2 Benefits of not losing weight?
What do you get to do that you enjoy doing? What do you avoid having to do?

- eat whatever I want
- dont have to exercise

4 Costs of not losing weight?
What unpleasant or undesirable effects are you likely to experience now or in the future? What are you likely to lose?

- rejection from others
- low self esteem
- poor health

FIGURE 3-1
Benefits and costs analysis applied to weight loss. This exercise helps put behavior change into the context of total lifestyle.

have been cherished. Familiar foods now missing from the diet may leave a void.

To deal with diet difficulties, positive **reinforcement** is critical.[1,7] This should be built into a diet plan. We deserve credit for attempting difficult tasks; we need rewards for hard work—perhaps a night at the movies, a new compact disc, an outing with friends, or a chance to sleep late. During this trial period, it is important to capitalize on success and learn how to derive psychological nourishment from conquering poor habits.

Finally, the person adopts and integrates the new behaviors into a total lifestyle. In the progression from becoming aware of a problem to adopting new behaviors, we can further take charge of our health. Now the possibilities for other improvements can be investigated, and the cycle repeated.[7]

CHARTING A PLAN FOR CHANGE

A good plan evolves over time. It is based on rational, deliberate decisions, coupled with trial and error experiences. Because a person can't know all possible strategies and tactics before beginning, a good plan incorporates all the information at hand.[7] Revisions will be necessary and should be expected.

If your goal is to control your weight, you should know that the typical restrictive diet not only fails to produce the desired results for most people but also can produce undesired results, such as fatigue and depression. Effective, long-range weight control programs encourage people to raise their activity levels and eat less fat, rather than to severely restrict their eating.[1] To discover more effective options, investigate some clinic programs and speak with registered dietitians. We will discuss the topic of weight loss in detail in Chapter 11.

BECOMING AWARE

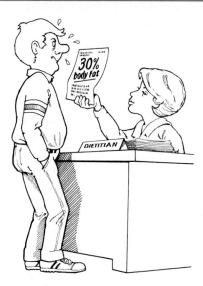

Alan is a 20-year-old male college student who has been steadily gaining weight since high school. At the YMCA a registered dietitian calculates that Alan stores about 50% more fat than is desirable. Alan is concerned about his long-term health and wants to correct his *overfat* problem before it leads to other health problems. Having seen his father change his diet and lose weight after a heart attack, Alan thinks that he too can make dietary changes with success.

Gathering baseline data

The next step in developing a personal plan for dietary change is to monitor eating behaviors, noting strengths and weaknesses.[4] Recording meals and snacks in a *food diary* may expose eating patterns previously unnoticed. Let's assume that you want to lower fat intake to help control your weight. You will have to adjust some habits, but which ones? In a diary, list any relevant behaviors, such as foods eaten, portion sizes, and amount of fat in the food eaten (Appendix D will help). Also, as you did in Chapter 1, record intensity of hunger; the time and location of the meal or snack; any other activity performed, such as watching TV; whether others were present; and your reasons for choosing that particular food (Figure 3-2). A blank form for recording this information is included in Chapter 1 and Appendix D.

A review of the diary might reveal how both your outside environment and internal cues influence your nutrition and health habits. This is the time to look for patterns—identify both positive behaviors and ones that need changes. The patterns might suggest which food habits would be easy to change and which might be more difficult to alter. Consider classifying food choices as "ones you can't give up" versus "ones you can live without." See if certain eating habits are paired with other activities. For example, you may find that you often eat while visiting with friends, in response to an angry mood, or perhaps after 6 PM.[4] Subtle associations that influence eating habits can provide a good starting point for behavior changes.

Food Diary • A written record of sequential food intake for a period of time. Details associated with the food intake are often recorded as well.

Let's assume information from your food diary, coupled with an evaluation of your current health status, reveals behaviors you need to change in order to establish better nutrition and health practices. You would like to take the next step, but are unsure of how to proceed. At this point a discussion with a physician or registered dietitian would be appropriate.

As we mentioned in Chapter 1, habit and sensory appeal—flavor, appearance, texture, and odor—usually determine both our intended and actual food choices. Of lesser importance in choosing foods to eat are health value, time

Time	Minutes spent eating	M or S*	H†	Activity while eating	Place of eating	Food and quantity	Others present	Reason for choice
7:10 a.m.	15	M	2	standing, fixing lunch	kitchen	1 c orange juice 1 c corn flakes ¼ c 2% milk 2 t sugar black coffee	—	health habit health taste habit
10:00 a.m.	4	S	1	sitting, taking notes	classroom	12 oz diet cola	class	weight control
12:15 p.m.	40	M	2	sitting, talking	union	1 chicken sandwich 1 pear	friends	taste health
2:30 p.m.	10	S	1	sitting, studying	library	12 oz regular cola	friend	hunger
6:30 p.m.	35	M	3	sitting, talking	kitchen	1 pork chop 1 baked potato 2 T margarine lettuce 1 oz ranch dressing 1 c whole milk 1 piece cherry pie	boyfriend	convenience health taste health taste habit taste
9:10 p.m.	10	S	2	sitting, studying	living room	1 glass mineral water	—	weight control

*M or S: Meal or snack.
†H: Degree of hunger (0 = none; 3 = maximum).

FIGURE 3-2
This activity can help one understand more about food habits.

constraints, social influence, energy value, and cost. After reevaluating your diary from Chapter 1, decide if this is true for you.

> **CONCEPT CHECK**
>
> In the process of changing behavior a person first becomes aware of a problem. Then the person studies the problem and develops a receptive frame of mind for making a change. He initiates a trial change. If he receives positive reinforcement, he may eventually incorporate the change into his lifestyle—he adopts it. Behavior change is most successful when tailored to specific personal needs. By carefully studying their own behaviors, people can more effectively change problem habits.

Setting attainable goals

What can we accomplish and how long will it take? Setting a realistic goal and allowing a reasonable amount of time to pursue it increases the likelihood of success.[7] For example, if one goal is to improve iron status, planning an iron-rich diet and taking iron supplements can show increased blood-iron levels within just a few months. Progress toward other types of goals, such as weight loss, might be apparent within a week and then progress from week to week. Seeing week-to-week progress can be the spark needed to continue moving ahead with a program.

If you aim to control a chronic disease, such as hypertension, diabetes mellitus, or heart disease, health professionals can supply specific behavior goals. A clinical examination will confirm your degree of success. If the goal is broader, for example, to maintain or improve overall nutritional health, the path is not as well defined. Chapter 2 offers some suggestions.

Considering all these possible goals, it is best to change only a few specific behaviors at first—for example, lowering fat intake, using more whole-grain products, and not eating after 7 PM. By attempting small and perhaps easier

If you're eating every dinner in fast-food restaurants and you want to change your habit, try a week of fixing one dinner a week at home. Consider this an experiment. Will it work for you?

BASELINE

To better understand his eating habits, Alan keeps a food diary. In it he tracks what and how much he eats, how quickly he eats, the time, the environment, and his feelings at the time of eating. From this record he finds a previously unnoticed pattern—he starts snacking after his 2 PM class and does not stop until dinner. He is alarmed that he consumes so many kcalories almost unconsciously. In addition, Alan notes that his lunches usually are high in fat and his days lack much physical activity.

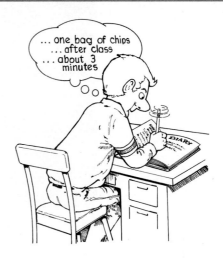

dietary changes first, you reduce the scope of the problem and increase the likelihood of success.[1]

> **Arthritis** • Inflammation at a point where bones join together. The disease has many possible causes.

Measuring commitment

The greater the personal commitment, the greater the chances of success. We need to examine the goals we set.[4] Are they worth pursuing? Are health benefits greater than the sacrifices to be made? Some people can ignore persistent **arthritis** in the knees, which is magnified by being overweight, because they derive great pleasure from eating. Others may love eating ice cream and chips and dips but finally realize that the price is too high. They realize that the benefit of keeping off unwanted pounds is greater than the momentary pleasure of immoderate snacking. They see that by changing eating habits, they feel better about themselves, move around more easily, feel less anxious in public, and most likely limit some future health problems.

People who are not strongly committed to changing a behavior often fail and become discouraged further. Usually, the more profound benefits from changing health and nutrition behaviors take time to achieve. This delayed success makes working toward long-term goals—improving fitness, lowering elevated blood pressure, and losing weight—difficult. As already noted, many long-term goals require a life-long commitment. Only the person who contemplates the change can determine whether the value of good nutrition and good health is worth the price.[7]

Working out the details

Once a person establishes goals and discovers personal strengths and weaknesses in pursuing them, it is time to set the details of the plan. To do this, we need to know something about nutrition. The information contained in this book is a good place to start. Again, if you feel unable to work out a plan, seek professional help from a registered dietitian or physician.

One goal, as we have often suggested, is to reduce fat intake. There are several means of doing this. You can eat less high-fat meat either by cutting your portion sizes or by eating meat less frequently. You might eat high-fat meats only twice a week instead of everyday. You can also search for new recipes and methods of preparation that use leaner and less meat—stir frying or broiling for example—to reduce fat intake (Table 3-1). Many more tactics for managing eating behavior exist (Table 3-2).[8] Once you control your consumption of high-fat meats, you can try other changes to help reach the overall goal.

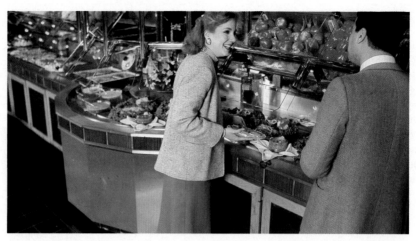

Salad bars contain both lowfat and high fat choices—proceed with caution.

TABLE 3-1

Healthy cooking methods

Microwave

Microwaving cooks foods faster that most other methods and is an excellent way to retain vitamins and color in vegetables.

Steam

Steaming is a good method for cooking vegetables without using fat. Try this method for frozen and fresh vegetables such as asparagus, broccoli, carrots, spinach, and summer squash.

Braise

Braising is used mainly for meats that need longer cooking times to become tender. Root vegetables are also good braised. Try using meat or poultry broth, cider, wine, or a combination of these for added flavor.

Barbecue

Roasting foods on a rack or a spit over coals is a fun, lower fat way to prepare meat, poultry, fish, and even vegetables. Barbecuing gives a distinctive smoked flavor to foods. If seasoning with a sauce, try one with less salt, sugars, and fat.

Broil

Broiling is a quick way of cooking foods under direct heat without added fat. It's great for poultry, fish, and tender cuts of meat. Use lemon juice, fruit juice, or broth for flavor. Vegetables like onions, zucchini, and tomatoes can also be broiled.

Stirfry

Quick and easy, stirfrying requires relatively little fat and preserves the crisp texture and bright color of vegetables. Add small pieces of vegetables such as broccoli, cauliflower, zucchini, sprouts, carrots, mushrooms, tomatoes, or green onions.

Roast or bake

Roasting takes somewhat longer than other methods, but requires little work on your part. Poultry and tender cuts of meat may be roasted. Potatoes, sweet potatoes, winter squashes, and onions are also good baked.

Boil or stew

Foods are cooked in hot liquids in these lowfat, low-salt methods. The liquid left after cooking can become a tasty broth or base of a sauce. Starchy or root vegetables such as potatoes, corn-on-the-cob, lima beans, and turnips are often boiled.

TABLE 3-2

Tactics for managing eating behavior

Many things can trigger inappropriate eating behavior. But effective tactics can be used to gain control of eating. You may want to incorporate the tactics suggested below into a behavior change strategy.

Buying and storing food

Avoid market aisles of problem foods.
Don't pretend it's for the children or company.
Store problem food out of sight, or don't buy it.

Cooking, preparing, and serving food

Broil, bake, or poach—don't fry.
Substitute lowfat and low-kcalorie ingredients for higher fat ones.
Don't sample while cooking.
Plan menus and measure portions.
Let others get their own snacks, desserts, and second helpings.

Eating food

Drink plenty of water but little or no alcohol.
Eat more starches and avoid high-fat foods.
Eat three meals a day.
Replace impulse snacking with planned, healthful snacks.

Coping with problem food

Make problem food temporarily off-limits, not forbidden forever.
Eat a little of a problem food when you aren't tempted to binge.

Eating out in restaurants

Choose a restaurant that allows healthful food choices.
Ask the waitress not to put bread and butter on the table before the meal.
Curb your appetite with an appetizer of broth-based soup.
Request no butter and no sauce on vegetables or entree.
Choose a broiled entree.
Request water with a meal.
Request salad dressing on the side or bring your own.
Don't look at the dessert list or dessert tray.

Coping with others

Ask coworkers not to offer food.
Instead of eating to be polite, say, "No, thank you, I've had enough. It was delicious, and I'm full."

Coping with emotions

Allow yourself an occasional treat; work it into your eating plan.
Avoid people and situations that upset you.
Go for a walk or use other exercise to unwind.
Lighten up, don't take it all so seriously.
Join a support group or seek counseling.

Managing your body

Exercise regularly.
Get adequate rest.

Adapted from Nash JD: *Maximize your body potential*, Palo Alto, Calif, 1986, Bull Publishing Co.

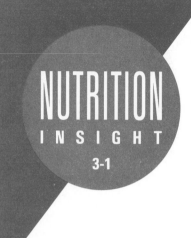

NUTRITION INSIGHT 3-1

EATING ON THE RUN

Choosing healthy foods is not that difficult in many of today's fast-food restaurants. While decadent desserts and skyscraper burgers aren't yet restaurant relics, such menu items may be passing their prime as some restaurants are trying to cater to their more health-conscious clientele. Today, many restaurants allow you to pursue a lowfat diet.[11] Consider substituting sauteed poultry for fried chicken, frozen yogurt for ice cream, and baked potatoes for French fries. Fast-food fare has evolved beyond hamburgers, French fries, and milk shakes to include a variety of vegetables, salad bars, and ethnic foods. Still, between 40% and 55% of the kcalories in most fast-food meals come from fat (Table 3-2). Thus many fast-food meal selections are high kcalorie options when compared to the amount of other nutrients provided.

People who eat regularly at fast-food restaurants should choose meals carefully to meet their nutrient needs without exceeding their energy needs. Because fast foods serve a need in our fast-paced society, they are probably a permanent part of the lifestyle of many North Americans.[10] Here is a list of nutritional selections among food choices in fast-food and other restaurants.

Breakfast

Before considering a local fast-food or a more formal restaurant for breakfast, decide whether you can make breakfast at home. Can breakfast be prepared the night before so that it is ready for the next morning? The effort might be as simple as putting bread next to the toaster or cereal on the counter with a bowl. Breakfast can be a relaxing time, and many of us need time away from the fast pace of daily life.

If you still prefer to eat breakfast out, we suggest a plain scrambled egg or an English muffin with no more than 1 teaspoon of margarine. Add orange juice for a good taste. For variety, substitute pancakes without the butter and minimal syrup for the egg and English muffin. Either way, you consume a lot less fat and kcalories than if you choose the typical meat, egg, and cheese-laden muffin or croissant. If you still want meat, consider Canadian bacon, a lean breakfast meat.

Lunch—with a fast-food emphasis

A good choice for lunch is a sandwich made with whole-wheat bread and some lean meat or tuna. Pizza is a good idea once or twice a week. If ordered with vegetable toppings—mushrooms, green peppers, and onion—pizza provides a very nutritious lunch for a moderate amount of kcalories. The cheese used is primarily a lowfat variety. The next best choice is probably a plain hamburger on a bun with lettuce, tomatoes, mustard, and a little ketchup. Be especially wary of mayonnaise, special sauces (like tartar sauce), melted cheese, bacon, fried onions, or other sources of added fat.[11] A fast-food restaurant will usually make a no-frills burger or fish sandwich at no extra cost, but expect a service delay. Chili is another good selection. It has less fat than a king-size hamburger, and the beans supply additional dietary fiber. Finally, soft burritos with beans or chicken are often low in fat. Cheese should be ordered on the side.

ANOTHER BITE Preparations that indicate less fat include grilling, broiling, stir-frying, roasting, poaching, and steaming. Terms like battered, fried, breaded, creamed, au gratin, escalloped, and hollandaise are clues that indicate higher fat content.

Bite-sized pieces of chicken should be made from chicken breast only and not from processed chicken, which can include ground chicken skin. Ask the restaurant manager what chicken parts are used to make the nuggets. Indicate your nutrition and health interests.[11] Broiled or baked chicken is healthiest. If fried, remove the coating along with the skin to minimize fat. The same principle applies to fish; remove the coating. Actually, chicken and fish start out as lowfat protein sources, but by the time they are deep-fat fried, their protein to fat ratio resembles that of a hamburger. You don't save much fat or many kcalories.

When selecting side dishes, consider portion sizes. Order a small rather than a large portion of French fries. Better yet, spice up a plain baked potato with plenty of chives and plain yogurt. Resist eating more than one pat of margarine. Stay away from sour cream, cheese, and other toppings—you can save as much as 300 kcalories.

At the salad bar, spare the cheese, bacon bits, and cheesy dressing. It's the lettuce and vegetables that contain rich sources of many nutrients and dietary fiber. Mayonnaise-based salads, such as macaroni and potato salad, and mayonnaise-based salad dressings are relatively high in kcalories.[11] To minimize saturated fat intake, try oil and vinegar dressing, French dressing, or lemon juice, rather than blue cheese dressing. Many fast food restaurants also supply low-kcalorie dressings. Salad bars also offer fresh fruits and vegetables, which can contribute to a healthy meal.

For beverages, consider lowfat (nonfat) milk, water, diet soft drinks, or ice tea. A typical milk shake contains about 350 to 400 kcalories. A cup of lowfat milk has only 120 kcalories.

Dinner—with a more formal emphasis

In more formal restaurants, it is important to be your own advocate. Restaurants do respond to customer demand. If you want lower-fat, healthier food, ask for it.[11] Request lowfat milk, margarine, broiled meats and fish, low-kcalorie salad dressings, or whatever else you want. If the restaurant does not offer a special menu section, look for a statement on the menu that encourages special requests.

For appetizers, choose fruit juice or a fruit cup instead of creamed soup. Vegetable juice and broth-based soups are good choices as well, but they can be high in sodium.

When selecting salads, limit the amounts of cheese and avoid chopped meats, bacon bits, marinated vegetables, potato salad, macaroni salad, and salad dressing. You can build a creative and tasty salad without relying on these products.

Find out how the main dish is prepared. Find an entree that is not fried, coated, or so hidden in a sauce that you can't tell what happened to it.

Ask for baked or mashed potatoes rather than French fries. Even with a small amount of butter or gravy added, both baked and mashed potatoes contain far fewer kcalories. Consider eating whole-grain breads, pita bread, bread sticks, Italian bread, or French bread instead of biscuits, croissants, and rich dinner rolls. Choose fresh fruit, fruit ices, frozen yogurt, gelatin, sherbet, or cake without frosting for dessert. Remove frosting from pastries to reduce kcalorie intake. For fruit pie, eat mostly the filling and keep serving size under control.

For beverages, if you drink alcoholic beverages, drink them in moderation. Alcohol can melt away good intentions and add numerous kcalories. Use lowfat or skim milk instead of cream in coffee or tea. When drinking milk, choose lowfat or skim milk instead of whole milk.

In all, focus on fat intake. Its 9 kcalories per gram adds up fast. It is easier to reduce fat intake in some restaurants than in others. Mexican and French menus are noted for many high fat choices, while Italian and Oriental menus offer many more lowfat alternatives. But by all means, enjoy eating out. Look at the total diet, not at whether one food or another is going to ruin your health. We should still think of eating as a pleasurable experience. There are some hurdles to clear, but once you learn the rules for eating on the run, you can find healthful, low-kcalorie meals even at fast-food restaurants.[10] ●

TABLE 3-3
Proceed with caution

	Kcalories	Percent Fat
Arby's		
deluxe roast beef sandwich	486	42
French fries*	211	34
ham 'n cheese sandwich	353	33
broccoli and cheddar potato	541	37
chocolate milk shake	384	26
Burger King		
Whopper with cheese	723	60
onion rings	274	53
apple pie	305	35
fish sandwich	488	50
chicken sandwich	688	52
scrambled egg platter	468	58
Kentucky Fried Chicken		
drumstick	147	55
center breast	257	49
buttermilk biscuit	269	47
potato salad	141	57
cole slaw	103	52
McDonald's		
Chicken McNuggets	323	59
Egg McMuffin	340	42
chocolate chip cookies	342	42
Taco Bell		
beef burrito	466	41
taco	186	39
tostada	179	40
Pizza Hut		
cheese pizza (2 slices)	492	33
medium pan pizza—pepperoni (2 slices)	540	37

*Hamburgers, French fries, milk shakes, etc. for fast-food outlets tend to have similar nutrient compositions. See Appendix A to evaluate your typical choices.

PLANNING THE DETAILS

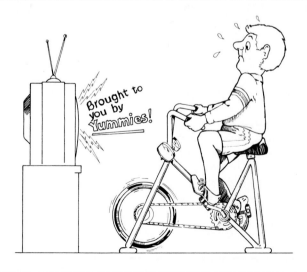

Brought to you by Yummies!

Alan addresses his overall weight problem in small steps. He plans to eat a better breakfast and lunch everyday so he won't feel ravenous by midafternoon. He will keep low-kcalorie snack foods, such as oranges, handy in the apartment—instead of the usual bag of chips or cookies. He will start packing his lunch and limit visits to fast-food restaurants to twice a week. In addition, at fast-food restaurants he will make wiser selections from the menu, opting for such choices as the "create your own hamburger bar." He will use lots of tomato slices for juiciness and then choose lowfat milk. He will try to avoid eating his usual double-cheeseburger, fries, and milkshake. Finally, he plans to increase activity by both walking to class instead of driving and purchasing an exercise bike to ride each night while watching sports on television.

Making it official

Drawing up a ***behavior contract*** often adds incentive to follow through with a plan. The contract could list goal behaviors and objectives, milestones for measuring progress, and regular rewards for meeting the terms of the contract (Figure 3-3). After finishing a contract, the person should sign it in the presence of some friends (Figure 3-4).[4] This aids commitment.

We need to remember that positive reinforcement for following the contract contributes more to successful behavior change than negative reinforcement.[7] Initially, plans need to reward positive behaviors and then focus on positive results. Positive behaviors, such as regular exercise, eventually lead to positive outcomes, such as weight loss. It may, however, take weeks to months to see the effects.

Behavior Contract • A written agreement that outlines intended behavior changes, plans for reinforcement, and witnesses to monitor progress.

Name _____

Goal

I agree to _____
(specify behavior)

_____

under the following circumstances _____
(specify where, when, how much, etc.)

_____

Substitute behavior and/or reinforcement schedule _____

_____

Environmental planning

In order to help me do this, I am going to (1) arrange my physical and social environment
by _____

_____

and (2) control my internal environment (thoughts, images) by _____

_____

Reinforcements

Reinforcements provided by me daily or weekly (if contract is kept):

_____

_____

Reinforcements provided by others daily or weekly (if contract is kept):

_____

_____

Social support

Behavior change is more likely to take place when other people support you. During the quarter/semester please meet with the other person at least three times to discuss your progress.

The name of my "significant helper" is: _____

This contract should include:

1. Baseline data (one week)
2. Well-defined goal
3. Simple method for charting progress (diary, counter, charts, etc.)
4. Reinforcements (immediate and long-term)
5. Evaluation method (summary of experiences, success, and/or new learnings about self).

FIGURE 3-3

Completing a contract can help provide commitment for behavior change.

Name *Alan Student*

Goal

I agree to *ride my exercise bike*

(specify behavior)

under the following circumstances *for 30 minutes, 4 times per week in the evening*

(specify where, when, how much, etc.)

Substitute behavior and/or reinforcement schedule *I will reinforce myself if I've achieved my goal after a month with a weekend off campus with my roommate.*

Environmental planning

In order to help me do this, I am going to (1) arrange my physical and social environment by *buying a new jogging suit at the local sporting goods store*

and (2) control my internal environment (thoughts, images) by *coordinating riding the bike with the first T.V. watching I do in the evening*

Reinforcements

Reinforcements provided by me daily or weekly (if contract is kept):
I will buy myself a new piece of clothing for off campus trip

Reinforcements provided by others daily or weekly (if contract is kept):
at the end of a month if I've completed my goal my parents will buy me a fitness club membership for winter.

Social support

Behavior change is more likely to take place when other people support you. During the quarter/semester please meet with the other person at least three times to discuss your progress.

The name of my "significant helper" is: *Mr. and Mrs. Student*

This contract should include:

1. Baseline data (one week)
2. Well-defined goal
3. Simple method for charting progress (diary, counter, charts, etc.)
4. Reinforcements (immediate and long-term)
5. Evaluation method (summary of experiences, success, and/or new learnings about self).

FIGURE 3-4

Alan's behavioral contract. What would your contract look like?

PSYCHING YOURSELF UP

While changing habits we are likely to get support from some friends, but others may prefer us the way we are. They may try to dissuade us from our plan. Even we may have moments when we want to abandon the plan. We all respond to others' opinions, especially about ourselves. We like approval, generally, and are influenced by others to behave in certain ways. No matter how committed we are to changing behaviors, we may need to mentally prepare ourselves to resist when others encourage behavior that defeats the desired goal.[7]

"Psyching yourself up" may enable you to pursue your goals in spite of others' expectations. Almost everyone benefits from some assertiveness training when it comes to changing behaviors. Here are a few suggestions:

- No one's feelings should be hurt if you say, "No, thank you," firmly and repeatedly, when others try to dissuade you from a plan. Rather, ask them—and yourself—why they want you to eat their way. Your needs are as important as someone else's.

- You don't have to eat a lot to accommodate anyone—your mother, business clients, or the chef. For example, going to a party with friends may make you feel like you have to eat a lot to participate, but you don't have to.[11] Also, ordering a lot just because someone else is paying for the meal is a trap.

- When entertaining, serve lighter, more healthful lowfat meals. Try some new recipes. This can be a useful step en route to changing your overall approach to cooking.

- Dealing with parties and social occasions built around food is difficult but possible. You can plan celebrations around a hike or a tennis court, rather than around chips, beer, and television. When you attend parties where food is everywhere, eat a lowfat salad (such as fruit salad) before you go, opt for pretzels or plain crackers,[13] converse far from the food table, and wear clothes that don't encourage you to overeat (Figure 3-5).

- Learn ways to handle "put-downs"—inadvertent or conscious. An effective response can be to communicate feelings honestly, without hostility. Tell criticizers that they have annoyed or offended you; that you are working to change your habits and would really like understanding and support from them.

- Fostering feelings of self-worth can empower you to change behavior. Ridding yourself of the habit of self-criticism requires strong self-restraint and retraining. Create and memorize lists of strengths, giving credit where it is deserved.[7] Practice forgiving yourself. Lower unrealistic expectations. Stop thinking negative thoughts about yourself; purposely switch to positive thoughts.

- If appropriate, persuade the cook to change the family or group diet. The best situation is when everyone wants to eat healthfully. The cook can influence healthy eating a great deal. It takes extra effort to find and develop new recipes and learn shortcuts and substitutions to cut fat

Why might people try to block your success in changing your food habits?

DRAFTING A CONTRACT

To motivate himself, Alan drafts his plan into contract form. In the contract, he outlines his behavior changes and his choice of positive reinforcement for carrying out the plan: a weekend off campus with his roommates. He introduces his roommates to the plan, and one of them even wants to join him, knowing that he too will benefit from exercise and weight loss. Alan posts a chart on the refrigerator to record the amount of time spent on the exercise bike each night and his weekly body weight.

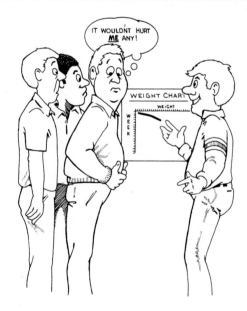

Behavior Chains • Activities linked together in a person's lifestyle, such as snacking while watching television.

and/or kcalories.[5] But the information can be found in cookbooks and newspaper recipes. Also, friends might have healthful recipes and food preparation tips.

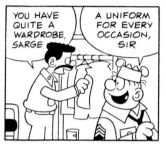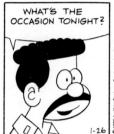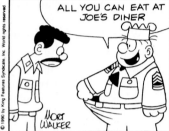

FIGURE 3-5
Beetle Bailey.

CONCEPT CHECK

To successfully change habits, a person needs to start by making small changes and providing rewards for sticking with the plan. At first, it is important to reward positive behaviors. Later, the focus switches to positive results, such as a loss of body weight or a lower blood cholesterol level. Before beginning a plan, one should determine the degree of commitment to it. Without commitment, changing habits can be a setup for failure.

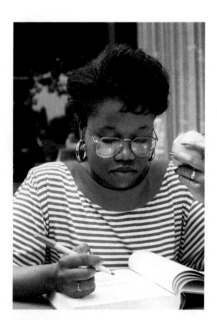

When snacking just can't be helped, fruit is an excellent choice.

PRACTICING THE PLAN

Once a person sets up a nutrition and health plan, the next step is to implement it. Start with a trial of at least 6 to 8 weeks. Thinking of a lifetime commitment can be overwhelming. Remember that we win the game one point at a time. Aim for a total duration of 6 months of new activities before giving up. It is difficult to overcome the habits of 5, 10, or 20 or more years.[4] More than once we may have to persuade ourselves of the value of continuing the behavior-change program. We may even backslide. That is not totally disastrous if we can learn to manage our thinking. Here are some suggestions to help keep a plan on track:

- Focus on reducing, but not necessarily extinguishing, undesirable behaviors—It is usually unrealistic to say "I will never eat a certain food again." Better to say "I will not eat that *problem* food as regularly as before."
- Monitor progress—Note progress in a diary and reward yourself according to your contract.[5] Regularly prove to yourself that you are following the plan. While conquering some habits and seeing improvement, you may find yourself quite encouraged, even enthusiastic, about the plan of action. That can be the impetus to move ahead with the program.
- Control environments—In the early phases of behavior change, try to avoid problem situations, such as parties, coffee breaks, and favorite restaurants (Figure 3-6).[4] Once new habits are firmly established, you can probably more successfully resist the temptations in these environments.
- Control related behaviors—These are known as **behavior chains** (Figure 3-7). If one goal is to reduce snacking, control linked behaviors that encourage snacking, such as skipping meals and watching television. Whatever is pushing you to deviate from your plan, substitute another behavior for it. Consider storing a list of alternative activities in a cookie jar.[4]

IMPLEMENTATION

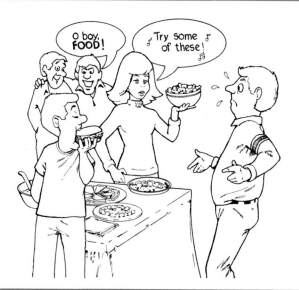

As Alan pursues his new practices, unexpected obstacles arise. Friday night parties are a challenge with their abundance of "munchies" and alcoholic beverages. Alan does not enjoy waking up earlier in the morning to pack his lunch, and he has to shop at the grocery store every few days for things he needs.

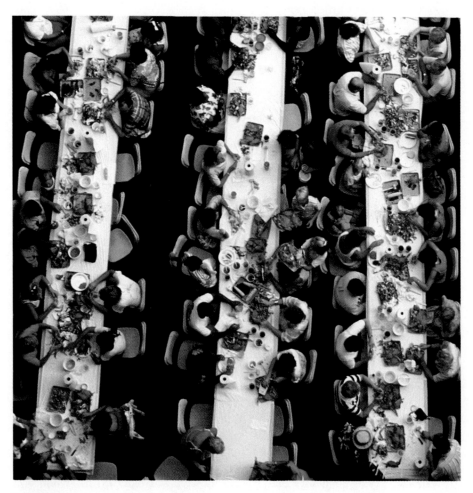

FIGURE 3-6
What would cause you to stop eating at this crab fest?

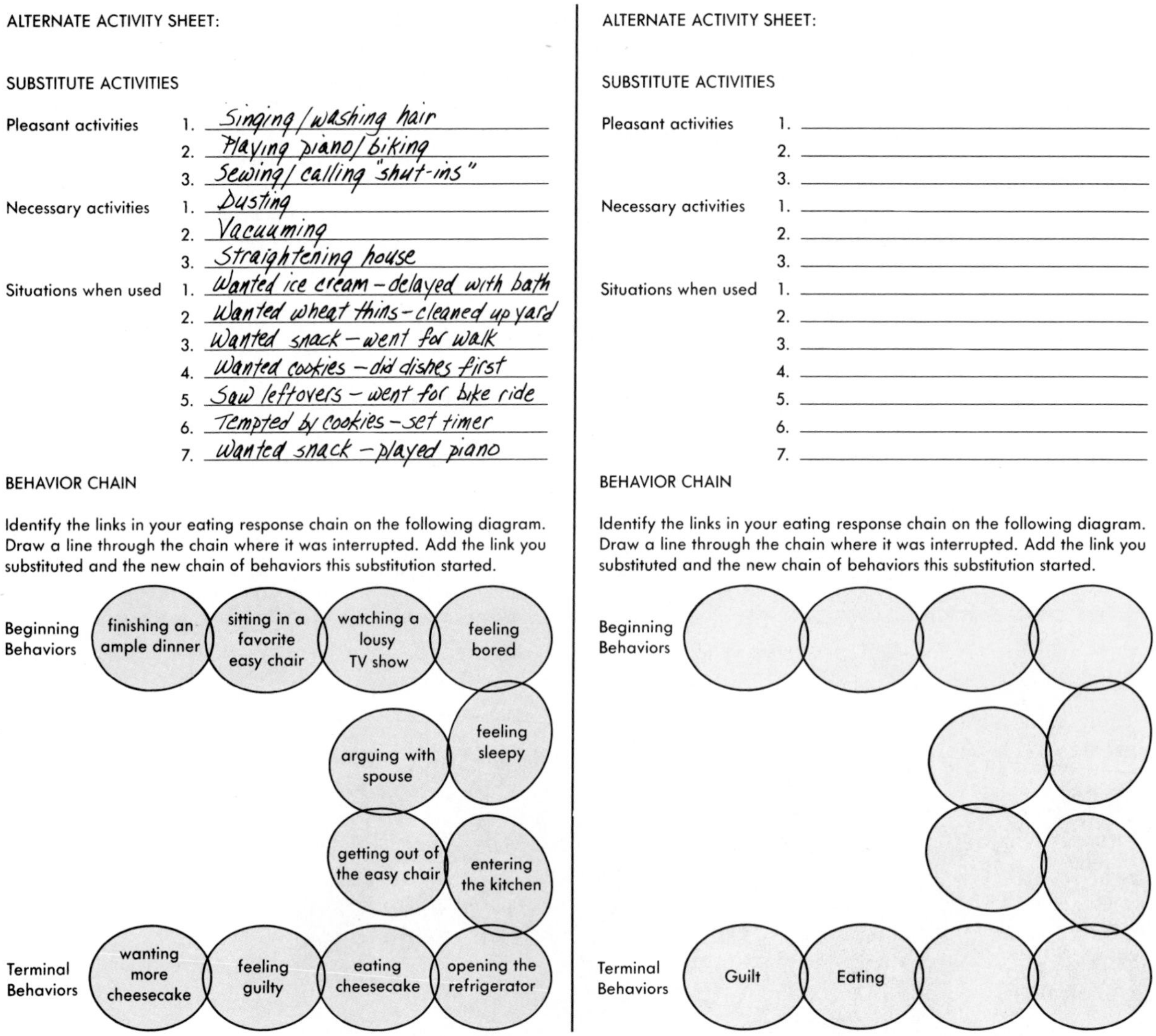

ALTERNATE ACTIVITY SHEET:

SUBSTITUTE ACTIVITIES

Pleasant activities 　1. _Singing/washing hair_
　　　　　　　　　　2. _Playing piano/biking_
　　　　　　　　　　3. _Sewing/calling "shut-ins"_

Necessary activities　1. _Dusting_
　　　　　　　　　　2. _Vacuuming_
　　　　　　　　　　3. _Straightening house_

Situations when used　1. _Wanted ice cream—delayed with bath_
　　　　　　　　　　2. _Wanted wheat thins—cleaned up yard_
　　　　　　　　　　3. _Wanted snack—went for walk_
　　　　　　　　　　4. _Wanted cookies—did dishes first_
　　　　　　　　　　5. _Saw leftovers—went for bike ride_
　　　　　　　　　　6. _Tempted by cookies—set timer_
　　　　　　　　　　7. _Wanted snack—played piano_

BEHAVIOR CHAIN

Identify the links in your eating response chain on the following diagram. Draw a line through the chain where it was interrupted. Add the link you substituted and the new chain of behaviors this substitution started.

ALTERNATE ACTIVITY SHEET:

SUBSTITUTE ACTIVITIES

Pleasant activities 　1. _____
　　　　　　　　　　2. _____
　　　　　　　　　　3. _____

Necessary activities　1. _____
　　　　　　　　　　2. _____
　　　　　　　　　　3. _____

Situations when used　1. _____
　　　　　　　　　　2. _____
　　　　　　　　　　3. _____
　　　　　　　　　　4. _____
　　　　　　　　　　5. _____
　　　　　　　　　　6. _____
　　　　　　　　　　7. _____

BEHAVIOR CHAIN

Identify the links in your eating response chain on the following diagram. Draw a line through the chain where it was interrupted. Add the link you substituted and the new chain of behaviors this substitution started.

FIGURE 3-7
Identifying behavior chains. This is a good tool for understanding more about your habits and pinpointing ways to change unwanted habits.

- Plan for failures—When faced with a situation or mood that may disrupt your plan, decide in advance what to do. If all else fails . . .
- Forgive and forget—Cultivate a long-term vision for a nutrition and health plan. Forgive occasional indiscretions. Focus on behaviors that have been established and performed day after day. Assume there will be setbacks, and work your way through them. An occasional lapse does not justify a relapse, and certainly not a collapse.[7]
- Recruit support from others—Have some family members, roommates, or friends witness your contract; educate them about the program and your needs. They can help prevent problem situations that encourage you to deviate from the plan.
- Watch for rationalization, the attempt to fool yourself—Distorting information and denying facts to support wishful thinking are ways we rationalize. Trying to justify backsliding by saying "I can't do it," when you have done it for 4 months already, is rationalizing. You won't fool even yourself.

- Be realistic—You cannot control every facet of your overall health. Genetic makeup and environment influence health. If you yearn for the body build of a sports hero or a movie star but have inherited other tendencies, reconsider. You may not achieve the shape you want, but can maintain a healthy body weight. Accept and like yourself for who you are.[7]

REEVALUATING A PLAN

After practicing a program for several months, a person needs to reevaluate it to clarify any issues. Does the plan of action actually lead to goals set? Are the goals in line with an overall nutrition and health plan? Reevaluation is especially in order if one's general lifestyle changes.

For example, as a person switches from a student lifestyle to that of a full-time worker, the level of physical activity may change drastically. A student may walk to classes and participate on intramural sports teams. But a job may require long hours at a desk. Though lifestyles change, the need for physical activity doesn't. Therefore the person may need to reevaluate plans for physical activity and adapt these to new situations.[12]

ANOTHER BITE Your friend whom you often study with makes a habit of eating potato chips during your study sessions. You frequently indulge yourself when offered the tempting snack. To stop this, think about buying an electric air-popper for a quick, almost no fat popcorn snack. This is a good alternative.

Changing some habits for a few days or even a few months may be easy. Changing them forever is tough, unless we learn to enjoy the changes and identify the new habits as our own. But a lifetime change can pay off.[7] Many who trim fat from their waistlines report a higher energy level. Having extra energy,

REEVALUATION

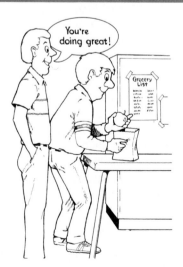

You're doing great!

Alan evaluates the obstacles he has encountered and brainstorms with his roommates to find ways to overcome them. He decides to cut back slightly on kcalories during the day on Fridays so at parties he can allow himself a limited number of snacks. He begins packing his lunch at night so he can grab it on the way to class and writes a complete grocery list that enables him to shop once each week.

Alan begins to notice how much more energy he has and so plans to continue the exercise program. He is even beginning to really enjoy it. He also realizes that he should move beyond his current food list so he doesn't get bored with his cooking and revert to relying on fast-food restaurants. After a month, he has not reached his desirable body weight, but friends are commenting on changes they see in him. This encouragement helps him to remain patient with his progress and focus on the ultimate goal, rather than the time needed to achieve it.

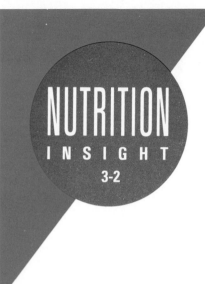

IS THERE ONE BEST ETHNIC DIET?

Based on research begun in the 1940s and 1950s, some scientists have developed a formula for a diet they consider to be one of the best overall. They found that the key is to eat simple foods, not rare and expensive treats. In many countries, inexpensive, traditional fare is the healthiest diet available—precisely the diet people abandon when they can spend more money on food.

The simple healthful diet, once probably a peasant diet, is the traditional food for people who live close to the land, such as people in Mexico and China. They eat a diet usually based on a grain (rice, wheat, or corn); fruits and vegetables; small amounts of dairy products or meat, fish, eggs; and a type of pea or bean. These diets are healthful because they are low in fat and high in dietary fiber, and most kcalories come from grains and peas or beans.

If you live in a society that has access to an abundance of rich foods, you must exercise willpower to keep your fat intake down. At a certain level of affluence, such as we have in the United States and Canada, people tend to eat less grains and beans in favor of more meats and cheeses—both high in kcalories and fat. The trick to finding healthy food is to look carefully at each dish and eat simply. No one food or one diet is all good or all bad.

Japanese foods

The traditional Japanese diet is built around a few lowfat foods: protein-rich soybean products (tofu and miso, made of fermented soybeans), fish, vegetables, noodles, and rice.[11] The Japanese eat little meat; it is used more as a garnish than as a main course. Seaweed, the Japanese lettuce, is high in nutrients. These basic foods have helped keep heart disease rates low in Japan. Life expectancy is the world's longest at 78 years, about 3 years longer than in the United States and 1½ years longer than in Canada.

But other foods in the traditional Japanese diet are salty, smoked, and pickled; foods that create Japan's two most serious public health problems—stroke and stomach cancer. Sodium (found in salted fish, pickled foods, and soy sauce) is linked to hypertension and risk of stroke. Salt and smoked foods contribute to Japan's high rate of stomach cancer.

Mexican foods

The Mexican diet is built around corn, beans, fish, chicken, and vegetables.[11] The food eaten in Mexican restaurants in the United States is not the same as that eaten in Mexico. The familiar fatty dishes—beef burritos swimming in melted cheese—aren't common in Mexico. Rich meat dishes generally only appear during holiday fiestas. Instead, corn and beans are the core of the Mexican diet. Corn is soaked in lime water, which increases the vitamin niacin, and is part of every meal. Corn is used in tortillas, steamed in corn husks to make tamales, or served as hot gruel. Beans provide the proteins that are missing in corn, and when corn and beans are eaten together, the body can synthesize any protein it needs. Hot chili peppers are excellent sources of vitamins A and C if you can "take the heat."

Traditional Eskimo foods

Although you may not find many Eskimo restaurants, Eskimo food habits are worth examination. One healthful Eskimo food habit is to eat fish regularly. Throughout the first half of this century, some Eskimo groups ate a diet that consisted almost entirely of seal, whale, and fish. Some caribou, berries, and other plant foods were also consumed. Overall, this diet is not desirable, but in Chapter 7 we note that a few fish dishes each week are a healthful part of a diet. Eating fish helps prevent heart attacks primarily by moderating the blood's capacity to clot. Blood clots in the vessels surrounding the heart are a key reason for heart attacks. Consider eating fish weekly, especially cold-water species—mackerel, salmon, tuna, herring, smelts, trout, and sardines.

The Chinese diet

Known for its variety, the average Chinese diet consists of about 69% carbohydrates, 10% protein, and 21% fat—proportions close to the diet that some experts recommend to reduce cancer risk. There is a richness and variety in the Chinese diet; as a population they use over 2000 different vegetables. The Chinese consume mostly vegetables in season, and in some regions they eat tubers, such as sweet potatoes, in generous quantities.

Rice is the core of the diet in the south; in the temperate north wheat is made into noodles, bread, and dumplings. Food prepared by quick frying in a lightly oiled hot wok and by steaming tends to keep its nutritional value.

Southern Italian diet

Southern Italy thrives on pasta, bread, olive oil, fruits, and vegetables. Pasta is the heart of the Italian diet. Italians still eat six times more pasta than North Americans eat. People in Mediterranean cultures eat at least three times as much bread as Americans, but it's rarely buttered.

What about the diet of early man?

Humans have walked the earth for about 40,000 years. For 30,000 of those years, humans survived by hunting wild animals and gathering plants. Early humans were constantly on the move, either pursuing wild game or following the seasonal ebb and flow of fruits and vegetables. Animal and plant foods obtained from successful hunting and gathering journeys spoiled quickly, so they had to be consumed within a short time. Very often, feasts were followed by periods of famine.

This led our early human ancestors to eat mostly a diet low in fat (especially lowfat wild game) and sodium but high in dietary fiber. Some researchers feel that we have, in a very short time, mistakenly left behind this diet—as it is the one we are ideally suited for. Even so, life expectancy has never been longer than it is in Western societies today, despite our penchant for fatty foods. Perhaps our ancestors did not live long enough to suffer the effects of their limited diets.[6] We know they lived a precarious life in which they probably faced alternating periods of food abundance and scarcity. In addition, their foods were not necessarily safe to eat, though they were free from pesticides and food additives. Parasites survived in their undercooked meats, grains were contaminated with mold, and toxic metals, such as lead, leached out of decorated pottery. Cyanide poisoning could even result from eating certain tubers and roots.[6]

We wouldn't turn back the clock that far, but moving toward a simpler diet is not a bad idea. ●

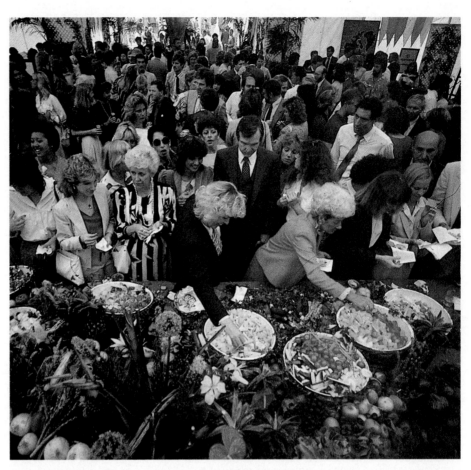

Behavior changes, such as choosing healthful food at a party, are one part of a successful weight loss plan.

feeling good, and looking better provide further motivation to continue to follow the new habits. For many people these assets are much stronger incentives than the less tangible goal of preventing disease.

Preventing relapse

Relapse often starts with a high-risk situation. Most people at first don't recognize the conditions that promote a relapse.[7] One *slip* sometimes snowballs into a series of lapses that lead to complete reversion into old behaviors. The first lapse could be caused by stress, interpersonal conflicts, or inability to cope adequately with everyday events. These factors signal a high-risk situation. One or two slips are not fatal. Healthful behavior can be recovered if the potential for relapse is planned in advance and even expected. Here are some suggestions:

- Identify high-risk situations—As a backslide begins, determine the factors that contributed to the slide and analyze what provoked the high-risk situation. By focusing on the risks inherent in a situation, you can both plan to avoid them in the future and avoid the trap of dwelling on self-defeating guilt feelings.
- Mentally rehearse a response to a backsliding behavior—Imagine backsliding and seeing yourself taking positive action to recover. Rehearse responses to as many potential lapses as you can think of.
- Remember your goals—Keep in mind the reasons for making the commitment to change behaviors and the hard work it took to achieve them.

CONCEPT CHECK

To implement a behavior-change plan, a person can write a contract that identifies behaviors to practice, behavior rewards, and the time frame for accomplishing the plan. While trying to change behaviors, it is important to control the environment (to discourage deviation from the plan) and to get support from others. A plan for problems is needed—problems should not be an excuse for a relapse. The person needs to invoke a strategy that will allow one to move ahead despite a few failures along the way. Problems may require reconsidering the action plan—this is to be expected.

SUMMARY

- Behavior change occurs in steps. First, a person becomes aware of a problem. Then the person openly receives new information about it, evolving a receptive framework for learning. That person then undertakes a trial period for the change, during which time positive reinforcement is critical. If an initial trial is successful, the person may permanently adopt new behaviors.

- Before charting a behavior-change plan, it is important to discover strengths and weaknesses regarding the intended behavior. A food diary kept for at least a week may show eating patterns and other behaviors that either contribute to or discourage new behaviors. The diary can reveal areas of one's outside environment that need to be altered to reduce temptation.

- When setting goals for a behavior plan, a key is to plan small steps that lead to the intended result and build in rewards to capitalize on achievements and maintain momentum.

- After setting a plan of action, drawing up a contract that lists intended tasks, the incentive rewards, and the time frame for the behavior change is helpful. The contract should at first reward positive behaviors and later reward ultimate objectives.

- Before embarking on the behavior-change program, a person needs to evaluate personal commitment. A plan, no matter how skillfully developed, will not succeed unless a person has a strong commitment to achieving the goals.

- When implementing a plan, the person needs to monitor progress and provide rewards. Controlling one's environment can reduce temptations to deviate from the plan. For example, deciding in advance to choose lowfat foods at a fast food restaurant is helpful. The person should expect small failures and not consider them an excuse to abandon change. A forgive-and-forget attitude can prevent collapse of the whole strategy.

- It is necessary to plan for the possibility of relapse. Most people revert to old behaviors during periods of stress or interpersonal conflict. Identifying problem behavior chains and ways to substitute better links is recommended. Strategies to recover from relapse include identifying high-risk situations and mentally rehearsing a response.

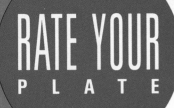

RATE YOUR
P L A T E

Here are five activity levels:

1. Sedentary
2. Mostly inactive
3. Moderately active
4. Active
5. Superactive

Each category is defined below.[12]

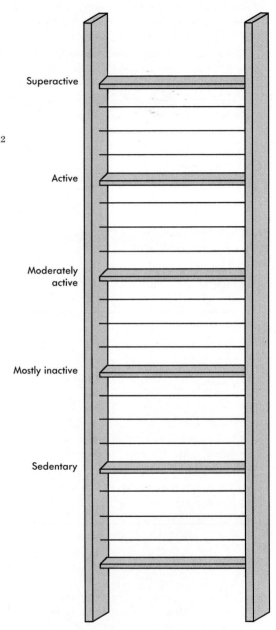

Superactive

Active

Moderately active

Mostly inactive

Sedentary

5. *Superactive*—1 hour of sustained activity at least 5 days per week. Examples are full-court basketball, mountain climbing, treadmill work, soccer, jogging, stair-climbing (machine included), biking (stationary bike included), swimming, walking briskly, cross-country skiing (NordicTrack included), and rowing (rowing machine included).

4. *Active*—20 minutes of sustained activity at least 5 days per week.

3. *Moderately active*—20 minutes of sustained activity at least 3 days per week or 10 to 15 minutes of sustained activity at least 4 days a week.

2. *Mostly inactive*—Sustained activity fewer than 3 days per week that involves mostly walking.

1. *Sedentary*—Most activity is limited to sitting or walking.

Your task is to track your activities for 3 weeks. Rate each week from 1 to 5 based on definitions given. Start on a Monday, for example, and estimate your activity level for the previous week. After 3 weeks, average the numbers by adding them and then dividing the answer by 3. This will result in a number between 1 and 5. Find your location on the physical activity ladder and circle your level of activity.

What kind of program would allow you to move up the ladder, if appropriate?

Use a behavioral contract to record your plan for improving or maintaining your level of activity (Figure 3-4). Fill out the contract completely including your goal, plan of activities, reinforcements, and social support. Make sure to share it with a significant other and have that person sign it as a witness to your contract. Start with trying to fulfill the contract for 1 week and then reevaluate its appropriateness.

REFERENCES

1. Brownell KD: *The LEARN program for weight control*, Philadelphia, 1989, KD Brownell.
2. Callaway CW and others: Statement on vitamin and mineral supplements, *Journal of Nutrition* 117:1649, 1987.
3. Council on Scientific Affairs: Vitamin preparations as dietary supplements and as therapeutic agents, *Journal of the American Medical Association* 257:1929, 1987.
4. Ferguson J: *Habits, not diets: the secret to lifetime weight control*, Palo Alto, Calif, 1988, Bull Publishing.
5. Frankle RT, Yang M: *Obesity and weight control*, Rockville, Md, 1988, Aspen Publishers.
6. Garn SM, Leonard WR: What did our ancestors eat? *Nutrition Reviews* 47:337, 1989.
7. Insel PM, Roth WT: *Core concepts in health*, ed 5, Mountain View, Calif, 1990, Mayfield Publishing.
8. Nash JD: *Maximize your body potential*, Palo Alto, Calif, 1986, Bull Publishing.
9. Read MH and others: Health beliefs and supplement use: adults in seven western states, *Journal of the American Dietetic Association* 89:1812, 1989.
10. Roberts C: Fast food fare, *New England Journal of Medicine* 321:752, 1989.
11. Sweet CA: Rethinking eating out, *FDA Consumer*, November, 1989, p 6.
12. Wood P: *California diet and exercise program*, Mountain View, Calif, 1983, Anderson World Books.
13. Weinstock CP: The grazing of America: a guide to healthy snacking, *FDA Consumer*, March, 1989, p 8.

HOW MUCH HAVE I LEARNED?

What have you learned from Chapter 3? Here are 15 statements about how to improve your diet. Read them to test your current knowledge. If you think the statement is true or mostly true, circle T. If you think the statement is false or mostly false, circle F. Use the scoring key at the end of the book to compute your total score. To review, take this test again later, and especially before tests.

1. T **F**   Behavior change is essentially a matter of willpower.
    Changing environment key to success
2. **T** F   People have different food preferences depending on their moods.

3. T **F**   If a goal is sufficiently worthwhile, a person will usually achieve it even when the commitment is weak.

4. T **F**   If you lapse while attempting to change your eating behavior, it is best to abandon that plan and try something else.

5. **T** F   Eating habits are difficult to overcome because people eat for pleasure. *find substitutes for food*

6. T **F**   If you aim for the best and try to attain a body type you most admire, you are more likely to achieve it. *aim to maximize personal potential*

7. **T** F   Behavior change involves measuring progress.

8. T **F**   For changing behavior, punishment works more effectively than reward.

9. T **F**   Midafternoon is routinely the toughest time for most dieters.
    evenings
10. T **F**   To control overeating it is best to keep as little food as possible in the refrigerator. *diet changes need to develop from restriction not starving*

? 11. T **F**   People should improve their diets by only eating foods they don't like.

12. T **F**   When beginning to change behavior, one should seek potential problem situations to test personal strength.

13. T **F**   Behavior changes are more successful if they simultaneously address all facets of a problem.

14. **T** F   Friends and relatives may oppose or sabotage attempts to change your dietary habits.

15. T **F**   Rewards should be given only when the final goal has been accomplished.

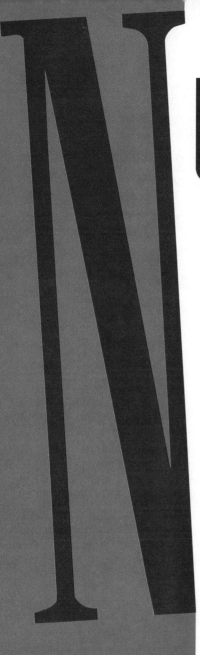

NUTRITION ISSUE

SHOULD YOU USE VITAMIN AND MINERAL SUPPLEMENTS?

In the early 1900s, vitamins were first a curiosity and then the subject of intense scientific scrutiny and research. Today, as many as 45% of adults in the United States consume vitamin and mineral supplements.[9] Most of this use is unnecessary. A balanced diet supplies necessary nutrients for most of us, as we noted in Chapter 2. Some health food enthusiasts and health food store owners would have us believe that high doses of vitamins are needed to prevent all kinds of illness. In fact, supplements are such big business that their sales more than doubled between 1976 and 1986 from $1.2 billion to $3.1 billion.

To determine whether you need to use supplements, first look closely at your diet. If your diet follows the Guide to Daily Food Choices discussed in Chapter 2, with emphasis on such nutrient-dense sources as whole grains, low-fat dairy products, leafy and dark green vegetables, fruits and vegetables that contain vitamin C, and a serving of vegetable oil, you are probably meeting your nutrient needs. However, some women with heavy menstrual flows may still need more iron to compensate for that lost in the blood. If you are still uncertain whether your diet provides enough vitamins and minerals, take a close look at what you eat for breakfast. Most breakfast cereals have extra vitamins and minerals added, some even matching the adult U.S. RDA.

What do the experts say?

Nutrition scientists generally agree with us that most people can obtain needed vitamins and minerals from a varied, balanced diet. We think you should start there first. Using the information in this chapter and Chapter 2 can help you improve your diet where needed. If you still think you need a supplement, talk to a registered dietitian and/or your physician. There is some risk from consuming even typical multivitamin and mineral supplements. For example, people who are genetically prone to a liver disease called ***hemochromatosis*** can easily develop iron toxicity. Women in the early months of pregnancy may risk birth defects from ingesting too much vitamin A (we discuss this further in Chapters 9 and 10).

Recently a panel of scientists from the American Institute of Nutrition and the American Society for Clinical Nutrition suggested specific cases in which vitamin and mineral supplements should be considered:[2]

- Women who bleed excessively during menstrual periods may need more iron.
- Pregnant or ***lactating*** women may need extra iron, calcium, and the vitamin folate.

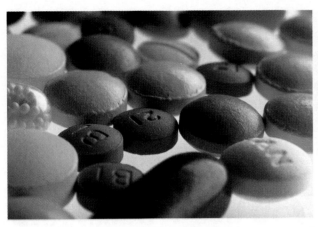 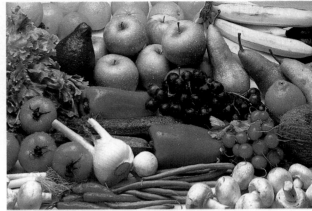

Before jumping to supplements, consider whether just eating better will be enough. Nutrition experts emphasize the latter option.

Hemochromatosis • A disorder of iron metabolism characterized by increased iron absorption and deposition in the liver tissue. This eventually poisons the liver cells.

Lactation • The period following childbirth during which milk is produced in the woman's breasts.

Diuretic • A substance that, when ingested, increases the flow of urine.

Megadose • Intake of a nutrient at levels greater than 10 times one's RDA value listed in the 1989 publication.

Do you take vitamin supplements? Why? If not, why not?

- People with low kcalorie intakes (1200 or less) need the range of vitamins and minerals. This can include elderly people who perform little physical activity.
- Some vegetarians may need extra calcium, iron, zinc, and vitamin B-12. Vitamin B-12 is found in reasonable amounts only in animal products.
- Newborns, under the direction of a physician, need a single dose of vitamin K to last until diet and synthesis by intestinal bacteria suffice.
- People with specific illnesses or diseases, and those on certain medications, may need supplementation of specific vitamins and minerals at the direction of a physician. Examples include extra potassium for someone using thiazide **diuretics** and possibly extra vitamin D for someone being treated for osteoporosis.

Supplementation during illness or drug therapy should be directed by a physician because some vitamins and minerals counteract the effect of certain medications. Vitamin B-6 can counteract the action of levodopa, a medication used to treat Parkinson's disease. Similarly, taking too much vitamin E can inhibit vitamin K metabolism and in turn increase the action of drugs designed to reduce blood clotting. By consuming many folate supplements, people with epilepsy who require anticonvulsant medication jeopardize their health; folate decreases the effectiveness of their medication. These examples illustrate the need for professional advice when you take vitamin and mineral supplements that exceed RDA levels. Only with professional advice can you appropriately evaluate whether supplementation is in your best interest.

Which supplement should you choose?

If you do decide to take a vitamin and mineral supplement, the Council on Scientific Affairs of the American Medical Association recommends taking no more than 50% to 150% of the adult U.S. RDA for vitamins.[3] For minerals, we suggest the same guidelines. These are typical supplemental doses, basically a one-a-day type of supplement, but always read the label to be sure. **Megadoses** are defined as greater than 10 times one's RDA. A moderate, balanced formulation in a multivitamin and mineral supplement is important because it minimizes the chances of vitamin and mineral competition, which can lead to an imbalance. For instance, a high amount of zinc in a supplement can inhibit copper absorption, and a large amount of the vitamin folate can mask the symptoms of a potentially life-threatening deficiency of vitamin B-12.

Buyer beware!

FDA does not regulate all vitamin and mineral supplements closely. The Proxmire Amendment to the 1938 Food, Drug, and Cosmetic Act prevents regulation of supplements unless they are known to be inherently dangerous or marketed with illegal claims. Therefore Americans cannot always depend on the federal government to protect them from vitamin and mineral supplement overuse. For health's sake, people should know what they are ingesting and preferably should seek the advice of physicians and registered dietitians. In cases where vitamin and mineral supplements are necessary, professional guidance is important. ●

SORTING NUTRITIONAL ADVICE
FACTS AND FALLACIES

Advice about foods to eat and avoid is overwhelming:

- Eat organic produce to avoid pesticides.
- Don't eat processed foods that contain preservatives.
- Take large doses of vitamin C to prevent colds.
- Eat foods that contain oat bran.
- Choose baked goods made with honey instead of sugar.
- Eat brown rice for perfect nutrition.
- Take large doses of laetrile (a compound found in apricot pits) to cure cancer.
- An apple a day keeps the doctor away.

Sound convincing? Have you heard these statements argued both ways? Contradictory advice can be confusing. How do you distinguish food fact from fiction? Many food products and legitimate businesses ride a nutritional bandwagon. Unfortunately, so do quacks.[1] This chapter presents popular nutrition myths and misconceptions. Familiarity with the claims and methods of quackery can help you distinguish between sound and unsound nutrition advice. If you can spot a myth, you can protect yourself from pretentious health claims and fraudulent food promotions and practices.[4,12] ●

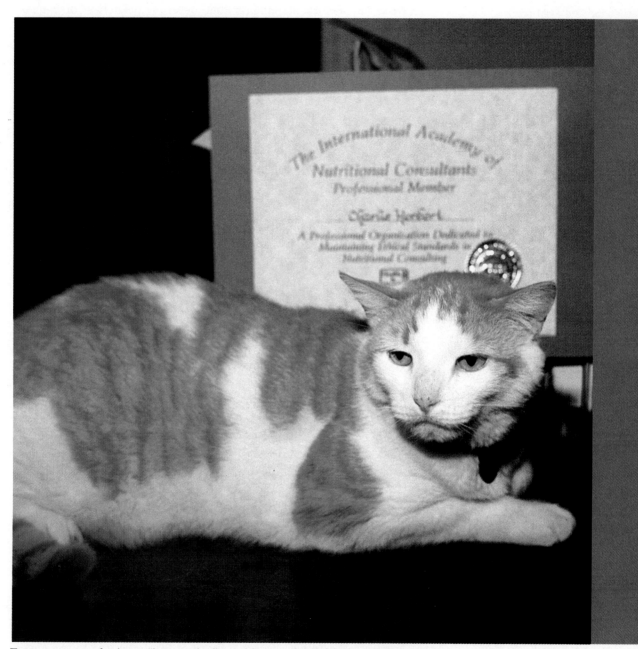

Even a cat can obtain an "impressive" nutrition credential from a mail-order firm.

Can You Spot a Quack?

Quacks are people who exaggerate health claims. Everyday, people fall prey to quackery. By following quack advice you can lose considerable money. You can also damage your health. Americans spend at least $10 billion a year on quackery. Protect yourself by knowing what to look for.

Put a "Q" in blanks preceding statements that describe behaviors of quacks. Write "E" before statements that describe behaviors of reliable nutrition experts.

__Q__ **1.** They use anecdotes and testimonials to support their claims. They refer to stories of people being cured of cancer or arthritis by using product X as proof of the effectiveness of the product.

__Q__ **2.** They promise quick, dramatic, miraculous cures.

__E__ **3.** They display credentials recognized by responsible scientists or educators.

__Q__ **4.** They say that most disease is caused by faulty diet and can be treated with "nutritional" methods.

__E__ **5.** They support the pros and cons of a claim with scientific studies and evidence.

__Q__ **6.** In literature they use or write, they cite few if any scientific studies to support the product or claims.

__E__ **7.** They claim that most food additives and preservatives are safe, however, some still require further testing and study.

__Q__ **8.** They claim that "natural" vitamins are better than synthetic ones.

__E__ **9.** They say you can get all foods necessary for a healthy diet from the supermarket.

__Q__ **10.** They tell you not to trust the medical community.

__E__ **11.** They tell you that no food is really good or bad, but that all foods provide some nutritional value, some more than others.

__Q__ **12.** They claim that modern food processing methods and storage remove all nutritive value from food.

__E__ **13.** They say that organically grown foods are not necessarily superior to plants grown using chemical fertilizers and pesticides.

__Q__ **14.** They claim that they are being persecuted by orthodox medicine and that their work is being suppressed because it is controversial.

__Q__ **15.** They recommend that everybody take vitamins, eat health foods, or both because diet alone does not supply enough nutrients.

INTERPRETATION

Characteristics of a quack: 1, 2, 4, 6, 8, 10, 12, 14, 15
Characteristics of an expert: 3, 5, 7, 9, 11, 13

Put the total number you answered correctly in this blank __15__

Were you able to tell the difference between a quack and a reliable expert?

Assessment adapted from Herbert V, Barrett S: Twenty-one ways to spot a quack, *Nutrition Forum*, September, 1986, p 65.

ASSESS YOURSELF

QUACKERY

Dictionaries define *quack* as "a pretender of medical skill; a charlatan" and "one who talks pretentiously without sound knowledge of the subject discussed." Quackery encompasses fraudulent actions, claims, and practices. These definitions suggest deliberate deception.[4] However, many promoters of ineffective and unproven remedies sincerely believe in their products. They may be victims of quackery themselves or may merely wish to believe in something they hope will make them better. In their naivete and enthusiasm they pass on misinformation.

Americans spend billions of dollars every year on quackery. Over $2 billion buys unnecessary vitamin and mineral supplements. Another billion buys false hope in unfounded cancer cures. Can you say you were never a victim of quackery? Health fraud and quackery fool many people, not just gullible or ignorant people. Quackery also preys on the unsuspecting.

Most fraudulent health claims cost only the money lost. But if trying a quack remedy delays needed medical treatment, the cost may be needless physical harm.[6] Until something bad happens, we usually don't recognize dishonest treatment. When we get "burned" by "hot" health frauds, a wiser skepticism results.

The elderly are particularly vulnerable to quackery.[6] The wish to relieve pain and heal a failing body can be a powerful force.[15] Hope of such relief offered with naive sincerity sells many useless, expensive cures to frightened and weary elders.

People tend to believe what they hear repeatedly. As with "brainwashing," a repeated claim can seem real even when it has no basis in fact. Nutritional brainwashing floods the media, the food shelves, and the conversations of those seeking good health. Quack ideas are everywhere, but repetition does not make them valid.[16]

> **Quack** • A person who pretends to have certain medical skills or knowledge.

ANOTHER BITE Can the government protect citizens from false advertising and misleading health claims? Despite its broad powers, it cannot. Only you possess that power. The following pages will alert you to a truer picture of reality:

"LET THE BUYER BEWARE"

Sources of nutrition quackery

Unsound nutrition claims enter your world daily through radio, television, newspapers, books, and magazines.[1,5] You need not seek fringe health sources for this false information. A well-meaning but poorly informed medical reporter on the nightly news may mislead you unknowingly. Separating fact from fiction can even stump health professionals. A product effective in relieving one ailment may be worthless for another. Often only intricate knowledge can tell fact from food fad. That's where nutrition studies come in.

Most medical schools offer minimal nutrition education. Physicians graduate with impressive skills in diagnosing and treating illnesses. But when patients need dietary advice, consultation with a registered dietitian may be advisable.[15] All in all, healthy skepticism may be our best guide in the often expensive arena of alternative food choices.

Miracle cures are myths (Table 4-1). If a cure has not been reported in a scientific journal and if physicians are not familiar with it, the cure is probably no miracle.[4,15] Most cures are discovered in steps, over long periods of time—rarely in a miraculous flash.

TABLE 4-1

Types of food fads and the behavior needs these practices serve

Victims	Need Served by Fad
Miracle-seeker	Seeks diets promising eternal youth in an attempt to believe in self-worth.
Rebel	Chooses foods that fit into antisocial belief system.
Mr. Atlas	Seeks diets promising to slow aging to fit with self-image of super strength and perfect health.
Skeptic	Rejects traditional medical and nutritional advice to establish appearance of control and independence.
Food Fashion Groupie	Buys into any popular diet to fit in and to gain approval and acceptance.
Ms. Know-It-All	Reads extensively and makes food choices to confirm own nutrition know-how.
Analyzer	Challenges all input to protect self from feared manipulation.
Worrier	Seeks certainty in food choices in attempt to find certainty and stability in the world.

Modified from Schafer R, Yetley EA: Social psychology of food faddism, *Journal of the American Dietetic Association* 66:129, 1975.

Let's now look specifically at the many forms of quackery and food fads. Has quackery infiltrated your daily life?

ALTERNATIVE FOOD CHOICES
Organically grown produce

Pesticide scares crop up in the news as regularly as a harvest season. One year we hear apples are unsafe; the next year it may be that grapes can kill. The public listens. To please the public, supermarket aisles are now stocked with produce once found only in health food stores. Today, organic food is a $3 billion industry. Though large, it still represents only about 1% of the United States' food production, partly because of its higher price.

Just what is organically grown food? Recently Congress passed a farm bill that called for a federal standard defining *organic*. But, until new laws are in place, no federal standard controls the production methods of such foods. *Organic* farmers usually reject **pesticides** and use natural soil improvers, such as compost instead of manufactured fertilizers.[19] They rotate crops to further enrich soil and may control pests with biological intervention. But still, even state requirements for *organic* foods are inconsistent. Currently some states require no pesticide use for 3 years before foods can be labeled organic. Other states require 1 year and some states have not delineated the time.

Organic food advocates claim these crops offer more nutrition and fewer health hazards than conventionally grown food. Nutrition scientists find such claims inherently misleading for the following reasons:

1. Surveys find similar pesticide levels in both organically and conventionally grown foods. Cross-contamination from wind and groundwater partly explains this. Washing fruits and vegetables removes some external pesticide residue from conventional foods. Still, according to the FDA, tiny amounts of pesticides that remain in conventional foods pose no significant health risk (see Chapter 17 for a detailed discussion). Most dangerous pesticides were banned in this country in 1973. Those currently used are regulated so that even if consumed over a lifetime, the chances of inducing cancer in a person would be less than one in a million.

2. Soil nutrients from natural fertilizers, such as manure, are no different from those in chemical fertilizers made in factories. Furthermore, nutrients

Fad is a shortened version of fiddle-faddle, which means to "play with" and then "cast aside."

Pesticide • A general term that signifies an agent can destroy bacteria, fungi, insects, rodents, or other pests.

However, dangerous pesticides may not be outlawed in other countries, and we may be consuming them in imported produce.

from organic fertilizers can't be absorbed until the organic material decomposes. The key issue is whether specific nutrients are present in a fertilizer—not which type of fertilizer is used.[4]

3. Genetic makeup determines a plant's nutrient content and needs. Plants thrive when soil offers a nutritious fare.[12] Long-term studies find no nutritional differences between organic crops and those grown under standard conditions.

4. Freshness, hereditary makeup, and harvest time determine a plant food's flavor. A large-scale study compared 25 types of organic foods with their ordinary supermarket counterparts for taste and eye appeal. In general, the ordinary produce won both the taste and the beauty contests.[7]

Organically grown produce costs more. Are you wasting your money? We suggest using your money to buy the freshest foods, which have the best taste and highest vitamin level. If eating organic food holds high value for you, then the extra dollars may give you peace of mind. If so, try to find out your store's standards for labeling foods *organic*. You may be paying more for an organic tomato that was actually grown very much like its counterpart on the next counter. Often a special label certifies the food as organic. Still, note again that most states do not have laws defining organic or legislative plans to enact any. So, when something is advertised as organic, it is not guaranteed to be free of pesticide residues or grown without chemical fertilizers.[19]

"Natural" foods

Decades ago a walk down your main street may have taken you past a health food store that offered mainly vitamins and other supplements. Today's health food industry goes beyond organic foods and herbal remedies and is much more visible. Like street corner "Mom and Pop" shops, health food stores offer produce and breads. Their proprietors promise *natural* products, which supposedly are minimally processed and have no additives or other artificial ingredients. But can a line be drawn between processed and unprocessed foods? Recall from Chapter 2 there are no labeling laws that restrict use of the word natural. Any food can claim to be so. What is your criteria for a natural food?

Consider for example a cracker. Making a single cracker requires grinding, mixing, boiling, baking, and pressing—a lot of processing. Yet health food crackers get a natural label (and price tag) because they contain no artificial coloring or **preservatives.** Is this fair? How natural are the ingredients once they become a cracker?

Ask questions when you see bold exclamations of natural foods.[4] Some natural food products are toxic: aflatoxins in grains, solanine in potatoes, goitrogens in some raw vegetables, and other poisons in mushrooms and herbs (see Chapter 17). In addition, some highly touted natural and health food snacks—while they may contain dietary fiber and other good things—are notoriously high in fat, particularly palm oils and other saturated fats. Therefore in health food stores, be on your guard.[4]

Are there true *health* foods?

We consider even the term *health food* inherently misleading. All foods eaten in moderation can be healthful in the context of a balanced diet.[12] And all foods, even Popeye's spinach, can be unhealthful when eaten in excess.

However, do some foods truly offer "super nutrition?" Though not the food of the gods, some foods such as brown rice and whole-wheat flour do offer more fiber, protein, and certain vitamins and minerals than their more highly processed counterparts. Still, most grocery stores stock these staples. Rice, wheat, and all grains—the seeds of grasses—have a germ (seed) surrounded by starch. The starch provides nourishment once the seed sprouts. A layer of bran and an outer, inedible hull protect the germ and starch. Edible whole grains, such as rice and whole wheat, contain everything but the hull.

Preservatives • Compounds that extend the shelf life of foods by inhibiting microbial growth or minimizing the destructive effect of oxygen and metals.

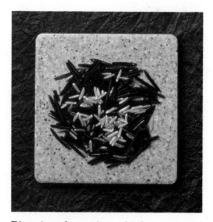

Rice is often given high status in health food circles.

Rancid • Having a disagreeable odor or taste, usually caused by fat breakdown.

Toxic • Poisonous; caused by a poison.

Most grain processing strips away this nutrition. The valuable dietary fiber of bran and the important nutrients of the germ are removed at the mill to produce the white rice and flour many desire. Food processors *enrich* some white rice and flour by adding the significant nutrients lost. And *converted* white rice can claim a few higher nutrient values than ordinary enriched rice. But both enriched and converted foods lack the fiber and some nutrients contained in the whole food. Overall, it is whole grains that offer us the good nutrition we should strive for.

However, food processing does not always mean removing healthful ingredients. Sometimes nutrients are added through fortification, which makes the food nutritious in some regards. Sometimes processing means safer food. For example, unprocessed (raw) milk can contain microorganisms that cause disease. Pasteurizing milk (heating it to high temperatures) kills microorganisms, such as toxic bacteria and viruses. Even when produced under high standards of cleanliness, raw milk is not safe. Each processed food, then, deserves a separate evaluation. As we said in Chapter 2, it is the total diet that deserves the main focus. How do your food choices fit into a diet plan to meet your nutrient needs?

What if a food contains additives?

The practice of commercially adding preservatives and other additives to foods tends to generate more heat than light. Preservatives retard growth of microorganisms, prevent off flavors in fat by reducing the incidence of **rancidity,** keep mixtures from separating, and retain food crispness. Some additives are nutrients or potentially beneficial—BHA and BHT may prevent cancer-causing chemicals from forming. Additives can raise the nutrient value, as they do in enriched rice, or they may enhance eye appeal and flavor (see Chapter 17).

FDA checks additive safety. But some people are skeptical. Having additive-free options means higher prices for the consumer.[19] But, even without additives, organic foods contain natural, yet potentially **toxic** substances, as we just pointed out. And our body's defense mechanisms help guard against harm from additives and other *foreign* compounds. Liver enzyme systems and the constant shedding mechanism of the intestinal tract are two of many means by which our bodies defend themselves.

Health food stores in perspective

Do some foods in the health food store serve important nutritional roles? Whole grain products, the most popular candidates, are followed in sales by fruits and vegetables, juices, yogurt, tofu, and nut butters. But you can buy these at your grocery store. And, one of three shoppers in health food stores spends money on dubious nutritional products. For example, digestive enzymes, amino acid supplements, bee pollen, ginseng, fiber, protein supplements, and primrose oil play no important nutritional role despite promotions as cures for all kinds of ailments[4,7] (Table 4-2). The same holds true for vitamin and mineral supplements for most people.

CONCEPT CHECK

Quackery is at work whenever the promises for a food or medical regimen go beyond its scientifically established benefits. The victim pays in dollars and cents and sometimes physical harm. Choosing organically grown and natural foods to avoid pesticides, chemical fertilizers, additives, and artificial ingredients costs more. Studies show no higher nutritional value in organic foods than in ordinary foods. In some cases, choosing processed foods buys safer nourishment. FDA, the nation's federal food regulatory watchdog, requires testing of all food additives when safety is questioned.

TABLE 4-2

Dubious claims for nutrition products

Food	Claims	Facts
Acidophilus milk (contains bacteria that ferment milk sugar)	Aids digestion; promotes health of digestive tract	Bacteria may not survive acidic stomach environment; of value to people who cannot readily digest milk sugar (lactose) or need to reestablish intestinal bacteria after long-term antibiotic therapy
Alfalfa sprouts	Have nutrients not available in other vegetables	Have less nutritional value than broccoli, carrots, and spinach; alfalfa tea can disturb digestion and respiration
Amino acid tablets	Help build muscle mass	Amino acids make up proteins. An abundant level is supplied by diets following the Guide to Daily Food Choices
Bee pollen	A perfect food; can help athletic and sexual performance; prevents cancer, infection, and allergy; prolongs life; promotes both weight loss and gain	Its nutrients are found in conventional foods; no evidence shows that it helps athletes; people allergic to specific pollens can develop severe allergic reactions after ingestion
Bioflavonoids ("vitamin P")	Essential for good health; provides resistance to colds and flu	Bioflavonoids are not vitamins or essential nutrients; no evidence suggests that they are useful for treating any health condition
Blackstrap molasses (less refined form of molasses)	Wonder food that can restore hair and cure anemia	Contributes to iron intake; has no effect on hair color and does not cure anemia
Bone meal	A rich source of calcium	Calcium in bone meal is poorly absorbed; can contain high levels of lead
Brewer's yeast	Excellent diet supplement	Good source of protein and several B vitamins, but adds nothing to a balanced diet; unsavory taste for some
Brown rice	Most perfect food; improves health even if eaten exclusively	A nutritious food, but lacks some needed nutrients; must be complemented by other foods to maintain health
Cider vinegar	Keeps body in balance; thins blood; aids digestion	No evidence to support these claims
Fertile eggs	Nutritionally superior to unfertilized eggs; have fewer unnatural hormones	Fertilization does not add to an egg's nutritional value; if hens are not given hormones, their eggs may have fewer unnatural hormones
Fish oil capsules	Lowers blood cholesterol levels	Can be used to lower some levels of blood fats (only cholesterol when given in very high doses), but can also make control of blood sugar in diabetes mellitus more difficult (see Chapter 7)
Garlic	Purifies blood; reduces high blood pressure; prevents diabetes and heart disease	Garlic and onion contain substances that help prevent blood cells from clumping into blood clots; garlic juice can lower blood sugar in diabetes; slows growth of fungi and mold that cause infections
Kelp (type of seaweed)	Good source of iodine; energy booster	A good source of iodine, but is more expensive than iodized salt
Lecithin	Reduces heart disease risk	Only flawed research supports lecithin's effectiveness in reducing heart disease; the body makes lecithin
Oat bran	Superior food ingredient for lowering blood cholesterol	Only effective in high doses (80-100 grams/day), while people usually eat much less; reducing saturated fat in the diet is a more reliable way to lower blood cholesterol levels (see Chapter 7)
PABA (para-aminobenzoic benzoic acid)	Oral doses can prevent or reverse graying in hair	PABA is a vitamin for bacteria but not for humans; useful ingredient in sunscreens
Spirulina (blue-green algae)	Helps you lose weight; helps people with diabetes, liver disease, ulcers	Good source of protein, but is more expensive than conventional foods; no evidence that it promotes weight loss or has medical value

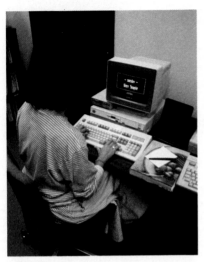

Make sure you need that vitamin supplement—analyze your typical intake first.

Vitamin and mineral supplements

If you check the grocery baskets of health food shoppers, you often find tucked amid the breads and grains bottles of vitamin/mineral supplements. The two most popular purchases are vitamin C and multiple vitamin/mineral products. People often buy these supplements, fearing that their normal diets fail to provide sufficient nourishment. You now know that this is not the case. In Chapter 2 you learned that a balanced diet offers the nutrition you need. Table 4-3 analyzes common sales pitches for vitamin supplements. Do any look familiar?

Nutrition experts believe that a diet following the Guide to Daily Food Choices provides the best diet for a healthy person.[11] This guide encourages a balanced diet containing a wide variety of foods, including some whole grains and fresh or frozen fruits and vegetables. Does your daily food intake meet the food guide standards? To find out, keep a record of every nibble, snack, and meal for a few days, as we suggested in Chapter 1. Then compare your choices with those in the food guide, or analyze your diet with the computer software available for this book. (Chapter 2 and Appendix D contain directions for completing a diet analysis.)

Some vitamin manufacturers advertise that stress raises vitamin needs. For these hucksters stress can mean physical demands, overwork, or mental burdens. A vitamin vendor might suggest you raise your intake around examina-

TABLE 4-3

Analysis of scare tactics used to promote vitamins

Claim	Comment
"Remember that the health of your eyes, teeth, bones, and internal systems depends on a sufficient intake of these vital nutrients"	Messages of this type, intended to make a person nutrient conscious, are true but misleading. They never say how to tell if a person is getting enough.
"Of the approximately 40 nutrients that are considered elemental in meeting daily body requirements, many cannot be manufactured or stored by the body. These nutrients must be ingested daily."	This claim subtly exaggerates the likelihood of deficiency. The body's storage of water-soluble vitamins is limited, but occasional low dietary intake poses no danger.
"How much of your vitamin C gets lost on the way to the table? Picking, packing, processing. All these plus transportation can lead to the destruction of part of the vitamin C in your foods."	The real issues are how much vitamin C remains in one's diet and whether it is enough. Following the Guide to Daily Food Choices ensures an adequate intake of vitamin C.
"No matter how hard you try, in our fast-food society, it's often difficult to make sure you're getting enough essential vitamins and minerals in the food you eat."	This claim exaggerates the difficulty of balancing one's diet.
"Most packaged foods have many, if not all, of the natural nutrients removed during processing and replaced with chemicals."	This statement greatly exaggerates the amount of nutrients lost in processing; exploits public fear that our foods contain too many chemicals.
"Our soils are depleted."	This claim falsely suggests that adequate nutrition can be obtained only by ingesting food supplements or special foods.
"I take my vitamins every day. Just to be on the safe side." (Said by man pictured climbing a steep mountain.)	This is a misleading comparison of the dangers of mountain climbing and of not taking daily vitamin pills.

From Cornacchia HJ, Barrett S: *Consumer health.* St Louis, 1989, Mosby–Year Book.

tion time or before a big date. Other supplement companies pursue athletes, homemakers, and busy executives by plugging products for each group's special needs.[4,7] Some companies make no health claims at all and rely on the product's name or fast-talking salesmen to sell it.

Stress vitamins typically contain several B vitamins and ten or more times the RDA for vitamin C. No scientific evidence demonstrates we have increased vitamin needs when enduring emotional stress. Though some physical conditions slightly raise the need for vitamins, rarely do needs exceed the RDA.[4]

Advertisements claim strenuous physical activity increases vitamin needs, implying the athlete or fitness enthusiast should shovel in supplements. A vigorous workout increases the need for kcalories, carbohydrates, and water. The body's natural instinct to eat will ensure that the nutrients are replaced. As we discuss in Chapter 12, extra vitamins do not provide extra energy.

ANOTHER BITE In 1985 E.R. Squibb & Sons, Inc. agreed to pay $15,000 to the state of New York and to stop making false claims for its Theragram Stress Formula. In 1986, Lederle Laboratories agreed to pay $25,000 and to stop suggesting that Stresstabs could reduce the effects of psychological stress or the ordinary stresses of life.

Natural versus synthetic vitamins

Are natural vitamins superior to the synthetic variety? No.[12] Vitamins are specific molecules. The slightly different structures of a few synthetic vitamins do not decrease their value inside the body. Your body cannot tell a natural vitamin from a synthetic one. The only real difference is price—natural vitamins cost more.

"ALTERNATIVE" THERAPIES
Meganutrient therapies

Nutrition therapy can occasionally fight a disease, but not most diseases. Touting nutrients as a cure for many diseases is quackery. About 35 years ago a few physicians began treating schizophrenic patients with megadoses of vitamins (quantities more than ten times the RDA). Today this approach is used by a tiny minority of physicians, who call it meganutrient, orthomolecular, or nutritional therapy.[4,7]

Will large doses of vitamin C cure your cold? Many households have supplemented morning orange juice with megadoses of vitamin C, a treatment touted by Dr. Linus Pauling. But as we pointed out in Chapter 3, excess vitamins and minerals can harm your body. While chemical imbalances in the body contribute to many diseases, meganutrient therapies have not been accepted as remedies to these imbalances.[4,7] Risk outweighs dubious benefits. In addition, high doses of vitamins A, D, and B-6 and minerals iron and copper—to name a few—all can cause harmful side effects.

Herbal therapies

Throughout history healers have gone to the garden, the forest, and the sea to seek herbal remedies. Largely by trial and error, certain roots, plants, barks, and seeds were found to possess medicinal properties.[20] As early as the second century B.C., the Egyptians used myrrh, cumin, peppermint, caraway, fennel, and clove oil for various ailments. In sixteenth-century Europe physicians began experimenting with sarsaparilla, the dried root of the smilax plant, in attempts to cure venereal disease. Later the root was gathered as a cure for chronic rheumatism and skin disease. When late-nineteenth-century physicians

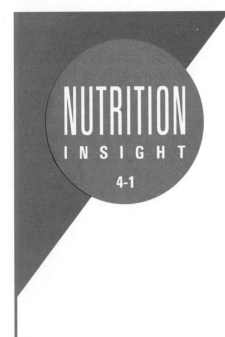

NUTRITION
INSIGHT
4-1

MEGAVITAMIN CLAIMS VERSUS FACTS: PAULING AND VITAMIN C

Widespread claims promise that very high doses of some vitamins and minerals miraculously cure or prevent many ailments. Dr. Linus Pauling, Nobel Prize winner in chemistry and professor emeritus of chemistry at Stanford University, gained great notoriety by claiming that vitamin C could do battle with the common cold.

His 1970 book, *Vitamin C and the Common Cold*, claims 1000 milligrams (1 gram) of vitamin C daily (about 15 times the RDA) will reduce the number of colds for most people by nearly half. A 1976 revision recommended still higher doses. Pauling has claimed to take a daily dose of 12,000 milligrams of vitamin C and raises the intake to 40,000 if he feels a cold coming on. As a result of the popularity of his books and the respectability of his credentials, millions of Americans supplement their diets with vitamin C.

But does it really work? Most medical and nutrition scientists strongly disagree with Pauling's views of vitamin C. Since the 1930s, medical investigators have rigorously explored the role of vitamin C in preventing infection. Numerous well-designed, double-blind studies have not shown vitamin C to reliably prevent colds, though it seems to slightly reduce cold symptoms.[4] Pauling's theories, based on the same studies, dispute the other scientists' results.

In 1979, a third Pauling book claimed high vitamin C doses may be effective against cancer. Pauling partly based his book on 1976 studies that he conducted with the Scottish physician Dr. Evan Cameron. The book claims a majority of 100 terminal cancer patients receiving 10,000 milligrams of vitamin C daily survived three to four times longer than similar patients receiving no vitamin C supplements.

Many cancer researchers challenge these conclusions, stating that control and experimental groups were not comparable. The experimental group had started tak-

abandoned belief in its medicinal powers, sarsaparilla found new life as a syrup for soft drinks.

In 1989 Americans spent an estimated $500 million for herbal teas, bulk herbs, and other herbal products. Many people choose herbal products for flavor; some choose them for healing. Today most plant substances, however, remain in the forest. They are replaced by medicines developed by pharmaceutical companies. For example, reserpine, found naturally in snakeroot (rauwolfia), was used effectively and extensively to treat high blood pressure during the 1950s and 1960s. Today synthetic drugs more effectively lower blood pressure. Companies run their synthetic drugs through rigorous FDA-approved tests to determine safety, effectiveness, and side effects. The controlled testing offers consumers information not available for herbal remedies.

Printed promotion for herbal therapies may be as simple as a cheaply printed flyer or as elaborate as an attractive, finely bound catalog. Don't be fooled by the cover.[7] Use your consumer knowledge to check the following points:

1. Like megavitamin recommendations, megaherb recommendations have no basis in fact. Hearsay, folklore, and tradition keep herbal-healing practices active. Some herbs have yielded valuable substances for modern medical care. However, scientific evidence that establishes their effectiveness, such as double-blind studies, is lacking for most herbal remedies.

2. Many claims are based on treatises written by the sixteenth-century herbalist John Gerard or the seventeenth-century apothecary-astrologer Nicholas Culpepper. Many herbs recommended by their writings contain cancer-causing compounds.

3. Though some herbs are dangerous, no warning labels accompany herbal remedies. Some herbalists claim that magical properties of a natural herb prevent it from harming people. No evidence supports this claim.

ing vitamin C when Dr. Cameron labeled them untreatable by other methods. The control group, under the care of other physicians, was labeled untreatable at a much later stage in their disease. Since this control group was nearer to death at the outset of the study, the experimental group naturally would be expected to live longer.

In 1979, the Mayo Clinic reported a double-blind study of 123 patients with advanced cancer. Half the patients received 10,000 milligrams of vitamin C daily, while the others received a placebo. Researchers found no difference between the two groups in survival time, appetite, weight loss, severity of pain, or amount of nausea and vomiting.

An almost identical result was obtained in a recent study by the North Central Cancer Treatment Group, composed of physicians from seven states and Canada. Survival rates for 71 patients who received 10,000 milligrams of vitamin C and 73 patients who received a placebo essentially overlapped. The placebo group actually survived an average of 1 week longer.

The Mayo Clinic conducted another controlled study of 100 patients with advanced colorectal cancer. Results showed once again that 10,000 milligrams of vitamin C offered no advantage over a placebo.[17]

These intricate studies have never supported Linus Pauling's claims that high doses of vitamin C prevent or cure disease. Nutrition research further warns the consumer that such doses can lead to toxic effects, such as diarrhea and iron toxicity (see Chapter 9). When seeking to reduce the severity of common cold symptoms, orange juice may be an option. But when looking for a cure for cancer, consult with your physician. ●

4. Many herbs contain hundreds or even thousands of chemicals that have not been completely cataloged. We may someday find that these chemicals serve useful medicinal purposes. But others could prove toxic.[10] Moreover, many conditions (such as diabetes mellitus and arthritis) for which herbs are recommended are not suitable for self-treatment.

If an herb contains a needed drug, pharmacists can provide the drug in a purer form and in a more controlled dosage than in herbal preparations or teas. With safe and effective medicines available, would you choose herbal treatment?

Promoters claim herbal teas offer therapeutic value. However these teas, often blends of up to 20 kinds of leaves, seeds, and flowers, can produce unpredictable and potentially serious side effects. The following substances in herbal teas can cause problems: juniper berries, shave grass, horsetail, buckthorn bark, senna leaves, burdock root, catnip, ginseng, hydrangea, lobelia, jimsonweed, wormwood, nutmeg, chamomile, licorice root, devil's claw root, sassafras root bark, Indian tobacco, mistletoe, and pokeweed (especially the root).[20]

The California-based company Herbalife International manufactures and markets a line of herb-based powders, pills, and other concoctions. In the past few years several legal actions have been taken against this company because of potentially harmful herbs present in its products. In 1982 Herbalife responded to an FDA "Notice of Adverse Findings" by removing two unsafe herbs, mandrake and pokeroot, from its products. FDA documented 100 cases of adverse reactions to Herbalife products. This example illustrates the danger of irresponsible herbal promotions.

Our knowledge of herbs is based largely on folklore and tradition rather than

Macrobiotics • A food plan that emphasizes vegetable foods over animal foods, often with heavy use of brown rice.

Rickets • A disease characterized by softening of the bones because of poor calcium deposition. This deficiency disease arises from lack of vitamin D activity in the body.

on reliable safety testing. The uses and dangers of these herbs is unexplored territory.[20] For treating serious illnesses we must consider that the poisons of some herbal substances can be dangerous.

Today the American public can buy herbs in pill form. Nature's Sunshine Products packages over 70 different herbs singly and encapsulates about 60 herbal combinations, some containing as many as 18 different herbs. The capsules have the safe appearance of traditional medicines. A little pill seems more legitimate than the mixing of magic potions. Same potions, different packages. Estimated 1989 sales of Nature's Sunshine Products exceeded $68 million.

Macrobiotics

Macrobiotics, a quasireligious/philosophical way of life founded by the late Japanese philosopher George Ohsawa, advocates a mainly vegetarian diet. Foods of animal origin get shifted from main course to condiment. Ohsawa outlined a 10-stage Zen macrobiotic diet with progressively more restrictive states. In the highest state followers consumed only brown rice and water. This eating plan was purported to overcome many illnesses attributed to excesses in diet. Though no scientific evidence supports the claims, proponents believe macrobiotics cures anemia, arthritis, appendicitis, cancer, cataracts, tuberculosis, diabetes, epilepsy, heart disease, hernia, leprosy, and schizophrenia.[21]

Today, under the leadership of Michio Kushi, Ohsawa's followers promote macrobiotics as a cancer cure. In fact, this diet can interfere with legitimate cancer treatment because patients lose their appetite as well as weight. Also, the diet may not meet the increased nutritional needs of some cancer patients.

To compare this food plan with a recommended vegetarian diet, see Chapter 8.

Current macrobiotic diets are less restrictive than earlier versions. Proponents now recommend whole grains (50% to 60% of each meal), vegetables (25% to 30% of each meal), whole beans or soybean-based products (5% to 10% of daily food), nuts and seeds (small amounts as snacks), miso soup, herbal teas, and small amounts of white meat or seafood once or twice weekly. Do you see any important foods missing from this diet?

The American Academy of Pediatrics cautions that a macrobiotic diet is especially hazardous to children. Recently some children following macrobiotic diets were diagnosed with *rickets.* This bone disease was linked in these cases to poor vitamin D and calcium intake.[8] Vitamin D–fortified milk in the diet would add these nutrients. This diet may also stunt growth by discouraging children from getting needed calories and protein. Children may not be able to eat enough of these bulky foods to meet their nutrient needs (see Chapter 15).

CONCEPT CHECK

We can meet vitamin and mineral requirements by eating a balanced diet. Mental stress does not create a need for nutritional supplements, nor do vitamins give extra energy.[4] Therapies based on herbs or megadoses of vitamins and minerals lack scientific endorsement and may be dangerous. Likewise, macrobiotic diets do not cure disease. Such diets can even harm children through inadequate nutrition.

HOW TO EVALUATE CLAIMS

The opening exercise in this chapter contains many tips for spotting quackery, as does reference 12. The following suggestions should help you make healthy and economically sound nutrition decisions:

1. Apply the basic principles of nutrition as outlined in Chapters 1 and 2 to any nutrition claim. Do you note any inconsistencies? Do reliable references support the claims? (See Appendix R for reliable sources of nutrition information.) Look closely for:

- testimonials about personal experience.
- disreputable publication sources.
- lack of evidence of supporting studies made by other scientists.

2. Examine the background philosophy of the individual, organization, or publication making a nutritional claim. Usually a reputable author is one whose educational background and/or present affiliation is with an accredited university or medical center that offers programs or courses in the field of nutrition, medicine, or a closely allied specialty. The philosophy will be based on scientific validation when possible.

3. Be wary of anyone who promotes the fads and fallacies identified in this chapter. Consider whether:

- the pros balance the cons. Are advantages and disadvantages discussed?
- conclusions are overstated. Are claims made about curing disease?
- extreme bias is aimed against the medical community or traditional medical treatments.
- fear-arousing techniques are used.
- the cure is quick and painless.
- the product promoted applies to a wide variety of diseases and conditions.
- the claim is touted as a new or secret scientific breakthrough.

4. Avoid practitioners who prescribe vitamin supplements for everyone or who sell them in connection with their practice.[3,4]

5. Examine product labels carefully. Be skeptical of any product promotion not clearly stated on the label. Remember, federal laws require that health

35 Pounds of Fat.

DR. EDISON'S OBESITY PILLS AND REDUCING TABLETS CURED MRS. MANNING.

No Other Remedies But Dr. Edison's Reduce Obesity— Take No Others.

SAMPLES FREE—USE COUPON.

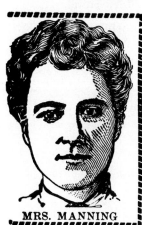

MRS. MANNING

Mary Hyde Manning, one of the best known of Troy's, New York, society women, grew too fleshy, and used Dr. Edison's Obesity Remedies. Read the letter telling of her reduction and restoration to health:—"In six weeks I was reduced 35 pounds, from 171 to 136, by Dr. Edison's Obesity Pills and Reducing Tablets. I recommend these remedies to all fat and sick men and women."

The following well-known men and women have been reduced by DR. EDISON'S OBESITY REMEDIES:

Mrs. H. Mershon, 156 South Jackson St., Lima, O., 148 lbs.
Mrs. Josephine McPherson, 7916 Wright St., Chicago, 42 lbs.
Rev. Edward R. Pierce, 410 Alma St., Chicago, 42 lbs.
C. C. Nichols, 145 Clark St., Aurora, Ill., 36 lbs.
Mrs. W. Davlin, Whitemore, O., 149 lbs.
W. H. Webster, 618 2d Ave., Troy, N. Y., 26 lbs.
J. M. McKinney, 4504 State St., Chicago, 30 lbs.
Mrs. J. M. McKinney, 4504 State St., Chicago, 33 lbs.
Mrs. A. Walker, 1104 Milton Place, Chicago, 20 lbs.

Quackery has been with us for ages. Even at the turn of the century, people wanted to believe that fat could be lost without changing habits or without much effort.

Consider reviewing the Nutrition Issue in Chapter 1 on applying the scientific method to nutrition.

products be truthfully labeled and carry adequate directions for use. A product is not likely to do something that is not specifically claimed on its label or package insert (which is legally part of the label).

6. Keep in mind that nutrition scientists normally report their studies in reputable scientific journals. Top-notch research journals require every article to be reviewed by other scientists. Follow-up studies are then demanded before hypotheses can be supported. Again, testimonials do not count as scientific evidence or support.[4]

HOW DO QUACKS PROMOTE QUESTIONABLE NUTRITION?
Skirting the law

How can freedoms of speech and press harm the consumer and protect the phony-food promoter? If you falsely promote a product but are not the actual vendor, you cannot be charged. Thus it would be illegal to label a vitamin as a cure for cancer, but a TV talk show guest could give unending testimonials to wonder cures without facing prosecution. Retailers can then refer to the talk show (or magazine article, etc.) and take advantage of misinformation. They can refer customers to more misinformation in popular literature or materials distributed by supplement manufacturers (Table 4-4).[7] Storekeepers attending seminars sponsored by trade organizations can gather these illegal claims and pass them on in the privacy of health food stores. Practitioners' offices and customers' homes also serve as pulpits for pandering such misinformation.[7]

Recognizing the quack

Beware of promoters who profess without scientific evidence that:[12]

1. particular foods can cure specific diseases.
2. many harmful foods should be eliminated from your diet.
3. only natural foods should be eaten.
4. modern processing methods strip the nutritional value from foods.
5. sugar is a deadly poison.
6. stress greatly increases your need for nutrients.

TABLE 4-4

Advertising ploys used to promote quack products and services

Product claims to have FDA approval:
Manufacturers are prohibited by law from claiming to have FDA approval.

Case histories and testimonials given are reliable and useful:
Such testimonials may come from people with chronic ailments who (1) have had a symptom-free period, (2) have had a spontaneous remission, (3) have experienced a placebo effect, or (4) have been misdiagnosed. Celebrities and sports heros often give testimonials in exchange for payment.

Persecution by the medical profession attempts to hide the truth:
The medical/scientific community uses the scientific method when testing validity of health claims. Double-blind studies prevent the results from being biased. The medical profession seeks truth, it does not bear grudges.

"Wondrous," "breakthrough," "ancient," "secret," "revolutionary" herald a reevaluation we should all consider:
True medical breakthroughs are never secret. They are reported in medical journals and the general media not in the back sections of magazines or in leaflets.

Claims that sound too good to be true:
No single product can be effective for a wide variety of ailments; any claim for a quick and painless cure is usually too good to be true.

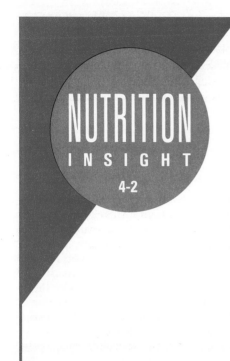

NOTHING TO LOSE

Acquired Immunodeficiency Syndrome (AIDS) was the diagnosis. A year earlier, confident and healthy, J.D. moved to Minneapolis for the security of a thriving gay community, which he had longed for. Now this dreaded disease pushed friends and family away. He had sought understanding and tolerance within this brotherhood, but now a deadly virus left him physically exhausted and spiritually abandoned.

Afraid and ultimately alone, J.D. joined a support group. The group offered the understanding he sought. With no medical hope for a cure, these dying young men sought other answers. Many began experimenting with the supposed healing powers of herbs and mineral salts. Angry with the unhalted course of his disease, J.D. tried every herbal remedy he encountered. He kept potions by his bedside when he was too weak to work and carried them in his car when he traveled to the revival tents of faith healers. He bought hope wherever he could find it.

In the terminal stages of the disease, J.D. sat with his physician, speaking of the miracles he had seen on his alternative course to healing. When his physician asked if the miracles had come his way as well, J.D. looked away.

"Faith is all I have left," J.D. sighed. "I need to believe in something. What good are the drugs if they offer me no hope? They are just a rip-off! I don't have much time . . . unless maybe these alternative therapies give me a miracle. Even placebos often work as well as treatment."

"J.D., it sounds like you spend a lot of your savings on these herbs, tonics, and vitamins," his physician quietly suggested. "I understand your need for hope, but I fear you are buying promises that can't be kept."

"What is money at this point? I have more money than I do time. What choice does a dying man have beyond betting his money on his life?" ●

Food faddists may be trying to use foods to achieve control over their life. Some aspects of food quackery evolve into social movements or rebellions against authority, society-at-large, or some imagined enemy, such as the medical profession or the government[6] (Table 4-1). Food faddism can take on an almost hysterical tone in reaction to fears of chemicals, pesticides, and preservatives in food. Although real health problems can arise from the use of certain foods, small unscientific groups guided by folklore, wishful thinking, and hearsay will not be the ones to separate fact from fiction. Choosing reliable sources and reading widely and skeptically will be your best guide to eating well.

Where do quacks find their victims? Enough people reject conventional medical and nutritional advice to create a booming market for alternative advice, alternative foods, and supplements.[14] Finding someone who seemingly listens and cares enough to try to help hooks many victims. Some quacks sincerely want to help. They offer their time along with their own innocence and ignorance. Alternative practitioners in one study spent about eight times as much time with their patients as did medical doctors. Consumers praise "the helpful people at the health food store because they take time to share the latest discoveries in the health field." Thus an important aspect of their success seems to be the "healer's" marketing of tender loving care.[6]

What motivates these scam peddlers? In many cases, particularly with mail-order crooks, it is profit—pure and simple. Quackery schemes are a very lucrative business. Quack practitioners connect with something basic in human nature. Beyond the quest for good health, people fall prey to scams in their search for a stable, predictable life pattern. By offering hope of good health and beauty, quacks play on what people want to believe. They repeatedly echo their

Acquired Immune Deficiency Syndrome (AIDS) • A disease characterized by poor function of one class of white blood cells (called helper T-lymphocytes). The resulting poor immune function leaves the person susceptible to infection, which can in turn result in rapidly failing health and death.

In the 1970s, laetrile promoters waged a vigorous and constant propaganda campaign, never feeling obligated to prove their claims for a cancer cure. Sales then peaked.[4]

sales pitch, knowing that what is repeated becomes truth in people's minds.[4,12]

Most of us are pushovers for hope. When the orthodox medical community offers no present hope for a cure to diseases, such as multiple sclerosis, acquired immune deficiency syndrome (AIDS), and advanced stages of certain cancers, an unorthodox "healer's" promises and attention seem very inviting. Feeling abandoned by personal physicians while living with pain and fear leaves patients vulnerable to quackery.[6]

If you felt left by the wayside and someone offered a magical drink of life for a price, would you choose to buy hope?

Let terms such as *alternative* and *holistic* serve as warning flags when they are used to promote treatments. Quacks are experts at "bio babble." Think twice when you hear buzzwords such as homeopath, naturopath, nutripath, clinical ecology, cytotoxic testing, and psychic surgeon. Worthless diagnostic methods and treatments include saliva tests, iridology (close examination of the eye), cellulite removal, applied kinesiology, metabolic therapy, hair analysis done by mail-order laboratories, coffee enemas, and colonic irrigation/detoxification.[4] Rigorous scientific testing has disproved the effectiveness of many of these.

Hair analysis is an experimental research tool used in mineral research. It has little or no place in clinical practice.[4]

Some quacks are impostors who purchase bogus credentials. Dr. Victor Herbert, a noted "quack buster" and nutrition scientist, purchased two diplomas—one from the American Association of Nutrition and Dietary Consultants, the other from the equally "prestigious" International Academy of Nutritional Consultants—by submitting the name and address of the applicant, along with a check for $50. The first certificate was inscribed with the name of Dr. Herbert's pet poodle, Sassafras; the other belongs to his cat, Charlie (see chapter photo, p. 95).[9]

Popular books

The health food industry's well-organized promotion machine capitalizes on popular books. *Life Extension*, a 1982-1983 bestseller, based its theme on the medically unacceptable premise that data from animal experiments can be generalized to help humans live to 150 years of age. According to the publisher's promotions, the authors appeared on national TV more than a dozen times. *Health Foods Business*, which reports industry trends, noted that sales of "antioxidants, moisturizers and anti-aging products" promoted by the book jumped after its publication. A number of companies even designed new products to take advantage of the book's popularity.[7]

Similarly, coinciding with public concern about AIDS, the 1985 publication of *Dr. Berger's Immune Power Diet* sparked the marketing of many health food products promising to boost the immune system. In fact, any aid beyond a balanced diet amounts to quackery.[21]

Sales pyramids

Many companies market food supplements, diet plans, and other health products using person-to-person sales. Anyone can become an *independent distributor*. Simply complete an application form, pay a small fee for a sales kit of product literature, and practice the pitch. Companies require no knowledge of nutrition or health care. Pitch the product with personal testimonials and persuade others to become distributors. This type of distribution system, known as a sales pyramid, is a typical get-rich-quick scam. When sales mount, distributors make money from a percentage of the sales of those below them in the

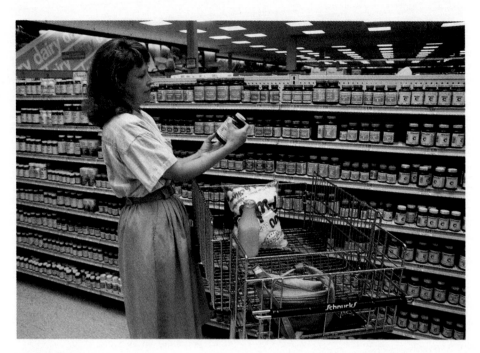

FIGURE 4-1
Health food stores sell billions of dollars in vitamin supplements each year.

pyramid. Like many such scams, promises of profits that continually multiply are rarely fulfilled.[7]

Health food stores

Health Foods Business estimated 1990 gross sales of the 7300 health food stores in the United States at $5 billion. This included $1.6 billion for vitamins and supplements (Figure 4-1). Although it is illegal for storekeepers to diagnose or prescribe, it is common for them to do both.[7] Investigators from the American Council on Science and Health uncovered the following practices in 1983 with 105 inquiries at stores in a three-state area:[2]

- When asked about eye symptoms characteristic of glaucoma, 17 of 24 storekeepers suggested a wide variety of products; none recognized that urgent medical care was needed.
- When asked over the telephone about a sudden, unexplained 15-pound weight loss in 1 month, 9 of 17 storekeepers recommended products sold in their store; only 7 suggested medical evaluation.
- Seven of 10 stores carried *starch blockers*, despite an FDA ban in 1982.
- Nine of 10 storekeepers recommended bone meal and dolomite, products considered hazardous from lead contamination.
- Nine stores made false claims for the effectiveness of bee pollen.
- Ten stores made false claims about RNA (ribonucleic acid, a common part of almost all cells).

The investigators concluded that most health food store clerks give advice that is irrational, unsafe, and illegal.

Pharmacists

Pharmacists play an important role in selling vitamin supplements. In 1985 reporters from *Consumer Reports* magazine visited 30 drugstores in Pennsylvania, Missouri, and California and complained of feeling tired or nervous. They asked whether a vitamin product would help. Nine of the 30 pharmacists correctly suggested consulting a doctor. The other pharmacists recommended vitamin products and, in one case, an amino acid preparation (amino acids are components of all proteins).[4] Pharmacists receive little training in nutrition and rarely discourage the use of the products they sell.

Organizations

Some organizations with scientific sounding names actually jeopardize public health with misleading nutritional information. One organization, the National Health Federation (NHF), promotes the gamut of alternative health methods with its theme of "freedom of choice" in health matters. Actually NHF just about locks out one choice—medically acceptable types of treatment. Their underlying message implies that anyone opposing NHF ideas is part of an anti-consumer conspiracy controlled by the government, organized medicine, and big business.[7]

NHF publications criticize such proven public health measures as pasteurizing milk, vaccinating for polio, and fluoridating water. This group, based in Monrovia, California, stretches its influence to Washington, D.C., filing lawsuits against government agencies and joining in the defense of people prosecuted for selling questionable "health" products or services.[7]

WHAT ACTIONS CAN YOU TAKE?

If you suspect false claims about a product or service, seek answers from reputable sources. Choices include:[5]

- the local public health department.
- medical societies.
- other professional organizations.
- registered dietitians in hospitals and private practice. (Nutrition Insight 2-3 discussed the RD's qualifications.)
- the medical or nutrition department of a university or college.

FDA also responds to inquiries about product claims. A local FDA office may be listed in the telephone book under Health and Human Services in the U.S. Government listings. False or misleading advertising about nutrition products is handled by the Federal Trade Commission (FTC), not FDA. In addition, the Postal Service can act against persons making false claims for products sold through the mail. Postal prosecution has been fairly effective in curbing this type of quackery.

You also can fight quackery through the media[5]—where it speaks loudest. If you notice a newspaper article, radio or television broadcast, or advertisement that contains health misinformation, complain to the source. Call the station or paper. Consider enlisting the help of the National Council Against Health Fraud, Inc. (Box 1276, Loma Linda, Calif, 92354). Some people fear that speaking out against quackery will put them in legal jeopardy. It won't if they stick to the facts and avoid name-calling. You need not label someone a "quack" to speak out against false claims for a product. Remember, if it sounds too good to be true, it likely is.[4]

CONCEPT CHECK

Quacks promote their ideas through salespeople and mainstream media—print, radio, and television. As long as people seek eternal health and quick cures, dubious health practitioners will thrive. Health food retailers often suggest remedies for illnesses best treated by a medical professional. Protect yourself by being an informed and skeptical consumer.

SUMMARY

- Though capable of causing bodily harm, quackery hits most people in the pocketbook. However, abandoning medical therapy for a quack remedy can have serious physical consequences.

- Organically grown and natural foods provide alternatives to foods that contain artificial ingredients and additives and to foods grown with chemical fertilizers and pesticides. But the nutritional benefits are few, if any.

- Quacks often suggest that the average diet lacks vitamins and minerals and should be supplemented with their products. Choosing whole grains, fruits and vegetables, and other selections from the Guide to Daily Food Choices provides excellent nutrition. An excess of certain vitamin and mineral supplements, such as vitamins A and D and the minerals iron and copper, can cause harm.

- Herbal remedies and megadose vitamin and mineral therapies seldom help and may be dangerous.

- Consumers who feel shortchanged by orthodox health care provide a large and willing market for those promoting questionable and dangerous nutritional advice. Before accepting alternative health products or suggestions, check for supporting evidence and reputable credentials. If in doubt, check with a physician or registered dietitian.

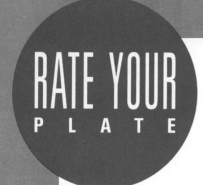

RATE YOUR PLATE

SHOULD I BAG THE BROWN FOOD?

Many articles in popular magazines have provocative titles such as:

"Newest Nutrition Breakthroughs"
"The Latest Secret to Weight Control"
"Exclusive Formula for Building Your Largest Muscles"
"The Only Diet to Conquer Chronic Fatigue"

Finding truth amid this hype is a challenge. Your powers to evaluate such claims should have been sharpened with this chapter. These consumer skills will save money, disappointment, and wasted time. The following article simulates those found in popular health and fitness magazines. Using information from this chapter, critically evaluate the article's claims and air of authority.

CONQUERING THE BLUES WITH BROWN FOOD
By Wilma Fuzzlenuts, N. D. C.

Do you often feel like you are living in slow motion? Are you always tired? Is fun the last thing on your mind? You might be suffering from what doctors now call Chronic Fatigue Syndrome—also called "Yuppie Flu." Many respectable scientists and doctors attribute the syndrome to a continual viral infection. Dr. Mickey Fibernugget, an endocrinologist, commented, "I was seeing so many tired patients in my practice that I knew it had to have some medical cause."

Would you like to have more energy? Feel sexier? Recapture that ambition to succeed in life? Well, a little known medical breakthrough may be the stroke of luck to lead you from your troubles. Recently discovered in a small laboratory and medical clinic in Bentenhausen, Norway, this miracle diet has not yet reached the desks of most physicians, nutritionists, and scientists.

When Dr. Val Hornwhipper, Ph.D., noted psychologist, fed his tired patients a diet of only brown food, their energy level and vigor vastly improved. Dr. Hornwhipper claims his Brown Food Empowerment Diet changes lives after only 2 weeks.

How does the brown food diet restore vigor? According to Dr. Nord Viplaugher, noted scientist of the Chocolate Guild in Norway, this exciting new diet speeds up your metabolic rate. You immediately feel energized. Viplaugher refers to this biochemical effect as "catalytic kinetics." In addition, brown food naturally causes your body's immune cells to destroy many different viruses.

By properly incorporating foods like brown rice, chocolate, brown bean soup, brown bread, and coffee, you can eliminate fatigue problems. Helen Howrowitz says, "After following the Brown Food Empowerment Diet for 1 week I felt like I could run a marathon." Vird Veerplank, world-class cross country skier, raved, "I've never performed like this in my sport." Over 20 psychologists and physicians now promote this exciting fatigue-buster.

Why feel tired for even 1 more day? Buy Dr. Hornwhipper's book, *The Brown Food Empowerment Diet* and begin waking up to high energy days. You have discovered a future your physician probably never dreamed of.

References

Hornwhipper V: *The brown food empowerment diet*, Springfield, Ohio, 1990, Bilbo Books, Inc.

Wilma Fuzzlenuts is a National Dietary Consultant for the Wambaugh Holistic Eating Center. She has run five marathons and has worked in nutrition for 10 years. Much of her knowledge comes from personally experimenting with foods to improve her athletic performance.

EVALUATION

1. Evaluate this article using characteristics of food faddhists (p. 98) and "How to Evaluate Claims" (p. 106). In your critique include aspects of the article that intrigued you and aspects that made you suspect.
2. After critiquing Fuzzlenut's article, would you buy Hornwhipper's book or follow his brown food diet?

REFERENCES

1. ADA Reports: Position of The American Dietetic Association: Identifying food and nutrition misinformation, *Journal of the American Dietetic Association* 88:1589, 1988.
2. Aigner C: Advice in health food stores, *Nutrition Forum* 5:1, 1988.
3. Barrett S: *The unhealthy alliance—crusaders for "health freedom,"* New York, 1988, American Council on Science and Health.
4. Barrett S: *Health schemes, scams, and frauds,* Mt Vernon, NY, 1990, Consumer Reports Books.
5. Barrett S: Fighting quackery, *Postgraduate Medicine* 81(7):13, 1987.
6. Beaven DW: Alternative medicine a cruel hoax—your money or your life, *New Zealand Medical Journal* 102:416, 1989.
7. Cornacchia HJ, Barrett S: *Consumer health,* ed 4, St Louis, 1989, Mosby–Year Book.
8. Dagnelie PC and others: High prevalence of rickets in infants on macrobiotic diets, *American Journal of Clinical Nutrition* 51:202, 1990.
9. Goldman B. American crusader brings message about health care fraud to Canada, *Canadian Medical Association Journal* 140:1189, 1989.
10. Haller JS: A short history of the quack's materia medica, *New York State Journal of Medicine,* September, 1989, p 521.
11. Harper AE: "Nutrition Insurance": a skeptical view, *Nutrition Forum Newsletter* 4:33, 1987.
12. Herbert V, Barrett S: Twenty-one ways to spot a quack, *Nutrition Forum Newsletter,* September, 1986, p 65.
13. Johnson GC, Gottesman RA: The health fraud battle, *Postgraduate Medicine* 85:289, 1989.
14. King L: Quackery, *Journal of the American Medical Association* 261:1979, 1989.
15. Kleiner SM: Beware of nutrition quackery, *Physician and Sportsmedicine* 18:46, 1990.
16. Mirkin G: Can bee pollen benefit health? *Journal of the American Medical Association* 262:1854, 1989.
17. Moertel CG and others: High-dose vitamin C versus placebo in the treatment of patients with advanced cancer who have had no prior chemotherapy, *New England Journal of Medicine* 312:137, 1985.
18. Richmond C: The campaign against health fraud, *Practitioner* 233:1329, 1989.
19. Simko MD, Jarosz L: Organic foods: are they better? *Journal of the American Dietetic Association* 90:367, 1990.
20. Tyler VE: *The new honest herbal,* Philadelphia, 1987, George F Stickley.
21. Yetiv J: *Popular nutrition practices,* Cleveland, Ohio, 1986, Popular Medicine Press.

HOW MUCH HAVE I LEARNED?

What have you learned from Chapter 4? Here are 15 statements about sorting nutritional advice. Read them to test your current knowledge. If you think the answer is true or mostly true, circle T. If you think the answer is false or mostly false, circle F. Use the scoring key at the end of book to compute your total score. To review, take this test again later, and especially before tests.

1. **(T)** **F**   There are no significant differences in health risks from pesticide levels in organic versus conventionally grown foods.

2. **T** **(F)**   Enriched white rice has the fiber replaced.

3. **T** **(F)**   Raw milk is as safe as pasteurized milk.

4. **T** **(F)**   Strenuous physical activity greatly increases the need for several vitamins. *increase need of calories, carbohydrates & H₂O*

5. **T** **(F)**   *Natural* foods are safer than processed foods.
    foods often contain natural toxin

6. **T** **(F)**   Most physicians support the use of large doses of supplementary nutrients to treat diseases.

7. **(T)** **F**   It is common for health food storekeepers to prescribe vitamins for symptoms of illness.

8. **T** **(F)**   It is likely that a product will do more than is claimed on its label.

9. **(T)** **F**   Vitamin C is of no value for treating colon cancer.

10. **(T)** **F**   Quackery is often promoted by victims of quackery.

11. **T** **(F)**   Quackery is not difficult to spot.

12. **T** **(F)**   Macrobiotic diets are useful in treating anemia.

13. **T** **(F)**   Natural herbal therapy is safe to self-prescribe.

14. **T** **(F)**   *Can be toxic* Most pharmacists are reliable sources of information about nutrition.

15. **(T)** **F**   Sales pyramids are a popular distribution method for promoting questionable nutrition products.

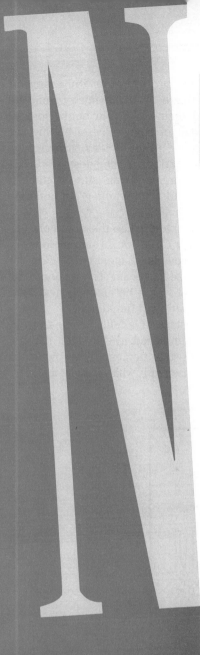

NUTRITION ISSUE

COLORFUL HUCKSTERS OF HEALTH FOOD

Chapter 6 introduces you to Sylvester Graham, of cracker fame, and to the rival cereal barons C.W. Post and the Kellogg brothers. Other men and women may not have left breakfast industries in their wake, but these men made waves worth noting. Each presented promises of health that captivated consumer food habits.[7]

James Caleb Jackson, a farmer turned doctor, attributed his health to gulping 30 to 40 glasses of water daily. In 1858 he opened a women's sanitarium that advocated frequent walks and naps, each minus the cumbersome corsets and petticoats of the times. Mealtime specialties included fresh fruit, whole-grain bread, Mr. Graham's crackers, and Mr. Jackson's own specialty, rock-hard bits of baked wheat softened in water. He called this appetizing mixture Granula, later marketing it through "Our Home Granula Company." Mr. Jackson's mixture is resurrected today as "granola."

Bernarr Macfadden, born in 1886, preached exercise. One hundred years later scientists agree with this basic concept. But most of Mr. Macfadden's beliefs were unfounded. He advocated:

- fasting to cure some 30 diseases, including heart disease.
- walking to work, preferably barefoot.
- eating a *perfect* diet of nuts and fruits.
- eating when hungry and drinking ½ gallon of water each morning to strengthen the heart and prevent constipation.
- exercising the teeth by eating hard crackers or zwieback.
- sleeping on the floor.

In 1890 Macfadden's *Physical Culture* magazine hit the newsstands. Within 2 years 100,000 subscribers were following his bare footsteps, and readership eventually ballooned to 1 million. By 1931 he had an estimated $31 million in revenues. He lived to the age of 87, still downing ½ gallon of water before breakfast.

Horace Fletcher, the high priest of mastication, chewed his way to fame and fortune. He believed large chunks of food interfered with digestion and advocated chewing until the food "swallowed itself." This meant approximately 30 to 70 chomps per mouthful, which reduced the food to near liquid form. Fletcher practiced what he preached, eventually taking nothing but liquids and purees. His death by heart failure in 1916 saddened many followers, including the editors of *The Ladies Home Journal.* Two years previously, in 1914, the popular magazine had begun promoting Fletcher's chew-your-food teachings to its readers.

Adelle Davis received a degree in dietetics from the University of California, Berkeley, and a master of science degree in biochemistry from the University of Southern California School of Medicine. Her four books sold 10 million copies. Davis accused the American diet of being excessively high in salt, loaded with refined sugar, and contaminated by pesticides, growth hormones, and preservatives. She claimed modern food processing destroyed vital nutrients. She advocated vitamin supplements, organic fruits and vegetables, wheat germ, certified raw milk, fresh stone-ground 100% whole grain bread or cereal, and many other health food products.

Three documented cases revealed harm to children when their mothers followed advice in Davis' book *Let's Have Healthy Children.* In one incident, a mother, following the book's recommendation, gave her 2-month-old infant liquid potassium for colic. Following the second dose he became listless and blue, stopped breathing, and was rushed to a hospital where he died the next day. High blood potassium levels interfered with proper heart function.[7]

After filing suit against the publisher, the estate of Adelle Davis, and the store where the potassium supplement was purchased, the infant's parents received a total of $160 thousand in out-of-court settlements. The publisher withdrew the book from the marketplace but reissued it with changes made by a physician aligned with the health food industry.

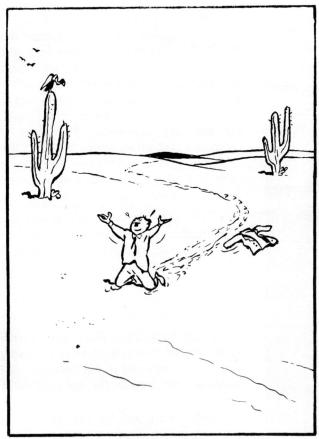

"Perrier! Perrier!"

FIGURE 4-2
Grin and Bear It.

Carlton Fredericks, described on his early book jackets as "America's Foremost Nutritionist," often diagnosed patients and prescribed vitamins to remove the aches and pains of illness. But according to FDA, Fredericks had virtually no nutrition or health science training. In 1945 he was charged with practicing medicine without a license. Fredericks pleaded guilty, paid a small fine, and went back to work. For 30 years, beginning in 1957, he hosted Design for Living, a daily radio show. For several years before his death in 1987, he performed nutrition consultations for $200 each in the offices of Robert Atkins, M.D. (author of *Dr. Atkins' Diet Revolution*). We discuss this fad diet in Chapter 11.[7]

The American diet changes when colorful figures such as these clamor their way to national attention. Hard crackers were big sellers at the turn of the century thanks to Bernarr MacFadden's belief in strong teeth. Chewing foods completely became a rage in the early 1900s when Horace Fletcher's teachings swept the homefront. Adelle Davis' devotion to organic foods changed the thrust of the health food industry in the 1960s. And people increased their intake of vitamin capsules when Carlton Fredericks' radio show echoed across the airwaves. Have any of your beliefs about nutrition been influenced by these popular trendsetters (Figure 4-2)? ●

2

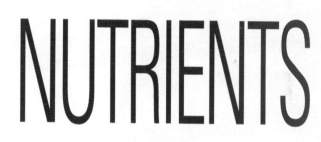

NUTRIENTS

**THE
HEART
OF
NUTRITION**

DIGESTION AND ABSORPTION
SUPPLYING NUTRIENTS TO CELLS

Merely eating food won't nourish you. You must first digest the food—break down the food into usable forms that can be absorbed into the bloodstream. Once nutrients are taken up by the bloodstream, they can be distributed to body cells.

We rarely think about, and certainly can't control, the digestion and absorption of foods. Except for a few voluntary responses, such as deciding what and when to eat, how well to chew food, and when to eliminate the remains, most digestion and absorption processes control themselves. We don't consciously decide when the pancreas will secrete digestive enzymes into the small intestine or how quickly to propel foodstuffs down the intestinal tract. Various hormones and the nervous system help control these functions.[12] Your only awareness of these involuntary responses may be a hunger pang right before lunch or a full feeling after eating that last slice of pizza. Nevertheless, countless reactions occur in your intestinal tract as you go about your daily routine of studying nutrition, walking home from classes, playing the piano, and eating lunch. Let's examine these processes. ●

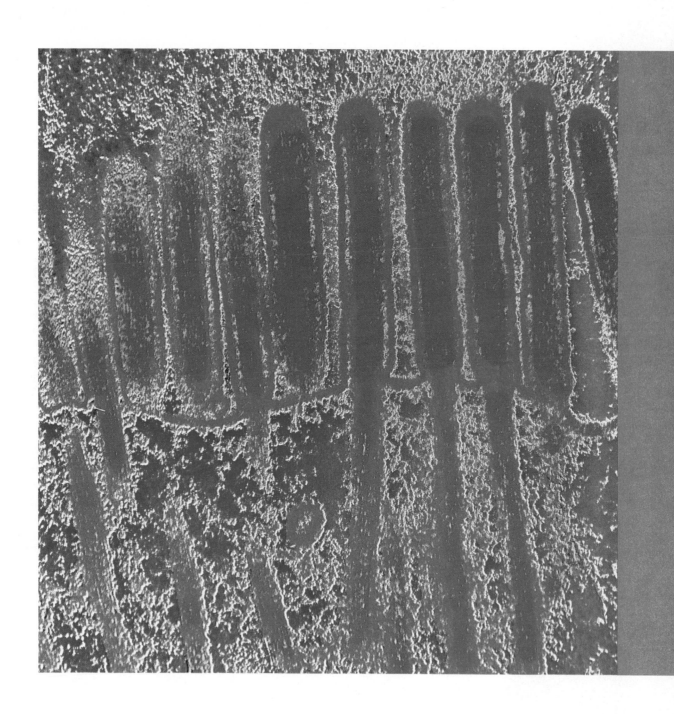

How Healthy Is Your Digestive Tract?

Humans rarely think about the health of their digestive tracts. There are symptoms we need to notice as well as habits we need to practice in order to keep our digestive tracts functioning appropriately. The following assessment allows you to examine your habits and symptoms associated with the health of your digestive tract. Put a "Y" in the blank to indicate a yes, and an "N" to indicate a no.

1. Are you currently experiencing greater than normal stress and tension? _____

2. Do you have a family history of digestive tract problems (e.g., ulcers, hemorrhoids, diverticulosis, constipation, lactose intolerance in parents or grandparents)? _____

3. Do you experience pain in your stomach region about 2 hours after you eat? _____

4. Do you smoke cigarettes? _____

5. Do you take aspirin frequently? _____

6. Do you experience the gnawing pain of heartburn in your upper chest at least once a week? _____

7. Do you frequently lie down after eating? _____

8. Do you drink alcoholic beverages with your meals at least two to three times per week? _____

9. Do you experience abdominal pain, bloating, and gas about 30 minutes to 2 hours after consuming milk products? _____

10. Are you Native American, Asian, Hispanic, of Mediterranean descent, or Black? _____

11. Do you often have to strain when having a bowel movement? _____

12. Do you drink less than 8 cups of water or fluid per day? _____

13. Do you exercise aerobically (jog, swim, walk briskly, row, climb stairs) less than 20 to 30 minutes, three times per week? _____

14. Do you eat a diet relatively low in fiber (a diet high in fiber contains liberal quantities of whole fruits, vegetables, legumes, nuts and seeds, whole-grain breads, and cereals)? _____

15. Do you frequently experience diarrhea? _____

16. Do you frequently use laxatives or antacids? _____

INTERPRETATION

Add up the number of yes answers you gave and record the total in the blank to the right. _____

If your score is from 8 to 16, your habits and symptoms put you at risk of experiencing digestive tract problems in the future. Take particular note of the habits you can use to cooperate with your digestive tract and prevent some of the conditions you have noted in this assessment.

ASSESS YOURSELF

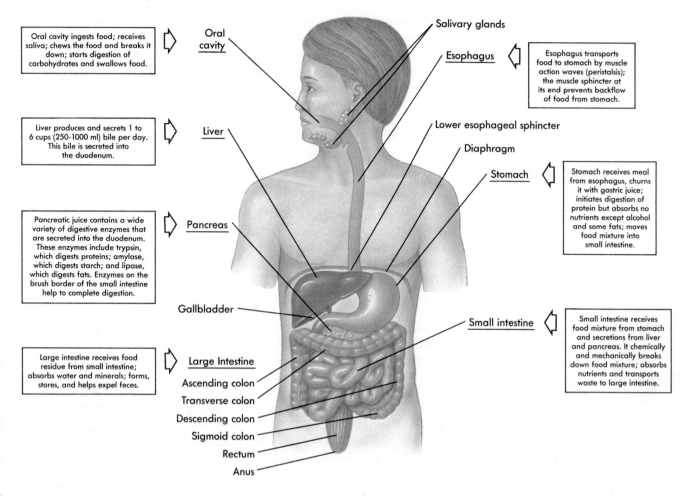

Oral cavity ingests food; receives saliva; chews the food and breaks it down; starts digestion of carbohydrates and swallows food.

Oral cavity

Salivary glands

Esophagus

Esophagus transports food to stomach by muscle action waves (peristalsis); the muscle sphincter at its end prevents backflow of food from stomach.

Liver produces and secrets 1 to 6 cups (250-1000 ml) bile per day. This bile is secreted into the duodenum.

Liver

Lower esophageal sphincter

Diaphragm

Stomach

Stomach receives meal from esophagus, churns it with gastric juice; initiates digestion of protein but absorbs no nutrients except alcohol and some fats; moves food mixture into small intestine.

Pancreatic juice contains a wide variety of digestive enzymes that are secreted into the duodenum. These enzymes include trypsin, which digests proteins; amylase, which digests starch; and lipase, which digests fats. Enzymes on the brush border of the small intestine help to complete digestion.

Pancreas

Gallbladder

Small intestine

Small intestine receives food mixture from stomach and secretions from liver and pancreas. It chemically and mechanically breaks down food mixture; absorbs nutrients and transports waste to large intestine.

Large intestine receives food residue from small intestine; absorbs water and minerals; forms, stores, and helps expel feces.

Large Intestine
Ascending colon
Transverse colon
Descending colon
Sigmoid colon
Rectum
Anus

FIGURE 5-1

The organization of the gastrointestinal (GI) tract. Many organs work in a coordinated fashion to digest food, absorb nutrients, and eliminate waste products.

THE PHYSIOLOGY OF DIGESTION

The *gastrointestinal (GI) tract*—also known as the *alimentary canal*—is a long tube stretching from the mouth to the anus (Figure 5-1). Nutrients from the food we eat must pass through the walls of this tube—in one side and out the other—to be absorbed into the bloodstream. The GI tract promotes digestion and absorption through a variety of functions.[12] It simultaneously moves and grinds foods (a process called motility). This is the *physical* phase of digestion. The GI tract also *secretes* chemical substances—like enzymes—to promote the breakdown of foods. This is the *chemical* phase of digestion. Finally, the GI tract eliminates any wastes. Throughout the process the GI tract additionally promotes nutrient production; the bacteria living in the intestine can make certain vitamins that we can use.

The flow of digestion

Let's review the major body parts used in digestion, starting with the mouth. Even before you put food into your mouth, you may experience a sudden rush of saliva in response to the sight or smell of food. This *saliva,* secreted by special glands in the mouth, contains *mucus* that envelops and lubricates each morsel, easing its passage down the GI tract. Saliva also contains specific substances called enzymes that break down large carbohydrates into small units. Chewing breaks food into small pieces, exposing more food surface to diges-

Digestion • The process where food is broken down into forms that can be absorbed by the GI tract.

Secrete • To produce and then release a substance from a cell into other cells.

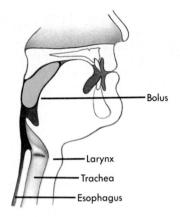

Bolus

Larynx

Trachea

Esophagus

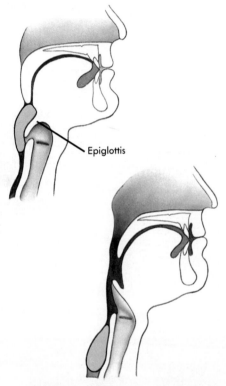

Epiglottis

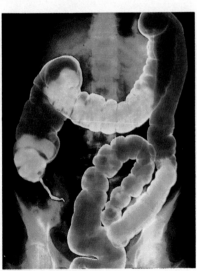

tive action. The more surface exposed, the more efficient digestion is in the mouth. This is true of the entire GI tract as well.

The tongue aids chewing and also contains taste sensors for sweet, salt, sour, and bitter. The sweet and salt sensors are near the tip of the tongue; the sour and bitter sensors are near the base.[11]

The mouth and stomach are connected by a tube called the esophagus. At its top is a flap of tissue (called the epiglottis) that prevents food from being swallowed into the trachea (wind pipe). During swallowing, food lands on the flap and folds it down to cover the opening of the trachea. Breathing also automatically stops. These responses, along with the lubricating mucus, muscular contractions, and gravity, ensure that swallowed food will only travel down the esophagus.

The food then enters the stomach, which is basically a 4-cup (1-liter) holding tank. Only proteins are significantly digested in the stomach. This protein digestion proceeds as the stomach secretes digestive acid and enzymes and slowly churns them into the food. A meal usually leaves the stomach within 2 to 3 hours after eating.[12] Solids take longer than liquids to leave the stomach, and a fatty meal usually leaves later than a meal that contains mostly protein or carbohydrate.

The stomach is connected to the small intestine. This is 10 feet in length and coiled inside the abdomen. The small intestine is considered "small" only because of its narrow diameter. Its 10-foot length provides ample opportunity for digestion to occur.

Constant muscular contractions mix the food in the small intestine. This churning enhances digestive action because more food surface is exposed to enzyme action. A meal remains in the small intestine about 3 to 10 hours. About 95% of a total meal has been digested by the time it leaves.[2] Most digestion is completed in the first half of the small intestine.

From the small intestine food moves into the large intestine, also called the **colon.** This organ is about 3½ feet long. Bacteria in the large intestine digest some leftover plant fibers; little else remains to be digested. The food remnants and wastes stay in the large intestine for about 24 to 72 hours before being eliminated.

The end of the large intestine connects to a cavity called the rectum, which is connected to the anus. These final sections work with the large intestine to prepare the feces for elimination.

Other organs associated with the GI tract aid digestion (Figure 5-1). The liver provides **bile** needed for fat digestion.[17] Bile helps suspend (**emulsify**) fat in the digestive mixture, making it more available to the digestive processes. The body stores bile in the gallbladder until it is needed. The pancreas also provides enzymes and other products that aid digestion. Ducts that lead from the pancreas and gallbladders merge, allowing the pancreatic juices and bile to blend as they are released into the duodenum for digestion. In this way the liver, pancreas, and gallbladder work with the GI tract but are not actually part of it.

GI tract control valves: sphincters

A variety of ringlike muscles form valves, called **sphincters,** all along the GI tract (Figure 5-2).[12] They retard or prevent backflow of partially digested food. These sphincters respond to various stimuli, such as impulses from the nervous system, hormones, and pressure that builds up around them. A sphincter in the lower esophagus is critical for preventing backflow of stomach contents up into the esophagus. If highly acidic stomach contents come in contact with the esophagus, they can cause pain, known as **heartburn.**[14] Coffee, alcohol, and nicotine can weaken the tension of this sphincter and cause heartburn in some people (see the Nutrition Issue on p. 146).

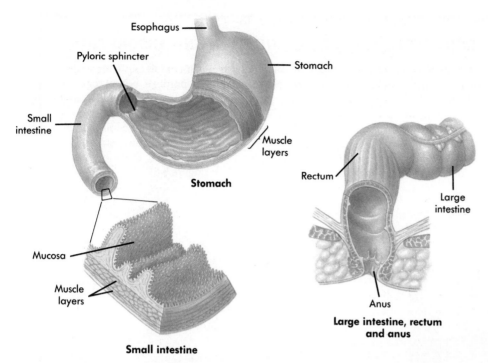

Esophagus

Pyloric sphincter

Stomach

Small intestine

Muscle layers

Stomach

Rectum

Large intestine

Mucosa

Muscle layers

Anus

Large intestine, rectum and anus

Small intestine

FIGURE 5-2

Close-up view of the intestinal tract—muscles, sphincters, and villi. These features of the GI tract perform key roles in digestion, absorption, and elimination.

The pyloric sphincter, located at the base of the stomach, controls flow from the stomach into the small intestine. About a teaspoon (a few milliliters) of acidic stomach contents squirt into the small intestine at a time. Such small amounts enable bicarbonate (essentially baking soda) from the pancreas to efficiently neutralize the acid. The neutralizing reduces the risk of acid injury to the small intestine and so decreases the chance of forming **ulcers** (again, see the Nutrition Issue on p. 146 for details).[5]

At the end of the small intestine another sphincter prevents the contents of the large intestine from reentering the small intestine. At the end of the large intestine are two final sphincters, both under voluntary control. Once a child is toilet-trained he can fairly well determine when these last two sphincters will relax and when they will stay rigid.

GI tract propulsion: peristalsis

Food is propelled down the GI tract mainly by a wavelike process called **peristalsis.** Groups of muscles encircle the GI tract, while other groups run along its length (Figure 5-2). When food is swallowed, coordinated squeezing and shortening by the muscle groups in the esophagus create two waves closely following each other.[12] In the stomach, the same muscle action creates a mixing and grinding motion as often as three times per minute during digestion. More active peristaltic waves occur in the small intestine, about every 4 to 5 seconds. In contrast, the large intestine has very sluggish peristalsis, using occasional large contractions, called **mass movements,** to help eliminate the feces.

Enzymes in digestion

As we noted, enzymes play a key part in digestion. Enzymes enhance digestion by making chemical reactions more likely to happen. Enzymes work by bring-

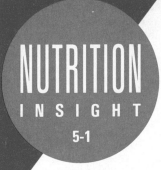

NUTRITION

I N S I G H T

5-1

BODY SYSTEMS USED IN DIGESTION AND ABSORPTION

The body is composed of millions of cells. Each is a self-contained, living entity. When cells of the same type work together for a common purpose, bound together by intercellular substances, they form tissues such as bone, cartilage, muscle, and nerve. Often two or more *tissues* combine in a particular way to form more complex *organs,* such as skin, kidneys, and liver. At still higher levels of coordination, several organs can cooperate for a common purpose to form an organ system, such as the respiratory system or the digestive system. The human body is a coordinated unit of many such organ systems, called an *organism* (Figure 5-3).

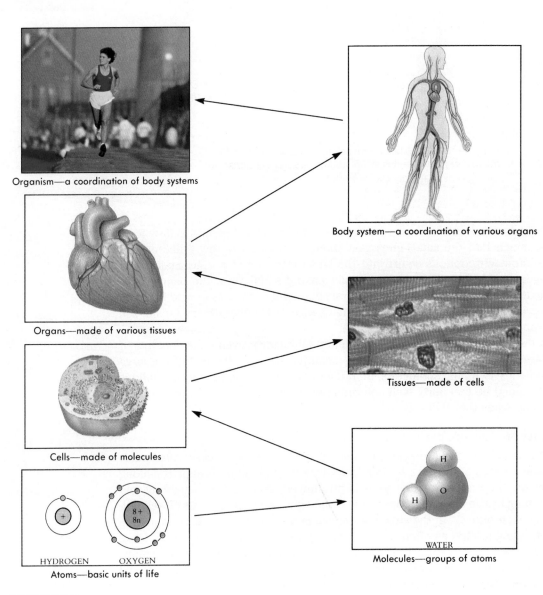

Organism—a coordination of body systems

Body system—a coordination of various organs

Organs—made of various tissues

Tissues—made of cells

Cells—made of molecules

HYDROGEN OXYGEN
Atoms—basic units of life

WATER
Molecules—groups of atoms

FIGURE 5-3
Levels of human biological organization. We are as simple as a collection of atoms and as complex as a whole organism.

Every cell in the human body performs a specialized job. A cell's master plan for work and for the necessary machinery are all encoded into the cell's genetic material—*DNA* (deoxyribonucleic acid). The DNA acts as a blueprint for synthesizing a specific protein—often an enzyme—required to perform a specific task. Even though most cells in the same organism contain the same DNA information, cells are programmed differently. As the embryo forms, different parts of the DNA become active in different cell types. For example, the intestinal cells make digestive enzymes while bone marrow cells make the oxygen-carrying protein hemoglobin.

Chemical reactions occur all the time in every living cell: the synthesis of new substances is balanced by the breaking down of other materials into smaller units. For these reactions to occur, the cell requires a continuous supply of energy, and most need oxygen. Cells also need water, the medium in which they live. They further need building blocks, especially the materials they can't make themselves—the essential nutrients supplied from food. These substances enable the tissues—composed of individual cells—to function properly.

An adequate supply of all nutrients to all body cells results from healthful nutrition. But to ensure optimal use of these nutrients by cells as well as the digestive system, the following systems must be healthy and work efficiently.

Urea • Nitrogen-containing waste product found in urine. Most nitrogen excreted from the body leaves in this form.

Adipose (Fat) Tissue • A grouping of fat-storing cells.

DNA • Site of hereditary information in cells. This directs the synthesis of cell proteins.

Circulatory system

The blood travels two basic routes. It circulates between the right side of the heart and the lungs (the pulmonary circuit) and between the left side of the heart and all other body parts (the systemic circuit) (Figure 5-4). The heart is a muscular pump that normally contracts and relaxes 50 to 90 times per minute while the body is at rest. This continuous pumping action keeps blood moving through the body.

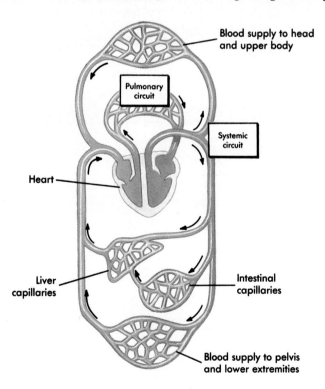

FIGURE 5-4

Blood circulation throughout the body. This drawing represents the route blood takes through the two circuits that begin and end at the heart. Red color indicates blood that is richer in oxygen; blue is for blood carrying more carbon dioxide.

Continued.

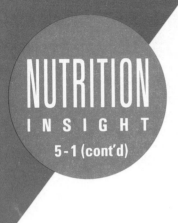

NUTRITION INSIGHT

5-1 (cont'd)

BODY SYSTEMS USED IN DIGESTION AND ABSORPTION

The circulatory system distributes nutrients from digestion and oxygen from the air we breathe to all body cells.[18] All blood goes to the lungs to pick up oxygen and release carbon dioxide. The oxygenated blood then returns to the heart to be pumped to all other body tissues. In the capillaries, cells exchange nutrients and wastes with the blood—cells empty their waste products into the blood and take nutrients from it. Capillaries—networks of tiny blood vessels—serve every region of the body via individual capillary beds, which are only one cell layer thick. Nutrients, gases, and other substances can pass through capillary cells both into and out of other body cells.

The lymphatic system is a second system of circulatory vessels that serves the body; it carries lymph, the clear fluid formed between cells. This fluid filters into tiny lymphatic vessels, which compose a one-way network that funnels lymph from all over the body into two large lymphatic vessels. These vessels empty lymph into major veins returning to the heart.[2] As you will see, lymphatic vessels that serve the small intestine have an important role in nutrition.

Excretory system

The kidneys, digestive tract, skin, and lungs all remove wastes from the body. For example, as blood passes through the kidneys, body wastes like *urea* are removed for excretion and put into the urine (Figure 5-5). Excess intakes of water-soluble nutrients and other substances are also filtered and excreted in this manner. For example, if the body already has enough vitamin C, the kidneys screen the extra amount out of the blood and redirect it into the urine. The skin excretes body wastes through the pores as part of perspiration. The lungs remove the carbon dioxide produced during metabolism of carbohydrates, fats, and proteins, and we exhale that into the air.

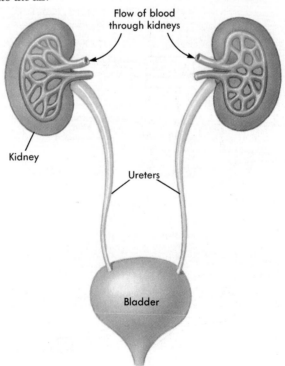

Flow of blood through kidneys

Kidney

Ureters

Bladder

FIGURE 5-5

The urinary tract. Blood enters the kidney by way of the arteries. The kidney filters waste from the blood and sends it as urine to the bladder. The bladder then periodically eliminates the urine.

Storage systems

The human body must maintain reserves of nutrients. Otherwise, we would need to eat continuously. Storage capacity varies for each different nutrient. Most fat is stored at sites designed specifically for this—*adipose (fat) tissue.* Short-term storage of carbohydrate occurs in muscle and liver, and the blood maintains a small reserve of amino acids. The many vitamins and minerals stored in the liver make animal liver a rich food source. Other nutrient stores are found in individual cells themselves.

During a period of deficiency some nutrients are obtained by breaking down a tissue that contains high concentrations of the nutrient. Calcium can be taken from bone and protein can be taken from muscle. But neither bones nor muscles are meant to act as nutrient reserves. Rather, nutrient losses in cases of deficiency harm these tissues.

Control systems

The hormonal and nervous systems form two control mechanisms that greatly influence nutrient use in the body.[13] The hormone insulin helps regulate blood glucose levels, and thyroid hormones help regulate the body's metabolic rate. Nerves influence acid secretion in the stomach and regulate GI tract muscle action. For example, the senses of sight, hearing, touch, smell, and taste all use nerve pathways to communicate information (e.g., the availability of food or the need for it) to the brain. Some nutrients are important in nerve functioning, especially the vitamins thiamin and niacin. ●

ing specific chemicals close together and then creating an environment that allows the chemicals to change forms (Figure 5-6). Almost every chemical process in the body—and especially digestive processes—requires an enzyme to hasten the event. Most digestive enzymes are produced by the pancreas and small intestine. A few are made by the mouth and stomach (Table 5-1).[12] Each type of enzyme can speed only one specific type of chemical process. For example, enzymes that recognize table sugar (sucrose) will ignore milk sugar (lactose).

Enzyme actions only occur under rather specific conditions. Besides the types of chemicals they process, enzymes are sensitive to acid and base conditions, temperature, and the types of vitamins and minerals they require. Digestive enzymes that work in the acid environment of the stomach do not work well in the alkaline environment of the small intestine.

TABLE 5-1

Examples of key digestive enzymes

Secretion Origin	Enzyme	Substrate	Major End Products
Salivary glands	Salivary amylase	Starch, glycogen	Maltose
Stomach glands	Pepsin	Proteins	Smaller proteins
Pancreas	Trypsin	Proteins	Peptides
	Chymotrypsin	Proteins	Peptides
	Pancreatic amylase	Starch	Maltose
	Lipase	Fats	Monoglycerides, free fatty
acids			
Intestinal wall	Peptidases	Peptides	Amino acids, smaller peptides
	Maltase	Maltose	Glucose
	Sucrase	Sucrose	Glucose, fructose
	Lactase	Lactose	Glucose, galactose

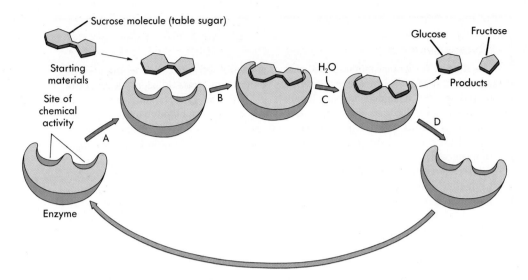

FIGURE 5-6
Model of enzyme action. With some enzymes, the reaction can go both ways.

ANOTHER BITE

When either the small intestine or the pancreas is diseased, it may not produce important enzymes in adequate quantities. The lack of enzymes can result in poor digestion and, consequently, very poor absorption of nutrients into the bloodstream. This is seen in many intestinal diseases. In such cases the foodstuffs travel into the large intestine, rather than mostly being absorbed into the bloodstream.[8] Once in the large intestine, bacteria metabolize the foodstuffs into acids and gas. A person with poor intestinal function often experiences abdominal discomfort from intestinal gas. Insufficient enzyme production or not enough time for complete enzyme action is often at the root of these problems.

CONCEPT CHECK

The gastrointestinal tract includes the mouth, esophagus, stomach, small intestine, large intestine (colon), rectum, and anus. Organs associated with the GI tract are the liver, gallbladder, and pancreas. Together these organs perform the digestion needed to extract nutrients from food and funnel them into the bloodstream. In the GI tract, peristalsis propels food from the esophagus to the anus. During this journey, digestion is aided by enzymes produced by the mouth, stomach, pancreas, and small intestinal cells. The lag time between eating food and eventually eliminating the undigestible remains is usually about 1 to 3 days.

DIGESTION—NUTRIENT BY NUTRIENT

A good way to study food digestion is to track a single food from its entry at the mouth until its parts are either absorbed into the bloodstream or eliminated in the feces. We will use banana bread as an example (Figure 5-7). As you will see, nutrients such as proteins, fats, and carbohydrates in the banana bread are digested at different sites in the GI tract and by different means. Specific enzymes do the work, while hormones and nerves mostly control the process.

But even before we eat a morsel of the banana bread (or many other foods), the work of digestion—breaking down foods into usable forms we can absorb—is often partially accomplished for us. Cooking or other preparations, such as marinating, pounding, or dicing, have often begun the process. Starch granules in foods swell as they soak up water during cooking, making them much easier to digest. Cooking also softens the tough connective tissues in meats and the fibrous tissue of plants, such as broccoli stalks. As a result, the food is easier to chew, swallow, and break down during later digestion.[12] As you will see in Chapter 17, cooking also makes many foods, such as meats, fish, and poultry, much safer to eat.

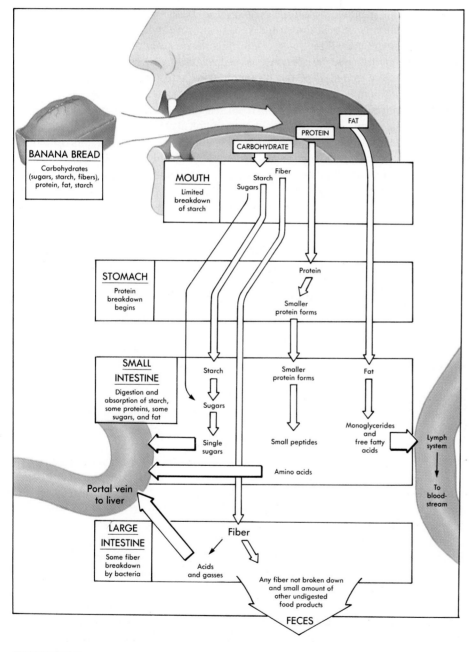

FIGURE 5-7
Digestion in practical terms. Many enzymes contribute to the digestion of foods. Water-soluble nutrients enter the bloodstream. Fat-soluble nutrients mostly enter the lymphatic system.

Pepsin • A protein-digesting enzyme produced by the stomach.

Autodigestion • Literally, self-digestion. The stomach limits autodigestion by covering itself with a thick layer of mucus and producing enzymes and acid only when needed for digestion of foodstuffs.

Chyme • A mixture of stomach secretions and partially digested food.

Trypsin • A protein-digesting enzyme secreted by the pancreas to act in the small intestine.

Peptides • A few amino acids linked together (often two to four).

Protein digestion

Let's begin with protein digestion, as this is the first nutrient digested in earnest by the GI tract. The digestion of protein in the banana bread, which comes mostly from the eggs and milk added, starts in the stomach. The stomach secretes *pepsin,* a major enzyme used for protein digestion. Pepsin attacks all proteins and breaks them down into shorter protein units. Pepsin is stored in its inactive form in the stomach cells. This prevents it from breaking down stomach cells while waiting to be secreted. When inactive pepsin enters the stomach's acidic environment, part of the substance is broken off, which in turn forms the active pepsin enzyme.[12]

The release of pepsin is controlled by the hormone *gastrin* (Table 5-1).[13] Just thinking about food or chewing food stimulates nerves in the brain that control special gastrin-producing cells in the base of the stomach. Gastrin release then signals cells in the stomach to begin producing pepsin.[7]

Gastrin also strongly stimulates other cells in the stomach to produce acid.[13] The acid-producing cells can likewise be stimulated by a breakdown product of proteins and by expansion of the stomach. The acid, which activates pepsin, also improves the absorption of the vitamin folate, iron, and calcium; keeps the stomach essentially free of bacteria (this lessens the risk of infections) and inactivates plant and animal hormones that might otherwise act in the body.

The stomach is protected from digesting itself—called *autodigestion*—in several ways. Since the hormone gastrin is released only when we eat or think about eating, acid production is limited to these times. Furthermore, as the stomach becomes strongly acidic, gastrin release stops. The stomach also protects itself by secreting a thick layer of mucus that lines and insulates it from the acid and pepsin produced for digestion.

Protein digestion continues in the small intestine

The partially-digested proteins then move with the rest of the nutrients in the banana bread from the stomach into the small intestine. The acidic mixture squirts at a slow rate through the pyloric sphincter, which separates the stomach from the upper part of the small intestine. All liquids consumed with the meal plus the stomach acid combine to form a very watery food mixture called *chyme.* As this chyme squirts into the duodenum, the acid in the chyme triggers the release of the hormone *secretin.*[12] That hormone stimulates the pancreas to release bicarbonate, which neutralizes the acid. Secretin also acts to reduce stomach peristalsis (motility)[13] (Table 5-2).

If the chyme is not neutralized, it corrodes the wall of the duodenum. This could quickly lead to an ulcer because, unlike the stomach, the small intestine lacks a protective layer of mucus.[16] This form of protection is impossible because it would impede nutrient absorption. Whereas only small amounts of alcohol and certain fats are absorbed in the mucus-protected stomach, the small intestine must absorb most products of digestion. The form of protection used by the small intestine is quick neutralization of the acidic chyme and the constant shedding of its cell lining.

Once in the small intestine, the proteins mix with other protein-digesting enzymes, such as *trypsin* and chymotrypsin. These are secreted by the pancreas.[13] The enzymes further digest the proteins into very short protein fragments called *peptides* and amino acids.[12] As with pepsin, these digestive enzymes are stored in their inactive forms in the pancreas. They are activated only when entering the intestine. Eventual digestion of all peptides into amino acids then occurs inside the absorptive cells that line the small intestine.

Fat digestion

The digestion of the fat from the vegetable oil and other ingredients in the banana bread mostly takes place in the small intestine. There the enzyme

TABLE 5-2

Some hormones that regulate digestion

Hormone	Origin	Stimulus to Secretion	Action
Gastrin	Pyloric region	Food and other substances in the stomach, especially proteins, caffeine, spices, alcohol; nerve input	Stimulates flow of stomach enzymes and acid
Cholecystokinin (CCK)	Upper small intestine	Food, especially fat and protein in upper small intestine	Causes contraction of gallbladder and flow of bile to duodenum; causes secretion of enzyme-rich pancreatic juice and bicarbonate-rich pancreatic juice
Secretin	Upper small intestine	Acid chyme; small proteins	Causes secretion of thin bicarbonate-rich pancreatic juice and reduces gastric motility

Lipase • Fat-digesting enzymes; lipase produced by the pancreas to act in the small intestine is the most important form used in digestion.

Monoglycerides • A breakdown product of a triglyceride consisting of one fatty acid linked to the carbohydrate glycerol.

Fatty Acid • Acids found in fats. These are composed of carbon atoms linked to hydrogen atoms with an acidic chemical group at one end.

Amylase • Starch-digesting enzymes produced by the salivary glands or pancreas.

lipase from the pancreas digests the fats into smaller products, called *monoglycerides* and *fatty acids*. Pancreatic lipase enters the small intestine at a concentration 1000 times in excess of that needed. This excess ensures very rapid and thorough fat digestion when bile is present to transform (emulsify) the fat in the watery chyme into globules called *micelles*. More details follow in a later section.

The hormone *cholecystokinin* (CCK) controls the release of enzymes—like lipase—from the pancreas and also the release of bile from the gallbladder (Table 5-2).[13] When food enters the small intestine, CCK is released from the wall of the upper small intestine into the bloodstream. This hormone then travels to the pancreas and gallbladder and causes these organs to release their products.

Fats and proteins in the chyme also stimulate the release of hormones that slow stomach emptying. One hormone is secretin.[12] This slowdown helps explain why fats in a meal cause a feeling of fullness: the chyme remains in the stomach longer, and so we feel full longer. On the other hand, hunger returns quickly after a lowfat meal—a common occurrence when one diets on lowfat foods to lose weight.

Carbohydrate digestion

Digestion of the large carbohydrates—starches—coming mostly from the flour in the banana bread begins as the starches mix with saliva during the chewing of food. Saliva contains an enzyme called salivary *amylase.* This enzyme converts starch—made of thousands of glucose units—into a smaller sugar form called maltose. (This is just one glucose linked to another glucose.) You can detect this starch to maltose conversion while chewing a saltine cracker. Prolonged chewing causes the cracker to taste sweeter as some starch is converted into the sweeter sugars.

Salivary amylase does not work in an acidic environment. Once food moves down the esophagus into the stomach, the stomach's acidity stops further starch digestion by deactivating salivary amylase.

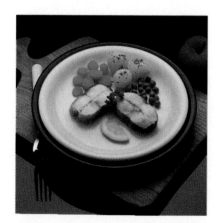

Despite what you read in popular health food books, the order in which these foods are eaten has no influence on the body's ability to digest them.

Absorptive Cells • A class of cells that line the villi (fingerlike projections in the small intestine) and participate in nutrient absorption.

Cystic Fibrosis • A disease that, among other effects, often leads to overproduction of mucus. Mucus can invade the pancreas, decreasing enzyme output. The lack of lipase enzyme output then contributes to severe fat malabsorption.

When the carbohydrates reach the small intestine starch digestion begins again as the pancreas releases its own form of amylase (pancreatic amylase). This continues the conversion of the starch into maltose. Specialized enzymes made by the **absorptive cells** of the small intestine then break down the many dietary sugars in the banana bread—mostly from the sucrose (table sugar) added—to single sugar forms, such as glucose and fructose. The enzyme maltase breaks maltose into two glucose molecules. The enzyme sucrase breaks down sucrose into glucose and fructose. The enzyme lactase breaks down lactose (milk sugar) into glucose and galactose.[12] These sugars are then absorbed, along with any glucose and fructose already present in the banana bread (Figure 5-7).

In **cystic fibrosis,** an inherited disease of infants, children, and sometimes adults, the pancreas is often affected. It develops thick mucous that blocks its ducts, and active cells die. As a result the pancreas is not able to effectively deliver its digestive enzymes into the small intestine. Digestion of carbohydrate, protein, and most notable fat is impaired because the enzymes amylase, trypsin, and lipase are not released. Often these enzymes must be given orally in capsule form with meals in order to digest the meal and to avoid abdominal discomfort from malabsorption. Recall if much undigested protein, carbohydrate, or fat makes it into the large intestine, bacteria found there make these into acids and gas.[8]

CONCEPT CHECK

In the broadest sense, digestion begins with cooking. Heat and moisture swell starch granules and soften tough fibrous tissues in plants. Enzymes produced in the mouth begin to digest starch. The stomach produces enzymes that digest protein. The small intestine is the major site of all digestion. There, proteins separate into smaller peptide forms and amino acids, carbohydrates yield sugars, and fats form monoglycerides and fatty acids. Fat digestion is aided by bile, which is produced by the liver and later released by the gallbladder. Peristaltic muscle contractions in the stomach and small intestine constantly mix the food, enhancing the digestive process. Enzymes used for digestion in the small intestine come from the pancreas and the cells lining the intestinal wall.

SMALL INTESTINE: SITE FOR MOST NUTRIENT ABSORPTION

As we said, most nutrient absorption occurs in the small intestine; little is absorbed in the stomach or large intestine. The small intestine can absorb about 95% of the kcalories it receives in the form of protein, carbohydrate, fat, and alcohol (Figure 5-8).[12] The mouth and/or stomach absorb only water, small

FRANK & ERNEST® by Bob Thaves

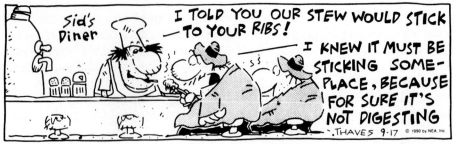

FIGURE 5-8
Frank and Ernest.

amounts of alcohol, certain types of minor fats, and some glucose. The large intestine absorbs some minerals, water, and some fat by-products (produced by bacterial action).

The enormous surface area of the small intestine aids efficient nutrient absorption. The wall of the small intestine is folded, and within the folds are fingerlike projections called *villi* (Figure 5-2). These fingers trap foodstuffs between each other to enhance absorption. Each villus (finger) is made up of numerous absorptive cells, and each of these cells has a highly folded cap known as the brush border or microvilli. All folds, fingers, and cell membrane indentations in the small intestine increase its surface area 600 times beyond that of a simple tube.[12] New absorptive cells are constantly produced and appear daily along the surface of each villus (finger).

Because absorptive cells are subjected to a harsh environment, their replacement every few days is an important adaptive mechanism for the body. Contact with various enzymes, bacteria, toxins, and even alcohol in the small intestine impairs the health of the absorptive cells. This makes constant renewal of the intestinal lining most likely a biological necessity.

ANOTHER BITE Cancer treatments often use medications (chemotherapy) to prevent rapid cell growth. Cancer cell growth is the intended target. But, although they can slow the growth of rapidly dividing cancer cells, the medications also affect other body cells that normally reproduce rapidly, such as the absorptive cells in the small intestine. This is why people undergoing chemotherapy often develop diarrhea as a side effect.

Types of absorption

In the small intestine absorption occurs by various processes. For some nutrients, like fats, the intestine is easily permeable to the nutrient. When the nutrient concentration is higher in the smaller intestine than in the absorptive cells, the difference in nutrient concentration drives absorption. The nutrients, such as fats, then enter the absorptive cells via *passive absorption* because nutrients naturally want to move from a higher to a lower concentration. Water and some minerals also are absorbed in this way.[12]

Another type of absorption uses a carrier as well as energy input to actively pump nutrients into the absorptive cells. In this way the body can take up nutrients even when they are not concentrated in the diet. Some sugars, for example, follow this route—called *active absorption.* In the case of the sugar glucose, it is much more concentrated in the absorptive cells than in the chyme in the small intestine. This is because the absorptive cells are bathed by the glucose-rich bloodstream. In order to get glucose into the absorptive cells, given the high concentration already present (uphill, so to speak), it must be pumped in using energy.[12]

Another type of *active* absorption occurs when the absorptive cells literally engulf compounds or liquids. A cell membrane can indent itself so that when particles or fluids move into the indentation, the cell membrane surrounds and engulfs them. This process is used when an infant absorbs immune substances from breastmilk (see Chapter 14).[6]

Portal and lymphatic circulation

Fluids and particles leaving the villi in the intestine drain into two different circulation systems. One is the bloodstream. The blood, laden with oxygen and nutrients, leaves the heart through arteries, travels to the intestine, and ends up in capillary beds inside the villi. The blood then passes through veins leaving

Villi • Fingerlike protrusions into the small intestine that participate in digestion and absorption of foodstuffs.

Passive Absorption • Absorption that requires permeability of the substance through the wall of the small intestine, as well as a concentration higher in the small intestine than in the absorptive cells.

Active Absorption • Absorption using a carrier and expending energy. In this way the absorptive cell can absorb nutrients, such as glucose, against a high concentration in the absorptive cells.

the capillary beds and collects in a large vein, called the ***portal vein*** (Figure 5-4). This vein leads directly to the liver. Most veins in the body double back directly to the heart. However, by going first to the liver, the portal vein enables the liver to process absorbed nutrients before they enter the general circulation of the bloodstream. Water-soluble products of digestion, as most of the nutrients are (e.g., glucose and amino acids), enter the bloodstream through the portal vein.[12]

The ***lymphatic system*** also drains the villi. Lymphatic vessels pick up products of fat absorption and other substances too large to enter the bloodstream directly. The lymphatic vessels from the intestine drain into a large duct that stretches from the abdomen to the neck. This duct connects with the bloodstream through a vein near the neck.[12]

Portal Vein • Capillary blood vessels from the intestine drain into a large portal vein that leads to the liver.

Lymphatic System • System of vessels that can accept large particles, such as products of fat absorption, and eventually pass them into the bloodstream.

Chylomicrons • Dietary fat surrounded by a shell of cholesterol, phospholipids, and protein. These are made in the intestine after fat absorption and travel through the lymphatic system to the bloodstream.

CONCEPT CHECK

The small intestine is the major site for nutrient absorption. Numerous folds and fingerlike projections create a large surface area for nutrient absorption. Absorptive cells have a life span of a few days, and so the lining of the small intestine is constantly renewed. These cells can perform passive types of absorption, promoted by a concentration difference, and more active forms of absorption, which overcomes the resistance of high concentration using a carrier and energy input. Another type of active absorption occurs when absorptive cells physically engulf compounds. Most products of absorption are water soluble. They pass into the portal vein and enter the liver. Fatty products from digestion mostly enter the bloodstream through the lymphatic system.

ABSORPTION—NUTRIENT BY NUTRIENT
Protein absorption

Small peptides and amino acids—breakdown products of the egg and milk proteins in the banana bread—are actively absorbed into the absorptive cells of the small intestine. The small peptides are then broken down into individual amino acids, as we mentioned earlier. The amino acids travel to the liver via the portal vein (Figure 5-7). There they are either combined into protein, converted into glucose or fat, used for energy needs, or released into the bloodstream.[12]

Fat absorption

Most of the products of fat digestion—mostly from the vegetable oil in the banana bread—are passively absorbed into the absorptive cells. These products are recombined into triglyceride forms, mixed with cholesterol and other substances, and coated with protein to form ***chylomicrons***. These chylomicrons then enter the lymphatic system and eventually the bloodstream (Figure 5-9).[2] Chapter 7 contains more details on this process.

Carbohydrate absorption

Finally, we come to the sugars. In the banana bread these occur naturally in the fruit, are added as table sugar, and are formed as by-products of earlier starch digestion in the mouth and small intestine. As we mentioned, glucose (and its close relative galactose) is then actively pumped into the absorptive cells of the villi. Fructose follows a type of passive absorption. Once the single sugar units enter the villi, they are transported via the portal vein to the liver.[12] The liver then exercises its metabolic options, which we will discuss in Chapter 6.

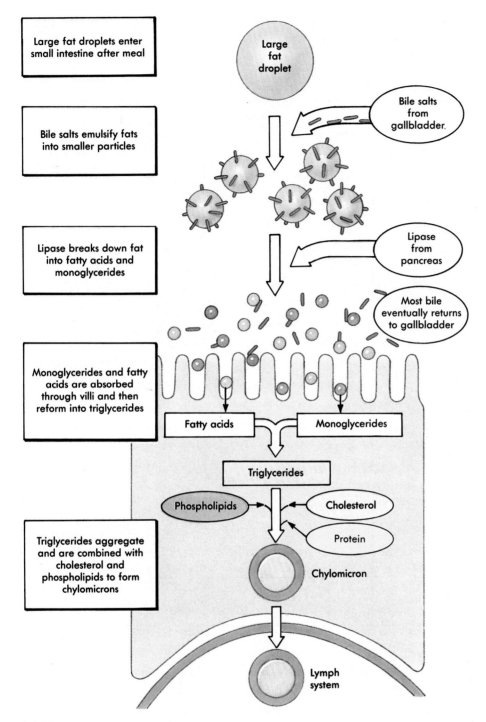

Large fat droplets enter small intestine after meal

Large fat droplet

Bile salts from gallbladder.

Bile salts emulsify fats into smaller particles

Lipase breaks down fat into fatty acids and monoglycerides

Lipase from pancreas

Most bile eventually returns to gallbladder

Monoglycerides and fatty acids are absorbed through villi and then reform into triglycerides

Fatty acids

Monoglycerides

Triglycerides

Phospholipids

Cholesterol

Protein

Triglycerides aggregate and are combined with cholesterol and phospholipids to form chylomicrons

Chylomicron

Lymph system

FIGURE 5-9

A simplified look at fat absorption. Triglycerides form primarily monoglycerides in digestion. These are absorbed using bile and reformed into triglycerides in the absorptive cells. Triglycerides are then formed into chylomicrons and enter the lymphatic system.

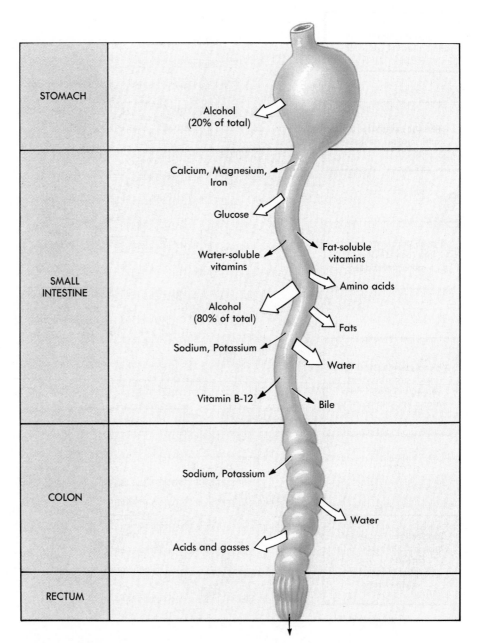

FIGURE 5-10

Major sites of absorption along the GI tract. Most absorption of nutrients is complete by the time the meal passes the midpoint of the small intestine.

The large intestine completes absorption

As the intestinal contents enter the large intestine, little of the original banana bread still remains. Only a minor amount (5%) of carbohydrate, protein, and fat have escaped absorption. Some water is still present since the small intestine absorbs only 85% to 90% of the fluid it receives, which includes large amounts of GI tract secretions produced during digestion. The remnants of the banana bread also include some minerals and food fibers.

In the first half of the large intestine, much of the remaining water and the minerals, mostly sodium and potassium, in the banana bread are absorbed (Figure 5-10). The unabsorbed water now amounts to only a few ounces.

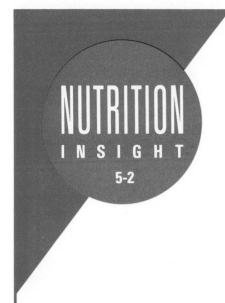

LACTOSE INTOLERANCE

A common intestinal problem is *lactose intolerance.* If *lactose*—milk sugar—is not digested by the enzyme lactase in the small intestine, the lactose then travels into the large intestine. There bacteria break down the lactose into acids and gas. About 30 minutes to 2 hours after consuming milk products, the person with lactose intolerance experiences abdominal distention and gas symptoms. This decrease in lactose digestion does not reduce calcium absorption from the milk, but it does create annoying problems.

Lactose intolerance is common in Native Americans, Asians, Hispanics, people of Mediterranean descent, and Blacks.[1] People that historically raised dairy herds, as did Northern Europeans, show the lowest rates. But even though lactose intolerance is more common in some races than in others, almost anyone is susceptible. Probably 70% of adults worldwide experience a large decrease in their abilities to synthesize lactase as they age. This loss of lactase activity is not due to disease; it happens naturally.

Ability to tolerate lactose is not "all or none." In addition, tolerance can be improved when food choices are changed appropriately. A person with lactose intolerance should not necessarily give up all milk and milk products because these are very good sources of calcium, the vitamin riboflavin, and the minerals potassium and magnesium. All four of these nutrients are present in other foods in the American diet, but there are groups of people who don't consume enough of them. Diet planning for these nutrients is much easier if one uses milk and milk products.

Better options for lactose-intolerant people include (1) consuming smaller servings of milk products and taking these with other foods. This often works because their digestive systems can digest some lactose but not large loads.[10] Fat in a meal also slows digestion, leaving more time for lactase action. (2) Affected people can eat cheese. Much lactose is lost when milk is made into cheese. And (3) yogurt can be eaten by lactose-intolerant people. The bacteria that make yogurt provide their own lactase activity, so the lactose in yogurt essentially digests itself. Note, however, that frozen yogurts, as currently manufactured, may have little remaining lactase activity.

In the last few years, manufacturers also have been producing low-lactose milk. To do this, they treat regular milk with lactase that has been isolated from yeast. Most of the lactose is digested into glucose and galactose. This milk tastes a bit sweeter, since the breakdown products—glucose and galactose—are together much sweeter than lactose. Low-lactose milk can be made at home by adding commercially available lactase to regular milk. Special lactase pills also can be purchased for use at meal times. ●

Lactose Intolerance • Lactose digestion is reduced as lactase production declines. Symptoms include gas and bloating after consuming dairy products.

Lactose • A sugar made up of glucose linked to another sugar called galactose.

Products from the metabolism of some plant fibers and small amounts of undigested starches are also absorbed.[3] The contents of the large intestine are semisolid by the time they have passed through the first two-thirds of it. The stool remains in the last third until muscular movements push it into the rectum for eventual elimination.

The presence of feces in the rectum stimulates elimination. This process involves powerful muscular reflexes in the large intestine and rectum, as well as relaxation of the anal sphincters. What remains in the feces, besides water, are undigestible plant fibers, tough connective tissues (from animal foods), and bacteria from the large intestine.[12]

CONCEPT CHECK

In protein absorption, peptides and amino acids are actively absorbed into the villi and are broken down into amino acid forms in the absorptive cell. The amino acids enter the portal vein en route to the liver. During fat absorption, the breakdown products are passively absorbed into the villi. These products are mostly resynthesized into triglycerides and formed into chylomicrons. Chylomicrons enter the lymphatic system and eventually the bloodstream. In carbohydrate absorption, some sugars, like glucose, are actively absorbed into the absorptive cells. Sugars travel via the portal vein to the liver. In the large intestine further water and mineral absorption occurs.

SUMMARY

- The gastrointestinal (GI) tract consists of the mouth, esophagus, stomach, small intestine, large intestine (colon), rectum, and anus. Most digestion and absorption of nutrients occurs in the small intestine.

- The liver, gallbladder, and pancreas participate in digestion and absorption. Products from these organs—enzymes and bile—enter the small intestine and play important roles in the digestion of protein, fat, and carbohydrates.

- Along the GI tract are ringlike valves (sphincters) that control the flow of foodstuffs. Muscular contractions, called peristalsis, propel the foodstuffs down the GI tract. A variety of nerves, hormones, and other substances control the activity of sphincters and peristaltic muscles.

- In digestion the mouth chews food to break it into smaller parts, thereby increasing the surface available for enzyme digestion. Starch digestion begins in the mouth. Much protein is digested in the stomach. In the small intestine, carbohydrate and protein digestion is finished and most fat digestion occurs. Some plant fibers are digested by the bacteria present in the large intestine; undigested plant fibers are eliminated in the feces.

- Digestive enzymes are secreted by the mouth, stomach, and wall of the small intestine and pancreas. Pancreatic enzyme release is controlled by the hormone cholecystokinin (CCK). The presence of food in the small intestine stimulates the release of this hormone. Bile needed for fat digestion is synthesized by the liver, stored in the gallbladder, and released in digestion, as directed by the action of CCK.

- The major absorptive sites consist of fingerlike projections called villi in the small intestine. Absorptive cells covering the villi have a life span of a few days. Thus the intestinal lining is continually renewed. Absorptive cells can perform passive and active forms of absorption, and they are able to absorb substances by physically engulfing them.

- The products of protein digestion—amino acids and peptides—are actively absorbed into the villi. Most end products of fat digestion are passively absorbed into the intestinal villi and rebuilt into triglycerides. Sugars from carbohydrate digestion are either actively or passively absorbed.

- Water-soluble compounds in the villi enter the portal vein and travel to the liver. Fat-soluble compounds are incorporated into chylomicrons and enter the lymphatic system, which eventually connects to the bloodstream.

- Final water and mineral absorption takes place in the large intestine. The absorption of products from bacterial breakdown of some plant fibers also occurs here. The presence of feces in the rectum provides a strong impetus for elimination.

THINK OF IT, NO DAIRY PRODUCTS

Let's say you are completely lactose intolerant (this is addressed in the Nutrition Insight on p. 141). You cannot consume milk or milk products. Also, assume you live where there are no special products available for lactose-intolerant people (e.g., milk with the lactose already digested). Without milk and milk products in your diet you most likely will not consume enough calcium riboflavin, potassium, and magnesium. Look at Tables 9-3 and 10-3, as well as the food composition table in Appendix A. Find nondairy foods that you could eat to compensate for the missing calcium, riboflavin, potassium, and magnesium in your diet (i.e., find specific foods rich in calcium, riboflavin, potassium, and magnesium). List three foods for each below, noting the kcalorie and appropriate nutrient content of each. Note that three glasses of 1% milk provide 900 mg of calcium, 1150 mg of potassium, 1.2 mg of riboflavin, and 102 mg of magnesium for only 305 kcalories.

Calcium	Riboflavin
(we need about 800-1200 mg)	(we need about 1.7 mg)

Potassium	Magnesium
(we need about 2000 mg)	(we need about 350 mg)

This exercise shows the great volume of food (and sometimes kcalories) one must consume to replace the nutrients provided by milk.

REFERENCES

1. Anonymous: Prevalence of lactose maldigestion, *American Journal of Clinical Nutrition* 48:1086, 1988.
2. Cashman MD: Principles of digestive physiology for clinical nutrition, *Nutrition in Clinical Practice* 1:241, 1986.
3. Cummings JH and others: The role of carbohydrates in lower gut function, *Nutrition Reviews* 44:50, 1986.
4. Donatelle EP: Constipation: pathophysiology and treatment, *American Family Physician* 42(5):1335, 1990.
5. Feldman M: Bicarbonate, acid, and duodenal ulcer, *New England Journal of Medicine* 316:408, 1987.
6. Gardner MLG: Gastrointestinal absorption of intact proteins, *Annual Reviews of Nutrition* 8:329, 1988.
7. Giduck SA and others: Cephalic reflexes: their role in digestion and possible roles in absorption and metabolism, *Journal of Nutrition* 117:1191, 1987.
8. Hermann-Zaidins MG: Malabsorption in adults: etiology, evaluation, and management, *Journal of The American Dietetic Association* 86:1711, 1986.
9. Kumar N and others: Effect of milk on patients with duodenal ulcers, *British Medical Journal* 293:666, 1986.
10. Martini MC, Savaiano DA: Reduced intolerance symptoms from lactose consumed during a meal, *American Journal of Clinical Nutrition* 47:57, 1988.
11. Mattes RD, Mela DJ: The chemical senses and nutrition, *Nutrition Today* May/June, 1988, p 19.
12. Mayes PA: *Nutrition, digestion, and absorption.* In Murray RK and others, editors: Harper's biochemistry, ed 22, East Norwalk, Conn, 1990, Appleton & Lange.
13. Nicholl CG and others: The hormonal regulation of food intake, digestion, and absorption, *Annual Reviews of Nutrition* 5:213, 1985.
14. Ohning G, Soll A: Medical treatment of peptic ulcer disease, *American Family Physician* 39(4):257, 1989.
15. Quimby GF and others: Active smoking depresses prostaglandin synthesis in human gastric mucosa, *Annals of Internal Medicine* 104:616, 1986.
16. Soll AH: Pathogenesis of peptic ulcer and implications for therapy, *New England Journal of Medicine* 322:909, 1990.
17. Thomson ABR: Intestinal aspects of lipid absorption, *Nutrition Today*, July/August, 1989, p 16.
18. Wilson JD and others: *Harrison's principles of internal medicine*, ed 12, New York, 1991, McGraw-Hill.

HOW MUCH HAVE I LEARNED?

What have you learned from Chapter 5? Here are 15 statements about digestion and absorption. Read them to test your current knowledge. If you think the answer is true or mostly true, circle T. If you think the answer is false or mostly false, circle F. Use the scoring key at the end of the book to compute your total score. To review, take this test again later, and especially before tests.

1. (T) F   Digestion primarily begins in the mouth. *for many foods digestion begins by 1st cooking them to make them soft.*

2. (T) F   Nutrients absorbed directly into the bloodstream from the digestive tract first go to the liver. *portal vein connects digestive tract to liver. Many nutrients must pass thru liver b/4 entering bloodstream*

3. (T) F   The small intestine is longer than 8 feet. *10 ft. 23 ft at autopsy*

4. (T) F   Mucus helps protect the stomach from acid.

5. (T) F   Colon is another name for the large intestine.

6. T (F)   Fruit and meat should not be eaten together. *digestive enzymes work well regardless of food combination*

7. (T) F   Many stomach enzymes work less efficiently in the small intestine. *stomach enzymes require acid conditions; sm. intestine is slightly alkaline*

8. (T) F   Hormones and nerves coordinate many digestive processes.

9. (T) F   As we age, our ability to digest lactose, a carbohydrate found in milk, often declines. *70% population*

10. T (F)   Stress often interferes with the absorption of nutrients. *not unless diarrhea results, stress doesn't affect digestion or absorption*

11. T (F)   Antacids should be taken after a large meal to prevent heartburn. *don't lie down after meal & don't eat so much*

12. (T) F   Glucose requires energy for its absorption, whereas fat does not. *w all is low - can passively be absorbed. glucose has high conc., so must expend energy if more is to enter intestinal cells from tract. fat concentration in intestinal*

13. (T) F   Peristalsis utilizes a coordinated muscle action. *muscles run lengthwise & circular*

14. (T) F   Gas produced in the large intestine results from partial malabsorption of food. *undigested foods entering colon are nutrient sources for bacteria there.*

15. T (F)   Most nutrient absorption takes place in the large intestine. *95% of nutrient absorption takes place in 1st half of small intestine*

WHEN THE DIGESTIVE PROCESSES GO AWRY

Ulcers

An unfortunate sign of success can be an ulcer. For some people, stress and tension greatly excite the nerves that control the stomach. This in turn increases acid secretion by the stomach's acid-producing cells. More tension means more acid. Eventually the acid erodes through the stomach's mucus layer into the stomach wall. Acid can also erode the wall of the upper small intestine. Either way, the result is an ulcer. Some people are more susceptible to ulcers than others because their stomach and intestinal cells can't sufficiently protect themselves from the acid. Recent research also links certain bacterial infections in stomach cells to ulcers.[16]

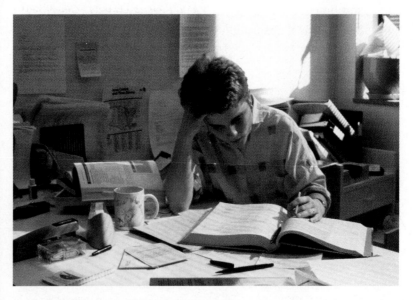

Stress can bring on an ulcer in some of us.

TABLE 5-3

Recommendations to prevent ulcers and heartburn from recurring

Ulcers
1. *Stop smoking, if you are now a smoker.*
2. Avoid aspirin, ibuprofen, and other aspirin-like compounds.
3. Avoid coffee, tea, and alcohol (especially wine).
4. Limit pepper, chili powder, and other strong spices, if this helps.
5. Eat nutritious meals on a regular schedule.
6. Chew foods well.
7. Lose weight if you are now overweight.

Heartburn
1. Wait about 3 hours after a meal before lying down.
2. Don't overeat at mealtime.
3. Observe the recommendations for ulcer prevention.

The typical symptom of an ulcer is pain about 2 hours after eating. Digestive acids that work on a meal irritate the ulcer after most of the meal moves down the small intestine.

The primary risk posed by an ulcer is that it can eat entirely through the stomach or intestinal wall. The GI tract contents could then spill into the body cavity, causing a massive infection. In addition, an ulcer may erode a blood vessel, leading to massive blood loss (hemorrhage).

In the past, milk and cream therapy was used to help cure ulcers. Today we know that milk and cream are two of the worst foods for an ulcer.[9] The calcium in these foods stimulates gastrin, the hormone that increases stomach acid secretion. Thus this therapy actually inhibits ulcer healing. Instead, antacid medications are the first line of medical treatment for ulcers. Added to these is a class of medicines that reduce stomach acid secretion. By decreasing stomach acidity, the medications greatly speed ulcer healing and so have greatly reduced the need for surgical treatment.

A person who is prone to developing ulcers should not smoke.[15] Minimizing the use of aspirin and other aspirinlike compounds also is important because these irritate the stomach.[14] This combination of therapies, along with the use of antacids and other anti-acid medications, has so revolutionized ulcer therapy that changing one's diet is of secondary importance (Table 5-3).

Heartburn

Some people are very susceptible to heartburn. The gnawing pain in the upper chest is caused by acid flowing back into the esophagus from the stomach.[18] Unlike the stomach, the esophagus has no mucus lining to protect it. The acid quickly erodes the esophageal wall, which causes pain.

An important dietary measure for avoiding heartburn is to eat smaller meals that are low in fat. Large meals containing much fat remain in the stomach longer than smaller, lowfat meals and create pressure in the stomach. This can force the stomach contents up into the esophagus. Someone who suffers from heartburn should not smoke, should not lie down after eating, and should avoid foods and other substances that can specifically contribute to heartburn, such as chili powder, onions, garlic, caffeine, alcoholic beverages, and chocolate. Each person must discover what foods are irritants and tailor the diet accordingly (Figure 5-11).

Certain physical conditions can lead to heartburn. For example, women who are pregnant and people who are obese have increased production of the hormones progesterone and/or estrogen. These hormones relax the sphincter in the esophagus, making backflow from the stomach into the esophagus more

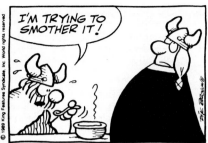

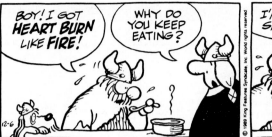

FIGURE 5-11
Hagar the Horrible.

likely. Pregnancy also increases pressures in the abdomen, which makes heartburn more likely. A pregnant woman may find it helpful to eat smaller, more frequent meals until she gives birth. An obese person can try to achieve a lower weight so that blood levels of these hormones decrease.

Heartburn that recurs several times a week for a month should be investigated by a physician.[18] Long-standing heartburn, especially when associated with difficulty in swallowing, painful swallowing, blood in the stool, or weight loss, may require aggressive medical therapy because it can lead to alteration in the cells of the esophagus. This increases the risk of a rare form of cancer.

Constipation and laxatives

Difficult or infrequent evacuation of the bowels is known as **constipation**.[4] It is caused by a slow movement of feces through the large intestine. The feces become dry and hard as fluids are increasingly absorbed during their extended time in the large intestine. Constipation can result from irregular elimination patterns that develop when people regularly inhibit their normal bowel reflexes for a long period of time. People tend to ignore normal urges when they don't want to interrupt occupational or social activities. Muscle spasms of an irritated large intestine can also slow the movement of feces and contribute to constipation. Even medications, such as antacids, can cause constipation.[4]

Constipation is difficult to diagnose. Normal stool frequency ranges from three to 12 times per week. However, definitions of normal vary from person to person. The best guide for recognizing constipation is the presence of unusually hard, dry stools at infrequent intervals—not a general prescription of once a day.[4] Any sudden, prolonged changes in stool frequency should be evaluated by a physician. This may be a warning that a more serious intestinal disorder is developing.[18]

Eating dietary fiber, such as that found in whole-grain breads and cereals, is the best alternative for treating typical cases of constipation (see Chapter 6 for a detailed discussion). Dietary fibers stimulate peristalsis by helping form a bulky stool. A person with constipation should also drink more fluids along with the dietary fiber. Eating dried fruits can also help. In addition, the person may need to develop more regular bowel habits; allowing the same time each day for a bowel movement can help train the large intestine to respond routinely. Finally, relaxation facilitates regular bowel movements, as does regular exercise.

Laxatives also can lessen constipation. They work either by irritating the intestinal nerve junctions in order to stimulate the peristaltic muscles or by drawing water into the intestine to enlarge the stool.[4] A larger stool stretches the peristaltic muscles, making them rebound and then constrict. Regular laxative use, especially of the irritating varieties, can decrease muscle action in the large intestine, causing future constipation. In time the GI tract can actually

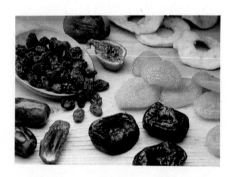

Eating dried fruit is another excellent way to increase your dietary fiber intake.

become dependent on laxatives for functioning. Thus it is unwise to use laxatives routinely, although people in certain circumstances—those who are bedridden or quite elderly—may need periodic help from laxatives to relieve constipation.

 ANOTHER BITE Perhaps you have heard that taking laxatives after overeating prevents fat gain from the excess kcalories. This erroneous and dangerous premise has gained popularity among followers of numerous fad diets. It is true that you may temporarily feel lighter after using a laxative. That is because laxatives hasten emptying of the large intestine and increase fluid loss. Note, however, that most laxatives do not actually hurry the passage of food through the small intestine, where digestion and most nutrient absorption take place. As a result, laxatives do not lessen fat gain compared with the fat gain you would have gotten from the same food without using the laxative.

Hemorrhoids

Hemorrhoids, also called piles, are swollen veins of the rectum and anus.[18] The blood vessels in this area are subject to intense pressure, especially during bowel movements. Added stress to the vessels from pregnancy, obesity, prolonged sitting, violent coughing or sneezing, or straining at the toilet can lead to a hemorrhoid.

Hemorrhoids can develop unnoticed until a strained bowel movement precipitates symptoms. These may include pain, itching, and bleeding. Itching, caused by moisture in the anal canal, swelling, or other irritation, is perhaps the most common symptom. Pain, if present, is usually aching and steady. Bleeding may result from an internal hemorrhoid and appear in the toilet or as a streak in the feces. The blood is bright red. Protrusion, or the sensation of a mass in the anal canal after a bowel movement, is symptomatic of an internal hemorrhoid that protrudes through the anus.[18]

Anyone can develop a hemorrhoid. Pressure from prolonged sitting or exertion is often enough to bring on symptoms, although diet, lifestyle, and possibly heredity play a role. If you think you have a hemorrhoid, you should consult your physician. Rectal bleeding, although usually caused by hemorrhoids, may also indicate other problems, such as cancer.[18]

A physician may also suggest a variety of self-care measures. Drinking liquids is important for maintenance of the digestive tract. Pain can be lessened by warm, soft compresses or sitz baths several times a day. A sitz bath requires sitting in a tub of warm water for 15 to 20 minutes. Over-the-counter remedies also can offer relief of symptoms. Americans spend an estimated $200 million annually on products to treat hemorrhoids. Ask a physician for advice.

The best treatment for hemorrhoids is prevention. The suggestions for relieving constipation may help prevent the formation of hemorrhoids. In addition:

- Maintain good anal hygiene. After each bowel movement gently clean the area.
- Do not strain to have a bowel movement. Straining causes unnecessary irritation to the rectal tissue.
- Keep your weight down. An overweight condition results in pressure on the blood vessels in and around the anus.
- Avoid tight undergarments. These can retain moisture and irritate the anal area. ●

CARBOHYDRATES

What did you eat to obtain the energy you are using right now? In the next three chapters we will examine this question by focusing on the nutrients the human body uses for fuel. These energy-yielding nutrients are mainly carbohydrates (4 kcalories per gram) and fats and oils (9 kcalories per gram). Not much protein (4 kcalories per gram) is used to fuel the body. Most people know that potatoes have carbohydrates and steak has fat and protein, but few people know what those terms signify. Knowing more about them both is exciting and helps you to choose appropriate foods for your needs.

You have probably eaten fruits, vegetables, milk, milk products, cereals, breads, and pasta. All these foods contribute to carbohydrate intake. Unfortunately, the benefits of these foods are often misunderstood. Many people think carbohydrate-rich foods are necessarily fattening—they are not. In fact, they are much less fattening than fats, pound for pound. Some people think sugars cause diabetes mellitus or hyperactivity—both highly unlikely. If you see carbohydrates as being unhealthy, it is unfortunate. In fact, carbohydrates, especially starches, have been the nutrient most promoted by diet recommendations in the last 10 years.[9] The link between fat—especially animal fat—and heart disease has prompted many nutrition scientists to urge Americans to switch their focus from high-fat foods to high-carbohydrate foods. ●

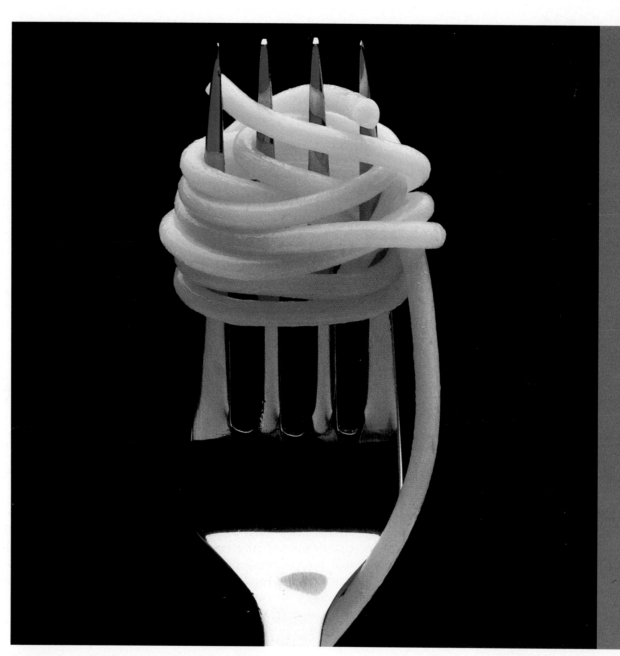

Carbohydrates help "power" most of the world's peoples.

Which Do You Choose More of, the Fluff or the Fiber?

Knowing your food preferences and habits, which of the two foods listed in each food pair would you choose? Answer the way you would really choose rather than what you think you should choose. Put a check mark (√) in the blank next to the food you would choose to eat normally.

1. _____ Whole wheat bread.   __√__ White bread.
2. _____ Brown rice.   __√__ White rice.
3. __√__ Baked potato with skin.   _____ Mashed potatoes.
4. __√__ Unpeeled apple.   _____ Applesauce.
5. __√__ Orange segments.   _____ Orange juice.
6. __√__ Whole grain cereals.   _____ Sweetened, refined cereals.
7. _____ Popcorn.   __√__ Potato chips.
8. _____ Bean dip.   __√__ Sour cream dip.
9. _____ Kidney beans on salad.   __√__ Bacon bits on salad.
10. __√__ Salad.   _____ French fries.
11. __√__ Fruit for snacks.   _____ Candy bars for snacks.
12. __√__ Baked beans or refried beans.   _____ French fries.

INTERPRETATION

The foods listed in the left column are those relatively high in fiber, while those in the right column have minimal fiber content. For every food you chose in the left column give yourself 1 point. When you total the points they should equal anywhere from 0 to 12.

Record your total points here _____

The higher your score the more high-fiber food choices you normally make. Do you generally make high-fiber choices? Do you eat a high-fiber or a low-fiber diet? Look back through the quiz and reflect on a relatively easy dietary change you could make to increase your fiber intake. Record it below:

_____

_____

As you read this chapter you will learn the health benefits of eating a high-fiber diet and practical ways to increase your diet's fiber content. Some people worry that if they increase their fiber intake they will have problems with intestinal gas. Initially this may be so, however, you will adapt to this diet. Over time you will notice progressively less gas production.

ASSESS YOURSELF

FORMS OF SIMPLE CARBOHYDRATES

Carbohydrates in our foods are made by green plants. Leaves capture the sun's heat and light in special areas of their cells and transform this to chemical energy. This energy then produces glucose from the carbon dioxide the leaves take from the air and the water the roots bring up from the soil. This complex process is called *photosynthesis.*[24]

As the name suggests, most carbohydrate molecules are composed of carbon, hydrogen, and oxygen atoms. Simple forms of carbohydrates are called sugars, while larger, more complex forms are called either starches or dietary fibers.

Monosaccharides—glucose, fructose, and galactose

Monosaccharides are single sugar forms (*mono* means one). Glucose is the major monosaccharide found in the body (Figure 6-1). Glucose is also known as dextrose or blood sugar, since it is the major sugar found in the bloodstream.

Monosaccharides

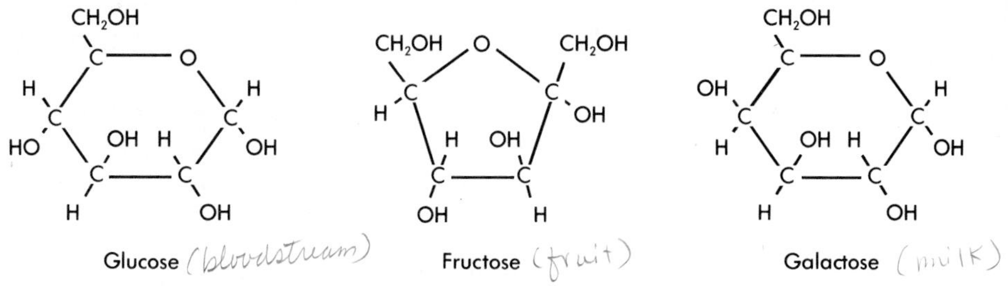

Glucose (bloodstream)   Fructose (fruit)   Galactose (milk)

Disaccharides

table sugar | Sucrose: glucose + fructose
milk | Lactose: glucose + galactose
beer | Maltose: glucose + glucose

FIGURE 6-1

Some common sugars. Sucrose and fructose are the most common sugars in our diets.

Fructose—also called levulose or fruit sugar—is another common sugar. After it is consumed, fructose is absorbed by the small intestine and then transported to the liver. There it is quickly metabolized; some turns into glucose while the rest goes on to form either a smaller carbohydrate, called *lactic acid,* or fat.[24]

The sugar galactose has nearly the same structure as glucose. It does not exist free in nature in large quantities. Instead, galactose usually is found attached to glucose in lactose, a sugar that is found in milk and other dairy products. After it is absorbed, galactose arrives in the liver. There it is either transformed into glucose per se, or further metabolized. Eventually it is stored as *glycogen,* a special storage form of glucose.[16]

Disaccharides—sucrose, lactose, and maltose

Disaccharides are formed when two monosaccharides combine (*di* means two). The most common disaccharides in foods are sucrose, lactose, and maltose.

Sucrose, which is table sugar, forms when the two single sugars glucose

Photosynthesis • Process by which plants use energy from the sun to synthesize energy-yielding compounds, such as glucose.

Monosaccharide • A single sugar, such as glucose, that is not broken down further during digestion.

Fructose • A monosaccharide with six carbons found in fruits and honey.

Lactic Acid • A three-carbon acid formed during cell metabolism; a partial breakdown product of glucose.

Glycogen • A carbohydrate made of multiple units of glucose containing a highly branched structure; sometimes known as animal starch. It is the storage-form of glucose, which is synthesized in the liver and muscles.

Disaccharides • Class of sugars formed by linking two monosaccharides.

Sucrose • Fructose linked to glucose.

6 carbon dioxides (CO_2) + 6 waters (H_2O) Æ the carbohydrate glucose ($C_6H_{12}O_6$) + 6 oxygens (O_2)

153

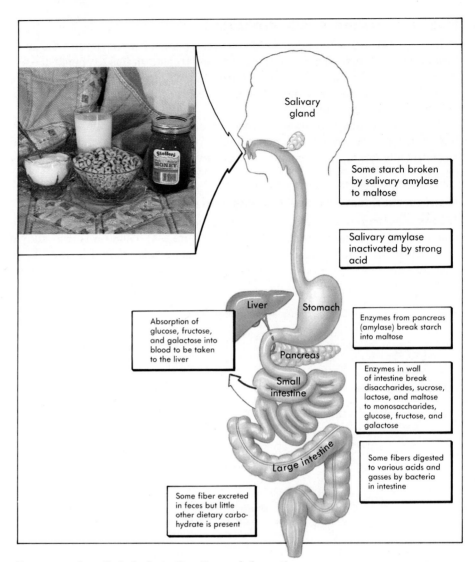

For your review. Carbohydrate digestion and absorption.

TABLE 6-1

Names of sugars used in foods

Sugar	Lactose
Sucrose	Mannitol
Brown sugar	Honey
Confectioners' sugar (powdered sugar)	Corn syrup or sweeteners
	High-fructose corn syrup
Turbinado sugar	Molasses
Invert sugar	Maple syrup
Glucose	Dextrose
Sorbitol	Fructose
Levulose	Maltose

and fructose join together. Sucrose is found in sugar cane, sugar beets, honey, and maple syrup. Animals do not make it.

Lactose forms when glucose joins with galactose. Again, our major food source for lactose is milk products. Chapter 5 discussed the problems that result when we can't readily digest lactose.

Maltose forms when two glucose molecules combine. Our major food source for maltose is produced when grains sprout (germinate). As the starch in grains breaks down during germination, maltose forms. To brew beer, grains are first germinated. The yeast can then metabolize the maltose, or malt, produced. We have few other sources of maltose in our diets.

Monosaccharides and disaccharides are often referred to as simple sugars since each contains few sugar units. Food labels sometimes lump all these sugars under one category, listing them as "sucrose and other sugars" (Table 6-1).

Maltose • Glucose linked to glucose.

Hyperglycemia • High blood glucose levels, above 140 milligrams per 100 milliliters of blood.

Hypoglycemia • Low blood glucose levels, below 40 to 50 milligrams per 100 milliliters of blood.

Insulin • A hormone produced by the beta cells of the pancreas. Insulin increases the synthesis of glycogen in the liver and the movement of glucose from the bloodstream into muscle and adipose cells, among other processes.

CONCEPT CHECK

Monosaccharides are single sugar forms. Important monosaccharides in the diet are glucose, fructose, and galactose (the latter as part of lactose). Disaccharides form when two single sugars combine. Important disaccharides in the diet are sucrose (glucose joined with fructose), maltose (glucose joined with glucose), and lactose (glucose joined with galactose). Once digested to monosaccharide forms and absorbed, most of these carbohydrates are transformed into glucose in the liver.

PUTTING SIMPLE CARBOHYDRATES TO WORK IN THE BODY
Producing energy

The main function of glucose is to supply energy for the body.[16] Certain tissues in the body, such as red blood cells, can use only glucose and other simple carbohydrate forms for energy. Most parts of the brain also derive energy only from simple carbohydrates, unless the diet contains almost none. Simple carbohydrates can also fuel muscle cells and other body cells, but many of these cells also use fat for energy needs.

In America carbohydrates supply about 45% of our dietary energy; sugars and starches contribute about equal amounts. Worldwide, however, carbohydrates account for about 70% of all kcalories consumed. In some countries this percentage climbs to as much as 80%. In North America and other industrialized areas where fat intake is high, carbohydrates supply a lower percentage of total kcalories.

Regulating this energy source. Under normal circumstances, a person's blood glucose level is regulated within a very narrow range. If blood glucose rises too high, the condition is called *hyperglycemia* (*hyper* means high and *emia* means in the bloodstream). Excess glucose then spills over into the urine.[16] This is what happens in people with poorly controlled diabetes mellitus (see the Nutrition Issue on p. 179). If blood glucose falls too low, a person feels nervous, irritable, and hungry, and may develop a headache. This is referred to as *hypoglycemia*[17] (*hypo* means low). It is not too surprising that a headache results since the brain is fueled almost entirely by glucose.

Recall that when carbohydrates are digested and taken up by absorptive cells of the intestinal villi, the portal vein then transports the resulting sugars to the liver. The liver is the first organ to screen the absorbed sugars. One of its roles is to guard against excess glucose entering the bloodstream after a meal.

The pancreas works with the liver to control glucose levels. As soon as eating begins, the pancreas releases small amounts of the hormone *insulin*. Once

In digestion, starches—also known as complex carbohydrates—are transformed into the single sugar glucose. Therefore, in the body, the main functions of most carbohydrates—both sugars and starches—are the same as they are for glucose itself. We cover starches in detail later.

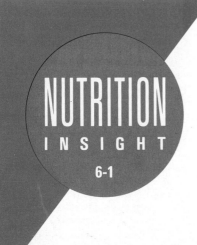

NUTRITION
INSIGHT
6-1

IS SUGAR BAD FOR YOU?

Many people think it is not healthy to consume sugar. Sugary foods may supply few, if any, vitamins, minerals, or proteins compared with the number of kcalories they supply. However, if you can afford to consume some extra kcalories, there is probably nothing wrong with eating sugar. Scientists think that sugar is mostly a problem when it is eaten in place of more nutritious foods. When this happens, a person could become deficient in vitamins and other important nutrients.

Dental caries (cavities) are the main problem associated with a high sugar intake.[1] They are formed when bacteria that live on the teeth metabolize sugars to acid. The acid then dissolves the tooth enamel and underlying structure (Figure 6-2). Starches in breads and cakes that stick to the teeth also can cause caries. These starches are metabolized to maltose by saliva in the mouth and then used by bacteria on the teeth.

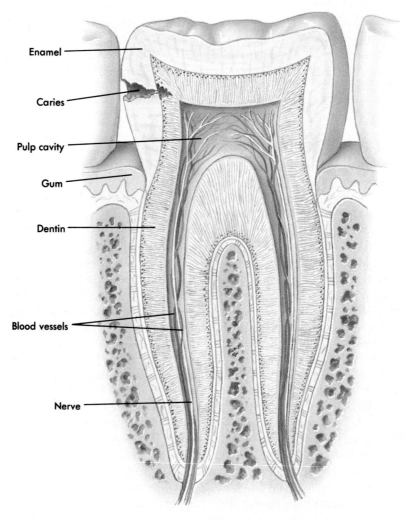

FIGURE 6-2

Dental caries. Bacteria can collect in various areas on a tooth. Simple sugars are used by the bacteria to create acid that can dissolve tooth enamel, leading to caries. The bacteria also produce plaque to adhere themselves to the tooth surface.

Tooth decay actually begins with dental plaque, the sticky film that continuously forms in the mouth. Bacteria that produce the plaque are also those responsible for the breakdown of food, particularly sugars, into acids.

 Research has indicated that certain foods, such as cheese, peanuts, or sugar-free chewing gum, actually can help reduce the amount of acid on teeth. Also, if one rinses after meals and snacks the acidity level in the mouth is reduced.

Sticky or gummy foods that are high in sugars, such as caramels and raisins, are the worst caries offenders, while liquid sugar sources, like fruit juices, are not nearly as bad. Snacking regularly on sugary foods allows the bacteria on the teeth to continually make acid. Thus the frequency of sugar consumption also affects dental health, in the absence of good dental hygiene. It is best to limit intake of sweets or eat them with meals, instead of between meals or by themselves. This way, other foods help to dilute and neutralize the acid that is produced.

In the last 15 years, dental-caries rates have decreased by 30% in the United States even though simple-sugar consumption has remained about constant.[1] This decline is primarily because of the addition of fluoride to water. When teeth develop in the presence of the mineral fluoride, they become much more resistant to acid (see Chapter 10).

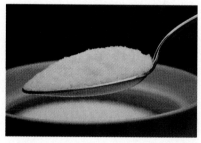

Sugar should be used in moderation, as it contains little else than a source of energy.

Are there risks besides dental caries?

No credible research supports claims that sugar causes heart disease, diabetes mellitus, and other problems. Many major scientific groups have examined the research surrounding sugar and basically have given sugar a clean bill of health, except for its tendency to cause dental caries.[1]

As for sugar's connection to hyperactivity, some researchers have suggested that sucrose affects behavior, especially in children. They claim that sucrose creates an excited, even antisocial, state, which may lead to violence and disruptive behavior. However, most researchers find that sucrose itself is not the villain. In addition, there is no adequate evidence to support the notion that reactive hypoglycemia caused by sugar consumption commonly causes violent behavior (see the Nutrition Issue on p. 179 for a discussion of hypoglycemia).[2] If there is a villain, it is probably the excitement or tension in situations where high-sucrose foods are prevalent, such as at parties and on Halloween. Any improvement in behavior that is seen when a child is put on a relatively sucrose-free diet is probably because of the extra attention received.

In the final analysis, use of sugar should follow the same advice given for many other food products—moderation. By regularly visiting the dentist and keeping blood sugar levels and weight under control, you can consume sugar in moderation by limiting it to about 10% of total kcalorie intake. That allows 10 teaspoons (50 grams) on a 2000 kcalorie diet. Table 6-2 advises how to reduce sugar intake if you think your intake exceeds this amount. ●

Glucagon • A hormone made by the pancreas that stimulates the breakdown of glycogen in the liver into glucose; this raises the blood glucose level. It also performs other functions.

Epinephrine • A hormone also known as adrenaline; it is released by the adrenal gland (located near the kidneys) and various nerve endings in the body. It acts to increase glycogen breakdown in the liver, among other functions.

TABLE 6-2

Suggestions for reducing sugar intake

At the supermarket
- Read ingredient labels. Identify all the added sugars in a product. Select items lower in total sugar when possible.
- Buy fresh fruits or fruits packed in water, juice, or light syrup rather than those in heavy syrup.
- Buy fewer foods that are high in sugar such as prepared baked goods, candies, sweet desserts, soft drinks, and fruit-flavored punches and soft drinks. Substitute vanilla wafers, graham crackers, bagels, English muffins, and diet soft drinks, for example.
- Buy nuts (dry roasted), sunflower seeds, and popcorn (use hot-air popper) to replace candy for snacks.

In the kitchen
- Reduce the sugar in foods prepared at home. Try new recipes or adjust your own. Start by reducing the sugar gradually until you've decreased it by one third or more.
- Experiment with spices such as cinnamon, cardamom, coriander, nutmeg, ginger, and mace to enhance the flavor of foods.
- Use home-prepared items (with less sugar) instead of commercially prepared ones that are higher in sugar, when possible.

At the table
- Use less of all sugars. This includes white and brown sugar, honey, molasses, and syrups.
- Choose fewer foods high in sugar such as prepared baked goods, candies, and sweet desserts.
- Reach for fresh fruit instead of a sweet for dessert or when you want a snack.
- Add less sugar to foods—coffee, tea, cereal, or fruit. Get used to using half as much; then see if you can cut back even more.
- Cut back on the number of sugared soft drinks and punches, you drink. Substitute water, fruit juice, or diet soft drinks.

Modified from USDA Home and Garden Bulletin No. 232-5, 1986.

much glucose enters the bloodstream, the pancreas releases more insulin. This insulin stimulates the liver to synthesize glycogen—the storage form of glucose in the body—and stimulates muscle cells, fat cells, and other cells to increase glucose uptake. By triggering both glucose storage in the liver and glucose movement out of the bloodstream into cells, insulin keeps glucose levels from rising too high in the blood.[16]

Other hormones have the opposite effects of insulin. When a person has not eaten for a few hours and the blood glucose level begins to fall, the pancreas releases the hormone **glucagon.** This hormone prompts the breakdown of glycogen into glucose, which is then released from the liver into the bloodstream. In this way glucagon keeps blood glucose levels from falling too low.[16]

A different mechanism increases blood glucose levels during times of stress. **Epinephrine** (adrenaline) is the hormone responsible for the "flight or fight" reaction. It is released in large amounts from the adrenal gland (located near the kidneys) and various nerve endings in response to a perceived threat, such as a car approaching head-on. Epinephrine causes glycogen in the liver to break down into glucose. The resulting rapid flood of glucose into the bloodstream helps promote quick mental and physical reactions.[16]

Other hormones, such as cortisol, growth hormone, and thyroid hormone also help regulate the blood glucose level. In essence, the action of insulin to decrease blood glucose is balanced by the actions of glucagon, epinephrine, and these other hormones as they increase blood glucose.

CONCEPT CHECK

Blood glucose levels are maintained within a very narrow range. When blood glucose levels rise after a meal, the hormone insulin is released in great amounts from the pancreas. Insulin acts to restore normal levels by increasing glucose storage in the liver and glucose uptake by muscles and adipose tissues. If blood glucose levels fall during fasting, then glucagon and other hormones increase the liver's release of glucose into the bloodstream to restore normal levels. In a similar way, the hormone epinephrine can make more glucose available in response to stress. It is the balance in hormone activity that maintains blood glucose levels within a healthy range.

Flavoring and sweetening foods

Even a young baby responds to sugars with a smile. On the tip of the tongue are sensors for tasting sweetness. The sensors recognize a variety of sugars, and even some noncarbohydrate substances. Some sugars are sweeter than others; per gram fructose is almost twice as sweet as sucrose under cold and acidic conditions, as found in soft drinks.[1] Glucose and lactose are much less sweet than fructose (Table 6-3).

Sparing protein

The importance of carbohydrate fuel for the body cannot be overstated. As a fuel for the brain and red blood cells, it is critical. If you don't eat enough car-

TABLE 6-3

The sweetness of sugars and alternate sweeteners[4]

Type of Sweetener	Relative Sweetness* (Sucrose = 1.0)	Typical Sources
Sugars		
Fructose	1.7	Fruit, honey, some soft drinks
Invert sugar†	1.3	Some candies, honey
Sucrose	1.0	Table sugar, most sweets
Glucose	0.7	Corn syrup
Maltose	0.4	Sprouted seeds
Lactose	0.2	Dairy products
Sugar alcohols		
Mannitol	0.7	Dietetic candies
Sorbitol	0.6	Dietetic candies, sugarless gum
Xylitol	0.9	Sugarless gum
Alternate sweeteners		
Saccharin (sodium form)	500	Diet soft drinks
Aspartame (NutraSweet, Equal)	200	Diet soft drinks, diet fruit drinks, sugarless gum, powdered diet sweetener
Acesulfame-K (Sunette)	200	Sugarless gum, diet drink mixes, powdered diet sweetener

*On a per gram basis.
†Sucrose broken down into glucose and fructose.

Ketone • Incomplete breakdown products of fat containing three or four carbons.

Ketosis • The condition of having high levels of ketones in the bloodstream.

Polysaccharides • Carbohydrates containing from hundreds to over 3000 or more glucose units; also known as complex carbohydrates.

Amylose • A straight-chain digestible polysaccharide made of glucose units.

bohydrates, your body is forced to make glucose from other nutrients, mainly the amino acids that make up proteins. But then some of the protein from your diet can't be used to make body tissues and perform other vital functions. Under normal circumstances, sugars in the diet are used by the brain and red blood cells for fuel.[16] Proteins then can be saved for their normal functions, like building muscles. Therefore, sugars are considered protein sparing.

During long-term starvation, proteins in muscles, heart, liver, kidneys, and other vital organs are broken down into amino acids, and these are turned into needed glucose. If the process occurs over weeks at a time, these organs become partially weakened. (See Chapters 8 and 18 for discussions of the specific effects of starvation.)

The life-threatening wasting of protein that occurs during long-term fasting has prompted companies who produce products used for rapid weight loss, like Optifast,* to include 30 to 100 grams of carbohydrate in the formulation. This significantly decreases protein breakdown, and so helps protect vital tissues and organs, including the heart.

———

*Most of these products are powders that can be mixed with different kinds of fluids, are consumed 5 to 6 times per day, and are very low in kcalories.

Preventing ketosis

When you don't eat enough carbohydrate, fats can't break down completely in the metabolic pathways. In essence, fats burn in a fire of carbohydrate. Without enough carbohydrate to spark the complete burning of fats, partial breakdown products of fats, called **ketones,** form.[24]

Ketone production is a normal metabolic response to starvation conditions, and it has survival value. The brain and other tissues can use ketones circulating in the bloodstream for fuel. Without this adaptive mechanism, the body would be forced to produce much more glucose from protein to support the brain's fuel needs than is usually seen in starvation. The resulting self-cannibalization would rapidly consume muscle, heart, and other organs, severely limiting the body's ability to tolerate starvation. Thus a person could not exist very long in a starvation state if the brain could not use ketones for energy. **Ketosis** overall is not desirable because by itself it can lead to health problems. But in starvation it is useful. The Nutrition Issue on p. 179 discusses other health problems that arise from ketosis.

To avoid ketosis, you need to eat at least 50 to 100 grams of carbohydrates per day. This ensures complete fat metabolism and prevents the body weakness that usually results from an insufficient carbohydrate intake. Typical adults in the United States need not worry. Our carbohydrate intakes usually exceed 150 grams.

CONCEPT CHECK

The major reason to consume carbohydrates is to provide glucose for the energy needs of red blood cells and parts of the brain. Eating less than 50 to 100 grams of carbohydrates per day forces the body to make glucose, using primarily amino acids from proteins found in vital organs. A low glucose supply in a cell also inhibits efficient fat metabolism, leading in turn to ketosis.

FORMS AND FUNCTIONS OF COMPLEX CARBOHYDRATES
Polysaccharides

Polysaccharides are very long carbohydrate chains composed of many monosaccharide units, mainly glucose (*poly* means many). Some polysaccharides have 3000 or more glucose units. The major digestible polysaccharides are called both starches and complex carbohydrates. These forms include *amylose* in plants and glycogen in animal tissues.

Amylose is a long, straight chain of glucoses (Figure 6-3). This forms much of the starch found in potatoes, beans, breads, pasta, and rice. As noted before glycogen (animal starch) is a storage form for glucose. This polysaccharide consists of a chain of glucoses with many branches. Enzymes that digest starches can start the digestion only at the ends of the molecule. The numerous branches of a glycogen provide many sites (ends) for enzyme action.[24] Therefore it is an ideal form for carbohydrate storage in the body as it can be quickly broken down.

The liver and muscles are the major storage sites for glycogen. Since only about 80 kcalories of glucose are available from the blood, these storage sites for carbohydrate energy, amounting to about 1800 kcalories, are extremely important. The 400 kcalories of liver glycogen can be turned into blood glucose, but the 1400 kcalories of muscle glycogen cannot.[16] Still, glycogen in muscles can supply glucose for muscle use, especially during high-intensity and

Simple

monosaccharides
glucose, fructose
galactose

↓

disaccharides
sucrose, lactose,
maltose

↓

polysaccharides
amylose, glycogen

Complex

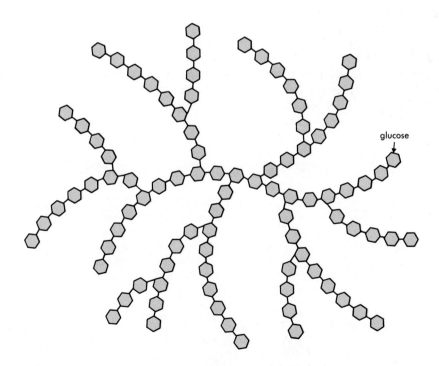

Amylose

Glycogen

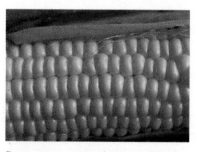

Sugars turn to starches as corn ages.

FIGURE 6-3
Some common starches. We consume essentially no glycogen. All that is found in the body is made by our cells, primarily liver and muscle.

Insoluble Fibers • Fibers that mostly do not dissolve in water and are not digested by bacteria in the large intestine. These include cellulose, some hemicelluloses, and lignins.

Soluble Fibers • Fibers that (1) either dissolve or swell when in water or (2) are metabolized by bacteria in the large intestine. These include pectins, gums, mucilages, and some hemicelluloses.

Crude Fiber • The remains of dietary fiber after acid and alkaline treatment. This primarily consists of cellulose and lignins.

Bacteria in the large intestine metabolize soluble dietary fibers into products such as acids and gases. These can cause intestinal gas (flatulence). Gas is not harmful but can be inconvenient. However, as we noted in the introduction, the body tends to adapt over time and produce less gas.

endurance exercise.[8] (See Chapter 12 for a discussion of carbohydrate use in exercise.)

Dietary fibers

Dietary fibers are primarily polysaccharides. They differ from starches in the links between the sugar units—even after cooking these links cannot be digested by human enzymes in the small intestine. This prevents absorption of the sugars that make up dietary fibers by the small intestine. Dietary fiber is not a single substance, but actually a group of substances with similar characteristics (Table 6-4).[13,22] The group consists of the carbohydrates *cellulose, hemicelluloses, pectins, gums,* and *mucilages,* as well as the noncarbohydrate *lignins,* which are alcohol derivatives.

Cellulose, hemicelluloses, and lignins form the structural parts of plants. A cotton ball is pure cellulose. Bran fiber is rich in hemicelluloses. The woody fibers in broccoli are partly lignins. Because none of these compounds readily dissolves in water, nor is metabolized by intestinal bacteria, they are called *insoluble fibers.*[22]

Pectins, gums, and mucilages are contained around and inside plant cells. These compounds either dissolve or swell when put into water. So they are called *soluble fibers.*[22] These exist as gum arabic, guar gum, locust bean gum, and various pectin forms in foods, especially in salad dressings, inexpensive ice creams, jams, and jellies.

Most foods contain mixtures of soluble and insoluble fibers.[13] A food listed as a good source of one type of fiber usually contains some of the other type of dietary fiber. So when adding fiber-rich foods to your diet, you usually get both types.[22]

Another term sometimes used for fiber is *crude fiber.* This term was coined in the 1800s to reflect the amount of indigestible foodstuff present in animal feed. Using acids and then alkalis to chemically digest the animal feed, the amount of crude fiber was determined by measuring what remained "undigested." This is mostly cellulose and lignins. Since the other types of dietary fibers are destroyed by this type of treatment, it is misleading to substitute the term crude fiber for dietary fiber. If you see the term crude fiber on food composition tables, keep in mind that values reported often bear little resemblance to dietary fiber values. This point is important. When nutrition scientists talk about fiber, they are referring to dietary fiber. Other terms for fiber, such as *roughage* and *bulk* are also no longer widely used.

We need much more data concerning the dietary fiber content of foods. In

TABLE 6-4

Classification of dietary fibers

Type	Component	Examples	Physiological Effects	Major Food Sources
Insoluble				
Noncarbohydrate	Lignins	Wheat bran	Uncertain	All plants
Carbohydrate	Cellulose	Wheat products	Increases fecal bulk	All plants
	Hemicelluloses	Brown rice	Decreases transit time	Wheat, rye, vegetables
Soluble				
Carbohydrate	Pectins, gums, mucilages	Apples Bananas Citrus fruits Carrots Barley Oats Kidney beans	Delays gastric emptying; slows glucose absorption; can lower blood cholesterol level	Citrus fruits, oat products, beans

fact, researchers still disagree on the best means for determining dietary fiber content.[22] In all analyses used today, some dietary fiber is lost. That explains the discrepancies that can be found between food tables and nutrition labels on foods concerning the amounts of dietary fiber present.

Why do we need dietary fiber?

Many types of dietary fiber absorb water and hold onto it in the intestine. When enough fiber is consumed, its water-retaining property helps enlarge and soften the stool, easing elimination.[23] Basically the larger stool size stimulates the intestinal muscles that promote peristalsis (see Chapter 5). Consequently, less pressure is necessary to expel the stool. This link between dietary fiber and the health of the intestine has interested people for hundreds of years.[6]

When too little dietary fiber is eaten, the opposite can occur; the stool may be small and hard. Constipation may result, requiring strong pressures to move the stool in the large intestine during elimination.[5] Hemorrhoids then may result from excessive straining. Also, the high pressures can force parts of the large intestine wall to pop out from between the surrounding bands of muscle. This forms small pouches, called *diverticula.* About 50% of elderly people have many of these pouches (Figure 6-4). Diverticula rarely occur in people in

Diverticula • Pouches that protrude through the outside wall of the large intestine. Diverticulosis is the condition of having many diverticula in the colon.

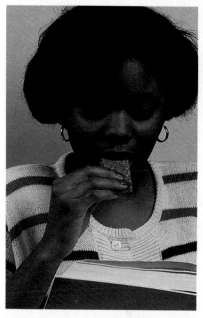

Make high-fiber food choices a regular part of your diet.

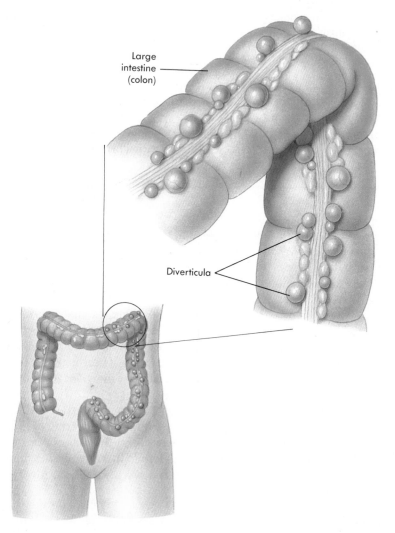

FIGURE 6-4
Diverticulae in the colon. A low-fiber diet increases the risk for their development.

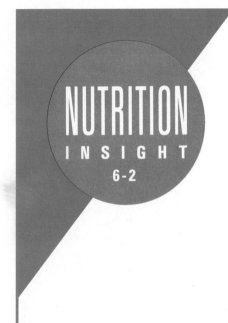

HISTORY OF FIBER IN AMERICA

Folklore surrounding dietary fiber has been a part of American culture since the 1800s. Food faddism flourished during this time.

Sylvester Graham, a minister, traveled up and down the East Coast extolling the virtues of fiber in the 1820s and 1830s.[6] Graham claimed that the true cause of disease was the removal of bran from flour during processing. The dark bread (brown bread) he recommended was later called Graham bread. Graham also believed that meat excited vile tempers and drove men to sexual excesses. He claimed that the bacterial infection cholera was the price for too much lewdness and eating chicken pie. He further claimed that people did not bathe enough and needed external applications of cold water at least weekly. Partly as a result of his advocacy, Saturday night baths and sitting-up exercises before open windows became common practices. His legacy to us is the Graham cracker. However, today's graham cracker bears little resemblance to the whole-grain product he promoted.

The next wave of fiber frenzy crested in the mid-1870s. Dr. John Harvey Kellogg was hired by the Seventh Day Adventist Church to manage their health sanitarium in Battle Creek, Michigan. Kellogg claimed that 90% of health ills centered in the stomach and bowels. He advocated ridding the digestive tract of "poisons" derived from meat-eating, drinking, smoking, condiments, and anything pleasurable. He believed that bowel eliminations should occur frequently. Tablespoons of sterilized bran were given to patients at every meal for laxative purposes. Lettuce and bran were commonly given at breakfast. Kellogg said, "Bran does not irritate, it titillates."

Adherents—including many famous people—came from all over the United States to "take the cure" at the sanitarium. Dr. Kellogg became the first person to earn a million dollars from "health foods," and he wrote more than 80 books.

One man who came for a cure in 1891, Charles W. Post, decided he could do what Dr. Kellogg was doing. He created the Post Toasted Cornflakes Company, started producing Postum Cereal Food Coffee, and developed a hard-baked wheat cracker, which he broke into small pieces and called Grape Nuts. Sold as a health food in 1898, it was advocated as a food for the brain and a cure for appendicitis, loose teeth, consumption, and malaria. Post netted $1 million from his products in 1901 alone.

Diverticulitis • An inflammation of the diverticula caused by acids produced by bacterial metabolism inside the diverticula.

Mortality • Synonymous with death; number of deaths.

Third World countries, probably because of their high dietary fiber intakes.[6] In contrast, people in Western countries often ingest only a small amount of dietary fiber in their diets.[14]

Diverticula are normally not noticeable. But, if the diverticula become filled with food particles, especially with hulls or seeds, bacteria can metabolize these food particles into acids and gases. This irritates the diverticula and may eventually cause inflammation, a condition known as *diverticulitis.* Treatment includes taking antibiotics, to counter the bacterial action, and eating a limited amount of dietary fiber, to reduce bacterial activity. Once the inflammation subsides, a high dietary fiber intake (but free of seeds) is begun to ease elimination and reduce the risk of a future attack.

Insoluble fibers, particularly certain types of hemicelluloses, are the best fibers for increasing stool size.[13] Again, bran, the fibrous covering of grain kernels, is rich in hemicelluloses. Since bran layers form the outer covering of all grains, whole grains are good sources of insoluble fiber. Increasing fluids and getting regular exercise to stimulate peristalsis are also helpful for intestinal health.[5]

Can dietary fiber play other roles in preserving health?

Dietary fiber may also play a key role in the prevention of colon cancer.[3,4] Among the deadly cancers, colon cancer ranks second only to lung cancer in occurrence and *mortality* in the United States. Dozens of epidemiological

Not to be outdone, William Kellogg, John Harvey Kellogg's brother, revived the Kellogg Toasted Corn Flake Company in 1906. Today both companies are active in the breakfast cereal market. True to form, the Kellogg Company is still promoting fiber to Americans.

Fiber finally received its scientific letters in the early 1970s.[6] Dr. Denis Burkitt, a noted British physician, observed that many "Western" diseases did not exist in Africa. These included diverticulitis, colon cancer, appendicitis, hemorrhoids, constipation, and other intestinal disorders. Burkitt surmised that the high-fiber intake of Africans was an important reason these diseases did not occur. He noticed that Africans had very large stools, almost twice the weight of stools from Westerners.

Many researchers followed Burkitt's lead. Soon studies showed that high-fiber intakes decreased the transit time of food through the GI tract. That is, the more fiber eaten, the less time needed to propel the undigested part through the intestinal tract to be eliminated. Researchers suggested that if the stool stayed in the colon for only a short time, less bacterial metabolism of the stool would occur. Thus probably fewer toxins and perhaps fewer carcinogens would form. This faster transit time is especially promoted by insoluble fibers.[23]

As we discussed in Chapter 2, the fiber argument sharpened in the mid-1980s when the Kellogg Company began promoting high-fiber cereals in the war against colon cancer. Actually, the company was following the lead of the National Cancer Institute. Scientists at the National Cancer Institute believed that a verifiable link existed between low-fiber diets and colon cancer and thought the public needed to be alerted.

The bold move by the Kellogg Company to promote fiber to Americans has been criticized as premature by many scientists. They believe that if a low-fiber intake is related to colon cancer, it is not a very strong association. Many scientists are still not convinced that a high-fiber diet will prevent enough colon cancer to justify giving fiber much publicity. Fiber is important for regular bowel habits (and is found in some laxatives for that reason). Soluble varieties can help lower blood cholesterol levels.[10] However, scientific research does not support the promotion of fiber to the average person much beyond that.[6] ●

studies have linked its occurrence to diets low in fiber and high in fat and excess kcalories. Still, researchers know little about how fiber might affect cancer development. There is good reason for suggesting that potential cancer-causing compounds in the intestinal contents are being diluted by fluid attracted to the fibers, bound to the fibers, and more rapidly excreted as fibers speed passage of feces through the intestinal tract.[3,4] Colon cancers have been prevented in laboratory animals by dietary fiber. Accumulating evidence also suggests that fat and total energy content of the diet, as well as dietary fiber, may be important causal factors.

Soluble fibers taken in high amounts in the diet can decrease blood cholesterol levels.[10] The dose, if oat bran is used, needs to be about 80 to 100 grams (about 3/4 of a cup) per day; not an easy feat. With cooked beans, about 150 grams (1 1/2 cups) is needed. The effect is partly caused by the binding of cholesterol-rich substances in the intestinal tract. These are pulled into the feces for elimination. Other mechanisms may be at work as well (see Chapter 7). Other rich sources of soluble fibers include fruits and vegetables in general, soybean fiber, rice bran, and psyllium seeds (found in many commercial fiber laxatives).

How much dietary fiber do we need?

A reasonable goal for dietary fiber intake is 20 to 35 grams per day.[13] The average intake for Americans is closer to half this amount.[14] Men's intakes of dietary fiber are greater on average than women's, partly because they eat more

TABLE 6-5

A 35-gram fiber diet for 1500 kcalories

Menu	Fiber
Breakfast	
1 orange	3.1
1 cup raisin bran cereal	6.0
½ cup 1% milk	—
2 slices whole-wheat toast	3.8
1 t margarine	—
coffee	—
Lunch	
2 oz lean ham	—
2 slices whole-wheat bread	3.8
⅓ cup cooked white beans	4.6
2 t mayonnaise	—
¼ cup lettuce	.2
1 pear (with skin)	4.3
Dinner	
3 oz broiled chicken (no skin)	—
1 baked potato including skin (medium)	3.6
1½ t margarine	—
½ cup frozen green beans	2.1
½ t margarine	—
1 cup 1% milk	—
1 apple (with peel)	3.0
TOTAL:	35 grams

kcalories. Increasing dietary fiber intake to 20 to 35 grams is not difficult to achieve (Table 6-5). This should prevent much diverticulosis, which typically develops in Western countries. Recall from Chapter 2 that the Guide to Daily Food Choices suggests we consume five to eight servings of fruits/vegetables and six to eleven servings of breads/cereals each day. All of these food choices can provide dietary fiber.

Increasing dietary fiber intake

Before increasing your dietary fiber intake, first calculate the amount of fiber you are already eating. If it is less than 20 to 35 grams per day, find some foods higher in fiber to substitute for those you already eat, or add some new ones (Table 6-6). Recall from Chapter 2 that eating a high-fiber cereal for breakfast is

TABLE 6-6

Increasing dietary fiber intake is not that hard to do

Try This:	Instead of This:
Whole-wheat bread	White bread
Brown rice	White rice
Baked potato in the skin	Mashed potatoes
Unpeeled apple (or applesauce made with unpeeled apples)	Regular applesauce
Orange segments	Orange juice
Whole-grain cereals (hot or ready-to-eat)	Sweetened cereals
Popcorn (lightly seasoned with butter or salt, if at all)	Potato chips
Bean dip	Sour cream dip
Kidney beans on salad	Bacon bits on salad
Fruit juice	Coffee or tea
Salad bar	French fries

a good idea. Also, don't remove edible peels from fruits or vegetables unless absolutely necessary.

We suggest whole food sources over bran supplement sources because foods provide a broader variety of nutrients. This is especially true for many natural high-fiber foods. Note also one should drink fluids with fiber-containing foods because fibers tend to bind with water.[23]

By eating **whole-grain** breads, beans, high-fiber cereals, and fruits and vegetables, it is easy to eat enough dietary fiber. However, some people may need to minimize their intake of foods made with refined flour—doughnuts, sweet rolls, coffee cakes, and white bread—to control kcalorie intake (Figure 6-5).

> **Whole Grains** • Grains containing the entire seed of the plant, including the bran, germ, and endosperm (starchy interior).

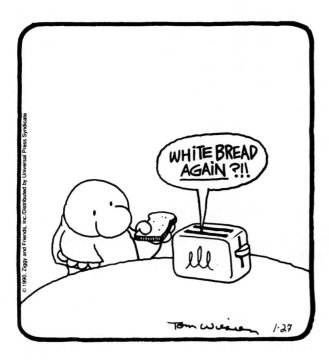

FIGURE 6-5

Read the label

We have already mentioned that a good place to look for dietary fiber is in whole-grain breads and cereals. To check for whole grains, read the label (Figure 6-6). Note that manufacturers often list enriched white flour as wheat flour on food labels. Most people think that if a product is labeled *wheat*, they are getting a whole-wheat product. However, if the label does not say whole-wheat flour in the ingredient list, it is not a whole-wheat product. Bread made from white (refined) flour lacks the bran that forms a protective coating around the wheat kernel. Bran makes flour coarser, but contains important nutrients, including dietary fiber.

In your search for dietary fiber, must you always avoid white bread, rolls, or fluffy, white pancakes? Must you always choose the whole-grain types? No. You don't have to give up favorite foods, as long as you frequently choose whole-grain alternatives. Again, the goal of 20 to 35 grams of dietary fiber a day is not that hard to attain.

INGREDIENTS: Corn, wheat, and oat flour; sugar; partially hydrogenated vegetable oil (one or more of: cottonseed, coconut, and soybean); salt; color added including yellow #6; natural orange, lemon, and cherry and other natural flavorings;
VITAMINS AND MINERALS: vitamin C (sodium ascorbate and ascorbic acid); niacinamide; zinc (oxide); iron; vitamin B$_6$ (pyridoxine hydrochloride); vitamin B$_2$ (riboflavin); vitamin A (palmitate; protected with BHT); vitamin B (thiamin hydrochloride); folic acid; and vitamin D.

CARBOHYDRATE INFORMATION

	Cereal	With ½ cup vitamins A & D skim milk
Complex carbohydrates, g	11	11
Sucrose & other sugars, g	13	19
Dietary fibers, g	1	1
Total carbohydrates, g	25	31

INGREDIENTS

Whole wheat, raisins, wheat bran, sugar, natural flavoring, salt, corn syrup and honey.

VITAMINS AND MINERALS

Vitamin A palmitate, niacinamide, iron, zinc oxide (source of zinc), vitamin B$_6$, riboflavin (vitamin B$_2$), thiamine mononitrate (vitamin B$_1$), vitamin B$_{12}$, folic acid and vitamin D.

CARBOHYDRATE INFORMATION

	Cereal	With skim milk
Dietary fiber	6g	6g
Complex carbohydrate	11g	11g
Natural sugar in raisins	7g	7g
Sucrose and other sugars	7g	13g
Total carbohydrate	31g	37g

FIGURE 6-6

Reading labels helps us choose more nutritious foods. Based on information from their nutrition labels, which cereal is the better choice for breakfast? Consider dietary fiber and sugars in each cereal. Did the ingredient list give you any clues (NOTE: Ingredients listed in descending order of weight)?

Problems with high-fiber diets

Very high dietary fiber intakes—for example, 60 grams per day—can pose some health risks. A high dietary fiber intake requires a high water intake. Not consuming enough water with the dietary fiber can leave the stool very hard, making it difficult and painful to eliminate. Intestinal blockage has occurred in people who consume great amounts of wheat bran and oat bran.[7] Large amounts of dietary fiber can also bind important minerals, especially calcium, zinc, and iron, making them less available to the body.[11] More studies are needed concerning the long-term effects of high-fiber diets on mineral status. High-fiber diets also contribute to intestinal gas. Finally, great amounts of dietary fiber can fill up a child before he or she eats enough food to meet energy needs. As with many practices, moderation with dietary fiber is the best approach (Figure 6-7).

CONCEPT CHECK

Dietary fiber has been the focus of human attention for centuries. Insoluble fiber forms a vital part of the diet by providing mass to the stool, which helps ease elimination and lessens the risk for developing diverticulosis. Fiber in the diet may also reduce the risk of colon cancer. Soluble fiber can aid in decreasing blood cholesterol levels. Whole grains, vegetables, and fruits are excellent sources of both types of dietary fiber.

GRIN & BEAR IT   By Wagner

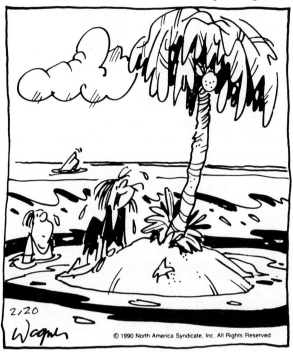

"Oh, good...roughage!"

FIGURE 6-7

RECOMMENDATIONS FOR CARBOHYDRATE INTAKE

No RDA for carbohydrate intake has been established. As we discussed before, it is important to consume at least 50 to 100 grams of carbohydrates per day to prevent ketosis. This assumes that the diet also contains enough total kcalories to meet energy needs. It is easy to consume 50 grams of carbohydrate. Just 3 pieces of fruit, 3 slices of bread, or a little more than 3 cups of milk suffice. In fact, it is difficult to follow a diet that will produce ketosis.

Beyond that need, carbohydrates provide important fuel for the body. The average American eats more than 150 grams of carbohydrates per day. This adds up to about 45% of all kcalories eaten. We noted in Chapter 2 that many health authorities recommend we boost carbohydrate intake to 55% of kcalories and reduce fat intake.[9]

Most carbohydrates in the American diet are consumed in the form of white breads, sugared soft drinks, baked goods, sugar itself, and milk. The Dietary Guidelines we discussed in Chapter 2 emphasize the importance of starch and fiber in the diet. We suggest that you eat at least one-third or more of your kcalories in the form of starches—35% to 45% of total energy intake is a reasonable goal. The diet listed in Table 6-5 illustrates one example of this approach.

About 125 pounds of simple sugars per American enter our food supply each year.[1] About three quarters of this comes from sucrose and one quarter from corn sweeteners. Most of these sugars are added to foods and beverages during manufacturing. The rest occurs naturally in foods or is added from the sugar bowl. Overall consumption of sucrose has dropped in the last 10 years, but consumption of corn sweeteners has increased. This is mostly because corn sweeteners are cheaper to use for food manufacturers than other forms of sugars.

ANOTHER BITE During processing of food, the sugar content often is increased. Usually, the more processed the food, the higher the sugar content. An apple has 0 grams of added sugar, canned apples in heavy syrup have 10 to 15 grams and ⅙ of a 9-inch apple pie has 30 grams of added sugar. For comparison purposes 1 teaspoon of sugar is 5 grams.

Although a desirable level of sugar intake has not yet been set, less than 10% of total kcalorie intake is considered a reasonable level.[1] As we mentioned before, this allows for 10 teaspoons a day on a 2000-kcalorie diet, including what is added to foods, such as cookies and soft drinks. Table 6-7 shows some common sources of sugars in our diets. Are these foods major players in your diet?

TABLE 6-7

Some sources of sugars

Food	Serving	Teaspoons of Sugar	Food	Serving	Teaspoons of Sugar
Beverages			**Jellies and jams**		
Cola drinks	1 (12 oz bottle or glass)	7	Apple butter	1 T	1
			Jelly	1 T	4-6
Cordials	1 (¾ oz glass)	1½	Orange marmalade	1 T	4-6
Ginger ale	12 oz	10	Peach butter	1 T	1
Orange-ade	1 (8 oz glass)	5	Strawberry jam	1 T	4
Root beer	1 (10 oz bottle)	4½	**Candies**		
Seven-up	1 (12 oz bottle)	7½	Av. chocolate milk bar (ex. Hershey)	1 (1½ oz)	2½
Cakes and cookies			Chewing gum	1 stick	½
Angel food	1 (4 oz piece)	7	Fudge	1 oz square	4½
Applesauce cake	1 (4 oz piece)	5½	Gum drop	1	2
Banana bread	1 (2 oz piece)	2	Hard candy	4 oz	20
Cheesecake	1 (4 oz piece)	2	Lifesavers	1	½
Chocolate cake (plain)	1 (4 oz piece)	6	Peanut brittle	1	3½
Chocolate cake (iced)	1 (4 oz piece)	10	**Canned fruits and juices**		
Coffee cake	1 (4 oz piece)	4½	Canned apricots	4 halv. / 1 T syr.	3½
Cupcake (iced)	1	6	Canned fruit juices sweetened	½ cup	2
Fruit cake	1 (4 oz piece)	5			
Jelly-roll	1 (2 oz piece)	2½	Canned peaches	2 halv. & 1 T syr.	3½
Orange cake	1 (4 oz piece)	4	Fruit salad	½ cup	3½
Pound cake	1 (4 oz piece)	5	Fruit syrup	2 T	2½
Sponge cake	1 (1 oz piece)	2	Stewed fruits	½ cup	2
Strawberry shortcake	1 serving	4	**Breakfast cereals***		
Brownies unfrosted	1 (¾ oz)	3	Cheerios	1 ounce	⅕
Chocolate cookies	1	1½	Special K	1 ounce	⅔
Fig newtons	1	5	Total	1 ounce	⅔
			Quaker 100% Natural	1 ounce	2
Dairy products			Sugar Frosted Flakes	1 ounce	2
Ice cream	⅓ pt (3½ oz)	3½	Sugar Smacks	1 ounce	3
Ice cream bar	1	1-7 accord. to size	Raisin Bran*	1 ounce	1½
			Cracklin' Oat Bran	1 ounce	1½
Ice cream cone	1	3½	Fruit Loops	1 ounce	2½
Ice cream soda	1	5	Cap'n Crunch	1 ounce	2½
Ice cream sundae	1	7	Rice Krispies	1 ounce	⅔
Malted milk shake	1 (10 oz glass)	5			
Frozen yogurt	3 ounces	3			

*Before milk is added.

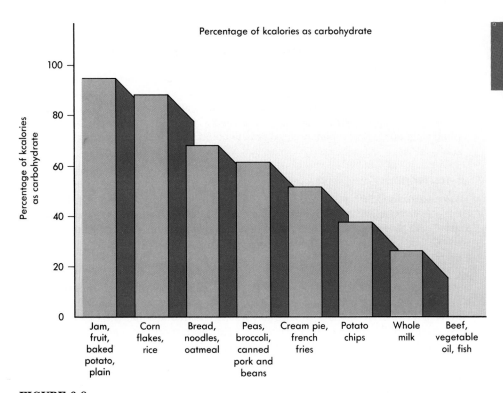

Percentage of kcalories as carbohydrate

FIGURE 6-8
Percent of kcalories as carbohydrates in foods. Jams, fruits, rice, and many breakfast cereals provide almost all kcalories as carbohydrates. Fruits, vegetables, and grains are often high in complex carbohydrates.

High Fructose Corn Syrup •
A corn syrup containing between 40% and 90% fructose.

CARBOHYDRATES IN FOODS

For foods in general, the greatest nutrient densities for carbohydrates are found in sugars, honey, jams and jellies, fruit, and potatoes. They contain essentially all their kcalories as carbohydrate (Figure 6-8). Corn flakes, rice, bread, and noodles all contain at least 75% of their kcalories as carbohydrates. Foods with moderate amounts of carbohydrates are peas, broccoli, oatmeal, pork and beans, cream pies, French fries, and skim milk. In these foods the overall carbohydrate concentration is reduced either by the ample protein content, as in the case of skim milk, or by fat, as in the case of a cream pie.

Chocolate, potato chips, and whole milk contain 30% to 40% of kcalories as carbohydrates. Again, the carbohydrate content of these foods is overwhelmed by either their fat or protein content. Foods with essentially no carbohydrates include beef, chicken, fish, vegetable oils, butter, and margarine.

Recall that the recommendation for a high-carbohydrate diet means a diet high in starches rather than high in simple sugars.[9] Figure 6-8 shows that a high-carbohydrate diet should emphasize potatoes, grains, pasta, and vegetables. A person cannot form a high-carbohydrate diet from chocolate, potato chips, and French fries because these foods contain too much fat.

Sweeteners in foods

Sucrose is the tried-and-true sweetener. A relatively new sweetener in food is **high-fructose corn syrup,** which contains 40% to 90% fructose.[1] It is made by treating corn starch with acid and enzymes. Much of the starch is broken down into glucose and then changed into fructose. The syrup is usually as sweet as sugar. Its major advantage is that it is cheaper and can be shipped in a more

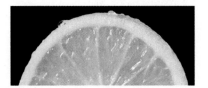

Fruits provide sugars in a balance with other nutrients, such as vitamins and minerals.

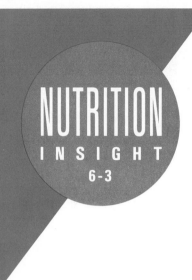

ALTERNATE SWEETENERS

Three major alternate sweeteners are available in the United States today—saccharin, aspartame, and acesulfame-K. Another alternate sweetener, cyclamate, was banned in 1970 by FDA because of its link with cancer and birth defects. New research has introduced some questions about the necessity of such a ban. Depending on this reexamination, cyclamate could be back on the grocery shelves soon.

Saccharin

Saccharin was first produced in 1879. Although widely used in soft drinks and table sweeteners, it has been recently linked with cancer. Laboratory animals have developed bladder cancer when given high doses of saccharin, especially animals in the second generation after exposure.[1] Arguments continue concerning the interpretation of data from these experiments.

In 1977 FDA attempted to ban saccharin because of this association with cancer. Many saccharin users protested a ban because it left them no low-kcalorie sweetener (the others were not available in 1977). Public pressure persuaded Congress to prevent FDA from banning saccharin. The current moratorium set by Congress expires in 1992; until then, FDA cannot act.[1] However, products containing saccharin must contain a label warning of the cancer risk.

Aspartame

In 1981 a new alternate sweetener, *aspartame,* became available. Its trade name is NutraSweet when added to foods and Equal when sold as powder. Aspartame is composed of the amino acids phenylalanine and aspartic acid, with the addition of methanol. Because amino acids are the building blocks of proteins, aspartame belongs more in the protein class than in the carbohydrate class. Aspartame yields energy—4 kcalories per gram—but is 180 to 200 times sweeter than sucrose. This means that much less aspartame yields the same sweetening potency as sucrose. Today aspartame is used in beverages, gelatin desserts, chewing gum, and other food items.[26]

Aspartame is in widespread use throughout the world. It has been approved for use by more than 70 countries, and its use has been endorsed by the World Health Organization, American Medical Association, American Diabetes Association, and American Academy of Pediatrics Committee on Nutrition.[26] Although aspartame never has been linked with cancer, individuals have filed complaints with FDA claiming adverse reactions to aspartame—headaches, dizziness, seizures, nausea, allergic reactions, and other side effects.

It is important for people who are sensitive to aspartame to avoid it. But the percentage of sensitive people is extremely small. Considering its wide use, the relatively small number of complaints made against aspartame to date suggest most people can use it.[18] In addition, careful research casts doubt on whether it causes headaches or mood swings.[21]

Saccharin • An alternate sweetener that yields no energy to the body; it is 500 times sweeter than sucrose.

Aspartame • An alternate sweetener made of two amino acids (part of proteins) and methanol; it is 200 times sweeter than sucrose (table sugar).

You may be left still feeling hungry after consuming an aspartame-sweetened beverage on an empty stomach.[19] This is because you essentially tried to quell hunger with carbonated water. Your usual sugared soft drink would have led to a rise in blood glucose levels and in turn reduced hunger (see Chapter 11 for a look at the glucose-hunger link). A possible solution is to combine these diet beverages with a small meal. This way you can save the kcalories that you would have consumed from the simple sugar-laden beverage and provide energy to quell your hunger from healthier foods.

Aspartame's high phenylalanine content concerns some people. They feel the blood levels of this amino acid may increase too much because aspartame is not balanced by the other amino acids normally found in protein foods. This situation can be easily avoided by consuming aspartame with protein foods. Some people also are concerned about aspartame's methanol content. However, the amount of methanol in a soft drink sweetened with aspartame is not more than is found in a cup of many fruit or vegetable juices.

Overall, the scientific community agrees that aspartame itself is safe; as we said numerous scientific and medical groups support its use. An acceptable daily intake set by FDA is equivalent to about 14 cans of diet soft drinks a day for an adult, or about 80 packets of Equal. Aspartame is safe for children and pregnant women to consume, but some scientists suggest cautious use by these groups.[15,26]

One final note about aspartame. A rare disease called *phenylketonuria* (PKU) prevents a person from metabolizing phenylalanine. We discuss PKU in Chapter 8. For now, note that you were tested for this disease as an infant, usually before leaving the hospital. Labels on products containing aspartame warn people with PKU against using the product. Individuals carrying only one PKU gene do not have the disease and can consume aspartame.[26] Only a person with two PKU genes has inherited the disease and should not use aspartame.

Acesulfame-K

The newest alternate sweetener in the United States, *acesulfame-K* (Sunette), was approved by FDA in July 1988. Acesulfame-K is 200 times sweeter than sucrose. Presently, it can be used in chewing gum, powdered drink mixes, gelatins, puddings, and nondairy creamers. It contributes no kcalories to the diet because it is not broken down by the body.

Some studies show that laboratory animals develop cancer after exposure to acesulfame-K. However, the FDA's analysis of these studies suggests that the tumors were not caused by acesulfame-K consumption. They were routinely seen in the untreated animal species studied. Therefore acesulfame-K has FDA approval. It is already used as a sweetener in foods and beverages in at least 20 countries. Acesulfame-K can be used in baking, whereas the current form of aspartame cannot because it breaks down when heated. So acesulfame-K may see wider uses. Currently, little information has been published about acesulfame-K. ●

A few other alternate sugars—single-sugar alcohols—appear in foods. Today the major one used is sorbitol. This is found in sugarless gum. It yields kcalories but is not readily metabolized by the bacteria in the mouth. Thus sorbitol does not promote dental caries (cavities).

Clostridium Botulinum • A bacterium that can cause a fatal type of food poisoning.

concentrated form than sugar. Also, it has better freezing properties because it doesn't encourage the formation of ice crystals. High-fructose corn syrups are used in soft drinks, candies, jams, jellies, other fruit products, and desserts.

In addition to sucrose and high-fructose corn syrup, brown sugar, turbinado sugar, honey, maple syrup, and other sugars are added to foods (see Table 6-1). Raw (unrefined) sugar cannot be sold in the United States because FDA considers it unfit for human consumption. A partially refined version of raw sugar that can be sold is turbinado sugar. This has a slight molasses flavor. Brown sugar is basically white sugar containing some molasses; either the molasses is not totally removed from the sugar during processing or it is added back to the sucrose crystals.

Maple syrup is made by boiling down the sap from sugar maple trees. Pancake syrup sold in supermarkets is sweetened mostly with corn syrup—not maple syrup.

To make honey, bees alter nectar from plants, breaking down the sucrose into fructose and glucose. Honey offers the same nutritional value as other simple sugar sources. A common misconception is that honey contains vitamins and minerals. It is a source of energy but little else (see Appendix A). Note that giving honey to infants is risky because it can contain spores of the bacterium, ***Clostridium botulinum.*** These spores can develop into bacteria that cause fatal food poisoning (see Chapter 17). Adults can safely consume honey because the acidic environment of an adult's stomach inhibits bacterial growth. An infant's stomach is not very acidic, leaving it susceptible to the risks this bacterium poses.

Only the sweetener molasses, a by-product of sugar production, contains any appreciable amount of minerals. However, our consumption of molasses in foods is very low.

CONCEPT CHECK

There is no RDA for carbohydrate; an intake of more than 100 grams, emphasizing starches, is advisable to about 55% of total kcalories. We should limit consumption of sugars to about 10 teaspoons per day. Most of these sugars are added to foods and beverages during manufacturing. The rest occurs naturally in foods or is added from the sugar bowl. To reduce simple sugar consumption one must reduce consumption of items that have had a lot of sugar added, such as some baked goods, certain beverages, and some breakfast cereals.

SUMMARY

- The monosaccharides in our diet include glucose, fructose, and galactose (the latter as part of lactose). Once absorbed via the small intestine into the liver, much of the fructose and galactose is turned into glucose.

- The major disaccharides are sucrose (glucose plus fructose), maltose (glucose plus glucose), and lactose (glucose plus galactose). When digested, these yield monosaccharide forms.

- The major digestible polysaccharides—starches—contain multiple glucose units linked together. Glycogen is animal starch and acts as a storage form of glucose in the liver and muscles.

- Carbohydrates provide energy (4 kcalories per gram), protect against needless metabolism of protein (during starvation), prevent ketosis, and provide flavor and sweetness to foods. They are not necessarily fattening. Simple carbohydrates can be metabolized to acids by bacteria on teeth. The acid can erode the tooth surface, leading to dental caries.

- Dietary fibers include the indigestible polysaccharides cellulose, hemicelluloses, pectins, gums, and mucilages, as well as the noncarbohydrate lignins. Dietary fiber, especially insoluble varieties, provides mass to the stool, thus easing elimination. It may also decrease the risk for colon cancer.

- There is no RDA for carbohydrate. An intake of 50 to 100 grams should prevent ketosis. If carbohydrate consumption is inadequate, the body can make what it needs to support cell metabolism. However, if inadequate carbohydrate intake continues for weeks at a time, the price is a loss of body protein, ketosis, and in turn a general weakening of the body.

- Diets high in complex carbohydrates are encouraged as a replacement for high-fat diets. A suggested goal is to consume 55% of total kcalories as carbohydrate, with an emphasis on starches. Foods to emphasize are potatoes, grains, pastas, and vegetables. Sugar intake should be limited to 10% of kcalories. Use of alternate sweeteners, such as aspartame, can help in limiting sugar intake.

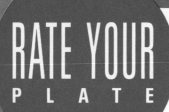

HOW DOES YOUR DIET RATE FOR CARBOHYDRATE AND FIBER?

Remember the nutritional assessment you completed at the end of Chapter 2? That activity includes some information to use for the following diet analysis:

1. Look at your analysis and find the total number of grams of carbohydrate you ate.

TOTAL GRAMS OF CARBOHYDRATE _____

   A. Did you exceed the minimum amount to avoid ketosis—50 to 100 grams?
   B. Calculate the percentage of kcalories in your diet from carbohydrate. You will need the total grams of carbohydrate from your assessment as well as the total kcalories you ate. Use this formula to calculate:

$$\frac{\text{Total grams of carbohydrate} \times 4}{\text{Total kcalories}} \times 100 = \% \text{ of kcalories from carbohydrate}$$

THE % OF KCALORIES FROM CARBOHYDRATE YOU ATE = _____

Did you approach 55% of kcalories from carbohydrate?
If you didn't, what could you do to increase your carbohydrate intake?

_____

_____

_____

2. Use the list of foods you cited in your nutrition assessment assignment, including the amounts, to calculate fiber consumption. Refer to the software printout for your dietary fiber intake or use the food composition table in Appendix A to look up the fiber content of each food you ate. Take the amount of that food you ate into account. Total the amount of fiber you ate for that day and record it in the blank provided below.

TOTAL AMOUNT OF FIBER CONSUMED _____ grams.

   A. Did you eat 20 to 35 grams as suggested in this chapter?
   B. If not, what could you do to increase your fiber intake? What foods could you substitute for some of the foods you ate?

_____

_____

_____

3. Finally, use Table 6-2 if you need to reduce your sugar intake, especially if you need to watch your total kcalorie intake to maintain an appropriate body weight.

REFERENCES

1. American Dietetic Association Reports: Position of The American Dietetic Association: appropriate use of nutritive and non-nutritive sweeteners, *Journal of The American Dietetic Association* 87:1689, 1987.

2. Bachorowski J and others: Sucrose and delinquency: behavioral assessment, *Pediatrics* 86:244, 1990.

3. Bright-See E: Dietary fiber and cancer, *Nutrition Today*, July/August, 1988, p 4.

4. Burkitt DP: Dietary fiber and cancer, *Journal of Nutrition* 118:531, 1988.

5. Castle SC: Constipation, *Archives of Internal Medicine* 147:1702, 1987.

6. Conner WE: Dietary fiber—nostrum or critical nutrient? *New England Journal of Medicine* 322:193, 1990.

7. Cooper SG, Tracey EJ: Small-bowel obstruction caused by oat-bran bezoar, *New England Journal of Medicine* 320:1148, 1989.

8. Costill DL: Carbohydrates for exercise: dietary demands for optional performance, *International Journal of Sports Medicine* 9:1, 1988.

9. Cronin FJ, Shaw AM: Summary of dietary recommendations for healthy Americans, *Nutrition Today*, November/December, 1988, p 26.

10. Demark-Wahnefried W and others: Reduced serum cholesterol with dietary change using fat-modified and oat bran supplemented diets, *Journal of The American Dietetic Association* 90:223, 1990.

11. Hallfrisch J and others: Mineral balance of men and women consuming high fiber diets with complex or simple carbohydrate, *Journal of Nutrition* 117:48, 1987.

12. Jenkins DJA and others: Metabolic effects of a low-glycemic-index diet, *American Journal of Clinical Nutrition* 46:968, 1987.

13. Kritchevsky D: Dietary fiber, *Annual Reviews of Nutrition* 8:301, 1988.

14. Lanza E and others: Dietary fiber intake in the U.S. population, *American Journal of Clinical Nutrition* 46:790, 1987.

15. London RS: Saccharin and aspartame: are they safe to consume during pregnancy, *Journal of Reproductive Medicine* 33:17, 1988.

16. Mayes PA: Regulation of carbohydrate metabolism. In Murray RK and others, editors: *Harper's biochemistry*, East Norwalk, Conn, 1988, Appleton & Lange.

17. Nelson RL: Hypoglycemia: fact or fiction, *Mayo Clinic Proceedings* 60:844, 1985.

18. Pivonka EE, Grunewald KK: Aspartame- or sugar-sweetened beverages: effects on mood in young women, *Journal of The American Dietetic Association* 90:250, 1990.

19. Rodin J: Comparative effects of fructose, aspartame, glucose, and water preloads on calorie and macronutrient intake, *American Journal of Clinical Nutrition* 51:428, 1990.

20. Saudek CD: Recurrent hypoglycemia, *Journal of the American Medical Association* 264:2791, 1990.

21. Schiffman SS and others: Aspartame and susceptibility to headache, *New England Journal of Medicine* 317:1181, 1987.

22. Slavin JL: Dietary fiber: mechanism or magic on disease prevention, *Nutrition Today*, November/December, 1990, p 6.

23. Stevens J and others: Comparison of the effects of psyllium and wheat bran on gastrointestinal transit time and stool characteristics, *Journal of The American Dietetic Association* 88:323, 1988.

24. Stryer L: *Biochemistry*, ed 3, New York, 1988, WH Freeman.

25. Wilson JD and others: *Harrison's principles of internal medicine*, ed 12, New York, 1991, McGraw-Hill.

26. Yost DA: Clinical safety of aspartame, *American Family Physician* 39(2):201, 1989.

HOW MUCH HAVE I LEARNED?

What have you learned from Chapter 6? Here are 15 statements about carbohydrates. Read them to test your current knowledge. If you think the statement is true or mostly true, circle T. If you think the statement is false or mostly false, circle F. Use the scoring key at the end of the book to compute your total score. To review, take this test again later, and especially before tests.

1. **T** F   Common table sugar is called sucrose. *glucose/fructose*

2. **T** F   Carbohydrates are obtained mostly from plants.
few carbs. present in animal foods

3. **T** F   Carbohydrates can cause dental caries (cavities). *simple sugars can be metabolized by acid on teeth*

4. **T** F   The primary role of carbohydrates is to supply energy for the body.

⟵ 5. T **F**   Dietary fiber and crude fiber are the same thing.

crude fiber represents only what remains after harsh chemical treatment

6. T **F**   There is an RDA for carbohydrates.

7. T **F**   The human body uses dietary fiber mainly for energy.
increase stool mass—eases elimination

8. **T** F   In practical everyday terms, milk is a good source of carbohydrates. *1 cup = min. carbo. need*

9. **T** F   Excess dietary carbohydrates can be converted into fat in the body. *when eaten in excess of energy needs, stored as glycogen & fat*

10. T **F**   Honey is a complex carbohydrate. *simple carbo.*

11. **T** F   No desirable level of sugar intake has been established, but intake by some people may be too high. *ea. person consumes 125 lbs/yr. should be 10% of total Kcal.*

infants don't have very acidic ⟵ 12. **T** F   Feeding honey to infants is risky.
stomachs. honey contains spores of bacterium. Clostridium botulinum which can grow & cause fatal food poisoning

13. T **F**   Diabetes mellitus is a disorder of low blood glucose levels. *high blood glucose levels*

14. **T** F   When people don't eat enough carbohydrate, as in starvation conditions, the body metabolizes protein to make needed glucose. *protein supplies carbon atoms needed to make glucose*

15. **T** F   Africans experience fewer intestinal disorders than North Americans. *observed by Dr. Burkitt*

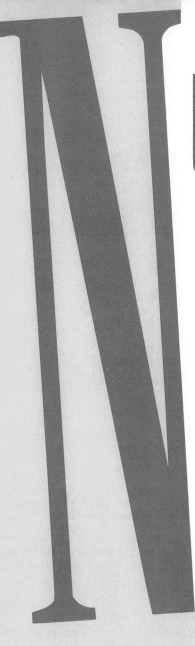

NUTRITION ISSUE

WHEN BLOOD GLUCOSE REGULATION FAILS

The major problem in regulating blood glucose seen in humans occurs when diabetes mellitus causes hyperglycemia, a high blood glucose level. The two forms of diabetes mellitus are *insulin-dependent* and *noninsulin-dependent.* The symptoms include fasting blood glucose levels above 140 milligrams per 100 milliliters of serum, frequent urination and thirst (diabetes mellitus essentially means output of much sweet urine), extreme hunger, rapid weight loss, blurred vision or a sudden change in vision, easy tiring, drowsiness, and general weakness.[16] Many of these symptoms may wax and wane or persist.

Insulin-dependent diabetes mellitus

The insulin-dependent form of diabetes mellitus often begins in late childhood, from the age of 8 years to the age of 12 years, but it can strike at any age. The hallmark of the disease is the tendency to develop ketosis.[25] Without sufficient insulin, glucose is not taken up by the cells that metabolize it. People with diabetes may have a full load of glucose in the bloodstream, but unless that glucose can get into the muscle and adipose cells, much of it cannot be used.[16] Much glucose then spills into the urine. Other hormone shifts cause the liver to respond by producing ketones.[16] In poorly treated insulin-dependent diabetes, the ketone level can rise excessively in the bloodstream. Ketones eventually spill into the urine and can lead to coma and even death. (Coma and/or death will not happen in ketosis caused by starvation because the ketone levels in the bloodstream do not rise as high.)

A viral infection may play an important part in the development of insulin-dependent diabetes.[25] Some infections are thought to trigger an immune response that attacks the pancreas, especially the cells that make insulin. The pancreas then gradually loses its ability to make insulin. When about 90% of the insulin-producing cells are lost, blood glucose levels are apt to rise very high after eating because not enough insulin is produced. Again, the excess glucose spills over into the urine. Figure 6-9 shows what typically happens when a person with diabetes mellitus eats glucose (glucose tolerance curve).

The disease is treated with diet therapy and insulin injections. The person must eat regular meals and snacks of a precise carbohydrate:protein:fat ratio and replace the missing insulin, either with injections (one to six times a day) or with an insulin pump. The pump dispenses insulin at regular intervals into the body, with higher amounts released after each meal. Regular meals are especially important for people with diabetes mellitus who use insulin, because insulin requires glucose in the bloodstream on which to act. Although these

Insulin-dependent Diabetes Mellitus • A form of diabetes prone to ketosis; it requires insulin therapy.

Noninsulin-dependent Diabetes Mellitus • A form of diabetes in which ketosis is not common and in which insulin therapy may be used but is often not required.

Atherosclerosis • A buildup of fatty material (plaque) in the arteries, including those surrounding the heart.

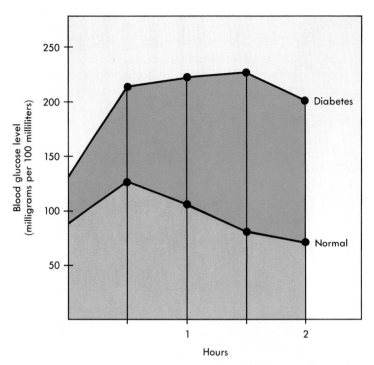

Typical responses seen after eating 50 grams (about 3 tablespoons) of glucose in normal and uncontrolled diabetic states.

FIGURE 6-9

Glucose tolerance test. These are typical responses seen after eating 50 grams of glucose in a healthy person and in a person with uncontrolled diabetes mellitus.

regimented activities may be inconvenient, they are necessary. If the person with diabetes doesn't eat, the injected insulin can cause severe low blood sugar levels—hypoglycemia—by acting on whatever little glucose is available.[16]

Noninsulin-dependent diabetes mellitus

The noninsulin-dependent form of diabetes mellitus usually begins in adulthood. It is the most common type of diabetes mellitus, accounting for about 90% of cases.[25] Most of these cases are associated with obesity; ketosis is not usually seen in this group. The large fat cells that develop in obese people cause an insulin resistance. The pancreas still makes some insulin, but body cells, especially the fat cells, resist insulin action. Therefore not much blood glucose is transported into fat cells, and the person develops hyperglycemia. If obesity is corrected, the diabetes often disappears.

People with noninsulin-dependent diabetes mellitus sometimes take oral medications that increase the capability of the pancreas to produce insulin. Regular exercise also helps because the muscles will take up more glucose. In addition regular meal patterns help minimize the high and low swing in blood glucose levels by spreading food intake throughout the day. Sometimes even insulin injections are used.

Although many cases of the noninsulin-dependent form of diabetes mellitus can be relieved by losing excess fat stores, many people are not able to lose weight. They continue to show symptoms of diabetes mellitus and suffer the consequences of both forms of this disease—blindness, loss of fingers and toes, kidney failure, and heart disease.[25] These problems are caused by nerve deterioration associated with high blood glucose levels and to a rapid progression of fatty buildup in blood vessels, which eventually chokes off the blood supply to nearby organs.

Hypoglycemia

Another carbohydrate disorder is low blood glucose levels, or hypoglycemia. Blood glucose drops to 40 to 60 milligrams per 100 milliliters of serum. This problem comes in two forms, reactive and fasting. ***Reactive hypoglycemia*** is characterized by irritability, nervousness, headache, sweating, and confusion 2 to 4 hours after eating a meal, especially one high in simple sugars.[17] Again, these symptoms make sense when you recall that the brain is particularly dependent on glucose for fuel. It is not clear what causes reactive hypoglycemia. It may be caused by the pancreas' overproduction of insulin in response to rising blood glucose levels.

A second type, ***fasting hypoglycemia,*** is usually caused by a cancer in the pancreas, which can lead to excessive insulin secretion.[20] Blood glucose falls to low levels after fasting for about a day. This form of hypoglycemia is very rare.

Some of us have bouts of hypoglycemia and never know it. To be diagnosed with hypoglycemia, both a low blood glucose level and the typical symptoms must appear together. People may think they have hypoglycemia, but few actually meet both criteria. Most hypoglycemic symptoms overlap with those of simple anxiety, stress, and depression. On a percentage basis, people complaining of fatigue, shakiness, occasional heavy sweats, and emotional instability rarely have documentable hypoglycemia.[17]

Nevertheless, if you sometimes feel you develop hypoglycemia, simple nutrition therapy is all that is often needed. Eat regular meals, make sure you have some protein and fat in each meal, and eat complex carbohydrates that contain ample soluble fiber—fruits and vegetables, for example. Fat, protein, and soluble fiber in the diet tend to moderate swings in blood glucose.[12] ●

Reactive Hypoglycemia ● Low blood sugar that follows a meal high in simple sugars, with corresponding symptoms of irritability, headache, nervousness, sweating, and confusion.

Fasting Hypoglycemia ● Low blood sugar that follows a day or so of fasting.

LIPIDS
FATS AND OILS

Your doctor informs you that "triglycerides are up." Your bill from a medical laboratory reads, "Blood lipid profile—$85." A health-food store advertisement suggests using omega-3 fatty acids to lower your blood cholesterol. Advertisers plug "lowest in saturated fat" or "cholesterol-free." We often hear these terms: triglycerides, blood lipids, omega-3 fatty acids, and cholesterol. What do they mean?

Lipids—better known as fats and oils—are probably the nutrients in our diets that concern us most. Fats (we will use this more familiar term in the chapter) contain more than twice as many kcalories as proteins or carbohydrates per gram. Eating too much saturated fat can boost a person's serum cholesterol over the desired level. This speeds the development of heart disease.[7] Perhaps you've been alarmed by newspaper reports that the leading cause of adult deaths in the United States is heart disease. That is disturbing news. But, does it mean you must stick to a boring regimen of cottage cheese and grapefruit? Read on and find out.

Although concern about fat is appropriate, certain varieties play very important roles in the body and in foods. Like many other nutrients, too much fat in the diet can cause problems, but not enough can devastate the body. Let's look at fats in detail—their functions, metabolism, food sources, and link to heart disease (again the number one killer of Americans). ●

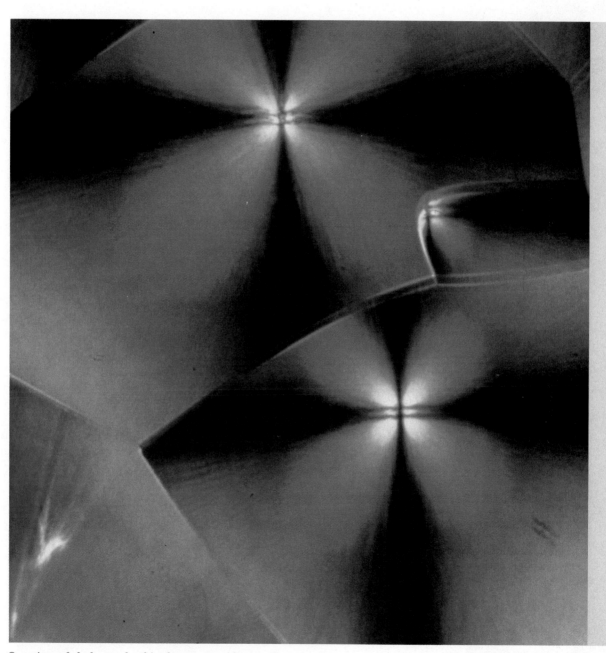

One view of cholesterol—this chapter provides another.

Are You Eating The "Clogged Channels" or "Open Tubes" Diet?

Instructions: Check the food you would typically select from the two choices you are given.

1. _____ bacon and eggs   ✓ ready to eat breakfast cereal
2. _____ doughnut or sweet roll   ✓ white or whole-wheat roll or bread, no margarine
3. _____ breakfast sausage   _____ fruit
4. _____ whole milk   ✓ lowfat milk
5. _____ cheeseburger   ✓ turkey sandwich, no cheese
6. _____ French fries   ✓ baked potato or salad with low-cal or no oil dressing
7. _____ meal including fried hamburger or fatty beef   ✓ meal including broiled lean hamburger (ground round), chicken, or fish
8. _____ creamed soup   ✓ clear soup (could have meat or vegetables in it)
9. _____ potato salad   ✓ baked potato plain
10. ✓ fruit or cream pie   _____ graham crackers
11. _____ ice cream   ✓ frozen yogurt, sherbet, ice milk
12. _____ butter or stick margarine   ✓ soft margarine in a tub

INTERPRETATION

The foods listed on the left are those that tend to be high in saturated fat, cholesterol, and total fat. Those on the right are low. If you want to follow a diet to reduce the risk of heart disease, choose the foods on the right.

ASSESS YOURSELF

FATS IN GENERAL

Fats are a diverse group of chemical compounds, but they share one main characteristic: they do not dissolve in water. When you compare the structures of two types of fats shown in Figure 7-1—a triglyceride (*E*) and cholesterol (*F*)— you will readily see how different they appear. Fats in general also contain fewer oxygens per carbon than do carbohydrates, protein, and alcohol.

FATTY ACIDS: THE SIMPLEST FORM OF FAT

The *fatty acid* is common to most fats both in the body and in foods. It is basically a long chain of carbons linked to hydrogens. If all the links (technically referred to as chemical bonds) between the carbons are single connections, a fatty acid is said to be *saturated* (Figure 7-1, *A*). In other words, it is filled with hydrogens, like a sponge saturated (full) of water.

Most saturated fatty acids remain solid at room temperature. Animal fats, for example, contain a high proportion of saturated fatty acids. The solid fat surrounding a piece of steak when it's at room temperature is a good example. Chicken fat, semisolid at room temperature, contains less saturated fat. Some saturated fats are suspended in liquid, as in milk, and so the solid nature of these fats at room temperature is not so apparent.

Fatty Acid • Acids found in fats. These are composed of a chain of carbon atoms linked by hydrogen atoms, with an acidic chemical group at one end.

Saturated Fatty Acid • A fatty acid with no carbon-carbon double bonds.

Recall from Chapter 1 the most common forms of lipids are called fats if solid at room temperature and oils if liquid at room temperature.

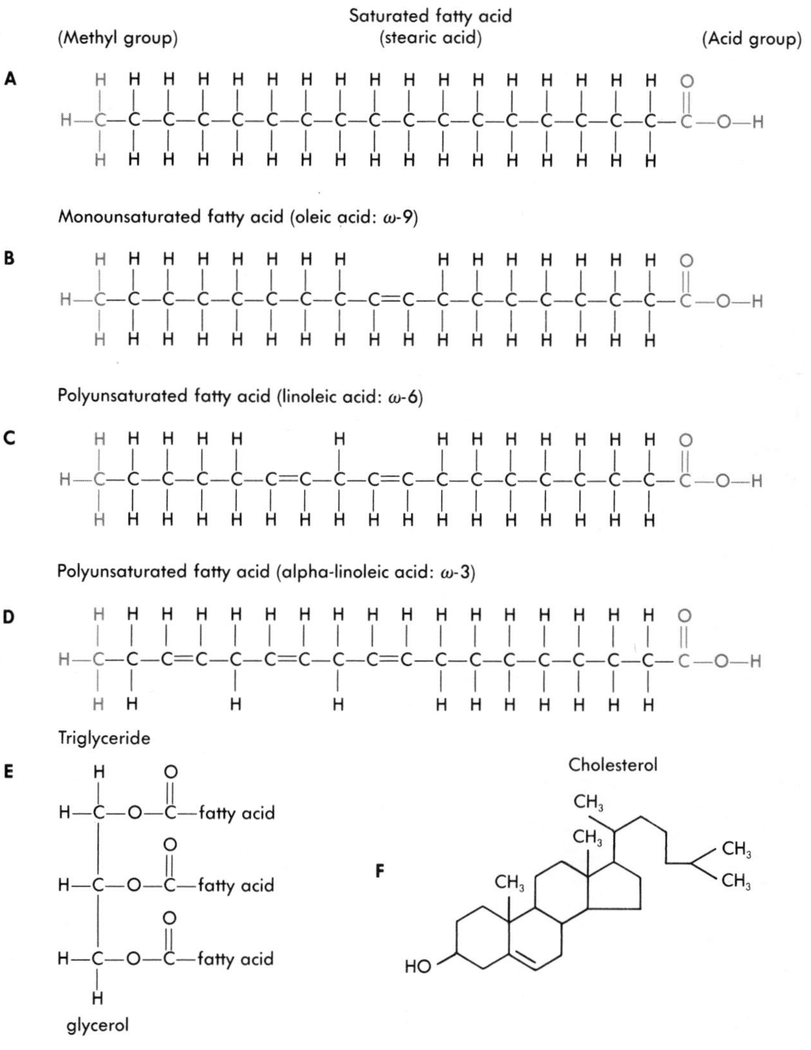

FIGURE 7-1
Examples of lipids (fats) found in foods.

If a fatty acid has one double bond between the carbons, it is **monounsaturated** (Figure 7-1, *B*). Olive and canola oils contain a high percentage of monounsaturated fatty acids. If two or more bonds between the carbons are double bonds, the fatty acid is **polyunsaturated** (Figure 7-1, *C* and *D*). Corn, soybean, and safflower oils are good sources of polyunsaturated fatty acids (Figure 7-2).

The point at which the double bonds begin in the fatty acid is important. If these double bonds start after the third carbon (counting from the end with a $-CH_3$ group), it is an **omega-3 (w-3) fatty acid.** If these bonds start after the sixth carbon, it is an **omega-6 (w-6) fatty acid,** and so on. **Alpha-linolenic acid** is the major omega-3 fatty acid found in food; **linoleic acid** is the major omega-6 fatty acid.

Essential fatty acids

Humans can't produce omega-3 and omega-6 fatty acids; we get them only by ingesting them.[5] That is why this structural distinction is important. These fatty acids are essential for us to eat, as they participate in immune processes and vision, help form cell membranes, and aid in the production of hormonelike compounds. Because we must get linoleic acid (omega-6) and alpha-linolenic acid (omega-3) from foods, they are called **essential fatty acids.**

We need to get about 1% to 2% of our total kcalories from linoleic acid. On a 2500 kcalorie diet that corresponds to 1 tablespoon of plant oil each day. We easily get that much—in mayonnaise, salad dressings, margarine, and other

Monounsaturated Fatty Acid • A fatty acid containing one carbon-carbon double bond.

Polyunsaturated Fatty Acid • A fatty acid containing two or more carbon-carbon double bonds.

Essential Fatty Acids • Fatty acids that must be present in the diet to maintain health; these consist of linoleic acid and alpha-linolenic acid.

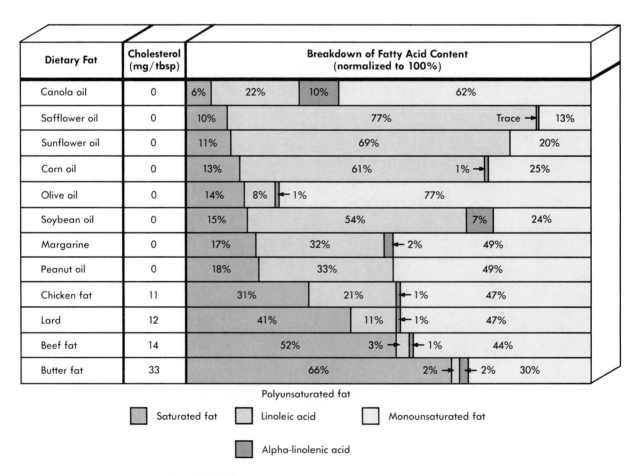

Dietary Fat	Cholesterol (mg/tbsp)	Breakdown of Fatty Acid Content (normalized to 100%)			
Canola oil	0	6%	22%	10%	62%
Safflower oil	0	10%	77%	Trace	13%
Sunflower oil	0	11%	69%		20%
Corn oil	0	13%	61%	1%	25%
Olive oil	0	14%	8%	1%	77%
Soybean oil	0	15%	54%	7%	24%
Margarine	0	17%	32%	2%	49%
Peanut oil	0	18%	33%		49%
Chicken fat	11	31%	21%	1%	47%
Lard	12	41%	11%	1%	47%
Beef fat	14	52%	3%	1%	44%
Butter fat	33	66%	2%	2%	30%

■ Saturated fat　　□ Linoleic acid (Polyunsaturated fat)　　□ Monounsaturated fat

■ Alpha-linolenic acid

FIGURE 7-2
Comparison of dietary fat for saturated fat, unsaturated fat, and cholesterol content.

foods—without even noticing. Barring these foods, regular consumption of whole grains and vegetables can also supply enough essential fatty acids.

Leading researchers also suggest that most diets should include a regular supply of either alpha-linolenic acid or its related omega-3 form, *eicosapentaenoic acid (EPA)*, which is found in high amounts in fatty, cold water fish.[17] To get this supply we need to eat either fish, such as salmon, tuna, and sardines every week, or regularly use canola or soybean oil. All are good sources of omega-3 fatty acids. We'll explore this idea further in the next few pages.

Effects of an essential fatty acid deficiency

If you don't consume enough essential fatty acids, your skin will become flaky and itchy, and diarrhea and other symptoms eventually develop.[5] But since our bodies need the equivalent of only about 1 tablespoon of polyunsaturated plant oil a day, even a lowfat diet, if it follows the Guide to Daily Food Choices, will provide this much.

> **Eicosapentaenoic Acid (EPA)** • An omega-3 fatty acid with 20 carbon atoms and 5 double bonds; present in fish oils.
>
> **Arachidonic Acid** • An omega-6 fatty acid with 20 carbon atoms and 4 double bonds; omega-6.
>
> **Eicosanoids** • Hormonelike compounds synthesized from polyunsaturated fatty acids; this class of compounds includes prostaglandins, thromboxanes, and leukotrienes.

CONCEPT CHECK

Fats are a group of compounds that don't dissolve in water. Fatty acids, the simplest forms of fats, differ from each other mainly in the number of double bonds between the carbons. Saturated fatty acids contain no carbon-carbon double bonds, monounsaturated fatty acids contain one, and polyunsaturated fatty acids contain two or more. If double bonds begin at the third carbon from the $-CH_3$ end of the chain, the fatty acid is an omega-3 fatty acid. If the double bonds begin at the sixth carbon, it is an omega-6 fatty acid. Humans can't make either omega-3 or omega-6 fatty acids, and so they are essential parts of a diet.

Putting fatty acids to work in the body

Once linoleic acid is in a cell, it can be lengthened with more carbons and have more double bonds added. This yields *arachidonic acid.* Alpha-linolenic acid can also be lengthened and have double bonds added to form EPA, the fish oil fatty acid. How fast humans can form EPA is still debatable, but body synthesis appears too inefficient to supply adequate EPA.[17]

Arachidonic acid and EPA are used for synthesizing a group of hormonelike compounds called *eicosanoids.* Prostaglandins are among these. Eicosanoids regulate vital body functions, such as blood pressure, contraction of certain types of muscles, blood clotting, immune responses, and stomach secretions. When cells make eicosanoids, they most often use the omega-6 fatty acid, arachidonic acid, because it is usually more plentiful in the body than EPA. However, in cells of people who eat a lot of fish, many eicosanoids are also made from EPA.[12]

The type of fatty acid used for synthesizing eicosanoids is important to consider. For example, minor differences in eicosanoid structure because of the type of fatty acid used profoundly affect the tendency of blood to clot. Overall, the omega-6 products made from arachidonic acid increase blood clotting, while the omega-3 products made from EPA decrease it. The differences between omega-3 and omega-6 eicosanoids can also affect blood pressure and inflammatory processes. Overall, the omega-3 forms show lower values/responses.[12]

Studies from Scandinavia, the Netherlands, and Japan show that people who eat fish about twice a week (8 ounces—240 grams—total weekly intake) run lower risks for heart attacks than do people who rarely eat fish. In these cases the omega-3 fatty acids in fish oil probably reduce blood clotting. In turn, the risk of heart attack decreases, especially for people already at high risk (see the

Nutrition Issue, p. 212, to learn about the link between blood clots and heart attacks).[17] Greenland Eskimos consume a lot of fish, seal, and whale, and also have a greatly reduced risk for heart attacks.

Should we be eating "Eskimo diets"?

Blood clotting is a normal body process. Eskimos who eat a lot of seafoods are more likely to have some types of strokes than other people because their blood does not clot readily enough. Too much omega-3 fatty acid intake could allow uncontrolled bleeding. A reduction in blood-clotting ability then can be seen as a two-edged sword. Because of the possibility of harm, we recommend not using fish oil supplements—stick to eating fish two to three times a week. Atlantic and Pacific herring, sardines, Atlantic halibut and salmon, lake trout, coho, pink and king salmon, blue fish, albacore tuna, and Atlantic mackerel are among the fish with the greatest omega-3 fatty acid contents. New research may soon add more types of fish to this list.

We also do not recommend consuming fish oil supplements (without a physician's advice) because they often contain high amounts of cholesterol, vitamins A and D, and uncommon fatty acids. Any of these substances taken in high amounts can lead to health problems. Current studies also show that consuming fish oil supplements can impede blood glucose regulation in people who have diabetes mellitus, and even raise cholesterol levels in people with high blood fat (triglyceride) levels.[12] This increase in blood cholesterol can speed development of heart disease (again see the Nutrition Issue, p. 212). Therefore it is better to eat fish than to emphasize fish oil supplements.

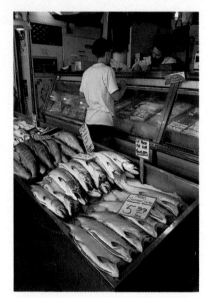

Eating fish regularly is linked to less heart disease in some groups of people, such as the Dutch and Japanese.

CONCEPT CHECK

When cells use omega-3 fatty acids to make hormonelike compounds called eicosanoids, the products differ markedly from those made from omega-6 fatty acids. In general, products made from omega-3 fatty acids tend to reduce blood clotting, blood pressure, and inflammatory responses in the body. Presently the recommendation to eat fish about twice a week is a good guide to provide omega-3 fatty acids for the body.

Chain length affects fatty acid characteristics

Fats in foods that contain primarily saturated fatty acids are solid at room temperature, especially if the fatty acids have a **long chain** (12 carbons or longer). **Medium-chain** saturated fatty acids (six to ten carbons long), such as those in coconut oil, produce liquid oils at room temperature. The shorter chain length overrides the effect of saturation. **Short-chain** saturated fatty acids (less than six carbons long) also form liquid oils at room temperature. Dairy fats are sources of these short-chain fatty acids. Fats containing primarily polyunsaturated or monounsaturated fatty acids are usually liquid at room temperature. These are not affected by chain length.[6]

The capability of some saturated fatty acids of short- or medium-chain lengths to form oils at room temperature is significant. You might assume—incorrectly—that nondairy creamers are a healthful substitute for cream because cream has a high percentage of saturated fat. However, many nondairy creamers contain coconut oil, which is also high in saturated fat. Lowfat milk is a much more healthful alternative to both. Manufacturers use coconut oil because it allows the product a long shelf life. You will understand why when we examine the issue of rancidity of fats in a later section.

Hydrogenation of fatty acids

In some food preparations such as pastry making, solid fats work better than liquid oils. To solidify vegetable oils for this and other uses into shortenings

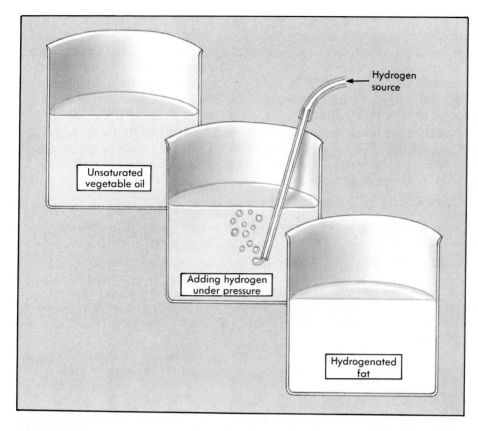

FIGURE 7-3
How liquid fatty acids become solid in margarine production. Unsaturated fat starts out in a liquid form. Hydrogen atoms are bubbled in (hydrogenation), changing double bonds to single bonds, as well as producing other changes in fatty acid structure. The hydrogenated product is now either semisolid or solid.

and margarines, the polyunsaturated fatty acids must become more saturated. In other words, more hydrogens must be added to turn double bonds between the carbons into single bonds. In the **hydrogenation** process, the hydrogens are added by bubbling hydrogen gas into liquid vegetable oils. As hydrogenation changes many carbon-carbon double bonds to single bonds, other structural changes in the fatty acid occur as well (Figure 7-3). Generally, the more hydrogenation that occurs, the harder the product is; stick margarine is more hydrogenated (saturated) than tub margarine, for example.[6] Note that if a liquid oil is listed before any hydrogenated oil on food labels, the food probably contains a greater amount of unsaturated than saturated fat.

Rancidity

Decomposing oils emit a disagreeable odor and taste sour and stale. As double bonds in fats break down, the by-products are said to be **rancid**. Ultraviolet rays of light, oxygen, and some chemicals can attack double bonds, break them, and in turn destroy the structure of polyunsaturated fatty acids. Saturated fats can much more readily resist these effects. Why?

Even though eating rancid oils can cause sickness, the odor and taste generally discourage us from eating enough to become sick. However, rancidity is a problem for manufacturers because it reduces a product's shelf life. Therefore manufacturers add hydrogenated plant oils to products to increase shelf life. This again explains why coconut oil—full of saturated fat—is added to nondairy creamers. Foods most likely to become rancid are fatty fish and fish

Hydrogenation causes some of the unsaturated fats to change shape, casting them in a so-called *trans* shape. This structural change also causes the fats to raise serum cholesterol levels like saturated fats do, providing another reason for us to limit intake of hydrogenated fat.

Antioxidant • A compound that can donate electrons to electron-seeking (oxidizing) compounds.

BHA and BHT • Butylated hydroxyanisol and butylated hydroxytoluene—two common synthetic antioxidants added to foods.

Glycerol • A 3-carbon atom alcohol used to form triglycerides.

oil, deep-fried foods, and foods with a large amount of exposed surface (such as powdered eggs or powdered milk).

Vitamin E helps protect foods against rancidity as it acts as an ***antioxidant.*** It guards against deterioration caused by various agents, such as metals found as impurities. The vitamin E that occurs naturally in plant oils inhibits the breakdown of double bonds in fatty acids. When food manufacturers want to prevent rancidity in polyunsaturated fats, they often add ***BHA and BHT.*** (Chapter 17 discusses the safety of these additives.) Look for these food additives in salad dressings, cake mixes, and other products that contain fat. They can even be added to a food's paper packaging. Manufacturers also tightly seal products and use other methods to reduce the presence of oxygen inside packages.

CONCEPT CHECK

At room temperature, saturated fatty acids tend to form solid fats, whereas polyunsaturated and monounsaturated fatty acids tend to form liquid oils. Hydrogenation is the process of turning carbon-carbon double bonds of fatty acids into single bonds by adding hydrogens. This solidifies the fat and reduces rancidity. The presence of vitamin E in oils naturally limits rancidity in unsaturated fatty acids.

TRIGLYCERIDES

Fats and oils in foods are mostly in triglyceride form. The same is true for fats found in body structures. Some fatty acids are found attached to proteins in the bloodstream as they are being transported, but fatty acids usually do not exist in the body as such. Instead, they form into triglycerides.

Triglyceride molecules contain a simple three-carbon alcohol, ***glycerol,*** which serves as a backbone for the three attached fatty acids (Figure 7-1, *E*). Removing one fatty acid from a triglyceride forms a diglyceride. Removing two fatty acids from a triglyceride forms a monoglyceride. Before dietary fats are absorbed in the small intestine, the upper and lower fatty acids are typically removed from the triglyceride molecules. This produces fatty acids, monoglycerides, and some glycerol molecules. These are absorbed into the intestinal cells. After absorption, the fatty acids and monoglycerides are mostly reformed into triglycerides.

Putting triglycerides to work in the body

Again, most key functions of fat in the body require the use of fatty acids in the form of a triglyceride. In the body, triglycerides are used for fuel, energy storage, and insulation, and for transporting fat-soluble vitamins. In foods, triglycerides impart the taste and texture we consider desirable, and they give us a feeling of satiety (fullness) after eating.

Providing energy for the body

The fatty acids supplied by triglycerides both in the diet and those stored in fat tissue are the main fuel for muscles while at rest and during light activity. Only in endurance exercises, such as long distance running and cycling, do muscles burn a lot of carbohydrate in addition to fatty acids. Other body tissues also use fatty acids for energy. Overall, about 40% of the energy used by the entire body at rest and during light activity comes from fatty acids. On a whole body basis the use of fatty acids by muscles is balanced by the use of glucose by the brain and red blood cells. Recall from Chapter 6 that all cells also need carbohydrate to use fatty acids for fuel; "fats burn in a fire of carbohydrate."

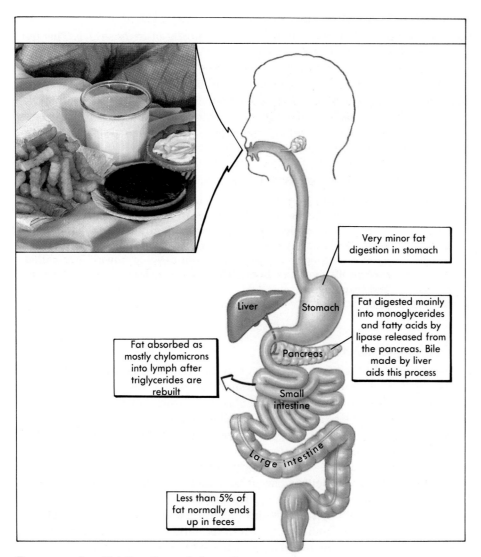

For your review. Fat digestion and absorption.

Storing energy

We store energy mainly in the form of triglycerides. The body's ability to store fat is essentially limitless. Its fat storage sites, adipose (fat) cells, can increase about 50 times in weight. If the amount of fat to be stored exceeds the ability of the cells to expand, the body can form new fat cells. (We will discuss this further in Chapter 11.)

When we store fats in fat cells, we store little else; fat cells are about 80% fat and only 20% water and protein. In contrast, if we stored energy as muscle tissue, we would need to store a lot of water, since muscle is about 73% water. The same is true for energy stored in the form of the carbohydrate glycogen. A 3-day supply of energy as glycogen would weigh about 14 pounds (6 kilograms). Think of the consequences if we stored energy as muscle tissue or glycogen.

Another advantage to storing triglycerides for energy is that they are energy dense. Recall that fats in the form of triglycerides yield 9 kcalories per gram, whereas proteins and carbohydrates yield only 4 kcalories per gram. In addition, extra energy is required to chemically convert glucose to store it as fat. Because fat requires fewer conversions before we store it, it costs less energy for the body to store energy as fat than as carbohydrate.

Insulating and protecting the body

The layer of fat just beneath our skin is made mostly of triglycerides. This fat tissue insulates and protects some organs—kidneys, for example—from injury. We usually don't notice the important insulating function of fat tissue because we wear clothes and add more as needed. But a layer of insulating fat is quite apparent in animals, particularly in those from cold climates. Polar bears, walruses, and whales all build a thick layer of fat tissue around themselves to insulate against cold-weather environments. The extra fat also provides energy storage for times when food is scarce.

 We can never be totally fat free because fat is an essential part of all cells. But people with *anorexia nervosa* often lose 25% or more of body weight and end up about as fat free as is biologically possible. In place of the layer of fat tissue under the skin, people with anorexia nervosa often develop downy hair called *lanugo* all over the body. These hairs insulate by standing up and trapping air.

Transporting fat-soluble vitamins

Triglycerides and other fats in foods carry fat-soluble vitamins to the small intestine and aid their absorption. If the small intestine is diseased, however, it may not be able to properly digest and absorb fat from foods. When this happens, the unabsorbed fat carries the fat-soluble vitamins—A, D, E, and K—into the large intestine. From there they are eliminated with the stool, and the body loses the benefits of the vitamins.

People who generally absorb fat poorly, such as those with the disease cystic fibrosis, are at risk for deficiencies of fat-soluble vitamins, especially vitamin K. A similar risk accrues from taking mineral oil as a laxative at meal times. Since the body cannot digest or absorb mineral oil, the undigested oil carries the fat-soluble vitamins from the meal into the large intestine where they are eliminated. This makes mineral oil a poor choice for a laxative.

Providing *satiety*

If you are fond of cheesecake, you know that a little goes a long way. It's the triglycerides in foods that help give us a full and contented feeling after a meal. The fat we eat triggers hormones that cause the stomach to retain foods longer than when we eat mostly carbohydrate or protein. This is why a high-fat meal allows us to feel full longer.

Many people who want to lose weight cut out much of the fat they eat. However, if dieters cut out too much fat, they lose its satiety value and get hungry quicker. Eating too little fat then actually defeats the intent to slim down (see Chapter 11 for further discussion).

Providing flavor and texture to foods

Triglycerides and other fats impart generally desirable textures and flavors to foods. Many flavorings dissolve in fat. Heating spices in oil intensifies the flavors of an Indian curry or Mexican dish far more than simply adding them at the table. Fat carries these flavors to the sensory cells that discriminate taste and smell in the mouth. We quickly associate *flavorful* with fatty foods. Foods that have had too much fat removed often lack taste and feel dry, as if they need something to bind them together.

If you have ever eaten a high-fat cheese or cream cheese, you probably agree that fat melting on the tongue feels good. This love of fat is universal. Western diets, Eskimo diets, and Mediterranean diets are all high in fat. Immigrants to Western cultures quickly embrace the high-fat diet.

> **Lecithin** • A phospholipid that contains two fatty acids, a phosphate group, and a choline (vitamin-like) molecule.

CONCEPT CHECK

Triglyceride is the major form of fat in the body and in food. Triglycerides in the body are used for and stored as energy; they are used to insulate and protect body organs, to transport fat-soluble vitamins, and to provide satiety to a meal. Triglycerides also add flavor and texture to foods.

PHOSPHOLIPIDS

Phospholipids are another class of lipid. Like triglycerides they are built on a backbone of glycerol. However, at least one fatty acid is replaced with a compound containing phosphorus (and often other chemical additions, such as ones containing nitrogen). Many types of phospholipids exist in the body, especially in the brain. They form important parts of cell membranes. **Lecithin** is a common example. It is found in cells and participates in fat digestion in the intestine. Egg yolks contain lecithin in abundance.

Some phospholipids, such as lecithin, function as emulsifiers. By breaking fat globules into small droplets, emulsifiers enable a fat to be suspended in water. The ability of a phospholipid to emulsify fat depends on whether it has various chemical groups. For example, the fatty acid end of lecithin attracts fat. The phosphorus and nitrogen at the other end of lecithin form an area that attracts water. When lecithin is added to an oil and water mixture, it then acts as numerous bridges that in turn form tiny oil droplets surrounded by thin shells of water. In an emulsified solution millions of tiny oil droplets are separated by shells of water (Figure 7-4).

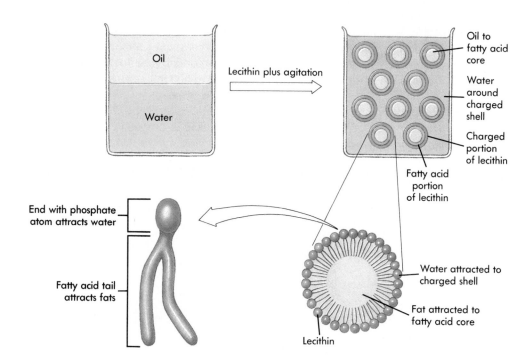

FIGURE 7-4

Emulsification and emulsifiers. Emulsifiers can organize oil and water to form droplets of oil surrounded by shells of water. Forming these droplets is a key step in fat digestion.

Bile • A substance that is made by the liver and stored in the gallbladder; it is released during digestion to aid in fat absorption.

Commercial salad dressings find practical use for emulsification; emulsifiers, such as Polysorbate 60, mono and diglycerides, and lecithin, are added to salad dressings and other fat-rich products to keep the vegetable oils and other fats suspended in the water. Eggs baked in cakes likewise suspend the fats in the fluid ingredients. Recall that emulsifiers are also crucial to complete the processes of digesting and absorbing dietary fats in the small intestine. The body's main emulsifiers, lecithin and **bile,** are produced by the liver and released into the small intestine via the gallbladder during digestion. By breaking up the fat globules, the emulsifiers create more fat surface for fat-digesting enzymes to act on.

Perhaps you've heard that it is important to take a lecithin supplement to maintain all your body cells. This health-food notion has been encouraged by some popular publications, but has no scientific basis. Eating lecithin isn't even an efficient way to obtain it for the body's use because the digestive system dismantles most of it before it even enters the bloodstream. All the lecithin you need for building cell membranes and other functions can be made by your body; in other words, lecithin is not an essential nutrient. Large doses of lecithin can even cause stomach upsets, sweating, salivation, and loss of appetite.

STEROLS

What do sterols have in common with the other fats we have discussed? Their multiringed structure makes them very different from the other fats you have seen. Consider the important sterol cholesterol (see Figure 7-1, *G*). This waxy substance doesn't look like a triglyceride—it doesn't have a glycerol backbone or any fatty acids. But since it doesn't dissolve in water, it is a fat.

Cholesterol is used to make some important hormones, such as the estrogens and testosterone. Cholesterol is used to make bile, a key emulsifier needed for fat digestion. Cholesterol is even incorporated directly into cell membranes, often bound to a fatty acid.[13] In other words, cholesterol is an essential part of life. We can get cholesterol into our bloodstream either from foods or by manufacturing it ourselves. Each day your liver makes about 700 milligrams of cholesterol, which circulates through the bloodstream to function as the body needs it. In comparison, we eat about 300 to 500 milligrams per day. When a diet doesn't contain enough cholesterol, the liver makes more.

Cholesterol is found only in the animal foods we eat (Table 7-1). An egg yolk contains about 220 milligrams of cholesterol. This is our main dietary source. However, humans can make all they need if they don't eat enough of it. Some

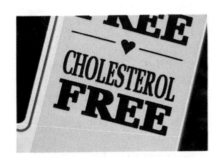

Choosing a diet lower in cholesterol is on many people's minds these days.

TABLE 7-1

Cholesterol content of common measures of selected foods (in ascending order).

Food	Amount	Cholesterol in Milligrams	Food	Amount	Cholesterol in Milligrams
Milk, skim	1 cup	4	Clams, halibut, tuna	3 oz	55
Mayonnaise	1 T	10	Chicken, turkey, light meat	3 oz	70
Butter	1 pat	11			
Lard	1 T	12	Beef,* pork*	3 oz	75
Cottage cheese	½ cup	15	Lamb, crab	3 oz	85
Milk, low fat, 2%	1 cup	22	Shrimp, lobster	3 oz	90-110
Half and half	¼ cup	23	Heart, beef	3 oz	164
Hot dog*	1	29	Egg, (egg yolk)*	1 each	213
Ice cream, ≈ 10% fat	½ cup	30	Liver, beef	3 oz	410
Cheese, cheddar	1 oz	30	Kidney	3 oz	587
Milk, whole*	1 cup	34	Brains	3 oz	2637
Oysters, salmon	3 oz	40			

*Leading contributors of cholesterol to the U.S. diet.

plants contain related sterols, but none we typically eat contains cholesterol. Manufacturers who advertise peanut butter, vegetable shortening, margarines, and vegetable oils as containing "no cholesterol" are taking advantage of uninformed consumers. Peanut butter and margarine never contain cholesterol—it is not part of their nature!

CONCEPT CHECK

Phospholipids differ from triglycerides: their glycerol backbone has fatty acids attached, but at least one fatty acid is replaced by another type of compound. Many phospholipids act as emulsifiers. These are compounds that suspend fat as small droplets in water. Phospholipids also form parts of cell membranes and other molecules of the body. Sterols are another class of lipids but are constructed quite differently than either triglycerides or phospholipids. Cholesterol, a sterol, forms hormones and bile and is found in cell membranes; it is essential to the body. Cholesterol is manufactured in the liver and if sufficient amounts are not ingested, the body makes up the difference. Of the foods we typically eat, cholesterol is found naturally only in those of animal origin.

CARRYING FATS IN THE BLOODSTREAM

Fat and water don't mix. This incompatibility presents a challenge in transporting fats through the watery mediums of blood and lymph systems.

Transporting dietary fats

Once dietary fat is digested and absorbed into the small intestine cells, triglycerides are reformed. These combine with phospholipids and cholesterol to form a chylomicron, which is a large droplet of fat (actually triglyceride) surrounded by a thin shell of protein, cholesterol, and phospholipid. This combination of fat (lipid) and protein is called a **lipoprotein**[13] (Figure 7-5). The shell around the chylomicron allows the fat inside to float freely in the water-based bloodstream. Some proteins in the shell also signal to other cells a chylomicron identity.

The chylomicron particle essentially emulsifies dietary fats before they enter the bloodstream. This process resembles the action of lecithin and bile in the small intestine when they emulsify dietary fats during digestion. The difference is that in digestion a layer of water—rather than one of protein and various fats—surrounds the fat droplets.

Chylomicrons enter the lymphatic system and travel into the bloodstream. Once there, the triglycerides in the chylomicrons are broken down into fatty acids and glycerol by the blood vessel enzyme **lipoprotein lipase.** Muscle cells, fat cells, and other cells in the vicinity then absorb most of the fatty acids. Cells can immediately use absorbed fatty acids for fuel or reform and store them as triglycerides. Muscle cells tend to burn the fatty acids, while fat cells tend to store them. When most triglycerides have been removed from a chylomicron, what remains is mostly cholesterol and protein. This *remnant* is taken up by the liver and metabolized (Figure 7-6).[10]

Transporting fats from nondietary sources

The liver produces more fats than any other body organ. When you eat too much protein, carbohydrate, or alcohol, your liver breaks them down and uses the resulting carbons, hydrogens, and energy to make things such as triglycerides and cholesterol. The liver then faces the same problem posed to the small intestine: how to equip newly synthesized fats so these can float in the water base of the bloodstream. To enable the fats to float, the liver coats the cholesterol and triglycerides with a shell of protein and fats. This is similar to

Lipoprotein • A compound found in the bloodstream containing a core of lipids with a shell of protein, phospholipid, and cholesterol.

Lipoprotein Lipase • An enzyme attached to the outsides of the cells that line the bloodstream; it breaks down triglycerides into free fatty acids and glycerol.

The whole process of clearing chylomicrons from the bloodstream after eating takes a few hours or longer. Because chylomicrons can affect results of blood tests, people often fast for at least 14 hours before undergoing certain tests.

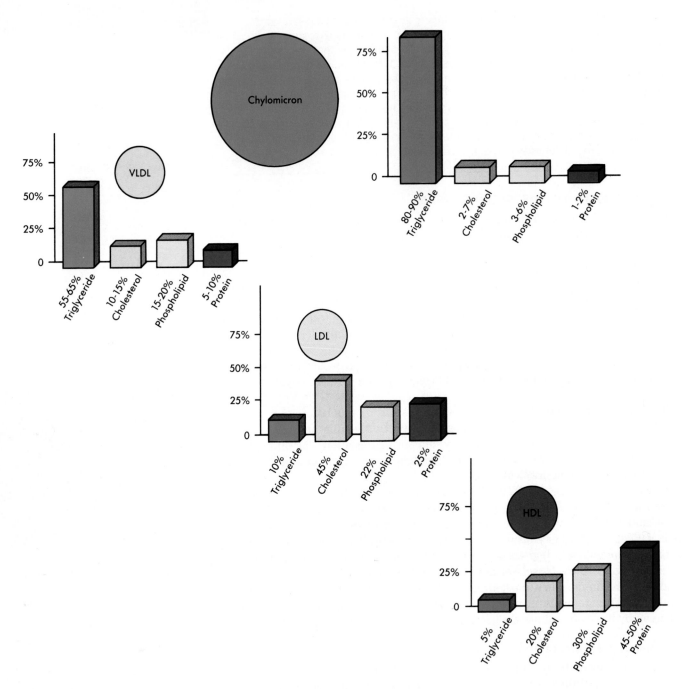

FIGURE 7-5
The structure and composition of the lipoproteins. This structure allows fats to circulate in the water-based bloodstream.

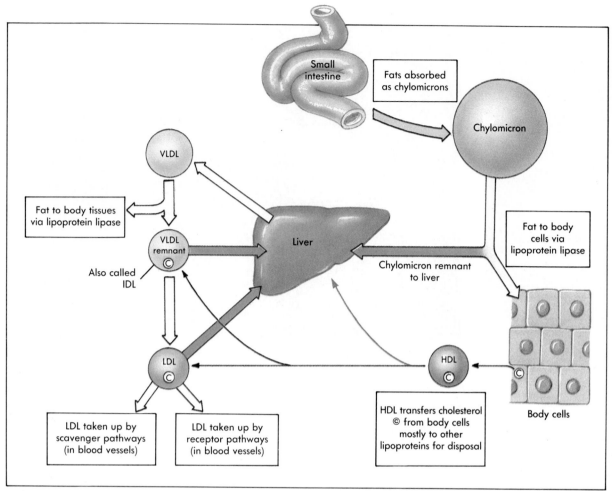

FIGURE 7-6

Lipoprotein interactions. Chylomicrons carry absorbed fat to body cells. VLDLs carry fat produced in the liver to body cells. LDLs arise from VLDLs and carry mostly cholesterol *to* cells. HDLs carry cholesterol *from* cells to other lipoproteins and the liver for excretion.

the packaging of a chylomicron. The liver's version of a chylomicron is called a ***very low density lipoprotein (VLDL).***[10]

When the VLDLs leave the liver, the enzyme lipoprotein lipase on the blood vessels breaks down the triglyceride in the VLDLs into fatty acids and glycerol. Because fats are less dense than water, VLDLs become much heavier—proportionately denser—as triglyceride is released. What remains of the VLDL then becomes an ***intermediate density lipoprotein (IDL).*** About two-thirds of the IDLs are taken up by the liver and the rest convert to ***low density lipoprotein (LDL).*** An LDL is composed primarily of cholesterol. It contains even less fat than an IDL and so is even heavier. For a cell to absorb an LDL, it needs a specific LDL port (technically known as a receptor) on its outer membrane to bind the main LDL protein, called ***apolipoprotein*** B.[10]

To review, VLDLs leave the liver with triglycerides and cholesterol. Enzymes on blood vessels then remove most triglycerides, changing VLDLs to IDLs. Some IDLs then become LDLs. The LDL particle in the bloodstream still contains the cholesterol that originally came from the liver. Cells with LDL receptors pick up the LDL particles in a process called the ***receptor pathway.*** When the LDL particles are received by a cell, they are broken down and their cholesterol and protein parts are transported throughout the cell. In this way

Very Low Density Lipoprotein (VLDL) • The lipoprotein that initially leaves the liver; it carries cholesterol and lipids newly synthesized by the liver.

Intermediate Density Lipoprotein (IDL) • The product formed after a very low density lipoprotein (VLDL) has most of its triglycerides removed.

Low Density Lipoprotein (LDL) • The product of the intermediate density lipoprotein (IDL) that contains primarily cholesterol; an elevated level is strongly linked to heart disease.

Apolipoproteins • Proteins imbedded in the outer shell of lipoproteins.

Receptor Pathway For Cholesterol Uptake • A process by which LDL molecules (cholesterol containing) are bound by cell receptors and incorporated into the cell.

Scavenger Pathway For Cholesterol Uptake • A process by which LDL molecules (cholesterol containing) are taken up by scavenger cells imbedded in the blood vessels.

Plaque • A cholesterol-rich substance deposited in the blood vessels; it contains various white blood cells, cholesterol and other lipids, and eventually calcium.

High Density Lipoprotein (HDL) • Lipoprotein synthesized by the liver and small intestine that picks up cholesterol from dying cells and other sources and transfers it to the other lipoproteins in the bloodstream. A low HDL level increases the risk for heart disease.

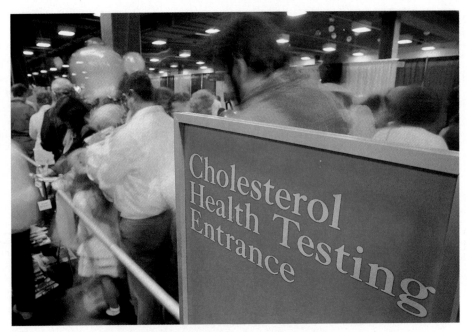

Every adult should know his or her own cholesterol level.

the cell absorbs the building blocks needed to make sex hormones and other compounds.

If LDLs are not rapidly taken up by body tissues, scavenger cells buried in blood vessels detect, alter (called oxidize), engulf, and digest the extra circulating LDL particles.[18] During this **scavenger pathway** for LDL uptake, the scavenger cell's alteration of the LDL molecule so that it cannot reenter the bloodstream is a key part of the process. Over time cholesterol inundates the scavenger cells.

 Some nutrients have antioxidant properties, as we cover in detail in Chapter 9. Fruits and vegetables are rich in many of these, such as beta-carotene and vitamins C and E. Eating fruits and vegetables regularly may then be one positive step we can take to slow the progression of heart disease. Recent research supports this hypothesis.[10]

When scavenger cells have collected and deposited cholesterol for many years at a heavy pace, cholesterol builds up on the inner blood vessel wall—in arteries especially—and **plaque** develops (Figure 7-7). The plaque eventually mixes with protein and is then covered with a cap of muscle cells and calcium. Atherosclerosis, hardening of the arteries, develops as plaque grows in the vessel.[19] This chokes off blood supply to organs, setting the stage for a heart attack and other problems (see the Nutrition Issue, p. 212).[7]

One important key to the rate of atherosclerosis buildup may lie in the liver. Because it contains about 75% of the LDL receptors in the body, the liver is the main regulator of blood cholesterol levels. For people who lack enough LDL receptors—genetic inheritance and a diet lush in saturated fat are two possible contributors—plaque build-up accelerates.

A final critical participant in this extensive process of fat transport is the **high density lipoprotein (HDL)**. Its high proportion of protein makes it the

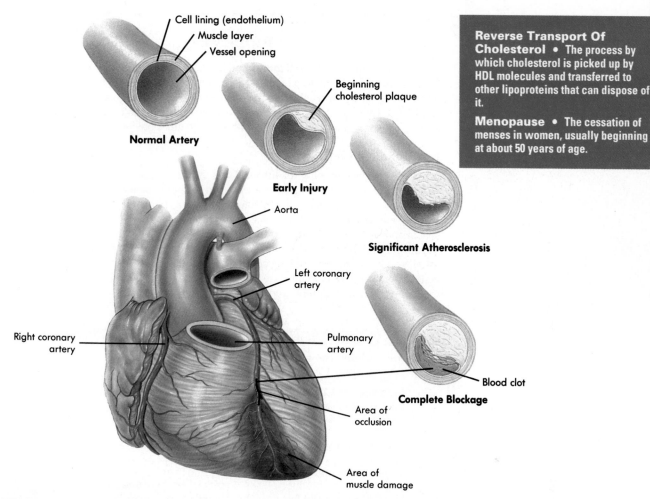

Normal Artery

- Cell lining (endothelium)
- Muscle layer
- Vessel opening

Early Injury

- Beginning cholesterol plaque

Significant Atherosclerosis

- Aorta
- Left coronary artery
- Right coronary artery
- Pulmonary artery
- Area of occlusion
- Area of muscle damage

Complete Blockage

- Blood clot

Reverse Transport Of Cholesterol • The process by which cholesterol is picked up by HDL molecules and transferred to other lipoproteins that can dispose of it.

Menopause • The cessation of menses in women, usually beginning at about 50 years of age.

FIGURE 7-7

The road to a heart attack. First an injury most likely causes initiation of the process. Then there is progression caused by buildup of plaque on the artery walls. The heart attack represents the termination of the process of atherosclerosis—in this case it resulted from blockage of the left coronary artery by a blood clot, the typical cause. The heart muscle that is serviced by the portion of the coronary artery beyond the point of blockage is damaged and may die. This can lead to a significant drop in heart function and often total heart failure.

heaviest (densest) lipoprotein. The liver and intestine produce HDLs that roam the bloodstream, picking up cholesterol from dying cells and other sources. The HDLs donate the cholesterol primarily to other lipoproteins for transport back to the liver for excretion (see Figure 7-6). This process is called ***reverse transport of cholesterol***.[7] Some HDLs may head back directly to the liver as well.

Large-scale studies clearly demonstrate that a person's HDL-cholesterol level can closely predict the risk for premature heart disease.[8] Increased risk arises if little blood cholesterol is transported back to the liver because of low HDL levels. If serum HDL-cholesterol level exceeds 60 milligrams per 100 milliliters, the risk of premature heart disease is likely to be low. If the HDL-cholesterol level is less than 35, the risk of developing premature heart disease increases.

Men's HDL-cholesterol levels often range from the high 30s to high 40s, while women's range from the low 50s to low 60s. The more desirable levels in women are one reason why, at least before ***menopause,*** they have a lower risk for heart attacks than men. The estrogen produced by women during child-bearing years appears to help keep HDL-cholesterol levels high.

We say *premature* heart disease because eventually everyone dies, often of heart disease. Heart-disease deaths of people in their 40s through 60s—this is about 10 to 30 years before statistics say they should die—are considered premature.

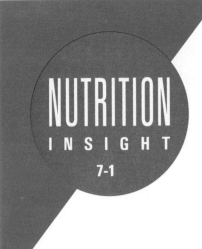

HIDDEN FAT

Some fat in food is obvious: butter on bread, mayonnaise in potato salad, and marbling in raw meat. Fat is less obvious in other foods that contribute much fat to our diets. Fat is hidden in whole milk, pastries, cookies, cake, cheese, hot dogs, crackers, French fries, and ice cream. When we try to cut down on fat intake, hidden fats need to be exposed and controlled, along with the more obvious sources.

Finding hidden fat

A place to begin searching for hidden fat is on the labels of foods you buy in the grocery store. Some words that can alert you to the presence of fat are chocolate; animal fats, such as bacon, beef, ham, lamb, meat, pork, chicken, or turkey fats; lard; vegetable oils; nuts; dairy fats, such as butter and cream; egg and egg-yolk solids; and hydrogenated shortening or vegetable oil. Conveniently, the label lists ingredients by order of weight in the product. If fat is one of the first ingredients listed, you know you are looking at a high-fat product. Whether or not to choose it depends on how you intend to use it in your diet: as a staple item, as an occasional treat, or as a garnish for other foods.

TABLE 7-2

Tips for avoiding too much fat and saturated fat

1. Steam, boil, or bake vegetables. For a change, stirfry in a small amount of vegetable oil. Consider buying an insert for a pot so you can easily steam your vegetables.
2. Season vegetables with herbs and spices rather than with sauces, butter, or margarine.
3. Try lemon juice on salad or use limited amounts of oil-based salad dressing.
4. To reduce saturated fat, use tub margarine instead of butter or stick margarine in baked products. When possible, use vegetable oil instead of either of these solid fats or hydrogenated shortenings.
5. Try whole-grain flours to enhance flavors when baking goods with less fat and cholesterol-containing ingredients.
6. Replace whole milk with skim or lowfat milk in puddings, soups, and baked products.
7. Substitute plain lowfat yogurt, blender-whipped lowfat cottage cheese, or buttermilk in recipes that call for sour cream or mayonnaise.
8. Choose lean cuts of meat. Limit bacon, ribs, and meat loaf.
9. Trim fat from meat before and after cooking.
10. Roast, bake, or broil meat, poultry, and fish so fat drains away as the food cooks.
11. Remove skin from poultry before cooking.
12. Use a nonstick pan for cooking so added fat will be unnecessary; use a vegetable spray for frying.
13. Chill meat or poultry broth until the fat solidifies. Spoon off the fat before using the broth.
14. Eat a vegetarian main dish at least once a week. Include fish (cooked without much added fat) in the diet every week.
15. Limit high-fat cheese intake.
16. Think about the balance of fats in your menu. If your meal contains whole milk, cheese, ice cream, a higher fat meat, or poultry with skin, use margarine and unsaturated vegetable oils for your spreads and dressings. Small amounts of butter, sour cream, or cream cheese can be included if other menu items are low in saturated fat.

TABLE 7-2

Tips for avoiding too much fat and saturated fat—cont'd

With an eye on dining out . . .

Appetizers

Best bets:	Vegetable juice, bouillon, fresh fruit, celery, radishes
Avoid	Deep-fried vegetables, creamed soups

Meat/Poultry/Fish

Best bets:	Roasted, baked, broiled—trim off excess fat
Avoid:	Fried, sauteed, breaded, gravy, ribs, fatty luncheon meats

Eggs (you may wish to limit as well)

Best bets:	Poached, boiled
Avoid:	Fried, scrambled

Potatoes/Rice/Pasta

Best bets:	Mashed, baked, boiled, steamed
Avoid:	Home fried, French fried, creamed, escalloped

Vegetables

Best bets:	Steamed, stewed, boiled
Avoid:	Creamed, fried, sauteed

Breads

Best bets:	Plain bread, toast, dinner rolls, or muffins
Avoid:	Sweet rolls, coffee cake, croissants, biscuits

Fats

Best bets:	Limited amounts of butter, margarine or reduced-calorie salad dressing, lowfat yogurt, lowfat cheeses
Avoid:	Gravy, cream sauces, fried foods, heavy-based dressings, sour cream, whole milk cheeses

Desserts

Best bets:	Fresh fruits, nonfat frozen yogurt, sorbet, angel food cake, split a dessert with a friend, new fat-free cake products
Avoid:	Pastries, custard, ice cream

Beverages

Best bets:	Water, coffee, tea, lowfat or skim milk, diet soft drinks
Avoid:	Chocolate milk, milk shakes, regular soft drinks, whole milk

Fast foods are notable for their content of hidden fat (see Table 3-3). Fast-food outlets often have nutritional information on their products, but you usually have to ask for it. This literature and your own common sense can help to reduce fat intake from these sources. When you can't find a nutrition label, remember that moderating portion size is a good way to keep fat intake down.

Trim meats before cooking to help reduce your fat intake.

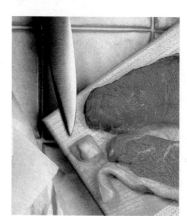

What to do

Overall, both visible and hidden sources of fat need to be examined when developing a plan to eat less fat. Consider the practical suggestions we provide in Table 7-2 for cutting down on visible and hidden fats. ●

Since a high HDL-cholesterol level slows the development of heart disease, the HDL form of cholesterol has been considered *good cholesterol*. By definition, then, the LDL form would be *bad cholesterol* because a high LDL-cholesterol level speeds the development of heart disease.

CONCEPT CHECK

Dietary fat is transported in the bloodstream in the form of chylomicrons. Fats synthesized by the liver are carried in the bloodstream as very low density lipoproteins (VLDL). After a VLDL has most of its triglycerides removed, it eventually becomes a low density lipoprotein (LDL). This is high in cholesterol. LDL particles are picked up by body cells, especially liver cells. Another type of lipoprotein is a high density form, or HDL. It picks up cholesterol from cells and delivers it to other lipoproteins for eventual transport back to the liver for excretion. An elevated LDL-cholesterol level speeds the development of heart disease, as does a low HDL-cholesterol level.

RECOMMENDATIONS FOR FAT INTAKE

Although we know a great deal about fats, there is no RDA. A good practice, suggested earlier, is to consume about 1 tablespoon of vegetable oil per day incorporated into foods, such as salad dressings, to obtain the essential fatty acids.

Americans eat about 38% of their total kcalories as fat. Vegetable and animal sources each supply about half the fat. Major sources of fat in the American diet can be found in beef products, luncheon meats, whole milk, and pastries.

The American Heart Association (AHA) recommends eating about 30% of your total kcalories as fat, using nearly equal amounts of saturated, monounsaturated, and polyunsaturated fatty acids, or a 1:1:1 ratio (Table 7-3). Eating equivalent amounts of the different fatty acids helps control saturated fat intake. Also, reducing fat to 30% of kcalorie intake helps reduce saturated fat consumption and also lowers the chances of creeping weight gain in adulthood. The AHA further recommends eating no more than 300 milligrams of choles-

TABLE 7-3

Dietary guidelines for healthy American adults. A statement for physicians and health professionals by the Nutrition Committee, American Heart Association (AHA)

1. Total fat intake should be less than 30% of kcalories.
2. Saturated fat intake should be less than 10% of kcalories.
3. Polyunsaturated fat intake should not exceed 10% of kcalories.
4. Cholesterol intake should not exceed 300 mg/day.
5. Carbohydrate intake should constitute 50% or more of kcalories, with emphasis on complex carbohydrates.
6. Protein intake should provide the remainder of the kcalories.
7. Sodium intake should not exceed 3 g/day.
8. Alcoholic consumption should not exceed 1 to 2 oz of ethanol per day. Two ounces of 100 proof whiskey, 8 oz of wine, or 24 oz of beer each contain 1 oz of ethanol.
9. Total kcalories should be sufficient to maintain the individual's recommended body weight.
10. A wide variety of foods should be consumed.

Chapter 2 compared the recommendations of the AHA with those of the Dietary Guidelines issued by the U.S. federal government.
From *Circulation* 77:721A, 1988.

TABLE 7-4

Menus containing 2000 kcalories and various percentages of fat

30% of Kcalories as Fat		20% of Kcalories as Fat	
Breakfast	**Teaspoons of fat**		**Teaspoons of fat**
1 cup orange juice	0	same	0
3/4 cup shredded wheat	1/5	same	1/5
1 toasted bagel	1/5	same	1/5
2 t margarine	1-3/4	same	1-3/4
1 cup 1% milk	1/2	1 cup nonfat milk	1/10
Lunch			
2 slices whole-wheat bread	1/2	same	1/2
2 oz lean roast beef	1	2 oz boiled ham	1/2
2 t mayonnaise	1-1/2	same	1-1/2
lettuce	0	same	0
1 sliced tomato	0	same	0
8 animal crackers	1/5	same	1/5
Snack			
1 apple	1/6	same	1/6
Dinner			
3 oz broiled lamb chop	2-1/3	3 oz broiled halibut	2/3
1-1/2 cup pasta	2/3	same	2/3
2 t margarine	1-3/4	1 t margarine	7/8
1/2 cup broccoli	0	1/2 cup	0
1 cup 1% milk	1/2	1 cup nonfat milk	1/10
		1 banana	1/10
Snack			
2 T raisins	0	1/4 cup	0
6 cups air-popped popcorn	1/2	same	1/2
with 2 teaspoons margarine	1-3/4	with 1 teaspoon margarine	7/8
TOTALS	14		8-1/2

terol a day. Lowering fat intake to 20% of total kcalories in cases where an elevated serum LDL-cholesterol level does not respond to the moderate recommendation is also advised (Table 7-4). One recent study even shows that lowering fat to 10% of kcalories causes plaque in arteries to regress.[16] More research on this is necessary before we advocate such a severe dietary change.

The National Cholesterol Education Program, established in 1985 in the United States, recommends reducing saturated fatty acids even further to 7% of kcalories if a high serum cholesterol level fails to respond to a 10% level (Appendix I).[7] Cholesterol intake should also fall below 200 milligrams per day. We currently eat about 15% of kcalories as saturated fat. Reducing total fat and saturated fat intake are suggestions that also fit in with the Dietary Guidelines for Americans we reviewed in Chapter 2.

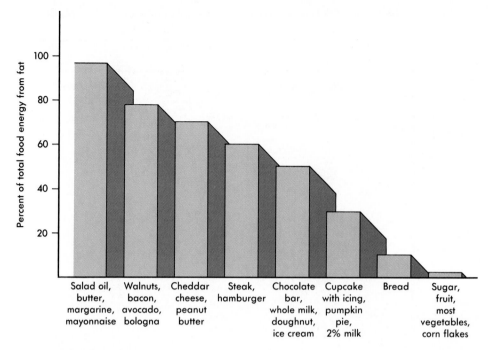

FIGURE 7-8
Percent of kcalories as fats in foods. Vegetable oils, butter, margarine, and mayonnaise provide almost all kcalories as fats.

FATS IN FOODS

Salad oils, butter, margarine, and mayonnaise all contain about 100% of kcalories as fat. In other words, they are loaded with fat (Figure 7-8). Walnuts, bologna, avocados, and bacon have about 80% of kcalories as fat. Peanut butter and cheddar cheese have about 75% of their kcalories as fat. Steak and hamburgers have about 60%, and chocolate bars, ice cream, doughnuts, and whole milk have about 50% of kcalories as fat. Pumpkin pie and cupcakes have 35%. Bread contains about 15% of its kcalories as fat. Cornflakes, sugar, and most fruits and vegetables have essentially no fat.

You read that a certain brand of hot dog is only 17% fat, or 83% fat-free. This might initially impress you. However, it means that the hot dog is 17% fat by weight, not in terms of kcalories. Remember that water makes up a significant part of the weight of many foods, including a hot dog. Actually, 53% of the kcalories come from fat. So don't be deceived by these kinds of statements. Read the label and calculate the percentage of fat to be sure (grams of fat per serving multiplied by 9 and divided by total kcalories in a serving).

We get most of our saturated fats from animal fats. They contain about 40% to 60% saturated fatty acids. Recent evidence suggests that saturated fatty acids with 12 to 16 carbons are the ones that raise serum cholesterol levels.[4,10] These problem saturated fatty acids make up about 25% to 50% of animal fats. Some plant products also contain significant amounts of *problem* saturated fatty acids; for example, cottonseed oil (27%), palm oil (46%), palm kernel oil (71%), and coconut oil (70%). The last 3 comprise what is often called tropical oils,

THE FAR SIDE   By GARY LARSON

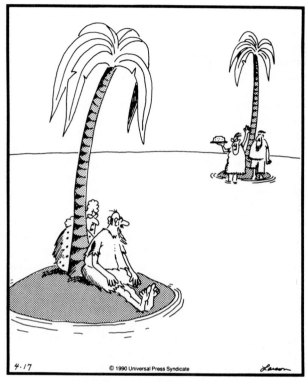

4-17   © 1990 Universal Press Syndicate   Larson

"Uh-oh. Carol's inviting us over for cake,
and I'm sure it's just loaded with palm oil."

FIGURE 7-9

based on their countries of origin (Figure 7-9). *Trans* fats in hydrogenated vegetable oils further add to the problem fatty acids, as we discussed earlier.

Plant fats contain mostly unsaturated fatty acids, ranging from 76% to 94% (excluding palm and coconut oils). Plant oils supply most of the essential fatty acids in our food supply. Olive oil, canola oil, and peanut oil contain a moderate to high amount of monounsaturated fatty acids (49% to 77%). Some animal fats are also good sources (30% to 48%) (see Figure 7-2). Corn, cottonseed, sunflower, soybean, and safflower oils contain mostly polyunsaturated fat; note that amounts vary (54% to 77%).

Many manufacturers and food growers are trying to devise products that are lower in fats generally, and particularly in saturated fats. During the past several decades, beef producers have altered breeding and feeding practices to increase muscle mass in beef cattle and decrease body fat.

CONCEPT CHECK

There is no recommended dietary allowance for fat. We need the equivalent of about 1 tablespoon of plant oils supplied by foods to provide essential fatty acids. Many health-related agencies recommend a diet containing no more than 30% of energy as fat, and a maximum of one third of that as saturated fat. The American diet contains about 38% of energy as fat. Foods high in fat (over 60% of total kcalories) include plant oils, butter, margarine, mayonnaise, walnuts, bacon, avocados, peanut butter, cheddar cheese, steak, and hamburger. Sources high in saturated fat include animal fats, coconut oil, and palm oil.

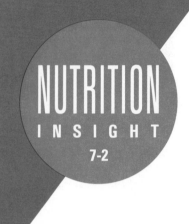

FAT REPLACEMENTS

For years manufacturers have used starch-derivatives to bind water in foods in an attempt to find a substitute that captures the feeling of fat in the mouth.[15] The goal is to create products that feel like ice cream melting on the tongue but contain few fat kcalories. Recently, public and scientific interest has focused on two newer fat replacements—olestra and Simplesse. Only Simplesse has been approved for use in foods.

Olestra is made by adding fatty acids to a sucrose (table sugar) molecule. Olestra with many fatty acids attached cannot be digested by either human digestive enzymes or bacteria that live in the intestine. Therefore it yields no kcalories to the body. As it leaves the body, it can even pull cholesterol-containing substances in the intestine with it, thereby lowering the person's serum cholesterol level.[11]

The product is quite versatile as an ingredient. The manufacturer feels it can replace up to 35% of the fat in salad dressings and cakes made at home, and it can be used for frying in food manufacturing.

Some problems are associated with olestra. It tends to bind the fat-soluble vitamin E, reducing its absorption. The manufacturer has proposed adding vitamin E to olestra in excess of the amount it could bind, to compensate.[11] Some years ago FDA would not permit the use of mineral oil in foods as a no-kcalorie fat because it bound up fat-soluble vitamins. Therefore it is unclear when this product will be available. If approved by FDA, olestra would reduce the fat content of many foods and permit us to eat rich desserts and fried foods and better control fat intake.

Simplesse is made from egg and milk proteins that are mixed together and heated in such a way that they produce microscopic, mistlike protein globules.[6] The minute globules feel like fat in the mouth, although fatty acids are not present in Simplesse. The texture changes suffice. While it yields energy, Simplesse has only about 1.3 kcalories per gram, much less than regular fat's 9 kcalories per gram. This low kcalorie value is partly because proteins contain 4 kcalories per gram and because of the amount of water incorporated into the product during processing; water accounts for much of its weight.

Currently Simplesse is approved by FDA for use in frozen desserts. It reduces kcalories by about one-half and fat content to a negligible amount in these prod-

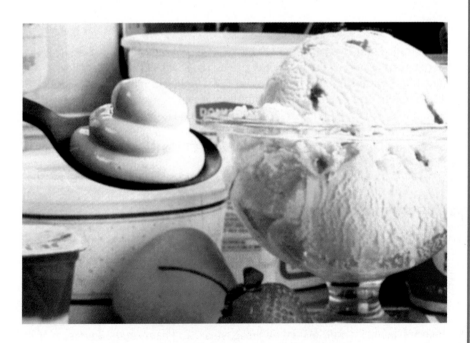

ucts.[15] Simplesse can also be used to replace fat in mayonnaise, salad dressings, yogurt, cheeses, and other dairy products, but the manufacturer must wait for FDA approval for use in these foods. Because high temperatures alter the structure of Simplesse so much that it no longer resembles fat, it cannot be used for cooking or frying. People who are allergic to milk and/or egg proteins should not consume Simplesse. With wide use, Simplesse could help reduce total fat intake.

Fat replacements in perspective

If you look at the 15 major contributors of total fat in the American diet listed below, you will understand why the effect of fat replacements will likely not be very substantial. They are not that versatile (Table 7-5). Many foods that are major fat contributors will remain so. The main benefit of using fat replacements will be cutting some fat from the diet, most importantly saturated fat and cholesterol. The actual kcalorie reduction will probably be less impressive because people tend to make up the lost energy by eating more of other foods.

TABLE 7-5

Leading contributors of fat in the American diet and the potential for fat replacements to replace much of that fat. A star (*) indicates a possible application

Food Source of Fat &	% of Total Fat in Diet	Applications for Olestra	Simplesse
hamburgers, cheeseburger, meatloaf	7.0	—	—
hot dogs, lunch meat	6.4	—	sausage, pate*
whole milk	6.0	—	—
doughnuts, cakes, cookies	6.0	shortenings, frying*	—
beef steaks, roasts	5.5	—	—
white bread, rolls, crackers	4.9	shortenings*	—
eggs	4.6	—	—
cheese	4.5	—	spreads*
margarine	4.5	—	spreads; not for cooking*
mayonnaise	4.3	—	*
pork	4.0	—	—
French fries, fried potatoes	2.7	frying*	—
salad and cooking oils	2.6	(?)*	—
butter	2.4	—	—
ice cream, frozen desserts	2.1	—	*!

*Based on NHANES II.
—no application as of yet.
NOTE: The use of Simplesse is limited mostly because it cannot be heated to high temperatures for a long period without losing its desirable properties.

We will always need balanced eating habits and moderation in food choice. A diet rich in fruits, vegetables, whole grains, and lean animal products still deserves the most attention. Fat replacements can reduce intake of saturated fat and cholesterol in popular foods Americans are unwilling to relinquish, such as ice cream. But we won't know the true impact of fat replacements on our diets until they are approved for more general use. For now they are of little significance. ●

SUMMARY

- Fats are a group of relatively oxygen-poor compounds that don't dissolve in water. Fatty acids can be grouped according to the type of bonds between the carbons: saturated fatty acids contain no double bonds; monounsaturated fatty acids contain one double bond; and polyunsaturated fatty acids contain two or more double bonds.

- If the double bonds in a fatty acid begin at the third carbon from the CH_3 end of the chain, the fatty acid is an omega-3 fatty acid. In omega-6 fatty acids the double bonds begin at the sixth carbon. Both omega-3 and omega-6 fatty acids are essential parts of a diet because our bodies don't produce them.

- When body cells use omega-3 fatty acids to synthesize compounds called eicosanoids, the products tend to reduce blood clotting, blood pressure, and inflammatory responses. Because many fish contain ample amounts of the beneficial omega-3 fatty acids, eating fish at least twice a week is a good dietary practice.

- Fats composed of saturated fatty acids tend to be solid at room temperature. Those with polyunsaturated fatty acids are usually liquid at room temperature. However, saturated fatty acids with short chain lengths—coconut oil, for example—are usually liquid. Hydrogenation is the process of adding hydrogens to fatty acids to turn double bonds into single bonds. Manufacturers hydrogenate (increase saturation of) fats to solidify vegetable oils for making shortenings and margarine and to reduce the breakdown of polyunsaturated fatty acids, which lessens rancidity.

- Triglycerides are the major form of fat in food and in our bodies. Besides supplying essential fatty acids to the body, triglycerides supply energy, allow efficient energy storage, insulate and protect the body, transport fat-soluble vitamins, provide satiety, and add flavor and texture to foods.

- Phospholipids are derivatives of triglycerides. They form important parts of cell membranes. Some act as efficient emulsifiers, allowing fats to disperse in water.

- Cholesterol is in the class of fats called sterols. It forms part of vital compounds, such as hormones, part of cell membranes, and bile. We eat cholesterol, and cells in the body make it.

- Fats are carried in the bloodstream by various lipoproteins: chylomicrons, very low density lipoproteins (VLDL), low density lipoproteins (LDL), and high density lipoproteins (HDL). The greater the amount of triglycerides in the lipoproteins, the less their density. Both an elevated LDL-cholesterol level and/or a low HDL-cholesterol level speed the development of heart disease.

- There is no RDA for fat. We need to eat the equivalent of about 1 tablespoon of plant oils daily in foods to get the needed essential fatty acids. Major contributors of fat to our diets include animal foods, whole milk, and pastries. The fat substitute Simplesse will allow us to eat some dairy products—frozen desserts, for example—without consuming much fat.

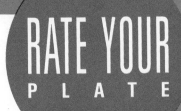
WHERE DO YOU STAND IN TERMS OF FAT?

How do your food practices compare to guidelines that have been suggested for fat, saturated fat, and cholesterol? Refer to the nutritional assessment you completed at the end of Chapter 2, and compare it to the guidelines issued by the American Heart Association and the National Cholesterol Education Program listed below:

- limit or reduce total fat intake to less than 30% of total kcalories.
- reduce saturated fat intake to 7% to 10% of kcalories or less.
- limit cholesterol to less than 200 to 300 milligrams per day.

To compare your nutritional assessment with these guidelines, the following pieces of information are needed from your assessment (write the numbers in the blanks given):

TOTAL KCALORIE INTAKE ___1814___

TOTAL GRAMS OF FAT ___62.7___

GRAMS OF SATURATED FAT ___10.15___

MILLIGRAMS OF CHOLESTEROL ___236.9___

Now complete the following steps:

1. Multiply your total grams of fat by 9 (kcals/gram of fat). Then divide the result by your total kcalorie intake. Next multiply this number by 100. THIS WILL GIVE YOU THE % OF KCALORIES YOU CONSUMED FROM FAT.

% OF KCALORIES FROM FAT ___31.1___

IS IT LESS THAN 30% OF YOUR TOTAL KCALS? YES _____ NO _X_

2. Multiply your grams of saturated fat by 9 (kcals/gram of fat). Divide the result by your total kcalorie intake. Now multiply this number by 100. THIS WILL GIVE YOU THE % OF KCALORIES YOU CONSUMED FROM SATU-RATED FAT.

% OF KCALORIES FROM SATURATED FAT ___5.0___

IS IT 10% OF YOUR KCALORIES OR LESS? YES _X_ NO _____

3. Look at your milligrams of cholesterol.

IS IT LESS THAN 300 MILLIGRAMS? YES _X_ NO _____

4. Look back at the foods you ate and notice the foods that contributed the most fat, saturated fat, and cholesterol. If you didn't meet one or more of the

guidelines, how could you change what you ate that day to improve your diet?

5. Now take the next step. Do you know your HDL- and LDL-cholesterol levels? If not, have them checked soon. All adults should know if their levels are in the abnormal ranges.

6. Finally, fill in the following assessment of your risk for developing premature heart disease. Decide today how you could modify your diet and lifestyle, if necessary, to reduce your risk.

Do you have . . .	YES	NO
a history of smoking?	___	___
high blood pressure?	___	___
a high LDL-cholesterol level?	___	___
a low HDL-cholesterol level?	___	___
diabetes mellitus?	___	___
a history of physical inactivity?	___	___
a family history of premature heart disease?	___	___
a history of obesity?	___	___

Other factors also could be considered, but this provides a good start for assessing your risk.

REFERENCES

1. Anderson JW, Gustafson NJ: Hypocholesterolemic effects of oat bran and bean products, *American Journal of Clinical Nutrition* 48:749, 1988.
2. Blumenthal D: Making sense of the cholesterol controversy, *FDA Consumer*, June, 1990, p 12.
3. Brunzell JD, Austin MA: Plasma triglyceride levels and coronary disease, *New England Journal of Medicine* 320:1273, 1989.
4. Bonanome A, Grundy SM: Effect of dietary stearic acid on plasma cholesterol and lipoprotein levels, *New England Journal of Medicine* 318:1244, 1988.
5. Das UN and others: Clinical significance of essential fatty acids, *Nutrition* 4:337, 1988.
6. Dziezak JD: Fats, oils and fat substitutes, *Food Technology*, July, 1989, p 78.
7. The Expert Panel: Report of the National Cholesterol Education Program Expert Panel on Detection, Evaluation, and Treatment of High Blood Cholesterol in Adults, *Archives of Internal Medicine* 148:36, 1988.
8. Gordon DJ, Rifkind BW: High density lipoprotein—the clinical implications of recent studies, *New England Journal of Medicine* 321:1311, 1989.
9. Grundy SM: Monounsaturated fatty acids and cholesterol metabolism: implications for dietary recommendations, *Journal of Nutrition* 119:529, 1989.
10. Grundy SM: Cholesterol and coronary heart disease: future directions, *Journal of the American Medical Association* 264:3053, 1990.
11. Harrigan KA, Breene WM: Fat substitutes: sucrose esters and Simplesse, *Cereal Foods World* 34(3):261, 1989.
12. Harris WS: Fish oils and plasma lipid and lipoprotein metabolism in humans: a critical review, *Journal of Lipid Research* 30:785, 1989.
13. Kris-Etherton PM and others: The effect of diet on plasma lipids, lipoproteins, and coronary heart disease, *Journal of the American Dietetic Association* 88:1373, 1988.
14. Nuovo J: Use of dietary fiber to lower cholesterol, *American Family Physician* 39:137, 1989.
15. Segal M: Fat substitutes: a taste for the future? *FDA Consumer*, December, 1990, p 25.
16. Ornish D and others: Can lifestyle changes reverse coronary heart disease? *Lancet* 336:129, 1990.
17. Simopoulus AP: Summary of the NATO advanced research workshop

on dietary w-3 and w-6 fatty acids, *Journal of Nutrition* 119:521, 1989.

18. Steinberg D and others: Beyond cholesterol: modifications of low-density lipoprotein that increase its atherogenicity, *New England Journal of Medicine* 320:915, 1989.

19. Steinberg D, Witztum JL: Lipoproteins and atherogenesis, *Journal of the American Medical Association* 264:3047, 1990.

20. Thompson PD and others: Modest changes in high-density lipoprotein concentration and metabolism with prolonged exercise training, *Circulation* 78:25, 1988.

HOW MUCH HAVE I LEARNED?

What have you learned from Chapter 7? Here are 15 statements about lipids. Read them to test your current knowledge. If you think the statement is true or mostly true, circle T. If you think the statement is false or mostly false, circle F. Use the scoring key at the end of the book to compute your total score. To review, take this test again later, and especially before tests.

1. T **(F)** Fats composed of long-chain saturated fatty acids are liquid at room temperature. *solid*

2. **(T)** F Fat has more kcalories per gram than carbohydrate. *9* *4 Kcal/g*

3. **(T)** F Cholesterol is naturally found only in the animal-derived foods we eat. *products advertised as cholesterol free may still contain saturated fat*

4. **(T)** F Animal fats are the major dietary factor that raises blood cholesterol levels. *are rich in saturated fat*

5. **(T)** F Triglycerides are the main form of fat found in foods. *& in body*

6. T **(F)** Fat is not absolutely necessary in our diet. *fatty acids used to make vital body compounds*

7. **(T)** F Hydrogenation makes vegetable oils more solid at room temperature. *prevents oils in peanut butter from separating during storage*

8. **(T)** F Fruits are essentially fat free.

9. **(T)** F Vitamin E helps protect foods from turning rancid. *protects against breakdown of double bonds in fatty acids*

10. **(T)** F The small intestine absorbs some vitamins better when dietary fat is present. *vitamins A, D, E, K are fat soluble; absorption enhanced by dietary fat*

11. T **(F)** A blood cholesterol test is not necessary if you are age 40 or less. *over age 20 should be tested; early detection of elevated LDL-cholesterol level is best*

12. **(T)** F Butter and margarine contain about the same amount of fat. *Butter contains more saturated fat tho than tub margarine*

13. T **(F)** High doses of fish oils in the diet pose no health problems. *can raise LDL cholesterol levels & disrupt glucose regulation in diabetes patients*

14. T **(F)** Nondairy creamers are healthier for you than lowfat milk. *creamers often contain coconut oil; high in saturated fat.*

15. T **(F)** The best way to use diet to lower a high blood cholesterol level is to follow a low cholesterol diet. *eat less saturated fat. eating more soluble fiber also helpful*

NUTRITION ISSUE

HEART DISEASE

When a heart attack hits, it can strike with the sudden force of a sledge-hammer. It can also sneak up on you at night, masquerading as indigestion with slight pain or pressure in your chest.

Heart disease is the major killer of Americans. Each year about 750,000 people die of heart disease in the United States, 60% more than cancer kills.[7] The overall male to female ratio is about 2 to 1. For each person in America who dies of heart disease, 10 more (over 6 million people) have heart disease symptoms. And about twice the number who die, 1.25 million, suffer heart attacks each year.

Heart disease is a chronic disease—it takes years to develop symptoms. Sometimes they do not appear until old age. Even men under the age of 20 show deposits of plaque in their arteries, as noted in autopsy data from the Korean and Vietnam wars.[7] Plaque buildup—atherosclerosis—actually begins in childhood and continues throughout life. It usually goes unnoticed for quite some time.

Preventing premature heart disease—that which appears before age 70 to 80—should be everyone's goal. Although we all die eventually, one key to a better life is to prevent premature death and live in optimal health until the entire body wears out. Heart attacks at ages 40 through 60 are closely linked to the risk factors listed below. For most people, there is a good chance to prevent premature heart disease by making some long-term changes.

Heart disease and strokes are associated with poor blood circulation. Blood supplies the heart muscle with oxygen and nutrients. When blood flow to the heart is interrupted, the heart muscle can be damaged. A heart attack— *myocardial infarction*—may result (Figure 7-7). This may cause the heart to beat irregularly or to stop altogether. If blood flow to parts of the brain is interrupted long enough, part of the brain dies, causing a *cerebrovascular accident,* or stroke. When a stroke causes loss of muscle control, death may occur.

Blood clots can stop blood flow to the heart or brain. Clots form more readily where cholesterol plaque has built up in the arteries that lead to the heart or brain.[19] Small doses of aspirin reduce blood clotting and are now used to treat people at risk for heart attack.

Plaque is probably first deposited to repair injuries in a vessel lining. Agents that lead to injury include the effects of hypertension, diabetes mellitus, and smoking. This repair is part of the *initiation phase.* The rate of further plaque deposition in the next phase—called the *progression phase*—partly depends on the amount of LDL-cholesterol in the bloodstream. The plaque thickens as layers of cholesterol, protein, muscle, and calcium are laid down. Arteries harden and narrow as plaque builds up, making them less elastic and so unable to expand to accommodate various blood pressures. Then arteries become further damaged as blood pumps through and pressure increases. Finally, in the *termination phase*, a clot or spasm in the plaque-clogged artery leads to the myocardial infarction or cerebrovascular accident.

What is your risk for heart disease?

The three most important risk factors for development of premature heart disease are smoking, hypertension (high blood pressure), and high LDL-cholesterol levels.[7] Family history is also important, particularly if a parent suffers a heart attack or stroke before age 60. Low HDL-cholesterol levels also increase risk, especially if the total cholesterol to HDL-cholesterol ratio exceeds 4.5. These factors should signal us to take aggressive early steps for prevention. Still significant, but less important, risk factors for the general public are diet, stress, inactivity, diabetes mellitus, serum triglycerides, and obesity. All these factors can contribute to heart disease. However, the most important contributors—smoking, hypertension, and a high LDL-cholesterol level—are the ones we should focus on first to prevent premature heart disease.

Do you smoke? Chemicals in smoke alter blood vessels, enabling plaque to build up faster. Smoking also makes blood more likely to clot. Do you have hypertension? If your **systolic blood pressure** is over 140 (millimeters of mercury) or higher or your **diastolic blood pressure** is 90 or more, you have hypertension. Do you have a high LDL-cholesterol level (over 130 milligrams per 100 milliliters) or total cholesterol level over 200? (If your cholesterol values come out high, have yourself tested at least two more times because the levels vary from day to day.) Is your HDL-cholesterol level low such that your total cholesterol to HDL-cholesterol ratio is high (greater than 4.5). If this is true or the HDL-cholesterol level alone is below 35 milligrams per 100 milliliters, you have increased risk for coronary heart disease. Add to this your family history and you can assess whether you are at risk.

LDL- and HDL-cholesterol levels and the total cholesterol to HDL-cholesterol ratio, rather than the total cholesterol level, are really the most important values to focus on. If a total cholesterol level is greater than 200 milligrams per 100 milliliters and the higher reading is primarily caused by a high HDL-cholesterol level, the ratio of the two may be lower than 4.5 and so the risk of heart disease is still about average or less. That is sometimes the case for women, especially before menopause. It is a good idea for women to have their HDL-cholesterol levels checked to see if this is why total blood cholesterol is elevated. Unfortunately, men with elevated total cholesterol levels usually have an elevated LDL-cholesterol level. Therefore the total cholesterol to HDL-cholesterol ratio is too high.

The National Institutes of Health in the United States encourage all people over age 20 to have their total cholesterol level checked.[7] We recommend having your HDL-cholesterol and triglyceride levels checked also. These values are used to calculate the LDL-cholesterol level and total cholesterol to HDL-cholesterol ratio. If you don't know your various cholesterol levels and ratio, you don't know your risk of developing premature heart disease. Keep in mind that you have remarkable potential for preventing premature heart disease if you are at risk, but first you must recognize your risk factors.

Lowering an elevated LDL-cholesterol level

If you discover that your LDL-cholesterol level is high, the first step is to consult a physician. Some diseases raise LDL-cholesterol levels, and treating the disease may remedy the LDL-cholesterol problem as well. If no other disease is present, diet change is necessary.[7]

Reducing saturated fat in your diet can lower an elevated LDL-cholesterol level. Although high blood cholesterol indicates risk for heart disease, the main food factor associated with a high cholesterol level is eating lots of saturated

Myocardial Infarction • Death of part of the heart muscle.

Cerebrovascular Accident (CVA) • Death of part of the brain tissue caused by a blood clot, also called a stroke.

Systolic Blood Pressure • The pressure in the bloodstream associated with the pumping of blood from the heart.

Diastolic Blood Pressure • The pressure in the bloodstream when the heart is between beats.

fat.[9] Eating less saturated fat is more important for most people than eating less cholesterol.

Almost everyone who minimizes saturated fat intake can lower an elevated LDL-cholesterol level by about 10% to 20%, especially if the person normally eats lots of foods that are high in saturated fats. About 10% of people have trouble lowering their blood cholesterol level with diet. On the other hand, about 10% can expect an even bigger drop in LDL-cholesterol levels. Lowering saturated fat in the diet is not that hard, as we point out in Table 7-2.

Only about 10% to 25% of people find that eating less cholesterol lowers their LDL-cholesterol level very much.[13] For some people, even eating six eggs a day for a month does not change their fasting blood cholesterol levels. Most people show minimal or no effect. Still, most authorities encourage us to eat less than 300 milligrams of cholesterol per day, partly to keep blood cholesterol levels right after eating as low as possible. This recommendation for cholesterol intake is close to what most women eat, but most men eat about 100 to 150 milligrams more.

Saturated fats from foods probably affect LDL-cholesterol levels by changing uptake of LDL-cholesterol by the liver.[10] When saturated fat intake is low, more LDL receptors appear in the liver, allowing more cholesterol to be cleared from the bloodstream and pulled into the liver for excretion as bile. This causes LDL-cholesterol levels to fall.

A reasonable goal is to eat no more than 7% to 10% of kcalories as saturated fats.[7] Currently we eat about 15%. Limit intake wherever you can, and pay close attention to what you eat. Find substitutes for fatty animal products, butter, coconut oil, palm oil, shortening, and other hydrogenated (solid) fats (see Tables 7-2 and 7-4). Make it a habit to read labels—saturated fats are often hidden in foods.

 Many people think they need to eliminate beef from their diets to moderate their saturated fat intake. That is not necessary if they choose the right cuts of beef and cook it appropriately, especially trimming the fat off before cooking. If *loin* or *round* is part of its name, the cut is relatively lowfat.

Eating right doesn't mean completely giving up favorite foods, even if they do contain higher-than-desirable levels of saturated fats. If you eat carefully most of the time, you can allow yourself latitude for occasional treats. If you indulge in a high saturated fat meal, it should be balanced by meals of lower-than-usual amounts of saturated fats.

To meet the AHA goals of no more than 300 milligrams of cholesterol per day, decrease the number of egg yolks to four or less per week; egg whites have no cholesterol. If you cook for yourself, it is easy to avoid egg yolks. In many recipes, such as those for pancakes, French toast, cookies, and cakes, you can substitute egg whites for whole eggs. Cholesterol-free eggs are also available in the grocery store. These are usually egg whites colored yellow, to which a small amount of fat has been added to improve the flavor. Note again it is the animal foods we eat that supply most of the cholesterol (see Table 7-1).

If fat is trimmed before and after cooking, a 3- to 4-ounce serving of chicken, beef, or pork has surprisingly little cholesterol, roughly a third to half of that in an egg. A 10 ounce serving of meat can contain 260 milligrams of cholesterol, slightly more than that in one egg. If meats have a reputation for being high in cholesterol, it is mainly because of an overgenerous portion size, rather than the amount of cholesterol in an ounce of meat—a mere 30 or so milligrams.

Monounsaturated and polyunsaturated fats

New observations show that monounsaturated fatty acids in the diet can lower cholesterol levels.[9] Until recently, polyunsaturated fatty acids were recommended as a substitute for saturated fatty acids in the diet in order to lower LDL-cholesterol levels. However, recent studies show that either monounsaturated or polyunsaturated fatty acids can be used. Note that there is nothing magic about any vegetable oil source of unsaturated fat—olive oil included. Each simply makes a good contribution to the fight against saturated fat.

Fiber and reduced heart disease

Another recent development, as we discussed in Chapter 6, is the connection between eating lots of soluble fiber—found in oatmeal, oat bran, beans, vegetables, and fruits—and lower LDL-cholesterol levels![14] Again, large amounts must be eaten to have a significant effect. Diets very high in overall fiber (50 to 60 grams per day), especially those that emphasize soluble fibers, work well. Some laxatives with psyllium fiber are also good sources of soluble fiber.

Although it is possible to follow a diet high in soluble fiber, extensive dietary changes would be necessary for most of us. Researchers also now are cautioning people against eating more than 35 grams of dietary fiber a day, primarily because of the potential to bind minerals in the diet. So, consult a physician if you are considering a very high-fiber diet. We think it is easier and safer to cut down on saturated fat than to raise soluble fiber intake dramatically.

Diets high in soluble fiber probably work by binding cholesterol and bile in the small intestine and carrying them into the large intestine for elimination. Removing bile from the body forces the liver to pull more cholesterol out of the bloodstream to make new bile. This action resembles that of some medications that lower LDL-cholesterol levels. Other mechanisms have also been suggested to account for the effects of soluble fibers.[1]

You've probably heard a lot about oat bran. Manufacturers were quick to realize the marketing potential of a product that might lower blood cholesterol levels. But oat bran is not the "magic bullet" manufacturers would have us believe (Figure 7-10). Recall from Chapter 6 that you would need to eat about a cup of it a day to reap the desired effect; an oat bran muffin alone won't do it.

FRANK & ERNEST® by Bob Thaves

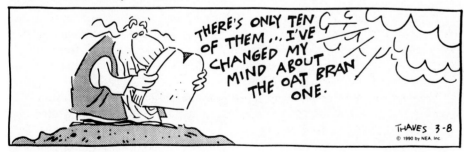

FIGURE 7-10

Raising the HDL-cholesterol level

An important step in lowering a LDL-cholesterol level is to keep the HDL-cholesterol level up at the same time. Exercising for at least 45 minutes four times a week can help protect the serum HDL-cholesterol level and may even raise it by about 5 milligrams per 100 milliliters.[20] Losing excess weight and avoiding smoking also helps to maintain or raise HDL-cholesterol levels.[7]

In addition, eating regularly (three balanced meals daily), matching the

Although drinking a lot of alcohol appears to raise a certain type of HDL-cholesterol, too many other risks—such as liver and heart muscle damage and accidents—are associated with heavy drinking to justify using it for this purpose.

Elevated blood triglycerides (greater than 150 milligrams per 100 milliliters of serum) mostly pose a heart health risk if linked to low HDL-cholesterol levels or diabetes mellitus. When serum triglycerides are 500 to 1000 another health risk arises—inflammation of the pancreas.[3]

amount of kcalories you eat with those you use up, and eating less total fat often help HDL-cholesterol levels by lowering triglyceride levels. Low triglyceride levels are often associated with high HDL-cholesterol levels. The reason for this is not clear. Nevertheless, the goal is to have fasting triglyceride levels below 150 milligrams per 100 milliliters. Certain medications also act to lower triglyceride levels. When this happens, HDL-cholesterol levels also often increase.

It is unfortunate that raising HDL-cholesterol levels is usually difficult. Lowering LDL-cholesterol levels is usually much easier.

Diet changes that work for one person may not work for another. Plan to make needed changes and then have your LDL-cholesterol and HDL-cholesterol levels rechecked in a month. Steady progress toward lowering your total cholesterol to HDL-cholesterol ratio by lowering LDL-cholesterol levels or raising HDL-cholesterol levels can mean a lower risk for developing premature heart disease.

MEDICATIONS TO LOWER SERUM CHOLESTEROL LEVELS

Medications are a last resort for treating high LDL-cholesterol or low HDL-cholesterol levels; most are expensive and all have side effects. But sometimes diet changes do not lower high LDL-cholesterol levels enough especially in people with strong genetic tendencies toward that problem. Current medications to lower LDL-cholesterol levels work in one of two ways. One group inhibits the liver from synthesizing some lipoproteins.[10] These medications include nicotinic acid, lovastatin, probucol, and gemfibrozil. Nicotinic acid and gemfibrozil are also notable for raising HDL-cholesterol levels. The side effects of these medications, however, necessitate a physician's careful evaluation. The other group of medications includes cholestyramine and colestipol; they bind bile in the small intestine and lead to its elimination,[10] forcing the liver to synthesize new bile. The liver pulls LDL cholesterol out of the bloodstream to do this.

All these medications work better when a proper diet is followed; they do not substitute for diet changes.

Exercise has been shown to moderately boost HDL-cholesterol levels in some studies.

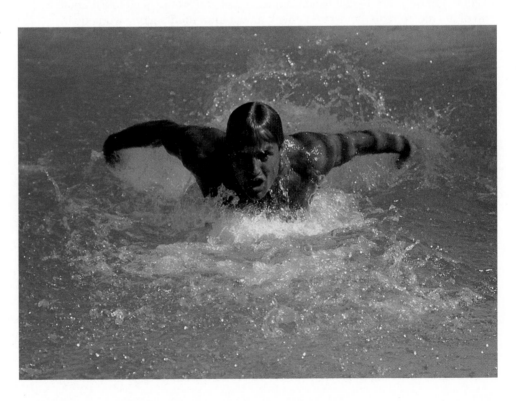

A controversy currently rages about using medications to combat heart disease.[2] The question is not whether a link exists between a high LDL-cholesterol level or a high total cholesterol to HDL-cholesterol ratio and an increased risk of a heart attack. The question concerns the point at which a person's risk is sufficient to warrant medical treatment. Diet changes are also criticized for the same reason. Still, the overwhelming sentiment of researchers in the heart disease arena is unanimous—change the diet and use medications (if needed) to lower an elevated LDL-cholesterol level and to get the total cholesterol to HDL-cholesterol ratio below 4.5. New research even shows that plaque regresses in arteries when LDL-cholesterol levels are aggressively lowered with surgery on the intestinal tract, diet plus medications,[10] and even with diet (albeit very low in fat)[16] alone.

What should one do?

To lower a high LDL-cholesterol level:

Action	Rationale
Eat less saturated fat and cholesterol.	This is the first method to employ and should be the overall major dietary focus.
Perform regular exercise.	This may protect HDL-cholesterol levels.
Eat regularly spaced meals, not one or two large ones.	The frequency of meals helps determine fasting triglyceride levels. One study shows this can even help reduce LDL-cholesterol levels.
Lose weight to attain a desirable body weight.	This helps reduce serum triglyceride levels (if elevated), lowers high blood pressure, and can increase HDL-cholesterol levels.
Eat more soluble fiber.	This binds cholesterol and bile in the small intestine to encourage their elimination via the large intestine rather than absorption into the bloodstream; other factors may affect the drop in LDL-cholesterol levels.
Eat less total fat.	This may help achieve the other goals, and it won't hurt anyone who eats the typical American diet.

A diet with 30% total kcalories from fat is an appropriate goal for children age 2 or older. Parents shouldn't go overboard with fat restrictions because children need about 30% fat in their diet to grow properly. We do not advise parents to feed fat-restricted diets to children under the age of 2 (see Chapter 15). ●

PROTEINS

Americans eat a lot of protein. For many of us protein translates into meat, poultry, fish, and eggs. Turkey, hamburger, cheese, and T-bone steak are some favorite animal protein foods in America. In contrast, our Stone Age ancestors obtained a greater percentage of their protein from vegetables.[5] They primarily picked and gathered their dietary protein, rather than hunted it. Not until *Homo erectus,* our immediate ancestors, emerged about 1.5 million years ago did meat displace other foods in primarily a vegetarian diet. Diets that are mostly vegetarian in nature still predominate in much of Asia and areas of Africa.

Few of us wish to exchange our comfortable modern lifestyles with those of our Stone Age ancestors, and yet we could benefit from eating more plant protein foods. It is possible—and desirable—to incorporate the most nutritious practices of both eras and enjoy the benefits of animal and plant protein. Let's see why. ●

CHAPTER

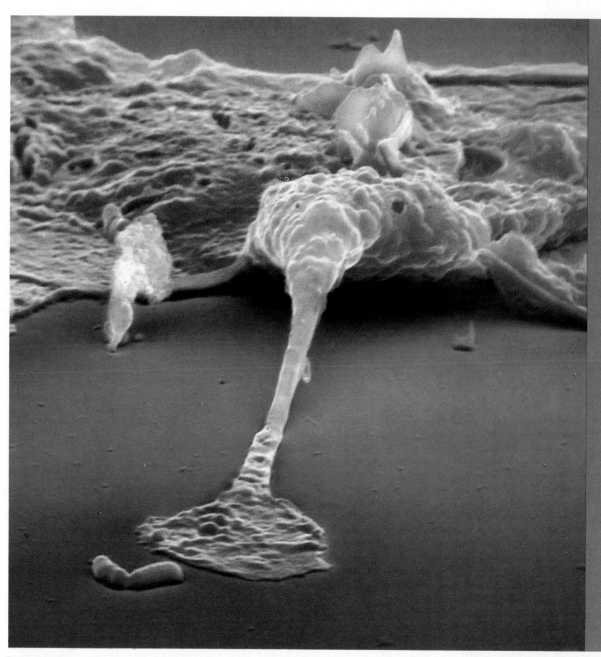

Proteins allow immune processes—like this white blood cell attacking a bacterium—to take place in the body.

What Are Your Protein Preferences?

Below is a list of various foods that are good sources of protein. Rank your preferences among them from 1 to 12. A ranking of 1 means you like that particular food the best; a ranking of 12 means you like it the least.

(A)   eggs _12_

*(P)   beans (e.g., kidney, pinto, navy, red, chick peas) _6_

*(A)   fish (e.g., salmon, halibut, swordfish, tuna) _6_

(A)   beef _4_

*(P)   grains (e.g., products made from wheat, corn, oats) _3_

*(A)   poultry (e.g., chicken, turkey) _8_

(A)   cheese _12_

*(P)   nuts and seeds (e.g., almonds, sunflower seeds) _8_

(A)   milk and milk products (e.g., ice cream, milk) _6_

(A)   pork _7_

(A)   processed meats (e.g., pepperoni, bologna, sausage) _10_

(A)   yogurt _3_

    As we pointed out in Chapter 3, today many rural societies consume more plant than animal sources of protein. This helps diets stay low in fat and cholesterol. In this respect it is healthier than the typical American diet because it helps prevent some chronic diseases. Where did the plant sources of protein rank in terms of your preference, high or low? Where did the sources that were either low in fat or cholesterol rank? Do you give excellent sources of plant proteins enough attention?

(A), Animal source; *(P)*, Plant source.
*By nature, the protein is low in either fat or cholesterol.

ASSESS YOURSELF

PROTEINS—A KEY LIFE FORCE

Thousands of various substances in the body are **proteins.** Aside from water, proteins form the major part of a lean human body, about 16% of body weight. Amino acids—the building blocks for these proteins—are generated by plants. By combining nitrogen from soil and air with carbon and other elements, plants form amino acids. They then form these into proteins. We ordinarily get enough nitrogen by consuming it in the amino acid form found in proteins. Proteins are very important because they supply nitrogen in a form we can readily use. This is something carbohydrates and fats cannot do.

Proteins provide a key life force. They are crucial to the minute-by-minute regulation and maintenance of our bodies. Vital body functions, such as blood-clotting, fluid balancing, hormone and enzyme production, visual processes, and cell repair, require specific proteins. Your body generates proteins in so many configurations and sizes that they can serve these greatly varied functions. All these proteins are made from the amino acids in protein foods you eat.[20]

If you don't regularly eat enough protein, many of your metabolic processes slow. The immune system, for example, no longer functions efficiently, increasing the risk of infections, disease, and eventually death.[15] Therefore, proteins truly deserve their name, which means "to come first."

Amino acids

Amino acids—again the building blocks of proteins—are formed mostly of carbon, hydrogen, oxygen, and nitrogen. Note that the key part of an amino acid is nitrogen. The marginal diagram shows what a typical amino acid looks like. In this case it is glutamic acid. The amino acids used to make protein show several different nitrogen-containing chemical backbones, all slight variations of the glutamic acid pictured.

Your body needs 20 different amino acids to function. Although they are all important, 11 of these amino acids are considered **nonessential dispensable**—it isn't essential to consume them because our bodies make them (Table 8-1).

Protein • Food components made of amino acids. Proteins contain the form of nitrogen most easily used by the human body.

Nonessential Amino Acids • Amino acids that can be synthesized by a healthy body in sufficient amounts; there are 11 nonessential amino acids. These are also termed dispensable amino acids.

glutamic acid

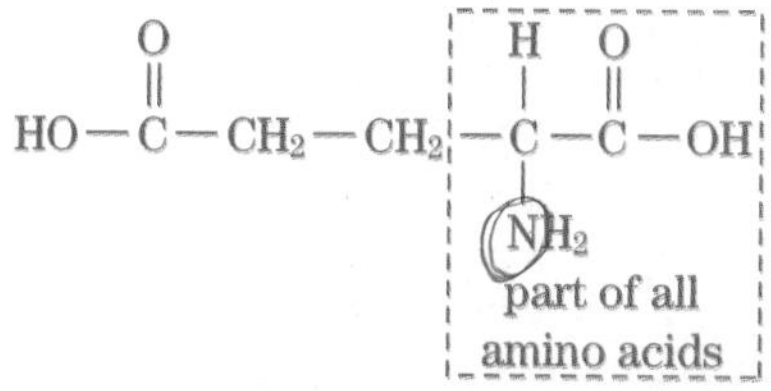

TABLE 8-1

Classification of amino acids

Essential (Indispensable) Amino Acids	Nonessential (Dispensable) Amino Acids
Histidine	Alanine
Isoleucine	Arginine
Leucine	Asparagine
Lysine[‡]	Aspartic acid
Methionine[†]	Cysteine[*]
Phenylalanine	(Cystine)
Threonine[‡]	Glutamic acid
Tryptophan[‡]	Glutamine
Valine	Glycine
	Proline
	Serine
	Tyrosine[*]

[*] These amino acids are also classed as semiessential. This means they must be made from essential amino acids if not enough is eaten. When that occurs, the body's supply of certain essential amino acids is depleted.

[†] In legumes and vegetables, the least concentrated amino acid when compared to our needs. You can consume legumes with grains, nuts, and seeds to improve the amino acid balance of protein at a meal if no animal protein is eaten.

[‡] In grains, nuts, and seeds, the amino acids in lowest concentration with respect to our needs. You can consume grains with legumes to improve the amino acid balance of protein at a meal if no animal protein is eaten.

The nine amino acids the body cannot make are known as **essential indispensable amino acids**—they must be obtained from foods.[21] Both nonessential and essential amino acids are present in foods that contain protein. If you don't eat enough essential amino acids, your body first struggles to conserve what essential amino acids it can.[18] However, eventually your body progressively slows production of new proteins until at some point you will break protein down faster than you can make it. When that happens, as we noted earlier, health deteriorates.

One way the body produces nonessential amino acids is by **transamination** (*trans* means across). In this process a nitrogen group (technically called an amino group) switches from one amino acid onto a carbon backbone. The nitrogen group comes from food proteins or body proteins. The carbon backbone comes from metabolic pathways, which are often fueled by glucose. Now a new amino acid is formed. What remains of the original amino acid after it loses its nitrogen group is a new carbon skeleton.[20]

Some amino acids simply lose their nitrogen group without transferring it to another carbon skeleton. This is called **deamination.** The process releases the nitrogen group, which is used to form urea in the liver. The kidneys then excrete the urea in the urine (Figure 8-1). About 80% of the nitrogen lost from the body normally travels this route. Once an amino acid breaks down to its carbon skeleton, the carbon skeleton can be burned for fuel or synthesized into other compounds, such as various fats and sometimes glucose (see Chapter 6).[20]

Essential Amino Acids • The amino acids that cannot be synthesized by humans in sufficient amounts and therefore must be included in the diet; there are nine essential amino acids. These are called indespensable amino acids.

Transamination • The transfer of an amino group from an amino acid to a carbon skeleton to form a new amino acid.

Deamination • The removal of an amino group from an amino acid.

Some nonessential amino acids must be made from essential amino acids if enough are not eaten. This use of essential amino acids depletes the body's supply. Scientists term these certain amino acids as semiessential since essential amino acids are the starting material for their synthesis. Researchers now suggest that some nonessential amino acids even assume an essential status at certain times when the body cannot readily generate them. This occurs in the premature infant and during some illnesses.

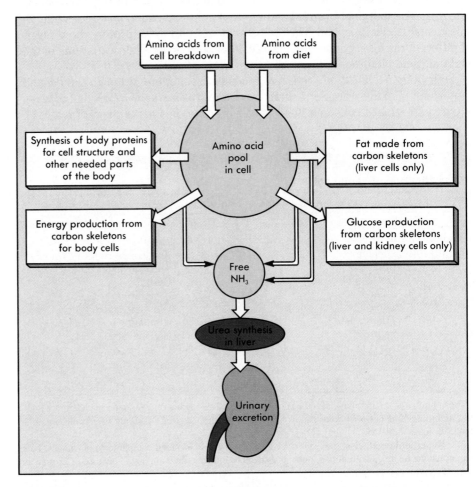

FIGURE 8-1
Amino acid metabolism. This yields a variety of products, from fat and glucose to urea.

PUTTING ESSENTIAL AMINO ACIDS INTO PERSPECTIVE
Physiological aspects

The disease *phenylketonuria* (PKU) illustrates the importance of both essential and nonessential amino acids. We discussed this disease in Chapter 6. Normally the body makes the amino acid tyrosine from the essential amino acid phenylalanine. However, enzymes in the liver of a person with PKU vary in their ability to do this. Liver enzyme activity may be grossly or mildly insufficient in converting phenylalanine to tyrosine. When the enzymes cannot synthesize enough tyrosine, both amino acids must be derived from foods. (Consumption of phenylalanine should be controlled because it can rise to toxic levels in the body.) Still, the key point here is that both amino acids are now *essential* in terms of dietary needs.

Dietary considerations

Animal and plant proteins can differ greatly in proportions of essential and nonessential amino acids. Animal proteins contain ample amounts of all nine essential amino acids. (Gelatin, made from the animal protein collagen, is an exception because it loses all of one essential amino acid during processing and is also low in other essential amino acids.) Plant proteins don't match our needs for essential amino acids as precisely as do animal proteins. Many plant proteins, especially those found in grains, are low in one or more of the nine essential amino acids.[13]

As you might expect, human tissue composition resembles animal tissue more than it does plant tissue. The similarities enable us to use proteins from animal sources more efficiently to support human growth and maintenance. Again, this is because animal proteins closely match the human pattern of essential amino acids. For this reason, animal proteins, except gelatin, are of high quality and considered **complete proteins**—they contain all the amino acids we need in sufficient amounts.[8] Plant proteins are of lower quality and are often considered **incomplete proteins** because their amino acid patterns are quite different from ours. Single plant proteins cannot easily support body growth and maintenance. To consume a sufficient amount of amino acids, very large quantities of plant proteins would need to be eaten because each protein lacks adequate amounts of one or more essential amino acids.

If you eat foods that contain low quality protein—that is, not an appropriate balance of all nine essential amino acids—you will need to eat much more to obtain enough of the essential amino acids needed for protein synthesis.[15,18] And, if any of the nine essential amino acids is used up, protein synthesis stops. Available amino acids present will be used instead for energy or converted to fat and stored as such. Because the absence of just one essential amino acid halts protein synthesis, the process illustrates the *all or none principle;* either all essential amino acids are available or none is used. The essential amino acid in shortest supply in a food or diet becomes the limiting factor (called the **limiting amino acid**) by limiting the amount of protein the body can synthesize.[21]

However, most of us eat large enough amounts and such a varied assortment of food proteins that we easily get a sufficient amount of all nine essential amino acids. That is, Americans eat a diet in which protein quality is high. This yields a *complete protein diet.* Even worldwide, most adults who eat sufficient protein get enough essential amino acids to yield a complete protein diet, even if protein from the diet is of low quality.[8] So healthy adults should have little concern about balancing proteins to obtain all nine essential amino acids (see the Nutrition Issue, p. 242, for more details).

Infants and preschool children, on the other hand, need much of their protein supplied by essential amino acids.[8] Consequently, food for young children must be more carefully planned to make sure enough proteins are present. If an infant drinks enough human milk or commercial formula to meet its protein

Complete Proteins • Proteins that contain ample amounts of all nine essential amino acids.

Incomplete Proteins • These lack an ample amount of one or more essential amino acids for human protein needs.

Limiting Amino Acid • The essential amino acid in lowest concentration in a food in proportion to body needs.

At the same time we need to eat enough kcalories so the proteins are not diverted to supply energy for the body.

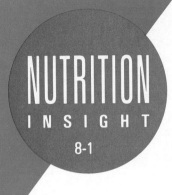

NUTRITION
I N S I G H T
8-1

AMINO ACID SUPPLEMENTS CAN BE POISONOUS

A rare blood disorder called eosinophilia-myalgia has been linked to the use of supplements of the amino acid tryptophan (L-tryptophan). A contaminant in the product was probably the real culprit.[3,10] In addition to marked changes in the blood, the condition leads to severe muscle and joint pain, swelling in the limbs, skin rash, and occasionally fever, which can run as high as 105° F. Deaths have been linked to the supplement as well. Of people who exhibit symptoms of this rare blood disease, 99% have been taking L-tryptophan. As of December 22, 1989, a total of 971 cases of toxicity accompanying L-tryptophan use had been reported to the Centers for Disease Control in Atlanta, Georgia. On March 23, 1990, the U.S. government ordered a recall of all L-tryptophan supplements.

Though this essential amino acid is normally supplied by protein in the diet, people use L-tryptophan supplements for a variety of problems, including insomnia, premenstrual syndrome, depression, and attention deficiencies in children. FDA has not approved it for these problems. Tryptophan is also found in many nonprescription and prescription nutritional products used in hospitals. Using these products poses no risk; it is the supplemental form that is linked to problems.[3,10]

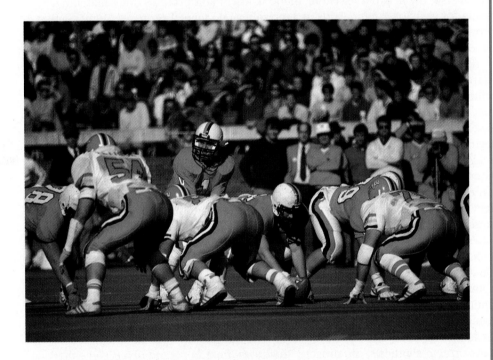

The main point here concerns not only the risk associated with taking tryptophan supplements. Amino acid supplements are not necessary because we can easily meet our protein needs through diet. This holds true for all of us, including athletes (see Chapter 12). The body is designed to handle whole proteins as a dietary source. As discussed in Chapter 5, the body breaks proteins into manageable pieces, then splits them a few at a time into amino acids, simultaneously absorbing amino acids into the bloodstream. When individual amino acid supplements are taken, they can overwhelm the absorptive mechanism, triggering amino acid imbalances in the body. These imbalances occur because groups of chemically similar amino acids compete for absorption into the bloodstream. An excess of one then can create such demand for a carrier that it hampers another amino acid from being absorbed.

Every amino acid taken in excess can be harmful. In some cases, excess amounts do not vary much above a normal daily intake. ●

needs, essential amino acid needs are likewise met. Famine situations, where often only one type of grain is available, pose the major health risk for children with respect to protein intake.[18] Famines increase the probability that children will not consume enough of some essential amino acids, leading to poor health. We discuss this in more detail later in the chapter.

CONCEPT CHECK

The human body uses 20 amino acids from foods. Because a healthy body can synthesize 11 amino acids, it is not necessary to get them from foods. The other nine must be consumed and so are termed essential amino acids. Foods that contain all nine essential amino acids in about the proportions we need are considered high quality and so are complete protein foods. Those low in one or more essential amino acids are lower in quality and so are considered incomplete protein foods. When different low quality protein foods are eaten together, the total intake of amino acids generally yields a high quality protein meal.

Peptide Bond • A bond formed to link amino acids in a protein.

Sickle Cell Disease • An anemia that results from a malformation of the red blood cell protein hemoglobin, which is caused by incorrect amino acid composition in its protein chains. The disease can lead to anemia and episodes of severe bone and joint pain, abdominal pain, headache, convulsions, paralysis, and even death.

Denature • Alteration of a protein's three-dimentional structure, usually because of treatment by heat, acid or alkaline solutions, or agitation.

PROTEINS—MANY AMINO ACIDS JOINED TOGETHER

Amino acids are joined by chemical links—technically called *peptide bonds*—to form proteins. These links are difficult to break. However, acids, enzymes, and other agents are able to break these links, as occurs during digestion.

Protein organization

By linking various combinations of the 20 types of amino acids, the body synthesizes thousands of different proteins. Amino acids are joined together in specific sequences to form distinct proteins. The sequential order of the amino acids determines a protein's configuration. The DNA in a cell directs this ordering during protein synthesis, as we noted in Chapter 5. The key point is that only correctly positioned amino acids can interact and fold properly to form the intended shape for the protein. The resulting unique three-dimensional form dictates the function of each particular protein (Figure 8-2). If it lacks the appropriate configuration, a protein cannot function.[20]

Sickle cell disease (also called sickle cell anemia) illustrates what happens when amino acids are out of order on a protein. Blacks are especially prone to this genetic disease. It originates in defective production of the protein chains of hemoglobin, a compound found in red blood cells. In two of its four protein chains a slight error in the amino acid strings occurs. This small error produces a profound change in hemoglobin structure: it can no longer form the shape needed to carry oxygen efficiently inside the red blood cell.[20] Instead of forming normal circular disks, the red blood cells collapse into crescent shapes. Health deteriorates, and eventually episodes of severe bone and joint pain, abdominal pain, headache, convulsions, and paralysis may occur.

These life-threatening symptoms are caused by a minute, but critical, error in the hemoglobin amino acid order. Why does this error happen? It results from a defect in a person's genetic blueprint, DNA, which is inherited through one's parents. A defect in the DNA can dictate that a wrong amino acid will be built into the sequence of body proteins. Many diseases stem from incorrect DNA information passed on in the body. Cancer, which we discuss in the next chapter, is an example.

Denaturation of proteins

Treatment with acid or alkaline substances, heat, or agitation can severely alter a protein's structure, leaving it unfolded and in a *denatured* state. The protein can no longer perform its function. For example, once an egg is cracked into a hot frying pan and solidifies, it can no longer produce a chicken. The same is

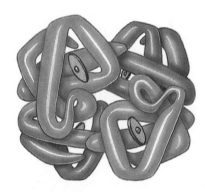

FIGURE 8-2

Proteins often form a coiled shape, as shown by this drawing of the blood protein hemoglobin. This shape is dictated by the order of the amino acids in the protein chain.

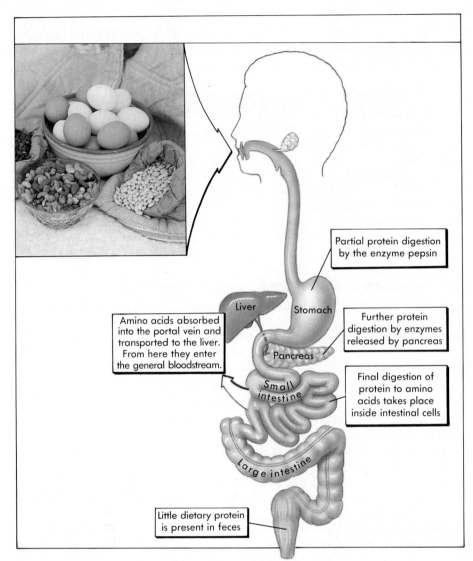

For your review. Protein digestion and absorption.

true for whipped egg whites. Once the bacteria in yogurt have synthesized enough acid and enzymes to precipitate some of the milk protein, the product solidifies irreversibly.

Destroying a protein's shape often destroys its normal functioning. That characteristic is useful for some body processes, such as digestion. When foods reach the stomach, stomach acid denatures some bacteria, plant hormones, many active enzymes, and other forms of proteins in foods. Cooking foods likewise denatures their proteins. These processes render the foods safer to eat and enhance our digestive processing. Denaturing proteins in some foods can also reduce their tendencies to cause allergic reactions. Recall that we need proteins in the diet to supply essential amino acids—not the active proteins themselves. We dismantle the proteins we get from foods and use the amino acids to assemble proteins we need.[20]

FUNCTIONS OF PROTEINS

As we have said, proteins function in a multitude of key roles in human metabolism and in the formation of body structures. We rely on foods to supply the amino acids needed to form these proteins. But again, only when we also eat enough carbohydrate and fat can food proteins be used most efficiently. If we don't consume enough kcalories to meet energy needs, some amino acids from proteins are broken down to produce needed energy, rather than used to make needed body proteins.[21]

Producing vital body constituents

Every cell contains protein. Muscles, connective tissue, blood-clotting factors, blood transport proteins, lipoproteins, enzymes, immune bodies, some hormones, visual pigments, and the support structure inside bones are mainly proteins. Measurements of the amounts of certain proteins, particularly some of those in the blood, are used as indicators of health or disease. Excess protein in the diet doesn't enhance the synthesis of body components, but eating too little can impede it.

Most vital body proteins are in a constant state of breakdown, rebuilding, and repair, especially in the bone marrow and the intestine. The GI tract lining is constantly *sloughed* off. The digestive tract treats sloughed cells just like food particles and absorbs the amino acids released during digestion. In fact, most protein breakdown products—amino acids—released throughout the body can be reused and are added to the pool of amino acids available for future protein synthesis (Figure 8-1).[20]

However, some protein breakdown products are lost rather than recycled. If a person habitually doesn't eat enough protein to replace this loss, the protein rebuilding and repairing process slows. For body growth and maintenance, amino acids must be supplied constantly from food. Otherwise, skeletal muscles, heart, liver, blood proteins, and other organs decrease in size or amount. Only the brain resists breakdown. To ensure good health a person must eat enough protein.

Maintaining fluid balance

Blood proteins—albumins and globulins—help maintain body fluid balance. Blood pressure in the arteries forces blood through blood vessels into capillary beds. The blood fluid then enters from the capillary beds into the spaces between nearby cells to provide nutrients to those cells (Figure 8-3). Proteins in the bloodstream are too large to move out of the capillary beds into the tissues. The presence of these proteins in the capillary beds attracts the fluid back to them, partially counteracting the force of blood pressure. This is especially true of the areas of the capillary beds right next to their venous connections (see Figure 5-4).

Unless enough protein is eaten, the level of proteins eventually decreases in the bloodstream. Excessive fluid then builds up in the tissues because the counteracting force produced by the smaller amount of blood proteins is too weak to pull much of the fluid back from the tissues into the bloodstream. As fluids pool in the tissues, the tissues swell. Clinical *edema* results.[15] Because edema sometimes leads to serious medical problems, the cause must be identified. In diagnosing the cause, an important step is to measure the level of blood proteins.

Contributing to chemical (ion) and acid-base balance

Proteins help regulate the degree of acidity—the acid-base balance—in the blood. Special proteins located in cell membranes act to pump chemical ions in and out of cells. The pumping action, among other things, works to keep the blood slightly alkaline. *Buffers*—compounds that maintain acid-base conditions within a narrow range—are another means used to regulate acid-base balance in the blood. Some blood proteins are especially good buffers for the body.[20]

Slough • To shed or cast off.

Edema • The buildup of excess fluid in extracellular spaces.

Buffer • Compounds that cause a solution to resist changes in acid-base balance.

Galactosemia • A disease characterized by the buildup of the single sugar galactose in the bloodstream because of the inability of the liver to metabolize it. If present at birth and left untreated, it results in severe growth and mental retardation.

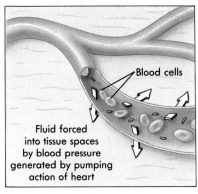
Arterial end of capillary bed

Blood cells

Fluid forced into tissue spaces by blood pressure generated by pumping action of heart

Blood pressure exceeds counteracting force of protein

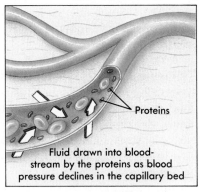
Venous end of capillary bed

Proteins

Fluid drawn into bloodstream by the proteins as blood pressure declines in the capillary bed

Blood pressure balanced by counteracting force of protein

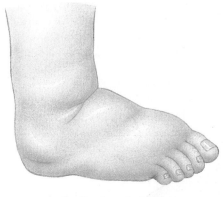
Swollen tissue (edema)

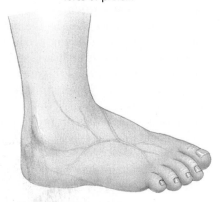
Normal tissue

FIGURE 8-3

Blood proteins are important for maintaining the body's fluid balance. Without sufficient protein in the bloodstream, edema develops.

Forming hormones and enzymes

Protein is required for the synthesis of many hormones—internal body messengers. Some hormones, such as the thyroid hormones, are made from only one or a few amino acids. Insulin on the other hand, is composed of 48 amino acids. These and other hormones classified as proteins perform important regulatory functions in the body, such as controlling the amount of glucose taken up from the bloodstream and the metabolic rate.[20]

 ANOTHER BITE Some hormone medicines from the protein class, such as the insulin used to treat some forms of diabetes mellitus, must be injected. If taken orally, insulin would be destroyed: the stomach and small intestine would digest the hormone, dismantling it into amino acids.

Enzymes are proteins.[20] Recall that enzymes are compounds that speed chemical reactions (see Chapter 5). Occasionally a cell lacks the correct genetic information to make needed enzymes. An infant, for example, suffering from the disease *galactosemia*, cannot make an enzyme needed to metabolize the single sugar galactose. This is much like what happens in PKU. If the infant is not put on a galactose-free diet soon after birth, its growth and mental development will be depressed. This example again demonstrates the crucial roles that enzymes, and thus proteins, play in cell function.[20]

Contributing to the immune function

Proteins make up key parts of the cells used by the immune system. Protein **antibodies** are produced by one type of immune cell. In an important immune response, the antibodies bind to foreign proteins in the body. Without enough protein from the diet, the immune system will eventually not produce enough of the cells and other tools needed to function properly.[15] However, eating more protein than is necessary doesn't boost immune function.

Forming glucose

In Chapter 6 we noted that the body must maintain a fairly constant level of glucose in the bloodstream to supply energy for red blood cells and nervous tissue. At rest, the brain uses about 35% of the body's energy requirements, and it gets most of that energy from glucose. If you don't eat enough carbohydrate to supply the glucose, your liver (and kidneys to a lesser extent) will be forced to make glucose from amino acids (see Figure 8-1). Many types of amino acids can by used for this purpose.[20]

Making some glucose from amino acids occurs normally. For example, when you skip breakfast and haven't eaten since 7 PM the preceding evening, glucose must be manufactured. Taken to an extreme, however, a constant need to convert amino acids into glucose, such as occurs in starvation, wastes much muscle tissue. This in turn reduces health.

Providing energy

Proteins supply about 10% of the energy the body uses (see Chapter 12 for information about the use of amino acids for energy during exercise). Most cells use primarily carbohydrates and fats for energy. Proteins and carbohydrates contain the same amount of usable energy, 4 kcalories per gram. However, proteins are a very costly source of energy, considering the amount of metabolism and processing the liver and kidneys must perform. The monetary cost of protein-rich foods is also a consideration.

CONCEPT CHECK

Amino acids are linked together in specific sequences to form distinct proteins. The amino acid order within a protein determines its ultimate structure. Destroying the shape or structure of a protein denatures it. Acid and alkaline conditions used in the body's digestive processes, heat, and other factors can denature proteins so that they lose their biological activity. Vital body constituents, such as muscle, connective tissue, blood transport proteins, enzymes, hormones, buffers, and immune bodies are mainly proteins. Proteins can also provide fuel for the body and be used for glucose production.

THE RECOMMENDED DIETARY ALLOWANCE FOR PROTEIN

How much protein (actually, amino acids) do we need to eat each day? People who aren't growing need to eat only enough protein to match whatever they lose daily from urine, feces, skin, hair, nails, and so on. In short, people need to balance protein intake with output. This maintains a state of protein equilibrium, as we discussed in Chapter 2.

When a body is either growing or recovering from an illness, it needs a positive protein balance to supply raw materials needed to build new tissues.[8] To

Antibody • Blood proteins that inactivate foreign proteins found in the body to prevent infections.

The more precise terminology is to refer to nitrogen balance. Recall proteins supply us with the form of nitrogen we use.

achieve this a person must eat more protein daily than he or she loses. This positive balance also requires an appropriate hormonal state. The hormones insulin, growth hormone, and testosterone all stimulate positive protein balance. Merely eating more protein does not guarantee a positive balance; building extra body tissues requires the right hormonal condition as well. Weight training also works by itself to enhance muscle mass.

Frequently during starvation or illness, the body loses much more protein than is replaced. The body then falls into a negative protein balance[15] (Table 8-2).

TABLE 8-2

Protein balance in practical terms

Protein equilibrium: body protein constant
Protein intake = Protein excretion
Positive protein balance: Increase in body protein
Protein intake > Protein excretion
Negative protein balance: decrease in body protein
Protein excretion > Protein intake

Positive protein balance	*Negative protein balance*
Growth	Inadequate intake of protein (fasting, intestinal tract diseases)
Pregnancy	Inadequate energy intake
Recovery stage after illness	Illnesses, such as fevers, burns, and infections
Athletic training*	
Increased secretion of hormones, such as insulin, growth hormone, and testosterone	Bed rest (days)
	Deficiency of essential amino acids
	Increased protein loss (as in some kidney diseases)
	Increased secretion of certain hormones, such as thyroid hormone and cortisol

*Only when additional lean body mass is being gained. Nevertheless, the athlete is probably already eating enough protein to support this extra protein synthesis: protein supplements are not needed.

For healthy people the amount of dietary protein needed to maintain nitrogen equilibrium (where intake equals output) can be determined by increasing protein intake until it just equals losses. Energy needs must be met so that amino acids are not diverted for energy use. Any protein intake above equilibrium also maintains a balance. But in order to estimate the requirement we need to determine the least amount of protein intake necessary to balance intake with output.[8]

Edward Smith, a British physician, studied energy and protein metabolism and in 1862 concluded that a physically active man would need 80 grams of protein daily. During the next 40 years, other estimates of protein needs, based on records of protein amounts consumed by healthy working men, ranged up to 150 grams per day. A controversy developed in the early 1900s after Russell Chittenden, an American chemist, concluded from studies on himself, his colleagues, and students at Yale that only 35 to 45 grams of protein daily was required for healthy adults.

Today the best estimate for the amount of protein required for nearly all adults is 0.8 grams of protein per kilogram of desirable body weight. This amount at least doubles during infancy. (We will discuss specific values for infants and children in Chapter 15 and the concept of desirable weight in Chapter 11.) Desirable weight is used as a baseline because excess fat storage doesn't contribute much to protein needs.

TABLE 8-3

The protein content of a 1200 and a 2400 kcalorie diet

This table illustrates how few kcalories can be consumed while still meeting the RDA for protein. It also shows how much protein we eat when we consume typical kcalorie intakes.

1200 Kcalories	Grams of Protein	2400 Kcalories	Grams of Protein
Breakfast			
1 cup skim milk	8	1 cup 2% milk	8
3/4 cup Cheerios	3	3/4 cup Cheerios	3
1 orange	—	2 soft-boiled eggs	12
		1 orange	—
Lunch			
2 slices whole-wheat bread	7	2 slices whole-wheat bread	7
2 oz chicken breast	18	2 oz chicken breast	18
1 t mayonnaise	—	2 oz provolone cheese	13
1 cup carrot sticks	1	1 t mayonnaise	—
1 fig	0.5	2 oatmeal raisin cookies	2
diet soda	—	2 figs	1
		diet soda	—
Dinner			
2 oz beef tenderloin	18	4 oz beef tenderloin	36
1 cup spinach pasta with 1 t garlic butter	7	1 cup spinach pasta with 1 t garlic butter	7
1/2 cup zucchini sauteed in 1 t oil	0.5	1/2 cup zucchini sauteed in 1 t oil	0.5
1 cup skim milk	8	1 cup 2% milk	8
1/2 toasted bagel	4	1 toasted bagel	7
1 t margarine	—	2 t margarine	—
	75 grams		**122 grams**

This recommended amount works out to about 56 grams of protein daily for a 70-kilogram (154-pound) man and about 44 grams of protein daily for a 55-kilogram (120-pound) woman. It is easy to eat this much protein each day, and even double this amount, given our typical kcalorie intakes (Table 8-3). American men typically consume about 90 grams of protein daily, while women typically consume 70 grams daily.

Recall that an RDA is an allowance, not a requirement. Some people need less than that amount of protein. Yet most of us get much more since we like many high protein foods and can afford to buy them. Excess protein eaten cannot be stored as such, so it is turned into glucose or fat and then either stored or burned for energy needs (see Figure 8-1).[20]

Pregnancy raises protein needs by about 6 grams daily averaged over the 9 months. However, mental stress, physical labor, and routine sports activity do not demand any extra protein allowance. To support either substantial gains in muscle tissue from high level sports activities or a large muscle mass acquired previously, increasing intake to about 1.3 to 1.5 grams per kilogram of body weight might be considered.[12] However, many Americans eat that much protein already. Adding extra dietary protein to normal adult diets, even for athletes, is usually not needed. In addition, there is no reason for athletes to take either protein or individual amino acid supplements—enough is available in whole foods (Table 8-3).

Does eating a mainly high-protein diet harm you?

The question is often asked whether the high protein intake of adults in America is harmful. (Getting too much protein can be very harmful to infants.

Canadians recommend 0.82 grams of protein per kilogram of body weight for adult men and 0.74 grams of protein per kilogram of body weight for adult women.

Instead of protein, it is most important for athletes to emphasize carbohydrate and fluid in the diet (see Chapter 12).

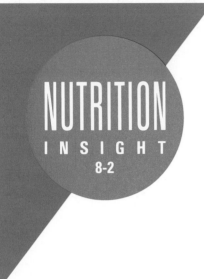

NUTRITION
I N S I G H T
8-2

DO YOU NEED TO REDISCOVER LEGUMES?

Legumes are a plant family with seed pods that contain one row of seeds: garden peas, green beans, lima beans, pinto beans, black-eyed peas, garbanzo beans, lentils, and soybeans. Dried varieties of the seeds—what we know as beans—yield an impressive contribution to the protein, vitamin, mineral, and dietary fiber content of a meal.[16]

Many people dismiss beans from their diets. This unfortunate oversight may be rooted in the Depression of the 1930s when people could afford little else. Beans are such a versatile food. They can anchor or blend into soups, salads, casseroles, sandwich spreads, and cracker dips. They can also be added in small quantities wherever extra body, texture, and/or nutritional value is desired. Incorporating them into your week's menu can add variety and new flavors (Table 8-4).

Most legumes, except lentils, need to be softened before cooking. Soak them overnight, or boil them uncovered for 2 minutes, remove from heat, cover, and let stand 1 hour. Dried beans double or triple in volume as they cook. Because legumes tend to soak up flavors during the cooking process, you can incorporate delicate flavors from combinations of herbs, spices, and broths.[16]

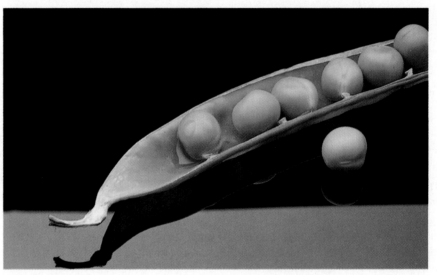

Peas are just one of the many legumes we can choose to eat.

We discuss this in Chapter 15.) The extra vitamin B-6, iron, and zinc that accompany protein foods is often beneficial, but the extra fat, especially saturated fat, found in many high protein animal foods is not. Research in the 1970s suggested that a high-protein diet might cause greater calcium loss in the urine. This worried researchers because they thought that protein caused calcium to leach out of the bones, setting the stage for osteoporosis, a severe bone disease (see Chapter 10). However, follow-up studies show that if extra phosphorus is also consumed, urine calcium does not increase so much.[19] Animal foods are excellent sources of both protein and phosphorus. So typical American protein consumption probably doesn't threaten calcium balance as long as it is part of a diet that also meets the RDA for calcium.

There is some concern that a diet high in protein may overwork the kidneys since they must excrete excess nitrogen (mostly as urea) into the urine. Laboratory animal studies show that getting just enough protein to meet nutritional needs preserves kidney function over time better than high-protein diets.

TABLE 8-4

Get to know the legumes

Type	Color	Use
Black beans	Black	Baked, soups, stews
Black-eyed peas	White with a black spot	Casseroles
Garbanzo beans (chickpeas)	Brown	Dips, casseroles, salads, soups, stews
Great northern beans	White	Baked, casseroles, chowder, soups, stews
Kidney beans	Red	Casseroles, chili, salads, soups
Lentils	Brown or green	Casseroles, salads, soups
Lima beans	White	Casseroles, soups
Navy beans	White	Baked, soups
Pinto beans	Pink	Baked, casseroles, soups
Red beans	Red	Casseroles, chili
Soybeans	Tan	Casseroles, salads
Split peas	Green or yellow	Soups

Adapted from Neiman, Butterworth, Neiman: *Nutrition*, 1990, William C Brown.

When you initially add legumes to your diet, they may cause intestinal gas. Split peas, limas, and lentils are less likely to do so than the others, so start with them. Take small servings at first and give your GI tract a few weeks to adjust. Many people have no trouble with legumes, but it's best to be cautious.

Like all foods, though, legumes do not offer every nutrient, and so they do not make a complete diet by themselves. They contain no vitamin A, vitamin C, or vitamin B-12, and their balance of amino acids needs to be improved by eating grains and other vegetables with them. Many traditional ethnic dishes combine legumes with grains and vegetables to yield a high quality protein balance: lentil curry on rice; pinto beans and corn tortillas; tofu (soybean curd) and rice; and corn and lima beans (succotash).[16] Try these combinations or create your own.

As you prepare foods or order them in a restaurant, look for beans—salad bars usually provide a few choices. Black bean and other bean soups, baked beans, chili, red beans and rice, and soy burgers are other possibilities. Regularly consuming vegetable proteins, as noted in Chapter 2, can add substantial amounts of nutrients to a diet. And as discussed in Chapter 7, the soluble fiber in them can help lower your blood cholesterol level as well. ●

Protecting kidneys is especially important for people with either diabetes mellitus or only one functioning kidney. Presently many medical centers in the United States are studying whether a conservative protein diet maintains kidney function better than the typical American protein intake for people with kidney disease. For people without diabetes the overall risk of kidney failure is low, and so the chances of a high-protein diet contributing to kidney disease in later life are slim.[2,17]

The importance of plant proteins

Vegetable sources of proteins deserve more attention from Americans. Many plant foods, in proportion to the amount of energy they supply, provide not only protein but also ample magnesium and dietary fiber, along with other benefits.[14] The vegetables we eat also contain no cholesterol and little saturated fat, unless these are added during processing. One or two daily servings of plant foods high in protein make a valuable addition to the Guide to Daily Food

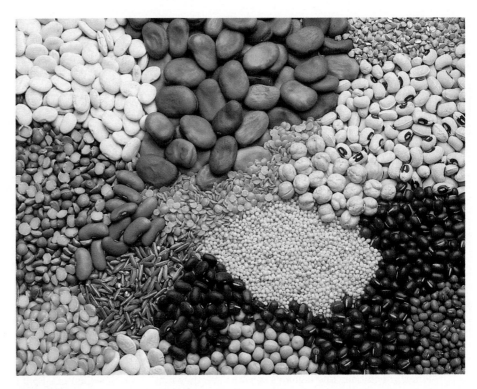

FIGURE 8-4
Legumes—another protein source that can meet a body's need. An added bonus is the many other nutrients also present in legumes.

Choices because they supply a variety of other nutrients. Presently concentrated sources of plant proteins are not very popular in America, except for maybe peanut butter, pork and beans, and refried beans. Should you give them a second look (Figure 8-4)?

CONCEPT CHECK

The Recommended Dietary Allowance for adults is 0.8 gram of protein per kilogram of desirable body weight. This adds up to 56 grams of protein daily for a 70-kilogram (156-pound) person. The average American man consumes about 90 grams of protein daily, and a woman consumes about 70 grams. So, typically, we eat more than enough protein to meet our needs. Aside from the fat present in most high protein diets, this excess poses no health risk for most of us.

PROTEIN IN FOODS

The most nutrient-dense source of protein is water-packed tuna, which has over 80% of kcalories as protein (Figure 8-5). Notice in Figure 8-5 that all foods with more than 20% of kcalories as protein are animal foods. They are also the major sources of protein in the American diet: we get over two-thirds of our protein from animal sources. Worldwide, 54% of the protein consumed comes from animal sources. In Africa and East Asia less than 25% of the protein eaten comes from animals.[15]

In the United States in 1988, red meat and poultry consumption reached an all-time high of 253 pounds per person per year, nearly 58 pounds above the 1960 figures. Beef still leads with an annual consumption of 104 pounds per per-

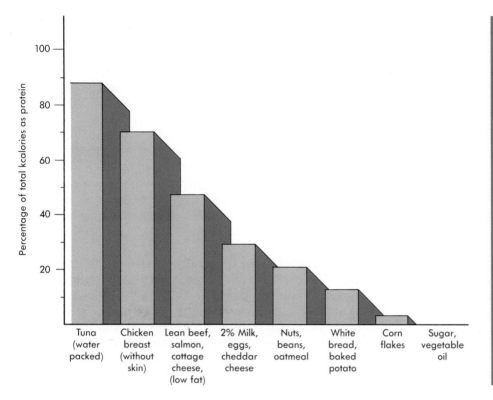

FIGURE 8-5
Percent of kcalories as proteins in foods. Water-packed tuna provides almost all kcalories as proteins. Notice all foods containing more than 20% of kcalories from protein are of animal origin.

son, but chicken is gaining fast, increasing from 28 pounds per person in 1960 to 64 pounds in 1988.

The amino acids most likely to be low in a diet are lysine, methionine, threonine, and tryptophan.[21] Table 8-1 lists plant foods characteristically low in these amino acids, although new strains of high-lysine and high-tryptophan corn are now available, along with other improved grains. These strains provide a better balance of amino acids. If a diet is low in an amino acid, we recommend finding a good food source to supply it. Forget about amino acid supplements—they can lead to problems, as we discussed earlier.

PROTEIN-ENERGY MALNUTRITION

In poorer areas of the world, people often eat diets low in kcalories and protein. This state of undernutrition stunts their growth in childhood and makes them more susceptible to disease throughout life.[15] (This state is a main focus of Chapter 18.) People who eat too little protein and energy food can go on to develop *protein-energy malnutrition* (PEM), also referred to as protein-calorie malnutrition (PCM). In its milder form, which is most common, it is difficult to tell if a person with PEM is eating too few kcalories or protein, or both. But if the nutrient deficiency, especially for kcalories, is quite severe, a deficiency disease called *marasmus* can result. On the other hand, when a poor nutrient intake, protein included, is added to other problems from concurrent diseases and infections, a disease called *kwashiorkor* can develop. These two diseases form the tip of the iceberg with respect to all states of undernutrition, and symptoms of these two diseases even can be present in the same person (Figure 8-6).

Kwashiorkor

Kwashiorkor is a word from Ghana that means "the disease that the first child gets when the new child comes." From birth the first child is usually breastfed. By the time the child reaches 1 to 1.5 years, the mother is probably pregnant or has already given birth again. Breastfeeding is no longer possible for the first child. That child abruptly switches from nutritious breast milk to native starchy roots and gruels. These foods have very low protein densities compared with total kcalories. The foods are also often so bulky and full of plant fibers that it is difficult for the child to eat enough of them. So these young children who have high nutrient demands for growth end up consuming some kcalories, but their protein needs are not met, especially when these needs are also raised by concurrent illnesses, infections, and an insufficient kcalorie intake.[15,18] Probably many vitamin and mineral needs also are far from being met. Feeding famine victims starchy roots, such as cassava (tapioca), creates the same problem.

The major symptoms of kwashiorkor are apathy, listlessness, failure to grow and gain weight, and withdrawal from the environment. These symptoms are often added to the results of other diseases present. Now measles—a condition that normally makes a healthy child sick for only a week or so—develops into a severely debilitating and even fatal disease. Further effects of kwashiorkor are changes in hair color, flaky skin, fat buildup in the liver, and massive edema in the abdomen and legs. The presence of edema, some visible fat stores, and only a moderate weight deficit are the hallmarks of this disease in children. In addition, a strange behavior among these children is that they hardly move. If you pick them up, they don't cry. When you hold them, you realize you are feeling the plumpness of edema, not lean body tissue.[15]

Edema with only a moderate deficit in body weight and maintenance of some fat tissue

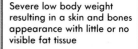

Severe low body weight resulting in a skin and bones appearance with little or no visible fat tissue

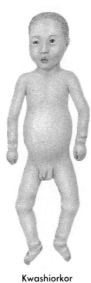

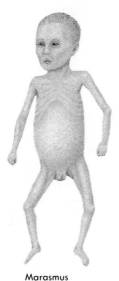

Kwashiorkor

Marasmus

FIGURE 8-6

A schema for classifying severe protein-energy malnutrition. The presence of visible fat (i.e., directly underneath the skin) and edema are the diagnostic keys. Infants and young children are generally the ones most severely affected in comparison to adults.

Although a variety of factors contribute to the clinical picture of kwashiorkor, we can explain some results of kwashiorkor based on what we know about proteins. Proteins play important roles in fluid balance, immune function, and production of tissues such as skin and hair. Children deprived of sufficient protein and energy cannot grow and mature normally. And they don't!

If a child with kwashiorkor is helped in time to address medical problems present and fed a diet ample in protein, kcalories, and other essential nutrients, the disease symptoms reverse. The child begins to grow again, and may even show no signs of the previous condition, aside perhaps from shortness of stature. However, by the time many of these children reach a hospital or care center, they already have severe infections. In spite of the best care, they still die. Or, if they survive, they return home only to repeat the cycle.

Marasmus

Marasmus is a disease that occurs when a child basically starves to death.[15,18] The word marasmus means "to waste away." Children do just that. They appear to be "skin and bones," like the figures on posters from relief agencies. Low body weight without edema or fat stores is the hallmark of the disease. A child with marasmus is usually under age 2 and was either not breastfed at all or breastfed for only a few months. In all probability, the weaning formula was improperly prepared, partly because of poor water supplies and partly because the parents couldn't afford enough formula for the child's needs. To stretch the formula out, the parents may have diluted it, providing less nutrients and more water for the child. The parents often have no other alternative.

Marasmus commonly occurs in the large cities of poverty-stricken countries. In the cities it is more common to bottle-feed. When people are poor and live in unsanitary conditions, bottle-feeding often leads to marasmus.[15,18] A child with marasmus requires large amounts of kcalories, protein, and other nutrients to attempt to recover from the disease.

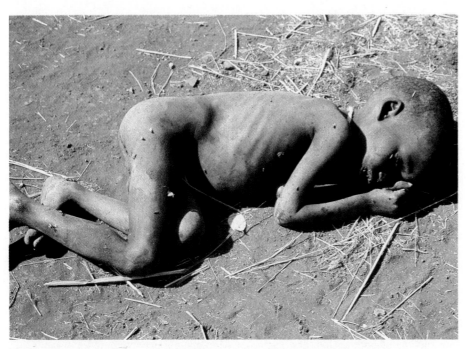

When undernutrition and people collide, human suffering is a typical result.

CONCEPT CHECK

Most undernutrition worldwide consists of mild deficits in kcalories, protein, and often other nutrients. If a person needs more nutrients because of disease and infection but consumes too few kcalories and too little protein, a condition known as kwashiorkor can develop. The person suffers from edema and weakness. Children around age 2 are especially susceptible to kwashiorkor, particularly if they already have other diseases. Famine situations where only starchy root products are available to eat can set up this problem. Marasmus is a condition where people—infants especially—essentially starve to death. Symptoms include muscle wasting, absence of fat stores, and weakness. Both an adequate diet and treatment of concurrent diseases must be promoted in poor countries to maintain nutritional health.

SUMMARY

• Amino acids are the building blocks of proteins. Amino acids contain a very useable form of nitrogen for us. Of the 20 types of amino acids found in food, nine are essential to consume and 11 can be synthesized by the body.

• High quality, also called complete, protein foods contain ample amounts of all nine essential amino acids. Animal foods typically supply all of them in approximately the right amounts. Low quality, also called incomplete, protein foods lack sufficient amounts of one or more essential amino acids. This is typical of plant foods, especially cereal grains. Plant foods eaten together often complement each other's amino acid deficits, in turn providing a high quality protein diet. Because supplementing the diet with large amounts of individual amino acids can lead to buildup of harmful levels, their use outside of medical therapy is not advised.

• Individual amino acids are linked together to form proteins. The sequential order of amino acids determines the protein's ultimate form and in turn function. If the three-dimensional shape of the protein eventually formed is unfolded—denatured—by treatment with heat, acid or alkaline solutions, or other processes, the protein loses its biological activity.

• Essential body components, such as muscles, connective tissue, transport proteins, visual pigments, enzymes, some hormones, and immune bodies are made of proteins. Proteins also provide carbon that can be used to synthesize glucose when necessary.

• RDA for protein for adults is 0.8 grams per kilogram of desirable body weight. For a 70-kilogram (156-pound) person this corresponds to 56 grams of protein daily. American men consume about 90 grams of protein daily and women consume closer to 70 grams. Thus the American diet generally supplies plenty of protein. The combined protein intake is also of sufficient quality so that most of what is present in the diet can be used for body functions.

• Animal meats are the most nutrient-dense sources of protein. Water-packed tuna contains over 80% of its kcalories as protein. These proteins show high values for biological value in that we have a great ability to turn them into body proteins. Plant foods generally contain less than 20% of their kcalories as protein; however, legumes provide much protein when regularly part of a diet and contribute to a high biological value for a meal if eaten with grain proteins.

• Undernutrition occasionally leads to kwashiorkor and marasmus. Kwashiorkor results primarily from a poor kcalorie and protein intake in comparison to needs, which in turn are often raised by concurrent disease and infections. Kwashiorkor often results when a child is taken off human milk and fed starchy gruels. Marasmus results primarily from starvation—a negligible intake of both protein and kcalories. Marasmus commonly occurs in famine conditions, especially in infants.

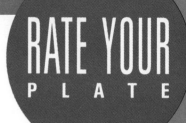

ARE YOU EATING ENOUGH PROTEIN?

How much protein do you eat in a typical day? Look at the nutrition assessment you completed at the end of Chapter 2. Review it closely. Find the figure indicating the amount of protein you consumed on that day, and write it in the space below:

TOTAL PROTEIN _____

Compare your protein intake to your RDA for protein. Find your desirable weight in pounds in Table 1-2, and choose a midrange value. Divide this number by 2.2 to reveal your desirable weight in kilograms. Next multiply by 0.8 grams per kilogram body weight. This will indicate your RDA. Write it in the space below:

RDA FOR PROTEIN _____

How does your consumption compare to your RDA?

_____

_____

_____

If you consumed either more or less than the RDA, what foods could you add, subtract, or eat more or less of? (Look at the foods you ate.)

_____

_____

_____

_____

Was most of your protein from animal or plant sources?

_____

_____

REFERENCES

1. ADA Reports: Position of the American Dietetic Association: Vegetarian diets, *Journal of the American Dietetic Association* 88:351-355, 1988.

2. Blum M and others: Protein intake and kidney function in humans: its effect on normal aging, *Archives of Internal Medicine* 149:211, 1989.

3. Belongia EA and others: An investigation of the cause of the eosinophilia-myalgia syndrome associated with tryptophan use, *New England Journal of Medicine* 323:357, 1990.

4. Dwyer JT: Health aspects of vegetarian diets, *American Journal of Clinical Nutrition* 48:712, 1988.

5. Eaton SB and others: *The Paleolithic prescription*, New York, 1988, Harper & Row.

6. Freeland-Graves JH: Mineral adequacy of vegetarian diets, *American Journal of Clinical Nutrition* 48:859, 1988.

7. Freeland-Graves JH and others: Health practices, attitudes and beliefs of vegetarians and nonvegetarians, *Journal of the American Dietetic Association* 86:913, 1986.

8. Fukagawa NK, Young VR: Protein and amino acid metabolism and requirements in older persons, *Clinics in Geriatric Medicine* 3:329, 1987.

9. Herbert V: Vitamin B-12: plant sources, requirements, and assay, *American Journal of Clinical Nutrition* 48:852, 1988.

10. Hertzman PA and others: Association of the eosinophilia myalgia syndrome with the ingestion of tryptophan, *New England Journal of Medicine* 322:869, 1990.

11. Jacobs C, Dwyer JT: Vegetarian children: appropriate and inappropriate diets, *American Journal of Clinical Nutrition* 48:811, 1988.

12. Meridith CN and others. Dietary protein requirements and body protein metabolism in endurance-trained men, *Journal of Applied Physiology* 66:2850, 1989.

13. National Institute of Nutrition (Canada): Risks and benefits of vegetarian diets, *Nutrition Today*, March/April, 1990, p 27.

14. Nieman DC and others: Dietary status of Seventh-Day Adventist vegetarian and non-vegetarian elderly women, *Journal of the American Dietetic Association* 89:1763, 1989.

15. Olson RE: World food production and problems in human nutrition, *Nutrition Today*, January/February, 1989, p 15.

16. Robertson L and others: *The new Laurel's kitchen*, Berkeley, Calif, 1986, Ten Speed Press.

17. Rudman D: Kidney senescence: a model for aging, *Nutrition Reviews* 46:209, 1988.

18. Scrimshaw NS: The phenomenon of famine, *Annual Reviews of Nutrition* 7:1, 1987.

19. Spencer H and others: Factors contributing to calcium loss in aging, *American Journal of Clinical Nutrition* 36:776, 1982.

20. Stryer L: *Biochemistry*, ed 3, New York, 1988, WH Freeman.

21. Young VR: Kinetics of amino acid metabolism: nutritional implications and some lessons, 1987 McCollum Award Lecture, *American Journal of Clinical Nutrition* 46:709, 1987.

HOW MUCH HAVE I LEARNED?

What have you learned from Chapter 8? Here are 15 statements about protein. Read them to test your current knowledge. If you think the statement is true or mostly true, circle T. If you think the statement is false or mostly false, circle F. Use the scoring key at the end of the book to compute your total score. To review, take this test again later, and especially before tests.

1. T (F) Most people have trouble assembling a diet containing all the essential amino acids.

2. (T) F An insufficient protein intake can stunt a child's growth. *protein important for building new tissues during growth.*

3. (T) F Most enzymes are proteins.

4. T (F) If only a few amino acids are rearranged in a specific protein, its function will not be affected.

5. (T) F The quality of protein can be measured by its biological value—nitrogen retention divided by nitrogen absorption. *Biological value represents body's ability to retain protein absorbed*

6. (T) F Milk provides higher quality proteins than most other foods. *milk proteins provide 1 of highest possible biological values from foods. Egg white has very best biological value*

7. T (F) The greatest need for protein occurs in the elderly years. *people require more protein per weight during growing years*

8. T (F) Athletes usually need at least double the amount of protein of nonathletes. Protein supplements are the preferred source. *protein supplements can be dangerous can get protein needs w/ basic foods*

9. (T) F Animal protein sources often contain high amounts of saturated fat. *Trimming fats off meat & broiling best*

10. (T) F Lack of energy can be a symptom of severe protein deficiency. *symptom of severe protein-energy malnutrition*

11. T (F) Gelatin supplements are ideal for strengthening the fingernails. *gelatin is an incomplete protein. lacks amino acid tryptophan. poor source for supporting any protein synthesis in body.*

12. (T) F Marasmus is a disease caused by starvation and often occurs in large cities of impoverished countries. *marasmus "waste away"*

13. T (F) There is little difference in nutrient content between animal and vegetable protein. *animal protein — most absorbable form of iron & almost all vitamin B₁₂ intake. plant protein — much dietary fiber & magnesium*

14. (T) F Water-packed tuna is almost pure protein. *80% protein*

15. (T) F Fruits contain very little protein. *mostly carbohydrate & water*

NUTRITION ISSUE

VEGETARIANISM

The practice of vegetarianism goes back to the time of the Greek philosophers, yet today it is new to many people. Throughout human history vegetarianism has evolved from a necessity into a personal option (Figure 8-7). Historically, vegetarianism was linked with specific philosophies, religion, or science. Today, vegetarianism in this country usually appeals to a younger segment of people.[7]

As nutrition science has grown, new information has enabled us to design adequate vegetarian diets. It is important for vegetarians to take advantage of this information because a diet of only plants can lead to various nutrient

THE FAR SIDE   By GARY LARSON

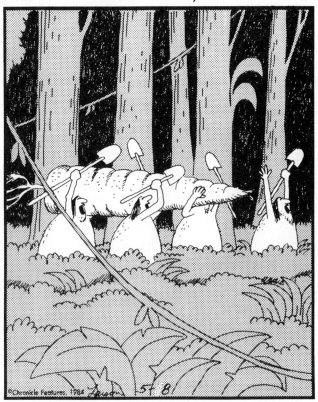

Early vegetarians returning from the kill.

FIGURE 8-7

deficiencies and poor growth in children. If you choose to eat a vegetarian diet, be confident that you can meet your nutritional needs by following a few basic rules. Recent studies even show that death rates from some chronic diseases are lower for vegetarians than for nonvegetarians. Healthful lifestyles (leanness, not smoking, abstinence from alcohol and drugs, and increased physical activity) and social class selection bias, in addition to the vegetarian diet, probably also all account for these findings.[7]

Why do people practice vegetarianism?

People choose vegetarianism for a variety of reasons. Some think it is more ethical not to kill animals for food. Hindus and Trappist monks eat vegetarian meals as a practice of their religion. In the United States many Seventh Day Adventists base their practice of vegetarianism on biblical texts and believe it is a healthier way to eat.[4]

A person might choose vegetarianism after realizing that animals are not efficient protein factories. Animals actually use much of the protein they eat just to maintain themselves, rather than using it to synthesize new muscle tissue. A cow eats 21 pounds of plant protein for every pound of meat protein it produces. The ratio for pigs is 8 to 1; for chickens 5 to 1. Food animals do sometimes eat grasses that humans cannot digest. However, many also eat grains humans can eat.

People might also practice vegetarianism because the diet encourages a high intake of carbohydrates, vitamin A, vitamin E, beta-carotene, vitamin C, magnesium, and dietary fiber, while limiting cholesterol and saturated fat intake.[4,7] This rationale produces a diet closely resembling that suggested in the Dietary Guidelines for Americans covered in Chapter 2. Studies confirm that vegetarians actually do eat nutritious diets.[14] Some people might pursue vegetarianism because meat is expensive.

Food planning for vegetarians

There are a variety of vegetarian styles. **Vegans** eat only plant foods. Fruitarians eat primarily fruits, nuts, honey, and vegetable oils. This plan is not recommended as it can lead to nutrient deficiencies in people of all ages. **Lacto-vegetarians** modify vegetarianism a bit—they include dairy products and plant foods. **Lacto-ovo-vegetarians** modify the diet even further and eat dairy products, eggs, and plant foods.[1] Actually, including these animal products makes food planning easier since they are rich in some nutrients missing or in low amounts in plants. Overall, the wider the variety of foods eaten, the easier it is to meet nutritional needs. Thus the practice of eating no animal sources of food significantly separates the vegans and fruitarians from all other semivegetarian styles.

Most people who call themselves vegetarians consume at least some dairy products, if not dairy products and eggs. A four-food-group plan has been developed for lacto-vegetarians (Table 8-5).[16] This plan's protein group includes nuts, grains, legumes, and seeds. There is also a vegetable group, a fruit group, and a milk and/or eggs group.

This plan differs a little from the typical Guide to Daily Food Choices for **omnivores**, but it shares some similarities. The key to this plan is seeking foods other than meats that supply the nutrients contained in meats. It's not nutritionally sound to just cut out meat and to eat everything else without making sure the body's needs are still met. One should eat good quality plant sources of nutrients to replace those that normally come from meat in the diet. Nuts, grains, legumes, and seeds supply ample nutrients when consumed together; they become the new "meat" group.[16] By following the food plan, a lacto-vegetarian should have no problem eating an adequate diet.

Vegan • A person who consumes no animal products.

Lacto-vegetarian • A semivegetarian food plan where milk products are consumed as well as vegetable products.

Lacto-ovo-vegetarian • A semivegetarian food plan where a person consumes plant products, dairy products, and eggs.

Omnivore • A person who consumes both plant and animal food sources.

TABLE 8-5

A four-food-group plan for lacto-vegetarians[6]

Group*	Servings	Key Nutrients Supplied
Grains, legumes, nuts, and seeds	6	Protein, thiamin, niacin, vitamin B-6, folate, vitamin E, zinc, magnesium, and fiber
Vegetables	3 or more (include one dark-green leafy)	Vitamin A, vitamin C, folate
Fruits	1 to 4	Vitamin A, vitamin C, folate
Milk	2 or more	Protein, riboflavin, vitamin D, vitamin B-12, and calcium

*Base serving size on those listed in the Guide to Daily Food Choices (see Chapter 2).

Following are examples of combinations of plant foods that, when eaten together, provide complete protein. These are often a legume-grain combination:
- rice and red beans
- rice and green peas
- barley and navy beans
- corn and pinto beans
- corn and green peas
- corn and lima beans (succotash)
- bulgur wheat and garbanzo beans
- soybeans and sesame seeds
- peanuts, rice, and black eyed peas
- sunflower seeds and green peas

The vegan

Eating a vegan diet requires some creative planning.[1] First, purchasing some vegetarian cookbooks will simplify the task. They provide numerous ideas for imaginative and nutritious ways to use plant foods. A real effort must be made to use grains and legumes to obtain good quality protein and other key nutrients. Then if one satisfies kcalorie needs, protein needs should also be met. A wide variety of protein sources, including the excellent ones just mentioned, should provide all amino acids needed for a complete protein diet. In other words, the essential amino acids deficient from one food protein are supplied by those of another protein in the same meal or in the next.

To get the benefit of a high quality protein diet, must vegans get all the essential amino acids from plant proteins within one meal? Can plant proteins complement each other's deficiencies if eaten at separate meals? Research demonstrates that all the essential amino acids can be effectively used even when eaten at separate meals in a day.[8] This is primarily because none of the meals will completely lack one or more of the essential amino acids.

The vegan diet also needs good sources of riboflavin, vitamin D, vitamin B-12, calcium, iron, and zinc (Table 8-6). Riboflavin can be obtained by eating green leafy vegetables, whole grains, yeast, and legumes. Most vegans eat these foods. Note that the major source of riboflavin in the American diet is milk, which is omitted from the vegan diet. Vitamin D can be obtained through regular sun exposure. Otherwise, a supplement containing vitamin D should be considered (see Chapter 9).

The vegan should find a reliable source of vitamin B-12, such as fortified soybean milk or special yeast grown on media rich in vitamin B-12 (check the label). Vitamin B-12 occurs naturally only in animal foods; plants can contain soil or microbial contamination that provides a trace amount of vitamin B-12.[9] Because the body can store enough vitamin B-12 for up to 4 years, it takes a long time for a deficiency to develop after someone has given up animal foods. If a deficiency develops, nerves can be damaged irreversibly. Therefore vegans need to prevent this vitamin B-12 deficiency (see Chapter 9).

To obtain calcium, the vegan can drink fortified soybean milk or fortified orange juice. Tofu, green leafy vegetables, and nuts also contain calcium but it

TABLE 8-6

Nutrients likely to be low in the diet of a total vegetarian (vegan)

Nutrient	Plant Sources
Vitamin D	Fortified margarines, fortified breakfast cereals
Riboflavin	Whole and enriched grains, leafy vegetables, mushrooms, beans, nuts, seeds
Vitamin B-12	Fortified breakfast cereals, fortified yeast, fortified soybean milk
Iron	Whole grains, prune juice, dried fruits, beans, nuts, seeds, leafy vegetables
Calcium	Fortified soybean milk,* tofu, almonds, dry beans, leafy vegetables, some fortified breakfast cereals, flours, and brands of orange juice*
Zinc	Whole grains, wheat germ, beans, nuts, seeds

*Fortified soybean milk and fortified orange juice are the best sources.

is either not well absorbed from them or not very plentiful. Calcium supplements are another option.

For iron the vegan can consume whole grains, dried fruits, and legumes. The iron in these foods is not absorbed as well as that found in animal foods, but a good source of vitamin C taken with these foods can greatly enhance iron absorption. Thus an excellent strategy is to consume vitamin C with every meal that contains adequate iron from plant foods.

The vegan can find zinc in whole grains and legumes.[6] Phytic acid in whole grains limits zinc absorption. Grains are most nutritious when leavened, as in bread, because this process reduces the influence of phytic acid.

Of all these nutrients, sufficient calcium is the most difficult to consume. Special diet planning is required (Table 8-6).

Veganism during childhood can pose problems.[11] The sheer bulk of a plant-based diet may make it difficult for a child to eat foods that supply enough energy to permit dietary protein to be used for synthesis of body proteins, rather than used for energy needs. Vegan children need concentrated sources of kcalories to avoid this problem.[1,13] Examples include fortified soybean milk, nuts, dried fruits, avocados, cookies made with vegetable oils, and fruit juices.

FRANK & ERNEST® by Bob Thaves

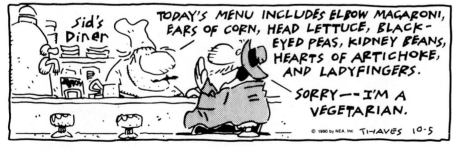

FIGURE 8-8

Anyone considering vegetarianism should realize that a healthful diet does not happen automatically. It takes planning and common sense (Figure 8-8). We keep stressing the importance of eating a wide variety of foods. This is especially important for the vegetarian. ●

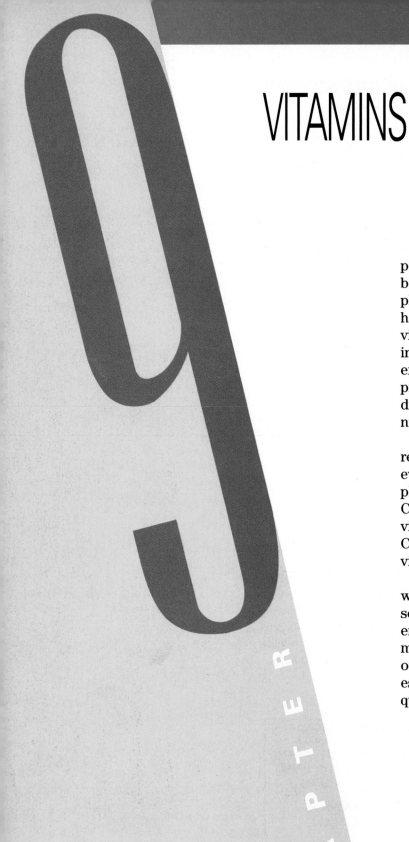

VITAMINS

W hen it comes to vitamins and minerals people often are told: If a little is good, more is better. This is a popular belief held by some people in their pursuit of better health. Today about half of the adults in some areas of the U.S. take vitamin supplements.[18] This fuels a $3 billion industry. The number of people who take extremely large doses in the belief that vitamins provide extra energy, health, and protection from disease is unknown, but sales suggest that the number is enormous.

In stark contrast, our total vitamin needs are really quite small, about 1 ounce (28 grams) for every 150 pounds (70 kg) of food we eat. Most plants can synthesize all the vitamins they need. Certain animal species can even synthesize some vitamins; cats and dogs make their own vitamin C. However, human bodies cannot make most vitamins, and so we rely on diet to supply them.

Who should take vitamin supplements and what dosage should be taken? What are the best sources of vitamins? Are there important differences between dietary sources of vitamins and man-made vitamins? How do vitamins work for our bodies? Can vitamins help prevent cancer, especially vitamins A, E, and C? These are some questions we address in this chapter. ●

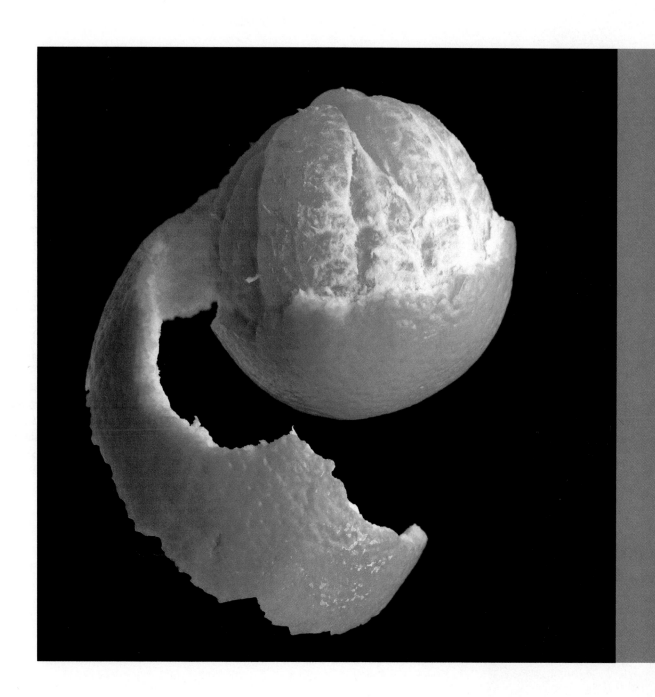

CHAPTER 9

What Do You Believe About Vitamin Supplements?

Below is a brief article about vitamins, typical of one you might find in a popular health and fitness or women's magazine. As you read it, it is your job to decide whether you think the claims being made are true or false. A blank is provided next to each claim to record your answers. Write "T" if you think the statement is true or "F" if you think it is false.

VITAMINS: OUR HEALTH PROMOTING ALLIES
BY DR. WILBERT GRUNTALOUD

Do you take vitamins? If not, you probably aren't doing all you can to promote your health. There are some hidden truths about vitamins that the medical community rarely discloses. Do you suffer from frequent colds and flu? Many people spend their hard earned dollars for cold medicines and lose a number of workdays because of these ailments. We now know that certain vitamin supplements can prevent colds and flu _F_.

Do you eat a relatively poor diet because of all the responsibilities you must handle? Vitamin supplements can completely make up for a poor diet _F_. Do you feel tired and fatigued frequently? You may be one of those people who requires very high intakes of vitamins to be healthy _F_. In addition, vitamin supplements will give you extra energy, especially during times of increased stress _F_. Most of us can't get all the vitamins we need from the food we eat because plants, potentially rich sources of vitamins, are vitamin deficient today because the soil is so depleted of the nutrients needed for healthy plant growth _F_. Worried about the negative health effects of chemical pollutants in our air and water? Vitamin supplements can protect you _F_.

See all the benefits vitamin supplements can bring you? Our Vitablast pack can provide you with all the vitamins you need. These vitamins are from natural sources and therefore safer and much better than synthetic ones _F_. We at Vitablast Distributors can provide you with a regular supply of vitamins and other supplements for a nominal fee.

Can you afford not to take vitamin supplements? Decide for yourself. Vitamin supplements are harmless, so taking extra amounts will just give extra benefits and security _F_. So what do you have to lose?

Check the answers you gave above with Table 9-1. Should you spend your money on vitamin supplements?

ASSESS YOURSELF

VITAMINS—A 20TH CENTURY PHENOMENON

Based on what we just said, **vitamins** can be defined as carbon-containing substances that the body must obtain, although in only small amounts, to maintain health. In this case *obtain* means either ingested or produced by the skin or bacteria in the intestine. The latter is true, however, in only a few cases. Vitamins are used by the body to help promote and regulate various chemical reactions and processes. Deficiency diseases arise when our bodies are deprived of a vitamin for a prolonged time. Furthermore, to be a *true* vitamin, it must cure the deficiency disease if resupplied in time. While vitamins do not directly yield energy, many do act as energy-yielding catalysts in processes such as body growth and development and energy production.

Scientists began to identify the substances we call vitamins around the turn of this century. Deficiency diseases, such as scurvy, beriberi, pellagra, and rickets, had been causing enormous suffering for centuries. Once scientists discovered that the problems arose because vital substances—vitamins—were missing from the diet, the diseases were dramatically cured. For the most part, as the vitamins were discovered, they were named alphabetically, A, B, C, D, E, and so on. Later many substances originally classified as vitamins were found not to be essential for humans and were dropped from the list. This explains

> **Vitamins** • Carbon-containing compounds that are needed in very small amounts in the diet to help promote and regulate chemical reactions and processes in the body.

TABLE 9-1

Myths and facts about vitamin supplementation

Most of us view scientific knowledge with awe, and we are quite justified, considering the scientific achievements of our age. Misconceptions about vitamins and their proper functions are understandable. Let's clear up some of these misconceptions:

Myth: Vitamins give you "pep" and "energy."

Fact: Vitamins yield no kcalories. They, of themselves, provide no extra pep or vitality beyond normal expectations, nor do they provide unusual levels of well-being.

Myth: Timing of vitamin intake is crucial.

Fact: There is no medical or scientific basis for this contention.

Myth: Some people need very high intakes of vitamins to be healthy.

Fact: A multitude of studies have shown that it is rare for anyone to need amounts higher than the RDA.

Myth: Vitamin supplements are necessary because today the soil is so depleted.

Fact: Crops can't grow in depleted soil. If a nutrient is low, the yield will be low, but the vitamin content will be normal.

Myth: Vitamins must be taken in precisely formulated amounts and ratios to each other in order to have best effects.

Fact: Intake should be adequate but not excessive for each. No precise ratios are required.

Myth: Organic or natural vitamins are nutritionally superior to synthetic vitamins.

Fact: Synthetic vitamins, manufactured in the laboratory, are identical to the natural vitamins found in foods. The body cannot tell the difference and gets the same benefits from either source. Statements to the effect that "Nature cannot be imitated" and "natural vitamins have the essence of life" are without meaning.

Myth: Vitamin C "protects" against the common cold.

Fact: Too bad, but extensive clinical research fails to support this.

Myth: The more vitamins the better.

Fact: Taking excess vitamins is a complete waste, both in money and effect. In fact, excess amounts of any of several different vitamins can be harmful.

Myth: You cannot get enough vitamins from the conventional foods you eat.

Fact: Anyone who eats a reasonably varied diet that includes animal products should normally not need supplemental vitamins.

Myth: Vitamin supplements are needed to protect against harmful chemicals and pollution.

Fact: Vitamin supplements do not have special abilities to ward off harmful agents.

Modified from Some facts and myths about vitamins, *FDA Consumer*, September, 1979.

Fat-soluble Vitamins •
Vitamins that dissolve in substances such as ether or benzene. These vitamins include A, D, E, and K.

Water-Soluble Vitamins •
Vitamins that dissolve in water. These vitamins include the B vitamins and vitamin C.

the many gaps in the alphabetical listing. Other vitamins, thought at first to be only one chemical form, turned out to be many forms, so the alphabetical name had to be broken down by numbers (B-6, B-12, etc.) (Figure 9-1).

Almost as soon as vitamins were identified, scientists began to synthesize them in laboratories or isolate them from plant or animal sources. This opened the door for vitamin supplements. Many people mistakenly assume that supplemental vitamins are somehow better than dietary vitamins. They are not. All work well in the body as they have the same chemical structures. This structure is the only thing the body cares about—not where the vitamin came from. Many other myths regarding vitamin supplementation also abound (Table 9-1). Learning the facts about vitamin supplementation is important because, as we will continually show in this chapter, taking doses of vitamins above the RDA is not without risk.

Consuming vitamin-rich foods daily is the ideal, but an occasional lapse in the intake of even one or more water-soluble vitamins should cause no harm. A typical healthy person takes 10 days to develop the first symptoms of a thiamin deficiency[17] and 20 to 40 days to develop symptoms of a vitamin C deficiency when these vitamins are completely lacking from the diet.[1] Therefore we can infer that we have reserves, although sometimes small, for all vitamins.

We conveniently class vitamins into two types—*fat soluble* and *water soluble.* They each behave differently in the body based on this difference. The water in cells dissolves water-soluble vitamins—the B vitamins and vitamin C—and easily flushes them out of the body via the kidneys. Fat-soluble vitamins—vitamins A, D, E, and K—are not readily excreted and rapidly can build

See the Nutrition Issue in Chapter 3 to reconsider whether you should take a vitamin supplement.

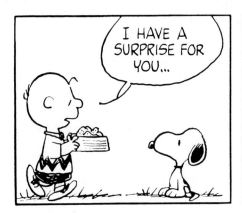
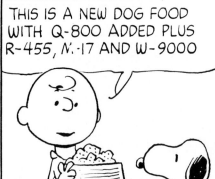
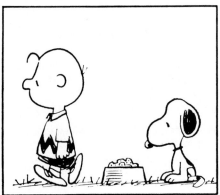
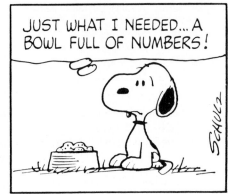

FIGURE 9-1

up in the body, causing toxic reactions. For that reason, we need to keep track of the amount of fat-soluble vitamins we ingest, especially vitamins A and D.

Have we found all the vitamins?

You may wonder if there are still more vitamins lurking in foods that have not been discovered. After all, the structure and chemical formula of the first known vitamin (thiamin) was not determined until 1937, and the last known vitamin (vitamin B-12) was characterized in 1948. Though some optimistic researchers hope to discover another vitamin, most scientists are confident that all vitamins needed by humans have been discovered. Evidence supports this assumption. For example, people have lived well for years on intravenous diets that consist of protein, carbohydrate, fat, all the known vitamins, and the essential minerals. With appropriate medical monitoring, these people continue not only to live, but also to build new body tissues, have babies, heal wounds, and fight existing diseases. They do not develop deficiency diseases or fail to thrive. Hence, we feel that no essential substance (vitamins included) remains undiscovered. Experiences with intravenous diets have also taught us that some lesser known vitamins, such as biotin, are still very important to health.

CONCEPT CHECK

Vitamins are carbon-containing compounds needed in small amounts that do not directly yield energy, but many are needed for energy-yielding reactions in the body. Vitamins A, D, E, and K are fat-soluble, while the B vitamins and vitamin C are water-soluble. In general, the fat-soluble vitamins are not readily excreted from the body and have the potential to build up rapidly to toxic levels. Water-soluble vitamins are much more readily excreted. Some people take vitamin supplements believing that they provide health benefits over dietary vitamins, but nutrition scientists agree that a well-chosen diet that includes animal products can almost always supply all the vitamins people need.

THE FAT-SOLUBLE VITAMINS—A, D, E, AND K

First, we will take a look at what we know about the fat-soluble vitamins—vitamins A, D, E, and K (Table 9-2).

Absorption of fat-soluble vitamins

Vitamins A, D, E, and K are absorbed along with dietary fat (see Chapters 5 and 7 for a refresher on fat absorption). These vitamins travel with dietary fats through the lymphatic system to reach the bloodstream. They then travel to body cells. Special carriers in the bloodstream help distribute vitamins A and K. Fat-soluble vitamins are mostly stored in the liver and fatty tissues.[23]

When fat absorption is efficient, about 40% to 90% of the fat-soluble vitamins are absorbed.[23] Anything that interferes with normal digestion and absorption of fats also interferes with fat-soluble vitamin absorption. People who use mineral oil as a laxative at mealtimes risk vitamin deficiencies since the intestine does not absorb mineral oil. Fat-soluble vitamins are simply eliminated with the mineral oil in the stool.

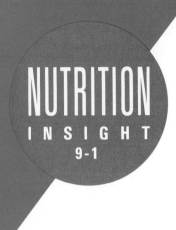

VITAMIN TOXICITY

Because fat-soluble vitamins are not readily excreted, some can build up in the body and cause toxic reactions. Vitamins A and D are especially likely to do so from heavy and regular consumption of supplements or foods such as liver. Regular use of a one-a-day type of multivitamin and mineral supplement will not cause toxicity problems if they yield less than two times the RDA. The possible exception to the safety of multivitamins is perhaps during pregnancy, and then only because of vitamin A content (see later discussion).

However, consuming too many vitamins, especially highly potent sources, can cause problems. In the 1930s some people took so much fish oil, particularly cod liver oil, that it caused vitamin toxicity because of its very high concentrations of vitamins A and D. Today major sources of vitamin toxicity are found in grocery, drug, and health food stores, where very concentrated forms of vitamin A and vitamin D are sold.

Isolated reports in the scientific literature show that vitamin E and the water-soluble vitamins niacin, vitamin B-6, and vitamin C also can be toxic but only when consumed in very high amounts (15 to 100 times the RDA). Therefore, except for excessive intake of vitamin supplements, these three vitamins are unlikely to cause toxic symptoms. In comparison, vitamins A and D can cause toxicity with long-term use at just five to ten times the RDA. Below we discuss the main vitamins with toxic potential.

Vitamin A

Toxicity problems occur only with excessive ingestion of preformed vitamin A. An intake of just 10 times the RDA for vitamin A can cause problems if taken for a prolonged time. Skin, hair, internal organs, and the central nervous system are affected. Most adverse effects disappear after the doses stop. Permanent damage to the liver, bones, and eyes, and recurrent joint and muscle pain, however, can occur.

A high vitamin A intake is especially dangerous during pregnancy because it may cause *fetal* malformations.[13] Birth defects and abortion caused by vitamin A toxicity have been clearly demonstrated in experimental animals. In humans excessive vitamin A intake has been associated with birth defects in infants.

The ingestion of large amounts of vitamin A–yielding carotenoids does not cause vitamin A toxicity. If someone consumes large amounts of carrots, or if infants eat a great deal of squash, or someone takes pills containing beta-carotene (more than 30 milligrams daily), high carotene levels can occur in the bloodstream. This can turn the skin yellow-orange. The palms of the hand and soles of the feet in particular become colored. This condition does not appear to cause any harm and disappears when the excess intake of carotenes decreases. The reasons that carotenes do not cause vitamin A toxicity are: (1) their rate of conversion into vitamin A is relatively slow and regulated, and (2) the efficiency of carotenoid absorption from the small intestine decreases markedly as the oral intake increases. Thus nature protects us from any serious toxic effects from dietary carotenoids.

Vitamin D

Vitamin D supplements are not necessary for normal healthy individuals, and in fact, they can be quite dangerous. Remember that vitamin D is poorly excreted; as little as four to five times the RDA taken regularly can create an overdose. Anyone who takes a dietary supplement should avoid a dosage higher than the RDA, 5 to 10 micrograms per day. Consuming more than 25 micrograms (1000 IU) of vitamin D per day requires close monitoring by a physician—above this level toxicity problems can occur, particularly overabsorption of calcium and eventual calcium deposits in the kidneys and other organs. The person also suffers the typical symptoms of high blood calcium levels—weakness, loss of appetite, diarrhea, vomiting, mental confusion, and increased urine output. Calcium deposits in organs cause metabolic disturbances and cell death.

Vitamin E

Vitamin E is relatively nontoxic. Some studies show that amounts in excess of approximately 500 milligrams (800 IU) per day of vitamin E can cause nausea, weakness, headache, diarrhea, and fatigue, as well as interfere with vitamin K metabolism. Antagonizing vitamin K metabolism can be especially dangerous if medications that decrease blood clotting are being used, because vitamin K has a major role in blood clotting. However, other studies show that intakes up to 2100 milligrams (3200 IU) may be safe for months. People with diseases such as phlebitis, in which blood clots form easily, sometimes benefit from large supplements of vitamin E, but should follow such a regimen under the careful supervision of a physician. Otherwise, hemorrhages may result.

Vitamin B-6

Intakes of 2 to 6 grams of vitamin B-6 per day for 2 to 40 months can lead to irreversible nerve damage. These high doses have usually been used by women with *premenstrual syndrome.* Symptoms of toxicity include walking difficulties and hand and foot numbness. Some nerve damage is probably reversible, but other nerve damage is probably permanent.[2] There is concern about toxicity from doses of vitamin B-6 as low as 50 to 500 milligrams per day. This concern deserves note. Since 500 milligram tablets of vitamin B-6 are available in health food stores, it is quite easy to take a toxic dose.

Niacin

Intakes of 100 milligrams or more of the nicotinic acid form of niacin can lead to increased blood flow to the skin, causing a general blood vessel dilation or *flushing* in various parts of the body. Headache and itching also may result. This excessive intake is sometimes used, under a physician's guidance, to lower elevated blood cholesterol levels.

Vitamin C

Vitamin C is probably not toxic when consumed in amounts less than 1 to 2 grams. Regularly consuming more than that can cause stomach inflammation, diarrhea, and iron toxicity (caused by overabsorption of iron. When the intake is abruptly reduced, a syndrome called *rebound* or *withdrawal* scurvy may result.[16] When receiving high doses of vitamin C, the body develops enzyme systems to rapidly metabolize it. If one abruptly reduces the intake to normal, the enzyme systems take a while to readjust, resulting in rebound scurvy. One may even find rebound scurvy in an infant born to a mother who consumed large amounts of vitamin C during pregnancy. When born, the child's daily dose of vitamin C drastically decreases. If a person has a history of a high vitamin C intake, gradually reducing it is recommended, rather than abruptly cutting down.

Most experts believe that consuming more than 100 to 200 mg/day of vitamin C yields no benefit. That much vitamin C can easily be obtained from the diet, making supplementation unnecessary. ●

Fetus • The developing human life form from 8 weeks until birth.

Premenstrual Syndrome • A disorder found in some women in the days surrounding menstrual periods that is characterized by depression, headache, bloating, and mood swings.

TABLE 9-2

Summary of the fat-soluble vitamins, their functions, deficiency conditions, and food sources

Vitamin	Major Functions	Deficiency Symptoms	People Most at Risk	Dietary Sources	RDA	Toxicity Symptoms
Vitamin A (retinoids) and pro-vitamin A (carotenoids)	1. Vision, light and color 2. Promote growth 3. Prevent drying of skin and eyes 4. Promote resistance to bacterial infection	1. Night blindness 2. Xerophthalmia 3. Poor growth 4. Dry skin (keratinization)	People in poverty, especially preschool children (still very rare)	Vitamin A Liver Fortified milk Provitamin A Sweet potatoes Spinach Greens Carrots Cantaloupe Apricots Broccoli	Females: 800 RE* (4000 IU†) Males: 1000 RE* (5000 IU†)	Fetal malformations, hair loss, skin changes, pain in bones
D (chole- and ergo-calciferol)	1. Facilitates absorption of calcium and phosphorus 2. Maintain optimum calcification of bone	1. Rickets 2. Osteomalacia	Breastfed infants, elderly shutins	Vitamin D–fortified milk Fish oils Tuna fish Salmon	5-10 micrograms (200-400 IU)	Growth retardation, kidney damage, calcium deposits in soft tissue
E (tocopherols, tocotrienols)	1. Antioxidant: prevent breakdown of vitamin A and unsaturated fatty acids	1. Hemolysis of red blood cells 2. Nerve destruction	People with poor fat absorption (still very rare)	Vegetable oils Some greens Some fruits	Females: 8 Alpha-tocopherol equivalents Males: 10 Alpha-tocopherol equivalents	Muscle weakness, headaches, fatigue, nausea, inhibition of vitamin K metabolism
K (phyllo- and mena-quinone)	1. Helps form prothrombin and other factors for blood clotting	1. Hemorrhage	People taking antibiotics for months at a time	Green vegetables Liver	60-80 micrograms	Anemia and jaundice

*Retinol equivalents.
†International units.

Retinoids • Chemical forms of preformed vitamin A; one source is animal foods.

Carotenoids • Pigment substances in plants that can often form vitamin A. Beta-carotene is the most active form.

VITAMIN A

The amount of vitamin A you consume is very important. Either too much or too little vitamin A can cause severe problems (Figure 9-2). Vitamin A is found in foods in a variety of forms. Retinol is one example. As a family, the various forms are called preformed vitamin A or **retinoids.** Vitamin A activity in the diet also occurs in the form of common plant pigments—*carotenoids*—such as the yellow-orange, beta-carotene pigment in carrots. Carotenoids are also called provitamin A because parts can often be turned into vitamin A. Over 600 carotenoids are found in nature; 50 of them serve as provitamin A. The most potent form is beta-carotene. The preformed vitamin A and the provitamin A carotenoids both make up what is generically referred to as vitamin A. Most vitamin A is stored in the liver in animals, which includes humans.

Functions of vitamin A

Vitamin A performs many important functions in the body. But although researchers have studied vitamin A since its discovery in 1913, its exact roles in

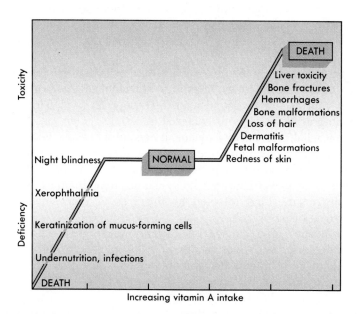

FIGURE 9-2

Consuming the right amount of vitamin A is critical to overall health. A very low (deficient) and a very high (toxic) vitamin A intake can produce damaging symptoms and even lead to death. The severity of effects and the intake range vary for individuals.

the cell are still baffling. Its importance to vision is perhaps its best-known role and the only role clearly understood at the chemical level. Researchers are investigating other ways that vitamin A functions in the body. Body changes that occur when vitamin A is lacking provide clues to its function.

Vision. The link between vitamin A and night vision has been known since ancient Egyptian times, when juice extracted from liver was used as a cure for night blindness. Vitamin A performs important functions in light/dark and color vision. It is a key part of the *visual cycle.* For a person to see in dim light, retinal, one form of vitamin A, is needed to start the chemical process that signals the brain that light is striking the eye. This allows the eye to adjust from bright light to dim light (such as after seeing the headlights of an oncoming car). Without sufficient dietary vitamin A, eventually the eye cannot quickly readjust to dim light. The condition is known as night blindness. An injection of vitamin A into the bloodstream can cure night blindness in a matter of minutes!

If night blindness is not corrected and vitamin A deficiency progresses, the cells that line the cornea of the eye (the clear outer window of the eye) also lose their ability to produce mucus.[4] The eye then becomes dry. Eventually, when dirt particles scratch the dry surface of the eye, bacteria infect it. The infection soon spreads to the entire surface of the eye and leads to blindness. This disease process is called *xerophthalmia,* which means dry eye.

Vitamin A deficiency is second only to accidents as a worldwide cause of blindness. Americans are at little risk because of generally good diets. However, people in less-developed nations, especially children, are very susceptible to vitamin A deficiency.[27] Poor dietary intakes and low stores of vitamin A fail to meet the children's high needs during rapid childhood growth. Over 500,000 children in poorer nations become blind each year because of vitamin A deficiency.[4]

Today, widespread deficiencies of vitamin A constitute one of the most important public health problems in developing countries. Worldwide, attempts to reduce this problem have included giving large doses of vitamin A twice yearly and supplementing sugar and monosodium glutamate with vitamin A. These food vehicles are used because they are commonly consumed by the populations of less-developed nations. In some countries this effort has proven effective.

Health of cells.   Vitamin A maintains the health of cells that line internal and external "skin" surfaces in the lungs, intestines, stomach, vagina, urinary tract, and bladder, as well as the eyes and skin.[28] These cells (called *epithelial cells*) serve as important barriers to bacterial infection. As we just noted for the eye, some epithelial cells secrete mucus, a needed lubricant. Without vitamin A, mucus-forming cells deteriorate and no longer synthesize mucus. Instead, the cells make a protein, typically found in the hair and nails, called keratin. This causes the cells to harden and crack, disabling them as barriers to invading microorganisms. First affected by this loss of mucus-synthesizing capacity are the eyes.

Vitamin A deficiency also causes insufficient mucus production in the intestines and lung cells and poor health of cells in general, all of which increase the risk of body infections. Vitamin A deficiency also reduces the activity of certain immune cells. Together, these effects leave the vitamin A-deficient person at a great risk for infections.[27]

Growth, development, and reproduction.   Vitamin A is necessary for cell growth and development. This is most easily demonstrated with laboratory animals, but human growth is also affected.[27] Resorbing old bone, which must occur before new bone can be deposited, requires bone cells that can be stimulated by vitamin A. Producing some components of bone also requires vitamin A. Vitamin A causes DNA in a cell's nucleus to increase its synthesis of cell proteins that stimulate proper growth and development. One consequence is that animals deficient in vitamin A cannot reproduce.

Cancer prevention?   Most forms of cancer arise from cells that are influenced by vitamin A. Coupled with its ability to aid immune system activity, vitamin A could be a valuable tool in the fight against cancer.[19] This is especially true for skin, lung, bladder, and breast cancers.[28] Scientists have been encouraged by research using animals. Human studies using various forms of vitamin A are now under way in many centers in America. However, until results of these studies are available, it is advisable to avoid personal experimentation, as toxicity can result. The Guide to Daily Food Choices remains the best guide for both obtaining all vitamins and potentially reducing cancer risk (see the Nutrition Issue, p. 286).

Forms of provitamin A, especially beta-carotene, may also help prevent cancer because they help protect the carbon-carbon double bonds present in the cells of the body.[6,19] Free oxygen atoms and other potentially toxic compounds most likely initiate the cancer process in some cells by destroying these bonds. Carotenes appear to limit this destruction. Some evidence shows that regular consumption of vegetables high in carotenes decreases risk of lung cancer in smokers. However, more investigation is needed in this area before specific recommendations can be made regarding carotenes and cancer prevention. The best advice is still to eat fruits and vegetables regularly and not smoke.

Vitamin A for acne.   The acne medication tretinoin (Retin-A) is made of one form of vitamin A. It has been used as a topical treatment (applied to the skin) for acne for more than 10 years. It appears to work by altering cell activity in the skin. Recently it has been popularized as a treatment for aging skin. Another derivative of vitamin A, 13-cis retinoic acid (Accutane), is an oral drug used to treat serious acne.

We know taking high doses of vitamin A itself would not be safe (see Nutrition Insight 9-1).[13] Even Accutane, a less toxic form, can induce toxicity symptoms. A person using either Retin-A or Accutane must also limit sun exposure because these drugs cause skin to sunburn easily. Furthermore, Accutane carries a very high risk for fetal malformations when used by pregnant women. Even the topical use of Retin-A is not recommended during pregnancy.

Vitamin A in foods

Vitamin A in foods exists in either the animal form (preformed vitamin A) or plant form (provitamin A). Preformed vitamin A is found in liver, fish oils, vitamin A–fortified milk, and eggs. Butter and margarine are also sources, as these are fortified with vitamin A. Provitamin A is mainly found in dark green and orange vegetables and some fruits. Carrots, spinach, squash, broccoli, papayas, and apricots are examples of sources. Beta-carotene contributes to the yellow-orange color of carrots. The yellow-orange color is often masked, however, by dark-green chlorophyll pigments in vegetables, such as in broccoli. Consuming a varied diet rich in green vegetables and carrots ensures sufficient sources for meeting vitamin A needs. About 50% of the vitamin A in the American diet comes from animal sources; the rest comes from plants.

Retinol equivalents (RE)

For vitamin A, the preferred unit of measurement is the retinol equivalent (RE). In this system all potential forms of vitamin A are scaled based on their activity. Most nutrient levels in foods, including vitamin A, were formerly expressed in less precise ***international units (IU)***. Some food labels still show the older IU values for nutrients because the U.S. RDA is based on the RDA from 1968, which used the IU system. The current RDA does not. Based on a mixture of preformed and provitamin A, 1 RE of vitamin A is equivalent to 5 IU of vitamin A. Otherwise, 3.3 IU of preformed vitamin A alone equals 1 RE.

RDA for vitamin A

The current RDA for vitamin A is 1000 RE for men and 800 RE for women. (Throughout this and the next chapter, refer to the inside cover for nutrient recommendations for other ages and to Appendix C for Canadian recommendations.) The recommendation approximates, but is often slightly above, the average intake for adult men and women in the United States. A higher intake of green vegetables could easily raise intakes to RDA levels.

In America, poor vitamin A status has been noted among preschool children who do not eat enough vegetables. This is especially true in Hispanic communities where typical food choices are not likely to provide adequate vitamin A. The urban poor, the elderly, and people who are alcoholics or who have liver disease (which limits vitamin A storage) also can show poor vitamin A status, especially poor vitamin A storage. Finally, children with severe fat malabsorption, as in cases of cystic fibrosis, may also show a vitamin A deficiency.

International Unit (IU) • A crude measure of vitamin activity, often based on the growth rate of animals. Today these units have been replaced by more precise milligram and microgram measures.

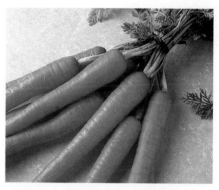

Carrots are a rich source of carotenes and vitamin A activity—good reasons to eat these regularly.

ANOTHER BITE Parents often encourage their children to eat vegetables. Besides contributing to good food habits, this practice helps children consume enough vitamin A. Parents provide important role models for children, and they can positively influence their children's eating interests by also eating their vegetables.

VITAMIN D

Vitamin D is not just a vitamin. It is also considered a hormone because the cells in the skin that convert a cholesterol-like substance to vitamin D using sunlight are different from those cells that mostly respond to vitamin D—bone cells and kidney cells (Figure 9-3).[21]

The amount of sun-time needed to produce vitamin D in skin cells depends on the darkness of the skin. Light-skinned people need approximately 15 min-

Recall from Chapter 5 that a hormone is a substance made in the body that travels through the bloodstream to act at a different site.

Calcitriol • The active hormone form of vitamin D (1,25-dihydroxyvitamin D)—not to be confused with calcitonin, a hormone that also affects calcium use.

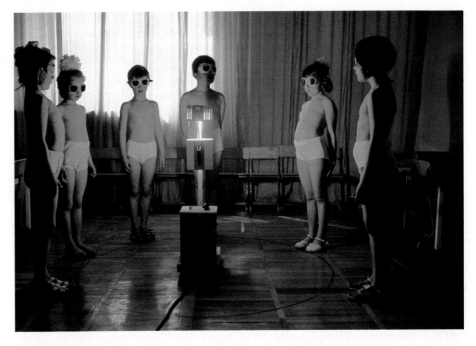

FIGURE 9-3

Who's got the tanning oil? Southern Russia endures a long winter. These Stavropol kids are exposed to a quartz lamp to provide the vitamin D synthesis they would normally experience from playing outdoors.

utes a day of direct sun exposure on the face and hands.[26] Dark-skinned people need more sun exposure. The process is also more efficient in younger people than in the elderly. The further you live from the equator and the more smog, fog, and smoke present, the greater the length of exposure needed to produce enough vitamin D. Anyone who does not receive enough sunlight to make sufficient vitamin D must consume vitamin D as well. Most Americans rely on the diet to help supply adequate vitamin D, particularly in winter.

As we noted, the starting product for vitamin D synthesis in the body is a cholesterol-like substance. Ultraviolet light is needed to convert this into vitamin D. Vitamin D toxicity does not result from tanning in the sun too long because the body regulates the amount made in the skin. The same cannot be said for dietary vitamin D sources. Its uptake into the body is not blocked when eaten at high doses.

Functions of vitamin D

Vitamin D first requires metabolism by the liver and then kidney to become the active hormone. The main function of the vitamin D hormone (called *calcitriol*) is to help regulate calcium and bone metabolism. In concert with other hormones, vitamin D closely regulates blood calcium levels to supply appropriate amounts of calcium to all cells. This overall task entails a variety of processes: the vitamin D hormone helps regulate absorption of calcium and phosphorus from the intestine, it reduces kidney excretion of calcium, and it helps regulate the deposition of calcium in the bones (Figure 9-4).[21] Even tissues in the brain, pancreas, and pituitary gland appear to be under the influence of the vitamin D hormone.

Rickets and osteomalacia

The net result of vitamin D hormone action is to increase calcium and phosphorus deposition in bones. Without adequate calcium and phosphorus, bones

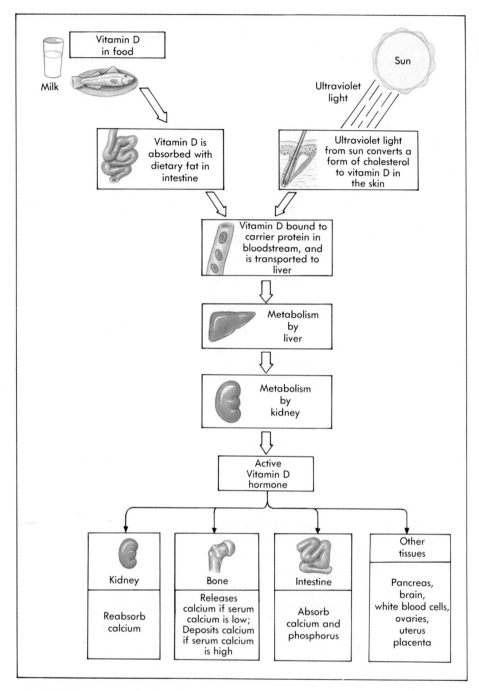

Rickets • A disease characterized by softening of the bones because of poor calcium content. This deficiency disease arises from lack of vitamin D activity in the body.

FIGURE 9-4

The many facets of vitamin D metabolism. Note that when made by the body using sunshine, vitamin D is actually a hormone.

weaken and bow under pressure. A child with these symptoms has the disease *rickets.* Symptoms also include enlarged head, joints, and rib cage and a deformed pelvis.[10]

Infant diets, especially those of breast-fed infants in their first 6 months of life, should contain a food or supplement source of vitamin D if sufficient exposure to sunlight is not possible to prevent rickets. Keep in mind supplements should be used very carefully to avoid vitamin D toxicity (see Nutrition Insight 9-1). Vitamin D fortification of milk has greatly reduced the risk of rickets in children. Today, rickets is most commonly associated with fat malabsorption,

Osteomalacia • Adult form of rickets. The weakening of the bones that is seen in this disease is caused by a poor calcium content. A reduction in the amount of the vitamin D hormone is the cause.

Be careful not to confuse this with osteoporosis, another type of bone disorder we discuss in Chapter 10.

such as occurs in children with cystic fibrosis.[10] Maximizing the amount of vitamin D these children make using sunlight is important.

An adult disease comparable to rickets is ***osteomalacia,*** which means soft bones. It results when calcium is withdrawn from the bones to make up for inefficient absorption in the intestine or poor conservation by the kidneys. Both of these problems can be caused by vitamin D deficiency. Bones then lose their minerals and become porous, weak, and easily broken. This leads to fractures in the hip, spine, and other bones.

Osteomalacia in adults most commonly occurs in people with kidney, stomach, gallbladder, or intestinal disease (especially when most of the intestine has been removed) and in people with cirrhosis of the liver. These diseases affect both vitamin D metabolism and calcium absorption. Adults with limited sun exposure may also develop the disease. In fact, concern exists that silent—undiagnosed—osteomalacia is common among the elderly. Combinations of sun exposure and/or vitamin D intake can help prevent this problem.

Vitamin D in foods and the RDA

When exposure to sunshine does not create sufficient vitamin D, fatty fish (and fish oils) and fortified milk serve as the most nutrient-dense sources. Because milk is not a naturally rich source of vitamin D, it is fortified in the United States by adding 10 micrograms (400 IU) of vitamin D to each quart. Milk is a good vehicle for vitamin D supplementation since it is also the main source of calcium for children. Eggs, butter, and liver contain vitamin D, but require too great a serving size to be considered significant sources. So few other foods contain vitamin D that food tables do not list sources.

The RDA for adults for vitamin D varies from 5 to 10 micrograms per day (200 to 400 IU per day). Recall that young light-skinned people are able to make this amount of vitamin D in about 15 minutes of sun exposure, and then on just the face and hands. Infants, children, and adolescents have higher RDA because of their growing bones.

As we noted, anyone who both stays inside most of the day and ingests little or no vitamin D is at risk for developing vitamin D deficiency. This includes infants who are fed only human milk, prisoners, and elderly people. These people need either a more predictable amount of sun exposure and/or a regular food source of vitamin D.

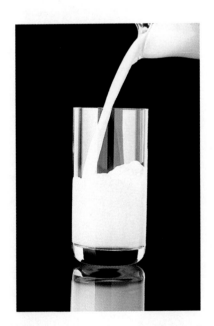

Milk is often fortified with vitamin D, which is important especially for people who receive little sun exposure.

CONCEPT CHECK

Vitamin A is found in foods as preformed vitamin A and as provitamin A carotenoids. The most understood function of vitamin A is its importance in vision. Blindness caused by vitamin A deficiency is a major problem in many parts of the world. Vitamin A is also needed to maintain health of many types of cells, to support the immune system, and to promote proper growth and development. Vitamin A may be important in preventing cancer. However, since taking supplements of preformed vitamin A can build up to a toxic level of it, the best recommendation is to eat plenty of provitamin A–rich foods, such as fruits and vegetables.

Vitamin D is a true vitamin only for people who fail to produce enough from sunlight. Using a cholesterol-like substance, people synthesize vitamin D by the action of sunlight on their skin. The vitamin D is later metabolized by the liver and kidneys to form the active hormone calcitriol. This hormone increases calcium absorption in the intestine and works with other hormones to maintain proper calcium metabolism in bones and other organs in the body. Significant food sources of vitamin D are fish oils and fortified milk. Dietary vitamin D can be quite toxic.

VITAMIN E

Vitamin E has been called the vitamin in search of a deficiency disease. A deficiency of vitamin E is unheard of in healthy humans who eat balanced diets.

Functions of vitamin E

Vitamin E, a fat-soluble antioxidant, mostly resides in cell membranes. As we discussed in Chapter 7, an antioxidant can form a barrier between a target molecule—an unsaturated fatty acid in a cell membrane, for example—and a compound seeking its electrons (Figure 9-5). The antioxidant donates electrons and/or hydrogens to the electron-seeking compound (called an *oxidizing compound*) to neutralize it. This protects other molecules or parts of a cell from having electrons nabbed. Note that vitamin C is a water-soluble antioxidant.

If vitamin E is not present, electron-seeking compounds can oxidize parts of cell membranes, DNA, and other electron-dense cell parts. Oxidization either alters the DNA, which may increase the risk for cancer, or destroys the cell membrane, causing cell death and possibly speeding of the aging process. After vitamin E donates two electrons, it is broken down itself and can no longer function. This breakdown product is then excreted in the urine.

 The mineral selenium can spare some of the body's need for vitamin E. Selenium enables an enzyme in cells to decrease the formation of certain oxidizing compounds. Thus an adequate dietary intake of selenium—from cereals, meats, and seafood—reduces the need for vitamin E, whereas low selenium intake in the diet increases it.

Oxidizing Compound • A compound capable of capturing an electron from another compound (or supplying an oxygen to another compound). The word oxidize literally means to loose an electron or gain an oxygen.

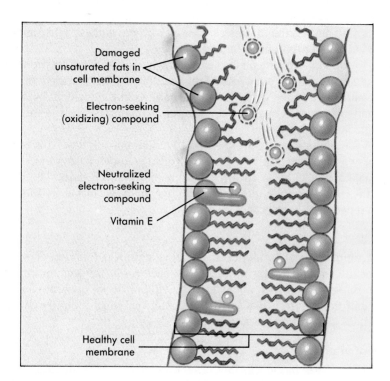

FIGURE 9-5

Vitamin E helps stop cell membrane damage. This needs to happen before much cell damage takes place.

Hemolysis • Destruction of red blood cells. The red blood cell membrane breaks down, allowing cell contents to leak into the fluid portion of the blood.

Tocopherols • The chemical name for some forms of vitamin E.

Prothrombin • A blood protein needed for blood clotting that requires vitamin K for its synthesis.

A deficiency of vitamin E causes cell membrane breakdown, especially in red blood cells of infants. Unsaturated fatty acids in the red blood cell membrane are very sensitive to attack by oxidizing compounds. Since vitamin E neutralizes these agents, it protects the red blood cell membrane from damage. Red blood cell breakage, called **hemolysis,** commonly occurs in premature infants because they did not receive sufficient vitamin E from their mothers. The rapid growth of premature infants coupled with the high oxygen concentration found in infant incubators, greatly increases the stress on red blood cells. This raises the risk of cell damage. Special formulas and supplements for premature infants are used to help compensate for lack of vitamin E.

Vitamin E can help improve vitamin A absorption if the dietary intake of vitamin A is low. In addition, vitamin E is used to metabolize iron in the cell and to help maintain nervous tissues and immune function.[12]

Note that popular health-food literature attests to many other benefits of vitamin E. None has been shown to be true for humans. A vitamin E deficiency in laboratory animals can result in muscular dystrophy, fetal death, and impotence. The link between vitamin E deficiency and fetal death in rats, noted in 1922, gave vitamin E its chemical name **tocopherol,** which means to bring forth birth. However, vitamin E supplementation in humans is unable to cure any of these conditions. Vitamin E has also been promoted as an antiaging vitamin. Unquestionably, consuming the RDA for vitamin E is important for minimizing cell destruction by oxidizing compounds and maintaining cell health. However, there is no evidence that supplementation beyond this amount stops aging.

Vitamin E in foods and the RDA

The most nutrient-dense food sources of vitamin E are plant oils, some fruits and vegetables, such as asparagus and green leafy vegetables, and margarine. Animal fats have practically no vitamin E. The actual vitamin E content of a food depends on how it was harvested, processed, stored, and cooked because vitamin E is very susceptible to destruction by oxygen, metals, light, and especially repeated use of oils in deep-fat frying.

Vitamin E content in plant oils is usually high, as it is used to protect the unsaturated fats found in plant oils. For healthy people, a varied diet that includes vegetable oils should supply sufficient vitamin E. Selenium in the diet, as mentioned, also spares the need for vitamin E by decreasing the formation of oxidizing compounds.

The RDA for adults for vitamin E is 8 to 10 milligrams per day. This is about the amount we eat each day. To convert from the older IU system, 10 milligrams equals about 15 IU. A variety of forms of vitamin E exist. The RDA is based on the alpha-tocopherol form. Amounts of other forms in foods are adjusted to reflect reduced activity.

VITAMIN K

A family of compounds known collectively as vitamin K is found in plants, fish oils, and meats. One form is synthesized by bacteria in the human intestine. These bacteria supply us with about half the vitamin K we absorb every day. The other half comes from diet. The amount in our diets alone is generally about five times higher than our needs.

Functions of vitamin K

Vitamin K is vital for blood clotting. The K stands for koagulation, as it is spelled in Denmark. This spelling is used because it was a Danish researcher who first noted the relationship between vitamin K and blood clotting. Vitamin K contributes to the synthesis of several blood-clotting factors, including **prothrombin** (Figure 9-6). A key effect is that vitamin K imparts a calcium-binding

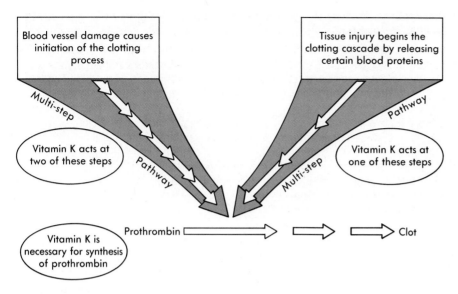

FIGURE 9-6
Forming a blood clot. This requires the participation of vitamin K.

potential to certain proteins, enabling them to participate in the process of blood clotting.[20]

A newborn's intestinal tract does not yet contain sufficient vitamin K–producing bacteria to allow for blood to clot effectively if the infant is injured. Therefore vitamin K injections are routinely given shortly after birth to bridge the gap until enough bacterial synthesis can take place. In adults a deficiency of vitamin K is most likely to occur when a person takes antibiotics for a long period of time or has severe fat malabsorption. Antibiotic use is a problem because it destroys many of the intestinal bacteria that normally account for half the vitamin K absorbed.

Physicians today often treat blood clotting disorders by using drugs whose structures resemble that of vitamin K. The drugs dicumarol and warfarin antagonize the action of vitamin K. Acting as potent anticoagulants, they are effective for people whose blood tends to clot excessively. However, people taking these drugs must be warned against consuming supplements of vitamin K and foods especially rich in vitamin K. This would reduce the action of the drugs.

Vitamin K in foods and the RDA

The most nutrient-dense food sources of vitamin K are green, leafy vegetables, other vegetables, such as peas and green beans, and liver. Vitamin K provides yet another reason to consume a diet rich in fruits and vegetables. Vitamin K is quite resistant to damage from heat and cooking.

The adult RDA for vitamin K is 60 to 80 micrograms per day. The average U.S. diet contains 300 to 500 micrograms per adult per day of vitamin K, again making a deficiency very unlikely.

Most vitamin K consumed in a day is gone by the next. This limits its toxic potential, even though it is fat-soluble. At the same time, vitamin K is so abundant in the diet that there is low risk of suffering a deficiency.

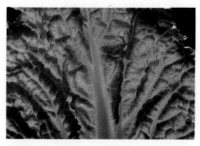

Green vegetables supply much vitamin K.

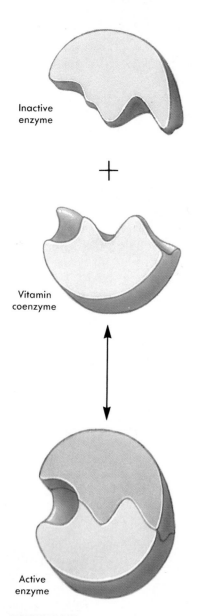

Inactive
enzyme

+

Vitamin
coenzyme

Active
enzyme

FIGURE 9-7
Coenzymes, formed from B vitamins,
activate enzymes.

Vitamin status can be tested by
measuring enzyme activities in
red blood cells that require
vitamins to function. Such
biochemical tests for enzyme
activity can be used to determine
thiamin, riboflavin, and vitamin B-
6 status.

CONCEPT CHECK

Vitamin E functions primarily as an antioxidant. It can donate electrons to electron-seeking (oxidizing) compounds. By neutralizing these compounds, vitamin E helps prevent cell destruction, especially the destruction of red blood cell membranes. The best sources of vitamin E are plant oils, but it occurs in a wide variety of foods.

Vitamin K plays a key role in efficient blood clotting; it imparts a calcium-binding ability to certain blood proteins, such as prothrombin. About half the vitamin K we absorb every day is synthesized by intestinal bacteria and about half comes from our diets. The amount in the diet alone is generally greatly in excess of our needs. Thus, except for newborns, a deficiency of vitamin K is unlikely, even though it is readily excreted from the body.

THE WATER-SOLUBLE VITAMINS—THE B VITAMINS AND VITAMIN C

Water-soluble vitamins are more readily excreted than fat-soluble vitamins. Any excess generally ends up in the urine or stool, so it is important to consume the water-soluble vitamins regularly. Because they dissolve in water, large amounts of these vitamins can be lost during food processing and preparation. A summary of much of what we know about water-soluble vitamins is presented in Table 9-3.

THE B VITAMINS

The B vitamins are thiamin, riboflavin, niacin, pantothenic acid, biotin, vitamin B-6, folate, and vitamin B-12. Since they often occur in the same foods, a lack of one B vitamin may mean other B vitamins are low as well. The B vitamins all are changed into **coenzymes,** small molecules that can interact with enzymes to enable enzymes to function. In essence, the coenzymes allow enzymes to take on *active* forms (Figure 9-7).

B vitamins play many key roles in metabolism. The metabolic pathways that link carbohydrates, fats, and amino acids together use B vitamins in their coenzyme forms. This makes many B vitamins interdependent since they participate in the same processes.[17] Their key roles in energy metabolism allows needs for some B vitamins to be expressed in terms of kcalories used, such as 0.5 milligrams of thiamin per 1000 kcalories. When setting the RDA, an estimate of kcalorie use by a person of a specific age and gender is made to yield the final value, such as of 1.1 to 1.5 milligrams of thiamin for adults.

After being ingested, B vitamins are first broken down from their coenzyme forms into free vitamins in the stomach and small intestine.[23] The vitamins are then absorbed, primarily in the small intestine. Typically, about 50% to 90% of B vitamins in the diet are absorbed. Once inside cells, the coenzyme forms are resynthesized. Because we make them when needed, we don't need to consume the coenzyme forms themselves.

THIAMIN

Thiamin (sometimes called vitamin B-1) is used to release energy from carbohydrate, to transmit nerve impulses, and to metabolize alcohol, among other things. Its coenzyme participates in reactions in which a carbon dioxide is lost from a larger molecule—a reaction that is particularly important in metabolizing glucose, the primary by-product of carbohydrate digestion (Figure 9-8).[17]

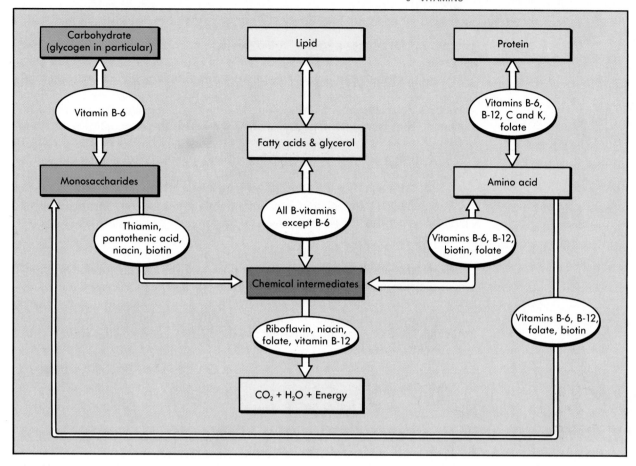

FIGURE 9-8

Examples of metabolic pathways for which vitamins are essential. The metabolism of
energy-yielding nutrients requires vitamin input.

Beriberi

The thiamin deficiency disease is called **beriberi,** a word which means "I can't,
I can't" in Sinhalese. The symptoms include weakness, loss of appetite, irritability, nervous tingling throughout the body, poor arm and leg coordination, and
deep muscle pain in the calves. A person with beriberi often develops an
enlarged heart and sometimes severe edema (*wet* beriberi).

Beriberi is seen where polished (white) rice, rather than brown rice, is a staple. In most parts of the world, brown rice has had its bran and germ layer
removed to make white rice. This makes it a poor source of thiamin. However,
thiamin is often replaced during the **enrichment** of white rice in the United
States (see Chapter 2).

Beriberi results when glucose, the primary fuel for brain and nerve cells, is
poorly metabolized. Since the thiamin coenzyme participates in glucose
metabolism, body functions associated with brain and nerve action quickly
show signs of a thiamin deficiency. Symptoms of depression and weakness can
be seen after only 10 days on a thiamin-free diet. This shows how limited the
body's stores of thiamin are and how important it is to consume thiamin-rich
foods daily.

Thiamin in foods and the RDA

Foods that contain a very high nutrient density of thiamin include pork products and sunflower seeds. Whole grains (wheat germ), enriched grains, green beans, organ meats, peanuts, dried beans, and other seeds are also good sources.

Major contributors of thiamin to the American diet are white bread and rolls, crackers, pork, hot dogs, luncheon meat, cold cereals, orange juice, and dairy products. White bread, bakery products, and cereals are usually enriched with thiamin. They serve as important sources because many people eat them so often.

Aside from pork products, there is really no one excellent source of thiamin in the American diet. The foods we eat tend to contribute small amounts of thiamin. Eating a wide variety of foods is the best way to obtain enough thiamin.

The adult RDA for thiamin is about 1.5 milligrams per day for men and 1.1 milligrams per day for women. The U.S. food supply yields approximately one-and-a-half times the RDA for thiamin per person per day, but that does not account for the thiamin lost in food preparation and in cooking.

Some groups of people, such as the poor and the elderly, probably barely meet their needs for thiamin. A diet dominated by highly processed and unenriched foods, sugar, fat, and alcohol also creates a potential for thiamin deficiency. Women should be especially careful to consume good sources of thiamin. Their average intake barely meets the RDA. Oral thiamin supplements are essentially nontoxic.

TABLE 9-3

A summary of the water-soluble vitamins, their functions, deficiency conditions, and food sources

Name	Major Functions	Deficiency Symptoms	People Most at Risk
Thiamin	Coenzyme involved with enzymes in carbohydrate metabolism; nerve function	Beriberi; nervous tingling, poor coordination, edema, heart changes, weakness	Alcoholism, poverty
Riboflavin	Coenzymes involved in energy metabolism	Inflammation of mouth and tongue, cracks at corners of the mouth, eye disorders	Possibly people on certain medications if no dairy products consumed
Niacin	Coenzymes involved in energy metabolism, fat synthesis, fat breakdown	Pellagra; diarrhea, dermatitis, dementia	Severe poverty where corn is the dominant food; alcoholism
Pantothenic acid	Coenzyme involved in energy metabolism, fat synthesis, fat breakdown	Using an antagonist causes tingling in hands, fatigue, headache, nausea	Alcoholism
Biotin	Coenzyme involved in glucose production, fat synthesis	Dermatitis, tongue soreness, anemia, depression	Alcoholism
Vitamin B-6, pyridoxine and other forms	Coenzyme involved in protein metabolism, neurotransmitter synthesis, hemoglobin synthesis, many other functions	Headache, anemia, convulsions, nausea, vomiting, flaky skin, sore tongue	Adolescent and adult women; people on certain medications; alcoholism
Folate (folic acid)	Coenzyme involved in DNA synthesis	Megaloblastic anemia, inflammation of tongue, diarrhea, poor growth, mental disorders	Alcoholism, pregnancy, use of certain medications
Vitamin B-12 (cobalamins)	Coenzyme involved in folate metabolism, nerve function	Macrocytic anemia, poor nerve function	Elderly because of poor absorption; vegans
Vitamin C (ascorbic acid)	Collagen synthesis, hormone synthesis, neurotransmitter synthesis	Scurvy: poor wound healing, pinpoint hemorrhages, bleeding gums, edema	Alcoholism, elderly men living alone

People with alcoholism are at great risk for thiamin deficiency because alcohol profoundly diminishes the ability to absorb and use thiamin. Furthermore, they often eat poorly. An alcohol-related thiamin deficiency can lead to a cluster of symptoms, including mental confusion, memory loss, and poor nervous system control of arms and legs.

Dermatitis • Inflammation of the skin.

RIBOFLAVIN

The name riboflavin comes from its yellow color—flavus means yellow in Latin. Riboflavin is sometimes referred to as vitamin B-2.

Functions of riboflavin

The coenzymes of riboflavin participate in many energy-yielding metabolic pathways. When cells form energy using oxygen or when fats are broken down and burned for energy, the coenzymes of riboflavin are used. Some vitamin metabolism also requires riboflavin.[17]

The symptoms associated with riboflavin deficiency include inflammation of the mouth and tongue, *dermatitis,* cracking of tissue around the corners of the mouth (called cheilosis), various eye disorders, sensitivity to the sun, and

Dietary Sources	RDA or ESADDI	Toxicity
Sunflower seeds, pork, whole and enriched grains, dried beans, peas, brewers yeast	1.1-1.5 milligrams	None possible from food
Milk, mushrooms, spinach, liver, enriched grains	1.2-1.7 milligrams	None reported
Mushrooms, bran, tuna, salmon, chicken, beef, liver, peanuts, enriched grains	15-19 milligrams	Flushing of skin at > 100 milligrams
Mushrooms, liver, broccoli, eggs; most foods have some	4-7 milligrams	None
Cheese, egg yolks, cauliflower, peanut butter, liver	30-100 micrograms	Unknown
Animal protein foods, spinach, broccoli, bananas, salmon, sunflower seeds	1.8-2 milligrams	Nerve destruction at doses > 100 milligrams
Green leafy vegetables, orange juice, organ meats, sprouts, sunflower seeds	180-200 micrograms	None, nonprescription vitamin dosage is controlled by FDA
Animal foods, especially organ meats, oysters, clams (not naturally in plant foods)	2 micrograms	None
Citrus fruits, strawberries, broccoli, greens	60 milligrams	Doses > 1-2 grams causes diarrhea and can alter some diagnostic tests

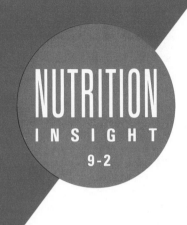

PRESERVING VITAMINS IN FOOD

Substantial amounts of vitamins in foods can be lost from the time the fruit or vegetable is picked until you eat it. The water-soluble vitamins, particularly thiamin, vitamin C, and folate, can be destroyed with improper storage and excessive cooking. Heat, light, exposure to the air, cooking in water, and alkalinity are all factors that can destroy vitamins. The sooner the food is eaten, the less chance of nutrient loss.[23]

In general, if the food is not to be eaten within a few days, freezing is the best method to retain nutrients. In fact, frozen vegetables and fruits are often better than supermarket *fresh* ones. Frozen foods are often processed immediately after harvesting. As part of the freezing process, vegetables are quickly blanched in boiling water. This destroys the enzymes that would otherwise degrade the vitamins. Fresh food often lingers in the grocery store or at home for a while before it is eaten.

Below are some tips to aid in preserving the vitamins in food:

- Keep fruits and vegetables cool. Enzymes in foods begin to degrade vitamins once the fruit or vegetable is picked. Chilling reduces this process, so refrigerating these foods until they are consumed is important.
- Refrigerate foods in moisture-proof containers. Nutrients keep best at temperatures near freezing, at high humidity, and away from exposure to air.
- Avoid trimming and cutting fruits and vegetables into small pieces as much as possible. The greater surface exposed speeds vitamin breakdown by oxygen. Keep in mind the outer leaves of lettuce and other greens have higher values of vitamins and minerals than the inner, tender leaves or stems. The skins of potatoes, apples, and carrots for example, are higher in vitamins and minerals than the center part.
- To retain the high levels of nutrients in vegetables, microwave cooking, steaming, or using a pan or wok with very small amounts of water and a tight-fitting lid are best. The less contact with water and the shorter the cooking time, the more nutrients retained. Whenever possible, cook fruits or vegetables in their skins.
- Minimize reheating food. This reduces the vitamin content.
- Don't add baking soda to vegetables to enhance the green color. The alkalinity destroys much vitamin C, thiamin, and other vitamins.
- Store canned goods in a cool place. To get maximum nutritive value from the canned goods, whenever possible, serve any liquid packed with the food. Canned foods vary in the amount of nutrients lost, largely because of differences in storage time and temperatures in the canning process.
- Keep milk cold, covered, and away from strong light. Riboflavin may be lost in direct light. ***Pasteurizing*** raw milk does not destroy the main nutrients that milk products provide—protein, riboflavin, and calcium, among others. ●

Microwave cooking provides many advantages as far as preserving nutrients during cooking. When cooking vegetables in a microwave little water is needed, decreasing the amount of vitamins that can be lost into the surrounding fluid. Also, microwave cooking exposes food to heat for shorter periods of time than conventional ovens or stoves.

confusion. The first symptoms of a deficiency are inflammation of the mouth and tongue. All of the symptoms associated with deficiency develop after approximately 2 months on a riboflavin-poor diet (consuming only one-fourth or less of the RDA).

Clinicians have great difficulty identifying true riboflavin deficiency because it shares symptoms with deficiencies of other B vitamins, such as thiamin, vitamin B-6, and folate. In addition, isolated riboflavin deficiencies probably do not exist. Instead, a riboflavin deficiency would occur with deficiencies of niacin, thiamin, and vitamin B-6, since these nutrients often occur in the same foods.

Riboflavin in foods and the RDA

Most riboflavin in the U.S. diet comes from one of its most nutrient-dense sources—milk and milk products. Including dairy products in your diet is the best guarantee for a sufficient riboflavin intake. The remainder of the U.S. riboflavin intake comes from enriched white bread, rolls, and crackers; meat; and eggs. For some people, high meat consumption partially offsets the low intake of dairy products in terms of riboflavin intake.

Riboflavin is very stable at temperatures used to pasteurize milk and reheat foods in a microwave. However, riboflavin breaks down rapidly when exposed to light. To protect milk products from light, paper and plastic cartons—not glass—work well.

The adult RDA for riboflavin is 1.4 to 1.7 milligrams per day for men and 1.2 to 1.3 milligrams per day for women. On average, people in the United States consume the riboflavin RDA. Athletes may need extra riboflavin because they use more fat for fuel and because their greater demand for energy taps many chemical pathways that require riboflavin. However, the RDA should still suffice. Overall, riboflavin deficiencies are rare, but some people, especially those who do not regularly consume milk and milk products, may be at risk. Athletic women should particularly take note of this. People with alcoholism risk riboflavin deficiency because they generally eat nutrient-poor diets.

We suggest that if you do not consume much milk or milk products, you should search for another adequate dietary source of riboflavin. Enriched breakfast cereals are a good choice.

NIACIN

Niacin is actually composed of a pair of related compounds. Both can function as niacin in the body. Niacin is sometimes referred to as vitamin B-3.

Functions of niacin

The coenzyme forms of niacin function in many cellular metabolic pathways. In general, when cell energy is being formed, a niacin coenzyme is used. Synthetic pathways in the cell—those that make new compounds—also often use a niacin coenzyme. This is especially true for fat synthesis.[17]

Pellagra

Since almost every cellular metabolic pathway uses a niacin coenzyme, a deficiency causes widespread changes in the body. The entire group of symptoms is known as pellagra, which means rough or painful skin. The symptoms of the disease are known as the *three Ds*—**dementia,** diarrhea, and dermatitis (especially on areas of skin exposed to the sun). Later, death often results. Early symptoms include poor appetite, weight loss, and weakness. Pellagra became epidemic in southern Europe in the early 1700s when corn became a staple food. It became a major problem in the southeastern United States in the late 1800s and persisted until the late 1930s when standards of living and diets improved. The pellagra epidemic in the United States in the early 1900s gave impetus to a federally sponsored program in 1941 to enrich grains. Since pellagra is extremely uncommon today, there is no general need for niacin supplements, especially since excess niacin can be toxic (see Nutrition Insight 9-1).

Niacin in foods and the RDA

The most nutrient-dense sources of niacin are mushrooms, wheat bran, tuna and other fish, chicken, asparagus, and peanuts. Most niacin in the American diet comes from enriched white bread, rolls, crackers, and breakfast cereals (to which niacin is added as part of the enrichment process); and beef, chicken, and turkey. Niacin is very heat stable, so little is lost in cooking.

Dementia • *A general loss or decrease in mental function.*

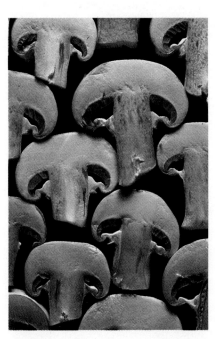

Mushrooms are rich in the B-vitamins: riboflavin, niacin, and pantothermic acid.

ANOTHER BITE Niacin in corn is bound by a protein. This hampers its absorption. Soaking corn in an alkaline solution such as lime water (water with calcium hydroxide) releases bound niacin and renders it more usable. Hispanic people traditionally soak corn in lime water before making tortillas. This treatment is one reason Hispanic populations never suffered much pellagra, in contrast to Europeans and white Americans. Spanish explorers, unaware of the importance of soaking the corn in lime water, failed to inform Europeans how to prepare corn properly when they brought it back from the New World. This inadvertently created widespread niacin deficiencies as corn gained popularity in Europe.

Besides the preformed niacin found in protein foods, each leftover 60 milligrams of the amino acid tryptophan—remaining from intake after protein synthesis—yields about 1 milligram of niacin. To estimate the number of milligrams of niacin supplied by dietary protein, just divide extra grams of dietary protein intake (intake exceeding the RDA) by 6. About half the niacin we use is produced by this process. Animal proteins (except gelatin) are especially rich in tryptophan.

The adult RDA for niacin is 15 to 19 milligrams per day for men and 13 to 15 milligrams per day for women. The difference in muscle mass between genders accounts for the different recommendations. The RDA is expressed as niacin equivalents to account for niacin received intact from the diet, as well as that made from tryptophan.

The average American diet contains 1.4 times the RDA per person per day, without considering the contribution from tryptophan. Note that tables of food values also ignore this contribution. Thus it is unlikely that you will develop a niacin deficiency when consuming a wide variety of foods. People with alcoholism are generally the only group to show a niacin deficiency.

CONCEPT CHECK

The B vitamins thiamin, niacin, and riboflavin are all important in the metabolism of carbohydrates, proteins, and fats. Energy metabolism in particular requires adequate amounts of coenzymes of these three vitamins. Enriched grains are adequate sources of all three vitamins. Otherwise, pork is an excellent source of thiamin, milk is an excellent source of riboflavin, and protein foods in general, such as chicken, are excellent sources of niacin. Deficiencies of all three vitamins can occur with alcoholism; a thiamin deficiency is the most likely.

PANTOTHENIC ACID

Like the other B vitamins, pantothenic acid helps release energy from carbohydrates, fats, and protein. By forming its coenzyme, called coenzyme A, pantothenic acid allows many important energy-yielding metabolic reactions to occur. Coenzyme A makes other molecules much more reactive. For example, coenzyme A must activate fatty acids before they can break down to yield energy. It is also used in the beginning steps of fatty acid synthesis.[22]

Pantothenic acid is so widespread in foods that a nutritional deficiency among healthy people who eat varied diets is unlikely. To study the possible consequences of a pantothenic acid deficiency, researchers must induce it in subjects by having them consume an antagonist to the vitamin. When antagonists are given, people suffer from general symptoms such as tingling hands, fatigue, headache, sleep disturbances, nausea, and abdominal distress.

Pantothenic acid in foods and the ESADDI

Pantothenic acid is present in all foods. Pantothen actually means from every side in Greek. Nutrient-dense sources of pantothenic acid are mushrooms, peanuts, and eggs. Other good sources are meat, milk, and many vegetables. Because pantothenic acid is not added to enriched grains, they are not especially good sources of the vitamin.

The *estimated safe and adequate daily dietary intake (ESADDI)* for pantothenic acid is 4 to 7 milligrams per day for adults. The average U.S. intake is about 6 milligrams of pantothenic acid per person per day. A deficiency of pantothenic acid might occur in alcoholism along with a very nutrient-deficient diet. However, the symptoms would probably be hidden among deficiencies of thiamin, riboflavin, vitamin B-6, and folate, so the pantothenic acid deficiency might be unrecognizable.[17] There is no known toxicity for pantothenic acid.

BIOTIN

Biotin exists in two active forms in foods. In the ultimate coenzyme form, biotin acts in fat and carbohydrate metabolism. Specifically, biotin assists the addition of carbon dioxide to other compounds. By doing so, it promotes the synthesis of glucose, fatty acids, and DNA, as well as helps break down some amino acids.

No accurate measure is available for assessing biotin status. Symptoms of biotin deficiency include a scaly inflammation of the skin, changes in the tongue and lips, decreased appetite, nausea, vomiting, anemia, depression, muscle pain, muscle weakness, and poor growth.[15]

Biotin in foods and the ESADDI

Cauliflower, egg yolks, peanuts, and cheese are the most nutrient-dense sources of biotin. Fruits are generally poorer sources. Intestinal bacteria synthesize and supply some biotin, making a biotin deficiency unlikely. We eat even less biotin than we eliminate in the stool. However, we still don't know what amount of biotin that is synthesized by bacteria in our intestines is actually absorbed.[15] Still, if the intestinal bacteria are not sufficient, as in people who are missing a large part of the small intestine or who need to take antibiotics for many months, special attention should be paid to eating good food sources of biotin.

A protein called *avidin* in raw egg whites can bind biotin and inhibit its absorption. Feeding many raw egg whites to animals leads to classic *egg white injury* deficiency symptoms, as described above. An occasional raw egg in eggnog is of no concern because it would take a regular daily consumption of 12 to 24 raw eggs to produce a biotin deficiency. In cases of alcoholism, however, biotin deficiency symptoms resulting from raw eggs have been reported in people with a regular consumption of just three raw eggs a day. These people probably had very poor diets. Nevertheless, consuming raw eggs is still a concern when you consider the increased risk for *Salmonella* bacteria food poisoning (see Chapter 17).

The estimated safe and adequate daily dietary intake (ESADDI) for biotin is 30 to 100 micrograms per day for adults. The average American diet is thought to contain 100 to 300 micrograms per person per day. It is important to avoid a biotin supplement that exceeds the ESADDI, unless a physician recommends it. We know very little about this vitamin, especially its potential for toxicity.

VITAMIN B-6

Vitamin B-6 is actually a family of three compounds. All can be changed to the active vitamin B-6 coenzyme. The general vitamin name is pyridoxine.

Estimated Safe and Adequate Daily Dietary Intake (ESADDI) • Nutrient intake recommendations made by the Food and Nutrition Board where a range for intake of some nutrients is given because not enough information is available to set an RDA.

Avidin • A protein found in raw egg whites that can bind biotin and inhibit absorption; cooking destroys avidin.

The vitamin B-6 coenzyme is important for the synthesis of hemoglobin, the oxygen-carrying part of the red blood cell. Vitamin B-6 is also necessary for the synthesis of white blood cells, which perform a major role in the immune system.[14]

Functions of vitamin B-6

The coenzymes of vitamin B-6 are needed for the activity of more than 50 enzymes involved in carbohydrate, protein, and fat metabolism. Because vitamin B-6 is needed in so many areas of metabolism, a deficiency results in widespread symptoms, such as depression, vomiting, skin disorders, irritation of the nerves, and impaired immune response.

The most important function of vitamin B-6 concerns protein because metabolizing any amino acid requires the vitamin B-6 coenzyme. By helping to split the nitrogen group ($-NH_2$) from an amino acid, the coenzyme participates in reactions that allow a cell to either synthesize some amino acids or to break them down for energy.[17] In normal circumstances, our bodies can synthesize 11 of the 20 types of amino acids we need. If vitamin B-6 were missing, every amino acid would become an essential amino acid—that is, an amino acid that has to be supplied by the diet.

The syntheses of many *neurotransmitters* require the vitamin B-6 coenzyme. Neurotransmitters allow nerve cells to communicate with each other and with other body cells. We noted above that deficiency of vitamin B-6 results in depression, headaches, confusion, and seizures. These results are predictable, given the importance of vitamin B-6 in the metabolism of key nervous system regulators. In the 1950s, infants fed oversterilized commercial formulas developed vitamin B-6 deficiency symptoms, particularly convulsions. Heat destroyed vitamin B-6 in the formulas, possibly contributing to the infants' decreased ability to synthesize a vital neurotransmitter. Today, manufacturers are more careful to maintain adequate vitamin B-6 levels in formulas.

The link between vitamin B-6 and neurotransmitters suggested to some researchers that vitamin B-6 might be helpful in the treatment of premenstrual syndrome (PMS). This disorder appears in some women associated with menstrual periods and is characterized by depression, headache, bloating, and mood swings. Researchers thought that increasing vitamin B-6 intake might increase synthesis of a neurotransmitter that controls mood, and in turn decrease the depression associated with premenstrual syndrome.

However, researchers now know that high doses of vitamin B-6 is not a reliable therapy for PMS.[25] In addition, vitamin B-6 has a great potential for toxicity (see Nutrition Insight 9-1). Some women have suffered toxic side effects of vitamin B-6 in attempting to treat themselves for PMS. The cause of PMS is not well understood, but a better approach to treatment is to eat a nutrient-rich diet; emphasize starches over fats; decrease alcohol, caffeine, nicotine, and salt to decrease symptoms of nervousness, depression, and bloating; and increase exercise to stimulate relaxation.[7] If nutrition-related therapy is not helpful, women with premenstrual syndrome should seek a physician's advice. They should definitely avoid the PMS *cures* widely available today. These are sold both in drug stores and by mail order.

Vitamin B-6 in foods and the RDA

The most nutrient-dense sources of vitamin B-6 are such fruits and vegetables as bananas, cantaloupe, broccoli, and spinach. But animal foods are the best sources because the vitamin B-6 present is often more absorbable than that in plant foods. Good animal sources include meat, fish, and poultry (vitamin B-6 is stored in muscles). Because vitamin B-6 is not added to foods as part of an enrichment process, breads, cakes, and cookies are not major sources as these are for some other B vitamins. Food tables listing vitamin B-6 are often incomplete because measuring this vitamin in foods is difficult.

The adult RDA for vitamin B-6 is 2 milligrams per day for men and 1.6 milligrams per day for women. The RDA is set high in response to high protein intakes (which leads to more protein metabolism) of people in the United States. Average consumption of vitamin B-6 in the United States approximately equals the RDA. Athletes may need more vitamin B-6 because they use more glycogen for fuel (glycogen metabolism requires vitamin B-6), use more amino acids for fuel, and eat a lot of protein. However, their usual dietary protein intake should easily supply any extra vitamin B-6 needed.

Numerous studies show that about 35% to 40% of adolescent, adult, and elderly women do not meet their RDA for vitamin B-6.[9] However, because vitamin B-6 values of many foods are not known, they are not counted.[14] True intakes, then, may be greater. Women also often eat less protein than that on which the RDA is based. Poor vitamin B-6 status can be found in women who use oral contraceptives. While this relationship has been known for the past 20 years, there is still no consensus about whether these women require vitamin B-6 supplements. Today, it is not possible to reliably separate adequate vitamin B-6 status from an abnormal or deficient state. Still, nutritionists are concerned that the vitamin B-6 status of many women is poor.

People with alcoholism are susceptible to a vitamin B-6 deficiency because acetaldehyde, a metabolite formed when ethanol (alcohol) is metabolized, can displace the vitamin B-6 coenzyme from its enzyme. This process increases the tendency for vitamin B-6 to be broken down. In addition, alcoholism decreases both the absorption of vitamin B-6 and its synthesis into the coenzyme form. Cirrhosis also disables liver tissue from actively metabolizing vitamin B-6. Cirrhosis often accompanies alcoholism (see Chapter 16).

Megaloblast • A large, immature red blood cell that results from the particular cell's inability to divide when it normally should.

Macrocyte • A greatly enlarged mature red blood cell; they have short life spans.

Anemia • Generally refers to a decreased oxygen-carrying capacity of the blood. This can be caused by many factors.

CONCEPT CHECK

Pantothenic acid and biotin both participate in metabolism of carbohydrate and fat. A deficiency of either vitamin is unlikely: pantothenic acid is found widely in foods, and our need for biotin is probably partially met by intestinal synthesis from bacteria. Vitamin B-6 is important for protein metabolism, neurotransmitter synthesis, and other key metabolic functions. Headache, anemia, nausea, and vomiting can result from a vitamin B-6 deficiency. Women should take particular care to consume a diet rich in vitamin B-6, emphasizing animal protein foods, broccoli, spinach, and bananas.

FOLATE

In the past, folate was known as folic acid and folacin. Today, the term folate is preferred because it encompasses the variety of food forms of the vitamin.

Functions of folate

Probably the most important role of the folate coenzymes is helping to form DNA.[3] The active coenzymes help in this synthesis by supplying or accepting single carbon compounds. The coenzymes also help metabolize various amino acids and their derivatives. One major result of a folate deficiency is that in the early phases of red blood cell synthesis, the immature cells cannot divide because they cannot form new DNA. The cells grow larger and larger because they can still synthesize enough protein and other cell parts to make new cells. But when it is time for the cells to divide, the amount of DNA is insufficient to form two nuclei. The cells then remain in a large immature form, known as a *megaloblast.* Megaloblasts can convert to abnormally large red blood cells, called *macrocytes.*

Since the bone marrow of a folate-deficient person produces mostly immature megaloblast cells, few mature red blood cells (called erythrocytes) arrive in the bloodstream. When fewer mature red blood cells are present, the blood's capacity to carry oxygen decreases, causing *anemia.* In short, a folate deficiency causes megaloblastic anemia.[11]

The changes in red blood cell formation occur after 7 to 16 weeks on a folate-free diet, depending on the person's folate stores. White blood cell formation is also affected but to a lesser degree. In addition, cell division throughout the entire body is disrupted. We focus primarily on red blood cells because they are easy to examine and have a relatively short life span. The need to continually replenish red blood cells leads to a great demand for folate, making anemia the first major symptom of folate deficiency. Other symptoms of folate deficiency are inflammation of the tongue, diarrhea, poor growth, mental confusion, and problems in nerve function.[11]

Some forms of cancer therapy provide a vivid example of the effects of a folate deficiency on DNA metabolism. A cancer drug, methotrexate, closely resembles a form of folate. Because of this resemblance, when methotrexate is taken in high doses, it hampers folate metabolism, preventing the formation of the active folate coenzymes. DNA synthesis—and consequently cell division—then decreases. Since cancer cells are among the most rapidly dividing cells in the body, they are among those affected first. However, other rapidly dividing cells, such as intestinal cells and skin cells, are also affected. Not surprisingly, typical side effects of methotrexate therapy are diarrhea, vomiting, and hair loss. These are also typical folate deficiency symptoms.

Folate in foods and the RDA

Green leafy vegetables (*folate* is derived from the Latin word *folium*, which means foliage), organ meats, sprouts, other vegetables, and orange juice are the most nutrient-dense sources of folate. In fact, 1 cup of orange juice contains about half of the RDA. While orange juice is promoted for its vitamin C content, an added benefit is its substantial folate contribution. The vitamin C in the juice also reduces folate destruction.

Food processing and preparation destroy 50% to 90% of the folate in food. Folate is very susceptible to destruction by heat. This underscores the importance of regularly eating fresh fruits and raw or lightly cooked vegetables. Vegetables retain their nutrients best when cooked quickly in minimal water—steaming, stir-frying, or microwaving.

The adult RDA for folate is 180 to 200 micrograms per day. These figures approximate the current folate content of the typical American diet without accounting for losses incurred during preparation and cooking. Folate deficiencies are possible during pregnancy. Pregnant women need extra folate to meet the greater cell division rate, and therefore greater DNA synthesis, for themselves and the fetus. One important reason why women need to see their physicians early in pregnancy is to find out if they need to increase their dietary folate sources (or start folate supplements). Some young women, especially those on oral contraceptives, also register low serum folate values.[8] It is important for women in general to seek good sources of folate in foods and to eat those foods regularly.

Folate deficiencies also often occur with alcoholism. Symptoms of a folate-related anemia can signal a physician to the possibility of alcoholism.

Legal limits are imposed on folate supplements

The FDA limits the amount of folate in a vitamin supplement to 400 micrograms. This measure is taken to prevent excess folate from masking a vitamin B-12 deficiency. The metabolism of folate and vitamin B-12 are linked, as we will soon discuss. For now, note that the major early detectable symptom of a vitamin B-12 deficiency is a change in blood cell formation, which results mainly in a folate-related anemia. However, this symptom does not occur if a large amount of folate is consumed regularly. Hence, a serious vitamin B-12 deficiency can exist silently.

A vitamin B-12 deficiency, for other reasons, can eventually result in paralysis and death. If a vitamin B-12 deficiency is developing in a person, it is important for a physician to diagnose and treat it early. Limiting folate in supplements aids in this goal.

VITAMIN B-12

Vitamin B-12 represents a family of compounds that contain the mineral cobalt. All vitamin B-12 compounds are synthesized by bacteria, fungi, and other lower organisms.

Absorption of vitamin B-12

The body's complex means of absorbing vitamin B-12 is unique among vitamins. Vitamin B-12 in food enters the stomach and is released from other materials by digestion, especially by stomach acid. The free vitamin B-12 then binds with a protein called **R-protein,** produced by salivary glands in the mouth (Figure 9-9). The R-protein/vitamin B-12 complex travels to the small intestine, where enzyme action removes the R-protein.

> **R-Protein** • A protein produced by the salivary glands that participates in vitamin B-12 absorption.

FIGURE 9-9
Absorption of vitamin B-12. Many factors and sites in the GI tract participate.

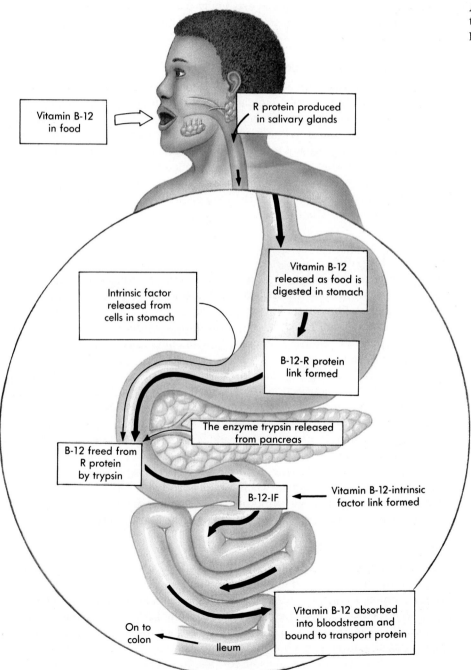

Vitamin B-12 in food

R protein produced in salivary glands

Vitamin B-12 released as food is digested in stomach

Intrinsic factor released from cells in stomach

B-12-R protein link formed

The enzyme trypsin released from pancreas

B-12 freed from R protein by trypsin

B-12-IF

Vitamin B-12-intrinsic factor link formed

Vitamin B-12 absorbed into bloodstream and bound to transport protein

On to colon

Ileum

Intrinsic Factor • A proteinlike compound produced by the stomach that enhances vitamin B-12 absorption.

Ileum • Essentially the area consisting of the last half of the small intestine.

Pernicious Anemia • The anemia that results from a lack of vitamin B-12 absorption; it is *pernicious* because of associated nerve degeneration that can result in eventual paralysis.

Once vitamin B-12 is free again, it binds to ***intrinsic factor,*** a type of protein made by the stomach's acid-producing cells. The resulting intrinsic factor/vitamin B-12 complex travels to the last portion of the small intestine, called the ***ileum.*** Ileum cells absorb vitamin B-12 and transfer it to a special blood transport protein.

Using this system, approximately 30% to 70% of dietary vitamin B-12 is absorbed, depending on the body's need for it. Any failure in this system results in only 1% to 2% absorption of dietary vitamin B-12.[11]

Vitamin B-12 absorption can be disrupted by such causes as inefficient synthesis of intrinsic factor, a genetic deficiency in R-protein synthesis, absence of the ileum or stomach, or tape worm infestations. Once a defect in absorption is established, the person usually takes regular injections of vitamin B-12 to bypass the need for absorption. About 95% of all cases of vitamin B-12 deficiencies in healthy people result from defective vitamin B-12 absorption rather than from inadequate intakes. This is especially true for elderly people. As we age the stomach loses its ability to synthesize the intrinsic factor needed for vitamin B-12 absorption.

Functions of vitamin B-12

Vitamin B-12 participates in a variety of cellular reactions. Probably its most important function is in folate metabolism. Vitamin B-12 is required to convert folate coenzymes to the active forms needed for important metabolic reactions, such as DNA synthesis. Without vitamin B-12, reactions that require certain active forms of folate do not take place in the cell. Thus a vitamin B-12 deficiency contributes to what amounts to a folate deficiency. Another vital function of vitamin B-12 is maintaining the myelin sheaths that insulate nerve fibers from each other.[5] People with vitamin B-12 deficiencies show patchy destruction of the myelin sheaths. This destruction eventually causes paralysis and perhaps death.[11]

Pernicious anemia

In the past the inability to absorb vitamin B-12 eventually led to death. Researchers in mid-nineteenth century England noted a form of anemia that caused death within 2 to 5 years of the initial illness, mainly because it destroyed the nerves. They called it ***pernicious anemia*** (pernicious literally means leading to death). Clinically, the anemia looks much like a folate deficiency anemia.

You can probably guess that the two types of anemia are similar—the folate/vitamin B-12 connection. Without vitamin B-12, folate can't convert to the active coenzymes needed to synthesize red blood cells. Because many macrocytes appear in the bloodstream, the vitamin B-12 anemia is called a macrocytic anemia. In pernicious anemia, symptoms of nerve destruction take about 3 years to appear. When a vitamin B-12 deficiency is caused strictly by a lack of the vitamin in the diet, it would take even longer for significant nerve damage to show up because whenever absorption is possible, tiny amounts suffice. Besides the anemia, symptoms of pernicious anemia include weakness, sore tongue, back pain, apathy, and tingling in the extremities.[11]

Vitamin B-12 in foods and the RDA

The most nutrient-dense sources of vitamin B-12 are clams, oysters, and hot dogs. Beef, pork, eggs, and milk are also good sources. Vitamin B-12 is present in large amounts only in animal foods. While plants can contain vitamin B-12, they do not make it. Any vitamin B-12 present in plants comes from contamination with organisms that can make it—soil organisms, stray bacteria, or yeast. This contamination can contribute some vitamin B-12 to the vegan's diet. However, these are not reliable sources (see Reference no. 9 in Chapter 8).

The RDA for vitamin B-12 for adults is 2 micrograms per day. The average diet in the United States includes approximately 8 micrograms of vitamin B-12 per person per day. This high intake provides the average meat-eating person with 2 to 3 years' storage of vitamin B-12 in the liver. Thus if you eat animal foods regularly and can absorb vitamin B-12, a vitamin B-12 deficiency is highly unlikely. It takes approximately 20 years of consuming a diet essentially free of vitamin B-12 for a person to exhibit nerve destruction caused by a diet deficiency. Vegans, who eat no animal products, should find a reliable source of vitamin B-12. As noted earlier, the elderly are at risk for developing pernicious anemia, and regular physical examinations should test for this possibility. Vitamin B-12 supplements are essentially nontoxic.

CONCEPT CHECK

Folate is needed for cell division mostly because it influences DNA synthesis. A folate deficiency results in anemia, as well as inflammation of the tongue, diarrhea, and poor growth—all signs of poor cell division. Folate is found in fresh vegetables and organ meats. It is important to emphasize fresh and lightly cooked vegetables, because much folate is lost during cooking. Folate needs during pregnancy are especially high.

Vitamin B-12 is necessary for the formation of the active coenzymes of folate. Without dietary vitamin B-12, folate deficiency symptoms, such as macrocytic anemia, develop. In addition, vitamin B-12 is necessary for maintaining the nervous system. Paralysis can develop from a vitamin B-12 deficiency. The absorption of vitamin B-12 requires a number of specific factors. If absorption is inhibited, the resulting deficiency can lead to pernicious anemia and its associated nerve destruction. Concentrated amounts of vitamin B-12 are found only in animal foods; meat eaters generally have a 3 to 5 year supply stored in the liver. Vitamin B-12 absorption may decline as we age. Monthly injections can make up for this.

VITAMIN C

Scurvy—the vitamin C deficiency disease—was long ago a constant threat to the health of sailors. Its symptoms include weakness, opening of previously healed wounds, slower wound healing times, bone pain, fractures, bleeding gums, diarrhea, and pinpoint hemorrhages around hair follicles on the back of the arms and legs.[1] On long sea voyages captains often lost half or more of their crew to scurvy. Epidemics of scurvy occurred in Europe from 1556 to 1857, and soldiers in the U.S. Civil War died of it. In 1740, the Englishman Dr. James Lind first showed that citrus fruits—two oranges and one lemon a day—could cure scurvy. Fifty years after Lind's discovery, rations for British sailors included limes to prevent scurvy. That is how the British earned the nickname limey—and one reason for their preeminence at sea during the nineteenth century.

Vitamin C (ascorbic acid) is a puzzling vitamin. It is found in all living tissues, and most animals synthesize their own from the simple sugar glucose. Only guinea pigs, monkeys, some birds, a few fish, and humans need vitamin C in their diets. What is strange is that animals who synthesize vitamin C often make quite a lot of it. For instance, a pig produces 8 grams per day (though we do not benefit from it when we eat pork, since it is lost in processing). This amount is over 130 times our human RDA of 60 milligrams, and even 60 milligrams appears to be quite a generous intake for humans. As little as 10 milligrams daily can prevent scurvy.

Why some animals make so much vitamin C while other animals, including humans, appear to need so little has fueled much controversy. Is the amount of vitamin C that prevents the disease scurvy the same amount that promotes optimal health? This question hasn't been fully answered.

Collagen • The major protein form found in connective tissue, cartilage, and bone. Vitamin C aids in its synthesis.

Vitamin C is also necessary for the synthesis of a number of hormones, neurotransmitters, and other vital compounds, such as bile acids and DNA. In animal studies vitamin C deficiency allows cholesterol to accumulate in the liver and lead to high levels in the blood.

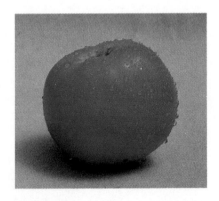

Tomatoes are a rich source of vitamin C.

Absorption of vitamin C

Absorption of vitamin C occurs in the small intestine. About 80% to 90% of vitamin C is absorbed when a person eats between 30 and 180 milligrams of it per day. If someone ingests 6 grams (6000 milligrams) per day, absorption efficiency drops to about 20%. A common side effect of high vitamin C intakes is diarrhea. The unabsorbed vitamin C stays in the small intestine and attracts water, finally causing diarrhea. Some health food enthusiasts even claim that the ideal dosage of vitamin C is one that produces diarrhea.

Functions of vitamin C

Collagen synthesis. The best understood function of vitamin C is its role in synthesizing the protein **collagen.** This protein is found in high concentrations in connective tissue, bone, teeth, tendons, and blood vessels. It is very important for wound healing. Vitamin C increases the cross-connections between amino acids in collagen, greatly strengthening the tissues it helps form.

When a person is deficient in vitamin C, widespread changes in tissue metabolism and structure occur. Most symptoms of scurvy are linked to a decrease in collagen synthesis. It takes about 20 to 40 days with no vitamin C intake for the first symptoms of scurvy to appear.[1]

Antioxidant. Vitamin C is one of the cell's water-soluble antioxidants. Recall that vitamin E is a fat-soluble antioxidant for the cell membrane. Using its antioxidant capabilities, vitamin C can reduce the formation of cancer-causing nitrosamines in the stomach and also keep the folate coenzymes intact, preventing their destruction. If vitamin C is found effective in preventing cancer, its effectiveness will probably be related to its antioxidant capabilities (see the Nutrition Issue, p. 286).

Enhancing iron absorption and the immune system. Vitamin C is important for iron absorption because it keeps iron in the most absorbable (ferrous) form. This renders the iron much more available in the small intestine's alkaline environment than for other forms of iron and thus increases iron absorption. To produce this effect, about 50 milligrams of vitamin C (about 4 ounces of orange juice) must be consumed at the same meal with the iron. Increasing vitamin C intake is very beneficial if one has poor iron stores. One symptom of vitamin C toxicity—seen in doses of 1 to 2 grams per day—can even be overabsorption of iron, with the potential of iron toxicity (see Nutrition Insight 9-1).

Vitamin C is vital for the function of the immune system, especially for the activity of certain cells in the immune system. Thus disease states can increase the need for vitamin C, but we don't know how much (if any) vitamin C intake above the RDA is needed.

Vitamin C in foods and the RDA

The most nutrient-dense sources of vitamin C are green peppers, cauliflower, broccoli, cabbage, strawberries, papayas, and romaine lettuce. Citrus fruits, potatoes, and other green vegetables are also good sources of vitamin C. The four servings of fruits and vegetables from the Guide to Daily Food Choices can easily provide enough vitamin C. The major contributors of vitamin C in the U.S. diet are orange juice, grapefruit and grapefruit juice, tomatoes and tomato juice, fortified fruit drinks, oranges, tangerines, and potatoes.

Vitamin C is easily lost in processing and cooking. Juices are good foods to fortify with vitamin C because their acidity reduces vitamin C destruction. Vitamin C is very unstable when in contact with heat, iron, copper, or oxygen.[23]

The adult RDA for vitamin C is 60 milligrams per day. The current RDA suggests that cigarette smokers consume 100 milligrams per day because they greatly stress their lungs with oxygen and toxic by-products of cigarette smoke. The average U.S. diet yields about twice the adult RDA (120 milligrams) of vitamin C per day. So probably almost all of us meet our daily need for vitamin C. Toxicity symptoms from excess vitamin C starts at doses of 1 to 2 grams.

Today vitamin C deficiency appears mostly in alcoholic people who eat nutrient-poor diets and in elderly men who live alone and also eat poorly. Men are more susceptible to vitamin C deficiency than women because, as a group, they tend to smoke more and are less apt to consume vitamin supplements. Studies show that 14% to 20% of adult and elderly men have low serum vitamin C levels. Overall, a diet with limited fruit and vegetable consumption puts a person at risk of deficiency. Worldwide, scurvy is associated with poverty. It is especially common in infants who are fed boiled milk (all forms of milk are poor sources of vitamin C) and not provided with a good food source of vitamin C or a supplement.

As we noted in Chapter 4, many different benefits—ranging from a cure for the common cold to a cure for cancer—have been attributed to large doses of vitamin C. By *large* doses we mean 2 grams (2000 milligrams) or more per day. Some people think that if 60 milligrams of vitamin C is enough for good health, then higher doses (megadoses) may produce even better health. But this assertion has not been demonstrated scientifically.[24] In fact, most vitamin C consumed in large doses just ends up in the stool or the urine. Only a small fraction of such large doses can be used. The body is totally saturated at intakes of 100 to 200 milligrams per day. This means that if more than 100 to 200 milligrams of vitamin C is ingested, it is very quickly excreted.

We don't believe that colds are severe enough or last long enough to merit vitamin C therapy. However, that is a personal decision. Consuming vitamin C may alleviate a cold's symptoms somewhat, so we see no reason to discourage people from drinking a few glasses of orange juice when they have a cold. If it doesn't help them physically, it may help them psychologically. Psychological effects often work wonders. However, as we said in Chapter 4, there is no striking evidence from double-blind studies that large amounts of vitamin C greatly decrease the severity or duration of a cold.[24] In addition, no credible evidence suggests that a dose even as high as 10 grams a day will cure colon cancer.

CONCEPT CHECK

Vitamin C is important in the synthesis of collagen, a major connective tissue protein. A vitamin C deficiency, known as scurvy, causes many changes in the skin and gums, such as small hemorrhages. This is mainly because of poor collagen synthesis. Vitamin C also improves iron absorption and is involved in synthesizing certain hormones and neurotransmitters. Citrus fruits, green peppers, cauliflower, broccoli, and strawberries are good sources of vitamin C. As with folate, it is important to eat fresh or lightly cooked foods since vitamin C loses a lot of its potency in cooking. At doses greater than about 15 times the RDA (1 gram), vitamin C can lead to diarrhea. These high doses do not prevent the common cold or cure cancer. However, consuming the RDA of vitamin C is part of the overall approach to good health.

Now that we have discussed the vitamins, review the Guide to Daily Food Choices in Chapter 2 and note how each group makes an important vitamin contribution.

VITAMIN-LIKE COMPOUNDS

A variety of vitamin-like compounds are found in the body. These include:

- choline
- carnitine

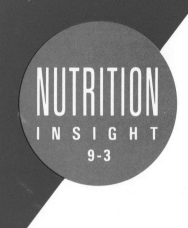

BOGUS VITAMINS

Health food enthusiasts promote a variety of compounds as vitamins even though these substances have no importance in human nutrition. Because some of these so called *vitamins* may cause increased growth in lower organisms, vitamin hucksters try to pass them off as necessary for humans (Figure 9-10). As these pseudovitamins continue to be represented as vitamins, sales profits mount to more than billions of dollars yearly.

The list of these pseudovitamins changes frequently. The following are some of the more persistent pseudos:[11]

- *Para-aminobenzoic acid (PABA):* Although this compound is part of the vitamin folate, we can't use it to make folate. Entrepreneurs represent PABA as "a member of the B complex family," omitting the words "for bacteria," so that they can sell it as a food supplement. If consumed along with sulfa antibiotics, it can defeat the effect of the antibiotic.
- *Laetrile:* This cyanide-containing compounds—wrongly labeled vitamin B-17—is promoted as a cure for cancer. FDA does not recognize it as a legitimate cancer therapy. Chronic cyanide intoxications from laetriles in the diet has produced thousands of cases of slowly progressing nerve damage with blindness, deafness, and muscle weakness the result.
- *Bioflavonoids:* These compounds—sometimes incorrectly called "vitamin P"—include rutin and hesperidin. They were originally thought to be more effective than vitamin C alone for treating fragile blood vessels in scurvy. Today there is no recognized nutritional or medical need for bioflavonoids, although they may enhance vitamin C absorption. Most flavonoids are concentrated in the skin, peel, and outer layers of fruits and vegetables. Beverages such as tea, coffee, wine, and beer also contain significant amounts.
- *Pangamic acid:* This bogus compound—wrongly labeled vitamin B-15—has no link to nutrition and deserves no attention. This includes athletes. Its roots are quackery, pure and simple.

Other compounds will surely come and go in the next few years. Again, since people have been maintained for years on intravenous feedings that contain all the known essential nutrients without developing deficiency symptoms, it is unlikely that any vitamin remains to be discovered. You can be sure that if a *new* compound has the potential to be a vitamin, the Food and Nutrition Board of the National Academy of Sciences will closely examine it. If it then appears with the rest of the nutrients that have an RDA or ESADDI, you can be confident the compound can be called a vitamin and is worth your attention. ●

- inositol
- taurine
- lipoic acid

All of these vitamin-like compounds are necessary to maintain proper metabolism in the body. They can be synthesized by cells using common building blocks, such as amino acids and glucose.

In disease states, synthesis of vitamin-like compounds may not meet needs, and so dietary intake can be crucial. The needs for choline, carnitine, and taurine in certain conditions, such as for premature infants, are currently being investigated. Although promoted and sold by health food stores, there is no concern that these vitamin-like compounds are needed by the average healthy adult (Figure 9-10). We make them each day. Some are present only in animal foods, and because vegans—who eat no animal products—show no evidence of deficiencies, body synthesis most likely suffices for us.

One Pack (3 tabs) Contains:		**%USRDA
VITAMINS		
Vitamin C (corn free)	1000 mg.	1666
Vitamin E (natural)	200 I.U.	666
Pantothenic Acid*	60 mg.	600
Niacinamide*	40 mg.	200
Choline (bitartrate)*	30 mg.	***
Inositol*	30 mg.	***
Vitamin B-1 HCl*	25 mg.	2500
Vitamin B-2*	25 mg.	1470
Vitamin B-6 HCl*	25 mg.	1250
PABA*		
(para-aminobenzoic acid)	15 mg.	***
Vitamin A (beta carotene)	10,000 I.U.	200
Folic Acid*	400 mcg.	100
Vitamin B-12*		
(from cobalamin)	200 mcg.	3333
Biotin*	100 mcg.	33
Vitamin D (calciferol)	400 I.U.	100
*Fortified with Rice Bran.		

MINERALS

Calcium (aminoate*)	200 mg.	20
Magnesium (aminoate*)	100 mg.	25
Potassium (a.a. complex*)	50 mg.	***
Iron (aminoate,* ascorbate)	18 mg.	100
Zinc (aminoate,* picolinate)	15 mg.	100
Manganese (aminoate*)	4 mg.	***
Copper (aminoate*)	0.5 mg.	25
Iodine (kelp)	150 mcg.	100
Selenium (aminoate*)	25 mcg.	***
Chromium (aminoate*)	20 mcg.	***
*Hypo-Allergenic Whole Brown Rice Chelate.		

BIOFLAVONOIDS

Lemon Bioflavonoid Complex	60 mg.
(citrus) (active flavonols, flavonones, flavones & naringen — 44%)	
Quercetin (saphora japonicas)	30 mg.
Rutin (saphora japonicas)	25 mg.
Hesperidin (citrus)	10 mg.
Eriocitrin (citrus)	3 mg.

NUCLEIC ACIDS (source: Spirulina)

RNA (ribonucleic acid)	21 mg.
DNA (deoxyribonucleic acid)	6 mg.

ENZYMES

Bromelain	
(pineapple, 600 GDU/grm)	40 mg.
Papain (papaya)	30 mg.
Betaine HCl (beet molasses)	25 mg.
Apple Pectin	20 mg.
Amylase (brown rice fermentation)	5 mg.
Lipase (brown rice fermentation)	5 mg.

PLANT PIGMENTS

Chlorophyll	7.5 mg.
Carotenoids	4 mg.

LIPIDS

Black Currant Seed Oil (with GLA)	50 mg.
Sunflower Oil, Supplying	
Linoleic Acid	54.1 mg.
Oleic Acid	9.3 mg.
Palmitic Acid	4.4 mg.
Stearic Acid	2.2 mg.

AMINO ACIDS (source: Spirulina)

L-Isoleucine	24.8 mg.	L-Aspartic Acid	38.6 mg.
L-Leucine	34.8 mg.	L-Cystine	4 mg.
L-Lysine	24 mg.	L-Glutamic Acid	53.6 mg.
L-Methionine	13 mg.	L-Glycine	20.8 mg.
L-Phenylalanine	23.8 mg.	L-Histidine	6.5 mg.
L-Threonine	25 mg.	L-Proline	17.8 mg.
L-Tryptophan	6.8 mg.	L-Serine	24 mg.
L-Valine	36 mg.	L-Cysteine*	10 mg.
L-Alanine	35 mg.	L-Carnitine*	10 mg.
L-Arginine	35.8 mg.	* Free Form Amino Acid	

HIGHLY ACTIVE NUTRIENT BASE

Spirulina	1000 mg.
Bee Pollen (Spanish)	100 mg.
Ginseng (Korean)	50 mg.
Octacosanol (wheat free)	200 mcg.

HERBAL BASE

Astragalus, Ligustrum, Schizandra, Young Barley Leaves, Echinacea, Irish Moss, Pau d'Arco, Thyme and Juniper Berry.

**United States Recommended Daily Allowance for Adults and Children 12 years and older.
***No USRDA has been established.

DIRECTIONS: As a dietary supplement, 3 tablets daily.

Do not take with sulfonamide since PABA interferes with the activity of the drug.

Manufactured with all natural fillers, binders, coatings and excipients including: Microcrystalline Cellulose, Vegetable Stearine, Silica, Protein Coating ...*and LOVE* ♥
Free from sugar, salt, starch, artificial colors and preservatives.
Free from the common allergens, yeast, wheat, corn, soy and milk.

VEGETARIAN FORMULA
KEEP TIGHTLY CLOSED IN A COOL, DRY PLACE.
KEEP OUT OF REACH OF CHILDREN.

Manufactured by
NATURE'S PLUS
10 Daniel Street, Farmingdale, NY 11735
Div. of Natural Organics, Inc.
PRODUCT NO. 3059
©NATURAL ORGANICS, Inc. 1986
All Rights Reserved

0 97467 03059 6

Also available in bottles of 30, 90, & 180 tablets and bottles of 90 & 180 capsules.

FIGURE 9-10

Health foods are noted for containing substances the healthy body does not need—vitamin-like compounds, such as inositol, and bogus vitamins, such as bioflavonoids.

SUMMARY

- Vitamins are compounds we generally need daily in small amounts from foods. They yield no energy, but many contribute to energy-yielding chemical reactions in the body and promote growth and development. Many vitamins act as coenzymes, which help enzymes function. Vitamins A, D, E, and K are fat soluble, while the B vitamins and vitamin C are water soluble.

- Vitamin A consists of a family of compounds that includes several forms of preformed vitamin A. Some carotenoids, such as beta-carotene, can also yield vitamin A. Vitamin A functions in vision, immune function, and cell development. Vitamin A is found in liver and fish oils; carotenoids are especially plentiful in dark green and orange vegetables. Vitamin A can be quite toxic even when taken at just 5 to 10 times the RDA. High vitamin A intakes are especially dangerous during pregnancy because they can lead to fetal malformations.

- Vitamin D is both a hormone and a vitamin. Human skin synthesizes it using sunshine and a cholesterol-like substance. If we don't spend enough time in the sun, foods such as fish oils and fortified milk must supply the vitamin. The active hormone form of vitamin D helps regulate blood calcium levels by influencing calcium absorption from the intestine. Children who don't get enough vitamin D may develop rickets, and adults with inadequate amounts in the body develop osteomalacia. Vitamin D is a very toxic substance. An intake just 2.5 to 5 times the RDA can cause problems.

- Vitamin E functions primarily as an antioxidant and is found in plant oils. By donating electrons to electron-seeking (oxidizing) compounds, it neutralizes them. This shields cell membranes and red blood cells from breakdown. Claims are made about the curative powers of vitamin E, but few are scientifically sound.

- Vitamin K helps blood clot. About half the vitamin K absorbed each day comes from bacterial synthesis in the intestine, and the other half comes from foods, primarily green leafy vegetables. Vitamin K is poorly stored in the body, but our dietary intake alone is usually sufficient. People who can't absorb fat well or who are on antibiotics for long periods of time may need extra vitamin K.

- Thiamin, riboflavin, and niacin play key roles as coenzymes in energy-yielding reactions. They help metabolize carbohydrates, fats, and proteins. Alcoholism and a poor diet can create deficiencies of these three nutrients. Enriched grain products are common sources of all three of these vitamins.

- Pantothenic acid, which participates in many aspects of cell metabolism, is widely distributed among foods. Biotin, which participates in glucose production, fat synthesis, and DNA synthesis, can be synthesized by bacteria in the intestine. We probably synthesize about half our requirement for biotin. The rest comes from foods such as eggs and cheese.

- Vitamin B-6 performs a vital role in protein metabolism, especially in synthesizing nonessential amino acids. It also helps synthesize neurotransmitters and performs other metabolic roles. Headaches, anemia, nausea, and vomiting result from a B-6 deficiency. Generally, women are more likely to have poor vitamin B-6 stores. Regular consumption of animal protein foods, cauliflower, and broccoli provides needed vitamin B-6. Taking high doses causes malfunction of the nervous system.

- Folate plays an important role in DNA synthesis. Symptoms of a deficiency are generally poor cell division in various areas of the body, anemia, tongue inflammation, diarrhea, and poor growth. Pregnancy puts high demands for folate on the body. A deficiency is most likely to occur in people with alcoholism. Excellent food sources are leafy vegetables, organ meats, and orange juice. Great amounts of folate can be lost in prolonged cooking.

- Vitamin B-12 is needed to metabolize folate and to maintain the insulation surrounding nerves. A deficiency results in anemia (because of its relationship to folate) and nerve degeneration. Elderly people often absorb vitamin B-12 inefficiently. If so, they benefit from monthly injections of the vitamin. For others, a deficiency is unlikely because vitamin B-12 is highly concentrated in animal foods, which constitute a major part of the American diet. Vitamin B-12 does not occur naturally in plant foods. Vegans need a supplemental source.

- Vitamin C is used mainly to synthesize collagen, a major protein for building connective tissue. A vitamin C deficiency results in scurvy, which is evidenced by poor wound healing, pinpoint hemorrhages in the skin, and bleeding gums. Vitamin C also enhances iron absorption and is needed for synthesizing some hormones and neurotransmitters. Fresh fruits and vegetables, especially citrus fruits, are generally good sources. Since the amount of vitamin C lost in cooking is high, a good diet should emphasize fresh or lightly cooked vegetables. Deficiencies can occur in people with alcoholism and in those whose diets lack sufficient fruits and vegetables. Smoking makes matters worse for people already at risk.

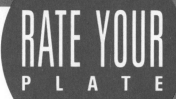

MEASURING YOUR VITAMIN INTAKE AGAINST THE RDA

This activity requires you to reexamine the nutritional assessment you completed in Chapter 2. You recorded the types of, the quantities of, and the amount of nutrients in the foods and drinks you consumed for one day. Then you assessed your intake by recording the total amounts of nutrient you consumed. You were then asked to compare your intake of nutrients to certain standards. Many of the standards you used were the 1989 RDA found on the inside cover of this book. Using your completed assessment, record your intakes of vitamins A, E, C, B-6, B-12, thiamin, riboflavin, niacin, and folate in the table below. Next, record the RDA for each of these nutrients off your assessment. Then, record the percentage of the RDA you had for each vitamin. Lastly, place a +, −, or = in the space provided reflecting an intake higher, lower, or equal to the RDA.

VITAMIN	INTAKE	RDA	% OF RDA	+,−,=
A *use IU*	4138	4000	103	+
E				
C	183	60	305	+
THIAMIN	1.26	.90	140	+
RIBOFLAVIN	1.40	1.08	130	+
NIACIN	14.49	11.88	122	+
B-6				
FOLATE				
B-12				

ANALYSIS

1. Which of your vitamin intakes equaled or exceeded your RDA?

   _____

2. Which of your vitamin intakes were below the RDA?

   _____

3. What foods could you eat to improve your dietary intake of vitamins? (Review sources of certain vitamins in the text.)

   _____

   _____

REFERENCES

1. Anonymous: Experimental scurvy in a young man, *Nutrition Reviews* 44:13, 1986.

2. Albin RL and others: Acute sensory neuropathy-neuronopathy from pyridoxine overdose, *Neurology* 37:1729, 1987.

3. Bailey LB: The role of folate in human nutrition, *Nutrition Today*, September/October, 1990, p 12.

4. Bauernfend JC: Vitamin A deficiency: a staggering problem of health and sight, *Nutrition Today*, March/April, 1988, p 34.

5. Beck WS: Cobalamin and the nervous system, *New England Journal of Medicine* 318:1752, 1988.

6. Burton GW: Antioxidant action of carotenoids, *Journal of Nutrition* 119:109, 1989.

7. Casey V, Dwyer JT: Premenstrual syndrome: theories and evidence, *Nutrition Today*, November/December, 1987, p 4.

8. Clark AJ and others: Folacin status in adolescent females, *American Journal of Clinical Nutrition* 46:302, 1987.

9. Driscoll JA and others: Longitudinal assessment of vitamin B-6 status in southern adolescent girls, *Journal of The American Dietetic Association* 87:307, 1987.

10. Feldman KW and others: Nutritional rickets, *American Family Physician* 42:1311, November, 1990.

11. Herbert VD: "Folic acid" and "vitamin B-12" and "pseudovitamins." In Shils ME, Young VR, editors: *Modern nutrition in health and disease*, ed 7, Philadelphia, 1988, Lea & Febiger.

12. Howard LJ: The neurologic syndrome of vitamin E deficiency: laboratory and electrophysiologic assessment, *Nutrition Reviews* 48:169, 1990.

13. Lammer EJ and others: Retinoic acid embryopathy, *The New England Journal of Medicine* 313:837, 1985.

14. Leklem JE: Vitamin B-6: of reservoirs, receptors and requirements, *Nutrition Today*, September/October, 1988, p 4.

15. Marshall MW: The nutritional importance of biotin—an update, *Nutrition Today*, November/December, 1987, p 26.

16. Maye ST and others: Rebound effect with ascorbic acid in adult males, *American Journal of Clinical Nutrition* 48:379, 1988.

17. McCormick DB: "Thiamin," "riboflavin," "niacin," "vitamin B-6," "pantothenic acid," and "biotin." In Shils ME, Young VR, editors: *Modern nutrition in health and disease*, ed 7, Philadelphia, 1988, Lea & Febiger.

18. Mederios DM and others: Vitamin and mineral supplementation practices of adults in seven western states, *Journal of the American Dietetic Association* 89:383, 1989.

19. Moon RC: Comparative aspects of carotenoids and retinoids as chemopreventive agents for cancer, *Journal of Nutrition* 119:127, 1989.

20. Olson RE: Vitamin K. In Shils ME, Young VR, editors: *Modern nutrition in health and disease*, Philadelphia, 1988, Lea & Febiger.

21. Reichel H and others: The role of the vitamin D endocrine system in health and disease, *The New England Journal of Medicine* 320:980, 1989.

22. Song WO: Pantothenic acid: how much do we know about this B-complex vitamin? *Nutrition Today*, March/April, 1990, p 19.

23. Sauberlich HE: Vitamins—how much is for keeps? *Nutrition Today*, January/February, 1987, p 20.

24. Truswell AS: Ascorbic acid, *New England Journal of Medicine* 315:709, 1986.

25. Van den Berg H and others: Vitamin B-6 status of women suffering from premenstrual syndrome, *Human Nutrition:Clinical Nutrition* 40C:441, 1986.

26. Webb AR, Holick MF: The role of sunlight in the cutaneous production of vitamin D, *Annual Reviews of Nutrition* 8:375, 1988.

27. West KP and others: Vitamin A supplementation and growth: a randomized community trial, *American Journal of Clinical Nutrition* 48:1257, 1988.

28. Willett WC: Vitamin A and lung cancer, *Nutrition Reviews* 48:201, 1990.

HOW MUCH HAVE I LEARNED?

What have you learned from Chapter 9? Here are 15 statements about vitamins. Read them to test your current knowledge. If you think the answer is true or mostly true, circle T. If you think the answer is false or mostly false, circle F. Use the scoring key at the end of the book to compute your total score. To review, take this test again later, and especially before tests.

1. **T F** If a vitamin is missing from your diet for 1 week, you are risking a vitamin deficiency.

2. **T F** People who use mineral oil as a laxative at mealtimes are susceptible to fat-soluble vitamin deficiencies.

3. **T F** Vitamin D improves calcium absorption.

4. **T F** Vitamin A is important for night vision.

5. **T F** Vitamin D is synthesized by sunlight.

6. **T F** Vitamin K is important for blood clotting.

7. **T F** Vitamin B-6 can prevent premenstrual syndrome by influencing neurotransmitter levels.

8. **T F** Thiamin needs are related to the amount of fat one eats.

9. **T F** Milk is a good source of riboflavin.

10. **T F** Using an amino acid, the body can make niacin.

11. **T F** A niacin deficiency causes severe skin inflammation.

12. **T F** The term folate comes from the word foliage.

13. **T F** Vitamin B-12 is concentrated only in animal foods.

14. **T F** Vitamin C enhances iron absorption.

15. **T F** High doses of vitamin C can prevent the common cold.

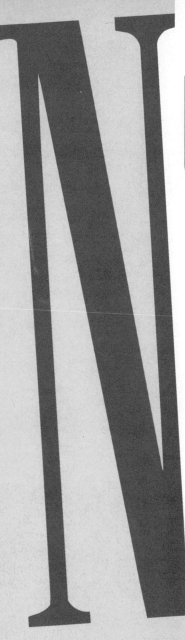

NUTRITION ISSUE

NUTRITION AND CANCER

Cancer is the second leading cause of death for adults in the United States. Cancer is actually many diseases; it affects different types of cells and arises from many different causes (Figure 9-11). Causes of skin cancer differ from the causes of breast cancer, and their treatments also differ. We need to look seriously at cancer in general and consider our risk of getting it.

Cancer occurs more in some families than in others; genetic background plays a role in the risk for cancer, especially colon cancer. However, lifestyle is also a critical factor. We know this because rates of cancer differ around the world. The Japanese, for example, have more stomach cancer and Americans have more colon cancer. When Japanese people immigrate to the United States, their rates of stomach cancer decrease but their rates for colon cancer increase. In addition, one third of all cancer cases in America is caused by smoking tobacco.

Cancer-causing mechanisms

To understand how to prevent cancer we first need to examine how cancer develops in the body. The process begins with an alteration in DNA, the genetic material in our cells. When the DNA is altered, the cell may no longer respond to normal body signals. The cell can then dictate its own rate of growth. It is not inhibited from growing at the expense of the cells around it.

Agents that alter DNA can cause cancer

There are many ways to alter DNA. A substance or phenomenon can directly alter DNA or lead to processes that in turn alter DNA. (Figure 9-12). DNA can be disrupted by these methods in time ranging from less than a second to days.

Radiation from the sun (ultraviolet form) can cause DNA to bind to itself or break into pieces. This is one way skin cancer begins. The altered skin cells may then begin to grow out of control. Cancer can result. X-rays, another type of radiation, readily damage the genetic material. Certain chemicals, both natural and man made, can alter DNA. These are often called *carcinogens.* Viruses alter DNA by inserting their *genes* into human cells. If the genes promote growth, the cell may begin to grow out of control.

Thus three common means of altering DNA are through radiation, certain chemicals, and viruses. However, having a cell with altered DNA does not mean cancer is inevitable. Special enzymes travel up and down the DNA to repair breaks and changes in it. The repair enzymes may fix alterations before the cell begins to grow out of control.

Altering DNA is not the only way to increase cancer risk

Compounds that increase cell division also are thought to promote cancer by either decreasing the time available for repair enzymes to act or by encouraging

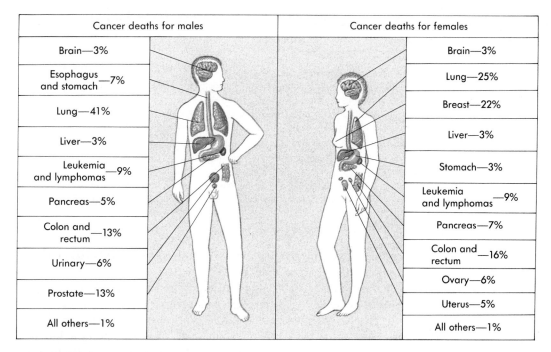

Cancer deaths for males	Cancer deaths for females
Brain—3%	Brain—3%
Esophagus and stomach—7%	Lung—25%
Lung—41%	Breast—22%
Liver—3%	Liver—3%
Leukemia and lymphomas—9%	Stomach—3%
Pancreas—5%	Leukemia and lymphomas—9%
Colon and rectum—13%	Pancreas—7%
Urinary—6%	Colon and rectum—16%
Prostate—13%	Ovary—6%
All others—1%	Uterus—5%
	All others—1%

FIGURE 9-11

Approximate cancer deaths by site and gender: 1990 estimate. Lung cancer is now the number one cancer killer in both men and women.

cells with altered DNA to develop and grow (Figure 9-12). Likely candidates are high levels of estrogen, alcohol, and probably dietary fat. Once a cell divides, any altered DNA will be reproduced along with the rest of the genetic material. Now the cell will follow its newly altered genetic instructions. Development and growth of these altered cells may take up to 20 years.

Once an altered cell has multiplied, there is still a chance that cancer won't result. First, the cell mass must increase until it can significantly affect body metabolism. During this initial stage of growth, the immune system may find the altered cells and destroy them. Or, the cancer cells may be so defective that their own DNA limits their ability to grow, and they die anyway.

Radiation • Literally energy that is emitted from a center in all directions. Various forms of radiation energy include x-rays, ultraviolet rays from the sun.

Carcinogens • Compounds that have the potential to cause cancer.

Genes • The genetic material on chromosomes that make up DNA. Genes provide the blueprints for the production of cell proteins.

If the cancer is left untreated, it can spread throughout the body. This makes death more likely. For this reason early detection is important. Aids to early detection include the seven warning signals of cancer:
1. a change in bowel or bladder habits
2. a sore that does not heal
3. unusual bleeding or discharge
4. a thickening or lump in the breast or elsewhere
5. indigestion or difficulty in swallowing
6. an obvious change in a wart or mole
7. a nagging cough or hoarseness

There are other ways to detect cancer early. Colon and rectum examinations for adults of both genders and pap tests and regular breast examinations for women are recommended by the American Cancer Society.

Diet and cancer

Besides a generally nutritious diet, other factors related to diet and lifestyle can reduce your risk of cancer (Table 9-4). For example, maintain a desirable body

Anticarcinogens • Compounds that can potentially inhibit the development of cancer.

TABLE 9-4

General dietary recommendations to reduce the risk of cancer*

1. Avoid obesity.
2. Reduce fat intake to 30% of total kcalories.
3. Eat more high-fiber foods, such as fruits, vegetables, and whole-grain cereals.
4. Include foods rich in vitamins A and C in the daily diet.
5. If alcohol is consumed, do not drink excessively.
6. Use moderation when consuming salt-cured, smoked, and nitrite-cured foods.

*The National Cancer Institute (U.S.) endorses all the above but warns not to exceed 35 grams of dietary fiber intake.

The American Cancer Society endorses all the above, but sets no percentage for fat intake.

The Canadian Dietetic Association generally endorses all of the above, but the specific language differs.

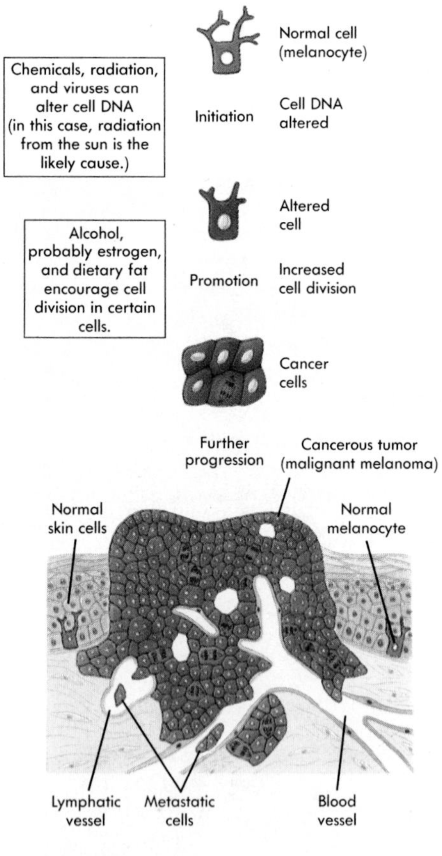

Chemicals, radiation, and viruses can alter cell DNA (in this case, radiation from the sun is the likely cause.)

Alcohol, probably estrogen, and dietary fat encourage cell division in certain cells.

Normal cell (melanocyte)

Initiation — Cell DNA altered

Altered cell

Promotion — Increased cell division

Cancer cells

Further progression — Cancerous tumor (malignant melanoma)

Normal skin cells

Normal melanocyte

Lymphatic vessel

Metastatic cells

Blood vessel

FIGURE 9-12

Progression from a normal skin cell to cancer. The ball of cells is a developing cancer tumor. As the mass of cells grows, it can invade surrounding tissues, eventually penetrating into lymph vessels and blood vessels. These vessels carry spreading (metastatic) cancer cells throughout the body, where they can form new cancer sites.

weight and practice regular physical activity. Both obesity and physical inactivity are linked to increased risk for many types of cancer.

In fact, obesity is related to all major forms of cancer except lung cancer. This includes breast cancer, colon cancer, endometrial cancer, and prostate cancer. The link probably occurs because adipose tissue synthesizes estrogen from other hormones in the bloodstream. High levels of estrogen in the bloodstream promote cancer. Habitual excessive over-eating, especially fatty foods, may also promote cancer. When animals are fed diets high in fat or total kcalories, they tend to experience more cancer, especially in the colon and breast.

The National Cancer Institute believes dietary fat is sufficiently linked to cancer, especially breast cancer, to warrant encouraging Americans to eat less fat. It recommends reducing dietary fat consumption to about 20% of total kcalories. Some nutritionists, however, believe that this agency has overreacted to the fat and cancer issue. Epidemiological evidence relates fat intake to cancer, but the evidence is not strong. The question of how much fat can be eaten while minimizing the risk of cancer is not settled.

Total kcalories eaten actually show an even stronger link to cancer in animals than fat intake. Rats with low kcalorie intake will have about a 40% reduction in tumor yield compared with rats consuming typical intake. The amount of fat in the diet is not important as long as the low kcalorie diet is about 70% of the animal's usual kcalorie intake. An altered hormonal balance probably orchestrates the effect of a lower kcalorie intake.

Can we use this evidence from animals? Americans want to avoid cancer, but very few of us are willing to settle for only 70% of our usual kcalorie intake. While a strong link ties some types of cancer and obesity, this evidence has failed to persuade many of us to slim down to desirable body weights. It is an even bigger task to reduce kcalories to 70% of usual intake. In addition, once cancer is present, kcalorie restriction is no longer helpful. Still, controlling fat intake and balancing energy intake with output is a wise recommendation.

Antioxidants may be anticarcinogens

Many single nutrients are promoted as keys to preventing cancer. They are called *anticarcinogens* (Table 9-5). The most important ones are beta-carotene (plant form of vitamin A), vitamin E, vitamin C, and selenium.[19, 28] All four of these nutrients function as, or contribute to, antioxidant systems in the body. These antioxidant systems help prevent DNA alteration by electron-seeking (oxidizing) substances. Recall that the antioxidant vitamin E also protects unsaturated fatty acids from oxidizing compounds. More research on the potential benefits of antioxidants in terms of cancer prevention is needed. For now, a diet rich in fruits and vegetables should provide enough of these nutrients to gain any possible benefit.

TABLE 9-5

Possible anticarcinogens in foods

Substance	Source	Action
Vitamin A	Liver, fortified milk, fruits and vegetables*	Encourages normal cell division and development
Vitamin E	Whole grains, vegetable oil, and green leafy vegetables	Antioxidant
Vitamin C	Fruits and vegetables	Antioxidant
Selenium	Meats and whole grains	Part of an antioxidant system (see Chapter 10)
Carotenes	Fruits and vegetables	Antioxidant
Indoles, phenols†	Vegetables, especially cabbage, cauliflower, and brussels sprouts	May reduce carcinogen activation
Dietary fibers	Whole grains, fruits, vegetables, and beans	May bind carcinogens in stool, decrease stool transit time
Calcium	Dairy products, green leafy vegetables	Slows cell division in the colon, binds bile acids and free fatty acids

*Fruits and vegetables contain caratones, many of which are converted to vitamin A.
†Chemical substances found in many plants.

Are dietary fiber or calcium anticancer agents?

In Chapters 5 and 6 we mentioned a possible role of fiber in preventing colon cancer. Fiber may do this by decreasing transit time so that the feces is in contact with the colon for a shorter period of time. This would reduce the contact of potential carcinogens with the colon wall. In addition, soluble fibers can bind bile acids. Bile acids are thought to promote cancer by irritating the colon cells, increasing cell division. However, the evidence regarding the importance of fiber in preventing colon cancer is still inconclusive. For now, the recommendation to eat 20 to 35 grams of fiber a day is probably best. Liberal intake of whole grains, fruits, and vegetables should suffice to yield this amount.

Dietary calcium is also linked to a decreased risk for developing colon cancer. As with fiber, the evidence is weak. Some studies show that calcium decreases the growth of colon cells. Therefore it probably decreases the risk of altered cells developing into a cancer. Calcium may also bind fatty acids and bile acids in the colon so they are less apt to interact with cells and cause cancer. We need more research before we can claim that calcium acts as a cancer-preventing agent. Nevertheless, there are many important reasons for consuming the RDA for calcium. We will discuss those in Chapter 10.

A bottom line?

Table 9-4 lists a variety of dietary changes you can make to reduce the risk of cancer. Start by controlling kcalorie and total fat intake and by increasing intake of fruits, vegetables, whole grains, beans, and lowfat dairy products. In other words, follow the Guide to Daily Food Choices. In addition, moderate the use of alcohol. Remember that 35% of all cancer cases are caused by cigarette smoking. Therefore a priority in avoiding cancer is to eliminate tobacco—even smokeless varieties (chewing tobacco). ●

Alcohol is toxic to cells. Resulting cell death creates a need for new cell division. In this way alcohol can increase cell division and therefore cancer risk.

WATER AND MINERALS

Water—the most versatile medium for all kinds of chemical magic—constitutes the major portion of our bodies. Without water, our life processes would cease in a matter of days. We operate on about 2 quarts (2 liters) of water daily, and it should be replenished daily because the body does not store water well. We experience this constant demand for water as thirst.

Because water dissolves many nutrients, it enables minerals and other chemicals to react in the body. Among other uses, it lubricates joints and serves as a vehicle to transport minerals and other substances throughout the body. In addition, water is a key means of controlling body temperature and removing waste products.

Minerals, like water, are vital to health. They are key players in body metabolism, muscle movement, body growth, and water balance, among other wide-ranging processes. Researchers are still defining what minerals the body requires and the quantities needed for good health. Based on the amount we need each day, minerals are categorized as major (requiring> 100 milligrams per day) or trace (requiring ≤ 100 milligrams per day). These categories do not reflect their importance to the body; deficiencies of some trace minerals can cause severe health problems. In this chapter you will see why the study of water and minerals is critical to understanding human nutrition. ●

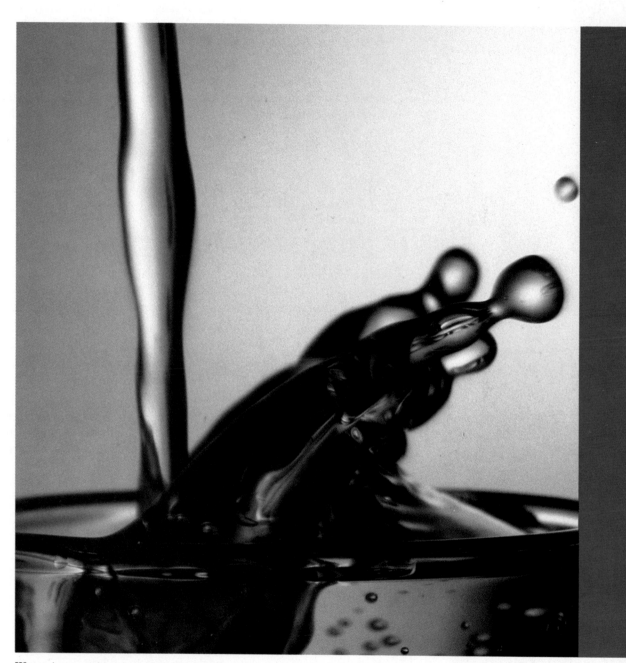

Water is a nutrient in a class by itself.

Working For Denser Bones

In this chapter you will learn important information about the disease, OSTEO-
POROSIS:

> Osteoporosis affects 20 to 25 million people in the United States One third of
> all women experience fractures because of it. It leads to 1.2 million bone
> fractures per year. In addition, 12% to 20% of all elderly people who suffer
> hip fractures die from complications.

This is a disease you can do something about. Some risk factors can't be
changed, but others can. To what degree are you doing the things that can help
prevent this debilitating disease? Answer "yes" or "no" to the following questions by placing an "X" in the appropriate blank:

	YES	NO
1. Do you average at least 30 minutes of sun exposure per day to at least your hands and face to get vitamin D or drink vitamin D–fortified milk regularly?	———	———
2. Do you regularly engage in weight-bearing exercise (jogging, walking, etc.)?	———	———
3. If you are a woman, do you experience regular menstruation?	———	———
4. Do you avoid smoking cigarettes?	———	———
5. Do you avoid regular consumption of large amounts (greater than two drinks) of alcohol?	———	———
6. Do you consume milk and cheese regularly, or substitute other foods to meet your RDA for calcium?	———	———

The more yes answers you have, the more you are actively preserving your
bone density for the future. Also, remember that this is not just a consideration
of women, because if men plan to live well into their 80s and 90s they are at
risk for osteoporosis.

ASSESS YOURSELF

WATER

To appreciate how minerals operate, we need to understand the nature of water and its characteristics. Water is the perfect medium for body processes because it enables chemical reactions to occur. It even participates directly in many of these reactions. Water forms the greatest component of the human body, making up 50% to 60% of its weight. Lean muscle tissue contains about 73% water.[20] Fat tissue is about 20% water. Thus as fat content increases (and the percentage of lean tissue decreases) in the body, total body water content declines toward 50%.

Depending on how much fat has been stored, an adult can survive for about 8 weeks without eating food but only a few days without drinking water. This occurs not because water is more important than carbohydrate, fat, protein, vitamins, or minerals, but rather because we can neither store nor conserve water as well as we can the other components of our diet.

Water in the body—intracellular and extracellular fluid

Water flows in and out of body cells through cell membranes. Water inside cells forms part of the intracellular fluid—that inside cells. When water is outside cells or in the bloodstream, water is part of the extracellular fluids—that outside cells (Figure 10-1). Because cell membranes are permeable to water, water shifts freely in and out of cells. For example, if blood volume decreases, water can move from the areas inside and around cells to the bloodstream to increase blood volume. On the other hand, if blood volume increases, water can shift out of the bloodstream into cells and the surrounding areas.[20]

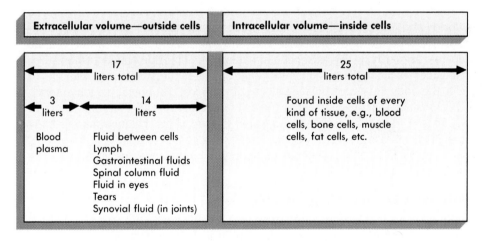

Extracellular volume—outside cells	Intracellular volume—inside cells

17 liters total	25 liters total
3 liters / 14 liters	Found inside cells of every kind of tissue, e.g., blood cells, bone cells, muscle cells, fat cells, etc.
Blood plasma / Fluid between cells, Lymph, Gastrointestinal fluids, Spinal column fluid, Fluid in eyes, Tears, Synovial fluid (in joints)	

FIGURE 10-1

The fluid compartments in the body. These can be broken down into two compartments—intracellular (within cells) and extracellular (outside cells).

The body controls the amount of water in the intracellular and extracellular compartments mainly by controlling ion concentrations. Ions have electrical charges. Water is attracted to ions such as sodium, potassium, chloride, phosphate, magnesium, and calcium. By controlling the movements of ions in and out of the cellular compartments, the body maintains the appropriate amount of water in each compartment. Where ions go, water follows.

Osmosis

Osmosis is the process that regulates and equalizes the proportion of water in cells and the bloodstream. Osmosis operates when fluid ion concentrations differ between compartments that are separated by a semipermeable membrane. In the body, for example, a semipermeable cell membrane separates cells from the fluid spaces (compartments) between cells. The semipermeable membrane

Examples that demonstrate osmosis are sugar pulling fluid from strawberries and a salty salad dressing wilting lettuce.

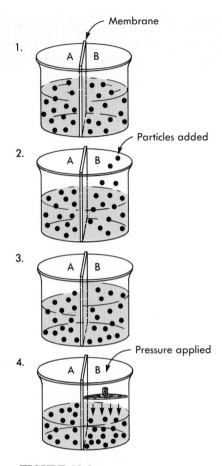

Membrane

1.

Particles added

2.

3.

4.

Pressure applied

FIGURE 10-2

A graphic representation of osmosis and osmotic pressure. *1.* Equal number of particles on both sides allows equal amounts of water. *2.* Now additional particles are added to *side B*, but the particles cannot flow across the membrane. *3.* Water can flow across the membrane, and so it flows to *side B* where there are more particles. The volume of water becomes greater on *side B*, causing the concentrations on *sides A* and *B* to again become equal. *4.* If physical pressure (such as a pump) compressed the fluid on *side B* to restore the original volume, that pressure would equal the osmotic pressure exerted by the added particles.

allows water to pass into cells but controls the flow of ions. If adjoining fluid compartments contain dissimilar concentrations of particles (have different total ion concentrations), it is water that flows through the cell membrane to equalize the particle concentrations in each compartment.

Figure 10-2 illustrates osmosis. Adding particles to the right compartment increases its particle concentration and, in turn, decreases its relative water concentration. This happens in the bloodstream when you eat sodium. Since particles cannot easily pass through the membrane depicted in Figure 10-2, water shifts from the compartment with a low particle concentration (the more diluted compartment) to the more highly concentrated one. To counteract a high sodium concentration in the bloodstream, one body response is to shift fluid from cells into the bloodstream.

Water and ions in the body—a balancing act

Adding water—instead of particles—to a compartment dilutes its particle concentration, and so the compartment tends to donate water to more concentrated compartments nearby. This happens when you drink water. Some of the water absorbed by the body moves from the bloodstream into body cells, which in turn equalizes the particle concentrations in the various body compartments. Therefore, because of the action of osmosis, water is forced to move across membranes to balance changes in particle—or ion—concentrations.[20]

Cells have pumping mechanisms that constantly draw potassium ions into the cell and pump sodium ions out. Other ions are exchanged as well. It is this pumping action, in effect, that leaves cell membranes semipermeable—that is, permeable to water but not to many ions. Ions, such as sodium, may cross into the cell, but the cell quickly pumps them back out.

Positive ions, such as sodium and potassium, pair with negative ions, such as chloride and phosphate. Intracellular water volume depends primarily on intracellular potassium and phosphate concentration. Extracellular water volume depends primarily on the extracellular sodium and chloride concentration.

Besides balancing ion concentrations between the inside and outside of cells, the body must also balance electrical charges.[20] If a negative ion enters a cell, a positive ion also must enter the cell or another negative ion must leave it. In addition, the body carefully regulates hydrogen ion balance among body compartments using a variety of responses. The goal is to maintain the blood's acid-base balance, which depends on hydrogen ion balance, just slightly on the alkaline side (pH 7.35 to 7.45).

Water contributes to temperature regulation

Water changes temperature slowly because it has a great ability to hold heat. It takes much more energy to heat water than it does to heat fat. Compare the time it takes to melt ice cubes with the time it takes to melt frozen butter in a microwave oven. Foods with high water content heat up and cool down slowly. Because water requires so much energy to change states—for example, from a liquid to a gas—it forms an ideal medium for removing heat from the body.

The body secretes fluids in the form of perspiration, which evaporates through skin pores. To evaporate water, heat energy is required. So, as perspiration evaporates, heat energy is taken from the skin, cooling it in the process. Each quart (liter) of perspiration evaporated represents approximately 600 kcalories of energy lost from the skin and surrounding tissues. For this reason, fever increases one's needs for kcalories.

However, to work efficiently, perspiration must be allowed to evaporate. If it simply rolls off the skin or soaks into clothing, perspiration doesn't cool us much. Evaporation of perspiration occurs readily when humidity is low. This is why humans often tolerate hot, dry climates far better than they do hot, humid climates.

Water helps remove waste products

Water is an important vehicle for ridding the body of waste products. Most unusable substances in the body can dissolve in water and leave the body in urine.

A major body waste product is **_urea._** This byproduct of protein metabolism contains nitrogen. The more protein we eat in excess of needs, the more nitrogen we excrete—in the form of urea—in the urine. Likewise, the more sodium we consume, the more sodium we excrete in the urine. Overall, the amount of urine a person produces is determined primarily by excess protein and sodium chloride (salt) intake. By limiting excess protein and sodium intakes it is possible to limit urine output—a useful practice, for example, in space flights. This type of diet is also used to treat some kidney diseases where the ability to produce urine output is hampered.

A typical urine volume is about 1 to 2 liters (1 to 2 quarts) per day, depending mostly on the amount of fluid intake. Somewhat more than that is fine, but less—especially less than 600 milliliters (2½ cups)—forces the kidneys to form a very concentrated urine. The heavy ion concentration increases the risk of kidney stone formation in susceptible people. Kidney stones are simply minerals and other substances that have precipitated out of the urine and accumulated in kidney tissues.

How much water do we need?

Adults need roughly 1 milliliter of water per kcalorie burned.[20] We consume about 1 liter (1 quart) of water a day in various liquids (Figure 10-3). Foods supply another liter of fluid; many fruits, vegetables, and beverages are more than 80% water. Water as a by-product of metabolism provides approximately 350 milliliters (1½ cups) of additional water. This yields a total of about 2.4 liters

> **Urea** • A byproduct of protein metabolism that contains nitrogen.

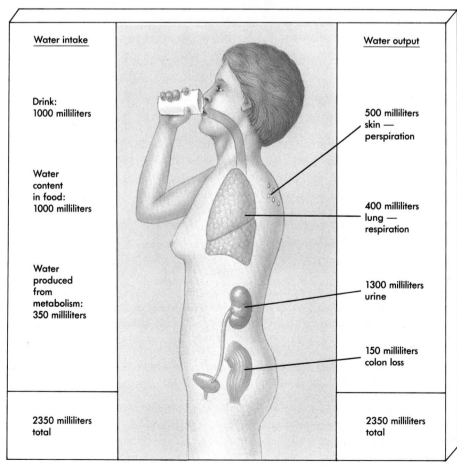

Water intake

Drink:
1000 milliliters

Water content in food:
1000 milliliters

Water produced from metabolism:
350 milliliters

2350 milliliters total

Water output

500 milliliters
skin —
perspiration

400 milliliters
lung —
respiration

1300 milliliters
urine

150 milliliters
colon loss

2350 milliliters total

FIGURE 10-3

Water balance—intake versus output. We maintain body fluids at an optimum level by adjusting water intake and output. Most water comes from the liquids we consume. Some water comes from the moisture in more solid foods, and the remainder is manufactured in metabolism. Water output includes that via lungs, kidneys, skin, and bowels.

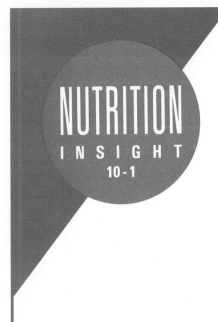

BOTTLED WATER

These days, it is common to see 5-gallon bottles of water being delivered to homes. Grocery store shelves are now stocked with all kinds of bottled waters—over 600 brands in the United States range from simple plastic milk jugs containing "pure spring water" to fancier, imported varieties of mineral water in glass bottles. In Europe bottled water is an institution, as popular as soft drinks are in the United States.

It is quite the fashion to order a bottle of Evian at a restaurant or bar. People are concerned not only with alternatives to alcoholic beverages and soft drinks, but also with the perceived health value or taste of bottled water. The bottled water industry does more than $2 billion a year in business.

Bottled waters vary, depending on the source, use, mineral content, and carbonation. All bottled waters must list the source of the water on the label. This can include wells, spas, springs, geysers, and quite often, the public water supply. Some bottled water companies add minerals such as calcium, magnesium, and potassium to give water a better taste. But the term *mineral water* is misleading because all water (except distilled and specially purified water) contains minerals. When carbon dioxide gas is present in the water source, it results in carbonation. Bottled waters from such sources are said to be *naturally sparkling*. Other carbonated waters have had carbon dioxide added during bottling.

Many people choose bottled water over tap water because they doubt the safety of public drinking water. The Environmental Protection Agency (EPA) is responsible for tap water quality. Under the Safe Water Drinking Act, all public drinking water supplies are monitored for contaminants, such as bacteria, various chemicals, and some toxic metals (such as lead and mercury). Some bottled water meets these same standards, but not all. FDA and private inspections of these products are less frequent than tests done on municipal utilities.

Insensible • In this case, not consciously noted by the person, such as water lost with each breath.

Antidiuretic Hormone (ADH) • A hormone secreted by the pituitary gland that acts on the kidneys to cause a decrease in water excretion.

(10 cups) of water for a 2400 kcalorie diet, or about 1 milliliter per kcalorie burned.

Of the 2.4 liters of water needed, about 1.4 liters is used to produce urine. The rest, about 1 liter, compensates for typical water losses through the lungs (400 milliliters), feces (150 milliliters), and skin (500 milliliters) (Figure 10-3). We are not normally aware of these *insensible* water losses. Note also that when we consider the large amount of water used to lubricate the gastrointestinal (GI) tract, the loss of only 150 milliliters of water a day through the feces is remarkable. About 8000 milliliters of water enter the GI tract daily via secretions from the mouth, stomach, intestine, pancreas, and other organs. Diet supplies an additional 2000 milliliters. The kidneys also conserve water by reabsorbing 97% of the water filtered from waste products.[20]

Too much water—whatever amount the kidneys are unable to excrete—can be toxic, but an excessive amount would have to approach many quarts (liters) each day. Most people have little risk of drinking too much water, but problems do accompany some disease states and mental disorders. When excessive water overwhelms the kidneys' capacity to excrete, blurred vision is one resulting symptom.

Thirst

If you don't drink enough water and total body water falls by 1% to 2%, your body often lets you know by signaling thirst. Your brain is communicating to

Water can be classified by whether it is hard or soft. Hard water generally comes from underground wells and characteristically contains calcium, magnesium, and iron. The harder the water the more minerals it contains. Soft water has a low content of these minerals and is often produced by replacing other minerals with sodium. The mineral content of hard water interacts with soap and detergents, inhibiting the chemical reactions that cause a soap lather to form. You know your water supply is hard if you must use a lot of soap to produce a good lather.

A recent EPA poll showed that 21 out of 50 bottlers surveyed revealed their source as the public water supply. This information, available on the label, indicates that many times bottled water is from the same source as the tap water found in many homes. On the other hand, bottled waters derived from springs and wells may lack potentially helpful minerals that many communities have in their drinking water (like fluoride, magnesium, and calcium) and also may be vulnerable to the same groundwater contamination as the public supply. Sometimes bottled water is simply filtered, and minerals are either removed or added for taste.

Keep in mind that, by most standards, bottled water ranges from moderately expensive to expensive. In many cases you are paying for water that is not much different from tap water. If you are concerned about the safety of your tap water, have it tested. A local testing laboratory or local health department can be of service. Compared to the cost of bottle water, the testing fee will be insignificant. ●

A recall in 1990 of Perrier water because of contamination of the water with benzene, a potentially cancer-producing chemical, has caused concern about the safety of bottled water. The source of the benzene was found and removed. The water is now safe.

you the need to drink. This thirst mechanism is not always reliable, however, especially during illness, in elderly years, and during vigorous exercise, such as in athletic events.[24] Athletes should weigh themselves before and after training sessions to determine their rate of water loss and thus their water needs. Two cups ($\frac{1}{2}$ liter) of water weighs about a pound (about half a kilogram) (see Chapter 12 for details on fluid use in athletics). Ailing children—especially those with fever, vomiting, diarrhea, and increased perspiration—and the elderly often need to be reminded to drink plenty of fluids. Long airplane flights are other situations that demand extra fluid intake: a traveler can lose about 6 cups (1.5 liters) of water during a 3-hour flight. The dehumidified air in an airplane is so dry that it induces excessive *insensible* perspiration and evaporation.

What if the thirst message is ignored?

Once the body registers a shortage of available water, it also increases fluid conservation. The pituitary gland releases ***antidiuretic hormone (ADH)*** to force the kidneys to conserve water. The kidneys respond by reducing urine flow. As fluid volume decreases in the bloodstream, blood pressure falls. This eventually signals the kidneys to retain more sodium and, in turn, more water.

However, despite mechanisms that work to conserve water, fluid is constantly lost via the *insensible* routes—feces, skin, and lungs. Those losses must be replaced. In addition, there is a limit to how concentrated urine can become. Eventually, if fluid is not consumed, the body becomes dehydrated and suffers ill effects.

Again, by the time a person loses 1% to 2% of body weight in fluids, he or she will be thirsty. At a 4% loss of body weight, muscles lose significant strength

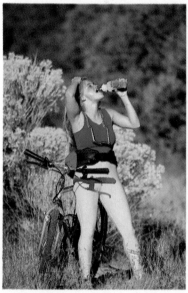

Water cools the body in more than one way—this includes perspiration.

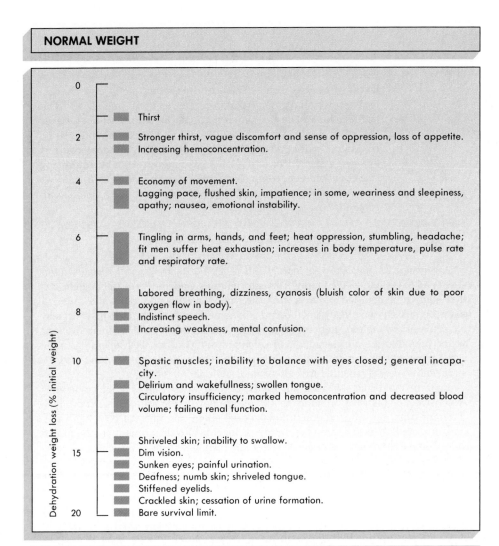

NORMAL WEIGHT

0	
	Thirst
2	Stronger thirst, vague discomfort and sense of oppression, loss of appetite. Increasing hemoconcentration.
4	Economy of movement. Lagging pace, flushed skin, impatience; in some, weariness and sleepiness, apathy; nausea, emotional instability.
6	Tingling in arms, hands, and feet; heat oppression, stumbling, headache; fit men suffer heat exhaustion; increases in body temperature, pulse rate and respiratory rate.
8	Labored breathing, dizziness, cyanosis (bluish color of skin due to poor oxygen flow in body). Indistinct speech. Increasing weakness, mental confusion.
10	Spastic muscles; inability to balance with eyes closed; general incapacity. Delirium and wakefullness; swollen tongue. Circulatory insufficiency; marked hemoconcentration and decreased blood volume; failing renal function.
15	Shriveled skin; inability to swallow. Dim vision. Sunken eyes; painful urination. Deafness; numb skin; shriveled tongue. Stiffened eyelids. Crackled skin; cessation of urine formation.
20	Bare survival limit.

Dehydration weight loss (% initial weight)

DEATH

FIGURE 10-4

The effects of dehydration. These range from thirst, as weight initially falls, to death.

Alcohol inhibits the action of antidiuretic hormone (ADH). One reason people feel so bad the day after heavy drinking is that they are very dehydrated. Even though they may have consumed a lot of liquid in their drinks, they have excreted even more liquid because alcohol has inhibited ADH.

and endurance. By the time body weight is reduced by 10% to 12%, heat tolerance is decreased and weakness results.[20] At a 20% reduction, coma and death may soon follow (Figure 10-4).

CONCEPT CHECK

Since the body can neither readily store nor entirely conserve water, we can survive only a few days without it. Water functions to dissolve substances, is a medium for chemical reactions, aids in temperature regulation, and is a lubricant. Water constitutes 50% to 70% of body weight and distributes itself all over the body: among lean and other tissues in both intracellular and extracellular fluids and in urine and other body fluids. Adults need about 1 milliliter of water for each kcalorie burned. Thirst is the body's first sign of dehydration. If this thirst mechanism is faulty, as it may be during illness or vigorous exercise, hormonal mechanisms also help conserve water by reducing urine output.

MINERALS

The metabolic roles of minerals vary considerably. Some minerals, such as copper and selenium, work as cofactors, which by definition enable enzymes to function. Minerals also contribute to important body compounds. For example, iodine is a component of the hormone thyroxine that comes from the thyroid gland. Iron is a component of hemoglobin in red blood cells. Sodium, potassium, and calcium aid in the transfer of nerve impulses throughout the body. Calcium is a key participant in muscle contraction. Body growth and development (i.e., bony skeleton) also depend on certain minerals, such as calcium and phosphorus. Water balance requires sodium, potassium, calcium, and phosphorus. At all levels—cellular, tissue, organ, and whole body—minerals clearly play important roles in maintaining body functions.

> **Bioavailability** • The degree to which the amount of an ingested nutrient is absorbed, and so available to the body.

Mineral bioavailability

Although foods contain and supply us with many minerals, our bodies vary in their capabilities to absorb and use available minerals. While minerals may be present in foods, they are not *bioavailable* unless a body can absorb them. The ability to absorb minerals from a diet depends on many factors.[5] A number listed in a food composition table for the amount of a mineral in a food is just a starting point for estimating the true contribution a food makes to our mineral needs. Spinach is a good example. It contains plenty of calcium, but only about 5% of it can be absorbed because of the vegetable's high concentration of oxalic acid, a calcium-binder.[11] Usually, about 20% to 40% of calcium is absorbed from foods by adults, with the higher figures coming from dairy products.

Minerals in the American diet come from both plant and animal sources. Overall, minerals from animal products are absorbed better because binders and dietary fiber (as we soon will discuss) are not issues. The mineral content of plants depends on mineral concentration in the soil. Animals, however, may consume foods from multiple soil conditions and eat a variety of plant products because they are often shipped across country during their growth, processing, and finishing in a feed lot. So soil conditions have less of an influence.

Generally the more refined a food—as in the case of white flour—the lower its content of minerals. The enrichment process adds only the mineral iron. The selenium, zinc, copper, and other minerals lost when grains are refined are not replaced.

Fiber-mineral interactions

Mineral bioavailability can be greatly affected by nonmineral substances in the diet. Components of fiber, especially phytic acid (phytate) in grain fiber, can greatly limit absorption of some minerals by binding to them.[5] Oxalic acid, mentioned before, is another substance found in plants that binds minerals and makes them less available to the body. High-fiber diets can decrease the absorption of iron, zinc, magnesium, and probably other minerals. An intake above the recommendation of 20 to 35 grams of dietary fiber per day can cause problems.

If grains are leavened with yeast, as they are in bread, enzymes produced by the yeast can break some of the bonds between phytic acid and minerals. This increases mineral absorption. The zinc deficiencies found among some Middle Eastern populations are attributed partly to low bioavailability of dietary zinc and partly to their consumption of unleavened breads. We discuss this in detail in a later section.

Mineral-mineral interactions

Many minerals are of similar sizes and chemical charges, such as magnesium, calcium, iron, and copper. Having similar sizes and the same chemical charge

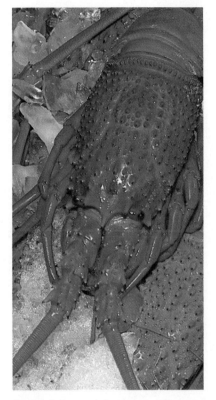

Seafood is a rich source of many trace minerals.

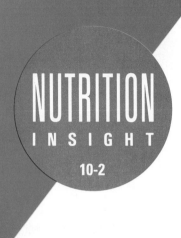

MINERAL TOXICITY

Minerals can be quite toxic, especially the trace minerals (see Tables 10-4 and 10-6). Toxicity is yet another reason to carefully consider the use of mineral supplements. Every year people poison themselves using mineral supplements, even though their intent is to maximize health. Many trace minerals are quite toxic at doses not much above the RDA or ESADDI. Mineral supplements exceeding 150% (1.5 times) of nutrient recommendations should be taken only under a physician's supervision since toxicity and nutrient interactions are possible. The trace minerals most likely to cause toxicity are discussed below.

Iron

Although iron deficiency is a common problem, an overabundance of iron can also be a serious problem. Even a large single dose of iron can be life-threatening. Iron pills and vitamin supplements that contain iron commonly poison children. Smaller doses (but still greater than what is needed) over a long period can also cause problems. A form of iron toxicity has been observed in an African tribe that brews beer in iron pots and in people of Mediterranean decent who often show a certain type of anemia.

In America, iron toxicity accompanies a genetic disease called **hemochromatosis.** People with this disorder over-absorb iron, and over a period of time the amount of iron in their bodies builds up to high levels, especially in the bloodstream and liver. If not treated, excess iron is deposited in inappropriate tissues, contributing to severe liver and heart damage. About 1 in 300 adults may have hemochromatosis.[7]

Many people with hemochromatosis are probably saved from experiencing serious effects of the disease because they consume such a low amount of iron. For many years some nutrition interest groups have recommended increasing iron enrichment in grain products to decrease the presence of iron-deficiency anemia. However, for people with hemochromatosis, that would probably increase the numbers who actually develop disease symptoms. How could we balance the interests of both groups?

Zinc

A high intake of zinc interferes with iron and copper absorption.[8] Over-supplementation with zinc can cause a copper deficiency. One study has shown that zinc supplements at approximately three to five times the RDA can reduce HDL—the good—cholesterol levels by about 15%.[3] This is disturbing for two reasons. First, you know low HDL-cholesterol levels are associated with an increased risk of developing heart disease. Second, it is common for people who take zinc supplements to consume this amount. So some adults, by unwittingly lowering their HDL-cholesterol levels, may be increasing their risk for developing heart disease—even though they think that supplementing zinc in the diet contributes to overall health.

causes these minerals to compete with each other for absorption, and so they affect each other's bioavailability.[5] We caution people against taking individual mineral supplements, unless a medical condition specifically warrants it. This is because an excess of one mineral influences the absorption and metabolism of other minerals. For example, the presence of a large amount of zinc in the diet decreases copper absorption. Calcium supplements can interfere with magnesium and iron absorption.

Vitamin-mineral interactions

Vitamin C improves iron absorption when the two are consumed together.[15] The active vitamin D hormone improves calcium absorption. In addition, many vitamins require minerals to enable them to perform their metabolic roles. For example, thiamin requires magnesium to function efficiently.

Again, this shows why mineral supplements should not be consumed except under a physician's supervision. Otherwise, more harm than good may result. Zinc intakes of over 2 grams daily also result in diarrhea, cramps, nausea, vomiting, and sometimes depression of immune system function.

Copper

Copper tends to cause vomiting at single doses greater than 10 to 30 milligrams.[12] When copper is used to treat a deficiency, it must be given in divided doses to limit this effect. An inherited condition called Wilson's disease results in accumulation of copper in the liver, brain, kidneys, and cornea of the eye. If recognized early, treatment that binds copper in the bloodstream and increases its excretion in the urine can prevent damage to these tissues and reduce the mental degeneration commonly seen in active cases.

Selenium

Selenium at daily intakes as low as 2 to 3 milligrams (35 times the RDA) can cause toxicity symptoms if taken for many months. These symptoms include a garlicky breath odor, hair loss, nausea and vomiting, and a general weakness. Rashes and cirrhosis of the liver may also develop. Selenium clearly illustrates the saying: "It's the dose that makes the poison."

Iodine

Reports in scientific literature raise concern about high iodide (the ion form of iodine) intake. Levels up to 1 milligram (6.6 times the RDA) per day appear to be safe.[19] However, when very high amounts of iodide are consumed, thyroid gland function is hampered. This can occur in people who eat a lot of seaweed, since some seaweeds contain much iodide; total iodide intake then can add up to 60 to 130 times the RDA.

Fluoride

A fluoride intake greater than 6 milligrams daily can *mottle* (stain) teeth during their development. High-fluoride intake in adults does not cause mottling. When fluoride intakes reach 20 milligrams daily during tooth development, the tooth structure is weakened and can crumble. This is called fluorosis and appears in humans and other animals. High doses of fluoride (20 or more milligrams per day) can also cause other side effects, such as stomach upset and bone pain.

The Guide to Daily Food Choices provides the most reliable food plan for meeting mineral needs. Supplemental intakes exceeding 150% (1.5 times) of recommendations are not in your best interest unless a medical condition warrants such therapy. ●

CONCEPT CHECK

Minerals are vital to the functioning of many body processes. Their bioavailability depends on many factors, including a mineral's interaction with fiber and other minerals. Animal products often yield better mineral absorption than plants. Still, both animal and plant sources help us meet our mineral needs. Taking an individual mineral supplement can greatly diminish the absorption and metabolism of other minerals. In addition, some minerals are potentially toxic. These are two good reasons to consider carefully any use of mineral supplements.

For your information, the chemical symbols for the minerals we discuss are given next to each mineral heading.

MAJOR MINERALS

We have discussed some general characteristics of minerals and how some of them interact with water in the body. Now let us review the individual properties of the *major minerals* in the context of the American diet. Recall that these are the minerals we need in excess of 100 milligrams each day (Figure 10-5).

Sodium (Na)

We both crave and fear sodium and its primary dietary source, table salt. Some of this fear is warranted, and some is not.

Functions of sodium. Almost all dietary sodium is absorbed. It then becomes the major positive ion in extracellular fluid and a key factor for retaining body water. Fluid balance throughout the body depends partly on varied sodium concentrations among the water-containing compartments in the body. Sodium ions also function in nerve impulse conduction.

A low-sodium diet, coupled with high perspiration losses, persistent vomiting, or diarrhea, can deplete the body of sodium. This state can lead to muscle cramps, nausea, vomiting, dizziness, and later to shock and coma.[20] Early kidney responses to a low sodium status, however, eventually trigger the body to conserve sodium. Thus even in cases of high rates of perspiration, sodium depletion in the body is unlikely.

Note that although perspiration tastes salty on the skin, sodium is not highly concentrated in perspiration. Rather, water evaporating from the skin leaves concentrated sodium behind. Perspiration contains about two-thirds the sodium concentration found in blood.

Sodium in foods and the minimum requirement for health. About one-third to one-half the sodium we consume is added during cooking or at the table.

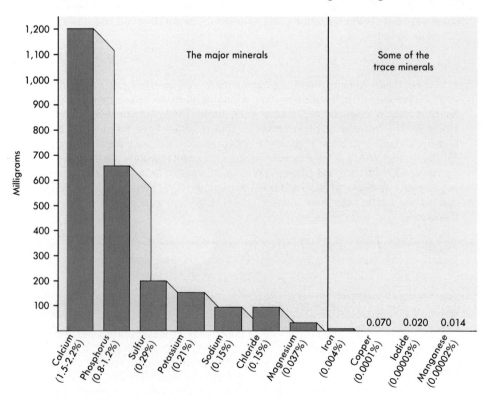

FIGURE 10-5

A list of minerals found in a 130-pound (60-kilogram) person. The percent figures represent percent of body weight. Other trace minerals of nutritional importance include chromium, fluoride, molybdenum, selenium, and zinc.

Most of the rest is added during food manufacturing. Almost all foods naturally contain little sodium; milk is one exception. The more home cooking one does, the more sodium control one has. Major contributors of sodium in the adult diet are white bread and rolls, hot dogs and lunch meats, cheese, soups, and spaghetti with tomato sauce, partly because these foods are eaten so often.[18] Other foods especially high in sodium are tomato-based products in general, salted snack foods, French fries and potato chips, and sauces and gravies. Many condiments also contain large amounts of sodium.

If we ate only unprocessed foods and added no salt, sodium intake would be about 500 milligrams per day. This is also the minimum sodium requirement for health in adults set by the current RDA. (See the inside cover for references to mineral needs for other age groups and Appendix C for Canadian recommendations.) Even this is a generous amount considering that we really need only about 100 milligrams.

If we compare 500 milligrams of sodium to the 3000 to 7000 milligrams typically eaten by adults, it is clear that food processing and cooking contributes most of our dietary sodium. As we discussed in Chapter 2, nutrition labels list a food's sodium content. When dietary sodium must be severely restricted, these labels become very helpful. In that case even contributions from tap water (especially from softened water), as well as medicines that contain sodium, must be considered.

Most humans can adapt to various dietary salt levels, though very high intakes can be toxic.[20] For most people who eat a typical diet, today's sodium intake is simply tomorrow's urine output. However, approximately 10% to 15% of adults are sodium sensitive. For these people, high sodium intakes contribute to hypertension, and lower sodium diets (about 2 grams daily) often correct their hypertension (see the Nutrition Issue, p. 332). Scientific groups suggest that all adults reduce intake to 2.4 to 3 grams, mostly to limit the risk of later hypertension (Figure 10-6). Table 10-1 helps you to examine your sodium habits.

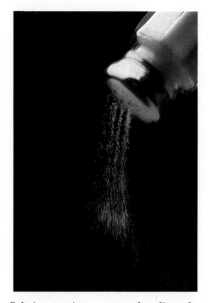

Salt is a major source of sodium for most of us.

Table salt is 40% sodium and 60% chloride. So the range of intake seen in adults of 3 to 7 grams of sodium per day translates to 7.5 to 18 grams of salt. A teaspoon of salt contains about 2 grams of sodium (2000 milligrams).

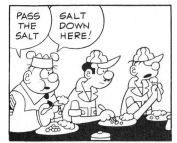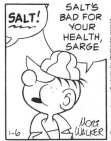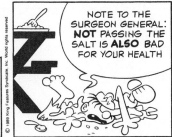

FIGURE 10-6

It is a good idea to have your blood pressure checked regularly. If you have hypertension, you should try to reduce your sodium intake and to determine what effect this can have. If you don't have hypertension, you might still consider slowly reducing your intake to build good habits for the future. If your daily sodium intake is already in the range of less than 3 grams, you are doing well.

Lowering your sodium intake. If you choose to lower your sodium intake, you can eventually adapt to a low-sodium diet. At first foods will taste quite bland, but eventually you will perceive more flavor as the tongue's salt receptors are triggered by less salt. By slowly reducing dietary sodium and substituting garlic, oregano, lemon juice, and other herbs and spices, you can eventually consume a diet that has only about 3 grams of sodium daily without sacrificing much flavor. Many new cookbooks offer excellent recipes for flavorful foods. Except for yeast breads, omitting salt from food preparation can still yield excellent products.

CONCEPT CHECK

Sodium is the major positive ion of the extracellular fluid. It is important for maintaining fluid balance and conducting nerve impulses. Sodium depletion is unlikely since the American diet has abundant sources and most sodium consumed is absorbed. The more foods we prepare at home, the more control we have over our sodium intakes. The minimum sodium requirement for health for adults is 500 milligrams per day. The average adult consumes 3000 to 7000 milligrams daily. About 10% to 15% of the population is sensitive to sodium. In these people hypertension can develop as a result of high-sodium diets. Scientific groups suggest that for all adults sodium intake should be limited to 2 to 3 grams per day.

Potassium (K)

Potassium performs many of the same functions as sodium, such as fluid balance and nerve impulse transmission. However, it operates inside of rather than outside of cells.[20] Intracellular fluids—those inside cells—contain 95% of the potassium in the body. Also, unlike sodium, potassium is associated with lower rather than higher blood pressure values.[13] We absorb about 90% of the potassium we eat.

TABLE 10-1

Examining your sodium habits

Examine how the foods you eat and the way you prepare and serve them affect the amount of sodium in your diet.

How often do you:	Less than once per week	1 or 2 times per week	3 to 5 times per week	Almost daily
1. Eat cured or processed meats, such as ham, bacon, sausage, frankfurters, and other luncheon meats?	☐	☐	☐	☐
2. Choose canned or frozen vegetables with sauce?	☐	☐	☐	☐
3. Use commercially prepared meals, main dishes, or canned or dehydrated soups?	☐	☐	☐	☐
4. Eat cheese?	☐	☐	☐	☐
5. Eat salted nuts, popcorn, pretzels, corn chips, and potato chips?	☐	☐	☐	☐
6. Add salt to cooking water for vegetables, rice, or pasta?	☐	☐	☐	☐
7. Add salt, seasoning mixes, salad dressings, or condiments, such as soy sauce, steak sauce, catsup, and mustard to foods during preparation or at the table?	☐	☐	☐	☐
8. Salt your food before tasting it?	☐	☐	☐	☐

The more checks you have in the last two columns, the higher your dietary sodium intake. However, not all of the items listed contribute the same amount of sodium. For example, many natural cheeses are relatively low in sodium. Most process cheeses and cottage cheese are higher.

To cut back on sodium intake, you can start by eating some items less often, particularly those you checked as "3 to 5 times a week" or more. This does not mean eliminating foods from your diet. You can moderate your sodium intake by choosing lower sodium foods from each food group more often and by balancing high-sodium foods with low-sodium ones. For example, if you serve ham for dinner, plan to serve it with fresh or plain frozen vegetables cooked without added salt, or use less salt when preparing other foods in the meal. Salt used in food preparation contributes greatly to sodium intake.

From USDA Home and Garden Bulletin No. 232-6, April 1986.

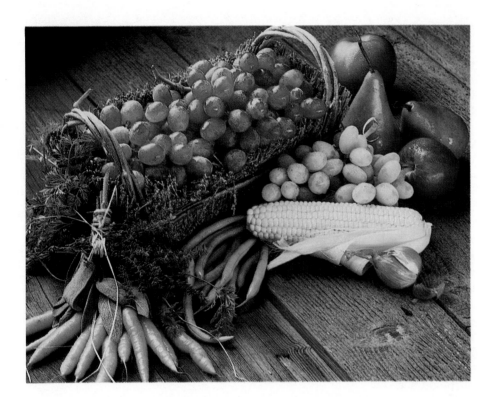

Many fruits and vegetables are high in potassium and low in sodium. This makes them an ideal food choice for people with hypertenison, as well as for all of us.

Results of a potassium deficiency. A low blood potassium level is a life-threatening problem. Symptoms often include a loss of appetite, muscle cramps, confusion and apathy, and constipation. Eventually, the heart beats irregularly, decreasing its capacity to pump blood.[20]

Potassium in foods and the minimum requirement for health. Generally, fruits and vegetables are nutrient-dense sources of potassium. Milk, whole grains, dried beans, and meats are also good sources. Major contributors of potassium to the adult diet include coffee, tea, milk, potatoes, orange juice, and animal products.[18] cola

The adult minimum potassium requirement for health set by the current RDA is 2000 milligrams (2 grams) per day. A typical adult's diet supplies enough potassium if a variety of foods is eaten. Americans average 2 to 3 grams per day, with women consuming amounts nearer the lower intake level.[18] If kidneys function normally, typical intakes of dietary potassium are not toxic; otherwise, high amounts in the body can lead to heart failure.

Bodies are more likely to be deficient in potassium than sodium because we generally do not add potassium to foods. Some *diuretics,* such as thiazides and furosemide, deplete body potassium. Water is excreted along with the potassium, in turn reducing blood volume and pressure. People who take such potassium-wasting diuretics need to monitor their potassium intakes carefully. High-potassium foods, such as fruits, fruit juices, and vegetables, are good additions to their diet, and perhaps potassium chloride supplements, if recommended by a physician.

A continual poor food intake, as may be the case in alcoholism, can also result in potassium deficiency. People with anorexia nervosa and bulimia, whose diets are poor and whose bodies are nutrient depleted from vomiting, are also at risk for potassium deficiency (see Chapter 13). In addition, people on very low calorie diets are at risk (see Chapter 11). All these people can compensate for potentially low body potassium levels by consuming potassium-rich food sources.

Tetany • A body condition marked by sharp contraction of muscles and failure to relax afterward; usually caused by abnormal calcium metabolism.

Chloride (Cl)

Chlorine is a very poisonous gas. Public water utilities often rely on it to kill bacteria in water supplies. Consequently many water-borne diseases are rare in America. In our bodies chloride, an ion form of chlorine, forms an important negative ion for the extracellular fluid. These ions are a component of the hydrochloric acid produced in the stomach and are also used during immune responses as white blood cells attack foreign cells. In addition, nerve function relies on the presence of chloride.[20] As is the case with sodium, most of the body's chloride is excreted by the kidneys; some is lost in perspiration.

A chloride deficiency is unlikely because our dietary sodium chloride (salt) intake is so high. Frequent and lengthy bouts of vomiting, if coupled with a nutrient-poor diet, can contribute to a deficiency because stomach secretions contain much chloride. From 1978 to 1979, insufficient chloride added to a brand of infant formula caused severe convulsions and other health problems in the infants who consumed it. This incident shows what can happen when the need for a nutrient normally abundant in our diets is not given adequate attention.

Chloride in foods and minimum requirement for health. A few fruits and some vegetables are naturally good sources of chloride. Chlorinated water also is a source. However, we consume most chloride as salt added to foods. If we know a food's salt content, we can predict closely its chloride content; salt is 60% chloride. Naturally occurring sodium or chloride won't significantly affect the prediction.

The minimum chloride requirement for health in adults set by the current RDA is 700 milligrams per day. Assuming that the average adult consumes at least 7.5 grams of salt daily, that yields 4.5 grams (4500 milligrams) of chloride, an abundance of this ion.

CONCEPT CHECK

Potassium performs functions similar to those of sodium, except that it is the main positive ion found inside, not outside, cells. Potassium is vital to fluid balance and nerve transmission. A potassium deficiency caused by poor intake, persistent vomiting, or use of some diuretics can lead to loss of appetite, muscle cramps, confusion, and heartbeat irregularities. Fruits and vegetables are generally rich sources of potassium. Potassium intake can be toxic if a person's kidneys do not function properly. Chloride is the major negative ion of extracellular fluid. Chloride also functions in digestion as part of hydrochloric acid and in immune and nervous system responses. Deficiencies of chloride are unlikely because we eat so much sodium chloride (salt).

Calcium (Ca)

All cells need calcium, but over 99% of the calcium in the body is used to strengthen bones and teeth. This calcium represents 40% of all the minerals present in the body and equals about 2½ pounds (1200 grams). As calcium circulates in the bloodstream, it supplies the calcium needs of all body cells. Growth and bone development in laboratory animals is closely tied to calcium intake. This link is seen in humans, too, but is not as strong.[1]

Functions of calcium. Forming and maintaining bones are calcium's major roles in the body, but it is important in many other processes as well. Calcium is essential for blood clotting and for muscle contraction. If the blood calcium level falls below a critical point, muscles cannot relax after contraction; the body stiffens and shows signs of *tetany.* In normal nerve transmission calcium works to release chemical messengers and permits the flow of ions in and out of nerve cells. Without sufficient calcium, nerve transmission fails, opening another path to tetany. Finally, calcium helps regulate cellular metabolism by influencing various enzyme activities and hormonal responses. It is the hormonal regulation of blood calcium levels that keep all these processes going even if you fail to eat enough calcium on a day-to-day basis.

Absorption of calcium. Calcium requires an acid environment to be absorbed efficiently.[5] Absorption occurs primarily in the upper part of the small intestine. The area tends to remain acidic because it receives the acidic stomach contents, which are eventually neutralized by fluids released from the pancreas. Calcium absorption in the upper small intestine depends on the active vitamin D hormone.

We absorb about 20% to 40% of the calcium in the foods we eat, but during times when the body needs extra calcium, such as in infancy and pregnancy, absorption might reach as high as 50% to 75%. Young people tend to absorb calcium better than do older people. Postmenopausal women generally absorb the least calcium, unless they receive supplements of the hormone estrogen. Estrogen therapy increases synthesis of the active vitamin D hormone, which aids calcium absorption (Table 10-2).[28]

Many factors end up enhancing calcium absorption: the acidic environment of the small intestine and the presence of the active vitamin D hormone, mentioned above; parathyroid hormone, dietary glucose, and lactose; and normal intestinal motility (flow). Factors limiting calcium absorption include large amounts of phytic acid in dietary fiber from grains; great excess of magnesium or phosphorus in the diet, and tannins in tea; a vitamin D deficiency; menopause; diarrhea; and old age.

One problem in setting an RDA for calcium is predicting how much calcium will be absorbed by the body. The RDA is based on an estimated 30% to 40% total calcium absorption. But calcium absorption efficiency varies among people. Those who absorb calcium less efficiently will need to consume more.

Because we have excellent hormonal systems to control blood calcium levels, a normal blood calcium level can be maintained despite poor calcium intake. The bones, however, pay the price. Bone loss caused by insufficient calcium intake proceeds slowly. Only after many years are clinical symptoms apparent. By not meeting the RDA for calcium, some people, especially women, are most likely setting the stage for future bone fractures.[28] However, because we don't know how efficiently each individual absorbs calcium, we often cannot predict who is at the highest risk.

TABLE 10-2

Absorption of calcium from the intestinal tract

Factors favoring absorption	Factors hindering absorption
Acid nature of upper intestinal tract	Alkaline state in lower intestinal tract
Normal digestive activity and motility of intestinal tract	Large amounts of dietary fiber
Dietary calcium and phosphorus in about equal amounts	Laxatives or any circumstances that cause diarrhea or rapid flow of the intestine
Vitamin D	*Great* excess of phosphorus or magnesium in proportion to calcium
Need for higher amounts by the body, as during pregnancy	Phytic acid, oxalic acid, and unabsorbed fatty acids: they all bind calcium in the intestine
Low calcium intake	Vitamin D deficiency
Parathyroid hormone (increases active vitamin D synthesis)	Menopause
Lactose	Old age
Glucose	Tannins in tea

Osteopenia • Decreased bone mass caused by cancer, hyperthyroidism, or other reasons.

Osteoporosis • Decreased bone mass where no outward cause can be found. Related to effects of aging, poor diet, and hormonal effects of menopause in women.

Osteoporosis. If bone mass is not maintained sufficiently, **osteopenia** (meaning little bone) eventually results. There are many contributors to bone loss, including osteomalacia, a condition where bones are poorly calcified (see Chapter 9), the use of certain medications, and cancer tumors. If all these causes of bone loss are ruled out, the diagnosis is **osteoporosis.** Osteoporosis is further classified as Type I (postmenopausal), which appears in the years right after menopause, and Type II (senile), which is found in people of advanced ages.[28] A long-standing poor calcium intake can contribute to both forms.

Bone composition in osteoporosis is essentially normal; basically there is just less bone mass throughout the body. Because the bones are not as dense as normal bones, osteoporosis can lead to a decrease in height, hip fractures in old age, and eventual loss of teeth (Figure 10-7).

Other possible benefits of calcium in the diet. Besides contributing to bone strength, dietary calcium may reduce the risk of colon cancer.[26] It appears that abundant calcium in the feces binds with the fats and bile acids there. These compounds, when free, tend to irritate the colon. Such irritation may increase cell turnover there, increasing the risk of cancer (see Chapter 9).

Another possible benefit of dietary calcium may be its effect on blood pressure. Consuming the RDA for calcium compared to much lower amounts can slightly decrease blood pressure (see the Nutrition Issue, p. 332).

Both these areas of calcium research—colon cancer and high blood pressure—are new. Practical dietary recommendations stemming from this research, aside from meeting the RDA for calcium, are not yet established.

Calcium in foods. Dairy products, such as milk, yogurt, and cheese, provide most of the calcium in the adult diet. Cottage cheese is an exception because most of its calcium is lost in production. White bread, rolls, crackers, and other

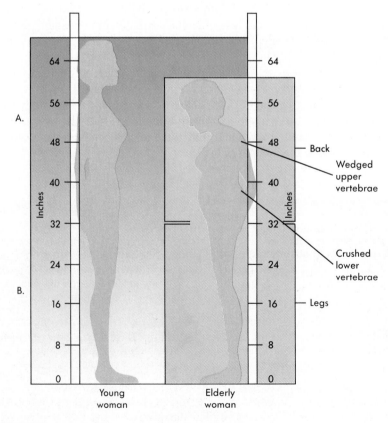

FIGURE 10-7

A loss of height and misshapen body are common results of osteoporosis. Monitor your adult height changes to detect early osteoporosis.

foods made with milk products are also contributors. Although green leafy vegetables are the most nutrient-dense calcium sources, their oxalic acid content prevents much of their calcium from being absorbed. Nonfat milk then provides the best overall source of calcium because of its high bioavailability. The new calcium-fortified versions of orange juice are close competitors. In addition, new high-calcium milks increase the calcium to kcalorie ratio for nonfat and lowfat dairy products even more. Soybean curd (tofu) is also a good source of calcium if it is made with calcium carbonate (check the label).

One reason the Guide to Daily Food Choices contains a milk, yogurt, and cheese group is to supply calcium to the diet. In addition, this group provides protein, vitamin A, vitamin D, riboflavin, potassium, and magnesium. People who do not like milk can use products made with milk, such as chocolate milk, yogurt, cheese, and ice cream. All forms of milk, yogurt, and cheese allow about the same degree of calcium absorption.[22] However, we hesitate to recommend either cheese or ice cream because they are usually high in saturated fat. Some lowfat cheeses and frozen desserts, such as yogurt and ice milks, are good calcium sources and have a low saturated-fat content. Bones found in canned fish, such as salmon and sardines, also supply calcium.

The target for calcium intake for most adults is 800 milligrams a day—for college-age students (to 25 years of age) the target is 1200 milligrams a day. Calcium supplements can be used by people who don't like milk or cannot tolerate adequate amounts of milk products or foods made with milk. However, before deciding on this option, estimate your calcium intake. Use the rule of 300s. Give yourself 300 milligrams to start with. This accounts for small amounts of calcium provided by a moderate kcalorie intake from foods scattered throughout a typical diet. Add to that another 300 milligrams for every 1 cup (0.25 liters) of milk or yogurt or 1.5 ounces (45 grams) of cheese.

If you eat a lot of tofu, almonds, or sardines, using Appendix A will give you a more accurate account of your calcium intake. Our shortcut method underestimates it, especially for people eating a strictly vegetarian diet. It is important for vegans to focus on eating good plant sources of calcium, as well as on the total amount of calcium ingested.

ANOTHER BITE Some calcium supplements are poorly digested because they do not readily dissolve. To test for this, put a supplement in 6 ounces of cider vinegar. Stir every 5 minutes. It should dissolve within 30 minutes.

We hesitate to encourage calcium supplement use, even though most supplements are absorbed about as well as milk calcium. Many people have difficulty adhering to a supplement regimen. Regular food habits can be integrated more easily into a routine than can remembering to take several pills a day. The major risk from taking excess calcium supplements is poor absorption of other minerals and possibly the development of kidney stones. Toxic products that are part of dolomite or oyster shell calcium supplements are also of concern.

RDA for calcium. As mentioned above, the RDA for calcium is 800 milligrams per day for most adults. But from ages 11 through 24 the recommendation increases to 1200 milligrams, with the intent that higher calcium intakes will help build a greater bone mass. Youth is the time to accumulate calcium and build strong bones[28]; the greater bone mass can then benefit the person for the rest of his or her life. At 800 milligrams a day, young adults have enough calcium to maintain bone, but some may not have enough to build their maximum level.

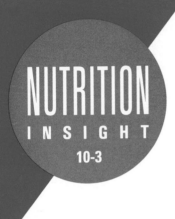

PREVENTING OSTEOPOROSIS

Widespread advertising has made it almost impossible for women to ignore osteoporosis. Its crippling effect on the elderly is now recognized as a medical emergency. The disease affects 20 to 25 million people in the United States, most of them women. About one third of all women experience osteoporosis-related fractures in their lifetimes.

Osteoporosis leads to approximately 1.2 million bone fractures per year, usually in the hip, spine, and wrist. The slender, inactive woman who smokes is most susceptible to osteoporosis, but any person who lives long enough can suffer from the disease. Table 10-3 lists many risk factors for the disease. As we age into our 80s and 90s, osteoporosis becomes the rule—not the exception. And it is not only debilitating, it can be fatal. Between 12% and 20% of all elderly persons who suffer hip fractures eventually die from fracture-related complications.

TABLE 10-3

Factors associated with bone maintenance versus bone loss

Maintenance	Loss	
Normal menses	Lack of menses	Excessive aluminum
Estrogen replacement	Early menopause	consumption
Black race	Glucocorticoid use	Alcoholism
Thiazide diuretics	Hyperparathyroidism	Cigarette smoking
Fluoride (1-6 milligrams/day)	Hyperthyroidism	Slender figure
Physical activity*	Thyroid hormone	Bed rest (months)
Dietary calcium	replacement	Dietary fiber (large
Body weight	Factors made by	amounts)
	white blood cells	Anorexia nervosa

*The degree of effect remains to be established.

Bone density at different ages

Rapid and continual bone growth and calcification occur throughout the adolescent years. Increases in bone density appear to continue through the ages of 20 to 30 years; scientists are not sure precisely when bone growth stops.[1] Women make less bone than men, lose it at a faster rate, and live longer. Thus women start their adult years with less bone and have a longer time to lose it. Also, bone density varies among adult women—some have much denser bone than others, perhaps because they built more bone when they were young. These women may more easily adapt to lower-calcium diets, allowing them to sustain greater bone loss without more fractures.

For women, bone loss begins around age 30 and proceeds slowly and continuously to menopause (approximately age 50). It often speeds up at menopause and continues at a high rate for the next 5 to 10 years. By age 65, the rate of bone loss falls to about the same rate as before menopause. In men, bone loss is slow and steady from around age 30.

Can bone loss be prevented?

Since 1985, hormone replacement therapy with estrogen has been widely recommended for women at menopause to prevent osteoporosis.[28] It is also used to reduce the symptoms of menopause. Studies show that estrogen replacement at menopause virtually stops further bone loss in women. Thus it is reasonable to assume that estrogen replacement therapy will eliminate risk for significant osteoporosis in women who begin treatment right after menopause and continue to take it. This therapy is thought to be very safe for most women but still must be closely supervised by a physician.[28] An added benefit of estrogen replacement therapy is a significant reduction of the risk of heart disease in women.

Is estrogen therapy the only answer?

Some women cannot take estrogen because they have estrogen-sensitive breast or uterine tumors. Other therapies, such as taking the active vitamin D hormone or the hormone calcitonin, are available and quite effective. However, will increasing calcium intake substitute for taking estrogen or other medications?

Studies from the United States and Denmark have found that taking as much as 2000 milligrams of extra calcium daily (equal to 7.5 glasses of milk) does not prevent bone loss in the spine, hip, or wrist after menopause as successfully as estrogen replacement does. Extra dietary calcium more effectively reduces bone loss in some bony areas better than doing nothing at all. But a high calcium intake may be no better for reducing bone loss in the spine than just meeting the RDA.[1]

Spinal fractures in women cause considerable pain and deformity and decrease physical ability. In addition, no reliable cure exists for osteoporosis. Therefore preventing these fractures is very important. Overall, for most women it is not a question of estrogen versus calcium, but estrogen plus calcium that constitutes one of the most effective treatments. Also, as women age 10 years beyond menopause, meeting the RDA for calcium leads to less bone loss throughout the body than consuming half that amount.

Will a nutritious diet in youth prevent osteoporosis later?

It appears that a good calcium intake builds a stronger bone structure than a poor intake. This is probably most beneficial during the years that bone density is increasing. Also, some less discussed mineral components of bone, such as copper, manganese, zinc, and fluoride, contribute to building and maintaining bones. Thus consuming a generally balanced and varied diet is wise for many reasons. Calcium's effect on bone development is a very active research area, and we expect more studies soon.[14] Until definite evidence is available, we think it is reasonable to assume that consuming calcium at the RDA for young women (1200 milligrams) may prevent or minimize much osteoporosis.

A plan for fracture prevention

As women mature, different strategies for preventing osteoporosis are needed based on risk factors present (Table 10-3). Young women should see a physician at any sign of irregular menstruation and should pursue an active lifestyle that includes sun exposure (to promote synthesis of vitamin D) and weight-bearing exercise (to stimulate bone building). In young women, regular menstruation is the overwhelming key to bone maintenance, as evidenced by poor bone density in non-menstruating female athletes and other women with irregular menstruation. Exercise cannot prevent the bone loss associated with irregular menstruation. It is also good to meet the RDA for calcium.[1] If foods from the milk and cheese group are not usually consumed, it is wise to find other calcium sources.

Smoking and excessive alcohol work against bone strength. Smoking lowers estrogen levels in women, increasing bone loss. Alcohol is toxic to all cells—this includes bone cells. Alcoholism is probably a major undiagnosed and unrecognized cause of osteoporosis today.

At menopause, women should discuss estrogen replacement therapy with a physician.[28] They also need to accurately track their height. A decrease of more than 1 inch from premenopausal values is a sign that significant bone loss is taking place. If a plan to prevent osteoporosis is not being pursued, a loss in height is the signal to see a physician and establish a plan.

Elderly men and women need to stay as physically active as possible and meet their RDA for calcium. This most likely limits bone loss in some areas of the body. They also need to minimize the risk for falls, especially by limiting their use of medications and alcohol that might disturb coordination. Getting regular sun exposure and consuming food sources of vitamin D are also good ideas. Securing throw rugs and liberal installation of hand rails in the house can help decrease the risk of falls and so fractures. ●

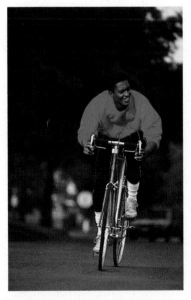

Exercise puts stress on bones, in turn contributing to their health.

311

A recent National Institutes of Health (NIH) committee also recommended that postmenopausal women who do not take estrogen replacements consume 1500 milligrams of calcium daily. Note that an intake up to 2500 milligrams per day is safe for adults. Still, as we discussed in the Nutrition Insight on preventing osteoporosis, even 1500 milligrams is not enough to prevent bone loss in the spine after menopause. Estrogen replacement is much more reliable.[28] Women who take estrogen at menopause still need calcium—about 800 to 1000 milligrams a day is recommended.

Unfortunately, the average calcium intake of adult women ranges from approximately 500 to 600 milligrams a day. For men the figure is 800 to 900 milligrams a day.[18] About 25% of women consume less than 300 milligrams per day. So women's diets tend to be deficient in calcium, while men's do not. Men eat more food in general to support their higher energy outputs, and that accounts for part of the difference. An easy way for women to consume more calcium is to increase their activity level and, in turn, to eat more in general.

CONCEPT CHECK

About 99% of calcium in the body is found in the bones. Aside from its critical role in bone formation and strength, calcium also functions in blood clotting, muscle contraction, nerve transmission, and cell metabolism. Calcium requires a slightly acid pH and the active vitamin D hormone for efficient absorption. Other factors that reduce calcium absorption include large amounts of dietary fiber, decreased estrogen levels, and excess levels of magnesium or phosphorus in the diet. Osteoporosis is bone loss caused by no other obvious condition. Women are particularly prone to osteoporosis because they make less bone than men, lose it faster, and live longer. Estrogen replacement at menopause for women and following a healthy diet remain the best methods of prevention. Dairy products and calcium-fortified orange juice are rich sources of calcium. Supplemental forms, such as calcium carbonate, are well absorbed. However, overzealous supplementation may interfere with the absorption of other minerals.

Phosphorus (P)

Phosphorus plays many important roles in the body. Although no disease is currently associated with a poor phosphorus intake, a deficiency may contribute to bone loss in elderly women. The body absorbs phosphorus quite efficiently and can increase absorption from 60% to 90% as body needs vary. This high absorption rate, plus the wide availability of phosphorus in foods, makes this mineral less important than calcium in diet planning. The active vitamin D hormone enhances phosphorus absorption, as it does for calcium. Kidney excretion primarily regulates phosphorus levels. This regulating mechanism differs from that of calcium, where changes in the rates of absorption are a more significant factor.

Functions of phosphorus.   Phosphorus is a component of enzymes, other key metabolic compounds, DNA (genetic material), all cell membranes, and bone. About 85% of the body's phosphorus is inside bone. The remaining phosphorus circulates freely in the bloodstream and functions inside cells.

Phosphorus in foods and the RDA.   Milk, cheese, bakery products, and meat provide most of the phosphorus in the adult diet. Cereals, bran, eggs, nuts, and fish are also good sources. About 20% to 30% of dietary phosphorus comes from food additives, especially in baked goods, cheeses, processed meats, and many soft drinks (about 75 milligrams per 12 ounce—$\frac{1}{3}$ liter—serving of soft drinks). Next time you have a soft drink, look for a listing of phosphoric acid on the label.

The same amount of phosphorus and calcium are recommended—800 milligrams per day for adults over age 24. Adults eat about 1400 to 1500 milligrams of phosphorus per day.[18] Thus deficiencies of phosphorus are unlikely in adults, especially because it is so efficiently absorbed.

Marginal phosphorus status can be found in premature infants, vegans, people with alcoholism, elderly people on nutrient-poor diets, people with long-term bouts of diarrhea, and people who use aluminum-containing antacids daily (these bind phosphorus in the small intestine).

Phosphorus does not appear to be toxic for healthy adults, but high amounts can lead to problems in people with certain kidney diseases. Early studies using animals led scientists to believe that a high phosphorus intake, coupled with a low calcium intake, contributed to bone loss. However, recent research casts doubt on the importance of the calcium to phosphorus ratio in a diet, as long as the RDA for calcium is met.[27] If calcium intake is not sufficient, a high phosphorus intake may compound the resulting bone loss.

Magnesium (Mg)

Magnesium is important for nerve and heart function and aids many enzyme reactions. It is found mostly in the plant pigment chlorophyll, where it functions in respiration. We normally absorb about 30% to 40% of the magnesium in our diets, but absorption efficiency can increase up to about 75% if intakes are low. The active vitamin D hormone appears to enhance magnesium absorption.

Functions of magnesium.   Bone contains 60% of the body's magnesium. The rest circulates in the blood and operates inside cells. Over 300 enzymes use magnesium, and many energy-yielding compounds in cells require magnesium to function properly.

Animals deficient in magnesium become very irritable, and with severe deficiency, eventually suffer convulsions and often die. In humans a magnesium deficiency causes irregular heart beat, sometimes accompanied by weakness, muscle pain, disorientation, and seizures. However, a magnesium deficiency develops very slowly because our bodies store it readily. A link between magnesium deficiency and sudden heart attacks has been observed.[21] However, since human magnesium status is difficult to measure, scientists have not been able to validate the relation of low magnesium levels to heart attacks.

Magnesium in foods and the RDA.   The best sources for magnesium are plant rather than animal products. Good food sources are whole grains (wheat bran), broccoli, squash, beans, nuts, and seeds. Milk and meats do supply some, however. Whole grains and vegetables are important parts of a diet partly because they are excellent magnesium sources. Dairy products, chocolate, and meats also contribute magnesium. Hard tap water—again, that containing a high mineral content—often contains a high concentration of magnesium.

The adult RDA for magnesium is 350 milligrams per day for men and 280 milligrams per day for women. Adult men consume an average of 300 milligrams daily, while women consume an average of 200 milligrams daily.[18] The low intake for women creates special concern because many of them are taking more calcium to offset the possibility of osteoporosis. Because calcium can interfere with magnesium absorption, we suggest women, and men too, find good sources of magnesium and eat them regularly.

Besides being a risk to women in general, poor magnesium status is found among users of certain diuretics; some diuretics increase magnesium excretion in the urine. In addition, perspiring heavily for weeks in hot climates and bouts of long-standing diarrhea or vomiting all cause significant magnesium loss. Alcoholism increases the risk of a deficiency because dietary intake may be poor, and alcohol increases magnesium excretion in the urine. The disorientation and weakness from alcoholism resembles that of people with low blood levels of magnesium. Magnesium toxicity occurs typically only in people with kidney failure.

Trace Mineral • A mineral vital to health that is required in the diet in amounts less than 100 mg per day.

Sulfur (S)

Sulfur is found in many important compounds in the body, such as some amino acids (like methionine) and the vitamins biotin and thiamin. Sulfur helps in the balance of acids and bases in the body and is an important part of the liver's drug-detoxifying pathways. Since proteins supply the sulfur we need, sulfur is naturally a part of a healthful diet. Sulfur compounds are also used to preserve foods (see Chapter 17).

CONCEPT CHECK

Phosphorus is an important component of bones and cell membranes and contributes to many chemical reactions throughout the body. Good food sources include dairy products, baked goods, and meat. The body absorbs phosphorus quite efficiently, especially in the presence of active vitamin D hormone. No clear deficiency symptoms caused by poor intake have been reported. Toxicity can occur in association with kidney disease. Magnesium is found mostly in the plant pigment chlorophyll where it functions in respiration. Magnesium is important to humans for nerve and heart function and is an activator of many enzymes. Women in general and people with alcoholism are at risk for a poor intake. Toxicity occurs mainly in people with kidney failure. Sulfur is a component of some vitamins and amino acids. Our diets supply sulfur as part of the protein and vitamins we normally consume.

See Table 10-4 for a review of the major characteristics of water and the minerals we have discussed so far.

TRACE MINERALS

Information about *trace minerals* is perhaps the most rapidly expanding area of knowledge in nutrition. With the exceptions of iron and iodine, the importance of trace minerals to humans has been recognized only within the last 30 years. Although we need only about 20 milligrams—or less—of each trace mineral daily, they are just as essential to good health as are major minerals. In some cases, discovering the importance of a trace mineral reads like a detective story. And the dramas are still unfolding.

As recently as 1961 researchers linked dwarfism in Middle Eastern villagers to a zinc deficiency. Other scientists recognized that a rare form of heart disease in an isolated area of China was linked to a selenium deficiency. In America, some trace mineral deficiencies were first observed in the late 1960s and early 1970s when the minerals were not added to synthetic formulas used for intravenous feeding.

It is difficult to define precisely our trace minerals needs because we need only minute amounts. Highly sophisticated technology is required to measure such small amounts in both food and body tissues.

Iron (Fe)

The importance of dietary iron has been recognized for centuries. The Persian physician Melampus in 4000 B.C. gave iron supplements to sailors to make up for iron lost from bleeding wounds during battles.[5] Today, iron deficiency is one of the most common nutrient deficiencies worldwide. Iron is the only nutrient for which adult women have a greater RDA than adult men. Iron is found in every living cell; adding up to about 5 grams (1 teaspoon) for the entire body.

Absorption and distribution of iron. The body uses several mechanisms to regulate iron absorption. Controlling absorption is important because our bodies cannot easily eliminate excess iron once it is absorbed. Iron absorption from foods varies from about 3% to 40%, depending on its form in the food, the body's need for it, and a variety of other factors (Table 10-5).[6,15]

TABLE 10-4

A summary of water and the major minerals

Name	Major Functions	Deficiency Symptoms	People Most at Risk	RDA or Minimum Requirement	Nutrient Dense Dietary Sources	Results of Toxicity
Water	Medium for chemical reactions, removal of waste products, perspiration to cool the body	Thirst, muscle weakness, poor endurance	Infants with a fever, elderly in nursing homes	1 milliliter per kcalorie* burned	As such and in foods	Probably occurs only in mental disorders: headache, blurred vision, convulsions
Sodium	A major ion of the extracellular fluid; nerve impulse transmission	Muscle cramps	People who severely restrict sodium to lower blood pressure (250-500 milligrams/day)	500 milligrams	Table salt, processed foods	High blood pressure in susceptible individuals
Potassium	A major ion of intracellular fluid; nerve impulse transmission	Irregular heart beat, loss of appetite, muscle cramps	People who use potassium-wasting diuretics or have poor diets, as seen in poverty and alcoholism	2000 milligrams	Spinach, squash, bananas, orange juice, other vegetables and fruits, milk	Slowing of the heart beat; seen in kidney failure
Chloride	A major ion of the extracellular fluid; acid production in stomach; nerve transmission	Convulsions in infants	No one, probably, when infant formula manufacturers control product quality adequately	700 milligrams	Table salt, some vegetables	High blood pressure in susceptible people when combined with sodium
Calcium	Bones and teeth strength; blood clotting; nerve impulse transmission; muscle contractions; cell regulation	Poor intake increases the risk for osteoporosis	Women in general, especially those who constantly restrict their energy intake and consume few dairy products	800 milligrams (greater than 24 years)	Dairy products, canned fish, leafy vegetables, tofu, fortified orange juice	Very high intakes may cause kidney stones in susceptible people
Phosphorus	Bones and teeth strength; part of various metabolic compounds; major ion of intracellular fluid	Probably none; poor bone maintenance possible	Elderly consuming very nutrient-poor diets; possibly total vegetarians and people with alcoholism	800 milligrams (greater than 24 years)	Dairy products, processed foods, fish, soft drinks	Hampers bone health in people with kidney failure; poor bone mineralization if calcium intakes are low
Magnesium	Bones strength; enzyme function; nerve and heart function	Weakness, muscle pain, poor heart function	People on thiazide diuretics, women in general	Men: 350 milligrams Women: 280 milligrams	Wheat bran, green vegetables, nuts, chocolate	Causes weakness in people with kidney failure
Sulfur	Part of vitamins and amino acids; drug detoxification; acid base balance	None	No one who meets their protein needs	None	Protein foods	None likely

*Just an approximation; best to keep urine volume greater than 1 liter (4 cups).

Hemoglobin • The iron-containing part of the red blood cell that carries oxygen to the cells and carbon dioxide away from the cells. It is also responsible for the red color of blood.

Myoglobin • Iron-containing compound that transports oxygen and carbon dioxide in muscle tissue.

Heme Iron • Iron provided from animal tissues as hemoglobin and myoglobin. Approximately 40% of the iron in meat is heme iron; it is readily absorbed.

Nonheme Iron • Iron provided from plant sources and animal tissues other than in the form of hemoglobin and myoglobin. Nonheme iron is less efficiently absorbed than heme iron.

TABLE 10-5

Dietary factors that affect iron absorption

Increase	Decrease
Vitamin C	Phytate fiber
Acid in the stomach	Oxalate
Heme iron	Tannins (in tea)
High body demand for red blood cells (blood loss, high altitude, physical training, pregnancy)	Full body stores
	Great excess of other minerals (Zn, Mn, Ca)
Low body stores	Lack of stomach acid
Meat protein	Some antacids

The form of iron in foods greatly influences how much is absorbed. About 40% of the total iron in animal flesh is in the form of **hemoglobin** (the same form as in red blood cells) and **myoglobin** (pigment found in muscle cells). This **heme iron** is absorbed more than twice as efficiently as the simple elemental iron, called **nonheme iron.** Nonheme iron is also present in animal flesh, as well as in eggs, milk, vegetables, grains, and other plant foods.[15]

About 10% to 15% of iron in the typical adult diet is heme iron and usually 25% to 35% is absorbed. Nonheme iron makes up the rest and usually 2% to 20% is absorbed.[15] Therefore animal flesh, especially red meat, is the best source of iron in the adult diet because of both its iron content and the amount in the heme form. Consuming heme iron and nonheme iron together increases nonheme iron absorption. A protein factor in meats also may aid nonheme absorption.[5,15] Overall, eating meat with vegetables and grain products enhances the absorption of all nonheme iron present.

Vitamin C can increase nonheme iron absorption. So when taking an iron supplement, consider drinking a glass of orange juice with it. Consuming more foods rich in vitamin C is particularly desirable if dietary iron is inadequate or serum iron levels are low. Iron use in the body is also aided by copper, as we explain in a later section.

Several dietary factors interfere with our ability to absorb iron.[15] Phytic acid and other factors in grain fibers and oxalic acid in vegetables can all bind iron and reduce its absorption. Tannins found in tea also reduce iron absorption. When trying to rebuild iron stores, it is a good idea to keep dietary fiber under 35 grams a day and to reduce tea consumption, the latter particularly at mealtimes. Zinc also interferes with iron by competing with it for absorption. Finally, high-dose calcium supplements can also bind iron—an important consideration when using calcium supplements as a substitute for dairy products.

The most important factor influencing iron absorption is the body's need for it.[6] In a deficiency state, nonheme iron absorption can increase about tenfold and heme iron absorption about twofold. When iron stores are inadequate, the main serum protein that carries iron, transferrin, readily binds more iron, shifting it from intestinal cells into the bloodstream. If iron stores are adequate and transferrin is fully saturated with iron, little will be absorbed from the intestinal cells. It stays bound as a ferritin protein in the intestinal cells.

By this mechanism, in normal circumstances, iron is absorbed only as needed. If not needed, when intestinal cells are shed at the end of their 2- to 5-day life cycle, the iron returns to the intestinal tract for excretion. This whole process is referred to as a *mucosal block* against excess iron absorption. High doses of iron can still be toxic (see Nutrition Insight 10-2), but absorption is carefully regulated under typical dietary conditions (Figure 10-8).

Most iron in the body is contained in the hemoglobin molecules of the red blood cells. Some iron is stored in the bone marrow, and a small portion goes

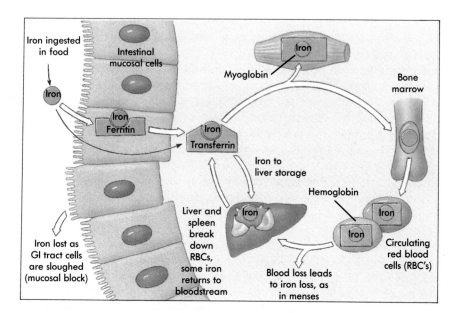

FIGURE 10-8

Iron absorption and distribution. Iron binds with a protein to form a protein called ferritin when stored in cells. If the intestinal absorption cells are shed before iron is absorbed from them, the iron is not absorbed into the bloodstream. This is one way the body can limit overabsorption of iron.

to other body cells, such as the liver, for storage. As iron is needed it can be mobilized from body stores. If dietary intake is inadequate, these iron stores become depleted. Only then do signs of an iron deficiency appear.

Functions of iron. We mentioned that iron forms part of the hemoglobin in red blood cells and myoglobin in muscle cells. Hemoglobin molecules in red blood cells transport oxygen (O_2) from the lungs to cells and return with carbon dioxide (CO_2) from cells to the lungs for excretion. In addition, iron is used as part of many enzymes, some proteins, and other important compounds that cells use in energy production. Iron is also needed for immune function and contributes to drug detoxification pathways in the liver.

Iron-deficiency anemia. If neither the diet nor body stores can supply the iron needed for hemoglobin synthesis, the number of red blood cells decreases in the bloodstream. Blood hemoglobin concentration also falls. When both the percentage of red blood cells falls (called the *hematocrit*) and the hemoglobin level falls, a physician would suspect iron deficiency. In severe deficiency, the hemoglobin and hematocrit levels fall so low that the amount of oxygen carried in the bloodstream is decreased. Such a person has anemia, defined as a decreased oxygen-carrying capacity of the blood. While there are many types of anemia, iron-deficiency anemia is the major type worldwide. About 30% of the world's population is anemic, and about half of those cases are caused by an iron deficiency. Probably about 8% of Americans have iron-deficiency anemia.

Iron-deficiency anemia most often appears in infancy, the preschool years, and at puberty for both males and females. Growth, with accompanying expansion of blood volume and muscle mass, increases iron needs, making it difficult to consume enough iron. Women are also very vulnerable during childbearing years when menstruation occurs. In addition, anemia is often found in pregnant women, as we will discuss in Chapter 14. Iron-deficiency anemia in adult men is usually caused by blood loss from ulcers, colon cancer, or hemorrhoids.

Clinical symptoms of iron-deficiency anemia primarily include pale skin, fatigue, poor temperature regulation, loss of appetite, and apathy. Insufficient iron for the synthesis of red blood cells and key cell compounds may cause the

A red blood cell has a life span of approximately 120 days. A rapid cell turnover such as this puts great nutrient demands on the body, and iron is one of those greatly demanded nutrients.

fatigue. Researchers suspect that poor iron stores may also decrease learning ability, attention span, work performance, and immune status even before a person is actually anemic (see Chapter 18).

More people have an iron deficiency than iron-deficiency anemia, especially in America. Probably about 30% of women have little or no iron stores. Their blood hemoglobin values are still normal, but they have no stores to draw from in times of pregnancy or illness.

To speed the cure of iron-deficiency anemia, a person needs to take iron supplements. A physician should also find the cause—a poor diet or a bleeding ulcer, for example—so that the anemia does not recur. A good diet may prevent iron-deficiency anemia, but supplemental iron is the only reliable cure. Recall that a vitamin C source consumed with an iron supplement enhances absorption.

Iron in foods. The most nutrient-dense iron sources are spinach, oysters, liver, clams, peas, and legumes. However, total iron content of foods and nutrient density are not the only considerations when choosing dietary iron sources. Serving size and bioavailability are probably more important. For example, although spinach is rich in iron, the body absorbs very little of it. Animal sources contain some heme iron, the most bioavailable form. These then are our best iron sources. Iron present in iron supplements also is absorbed well. The major iron sources in the adult diet are animal and grain products.[18] Most of the iron in bakery products has been added to refined flour in the enrichment process.

The use of iron-fortified formulas and cereals in the Special Supplemental Food Program for Women, Infant, and Children Program (WIC) in the United States is probably a major contributor to decreasing rates of iron-deficiency anemia in preschool children (see Chapters 14 and 15). Another possible iron source is cooking utensils. When acidic foods, such as tomato sauce, are cooked in iron pots and frying pans, some iron from the cookware is taken up by the food.

Milk is a very poor source of iron. A common cause of iron-deficiency anemia in children is an over-reliance on milk, coupled with an insufficient meat intake. Total vegetarians (vegans) are particularly susceptible to iron-deficiency anemia because of their lack of dietary heme iron.

RDA for iron. The daily adult RDA for iron is 10 milligrams for men and 15 milligrams for women. The RDA value assumes that about 10% of dietary iron is absorbed. If iron absorption exceeds that, less dietary iron is needed.

The higher RDA for women is primarily because of menstrual blood loss. Women who menstruate more heavily and longer than average may need even more dietary iron, and those who have lighter and shorter flows may need less iron. The variation in menstrual blood loss, and hence, loss of iron, makes it difficult to set an RDA for iron for women.

By recording dietary intakes from a variety of women, we find that most women do not consume 15 milligrams of iron daily. The average daily value is closer to 11 milligrams.[18] Of course, not all women need 15 milligrams of iron daily because the RDA is set high enough to allow for variations in menstrual flow and absorption rates. Whether male or female, if you are not consuming the RDA for iron, you should be concerned, but not alarmed. Try to consume a diet that meets the RDA for iron. It is difficult to tell whether a lower iron intake is actually harmful. Although we have very sensitive measures of iron stores in the body, we lack the knowledge to reliably predict health status when people register low values.

As stated earlier, an iron deficiency is most common when iron needs are greatest—during infancy, preschool years, puberty, and during childbearing years for women. Pregnancy and disease also increase iron needs, setting the stage for iron deficiency. Women who experience repeated pregnancies may have difficulty maintaining adequate iron stores.

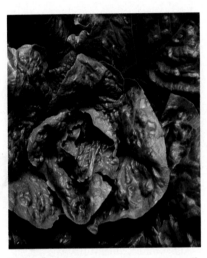

Spinach is rich in iron, but the bioavailability of iron from spinach is low.

ANOTHER BITE The adult human body contains about 21 cups (5 liters) of blood. Blood donations are generally 2 cups (500 milliliters). Thus a blood donor gives about a tenth of his or her total supply. Healthy people generally can donate blood four times a year without harmful consequences. As a precaution, blood banks first screen potential donors' blood for the presence of anemia.

The adult diet contains about 5 to 7 milligrams of iron per 1000 kcalories. Thus men generally achieve a good iron status because a daily energy intake of 2000 to 3000 kcalories meets their RDA for iron. By these criteria, most women would have to eat 3000 kcalories daily in order to meet the RDA of 15 milligrams of iron. For women with typical activity levels, it would be difficult to maintain desirable weight while eating so much. One way to resolve this problem is to eat nutrient-dense forms of iron, such as those found in fortified breakfast cereals, with an accompanying glass of orange juice to improve absorption of the iron. If that is not sufficient, a supplement can be used. Poor iron stores and iron-deficiency anemia do not develop only in the poor; they cut across all levels of society. Keep in mind also that although iron deficiency is a common problem, an intake of too much iron is toxic (see Nutrition Insight 10-2).

CONCEPT CHECK

Iron absorption depends on its form (heme iron is best) and the body's need for it. Iron absorption increases in the presence of vitamin C and decreases in the presence of calcium and some components of grain fiber, such as phytic acid. Iron is most important in forming hemoglobin and myoglobin and in supporting immune function. An iron deficiency can cause decreased red blood cell synthesis, which can lead to anemia. It is particularly important for women of childbearing age to consume adequate iron, primarily to replace that lost in menstrual blood. Good sources include meat, enriched grains and cereals, and seafood. Large doses of iron can lead to toxicity.

Zinc (Zn)

Although zinc has been recognized as an essential nutrient in animals since the early 1900s, zinc deficiency was first recognized in humans in the early 1960s in Egypt and Iran. Zinc deficiencies were determined to cause growth retardation and poor sexual development in some groups of people, even though the zinc content of their diets was fairly high. However, the customary diet contained almost exclusively unleavened bread and little animal protein. Unleavened bread is very high in phytic acid and other factors that decrease zinc bioavailability. Parasite infestation and the practice of eating dirt also probably contributed to the severe zinc deficiency.

In America zinc deficiencies were first observed in the early 1970s in hospitalized patients fed only intravenously. Zinc was not added to solutions used before this time, but the protein source in the solutions was based on milk protein or a blood protein, which are both naturally rich in zinc. When the solutions were changed to include mostly individual amino acids as the protein source, deficiency symptoms quickly developed. This source of protein is very low in zinc.

Symptoms of adult zinc deficiency include an acne-like rash, diarrhea, lack of appetite, reduced sense of taste and smell, hair loss. In children and adolescents, poor growth, poor sexual development, and poor learning ability may also result.

Like iron, zinc absorption is influenced by foods ingested. About 25% to 40% of dietary zinc is absorbed; the higher figure is more likely when animal protein sources are used and when the body needs more zinc. Supplementary iron competes with zinc for absorption and vice versa—again exhibiting a toxic potential for both minerals. Toasting cereals also reduces zinc absorption. Most people worldwide rely on cereal grains (low in zinc) for their source of protein, kcalories, and zinc. This makes consuming adequate zinc a problem.

Functions of zinc. Over 200 enzymes require zinc for optimum activity. Adequate zinc intake is necessary to support many bodily functions, such as:

- DNA and protein metabolism, wound healing, and growth.
- proper immune function (taking more than the RDA does not provide extra benefit to immune function).
- proper development of sexual organs and bone.
- storage and release of the hormone insulin.
- alcohol metabolism.
- taste sensation.

A recent study emphasizes the importance of zinc for growth. Children recovering from semistarvation gained weight much faster when they consumed zinc supplements, containing approximately three times the RDA, under a physician's guidance.

Zinc in foods and the RDA. In general, protein-rich diets are also rich in zinc. Animal foods supply almost half our zinc intake; their cost makes zinc a very expensive nutrient. The most nutrient-dense sources of zinc are oysters, shrimp, crab, lean beef, lamb, turkey, beans, and mushrooms. As with iron, nutrient density is not the only issue; bioavailability is probably more important. Animal foods are again our best sources because zinc from animal sources is not bound by phytic acid.[16,18] However, good plant sources of zinc—such as whole grains, peanuts, and beans—should not be discounted. Studies show they can deliver substantial amounts of zinc to body cells.

The daily adult RDA for zinc is 15 milligrams for men and 12 milligrams for women. The average daily U.S. adult intake of zinc is 9 to 16 milligrams, with men showing the higher values.[18] This raises concern that many women do not consume enough. Still, there are no indications of moderate or severe zinc deficiencies in an otherwise healthy adult population. Probably many Americans have only marginal zinc status—especially women in general, poor children, vegans, the elderly, and people with alcoholism. However, because we lack a sensitive marker for zinc status, a body must be very zinc-depleted for clinical tests to register a deficiency.

Zinc is not part of the enrichment process, so refined flours are not a good source.

Selenium (Se)

Selenium exists in many forms that are readily absorbed. Selenium's best understood role is aiding in the activity of an enzyme that participates in reducing the damage that electron-seeking (oxidizing) compounds can do to cell membranes.

In Chapter 9 we saw that vitamin E helps prevent attacks on cell membranes by electron-seeking compounds. Thus vitamin E and selenium work together toward the same goal. In Chapter 9 we also discussed how electron-seeking compounds can possibly cause cancer. But although selenium could prove to have a role in cancer prevention, it is premature to recommend selenium supplementation for this purpose. Animal studies in this area are encouraging, and in human studies scientists are presently working to clarify selenium's role, if any. Selenium may have yet other metabolic functions, but none has been firmly established.

Selenium deficiency symptoms in farm animals and humans include muscle pain, muscle wasting, and heart disease.[23] Farm animals in areas with low selenium soil concentration, such as New Zealand, and humans in some areas of China develop characteristic muscle and heart disorders associated with poor selenium intake. Other factors probably also contribute.

Selenium in foods and the RDA. Fish, meats (especially organ meats), eggs, and shellfish are good animal sources of selenium. Grains and seeds grown in soils containing selenium are good plant sources. Major selenium contributors to the adult diet are animal and grain products.[18] Since we eat a varied diet of foods supplied from many geographic areas, it is unlikely that low soil levels of selenium in a few locations will mean inadequate selenium in our diets.

The RDA for selenium is 55 to 70 micrograms for adults. In general, adults meet the RDA, consuming on average 60 to 110 micrograms of selenium each day.[18] High amounts can be toxic to animals and humans (see Nutrition Insight 10-2), so supplements are not advised unless supervised by a physician.

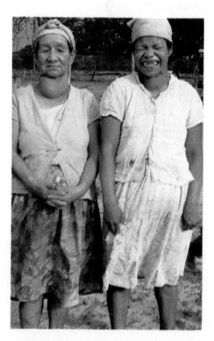

Goiter • An enlargement of the thyroid gland; this is often caused by a lack of iodide in the diet.

CONCEPT CHECK

Zinc functions as a cofactor for many enzymes and is important for growth, immune function, and sense of taste. Beef, seafood, and whole grains are good food sources. As in the case of iron, the intestinal cells regulate zinc absorption subject to the body's needs for the mineral. If taken in excess amounts, copper and iron compete with zinc for absorption. Selenium activates an enzyme that helps change electron-seeking (oxidizing) compounds into less toxic compounds, so these do not attack and break down cell membranes. By helping to dismantle the electron-seeking compounds, selenium works to the same goal as vitamin E. A selenium deficiency results in muscle and heart disorders. Animal products and grains are good selenium sources; however, the selenium content in plants depends on the selenium concentration in the soil.

Iodine (I)

Iodine in foods is actually found in the ion form, called iodide. During World War I, a link was discovered between a deficiency of iodide and the production of a *goiter,* an enlarged thyroid gland (Figure 10-9). Men drafted from the Pacific Northwest and the Great Lakes Region of the United States had a much higher rate of goiter than men from other areas of the country. The soils in these areas have very low iodide contents. In the 1920s, researchers in Ohio found that low doses of iodide given to children over a 4-year period could prevent goiter. That finding led to the addition of iodide to salt beginning in the 1920s.

Today, many nations require iodide-fortification of salt. In the United States, salt can be purchased either iodized or plain. Check for this on the label of a package of salt next time you are in a grocery store. By law, the label on a salt container sold in the United States must clearly state if iodide is present or not. Some areas of Europe, such as northern Italy, have very low soil levels of iodide, but have yet to adopt the practice of fortifying salt with iodide. People in these areas, especially women, still suffer from goiter, as do people in areas of Central America, South America, and Africa.

Function of iodide. The thyroid gland actively accumulates and traps iodide from the bloodstream to support its hormone synthesis. Thyroid hormones, such as thyroxine, are synthesized using iodide. These hormones help regulate metabolic rate, growth, and development; in addition they promote bone and protein synthesis.

If a person's iodide intake is insufficient, the thyroid gland enlarges as it attempts to take up more iodide from the bloodstream. This eventually leads to

FIGURE 10-9

Goiter and cretinism in Bolivia. The mother on the left is goitrous, but otherwise normal. The daughter is goitrous, mentally retarded, and a deaf mute.

Cretinism • Stunting of body growth and poor mental development that results from inadequate maternal intake of iodide during pregnancy.

Goitrogens • Substances in food that interfere with the absorption and use of iodide. They therefore may cause goiter if consumed in large amounts.

goiter. Although iodide can prevent goiter formation, it does not shrink a goiter once it has formed. Goiters have been described in people—usually women—as far back as 3000 B.C.

Goiters are sometimes found in people who consume large amounts of raw turnips and rutabagas. These vegetables contain compounds called *goitrogens*, which inhibit the function of the thyroid gland and, in turn, thyroid hormone synthesis. However, goitrogens are generally not an important cause of goiter because the cooking process destroys them, and turnips and rutabagas are not typically staples in human diets.

If a woman consumes an iodide-deficient diet during the early months of her pregnancy, the fetus suffers iodide deficiency because the mother's body uses up the available iodide. The infant then may be born with growth failure and develop mental retardation. This stunted growth is known as *cretinism*. Cretinism appeared in America before iodide fortification of table salt began. Today, cretinism still appears in Europe, Africa, Latin America, and Asia.

Food sources of iodide and the RDA. Saltwater fish, seafood, iodized salt, dairy products, and grain products contain various forms of iodide. Sea salt found in health food stores, however, is not a good natural source, since the iodide is lost during processing.

The RDA for iodide for adults is 150 micrograms. A half teaspoon of iodide-fortified salt (about 2 grams) supplies that amount. Most adults consume much more iodide than the RDA—an estimated 240 to 400 micrograms daily.[18] This extra amount adds up because dairies and fast-food restaurants use it as a sterilizing agent, bakeries use it as a dough conditioner, food producers use it as part of food colorants, and it is added to salt. Because it is potentially toxic in high amounts,[19] manufacturers are currently working to reduce unnecessary iodide use in dairies, restaurants, and bakeries.

Copper (Cu)

Copper is a critical element in metabolizing iron; it operates in processes that form hemoglobin and transport iron. A copper-containing enzyme, ceruloplasmin, appears to help aid in release of iron from storage.[12]

Copper is needed by enzymes that create cross-connections in collagen and elastin, connective tissue proteins. In laboratory animals with copper deficiencies, blood vessels rupture because collagen is unavailable to form the important connective tissue network that strengthens blood vessels.

Copper also is needed by other enzymes, such as those that defend the body against electron-seeking (oxidizing) compounds and those that act in the brain and central nervous system. In addition, copper also performs in immune system function and blood clotting. Symptoms of copper deficiency include anemia, low white blood cell count, bone loss, poor growth, and some forms of heart disease.[4]

Copper in foods and the ESADDI. Copper is found primarily in liver, cocoa, legumes, nuts, dried fruits, and whole-grain breads and cereals. It is not added to breakfast cereals since it speeds fat breakdown in the product. Milk is also a very poor source of copper. Overall, we need whole grains, nuts, and legumes to supply our copper needs. We absorb about 25% to 40% of dietary copper.

The estimated safe and adequate daily dietary intake (ESADDI) for copper is 1.5 to 3 milligrams daily for adults. The average adult intake is about 0.9 to 1.2 milligrams per day.[18] Women generally consume the lesser amount. Even so, the copper status of adults appears to be good, though we lack sensitive measures for copper status. We suggest you regularly eat good sources of copper.

The groups most likely to develop copper deficiencies are premature infants, infants recovering from semistarvation on a milk-dominated diet (which is a poor source of copper), and people recovering from intestinal surgery (during which time copper absorption decreases).

Recall that a copper deficiency can result from overzealous supplementation of zinc, since zinc and copper compete with each other for absorption (see Nutrition Insight 10-2). Vomiting and other symptoms of toxicity result from single doses of copper greater than 10 to 30 milligrams.

Fluoride (F)

Dentists in the early 1900s noticed a lower rate of dental caries (cavities) in the southwestern United States. These areas contained high amounts of fluoride in the water. The levels were sometimes so high that small spots on the teeth, called mottling, appeared. Even though mottled teeth were quite discolored, they contained very few dental caries. After experiments showed that fluoride in the water did indeed decrease the rate of dental caries, controlled fluoridation of water in parts of the United States began in 1945.

Those of us who grew up drinking fluoridated water generally have 50% to 70% fewer dental caries than people who did not drink fluoridated water as children. Dentists can provide fluoride treatments, and schools can provide fluoride tablets, but it is much less expensive and more reliable to simply add fluoride to a community's drinking water. State and private water sources do not always contain enough fluoride, however. When in doubt, contact your local water plant or have the water in your home analyzed for fluoride content. If it is less than 1 part fluoride per million parts of water (1 ppm), talk to your dentist about the best means for your children to obtain the needed fluoride.

Functions of fluoride.   Dietary fluoride consumed during childhood, when bones and teeth are developing, aids the synthesis of tooth crystals that strongly resist acid. Therefore teeth become very resistant to dental caries. Fluoride also inhibits the growth of bacteria that cause dental caries (Chapter 6 reviews the development of dental caries).

Dietary fluoride has also been shown to improve growth rate in mice, but scientists are not sure if fluoride is actually necessary for growth in humans.

Fluoride in foods and the ESADDI.   Tea, seafood, seaweed, and some natural water sources are the only good food sources of fluoride. Most fluoride consumed in America comes from water-fortification, toothpaste, and fluoride treatments performed by dentists. No evidence shows that water fluoridation is harmful at levels currently used in the United States.

The estimated safe and adequate daily dietary intake (ESADDI) of fluoride for adults is 1.5 to 4 milligrams. This amount provides resistance to dental caries without causing mottling of the teeth or other toxicity symptoms. Adults generally meet this level of intake.

CONCEPT CHECK

Iodide is vital for the synthesis of thyroid hormones. A prolonged insufficient intake causes the thyroid gland to enlarge, resulting in a goiter. The use of iodized salt in America has virtually eliminated this condition. Copper functions mainly in iron metabolism and in the cross-bonding of collagen. A deficiency can result in an iron-deficiency type of anemia. Good food sources of copper are seafoods, legumes, nuts, dried fruits, and whole grains. Fluoride aides in tooth and bone development. When incorporated into the diet during development, fluoride makes teeth resistant to acid and bacterial growth, in turn reducing development of dental caries. Most adults get adequate amounts of fluoride via water fortification and in toothpaste.

Chromium (Cr)

The importance of chromium in human diets has been recognized only in the past 20 years. There is much we do not understand about this mineral, but chromium deficiency may be related to both diabetes mellitus and coronary heart disease.

Functions of chromium. Chromium helps with glucose entry into cells, but the mechanism by which it works continues to puzzle researchers. In both laboratory animals and humans, a chromium deficiency results in impaired glucose clearance from the bloodstream and elevated blood cholesterol levels. We don't know how chromium influences cholesterol metabolism either, but the mechanism may involve enzymes that control cholesterol synthesis. Chromium deficiency appears in people maintained on intravenous feedings not supplemented with chromium and in children during semistarvation. Since sensitive measures of chromium status are not available, marginal chromium deficiencies can go undetected.

Food sources of chromium and the ESADDI. Overall, we have little information about chromium values of foods. Egg yolks, whole grains, and meats are good sources. Poor sources are fruits, vegetables, many seafoods, highly processed foods, and drinking water. The ultimate chromium level in foods is closely tied to soil content, which varies with locality. To provide yourself with good chromium sources, eat mostly whole—not refined—forms of grains.

The estimated safe and adequate daily dietary intake (ESADDI) of chromium is 50 to 200 micrograms. We eat about 25 to 90 micrograms per day. Marginal to low chromium intakes in the elderly may contribute to an increased risk for developing diabetes mellitus. Some research shows that an intake at the high end of the ESADDI, or slightly above, raises blood HDL-cholesterol levels, that is, the *good* cholesterol. More research is needed on this effect. Chromium toxicity has been reported in people exposed to industrial waste and in painters using art supplies with a very high chromium content. Liver damage and lung cancer can result.

Manganese (Mn)

It is easy to confuse the mineral manganese with magnesium. Not only are their names similar, but they also often substitute for each other in metabolic processes. Manganese is needed by some enzymes, such as those used in carbohydrate metabolism. Manganese is also important in bone formation.[9]

No human deficiency symptom is associated with a low manganese intake. Animals on manganese-deficient diets suffer alterations in brain function, bone formation, reproduction, and blood glucose regulation. If human diets were low in manganese, these symptoms would probably appear as well. As it happens, our need for manganese is very low, and our diets tend to include a lot of manganese.

Good food sources of manganese are nuts, rice, oats and other whole grains, beans, and leafy vegetables. The estimated safe and adequate daily dietary intake (ESADDI) of manganese is 2 to 5 milligrams. Manganese is toxic at high doses, so be cautious with supplements that exceed our needs.

Molybdenum (Mo)

Molybdenum interacts with iron and copper, especially to inhibit copper absorption. Several human enzymes use molybdenum. No molybdenum deficiency has been noted in people who consume normal diets, though deficiency symptoms have appeared in people maintained on intravenous feedings. These symptoms include increased heart and respiration rates, night blindness, mental confusion, edema, and weakness.

Good food sources of molybdenum include beans, whole grains, and nuts. The estimated safe and adequate daily dietary intake (ESADDI) for molybdenum is 75 to 250 micrograms. When consumed in high doses, symptoms of molybdenum toxicity in laboratory animals include weight loss and decreased growth.

OTHER TRACE MINERALS

Although a variety of other trace minerals is found in humans, many of them have not yet been shown to be required. The list of minerals in this category includes boron, nickel, vanadium, arsenic, lithium, silicon, tin, and cadmium.[17] Widespread deficiency symptoms in humans have never been noted, probably because typical diets provide adequate amounts and they are needed by very few enzymes and metabolic systems. Their potential for toxicity should make one question any supplementation not supervised by a physician.

These trace minerals may achieve more importance as more research is reported. See Table 10-6 to review what we have discussed about the trace minerals.

TABLE 10-6

A summary of key trace minerals

Mineral	Major Functions	Deficiency Symptoms	People Most at Risk	RDA or ESADDI	Nutrient Dense Dietary Sources	Results of Toxicity
Iron	Part of hemoglobin and other key compounds used in respiration; used for immune function	Low serum iron levels; small, pale red blood cells; low blood hemoglobin values	Infants, preschool children, adolescents, women in child-bearing years	Men: 10 milligrams Women: 15 milligrams	Meats, spinach, seafood, broccoli, peas, bran, enriched breads	Toxicity is seen when children consume 200-400 milligrams in iron pills and in people with hemochromatosis; in this latter case people overabsorb iron
Zinc	Over 200 enzymes need zinc, including enzymes involved in growth, immunity, alcohol metabolism, sexual development, and reproduction	Skin rash, diarrhea, decreased appetite and sense of taste, hair loss, poor growth and development, poor wound healing	Vegetarians, women in general, the elderly	Men: 15 milligrams Women: 12 milligrams	Seafoods, meats, greens, whole grains	Reduces iron and copper absorption; can cause diarrhea, cramps, and depressed immune function
Selenium	Part of antioxidant system	Muscle pain, muscle weakness, heart disease	Unknown	55-70 micrograms	Meats, eggs, fish, seafoods, whole grains	Nausea, vomiting, hair loss, weakness, liver disease
Iodide	Part of thyroid hormone	Goiter; poor growth in infancy when mother is deficient in pregnancy	None in America, as salt is usually fortified	150 micrograms	Iodized salt, white bread, saltwater fish, dairy products	Inhibition of function of the thyroid gland

TABLE 10-6—CONT'D
A summary of key trace minerals

Mineral	Major Functions	Deficiency Symptoms	People Most at Risk	RDA or ESADDI	Nutrient Dense Dietary Sources	Results of Toxicity
Copper	Aids in iron metabolism; works with many enzymes, such as those involved in protein metabolism and hormone synthesis	Anemia, low white blood cell count, poor growth	Infants recovering from malnutrition, people who use overzealous supplementation of zinc	1.5-3 milligrams	Liver, cocoa, beans, nuts, whole grains, dried fruits	Vomiting; nervous system disorders
Fluoride	Increases resistance of tooth crystal to dental caries	Increased risk of dental caries	Areas where water is not fluoridated and dental treatments do not make up for this lack of fluoride	1.5-4 milligrams	Fluoridated water, toothpaste, dental treatments, tea, seaweed	Stomach upset, mottling (staining) of teeth during development
Chromium	Enhances blood glucose control	High blood glucose levels after eating	People on total parenteral nutrition, and perhaps elderly people with noninsulin-dependent diabetes mellitus	50-200 micrograms	Egg yolks, whole grains, pork	Due to industrial contamination, not dietary excess
Manganese	Aids action of some enzymes, such as those involved in carbohydrate metabolism	None in humans	Unknown	2-5 milligrams	Nuts, rice, oats, beans	Unknown in humans
Molybdenum	Aids action of some enzymes	None in humans	Unknown	75-250 micrograms	Beans, grains, nuts	Unknown in humans

CONCEPT CHECK

Chromium acts to maintain normal glucose uptake into cells. The amount of chromium found in food depends on soil content. Meats, whole grains, and egg yolks are some good sources. Manganese is a component of bone and used by many enzymes, including those involved in glucose production. Since our need for it is low, deficiencies are rare. Nuts, rice, oats, and beans are good food sources. Molybdenum is another trace mineral required by a few enzymes. Deficiencies appear only with intravenous diets. The needs for some other trace minerals, such as boron, nickel, arsenic, and vanadium, have not been fully established in humans. If required, they are needed in such small amounts that our current diets are probably adequate sources of them.

SUMMARY

- Water constitutes 50% to 70% of the human body. Its unique chemical properties enable it to dissolve substances, as well as serve as a medium for chemical reactions, temperature regulation, and lubrication. Water also helps regulate the acid-base balance in the body. For adults, daily water needs are estimated at 1 milliliter per kcalorie burned.

- Many minerals are vital for sustaining life. For humans, animal products are the most bioavailable sources of most minerals. Supplements of minerals exceeding 150% of the U.S. RDA should be taken only under a physician's supervision since toxicity and nutrient interactions are a likely possibility.

- Sodium, the major positive ion found outside cells, is vital in fluid balance and nerve impulse transmission. The American diet provides abundant sodium through processed foods and table salt. About 10% to 15% of the adult population is sodium-sensitive and is at risk for developing hypertension from consuming excessive sodium.

- Potassium, the major positive ion found inside cells, functions similarly to sodium. Milk, fruits, and vegetables are good sources. Chloride is the major negative ion found outside cells. It is important in digestion as part of gastric hydrochloric acid and in immune and nerve functions. Table salt supplies most of the chloride in our diets.

- Calcium forms a vital part of bone structure and is also very important in blood clotting, muscle contraction, nerve transmission, and cell control. Calcium absorption is enhanced by stomach acid and the active vitamin D hormone. Dairy products are important calcium sources. Bone loss in osteoporosis is linked to low calcium intake. Women are particularly at risk for this condition and should get plenty of calcium and exercise regularly. Estrogen replacement at menopause is currently the most accepted way to stop significant adult bone loss in women after menopause.

- Phosphorus aids enzyme function and forms part of energy-containing molecules, cell membranes, and bone. It is efficiently absorbed, and deficiencies are rare, although there is concern about the intake by elderly women. Good food sources are dairy products, bakery products, and meats. Sulfur is incorporated into certain vitamins and amino acids. Magnesium is a mineral found mostly in plants. It is important for nerve and heart function and as an activator for many enzymes. Whole grains (bran portion), vegetables, nuts, seeds, milk, and meats are good food sources.

- Iron absorption depends mainly on the form of iron present and the body's need for it. Heme iron from animal sources is better absorbed than the nonheme iron obtained primarily from plant sources. Consuming vitamin C simultaneously with iron will increase nonheme absorption. Iron operates mainly in synthesizing hemoglobin and myoglobin and in the action of the immune system. Women are at great risk for developing iron deficiency, which decreases blood hemoglobin level and red blood cell number. When this condition is severe enough to decrease the amount of oxygen carried in the blood, iron-deficiency anemia develops. Iron toxicity usually results from a genetic disorder called hemochromatosis. This disease causes overabsorption and accumulation of iron, which can result in severe liver and heart damage.

- Zinc functions aid in the action of over 200 enzymes that are important for growth, development, immune function, wound healing, and taste. A zinc deficiency results in poor growth, loss of appetite, reduced sense of taste and smell, hair loss, and a persistent rash. Zinc is best absorbed from animal sources. The most nutrient-dense sources of zinc are oysters, shrimp, crab, and beef. Good plant sources are whole grains, peanuts, and beans. Copper is important for iron metabolism, collagen cross-linking, and other functions. A copper deficiency can result in an iron-deficiency type anemia. Copper is found mainly in liver, cocoa, legumes, and whole grains. Milk is a poor source.

- An important role of selenium is decreasing the action of electron-seeking (oxidizing) compounds. In this way selenium acts along with vitamin E. Muscle pain, muscle wasting, and heart disease may result from a selenium deficiency. Meats, especially organ meats, eggs, fish, and shellfish are good animal sources of selenium. Good plant sources include grains and seeds. Selenium is potentially toxic in high doses. Iodide forms part of the thyroid hormones. A lack of dietary iodide results in the development of an enlarged thyroid gland or goiter. Iodized salt is a good food source. Fluoride incorporated into dietary intake during development makes teeth resistant to dental caries. Most Americans receive the bulk of their fluoride from fluoridated water and toothpaste.

- Chromium appears to help regulate glucose uptake by cells. Egg yolks, meats, and whole grains are good sources of chromium. Manganese and molybdenum are used by various enzymes. Deficiencies are rarely seen for any of these three nutrients. Human needs for other trace minerals are so low that deficiencies are uncommon.

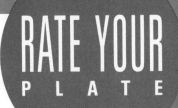

HOW DOES YOUR MINERAL INTAKE MEASURE UP AGAINST VALUES FROM THE CURRENT RDA?

To complete this activity you must reexamine your nutritional assessment from Chapter 2. Compare your intake of selective minerals to the RDA (or other standards given). Use your completed nutritional assessment to complete the table below. For each mineral, record your intake, the RDA, the percentage of the RDA you consumed, and a +, −, or = to indicate an intake higher, lower, or equal to the RDA. Note that for sodium and potassium minimum requirements of health are designated and are already recorded in the table (these also can be found on the inside front cover of the book). RDA have not been established for these two minerals.

Mineral	Intake	RDA	% of RDA	+, −, =
Calcium	452	800 mg	57%	−
Phosphorus		800 mg		
Sodium	2534	500 mg 2200	115%	+
Potassium	3,009	2000 mg 3750	80%	−
Iron	28.83	18 15 mg	160%	+
Zinc		15 mg		

ANALYSIS

1. Which of your mineral intakes equaled or exceeded the RDA (or other standard given)?

   Sodium + Iron

2. Which of your intakes were below the RDA (or other standard given)?

   Calcium + Potassium

3. What foods or cooking practices could be emphasized or deemphasized to modify your weaknesses?

   I could increase milk consumption to increase my cal. intake, (which I am currently trying hard to improve) Or I could eat more milk products like yogurt & cottage cheese. Increasing my milk consumption would also help to improve my potassium intake, or I could either increase serving size or consume on a more regular basis fruits & veg. (kiwis, oranges, bananas, spinach, squash)

329

REFERENCES

1. Anderson JB: Dietary calcium and bone mass throughout the life cycle, *Nutrition Today*, March/April, 1990, p 9.
2. Australian National Health and Medical Research Council: Fall in blood pressure with modest reduction in dietary salt intake in mild hypertension, *Lancet* 1:399, February 25, 1989.
3. Black MR and others: Zinc supplements and serum lipids in young adult white males, *American Journal of Clinical Nutrition* 47:970, 1988.
4. Castillo-Duran C, Uauy R: Copper deficiency impairs growth in infants recovering from malnutrition, *American Journal of Clinical Nutrition* 47:710, 1988.
5. Clydesdale FM: The relevance of mineral chemistry to bioavailability, *Nutrition Today*, March/April, 1989, p 23.
6. Cook JD: Adaptation in iron metabolism, *American Journal of Clinical Nutrition* 51:301, 1990.
7. Edwards CQ and others: Prevalence of hemochromatosis among 11,065 presumably healthy blood donors, *New England Journal of Medicine* 318:1355, 1988.
8. Fosmire GJ: Zinc toxicity, *American Journal of Clinical Nutrition* 51:225, 1990.
9. Freeland-Graves JH: Manganese: an essential nutrient, *Nutrition Today*, November/December, 1988, p 13.
10. Garraway WM, Whisnant JP: The changing pattern of hypertension and the declining incidents of stroke, *Journal of the American Medical Association* 258:214, 1987.
11. Heaney RP and others: Calcium absorbability from spinach, *American Journal of Clinical Nutrition* 47:707, 1988.
12. Johnson MA, Kays SE: Copper: its role in human nutrition, *Nutrition Today*, January/February, 1990, p 6.
13. Kaplan NM, Ram CUS: Potassium supplements for hypertension, *New England Journal of Medicine* 322:623, 1990.
14. Mazess RB, Barden HS: Bone density in premenopausal women: effects of age, dietary intake, physical activity, smoking, and birth-control pills, *American Journal of Clinical Nutrition* 53:132, 1991.
15. Monsen ER: Iron nutrition and absorption: dietary factors which impact iron bioavailability, *Journal of the American Dietetic Association* 88:786, 1988.
16. Moser-Veillon PB: Zinc: consumption patterns and dietary recommendations, *Journal of the American Dietetic Association* 90:1089, 1990.
17. Nielsen FH: Nutritional significance of the ultratrace elements, *Nutrition Reviews* 46:337, 1988.
18. Pennington JAT, Young BE: Total diet study nutritional elements, 1982-1989, *Journal of The American Dietetic Association* 91:179, 1991.
19. Pennington JAT: A review of iodine toxicity, *Journal of the American Dietetic Association* 90:1571, 1990.
20. Randal HT: Water, electrolytes, and acid-based balance. In Shils ME, Young VR, editors: *Modern nutrition in health and disease*, Philadelphia, 1988, Lea & Febiger.
21. Rasmussen HS and others: Influence of magnesium substitution therapy on blood lipid composition in patients with ischemic heart disease, *Archives of Internal Medicine* 149:1050, 1989.
22. Recker RR and others: Calcium absorbability from milk products and imitation milk and calcium carbonate, *American Journal of Clinical Nutrition* 47:93, 1988.
23. Robinson MF: Selenium in human nutrition in New Zealand, *Nutrition Reviews* 47:99, 1989.
24. Rolls BJ, Phillips PA: Aging and disturbance of thirst and fluid balance, *Nutrition Reviews* 48:137, 1990.
25. Schottee DE, Stunkard AJ: The effects of weight reduction on blood pressure in 301 obese patients, *Archives of Internal Medicine* 150:1701, 1990.
26. Sorenson AW and others: Calcium and colon cancer: a review, *Nutrition and Cancer* 11:135, 1988.
27. Spencer H and others: Do protein and phosphorus cause calcium loss? *Journal of Nutrition* 118:657, 1988.
28. Wardlaw GM, Barden HS: Osteoporosis—summary of the 19th Steenbock Symposium, *Nutrition Today*, September/October, 1989, p 30.

HOW MUCH HAVE I LEARNED?

What have you learned from Chapter 10? Here are 15 statements about water and minerals. Read them to test your current knowledge. If you think the answer is true or mostly true, circle T. If you think the answer is false or mostly false, circle F. Use the scoring key at the end of the book to compute your total score. To review, take this test again later, and especially before tests.

1. T **(F)** Major minerals are more important to health than trace minerals.

2. **(T)** F Vitamins often need minerals to help perform metabolic reactions.

3. T **(F)** Plant foods are usually the best sources of minerals.

4. **(T)** F When water evaporates from your skin, you feel cooler because evaporating water takes heat with it.

5. **(T)** F Sodium is often added to processed foods.

6. T **(F)** Calcium supplements can prevent osteoporosis.

7. T **(F)** Salt is bad for most people.

8. **(T)** F Trace mineral deficiencies are difficult to detect.

9. **(T)** F Some trace minerals interfere with the absorption of other minerals.

10. **(T)** F Iron is the only nutrient with a higher RDA for adult women than for adult men.

11. T **(F)** Iron is easily excreted from the body when consumed in excess.

12. **(T)** F Zinc is important to the growth of children.

13. **(T)** F An iodide deficiency can result in a goiter.

14. **(T)** F Copper plays a role in iron metabolism.

15. **(T)** F Fluoride inhibits the growth of the bacterium that causes dental caries.

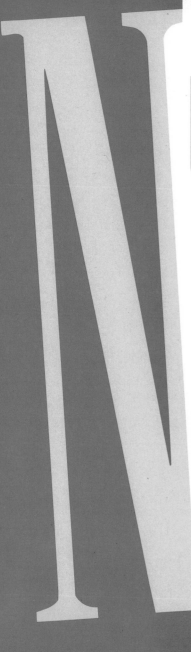

MINERALS AND HYPERTENSION

Blood pressure is expressed by two different numbers. The higher number represents systolic blood pressure, the pressure in the arteries when the heart actively pumps blood. The second value is diastolic pressure, the pressure in the arteries when the heart is relaxed. Normal systolic blood pressure values vary from 100 to 140 millimeters of mercury (mm Hg). Normal diastolic blood pressure values vary from 60 to 90 mm Hg.

Hypertension is defined as sustained high blood pressure, usually with systolic pressure exceeding 140 mm Hg or diastolic blood pressure exceeding 90 mm Hg. Most hypertension (90% to 95%) has no apparent cause. It is called primary or *essential* hypertension. Kidney disease often causes the other 5% to 10% of cases.

About 30% of adults have essential hypertension. This is called a *silent* disease because, unless blood pressure is measured periodically, no one knows it is developing. A physician usually does not treat hypertension with medication until the diastolic blood pressure measures at least 95 mm Hg on three or more occasions. But any value over 90 mm Hg is actually too high and deserves dietary and lifestyle interventions.

Why control hypertension?

Hypertension needs to be controlled mainly to prevent heart disease, kidney disease, and strokes. All three diseases are much more likely to be found in people with hypertension than in those with normal blood pressure. People with hypertension should be diagnosed and treated as soon as possible. We now know the value of aggressively treating hypertension; in the last 20 years, blood pressure values have fallen, along with strokes and heart attacks.[10]

Causes of high blood pressure

A variety of factors affect blood pressure. Blood pressure usually increases as a person ages. Atherosclerosis causes some increase (see Chapter 7). As plaque builds up, arteries become less flexible and cannot expand as the heart pumps. When vessels remain rigid, blood pressure remains high. Eventually the plaque begins to choke off blood supply to the kidneys, decreasing their ability to control blood volume and, in turn, blood pressure.

Obesity is associated with high blood pressure, especially in men. Inactivity also increases the risk for high blood pressure. If an obese person can lose weight and become more physically active by exercising three to four times a week, blood pressure often returns to normal values. A weight loss of as little as 10 pounds can help, especially in men.[25] Often a minor change in lifestyle can greatly reduce, or even eliminate, the need for medications.

Blacks are more likely to have high blood pressure than are whites. In addition, alcohol has a greater tendency to raise blood pressure in blacks than it does in whites. However, both races should moderate alcohol intake, especially men, to control blood pressure. Various blood enzymes and hormonelike compounds also affect blood pressure.

Sodium and blood pressure

Sodium tends to increase blood pressure in some people. The average adult intake of 3 to 7 grams can elevate blood pressure, particularly in those who are sensitive to its effects. However, not all of the 30% of Americans with hypertension are very sensitive to sodium. Therefore sodium in the diet is not a problem for everyone, even among people with hypertension. Nevertheless, in populations that eat 1.5 grams or less of sodium daily, hypertension is rare. A decrease in blood pressure usually appears when sodium is restricted to a level of approximately 2 grams a day.[2] Although some experts recommend that all people with hypertension reduce sodium intake, ideally, we feel dietary advice should be given on an individual basis once a response to treatment is verified.

Calcium and blood pressure

Since 1983 there has been debate concerning whether calcium intake can affect blood pressure. Careful studies show that some people register slightly lower blood pressures when they consume the RDA for calcium compared to a poor intake. Systolic blood pressure is affected more than diastolic blood pressure. It is reasonable for a person with hypertension to experiment, in consultation with a physician, by increasing calcium intake to see if that produces a benefit worth the trouble and expense.

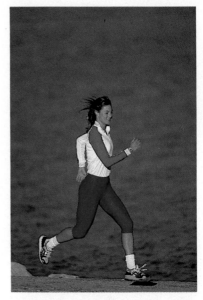

Add regular exercise to your efforts to keep blood pressure under control.

Preventing hypertension

Hypertension develops in many adults, especially in those with family histories of hypertension. To prevent hypertension, we recommend maintaining an active lifestyle and a desirable body weight. Regular exercise is a key component. Limiting alcohol use is also very important. A reduction in stress adds to the list of preventive measures. Population studies suggest that a low-sodium diet may lead to less hypertension later in life. But many people never develop hypertension, regardless of their sodium intake. As we saw with dietary cholesterol in Chapter 7, sodium appears to be a villain only for some of us. If you have hypertension or a family history of hypertension, it is a good idea to reduce sodium intake. The American Heart Association suggests that you keep your sodium intake under 3 grams per day. Some people may choose to limit their sodium only if hypertension develops. As we said before, most of us need to be prudent—not paranoid—about dietary sodium.

In addition, we suggest consuming a diet rich in dairy products, fruits, and vegetables. This provides ample potassium, calcium, and magnesium—all of which may contribute to a lower blood pressure.[13] Even if drugs are needed, a proper diet and lifestyle approach can often reduce the necessary dosage and, in turn, reduce the expense and side effects of medications. Nutritional therapy is a key to treating hypertension. ●

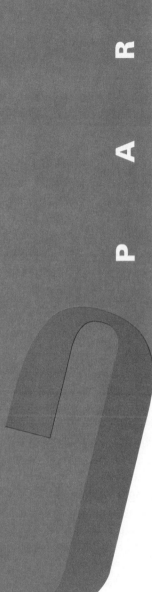

ENERGY

**BALANCE
AND
IMBALANCE**

WEIGHT CONTROL

Imagine a magic pill or potion melting away unwanted pounds. No sweat or starvation, just a sleek body in a few quick swallows. Many *magical* drinks, drugs, and diet programs claim they eliminate excess fat forever. Unfortunately, many people trust in these too good to believe offers.

Consumers presently pour $33 billion into the diet industry, a business predicted to increase $20 billion within 5 years. The diet industry digests dollars, and consumers lose not only pounds. They often lose cash needlessly—and sometimes good health.

Of people you see on the street, one fourth of the men and nearly half the women you see will be struggling to control weight.[24] But for all the struggles, the ranks of the obese in America are still bulging. With the bulge comes a hefty increase in diet-of-the-century books. Nonetheless, most diets fizzle before bodies become slim. Monotonous, ineffective, and confusing, diets endanger some populations, such as children, teenagers, pregnant women, and people with various health disorders.

The secret to weight loss is actually as simple as one, two, three: (1) eat less, (2) exercise more, and (3) change problem eating behaviors.[6] This chapter discusses these recommendations to help you understand obesity's causes, treatments, and effects. You will explore how obesity is linked to environment and heredity and how these factors make the battle of the bulge harder for some than for others. You will learn how to take charge of a weight problem by replacing fad diets with the three key recommendations mentioned above. ●

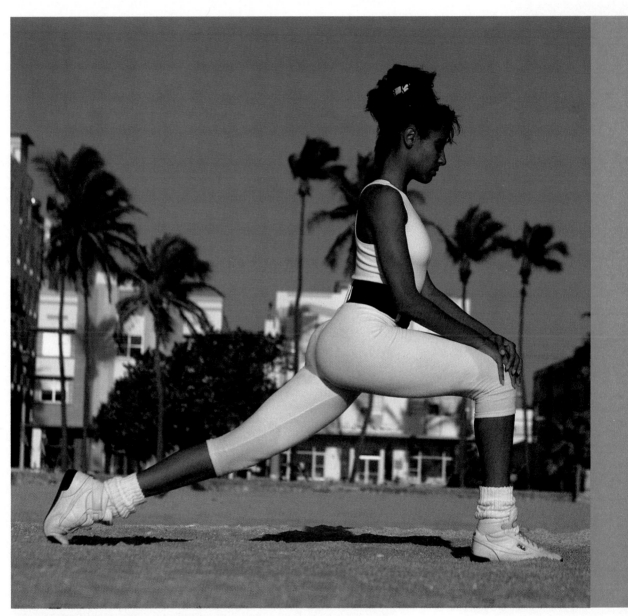

Physical activity is one of the three classes of energy use by the body.

Is The TTFV Lipoloss Weight Loss Plan For You?

Read the following discussion of the TTFV Lipoloss Weight Loss Plan. See if it is one you would want to follow.

Do you want to turn your body into a high-powered fat burner? Try the TTFV Lipoloss Weight Loss Plan, scientifically proven to be the quickest and most permanent fat loss miracle in America. The nutritional part of the TTFV Plan consists of eating 800 kcalories of delicious tuna, turkey, fruits, and vegetables. Combine the fruits with the turkey and the vegetables with the tuna to achieve the greatest lipoloss effect (remember, lipo means fat).

We encourage at least 30 minutes of aerobic exercise—brisk walking, jogging, swimming, or biking—three to five times per week. And we haven't forgotten those diet-wrecking urges and cravings. Fight them with our high fiber Urgesmasher Wafers. These wafers fill you up, fighting the gnaw of hunger.

If you have any health problems, see your physician for approval and clearance for regular exercise. Overall, with the TTFV LipoLoss Plan you can lose 3 to 5 pounds each week and enjoy a variety of tasty food.

Now rate this diet based on the following questions; a perfect score of 100 points indicates a good weight loss plan.

1. Will the diet meet all nutritional needs with a wide variety of foods? IF NOT, SUBTRACT 10 POINTS.
2. Does the program stress slow and steady weight loss of about 1 to 2 pounds per week rather than rapid loss? IF NOT, SUBTRACT 10 POINTS.
3. Is the diet tailored to individual habits and tastes, diminishing feelings of deprivation? IF NOT, SUBTRACT 10 POINTS.
4. Does the plan avoid rigid rituals such as eating fruits only in the morning or not eating meat after milk products? IF NOT, SUBTRACT 10 POINTS.
5. Does the diet minimize hunger and fatigue by containing at least 1000 kcalories per day? IF NOT, SUBTRACT 10 POINTS.
6. Does the diet include readily obtainable foods, with no special products to buy to speed weight loss? IF NOT, SUBTRACT 10 POINTS.
7. Is the diet socially acceptable, allowing the dieter to attend parties, eat at restaurants, and participate in normal daily activity? IF NOT, SUBTRACT 10 POINTS.
8. Does the plan promote changes in eating habits and lifestyle so that weight maintenance will be possible? IF NOT, SUBTRACT 10 POINTS.
9. Does the plan emphasize regular physical activity? IF NOT, SUBTRACT 10 POINTS.
10. Does the plan encourage the dieter to see a physician before starting if the person has existing health problems, wants quick weight loss, is over 35 years of age, or plans to perform vigorous physical activity? IF NOT, SUBTRACT 10 POINTS.

Now, having assessed the TTFV Lipoloss Weight Loss Plan, how many points would you give it?   SCORE _____

Would you choose this weight loss plan if you were attempting to lose fat and keep it off?   YES _____   NO _____

To assess the legitimacy of any weight loss plan, ask yourself questions like those above. With so many competing diet plans available, you can save yourself money, disappointment, effort, and time by asking the right questions.

ASSESS YOURSELF

ENERGY INTAKE: THE FIRST HALF OF ENERGY BALANCE

Does your weight yo-yo up and down while you aim for your ideal? If the scales keep you emotionally off balance, consider another scale—that of energy balance. This balance depends on kcalorie input and kcalorie output. Excesses or

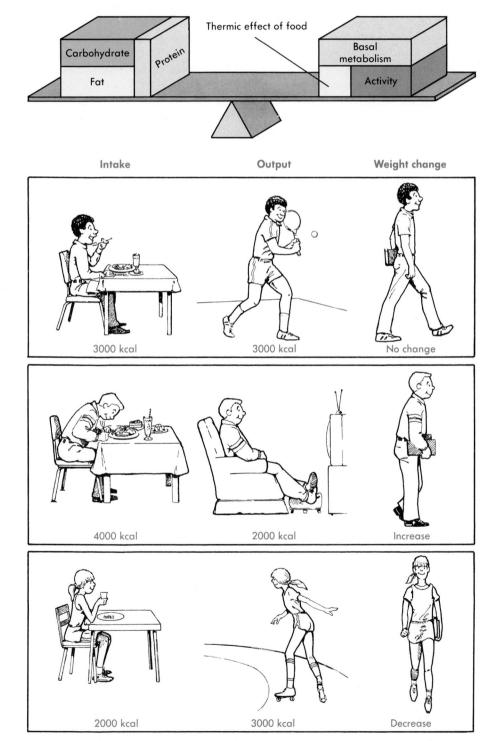

FIGURE 11-1

A model for energy balance. This model incorporates the major variables that influence energy balance. Overall, to maintain weight we need to use roughly the same number of kcalories we consume. It's a simple equation, but an unforgiving one if we deviate either way.

Hunger • The physiological drive to find and eat food.

Appetite • The psychological drive to find and eat food, often in the absence of hunger.

Satiety • A state in which there is no longer a desire to eat.

Hypothalamus • A grouping of cells at the base of the brain. These cells participate in many body functions, such as in the regulation of hunger.

deficits in this balance go on to influence energy stores, primarily in adipose (fat) tissue (Figure 11-1). Let's look at the factors affecting this balance.

Two drives influence our desire to eat, **hunger** and **appetite.** These differ dramatically. Hunger is our physiological drive to eat; appetite is our psychological drive to eat. Fulfilling both drives normally brings a state of **satiety,** temporarily halting the desire to eat.[18]

The hypothalamus: a satiety regulator

The **hypothalamus,** a portion of the brain stem, helps regulate satiety. When stimulated, cells in the *feeding center* of the hypothalamus signal us to eat. Hunger decreases—and we are likely to stop eating—when cells in the *satiety center* of the hypothalamus are stimulated.[26] Blood glucose levels probably stimulate both of these centers. When glucose levels drop, we eat. Other cues to eat likely come from amino acids and fatty acids in the bloodstream and from various hormones and other substances.

Chemicals, surgery, and some cancers can destroy the feeding and satiety centers in the hypothalamus. Without satiety center activity, laboratory animals (and humans) eat their way to obesity. Without feeding-center activity, animals eat little and eventually lose weight.

Satiety is regulated at other body sites

Satiety is actually controlled by a complex network of body sites that regulate the desire to either eat or avoid food. The satiety and feeding centers in the hypothalamus especially communicate and interact with other decision points in the brain and in the liver.[18]

Hormones regulate satiety

Endorphins, the body's natural painkillers, and hormones, such as high amounts of cortisol, can prod us to eat. On the other hand, other hormones, hormone-related compounds, and still other chemical factors in the body can contribute to the feeling of satiety.[8] With eating, blood concentrations of some digestive hormones—cholecystokinin (CCK), secretin, gastrin, and others—increase. This increase, combined with stomach distention, helps shut off hunger.[26] Certain arms of the nervous system also contribute to this satiety.

Does appetite regulate what we eat?

Various feeding and satiety messages from body cells do not singlehandedly influence what we eat. Almost everyone has encountered a mouthwatering dessert and devoured it, even on a full stomach (Figure 11-2).

We often eat because food confronts us. It smells good, tastes good, and looks good. We might eat because it is the right time of day, we are celebrating, or are trying to overcome the blues. Appetite may not be a biological process,

FIGURE 11-2
The Middletons.

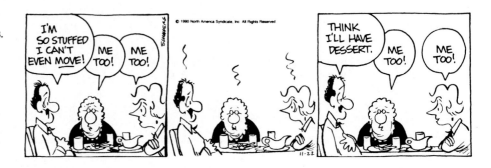

but it does influence food intake. After a meal, memories of pleasant tastes and feelings reinforce appetite. If stress or depression sends you to the refrigerator, you are mostly seeking comfort, not energy.

American prosperity and ample food supply set the stage for a population that eats primarily from appetite and habit, not hunger. If you rarely feel real hunger, you probably reach for food mostly as a reflex (Figure 11-3).

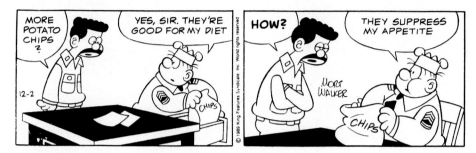

And later . . .

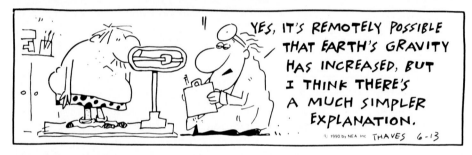

FIGURE 11-3
Beetle Bailey and Frank & Ernest.

Putting hunger and appetite into perspective

The next time you pick up a candy bar or ask for second helpings, remember the physiological and psychological influences on eating behavior (Figure 11-4). Body cells (brain, mouth, stomach, intestine, liver, and other organs), hormones (like cortisol), and social customs all influence food intake. Where food is ample, appetite, not hunger, mostly triggers eating. Keep track of what triggers your eating for a few days. Is it primarily hunger or appetite?

CONCEPT CHECK

Hunger is the physiological drive to find and eat food. Appetite is the psychological drive to find and eat food. Appeasing them both typically leaves us satiated. This state of satiety depends on messages from cells in the brain, liver, other organs, various hormones, other chemical substances in the body, and nervous system activity. Appetite is affected by social custom, habit, time of day, food availability, palatability, and other factors. Americans probably respond to appetite cues more than hunger cues for choosing when to eat.

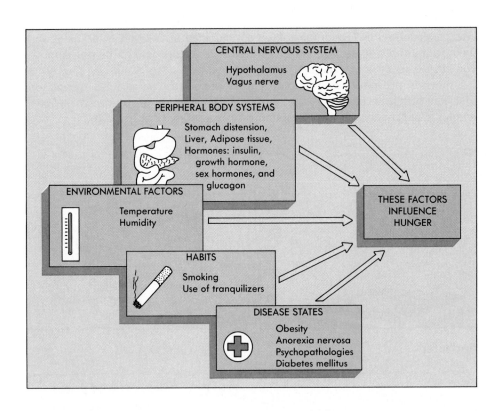

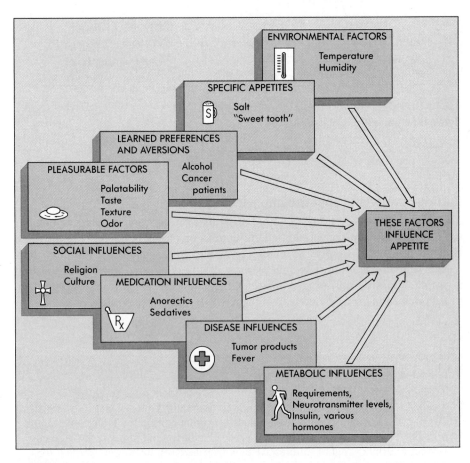

FIGURE 11-4

A model incorporating many factors that influence hunger and appetite. Together these influences regulate satiety.

ENERGY USE: THE OTHER SIDE OF ENERGY BALANCE

We have examined some factors that encourage energy intake. Now let's look at the other side of the relationship—energy output.

Energy use by the body

The body uses energy for three general purposes: basal metabolism, physical activity, and the thermic effect of food (Figure 11-1). Shivering, the body's reflex to cold, demonstrates another minor form of energy turned into heat production.

Basal metabolism

Basal metabolism represents the minimum energy expended to keep a resting, awake body alive. This requires about 60% to 70% of total kcalorie use by the body. The processes involved include maintaining a heartbeat, respiration, temperature, and other functions. It does not include energy used for physical activity or digesting foods. Basal metabolism accounts for about 1 kcalorie per minute or about 1450 kcalories per day.

Energy used in basal metabolism depends primarily on lean body mass. The participating tissues, such as muscles and liver, show high metabolic activity and have high kcalorie needs. Other influences that determine basal metabolism are:

- the amount of body surface (the greater the area the greater the heat loss).
- gender (males average higher energy rates because of greater lean body mass).
- body temperature (fever increases metabolic rate).
- thyroid hormone levels (higher levels increase metabolic rate).
- aspects of nervous system activity.
- age (metabolic rate falls as we age through adulthood).
- nutritional state (eating less slows metabolic rate).
- pregnancy (metabolic rate increases).
- caffeine and tobacco use (metabolic rate increases).

A low-kcalorie intake decreases the basal metabolic rate (BMR) about 10% to 20%, or about 150 to 300 kcalories per day.[24] This lowered BMR makes losing weight difficult. In addition, the effects of aging make weight maintenance hard. BMR declines about 2% each decade past age 30 as actively metabolizing cells slowly and steadily decrease. However, because physical activity helps maintain lean body mass, remaining active as one ages helps maintain a high basal metabolism and, in turn, aids weight control.

Energy for physical activity

Physical activity demands about 25% to 40% of total energy output. In choosing to be inactive or active, we determine our energy expenditure. Unlike basal metabolism, this expenditure varies widely among people. Basal metabolism uses roughly the same proportion of energy in most people (usually ± 25% to 30%).

Climbing stairs rather than riding the elevator, walking rather than driving to the store, and standing in a bus rather than sitting increase physical activity and, hence, energy use. Recent studies show that people who fidget and can't sit still use more energy (an extra 100 to 800 kcalories daily in one study) than those who readily relax.

The alarming rate of obesity in America is caused by our inactivity.[6] We eat little more than people did at the turn of this century, but we are less active. Jobs demand less physical activity, and leisure time usually is spent slouched before a television. What are the alternatives to obesity and inactivity? One answer is *movement!*

Basal Metabolism • The minimum energy the body requires to support itself when resting and awake. It amounts to roughly 1 kcalorie per minute, or about 1400 kcalories per day.

While a person is resting, the brain and liver together use about 60% of body energy, muscle uses about 20%, and fat tissue about 2% to 5%.

343

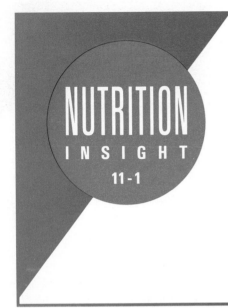

THE TRUE ENERGY VALUE OF FAT

In the bomb calorimeter, fats produce about 9 kcalories per gram. However, when stored for energy, fats function very efficiently. Dietary fats induce little thermic effect of food because most fat consumed bypasses the liver on its way to the bloodstream and ultimately to body cells. Thus because no energy is used to metabolize it in the liver, very little energy in fat is lost when it transfers from food directly to fat storage.

In contrast, all carbohydrate and protein eaten must pass through the liver, the latter as amino acids. We have an especially limited ability to store carbohydrate.[3] Excess amounts generally are metabolized into various fats and go on to the bloodstream. This includes excess protein intake as well. Metabolic changes demand about a quarter of the energy content of carbohydrates or proteins.

Scientists note that, fed equal amounts of kcalories, growing rats on high-fat diets gain more weight than rats on lowfat diets. If fats use fewer kcalories per gram during their initial distribution in the body, it follows that high-fat diets will cause greater weight gain. Overall, high-fat foods tend to make us fat. In cutting kcalories, eliminating fat first is the best policy. ●

Thermic Effect of Food • The increase in metabolism occurring during the digestion, absorption, and metabolism of energy-yielding nutrients. This represents 5% to 10% of kcalories consumed.

Direct Calorimetry • A method to determine energy use by the body by measuring heat that emanates from the body.

Thermic effect of food

In addition to basal metabolism and physical activity, the body uses energy to digest, absorb, and further process food nutrients.[20] Energy used for these tasks contributes the *thermic effect of food*. The energy cost of this thermic effect is analogous to a sales tax. It is like being taxed about 5% to 10% for the total kcalories you eat. The charge covers the cost of processing those kcalories. To supply the body with 100 kcalories for basal metabolism and physical activity, a person must then eat between 105 and 110 kcalories. The processes of digestion, absorption, and metabolism use the extra 5 to 10 kcalories to modify the energy-yielding nutrients for use. Given a daily kcalorie intake of 3000, the thermic effect of food would use 180 to 300 kcalories. The total amount used varies little between individuals.

CONCEPT CHECK

The body uses energy for three main purposes.

- Basal metabolism represents the minimum amount of energy needed to maintain a body in a resting state. The rate of a person's basal metabolism depends greatly on the amount of lean body mass, the amount of body surface, thyroid hormone levels, and other hormone levels.
- Physical activity represents energy use for total body cell metabolism above what is needed during rest (i.e., basal metabolism).
- The thermic effect of food represents the energy needed to digest, absorb, and process absorbed nutrients. This corresponds to about 5% to 10% of energy used for basal metabolism and physical activity.

In a sedentary person, most energy (60% to 75%) is used for basal metabolism combined with the thermic effect of food.

MEASURING ENERGY USE BY THE BODY
Direct and indirect calorimetry

The amount of energy a body uses can be measured by both direct and indirect calorimetry. To understand *direct calorimetry,* imagine a science fiction film in which a creature is submerged in ice water. The creature gradually raises the water temperature to a tropic warm simply by releasing body heat. Direct calorimetry uses this concept to measure the body heat released by a person. The subject is put into an insulated chamber, often the size of a small bedroom, and body heat released raises the temperature of a layer of water surrounding the chamber. A kcalorie, recall, is the amount of heat required to raise the temperature of 1 liter of water 1 degree Celsius. By measuring the water temperature in the direct calorimeter before and after the body releases heat, scientists can determine the number of kcalories expended.[20] This method resembles the bomb calorimeter's method for measuring the kcalorie content in food (see Figure 1-2).

Indirect Calorimetry • A method to estimate the energy use by the body by measuring oxygen uptake and then using formulas to convert that gas usage into kcalorie use.

Today, scientific journals often express energy intake and output in kjoules, rather than kcalories. A kjoule is a measure of work, not heat. It is the amount of work involved in moving 1 kilogram for 1 meter with the force of 1 newton. Heat and work are just two forms of energy. Energy expressions in the form of either heat or work can be exchanged for each other; 4.18 kjoules equals 1 kcalorie.

Direct calorimetry works because all the energy used by the body eventually leaves as heat. However, few studies use direct calorimetry, mostly because of its expense and complexity.

In *indirect calorimetry,* instead of measuring heat output, a technician measures the amount of oxygen a person uses (Figure 11-5). A predictable relationship exists between the body's use of energy and oxygen. For example, when burning a mixed diet of carbohydrate, fat, and protein—a typical blend of nutrients we use—the human body needs 1 liter of oxygen to burn about 4.85 kcalories.[20]

Instruments used to measure oxygen consumption for indirect calorimetry have great versatility. They can be mounted on carts and rolled up to a hospital bed or carried in backpacks while a person plays tennis or jogs. Tables showing energy demands of various exercises rely on information gained from indirect calorimetry studies (see Appendix M).

Estimating energy needs

The RDA provides rough estimates of total energy needs for people who perform light activity (see inside cover). Another rough estimate uses a person's weight and activity level. Total energy needs for a sedentary person are set at 9 kcalories per pound (20 kcalories per kilogram). The value is then decreased by 100 kcalories for every 10 years of age over age 30. People performing light activity such as routine walking start with 13 kcalories per pound (30 kcalories per kilogram); regularly performing heavy activity, as required in some sports play, starts at 20 kcalories per pound (45 kcalories per kilogram). These values are then adjusted for age as mentioned above. For example, a 150-pound, 40-year-old woman performing light activity needs to eat about 1850 ([13 × 150]−100) kcalories to meet total energy needs.

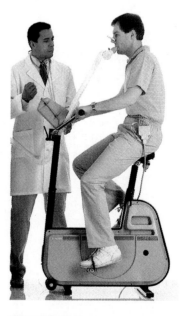

FIGURE 11-5

Indirect calorimetry. This method can be used to measure energy output during daily activities.

CONCEPT CHECK

Energy use by the body is measured by direct calorimetry as heat given off and by indirect calorimetry as oxygen used. Total energy needs can be estimated based on the RDA using a person's weight, age, and activity level.

Obesity • A condition characterized by excess body fat, usually defined as weighing 20% above desirable weight.

ENERGY IMBALANCE

Problems associated with *obesity*—the major type of energy imbalance in America—go far beyond any social stigma (Table 11-1). Since 1948 the Framingham Heart Study has medically tracked several thousand residents of Framingham, a small Massachusetts town. The study has observed that carrying an excess of 20% or more of one's desirable weight poses health risks. This supports other studies that show excess weight raises risk for:[6,17]

- surgical complications
- adult-onset (noninsulin-dependent) diabetes mellitus
- hypertension
- heart disease
- arthritis
- gallstones
- various forms of cancer—colon, rectal, and prostate cancer in men and breast, uterine, and ovarian cancer in women
- pregnancy risks
- early death

Numerous studies indicate that a significant number of people with hypertension, noninsulin-dependent diabetes mellitus, and osteoarthritis can reverse the conditions through weight loss. Table 11-1 lists possible explanations of why obesity causes some of these disorders.[19]

TABLE 11-1

Health problems associated with excess body fat

Health problem	Partially attributed to:
Surgical risk	Increased anesthesia needs and greater risk of wound infections
Pulmonary disease	Excess weight over lungs
Adult-onset diabetes mellitus (NIDDM)	Enlarged fat cells, which then poorly bind insulin and also poorly respond to the message insulin sends to the cell
Hypertension	Increased miles of blood vessels found in the fat tissue; however, no validated cause is yet known
Coronary heart disease	Increases in serum cholesterol and triglyceride levels, as well as a decrease in physical activity
Bone and joint disorders	Excess pressure put on knee, ankle, and hip joints
Gallbladder stones	An increase in cholesterol content of bile
Skin disorders	The trapping of moisture and microbes in fat folds
Various cancers	Estrogen production by fat cells; animal studies suggest excess energy intake encourages tumor development
Shorter stature (in some forms of obesity)	An earlier onset of puberty
Pregnancy risk	More difficult delivery and increased anesthesia needs (if the latter is used)
Early death	A variety of risk factors for disease listed above

The greater the degree of obesity, the more likely and the more serious these health problems generally become. They are much more likely to appear in people who are greater than twice their desirable body weight.

Defining obesity

Obesity can be defined along the dimensions of body weight, body fat, fat distribution, and age of onset (Figure 11-6).

Using body weight. Overweight can be defined as weighing at least 10% more than desirable body weight. Obesity weighs in at 20% more than desired weight.[19] Body weight is actually a crude measure of obesity because it can miss the critical factor—being overfat. However, with the exception of the husky athlete, overfat and overweight (obese) conditions generally appear together. The focus is on body weight because it is easier to measure.

Medical literature currently uses the term desirable rather than ideal when referring to body weight.

As the following chart shows, obesity comes in degrees. While mild obesity carries little risk, morbid obesity raises overall health risk twelve fold.[2]

Degrees of obesity

% Over desirable body weight	% Of cases	Form of obesity
20 to 40	90%	MILD
41 to 99	9.8%	MODERATE
100+	0.2%	SEVERE (MORBID)

To determine desirable body weight, most physicians, registered dietitians, and research scientists use the current (1983) Metropolitan Life Insurance Table (Table 11-2).[19] This tool estimates weights that enable people to lead a long life. The weight range is based on height, age, and frame size. Methods of estimating frame size use measurements of wrist width or elbow breadth (see Appendix K). The weight range listed does not, however, necessarily tell which weight offers optimal health. If you have good health and weigh slightly more or less than the chart range indicates, you need not be concerned.

The Metropolitan Life Insurance Table does not offer weight estimates for people over 60 years of age. It is not clear if the condition of overweight or obesity in elderly people follows the same pattern of association with disease as it does in younger people. An obese, elderly person may have already avoided the

DEGREE OF CONFIDENCE	METHOD	CUT OFF VALUE
Rough estimate	% of desirable weight (Current wt. − desirable wt.) x 100 / Desirable weight	Mild: >20% Moderate: >40% Severe: >100% (morbid)
↓	Body mass index (wt (kg)/ht² (m))	Mild: 25-30 Moderate: 30-35 Severe: 35-40
↓	Total body fat from skinfold thicknesses/bioelectrical impedance/infrared measurements or Loss of weight while underwater (hydrostatic weighing)	Men: >25% of body weight Women: >30% of body weight
Sensitive estimate of obesity—related health risk	Upper body distribution of fat stores	Ratio of waist to hip circumference: Men: >0.9 Women: >0.8

FIGURE 11-6

Diagnosing the extent of obesity to predict health risk. If one is obese by any of these measures and has an upper body distribution of fat stores, the risk of complications is more likely than if the fat distribution is primarily in the lower body.

Body Mass Index • Weight (in kilograms) divided by height squared (in meters); a value of 30 or more indicates obesity.

typical causes of death, such as stroke, heart disease, and cancer, to which obesity contributes. The fact that they have survived into their 70s and 80s could suggest that they are more resistant to the effects of obesity than people who have already died.

The *pounds per inch of height* method for estimating desirable body weight offers another measurement. For women allow 100 pounds for the first 5 feet, and add 5 pounds for every inch thereafter. To estimate a man's desirable body weight, allow 106 pounds for the first 5 feet and then add 6 pounds for each inch thereafter. A 6 foot tall man then should weigh about 178 pounds (106 + [12 × 6]) based on this system.

Using body mass index. *Body mass index* offers an alternative way to define obesity.[2] To calculate body mass index, divide a person's weight in kilograms by height in meters squared. Figure 11-7 does this calculation for you. A 70-kilogram (154-pound) man who is 1.78 meters (70 inches) tall has a body mass index of 22 ($70/[1.78]^2$).

TABLE 11-2

1983 Metropolitan Life Insurance Co height and weight table

Height	Small Frame	Medium Frame	Large Frame
		Weight in pounds	
Men[*]			
5′ 2″	128-134	131-141	138-150
5′ 3″	130-136	133-143	140-153
5′ 4″	132-138	135-145	142-156
5′ 5″	134-140	137-148	144-160
5′ 6″	136-142	139-151	146-164
5′ 7″	138-145	142-154	149-168
5′ 8″	140-148	145-157	152-172
5′ 9″	142-151	148-160	155-176
5′10″	144-154	151-163	158-180
5′11″	146-157	154-166	161-184
6′ 0″	149-160	157-170	164-188
6′ 1″	152-164	160-174	168-192
6′ 2″	155-168	164-178	172-197
6′ 3″	158-172	167-182	176-202
6′ 4″	162-176	171-187	181-207
Women[†]			
4′10″	102-111	109-121	118-131
4′11″	103-113	111-123	120-134
5′ 0″	104-115	113-126	122-137
5′ 1″	106-118	115-129	125-140
5′ 2″	108-121	118-132	128-143
5′ 3″	111-124	121-135	131-147
5′ 4″	114-127	124-138	134-151
5′ 5″	117-130	127-141	137-155
5′ 6″	120-133	130-144	140-159
5′ 7″	123-136	133-147	143-163
5′ 8″	126-139	136-150	146-167
5′ 9″	129-142	139-153	149-170
5′10″	132-145	142-156	152-173
5′11″	135-148	145-159	155-176
6′ 0″	138-151	148-162	158-179

[*]Weights at ages 25 to 59, based on lowest mortality. Weight in pounds according to frame (in indoor clothing weighing 5 lb, shoes with 1″ heels).
[†]Weights at ages 25 to 59, based on lowest mortality. Weight in pounds according to frame (in indoor clothing weighing 3 lb, shoes with 1″ heels).
See Appendix K for methods to determine frame size.
Courtesy of Metropolitan Life Insurance Company.

When the body mass index exceeds 25, obesity-related health risks begin for men and women (Figure 11-7). At a value of about 27, the risk for diabetes mellitus or hypertension is three times greater than normal and the risk for a high serum cholesterol level (greater than 240 milligrams per deciliter) is two times normal. A body mass index above 30 poses even greater health risks. About 10% of Americans exceed this value. A body mass index above 40 represents a severe health risk. These body mass index values for health risk are the same for both men and women.

Using body fat. Remember, risks of being overweight apply mostly to people who are overfat. Men with over 25% body fat and women with over 30% body fat run health risks.[2] Dropping body fat to about 15% for men and 25% fat for women also drops risk. Women need more body fat than men because some sex-specific fat is needed for reproductive functions. Because this extra fat in women is needed, it is factored into calculations of body composition.

Various methods are used to determine body fat levels. Underwater weighing, the most accurate method, works because fat tissue is less dense than lean tissue; since fat floats, the more fat tissue present, the less a person weighs when submerged. Because this procedure requires a trained technician and forces the subject to be submerged, it is primarily used as a research tool.

The method most widely used to estimate total body fat is skinfold thickness. Clinicians use special calipers to measure the fat layer directly under the

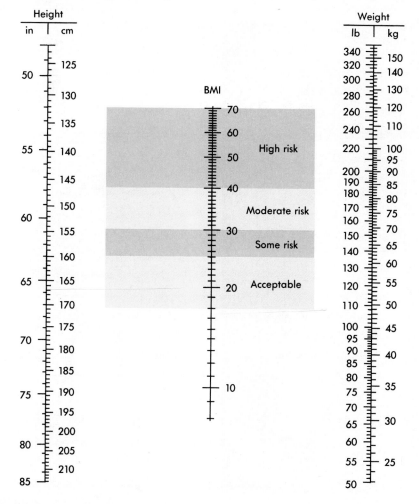

FIGURE 11-7

A quick way to determine body mass index (BMI). Mark your height and your weight on the corresponding scales. Using a ruler, draw a line connecting those two points. Read your BMI from the middle scale.

skin. This 20-minute test works because more than half of all body fat lies directly under the skin (Figure 11-8).

Clinicians have recently begun measuring total body fat using *bioelectrical impedance.* This technique sends a painless, low-energy electrical current to and from the body via wires and electrode patches. Because fat resists electrical flow, more fat per inch of height means greater electrical resistance. Within a few minutes bioelectrical impedance analyzers convert body electrical resistance into an estimate of total body fat.

Another new method for estimating total body fat exposes the biceps to infrared light, assessing the interactions with the fat and protein in arm muscle. After only 2 seconds this flashlight-size device can give an estimate.

Using body fat distribution. Where we store fat—as well as how much— can predict health risks.[1] Some people store fat in upper body areas. Others hold fat low. Each storage space has risks. Fat deposited in the lower body resists being shed. However, *upper body obesity* is related to more heart disease, hypertension, and diabetes mellitus.

High testosterone (a male hormone) levels apparently encourage upper body obesity. This characteristic male pattern of fat storage appears in the "apple-on-a-stick" shape (large abdomen [pot belly] and small buttocks and thighs). A ratio of waist circumference (at the level of the umbilicus) to hip circumference more than 0.9 in men and 0.8 in women indicates upper body fat storage.

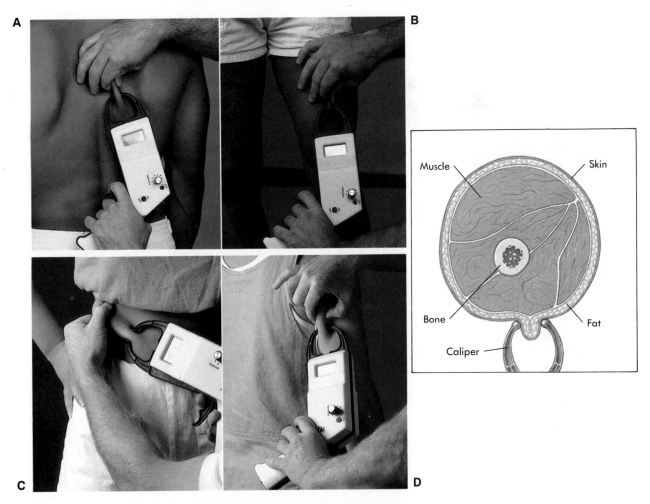

FIGURE 11-8
Skinfold measurements. Using a proper technique, calibrated equipment, and standards, skinfold measurements can be used to accurately predict body fat content in about 20 minutes. Commonly measured skinfolds are: **A,** subscapular, **B,** thigh, **C,** suprailiac, and **D,** triceps.

Progesterone (a female hormone) encourages lower body fat storage and so *lower body obesity*—the typical female pattern. The familiar small abdomen and much larger buttocks and thighs give a pear-shape appearance.

ANOTHER BITE In the future we may have obesity standards that apply more strictly to upper body fat distribution and more leniently to lower body fat distribution. Excess abdominal fat is more harmful to health than excess fat in the buttocks and thighs.

Using age of onset. Obesity can be classified as juvenile-onset or adult-onset. When obesity develops in infancy or childhood, numerous adipose (fat) cells develop, each with the ability to grow larger. In adult obesity, fewer fat cells are usually present, but these contain an excess amount of fat.

Juvenile-onset obesity presents concern because the greater number of fat cells may increase the body's resistance to cutting down fat stores. Fat cells have a long life span, which makes the battle to eliminate them difficult. Additionally, fat cells appear to need to store some fat. If more fat cells automatically require more fat storage, reducing total body fat becomes a tough task. Though still a puzzle, it appears long-term obesity makes losing weight more difficult.

THE MULTIPLE CAUSES OF OBESITY

Obesity is a very personal disorder. It may be measured many ways, but statistics aside, each person has unique characteristics and problems.[4] Treatment needs to consider current energy expenditure, fasting blood glucose levels, family history of obesity, and the extent of erroneous nutrition beliefs. Each individual faces possible complications requiring individual treatment plans.

A history of *yo-yo dieting,* the repeated loss and regain of weight, also bears consideration.[4] This can predispose a person for subsequent failure with dieting. Some experiments show that in a second bout of weight loss and gain, laboratory animals regain the lost weight in half the time it took to regain it the first time. Basal metabolism appears to dive to low levels during a second dieting phase, creating a system that expends little energy. This energy-thrifty system hoards fat stores and greedily seeks to regain weight.

No data yet suggests how long yo-yo cycles of dieting affect future attempts at weight control. Researchers are studying this puzzle. If you've been a yo-yo dieter in the past, you can still take control of your weight. It may just take a little more effort, a little more patience, and a greater emphasis on physical activity the next time around.

> **Lower Body Obesity •** The type of obesity, also called gynoid, in which fat storage is primarily located in the buttocks and thigh area.
>
> **Yo-Yo Dieting •** The practice of losing weight and then regaining it, only to lose it and regain it again. This practice in animals (and probably humans) makes it more difficult to succeed in further attempts to lose weight.

CONCEPT CHECK

Obesity refers to a state of excessive body fat storage. Obesity exists when:

- scale weight is 20% above desirable body weight as predicted by the 1983 Metropolitan Life Insurance Table.
- body mass index is over 30 (calculated as weight in kilograms divided by height in meters squared).
- a man's percent of body fat exceeds 25%; a woman's exceeds 30%.

Body fat storage can be estimated using skinfold thickness or bioelectric impedance. Fat storage distribution further defines an obese state as upper body or lower body. Obesity leads to an increased risk for heart disease, some types of cancer, hypertension, adult-onset diabetes mellitus, bone and joint disorders, and some digestive disorders. The risks for some of these diseases are especially high with upper body fat storage.

Identical Twins • Two infants that develop from a single ovum and sperm and consequently have the same genetic makeup.

Thrifty Metabolism • A metabolism that characteristically conserves more kcalories than normal, such that it increases the risk of weight gain and obesity.

Fraternal Twins • Infants that develop from two separate ova and sperm and therefore have separate genetic identities, although they develop simultaneously in the mother.

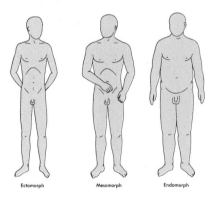

Ectomorph, mesomorph, and endomorph body shapes.

WHY SOME PEOPLE ARE OBESE—NATURE VERSUS NURTURE

Both genetic traits and psychological factors can increase the risk for obesity. These diverse influences spark controversies concerning which factor yields the greater influence.

How does nature contribute to obesity?

Identical twins raised apart tend to show similar weight gain patterns, whether lean or obese. It appears nurture—what we learn about eating habits and nutrition, which varies with twins who were raised apart—has less to do with obesity than do one's genes. In fact, research suggests genetic background accounts for about 70% of weight differences between people. Twins even tend to accumulate fat in the same body sites. Our genes help determine rates of metabolism and differences in brain chemistry. Both affect weight.

We also inherit specific body types, such as pencil-thin or muscular. The specific body types, known as endomorphs, mesomorphs, and ectomorphs greatly determine human size and shape. Endomorphs, with their stocky builds, have short, stubby bones, short trunks, round heads, wide chest and hips, and very short fingers. Ectomorphs, like Abraham Lincoln, are tall and slender with long, thin bones, and narrow chests, hips, heads, and fingers. Mesomorphs exhibit a medium, muscular build.

Ectomorphs appear to have an inherently easier time maintaining body weight. Basal metabolism increases as body surface increases. Tall people have more body surface (based on body weight comparisons) than short, stubby people. Therefore, even when resting, taller people use more energy than do shorter ones.

You've heard of fat cats, but have you heard of fat rats? Some rats and mice have a genetic predisposition to obesity. They inherit a *thrifty metabolism,* one that uses energy frugally.[21] This enables them to store fat more readily than the typical animal. Some people probably inherit a thrifty metabolism as well. Farmers once bred cows and hogs based on their ability to acquire fat. Today, because we know that eating too much animal fat can increase the risk for heart disease, farmers breed leaner animals.

A thrifty human metabolism requires less energy to get through the day. In earlier times, when food supplies were scarce, a thrifty metabolism helped protect against starvation. With today's general abundance of food, operating in this low gear requires high energy output and wise food choices to prevent obesity.

We cannot measure small differences in energy efficiency among humans. In the long run, however, even a 1% or 2% difference in metabolic rate may be a decisive factor between massive weight gain and healthy weight maintenance. Resting metabolic rates of family members tend be more similar than a comparison with the general population. Families with lower resting metabolic rates have higher rates for obesity. Even after adjusting for the amount of body fat, research shows that resting metabolic rate varies as much as 30% between leaner and more obese families. Some Native American tribes also show a high rate of obesity, linked in part to lower metabolic rates.[21]

If you think your metabolism promotes weight gain, you probably inherited a thrifty metabolism to some extent. A child with no obese parent has only a 10% chance of becoming obese. A child with one obese parent has a 40% risk, and one with two obese parents an 80% risk. It can be argued that these probabilities are related, in part, to the eating behaviors a child learns. *Fraternal twins* vary less in weight than two unrelated people. That pattern supports the theory that environment, or nurture, affects obesity. Still the close association of body weights between identical twins strongly supports the genetic explanations. This varied evidence shows how complicated it is to separate nature from nurture when searching for the causes of obesity.

Does nurture have a role?

Genetic factors determine some differences in energy metabolism and explain certain weight gain variations among people. However, environmental factors, such as high-fat diets and inactivity can literally shape us as well. Family members often have similar eating habits and choose similar foods. Even husbands and wives—who have no genetic link—may behave similarly toward food and eventually assume similar degrees of leanness or chunkiness.[12] Therefore the family that bonds at the fast-food counter can influence each other's eating habits and, ultimately, fatness.

Does being poor make you fat? By a peculiar twist of irony, the answer is often yes. In America people of lower socioeconomic status, especially females, are more likely to be obese than those in upper socioeconomic groups. Are cultural expectations the cause of this?

Adult obesity in women is often rooted in childhood obesity. In addition, periods of stress and boredom and excess weight gain in pregnancy contribute to female obesity. These patterns have stronger social than genetic links. Male obesity, however, is not strongly linked to childhood obesity and instead tends to appear after age 30. In part, a working life encourages a sedentary life for men. This powerful and prevalent pattern reinforces the critical role of nurture in obesity. If nature were the key cause of obesity in men, obesity would appear much earlier in life.

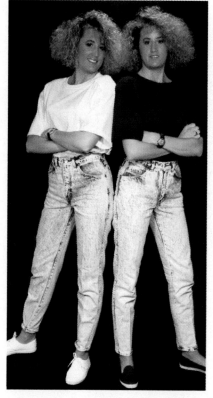

Nature or nurture—what causes these twins to have similar body weights?

ANOTHER BITE Early research suggested that infant feeding practices, such as introducing solid foods and bottle feeding before age 6 months, encourages infant weight gain and higher risk of obesity later in life. However, many recent studies reexamining this issue show very little relationship between infant feeding practices or obesity and childhood obesity. The exception could be the infant who gains weight very rapidly in the first 6 weeks of life. Most overweight or obese infants become normal-weight schoolchildren. However, if a child has become obese by 5 years of age, immediate attention is necessary. Obesity in childhood is strongly related to obesity in adulthood.

Nature and nurture together

Evidence suggests that both nature and nurture influence the tendency toward obesity (Figure 11-9). Consider the possibility that obesity is nurture allowing nature to express itself, like an accident waiting to happen. Some people begin with a slower metabolism. Put these people into an inactive environment, feed them high-kcalorie foods, and praise them for eating. They, like any of us, can be nurtured into gaining weight, allowing their natural tendency for obesity to blossom. Weight gain in adulthood often alternates with periods of weight maintenance. This suggests that for some of us a natural tendency to gain weight persists, and that changes in our nurturing environment cause spurts of weight gain.

If your parents are obese, you're likely to be at risk for obesity all your life. To avoid it will require eternal vigilance. Eat the right foods at the right times for the right reasons. Remember as well, genes are not destiny. With increased exercise and decreased food consumption, even those of us with a genetic tendency toward obesity can maintain a healthy body weight.

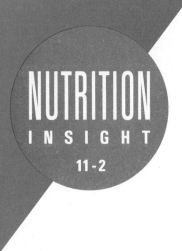

A SET POINT FOR BODY WEIGHT?

Some scientists suggest that in humans and laboratory animals, cells in the brain continually monitor the amount of body fat. This self-regulating fat level or *set point* supposedly reacts when weight shoots up or edges down. A protein produced by fat cells, called *adipsin*, may form the regulating (communication) link between fat cells and the brain.[16]

Researchers compare set point to the tight regulation of blood pressure and body temperature. One researcher described the set point as a coiled spring: the further you stray from your set weight, the stronger the force pulls you back.

Sound evidence suggests that the body tends to maintain a set weight. After an illness most people regain the lost weight. Conversely, if you just eat less, the blood level of a thyroid hormone falls, decreasing metabolic rate.[24] Your body begins to resist further weight loss. These findings suggest that adjustments in energy output are important in regulating body weight. They present evidence for the set-point theory of body-weight regulation. In addition, weighing less results in burning less energy during activity. And because total lean tissue decreases, total energy use decreases. Furthermore, the enzyme used by fat cells and muscle cells to pull in fat from the bloodstream can grow more active as one tries to lose weight.

Putting some numbers on set point

You will eat about 35 tons of food in about as many adult years. Daily energy intake varies from about 20% below to 20% above a monthly average (about ± 400 kcalories). But a 2% (40-kcalorie) over-consumption of energy per day, if continued for 20 years, adds up to an 82-pound weight gain.[18] Still, people tend to gain only 15 to 20 pounds between the ages of 18 and 54 years. The significant gain possible from such a small error—far in excess of what we usually see—suggests some degree of set point exists. Considering that 35 tons of food equals about 30 million kcalories, your body's regulation of that tonnage, though imperfect, is still quite impressive.

Will exercise or a lowfat diet lower your set point? Popular books and magazines suggest so. Science hasn't decided. Whether a set point exists is even immaterial. With or without it you need to consider: (1) exercise is important for weight maintenance, (2) a high-fat diet is often very high in kcalories, and (3) dieting is very difficult. If these phenomena are easier to understand using the concept of set point, use it. However, very little valid evidence shows how set point operates. We must remember to eat moderately, stay active, and face the fact that—even with a set point helping us—we must stay vigilant against creeping weight gain in adulthood.

Beyond set point

Perhaps it's time for a radical idea. Instead of focusing on what we should weigh, we could let our lifestyles guide us. Shift focus from a particular weight or set point. Focus instead on moderate intake of healthful foods, plenty of exercise, positive thinking, and learning to cope with stress. Let the pounds fall where they may. For most people, the result will be close to the recommended weight ranges discussed earlier. For some people, weight will be somewhat higher than societal norms—but right for them (and their set point?). By focusing on healthy lifestyle for weight control, we might shift our fixation (and that of the nation) away from dieting hysteria.[7] ●

Set Point • The close regulation of body weight. It is not known what cells control set point or how it actually functions in weight regulation. There is no doubt, however, that there are mechanisms that help regulate weight.

Adipsin • A protein that appears to be made by fat cells and acts as a communication link between these cells and the brain.

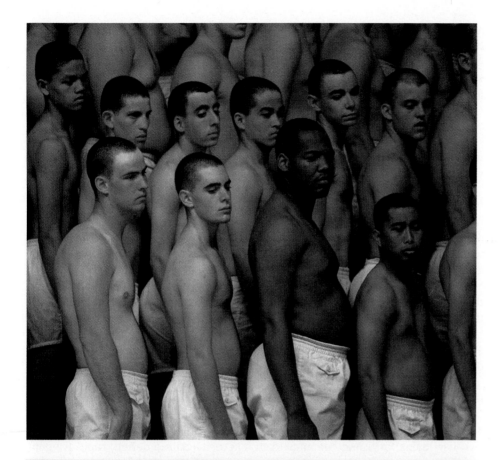

FIGURE 11-9
Is the difference in body fat in these Marine recruits caused by nature, nurture, or both?

CONCEPT CHECK

Genetic background plays a role in obesity, body shape, and rate of basal metabolism. Nurture is exhibited in similar eating habits, activity levels, and degrees of fatness in families. In addition, men's tendency to develop obesity after age 30 and women's pattern of having both childhood and adult roots for obesity suggest the powerful influence of nurture in men. Since both factors have an impact, we speculate that a nurturing state may serve as a catalyst for expressing or denying a genetic tendency toward obesity.

TREATMENT OF OBESITY

If a *secret formula* to weight loss or weight control exists, it is, as we said before, to practice eating a moderate amount of total kcalories, minimize fat kcalories, and stay physically active.[6,11] Unfortunately, this simple formula hasn't the glamour or hype of the latest fad diet nor does it promise effortless slimness. If only kcalories didn't count or a beautifully proportioned body could be had with just moments of exercise. Then the continuing assault of diet books, special programs, dietary supplements, and medical procedures for weight loss might disappear. Obesity would vanish as a public health problem and a common cause of great personal agony. Don't hold your breath.

Some basic premises

Let's focus on three other important principles concerning weight loss for adults: (1) the body naturally resists weight loss, (2) preventing obesity is key, and (3) weight should be lost from fat storage.

First, the body resists weight loss. Thyroid hormone levels, and consequently basal metabolism, drop during weight loss. The rate returns to prediet values when the diet stops.[24] But BMR stays lower if the person has lost lean body mass, making it difficult to keep losing weight or maintain a lower weight. Recent studies show that a fat storage enzyme increases its activity in fat cells after weight loss.[14] So after dieting, the body more efficiently takes up and stores fat from the bloodstream. This is a good reason to stay on a lowfat diet for weight maintenance.

Second, prevent obesity.[5] Reversing it is a demanding battle. Only about 5% of those who diet actually lose weight and keep it off. A weight-loss program should be considered successful only when participants remain at their lower weight for 3 to 5 years. The overall statistics for maintaining this degree of weight-loss are grim.[15]

From ages 25 to 34 a weight gain danger zone exists, especially for women. If weight gain has plagued you, practice particular prudence in this decade. Childhood and adolescent years also deserve special focus. Rapid weight gainers should closely monitor food intake and activity level. In addition, we need to avoid the trap of today's crash diet setting the stage for next month's weight gain. This cycle of yo-yo weight swings often promotes weight gain.

Third, the goal is to drop weight from fat storage, not muscle and other lean tissues. Quick weight loss fools those who follow fad diets. Weight drops, but little of it is fat loss. Rapid, initial weight loss often represents fluid lost because of decreased salt intake and glycogen lost from the liver and muscles. Much muscle tissue drops as well. As the diet continues, weight loss slows down. As a result, dieters often believe their efforts have failed. They give up, not realizing that smaller losses later in a diet are actually better because, unlike the initial big losses, they represent mostly fat losses.

Wishful shrinking—why can't we lose mostly fat?

Because losing fat tissue demands such a severe kcalorie deficit, rapid weight loss must necessarily be caused by depletion of other tissues. Fat storage—adipose tissue plus lean support tissues such as connective tissue—represents approximately 2700 kcalories per pound.[20] The fat itself holds about 3500 kcalories per pound. To lose 1 pound of fat storage each week, energy intake must be cut by about 400 to 500 kcalories a day. Cutting about 1000 kcalories a day for 6 weeks, while keeping activity the same, would then yield about a 12 pound fat loss. Diets that promise 10 to 15 pounds weight loss every week cannot promise weight loss from fat storage alone. One would have to cut about 5000 kcalories a day for that 10 pound loss of fat, a feat neither practical nor healthy.

A SOUND WEIGHT-LOSS PROGRAM—WHAT TO LOOK FOR

A sound weight-loss program addresses the three key issues we have stressed: controlling kcalorie intake, changing problem food habits, and increasing physical activity. Cutting back on kcalories is important. Unfortunately, 100 kcalories is a trivial amount of food, but a large amount of exercise, given our lifestyles. We need also to look for the following characteristics in a weight-loss program:[6,22]

1. The plan should meet nutritional needs, except for kcalories. This means following the Guide to Daily Food Choices, emphasizing lower fat choices among a wide variety of foods.
2. The plan should stress gradual—not rapid—weight loss. Look for a fat storage loss of 1 to 2 pounds per week.
3. The plan should adapt to habits and tastes. This will diminish discouraging feelings of deprivation, food binges, and rebound weight gain—all hallmarks of relapse. We should avoid plans that support practices such as eating fruits only in the morning or not eating meat after milk products. No rigid rituals should be required.

4. The plan should minimize hunger and fatigue while ideally supplying at least 1500 kcalories per day. With a daily intake of only 1200 to 1500 kcalories, young women especially may become iron deficient. These lower kcalorie regimens should recommend either fortified foods (breakfast cereals, for example) or a vitamin and mineral supplement (see Chapter 3 for advice on using supplements).

5. The plan should include a range of readily obtainable foods. No magical food speeds weight loss. If a plan promotes a particular food's *extraordinary* properties—whether ginseng, tofu, or garlic—look elsewhere for advice.

6. The plan should be socially acceptable, allowing the dieter to attend parties, eat at restaurants, and participate in normal daily activities. There is also no need for it to be expensive to follow.

7. The plan should help reshape lifestyle and problem eating habits to make weight loss and later maintenance possible.

8. The plan should improve overall health. It should emphasize regular physical activity, proper rest, stress reduction, and other healthy changes in lifestyle.

9. The plan should require physician approval if the dieter:
   - has existing health problems,
   - intends to lose weight as quickly as possible, or
   - is over 35 years of age and intends to perform substantially greater than usual physical activity.

CONTROLLING ENERGY INTAKE

Women often need to reduce kcalories to about 1200 per day and men to about 1500 to lose 1 to 2 pounds of fat storage per week. We need to eat at least 1000 kcalories to keep hunger at bay. When weight loss slows, a person should increase activity level, which allows one to eat enough kcalories to satisfy the need to take in nutrients.

High-carbohydrate foods such as spaghetti, rice, and whole-wheat bread (minus the butter) fill us up with few kcalories. We can replace pizza toppings like pepperoni, sausage, and extra cheese with vegetables. Carbohydrates provide less than half as many kcalories as fat. Eating at least 150 grams (600 kcalories) of carbohydrate daily promotes normal metabolism and reduces the risk of eating binges, particularly on sweets, because of intense hunger.

Avoiding hunger is crucial. A regular meal pattern decreases extreme hunger, one roadblock to weight control. Eating breakfast is one excellent suggestion. Sticking with a diet is easier when we make small, daily changes, and include a variety of foods.

A person should not reduce the fat content of a diet below 20% of kcalorie intake. A diet very low in fat produces little satiety, so hunger returns quickly after eating. A diet with 30% kcalories as fat permits most commonly eaten foods. To lose weight and keep it off, dietary changes must fit daily life for years to come.

Many other appealing foods can keep us lean. Healthy, lowfat substitutes can replace the worst high-fat offenders (Table 11-3). Tomato sauce on pasta instead of a creamy alfredo sauce is one idea; substituting fresh fruit or frozen yogurt for ice cream and pie is another. In some cases, minor switches help, like leaving the cheese off a hamburger.

Most people need to lose fewer than 50 pounds. By consuming a lower-kcalorie diet, that goal can be reached within 1 year or less. Weight is gained slowly and should come off at the same steady pace. This helps make the overall weight loss attempt a long-term success.

A good idea is to keep lowfat snack foods close at hand, especially during peak snacking periods. Reaching for fruit by the refrigerator may stop you from snacking on fat-laden foods. While it would be desirable to have the willpower to not eat high-fat foods, most people find that the best alternative is to avoid the temptations.

TABLE 11-3

Choosing "thin" foods

The chart below can help you plan your meals while following the simple guidelines for healthy eating. When you select a variety of foods from those listed in the far right column, you'll be eating foods that are low in fats and/or high in fiber.

Types of Food	Select Most Often	Select Moderately	Select Least Often
Animal protein	Lean cuts of beef/pork Salmon, halibut, (broiled) Canned tuna in water Poultry (without skin) Egg Crab	Untrimmed beef and pork Canned tuna in oil Poultry (with skin) Lobster, shrimp Canadian bacon	Fatty beef, lamb, pork Luncheon meats/hot dogs Fried chicken Fried fish Liver, kidneys Bacon
Dairy	Nonfat yogurt Nonfat milk (or ½%) Nonfat dry milk Nonfat frozen yogurt	Reduced fat and part-skim cheeses Lowfat cottage cheese Lowfat milk Lowfat yogurt 95% Fat-free frozen yogurt	Whole milk cheese (cheddar, muenster) Whole milk Sour cream, ice cream Cream, half and half
Vegetable proteins	Dried beans and peas (kidney, lima, and soy beans; lentils, split peas) Tofu (bean curd)	Raw or dry-roasted nuts and seeds Peanut and other nut butters (moderate amounts)	Oil-processed nuts and seeds
Vegetables	Raw, fresh vegetables Fresh or frozen, slightly cooked vegetables	Canned vegetables Canned tomato or vegetable juice	Vegetables in cream or butter sauces Fried vegetables
Fruits	Fresh, raw fruit Dried fruit Frozen and fresh fruit juices	Canned fruit packed in juice Canned fruit juices Frozen fruit	Fruit-flavored beverages Canned fruit packed in syrup Avocados Olives
Grain products	Shredded wheat, oats Whole-grain cereals Whole-grain breads Brown rice Wheat bran, oat bran Bagels Fig bars	Refined cereals Enriched white breads Refined pastas White rice Granolas Toast w/margarine Plain cookies	Cookies, cakes, pies Sweetened cereals Tortilla chips Donuts Oil-processed crackers Cream-filled cookies Croissants, doughnuts
Other (still limit quantity)	Popcorn (air popped) Soft-tub margarines Canola and olive oils Corn oil Safflower oil Sunflower oil	Salad dressings Mayonnaise Stick margarine Pretzels	Hydrogenated shortenings, butter Lard, salt pork, bacon Gravies, cream sauce Alcohol Potato chips

CONCEPT CHECK

Dieting deserves consideration of these points:
1. the body resists weight loss,
2. prevent obesity; reversing the condition is much harder, and
3. lose weight from fat stores, not from lean tissues.

Good weight loss diets:
1. meet nutritional needs (you can evaluate this by referring to the Guide to Daily Food Choices),
2. accommodate the dieter's habits and tastes,
3. include a range of readily obtainable foods,
4. promote changing habits that lead to overeating, and
5. encourage an increase in physical activity.

BEHAVIOR MODIFICATION—WHAT MAKES US TICK?

Does dieting test your self-control? Do you know what habits sabotage your good intentions? Controlling food intake, so important to weight loss, means modifying *problem* behaviors.[11,13] Only you can decide what behaviors keep you reaching for the wrong foods at the wrong times for the wrong reasons. And only you can modify those behaviors. What events start (or stop) your eating? What factors influence food choices? Psychologists often use terms like *chain-breaking, stimulus control, cognitive restructuring, contingency management,* and *self-monitoring* when discussing behavior modification (Table 11-4). This terminology, introduced in Chapter 3, helps place the problem in perspective and organize the intervention strategy into manageable steps.

Chain-breaking separates behaviors that tend to occur together; for example, snacking on chips while watching television. While these activities do not have to occur together, they often do. We need to break the chain reaction (see Figure 3-7).

Stimulus control puts us in charge of temptations. You might want to push tempting food to the back of the refrigerator, remove fat-laden snacks from the kitchen counter, or avoid the path by the vending machines. Provide positive stimulus by keeping low kcalorie snacks ready to satisfy hunger/appetite. Note alcohol and foods offer quick, easy stress relief. We need to plan healthy alternatives.

Cognitive restructuring changes our frame of mind. For example, after a hard day, respond with a walk or satisfying talk with a friend instead of a binge. Replace eating reactions to stress with healthy, relaxing alternatives.

Decreeing some food off limits sets up an internal struggle to vigilantly resist the urge to eat that food. This hopeless battle can keep us feeling deprived. We lose the fight. It is best to manage food choices with the principle of moderation. If a favorite food becomes troublesome, place it only temporarily off limits until you can face it frugally.

Contingency management prepares us for potential pitfalls and high-risk situations. You might rehearse ahead responses to pressure—like food being passed at a party.

Did you keep a record of what you ate and what catalysts urged you to pick up the fork or put it down as we suggested in Chapter 1? If so, you already know one key tool in modifying behavior, self-monitoring. A self-monitoring record can reveal patterns—such as unconscious overeating—that may explain problem eating habits (see Figure 3-2). This record can encourage new habits to counteract unwanted behaviors.

New habits often need to replace defeating ones. For example, limiting eating to a single room in the house might eliminate television snacking. Eating rapidly, holding an ever-ready forkful of food while chewing, outpaces the natural satiety response. It takes about 20 minutes for the brain to register satiety. Put down the fork! Since appetite, not physical hunger, often opens the mouth, one may need to simply stop purchasing irresistible foods.

Studies show that people inaccurately estimate portion sizes. During the first week of self-monitoring, it is best to measure food as precisely as possible. Including estimated amounts of toppings, gravies, and garnishes is important. If an eating plan allows only three ounces of skinless chicken breast, we need to know what a three-ounce portion looks like on the plate. It's not much bigger than a pack of playing cards, or the palm of your hand. Investing in a kitchen scale may serve us as well as the one in the bathroom.

Overall, we need to analyze shortcomings that make dieting difficult. Address specific problems, such as snacking, compulsive eating, or mealtime overeating. Table 3-2 provided options for changing shopping and eating behaviors. Figure 3-4 showed how to set up a contract with goals, as well as activities

Chain-Breaking • Breaking the link between two or more behaviors that encourage overeating, such as snacking while watching television.

Stimulus Control • Altering the environment to minimize the stimuli for eating, for example, removing foods from sight and storing them in kitchen cabinets.

Cognitive Restructuring • Changing one's frame of mind regarding eating, for example, instead of using a difficult day as an excuse to overeat, substituting other pleasures for rewards, such as a relaxing walk with a friend.

Contingency Management • Forming a plan of action to respond to an environment where overeating is likely, such as when snacks are within arm's reach at a party.

Self-Monitoring • A process of tracking foods eaten and conditions affecting eating; actions are usually recorded in a diary, along with location, time, and state of mind. This is a tool to help a person understand more about his or her eating habits.

TABLE 11-4

Behavioral principles of weight loss

Stimulus control

Shopping

1. Shop for food after eating—buy nutritious foods
2. Shop from a list; do not buy irresistible "problem" foods
3. Avoid ready-to-eat foods; let others who want them buy them and store them
4. Put off shopping until absolutely necessary

Plans

1. Plan to limit food intake as needed
2. Substitute exercise for snacking
3. Eat meals and snacks at scheduled times; don't skip meals

Activities

1. Store food out of sight, preferably in the freezer so that impulsive eating is discouraged
2. Eat all food in the same place
3. Keep serving dishes off the table, especially sauces and gravies
4. Use smaller dishes and utensils

Holidays and parties

1. Drink fewer alcoholic beverages
2. Plan eating habits before parties
3. Eat a low-calorie snack before parties
4. Practice polite ways to decline food
5. Don't get discouraged by an occasional setback

Eating behavior

1. Put fork down between mouthfuls
2. Chew thoroughly before taking the next bite
3. Leave some food on the plate
4. Pause in the middle of the meal
5. Do nothing else while eating (read, watch television)

Reward

1. Solicit help from family and friends
2. Help family and friends provide this help in the form of praise and material rewards
3. Utilize self-monitoring records as basis for rewards
4. Plan specific rewards for specific behaviors (behavioral contracts)

Self-monitoring

Diet diary

1. Note time and place of eating
2. List type and amount of food eaten
3. Record who is present and how you feel
4. Use diet diary to identify problem areas

Cognitive restructuring

1. Avoid setting unreasonable goals
2. Think about progress, not shortcomings
3. Avoid imperatives like "always" and "never"
4. Counter negative thoughts with positive restatements

See Chapter 7 for lowfat methods of cooking.

Modified from Frankle RT, Yang M: *Obesity and weight control*, Rockville, MD, 1988, Aspen Publishers.

to meet these goals. A written plan shared with a friend or spouse can help meet goals. Rewards for following the plan add incentive when focused on both short-term and long-term successes. In all, consult Chapter 3 again for a more detailed discussion of how to develop a plan to change behavior.

ANOTHER BITE

People carry on an internal dialogue—self-talk—to sort out their own truth, beliefs and attitudes, and responses to events around them. Positive self-talk leads us kindly through changes, like choosing to lose weight. We praise ourselves for success. Negative self-talk is different. Praise is replaced with self-deprecating remarks; self-blame; and angry, guilt-producing put-downs. Negative self-talk undermines efforts at self-control—dieting included—and leads to anxiety and depression. Beliefs and self-talk influence how we interpret events of today and expectations of the future, as well as how we feel and react. Positive self-talk and problem-solving efforts and realistic beliefs and goals lead us to a healthy, self-caring lifestyle.

A dieter can tolerate an occasional lapse. Plan for lapses. Encourage calm when you slip, but take charge immediately. As noted in Chapter 3, change responses like "I ate that cookie; I'm a failure," to "I ate that cookie, but I did well to stop after only one!" An occasional cookie is fine; a pound of cookies in an afternoon deserves reconsideration. When a dieter lapses from the diet plan, newly learned food habits should steer one back toward the plan. This should enable the dieter to avoid the lapse-relapse-collapse trap. Without a strong behavioral plan, a lapse frequently turns into a relapse. Once a pattern of poor food choices begins, the dieter feels like a failure and strays further from the plan. As the relapse lengthens, the diet plan collapses, and the person falls short of the weight-loss goal. Even with a good behavioral plan, a person may fail at a diet. Losing weight is difficult.

CONCEPT CHECK

We should consider the following changes when dieting: (1) Modify behavior to improve conditions for losing weight. (2) Break habit chains that encourage overeating, such as snacking while watching television. (3) Reduce temptations by not buying irresistible foods and by storing foods out of sight. (4) Preplan how to refuse food temptations at a party. (5) Rethink the role of food, replacing food with relaxing activities as a reward for coping with stress. (6) Carefully observe and record eating habits to reveal subtle behaviors that lead to overeating.

PHYSICAL ACTIVITY—ANOTHER KEY TO WEIGHT LOSS

Exercising—until recently a relatively neglected strategy in weight control—causes us to expend far more energy than when we rest (Figure 11-10). Burning only 200 to 300 extra kcalories a day—above and beyond the normal activity level—can eliminate about a half pound of fat storage per week: that's about 25 pounds of fat in a year.

Walking and riding bicycles, transportation for much of the world, offers an easy way to increase daily physical activity. Experts recommend an hour or so of brisk walking every day as one option.

Exercise also reduces the stress and boredom of a diet. A walk takes the dieter out of the house and away from temptations. Regular exercise gradually increases muscle mass as well. More lean tissue raises basal metabolism so that we burn more energy, even while we are sitting still. A higher ratio of lean tissue to fat gives us a "losing" advantage.

FIGURE 11-10
Exercise improves any diet. Weight loss will occur because we burn more kcalories than at rest.

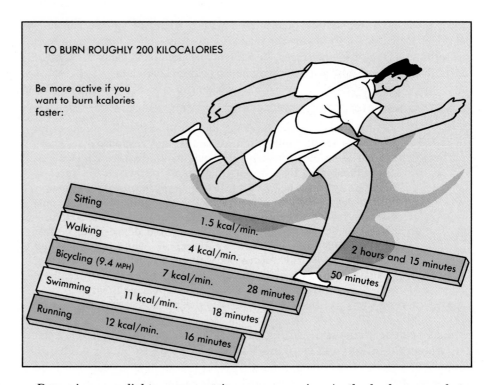

TO BURN ROUGHLY 200 KILOCALORIES

Be more active if you want to burn kcalories faster:

Sitting	1.5 kcal/min.	2 hours and 15 minutes
Walking	4 kcal/min.	50 minutes
Bicycling (9.4 MPH)	7 kcal/min.	28 minutes
Swimming	11 kcal/min.	18 minutes
Running	12 kcal/min.	16 minutes

Gastroplasty • Surgery on the stomach to limit its volume to approximately 50 milliliters, which is the size of a shot glass.

Becoming even lighter may require more exercise. As the body responds to exercise, weight loss usually slows; the lighter body weight reduces the energy cost of activity. The metabolic rate also slows as the body loses lean tissue along with fat tissue during dieting. Walking 15 minutes more each day to help receive the same exercise benefit during efficient energy use is one response. The goal is to keep exercising.[23] A lifelong commitment to exercise promises leaner bodies and better health for all.

PROFESSIONAL HELP FOR WEIGHT LOSS

See your family physician or student health service professionals for advice about a weight-loss program. Doctors, trained to assess overall health and the appropriateness of weight-loss, can refer you to a registered dietitian. With their knowledge of food composition and how people use foods to cope with psychological challenges, registered dietitians can answer diet-related questions and design a specific weight-loss plan.

Self-help weight-loss organizations, such as Take Off Pounds Sensibly (TOPS) and Weight Watchers, offer sensible guidance and support. Other programs, such as Nutri-System, Jenny Craig, Diet Center, and Physicians Weight Loss Center, among others, are often less helpful for the average dieter. These are generally expensive because of the intense counseling and/or mandatory diet foods and supplements required.

Many programs unfortunately pay only lip service to maintenance. Weight Watchers, an exception, offers free meetings as long as one stays within the goal weight range. People generally need 18 to 24 months in an organized maintenance program to incorporate the lifestyle changes that keep weight off. If the program doesn't encourage exercise, take our advice—stay active.

Treating morbid obesity

Morbid obesity—weighing at least 100 pounds over desirable body weight, or twice the desirable body weight—requires professional treatment. Because of the severe health problems related to morbid obesity, drastic treatment measures are often necessary.

Stomach surgery. *Gastroplasty*, or stomach stapling, is the most common surgical procedure for treating morbid obesity.[10] The procedure relies on physi-

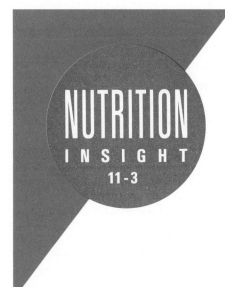

NUTRITION INSIGHT 11-3

DIET PILLS

Over-the-counter medications that claim to help weight loss sell briskly. Though some can be effective, none matches diet moderation and physical activity for weight loss. Diet aids include caffeine, fiber pills, phenylpropanolamine, and benzocaine. Caffeine tends to blunt appetite. Benzocaine numbs the tongue and affects the sense of taste, so a person tends to eat less. Fiber pills can increase bulk in the stomach and ideally lead to satiety. A typical side effect is significant intestinal gas. Can you guess why? (See Chapter 5.)

Phenylpropanolamine is an epinephrine-like drug that can cause a slight decrease in food intake.[11] At a typical dose of 75 milligrams per day, the degree of appetite suppression varies among people. FDA recommends phenylpropanolamine be used with caution in people with hyperthyroidism, cardiovascular disorders (including hypertension), and diabetes mellitus. Adverse reactions may also occur among those taking various other medications at the same time.

Prescription medications

Physicians sometimes prescribe amphetamines for weight loss.[25] Amphetamines decrease appetite, but they can have a hook: addiction. In addition, amphetamines can increase heart rate and nervousness and lead to insomnia. Thyroid hormone preparations, once popular, caused significant loss of lean tissue.

Fenfluramine and fluoxetine have been prescribed by physicians to promote weight loss. By increasing the action of a neurotransmitter in the brain, they may lead to less food craving, especially for high-carbohydrate foods. Note some people complain of rapid weight gain after discontinuing the drug, and fenfluramine worsens depression in those people who already show signs of this disorder.

The experimental medications naloxone and naltrexone significantly decrease food intake in laboratory animals. Results from human studies, however, have proved discouraging. Development of related drugs is continuing.

Overall, in skilled hands, prescription medications can aid weight loss when coupled with diet control[11]; however, they do not substitute for the more conservative approaches of reducing kcalorie intake, modifying problem behaviors, and increasing physical activity.

Useless medications

The hormone cholecystokinin (CCK) may regulate food intake within the body, but bought in a bottle, it wastes money. It is widely available in health-food stores in the form of ground up animal intestines (recall CCK is produced in the small intestine). However, the amount of CCK in each pill is almost too small to detect, let alone suppress appetite. In addition, CCK is a protein and so is destroyed by digestion in the stomach; little is absorbed as such from an oral dose. It must be injected to be effective,[11] and you can't buy a form that is safe to inject.

Another class of useless and potentially harmful diet aids is diuretics or "water pills." They have a legitimate medical use in the treatment of hypertension, but they cannot control body fatness. Obesity is not primarily caused by excess water accumulation in healthy people. ●

cal restriction of eating. By reducing the stomach to the size of a shot glass, about 50 milliliters (2 ounces), overeating of solid foods is less likely. Rapid vomiting would result. The smaller stomach also promotes more rapid satiety. With the enforced food reduction, about 75% of people with morbid obesity eventually lose 50% of excess body weight. The surgery's success at long-term loss maintenance often leads to dramatic health improvements, such as reduced blood pressure and correction of adult-onset diabetes mellitus. Risk of death from the surgery itself is about 1%.

Stomach stapling has disadvantages. It is costly and often not covered by medical insurance. Months of difficult emotional adjustments face the dieter

Phenylpropanolamine • An over-the-counter stimulant that has a mild appetite-reducing effect.

Lipectomy • Surgical removal of body fat; also known as liposuction.

Very Low Calorie Diet (VLCD) • Also known as a protein-sparing modified fast (PSMF), this diet allows the consumption of 400 to 700 kcalories per day in liquid form. Of this, about 30 to 45 grams are made up of carbohydrate; the rest is protein.

Very low calorie diets should not be used by infants, children, teenagers, pregnant women, or the elderly.

while enduring this drastic approach to weight loss. This surgery is not reversed, even after reaching a desired weight. Thus, though successful for weight loss, it requires major lifetime lifestyle changes.

Lipectomy, surgically removing localized fat deposits from humans, is a cosmetic choice for diet resistant areas. A pencil-thin tube inserted through an incision in the skin suctions off fat tissue from the buttocks, thighs, and similar areas. Risks include infection, large, lasting skin depressions, and blood clots that can lead to kidney failure. This often painful surgery requires an experienced physician. Over 100,000 procedures were performed in 1988, with women receiving 85% of them.

Very low calorie diets. Physician-supervised *very low calorie diets (VLCD)* offer an alternative for morbidly obese people who prefer no temptations from conventional food.[9] These 400 to 800 kcalories per day diets, usually in liquid form, were earlier called protein-sparing modified fasts. They provide about 30 to 120 grams of carbohydrates. The remainder, about 50 to 100 grams, is high quality protein, such as is found in egg whites, chicken, turkey, and lean beef. The diets include vitamin and mineral supplements. The minimal kcalories and absence of food choice can usually produce about a 3 to 5 pound loss per week. On these diets men tend to lose weight faster than women.

Some researchers support use of VLCD therapy with people who have body weights greater than 30% to 40% above desirable weight. However, a recent study showed few people can maintain the weight loss after following a VLCD. Changing behavior and exercising regularly still are key parts of long-term therapy. These concepts are given attention in the latest commercial VLCD programs. In addition, losing weight too rapidly on a VLCD can cause gallstones as well as a significant loss of heart tissue, which has occasionally led to sudden death from heart attack. These risks demand we use careful, physician-guided consideration when choosing and while following VLCD therapy.

VLCD therapy has other less serious side effects, such as cold intolerance, fatigue, light-headedness, nervousness, euphoria, constipation, diarrhea, dry skin, thinning reddened hair, anemia, and menstrual irregularities.

CONCEPT CHECK

Morbid obesity's high failure rate with conservative weight loss strategies suggests a need for other interventions. Two options include surgery to reduce stomach volume to about 50 milliliters or a very low calorie diet consisting of 400 to 700 kcalories per day. Both require careful monitoring by a physician to evaluate health risks. Behavior modification and exercise should be included to maintain weight loss and overall health.

PUTTING WEIGHT LOSS INTO PERSPECTIVE

Have you known anyone who has lost and regained the same 10 pounds—plus some—many times? It appears that dieting actually promotes obesity. Can you imagine the time and trouble that went along with each lost pound? The emotional demands of dieting require strong motivation and strong social support to sustain the loss. We need to put supports in place first. Weight loss and subsequent weight maintenance demand ongoing attention.

If this lifelong commitment will be a struggle for you, make dieting choices wisely so that each pound lost is lost forever. You deserve not to repeat your struggling steps. If you have healthy, acceptable body weight, simple maintenance is a positive step.

Disease-free bodies that do not weigh 20% over desirable body weight standards do not require weight loss for health's sake. These people would be better served if our culture simply rethought its obsession with slimness.[7] For people who are at least 30% over desirable body weight or who have heart disease, hypertension, diabetes mellitus, arthritis, or another disorder that is clearly worsened by obesity, weight loss is recommended.

Your own strengths and weaknesses will determine which weight loss techniques work for you. A true measure of diet success is improved health and self-esteem as weight is lost.

TREATING THE UNDERWEIGHT PERSON

Sometimes being underweight requires medical intervention. A physician should be consulted to rule out hormonal imbalances, depression, and other hidden disease, such as anorexia nervosa or bulimia. Risks associated with being underweight include complications in surgery and slow recovery after illness. Underweight women may have menstrual irregularities, stop menstruating altogether (which is associated with bone loss—see Chapter 10), and deliver low birth weight newborns.

One approach for treating underweight adults is for them to gradually increase their consumption of energy-dense foods, especially those higher in vegetable fat. Italian cheeses, nuts, and granola are good kcalorie sources with low saturated fat content (read the label to see if the product is high in mostly unsaturated fat). Dried fruit and bananas provide other higher kcalorie fruit choices. If eaten at the end of a meal, they don't cause early satiety. Underweight people should replace such foods as diet soft drinks with good energy sources, like fruit juices. Keeping a daily food record for weekly review can help point one toward wise high-kcalorie food choices (the right side of Table 11-3 lists some possible choices).

A physically active underweight person could reduce activity. If weight stays low, a weight-lifting program might add muscle mass.

If these efforts fail to achieve the desired weight, they should at least prevent health problems associated with being underweight. After achieving that, the person may have to accept his or her very lean frame.

SUMMARY

- Hunger, the physiological drive to find and eat food, is triggered partly by cells that form satiety and feeding centers in the hypothalamus. Destroy the satiety center in animals or humans and overeating with eventual obesity results. Destroy the feeding centers and semistarvation results. These centers monitor and respond to blood glucose and other nutrients. Hormones and other compounds made by cells also help regulate satiety.

- Appetite, the psychological desire to find and eat food, is affected by time of day, food availability and palatability, and social custom. Because food is so readily available in America, appetite, not hunger, is often the catalyst for food intake.

- To some extent, body weight tends to regulate itself naturally. Does a set point for weight level exist? Trusting a set point to maintain a desirable weight isn't reliable; adults tend to gain 15 to 20 pounds between the ages of 18 and 54.

- Basal metabolism, the thermic effect of food, and physical activity account for most of the body's energy use. Basal metabolism, the minimum energy needed to keep the resting body alive, is primarily determined by lean body mass, amount of body surface, and thyroid hormone levels. The thermic effect of food is energy the body uses to digest, absorb, and process nutrients recently consumed. Unused energy intake is stored as fat.

- We measure the body's energy use directly, from heat output, or indirectly, from oxygen uptake. Formulas based on various combinations of body weight, height, and age estimate the body's energy needs.

- Obesity can be defined along several dimensions:
  - weighing 20% more than desirable body weight (based on the Metropolitan Life Insurance Table, published in 1983)
  - a body mass index value (weight in kilograms divided by height in meters squared) over 30
  - a total body fat exceeding 25% in men and 30% in women; body fat is most often measured by skinfold thickness

- Fat distribution predicts health risks linked to obesity. Upper body obesity (characterized by a large abdomen and small buttocks and thighs) means higher risks of hypertension, heart disease, and diabetes mellitus than lower body obesity (characterized by small abdomen and larger buttocks and thighs).

- Genetic factors influence basal metabolism and body shape, and so influence the tendency to obesity. How one is raised (or nurtured) also influences obesity, since family members often develop similar eating habits and activity patterns. Obesity may essentially be nurture allowing nature to express itself.

- When considering a treatment for obesity, remember (1) the body resists weight loss; (2) since obesity is difficult to reverse, the goal is prevention; (3) lose weight from fat storage, not from muscle and other lean tissues.

- A sound weight-loss diet should meet a dieter's nutritional needs by following the Guide to Daily Food Choices. A good plan should adapt to the person's habits, encourage readily obtainable foods, strive to change poor eating habits, and promote regular physical activity. It should also insist that the dieter see a physician if weight is to be lost rapidly or if the person is over 35 years of age and plans to perform substantially greater physical activity than usual.

- A pound of fat tissue—gained or lost—represents approximately 2700 kcalories. If energy output exceeds energy intake by 400 to 500 kcalories per day, one can lose a pound of fat storage in a week. We can best cut kcalories by decreasing high-fat foods.

- Behavior modification helps weight-loss programs because current habits may encourage overeating and discourage weight maintenance. Specific behavior modification techniques, such as stimulus control and self-monitoring, help change problem behaviors.

- Increasing physical activity sheds pounds. A good goal is to expend an extra 200 to 300 kcalories in activity each day.

- Morbid obesity, defined as weighing at least 100 pounds over desirable body weight or twice the desirable body weight, may require: (1) stomach surgery to reduce stomach volume to approximately 50 milliliters, or (2) very low calorie diets, containing 400 to 700 kcalories per day. Only people who fail at more conservative approaches to weight loss should use these procedures.

- Over-the-counter weight loss medications include caffeine and other mild stimulants and fiber pills. None of these, however, replaces a good diet, behavior changes, and exercise.

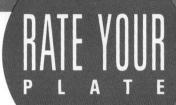
AM I A CANDIDATE FOR WEIGHT LOSS?

Determine the following two indices of your body status: Body mass index and waist to hip ratio

BODY MASS INDEX

Record your weight in pounds: _____ lbs.

Divide your weight in pounds by 2.2 to determine your weight in kilograms: _____ kg.

Record your height in inches: _____ in.

Divide your height in inches by 39.3 to determine your height in meters: _____ m.

Calculate your Body Mass Index using the following formula:

$$BMI = Weight\ (kg) / height\ (m)^2$$

$$BMI = \underline{\hspace{2cm}} kg / \underline{\hspace{2cm}} m^2 = \underline{\hspace{2cm}}.$$

WAIST TO HIP RATIO

Take a tape measure and measure the circumferences of your waist (at the belly button) and hips (widest point).

Circumference of waist (umbilicus) = _____ in.

Circumference of hips = _____ in.

Calculate your waist to hip ratio using the following formula:

Circumference of waist/circumference of hips

Waist to hip ratio = _____ in / _____ in = _____.

INTERPRETATION

1. When BMI is greater than 25, health risks from obesity begin. It would be advisable to attempt weight loss if your BMI exceeds this.

Does yours exceed 25? Yes _____ No _____

2. When a person is obese (greater than 20% above desirable weight), a waist to hip ratio greater than 0.9 in men and 0.8 in women indicates upper body obesity. This is associated with an increased risk of heart disease, hypertension, and diabetes mellitus.

If appropriate, does your ratio exceed the standard appropriate for your gender? Yes _____ No _____

3. Do you feel you need to pursue a program of weight loss?
Yes _____ No _____

APPLICATION

From what you've learned in this chapter, what changes in eating and exercise habits could you make to lose weight and help ensure you maintain the loss?

_____

_____

_____

_____

REFERENCES

1. Bjorntorp P: Classification of obese patients and complications related to distribution of surplus fat, *Nutrition* 6:131, 1990.
2. Bray GA: Nutrient balance and obesity: classification and evaluation of the obesities, *Medical Clinics of North America* 73:29, 1989.
3. Bray GA: Treatment for obesity: a nutrient balance/nutrient partition approach, *Nutrition Reviews* 49:33, 1991.
4. Brownell KD: Obesity and weight control: the good and bad of dieting, *Nutrition Today*, May/June, 1987, p 4.
5. Canadian Dietetic Association: Obesity: a case for prevention, *Journal of the Canadian Dietetic Association* 49:11, 1988.
6. Council on Scientific Affairs, American Medical Association: Treatment of obesity in adults, *Journal of the American Medical Association* 260:2547, 1988.
7. Czajka-Narins DM, Parham ES: Fear of fat: attitudes toward obesity, *Nutrition Today*, January/February, 1990, p 26.
8. Fernstrom JD: Tryptophan, serotonin, and carbohydrate appetite: will the real carbohydrate craver please stand up? *Journal of Nutrition* 118:1417, 1988.
9. Fisler JS, Drenick EJ: Starvation and semi-starvation diets in the management of obesity, *Annual Reviews of Nutrition* 7:465, 1987.
10. Forse A and others: Morbid obesity: weighing the treatment options—surgical intervention, *Nutrition Today*, September/October, 1989, p 10.
11. Frankel RT, Yang M: *Obesity and weight control*, Rockville, Md, 1988, Aspen Publishers.
12. Garn SM: Family-line and socioeconomic factors in fatness and obesity, *Nutrition Reviews* 44:381, 1986.
13. Holli BB: Using behavior modification in nutrition counseling, *Journal of the American Dietetic Association* 88:1530, 1988.
14. Kern PA and others: The effects of weight loss on the activity and expression of adipose tissue lipoprotein lipase in very obese humans, *The New England Journal of Medicine* 322:1053, 1990.
15. Kramer FM and others: Long-term follow-up of behavioral treatment for obesity: patterns of weight regain among men and women, *International Journal of Obesity* 13:123, 1989.
16. Leibel RL, Hirsh J: Metabolic characterization of obesity, *Annals of Internal Medicine* 103:1000, 1985.
17. Manson JE and others: Body weight and longevity, *Journal of the American Medical Association* 257:353, 1987.
18. Martin RJ, Mullen BJ: Control of food intake: mechanisms and consequences, *Nutrition Today*, September/October, 1987, p 4.
19. National Institutes of Health Consensus Development Conference Statement: Health implications of obesity, *Annals of Internal Medicine* 103:1073, 1985.
20. Owen OE: Regulation of energy and metabolism. In Kinney JM and others, editors: *Nutrition and metabolism in patient care*, Philadelphia, 1988, WB Saunders.
21. Ravussin E and others: Reduced rate of energy expenditure as a risk factor for body-weight gain, *The New England Journal of Medicine* 318:467, 1988.
22. Rock CL, Coluston AM: Weight-control approaches: a review by the California Dietetic Association, *Journal of the American Dietetic Association* 88:44, 1988.
23. Simms EAH: Storage and expenditure of energy in obesity and their implications for management, *Medical Clinics of North America* 73:97, 1989.
24. Wadden TA and others: Long-term effects of dieting on resting metabolic rate in obese patients, *Journal of the American Medical Association* 264:707, 1990.
25. Weintraub M, Bray GA: Drug treatment for obesity, *Medical Clinics of North America* 73:237, 1989.
26. York DA: Metabolic regulation of food intake, *Nutrition Reviews* 48:64, 1990.

HOW MUCH HAVE I LEARNED?

What have you learned from Chapter 11? Here are 15 statements about weight control. Read them to test your current knowledge. If you think the statement is true or mostly true, circle T. If you think the statement is false or mostly false, circle F. Use the scoring key at the end of the book to compute your total score. To review, take this test again later, and especially before tests.

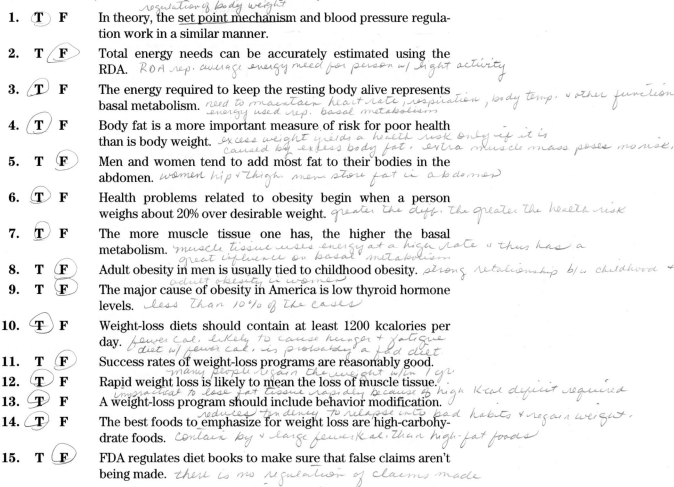

1. (T) F   In theory, the set point mechanism and blood pressure regulation work in a similar manner. *regulation of body weight*

2. T (F)   Total energy needs can be accurately estimated using the RDA. *RDA rep. average energy need for person w/ light activity*

3. (T) F   The energy required to keep the resting body alive represents basal metabolism. *need to maintain heart rate, respiration, body temp. & other functions energy used rep. basal metabolism*

4. (T) F   Body fat is a more important measure of risk for poor health than is body weight. *excess weight yields a health risk only if it is caused by excess body fat. extra muscle mass poses no rise.*

5. T (F)   Men and women tend to add most fat to their bodies in the abdomen. *women hip & thigh. men store fat in abdomen*

6. (T) F   Health problems related to obesity begin when a person weighs about 20% over desirable weight. *greater the diff. the greater the health risk*

7. (T) F   The more muscle tissue one has, the higher the basal metabolism. *muscle tissue uses energy at a high rate & thus has a great influence on basal metabolism*

8. T (F)   Adult obesity in men is usually tied to childhood obesity. *strong relationship b/w childhood & adult obesity in women*

9. T (F)   The major cause of obesity in America is low thyroid hormone levels. *less than 10% of the cases*

10. (T) F   Weight-loss diets should contain at least 1200 kcalories per day. *fewer cal. likely to cause hunger & fatigue diet w/ fewer cal. is probably a fad diet.*

11. T (F)   Success rates of weight-loss programs are reasonably good. *many people regain the weight w/in 1 yr.*

12. (T) F   Rapid weight loss is likely to mean the loss of muscle tissue. *impractical to lose fat tissue rapidly because of high kcal deficit required*

13. (T) F   A weight-loss program should include behavior modification. *reduces tendency to relapse into bad habits & regain weight.*

14. (T) F   The best foods to emphasize for weight loss are high-carbohydrate foods. *contain by & large fewer kcal. than high-fat foods*

15. T (F)   FDA regulates diet books to make sure that false claims aren't being made. *there is no regulation of claims made by fad diets, only concerned when products are suspected of causing serious harm*

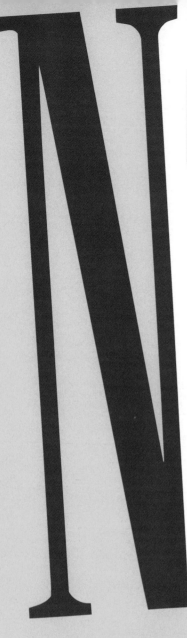

NUTRITION ISSUE

FAD DIETS—WHY ALL THE COMMOTION?

Bowker's *Books in Print* lists an astounding 455 titles under diet books. Diet quacks probably make more unreasonable, unproven, and dangerous claims for fat loss treatments than for any other products. So-called cures show up everywhere—television, magazines, newspapers. As we noted in Chapter 4, dieting quackery has existed for years. Today, advertisers push pills, hypnosis, and wonder diets, all promising fewer fat cells, just like magic. But any dieter should know magic can't do the trick.

Still, many overweight people attempt to turn fad diet books into self-treatment. As you will see, most of these diets provide no special help, and some can do harm (Table 11-5).

Why do fad diet books still exist? Why doesn't the government ban them? Many contain obvious misinformation. FDA gets tough only when products threaten serious harm. FDA's heavy demands prevent it from pursuing every new fad diet. So the ancient advice still applies: *Let the buyer beware.* Authors and publishers seeking success may shirk their responsibility to the reader with little risk. Outrageous claims sell more books than telling people to eat less fat and exercise more.

How to recognize a fad diet

Fad diets typically share some common characteristics. We list a few here:[4,22]

1. They promote quick weight loss, but it is primarily through glycogen, sodium, and muscle mass depletion. All lead to a loss of body water. Little fat is lost.
2. They limit food selections and dictate specific rituals, such as eating only fruit for breakfast.
3. They use testimonials from famous people and tie the diet to celebrity cities, such as Beverly Hills and New York.
4. They bill themselves as cure-alls. Whatever the type of obesity or whatever a reader's specific strengths and weaknesses, these diets claim to work for everyone.
5. They often recommend expensive supplements. Some supplements can be harmful, such as high doses of vitamin A, vitamin D, niacin, or vitamin B-6.
6. No attempts are made to change eating habits permanently. The dieter follows the diet until reaching the desired weight, then reverts to old eating habits. Eat rice for a month, lose weight, and then return to old habits.
7. The authors generally criticize the scientific community, suggesting physicians and registered dietitians do not really want people to lose weight. They encourage dieters to seek advice outside the medical and scientific establishment.

TABLE 11-5

Summary of popular dietary approaches to weight control

Approach and Examples	Characteristics and Possible Negative Health Consequences
Moderate caloric restriction	
The Setpoint Diet	Usually 1000-1800 kcal per day
Slim Chance in a Fat World	Reasonable balance of macronutrients
Weight Watcher's Diet	Encourage exercise
The American Heart Assoc. Diet	May employ behavioral approach
Mary Ellen's Help Yourself Diet Plan	
The Beyond Diet	Weaknesses; none if vitamin and mineral supplement used and permission of family physician is granted
Macronutrient restriction	
Low carbohydrate:	
Atkins' Diet Revolution	Less than 100 grams carbohydrate per day
Calories Don't Count Diet	
Wild Weekend Diet	
Miracle Diet for Fast Weight Loss	Weakness ketosis; poor exercise capacity due to poor glycogen stores in the muscles; excessive animal fat intake
Drinking Man's Diet	
Woman Doctor's Diet for Women	
The Doctor's Quick Weight Loss Diet (Stillman's)	
The Complete Scarsdale Medical Diet	
Four Day Wonder Diet	
Lowfat:	
The Rice Diet Report	Less than 20% of calories from fat
The Macrobiotic Diet (some versions)	Limited (or elimination of) animal protein sources, all fats, nuts, seeds
The Pritikin Diet	
The Tokyo Diet	
The Palm Beach Lifelong Diet	Weakness; little satiety; flatulence, possibly poor mineral absorption from excess fiber; limited food choices → deprivation
The James Coco Diet	
The 35+ Diet	
7-Week Victory Diet	
Fat to Muscle Diet	
T-Factor Diet	
Fit or Fat	
Two Day Diet	
Complete Hip and Thigh Diet	
The Maximum Metabolism Diet	
The Pasta Diet	
The McDougall Plan	
Novelty diets	
Dr. Abravanel's Body Type and Lifetime Nutrition Plan (or his other books)	Promote certain nutrients, foods, or combination of foods as having unique, magical, or previously undiscovered qualities
Dr. Berger's Immune Power Diet	
Fit for Life	
The Rotation Diet	Weaknesses; malnutrition; no change in habits → relapse; unrealistic food choices → leading to possible bingeing
The Hilton Head Metabolism Diet	
The Junk Food Diet	
The Beverly Hills Diet	
Dr. Debetz Champaign Diet	
Sun Sign Diet	
F-Plan Diet	
Fat Attack Plan	
The Ultrafit Diet	
The Princeton Plan	
The Diet Bible	
Bloomingdale's Diet	
The Love Diet	
Eat to Succeed	
The Underburner's Diet	
Eat to Win	

Continued.

TABLE 11-5

Summary of popular dietary approaches to weight control—cont'd

Approach and Examples	Characteristics and Possible Negative Health Consequences
Very low calorie diets	
Optifast	Less than 800 kcalories per day
Cambridge Diet	Also known as protein-sparing modi-
The Last Chance Diet	fied fasts
Genesis	
Medifast	Weakness; organ tissue loss—especial-
New Directions	ly from the heart; low serum potassi-
HMR	um level → heart failure; expense →
	must be under close physician
	scrutiny; gallstones; gout
Formula diets	
U.S.A. (United Sciences of America), Inc.	Can help people who find it easier not to eat whole foods while dieting to
Optifast	lose weight
Genesis	Based on formulated or packaged
Cambridge Diet	products
Herbalife	
The Last Chance Diet	Weaknesses: many are very low-calo- rie diet regimens (see above)
Slimfast	No change in habits → increased chance of relapse; expensive; consti- pation
Premeasured diets	
Nutri-System	Most food supplied in premeasured
Jenny Craig	servings to take much of the deci- sion-making out of the process of eating
	Weaknesses: expensive; may not allow for easy sound eating later

Diets may be listed in more than one category if multiple characteristics apply.

Fad diets fail. Most cruelly, dieters are left to assume the guilt and burden, believing they are failures. Fad diets are built for the quick fix. They often don't address problem eating habits (Figure 11-11). They can severely limit food selection, dooming the dieter to quit within a few weeks. But the hook comes with quickly vanishing pounds. Although dieters assume they have lost fat, they actually lose mostly water and lean tissue mass. When normal eating resumes, the lost water and tissue return. In a matter of weeks, most of the lost weight returns, too. This whole scenario sets up an emotionally damaging cycle of hope, discipline, failure, and guilt. Professional help, which fad diets rarely offer, is preferable.

Types of fad diets

Low-carbohydrate approaches. The most common form of fad diet, the low-carbohydrate diet, forces the liver to produce the glucose vital to such cells as red blood cells (see Chapter 8 for a review). Muscle and other lean tissue generate the carbons used to make new glucose. Thus a low-carbohydrate diet depletes muscle tissue. Since muscle tissue is mostly water, the person loses weight very rapidly. When a normal diet is resumed, the muscle tissue is rebuilt and weight quickly returns.

Low-carbohydrate dieting does not guarantee weight loss. Restricting kcalories is what helps. A low-carbohydrate diet by itself results in no more weight loss than other diets. Low-carbohydrate diets include Dr. Atkins' Diet Revolution, Dr. Stillman's Calories Don't Count Diet, the Scarsdale Diet, the Drinking Man's Diet, Four Day Wonder Diet, and the Air Force Diet. Check new fad diets for carbohydrate levels. Extremely limited amounts of breads, cereals, fruits, and vegetables indicate a low carbohydrate diet.

Lowfat approaches. Lowfat diets, though not harmful, generally fail because fat restrictions (as low as 5% to 10% of kcalories) generate eventual cravings for foods rich in fat. Overall, the very lowfat diet—the Pritikin Diet, for example—turns out to be a very high carbohydrate diet. The dieter primarily eats grains, fruits, and vegetables. The rigid restrictions lead dieters to a lapse, then a relapse, and probably a collapse. These diets are too far removed from our usual diets for most of us to follow consistently.

Novelty diets. Gimmicks sell many diets. The Rotation Diet, for example, rotates the total amount of kcalories every few days, attempting to prevent dieting's usual drop in metabolic rate. No scientific data show that this diet works or even how it might work. We label this a fad diet because, in suggesting fewer than 1000 kcalories for some phases, it has a low nutrient content.

Some novelty diets suggest gorging on particular foods or food groups. An egg diet suggests swallowing all the eggs you can eat. The Beverly Hills Diet promotes dining almost exclusively on fresh fruit. A rice diet, designed in the 1940s to lower blood pressure, recently resurfaced for weight loss. More fruit; lots of rice; useless in the long run.

The rationale behind these diets is that you can eat only eggs, or fruit, or rice for so long. You will soon become bored and, in theory, reduce your energy intake. These diets are based on fake science. And, chances are that you will abandon the diet entirely before you lose much weight.

In the 1960s diet aids were introduced. For appeal, the popular grapefruit diet enlisted help from some aids: lecithin to help release fat from the tissues, vitamin B-6 to act as a diuretic, vinegar to provide potassium, and kelp to stimulate the thyroid gland. These aids don't deliver what they promise. In the 1980s we had an entirely new product, Herbalife. The aid in Herbalife is herbs high in caffeine; caffeine stimulates the metabolic rate. None of these diet aids can substitute for moderating food intake, modifying behavior, and increasing activity.

The most bizarre of the novelty diets propose that "food gets stuck in your body." Fit for Life and the Beverly Hills Diet suggest that food gets stuck in the intestine, putrifies, and creates toxins that invade the bloodstream and cause disease. This is utter nonsense. Nevertheless, health-food books have proposed this chain of events since the 1800s. Today, Fit for Life suggests meat eaten with potatoes will not be digested and that only fresh fruit should be consumed before noon. These recommendations are absurd. These supposedly controversial gimmicks are really designed to sell books. If weight loss does occur, it is because the books combine such complicated rules and rituals that, by the time you have figured out what you can eat, it is the wrong time to eat!

Does your food make you sick? One scheme suggests 30% of us have food allergies that in turn cause most current disease. Find the food allergy, treat it, and, like magic, disease will be waved away; obesity as well. This theory of the early 1980s was made popular by Dr. Berger's Immune Power Diet Book. However, we know of no research that supports Dr. Berger's claim that 30% of people have food allergies.

Now in the 90s there are diets to hook everyone: if astrology guides you, follow the Sun Sign Diet; if you need a drink, celebrate with the Champagne Diet; or match your "dominant" gland with the Body Type and Lifetime Nutrition Diet. Quackery never sleeps, so keep on your toes. ●

cathy®   **by Cathy Guisewite**

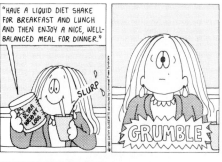
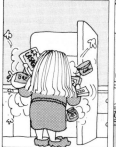
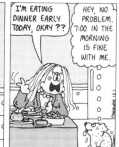

FIGURE 11-11

NUTRITION
ATHLETICS AND FITNESS

We have integrated a variety of concepts into this chapter on nutrition and fitness. To begin, many chemical processes in the body release energy. Your muscles and other organs use the energy to do work. Understanding where this energy comes from and how it is used is fascinating even if you don't compete in sports.

Once your muscles have energy available to them, what determines the type of fuel they use? You do, to an extent, depending on how physically fit you are and how hard you perform. Physical fitness—defined as the ability to do moderate to vigorous activity without undue fatigue—affects your fuel use. Diet also has an effect. We will discuss this in detail later in the chapter.

Finally, you will discover how physical fitness benefits the entire body: it is an essential ingredient in achieving maximal health.[3] Benefits include improvement of heart function, less injury, better sleep habits, and improvement in body composition (less body fat and more muscle mass). Exercise also positively affects blood pressure and blood sugar regulation. Another basic reason to be physically fit is, of course, it's fun and it feels good. Some people are active not because they're thinking about health benefits, but simply because they're enjoying it, whether they're skiing, swimming, hiking, playing basketball, or engaging in any of innumerable other activities. Let's now look at these concepts further. ●

CHAPTER

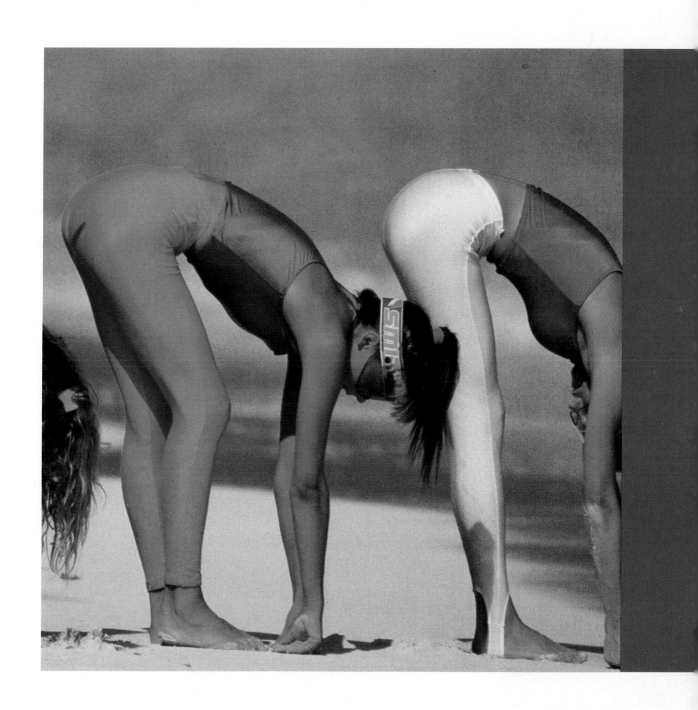

How Active are You?

The following questions will help you determine your level of physical activity. Place a "Y" in the space indicating yes, or an "N" for no.

_____ 1. Do you walk to school or work, at least ½ mile each way? | 1 point

_____ 2. Do you usually take the stairs rather than the elevator or escalator? | 1 point

_____ 3. Do you spend most of your day walking briskly or many hours shoveling or lifting? | 5 points

_____ 4. Do you do several hours of gardening or lawn work each week? | 1 point

_____ 5. Do you do an hour or more of vigorous dancing at least once per week (in a club; at a dance; square, folk, or modern dancing)? | 1 point

_____ 6. Do you play golf without a cart at least once per week when the weather is right? | 1 point

_____ 7. Do you often walk for recreation? | 1 point

_____ 8. Do you use exercise to relieve stress? | 1 point

_____ 9. Do you do calisthenics (situps, pushups, jumping jacks) at least two times per week? | 3 points

_____ 10. Do you regularly perform stretching exercises for at least 5 minutes each time you exercise? | 2 points

_____ 11. Do you participate in active recreational sports (basketball, racquetball, tennis, handball, squash) at least twice per week? | 5 points

_____ 12. Do you perform vigorous physical activity (jogging, biking, swimming, brisk walking, stairmaster, rowing) for at least 20 minutes per session, 3 times per week? | 10 points

_____ 13. Do you perform weight lifting at least 2 times per week? | 3 points

INTERPRETATION

Look at the point values to the right of each question. Total the points for each yes answer and write the total in the blank:

TOTAL POINTS _____

If YOU SCORED:

> Less than 12—You are inactive to moderately inactive. Try to work to improve your fitness level.
> 12 or greater—You are active to very active. Keep up the good work.

ASSESS YOURSELF

METABOLISM

Muscle cells, like all cells, need energy to perform. Cells need to capture this energy and then release it to do work.

Our discussion of this process—energy *metabolism*—must start with the definition of metabolism. This term refers to all chemical processes that take place in the body. Any sequence of a chemical process from beginning to end—for example, burning glucose for fuel—is called a *pathway.*

Metabolic pathways can produce both *anabolic* and *catabolic* results. Anabolic pathways build compounds. In these pathways the typical building blocks used to form new, larger compounds are oxygen (O_2), water (H_2O), and carbon dioxide (CO_2). These parts can be made up to form a fatty acid, glucose, or even the complex cholesterol molecule. The process of building requires energy input to make it go.[21]

Conversely, catabolic pathways, which break down compounds into smaller units, often release energy. Glucose and fatty acids, for example, are catabolized when broken down into carbon dioxide and water. Energy is released as a by-product. Anabolic and catabolic pathways take place simultaneously in cells.

Overall, the catabolism for the ultimate energy production from foodstuffs occurs in two stages. In the first stage large compounds in food—proteins, starches, and triglycerides—are broken down during digestion into smaller units, such as amino acids, simple sugars, and fatty acids. These units are then delivered to working cells, like muscle cells, via the bloodstream. In this second stage these compounds are eventually broken down into carbon dioxide and water inside the cell. During this second process, large amounts of energy are released to power the cell.[21]

Energy a cell can use

The energy that runs the body originates as solar energy. Plants capture this energy through a process called *photosynthesis.* Plants use the energy to produce carbohydrates, proteins, and fats. In essence, plants trap solar energy and store it as chemical energy in these nutrients. Every amino acid, glucose, and fatty acid molecule has numerous sites where chemical energy is stored for our use.

One key function of metabolism is to convert energy stored in foodstuffs to a form human cells can use. Overall, each cell must first break down glucose or other energy-rich sources to release stored energy and then convert that energy into usable and smaller energy packets.

Adenosine triphosphate (ATP)

As you may have guessed from our previous discussion, cells can't directly use the energy released from breaking down glucose or fat. Rather, the energy must first be stored in a special form. This is called *adenosine triphosphate (ATP).* To store chemical energy, our cells make ATP. Again, the cells are using the energy obtained from foodstuffs. Conversely, to release energy from ATP, cells partially break down ATP. This releases usable energy for cell functions.

Essentially, ATP is the immediate source of energy for body functions. This includes locomotion.[21] The overall goal of any fuel use—carbohydrate, fat, or protein—is to make ATP. A resting muscle cell only has a small amount of ATP that can be used. If no resupply of ATP were possible, this stored ATP could keep the muscle working maximally for only about 2 to 4 seconds. Fortunately, there are several types of chemical compounds—*phosphocreatine (PCr)*, carbohydrates, fats, and proteins—that can be broken down to release enough energy to make more ATP. Cells actually must constantly use and then reform ATP, over and over again.

Metabolism • Chemical reactions that occur in the body, enabling cells to release energy from foods, convert one substance into another, and prepare end products for excretion.

Pathway • A metabolic progression of individual steps from starting materials to ending products, like glucose → → → CO_2 + H_2O.

Anabolism • The process of building compounds.

Catabolism • The process of breaking down compounds.

Photosynthesis • The process by which plants use energy from the sun to produce energy-yielding compounds, such as glucose.

Adenosine Triphosphate (ATP) • The main energy currency for cells. ATP energy is used to promote ion pumping, enzyme activity, and muscular contraction.

Phosphocreatine (PCr) • A high energy compound that can be used to reform ATP.

Almost every step in any metabolic pathway depends on input from an enzyme to allow the step to take place.

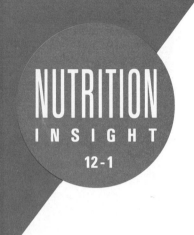

WHAT CAN A PHYSICALLY ACTIVE LIFESTYLE PROMISE?

Was your New Year's resolution to start exercising? Do you often wish that you could be healthier and more physically fit? Today, the interest in physical fitness that blossomed into a full-fledged movement nearly 20 years ago shows no signs of fading. Experts in medicine and nutrition support this trend (Figure 12-1).[17] More people than ever engage in a wide range of activities, from mall walking to stair climbing and triathalons. This interest in physical activity, particularly as an integral component of overall health and wellness, is evident by the explosion in the number of health clubs nationwide.

To counteract widespread heart disease, diabetes mellitus, obesity, and osteoporosis, many people have become interested in the potential health benefits of regular physical activity. Increasing evidence suggests that physical activity may delay the onset and/or help treat these diseases.[14] Although an increase in physical activity is hardly a magic bullet, many people change their habits in hopes that moderate exercise will improve their chances of living longer. This hope is not without scientific support. Regular physical activity also can help reduce stress and increase self-esteem. Best of all, you don't have to be a marathon runner to reap the benefits of exercise. Moderate or leisure-time physical activities, if done frequently and for a sufficient duration, many offer the same benefits as more rigorous activities.

FRANK & ERNEST® by Bob Thaves

FIGURE 12-1

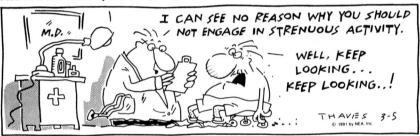

Overall exercise fitness

Repeated aerobic exercise produces beneficial changes in the heart and in blood vessels responsible for delivering oxygen to the muscles. Because it uses more oxygen, the body responds to training by producing more red blood cells and increasing total blood volume. The heart, a muscle itself, enlarges and strengthens. Each contraction empties the heart's chambers more efficiently, enabling more blood to be pumped with each beat. Exercise increases the heart's efficiency by lowering its rate of beating at rest and during submaximal exercise. This is an index of fitness—the heart rate lowers as fitness increases. In addition, oxygen can be delivered more easily throughout the muscles because the number of capillaries in the muscles increases after exercise training.

After a period of aerobic training, the muscles can more efficiently fuel themselves from fatty acid stores. Changes caused by aerobic exercise eventually allow muscle cells to produce more ATP using oxygen-requiring pathways. This includes the pathway used to burn fat for fuel. This in turn allows for greater intensity during aerobic exercise and harder and longer training at an aerobic pace.[6]

Heart disease

How can a physically active lifestyle reduce the risk of coronary heart disease? Exercise can improve **cardiovascular** fitness, help maintain weight, regulate blood pressure, and often modestly boost HDL-cholesterol (good cholesterol) levels.

Based on a review of many studies, for heart health the American College of Sports Medicine recommends at least 15 to 60 minutes of aerobic exercise, 3 to 5 days per week, with a heart rate elevation of 60% to 90% of one's age-dependent maximal heart rate (220 minus current age). Still, even moderate or leisure-time physical activity, such as walking, can benefit the cardiovascular system. And, significantly, we are more likely to persevere in moderate—rather than more rigorous—physical activities. Daily, routine stair climbing is one easy way to get moderate aerobic stimulation. For sedentary and middle-aged people who have not maintained a physically active lifestyle, brisk walking and moderate activities are preferable at the start to jogging and more rigorous types of activities.

Diabetes mellitus

Exercise contributes to weight loss in obesity, which, in turn, enhances the action of the hormone insulin. Poor insulin action is the main short-term problem resulting from the major form diabetes mellitus. Enhancing insulin sensitivity also improves glucose removal from the bloodstream and potentially allows insulin dosage to be reduced for those who use it. A person with diabetes mellitus must work with a physician to make the correct alterations in diet and medications to perform exercise safely. This is because physical activity can adversely affect some people with diabetes mellitus (by inducing low blood sugar, for example). These people need to be aware of their blood glucose response to exercise. To determine this response, they can self-monitor their blood glucose levels before, during (if exercise is prolonged), and after physical activity. The benefits of exercise on insulin action appear to be short-lived, so regular moderate physical activity is encouraged.

Obesity

As a means of losing or controlling weight, a physically active lifestyle offers several benefits, as noted in Chapter 11. In review, first, by increasing energy use, exercise may allow a person to lose weight while eating more than normal. More food and greater variety can then allow better overall nutrient intake. Losing weight by dieting usually entails losing lean tissue as well as body fat. Performing regular physical activity along with dieting spares some of this lean tissue loss, while promoting the loss of fat tissue. Furthermore, physical activity, especially if it helps someone lose fat, may also help reverse some risk factors associated with obesity, such as diabetes mellitus, hypertension, and premature cardiovascular disease.[8]

At moderate levels of activity, exercise increases one's resting metabolic rate, but only for a short time after exercise ceases. Therefore, to get a regular boost in kcalorie burning, exercise should be a daily routine for an obese person, and for that matter, all of us. Note that little bursts of activity can mount up to a lot of daily activity.

Osteoporosis

Osteoporosis is a disease that leads to a high risk for bone fracture caused by bone loss. Each year osteoporosis leads to over 1 million bone fractures in people over 45 years of age, most of whom are women. Both genetic and environmental factors are implicated as causes. Estrogen deficiency at menopause is a major factor. Regularly getting too little calcium may be another contributor. Physical activity, particularly moderate weight-bearing exercise, can help to prevent osteoporosis.[17]

An extremely sedentary lifestyle causes bone loss. Bone loss occurs under extreme conditions of prolonged bed rest or weightlessness, as astronauts experience in space. Experts agree that regular moderate exercise is important for bone health. Regular physical activity may offer even more benefits for the elderly, who are at great risk of osteoporosis. The agility and strength from activity can reduce both the likelihood of falls and/or injuries caused by falls.

Maintaining ones drive

Even a minimal amount of exercise—a brisk half-hour walk a few times a week—is important for promoting cardiovascular fitness, as well as forestalling disease from a wide range of other causes. People who exercise even a little bit tend to live longer. ●

Cardiovascular • Pertaining to the heart and blood vessels.

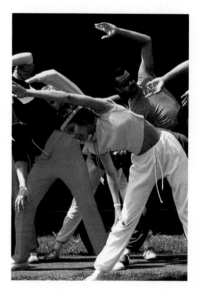

Stretching before exercise warms the muscles. This lessens the risk of later injury.

Chapter 3 lists many guidelines for setting goals and sticking to them. These suggestions are quite applicable to a goal of performing regular exercise.

ANOTHER BITE Think about ATP the next time you race after a bus. When you finally sit down, you are exhausted, you breathe hard, and your heart races. Your muscle cells have used up most of their ATP and other high energy compounds. While you rest, muscle cells begin to resynthesize the ATP used up during your run. Reforming ATP requires energy. Again, cells can get this energy from foodstuffs. If you sit long enough, you can then race off to class using some of the newly formed ATP.

Phosphocreatine is the first line of defense for resupplying ATP in muscles

The instant that breakdown products of ATP begin to accumulate in the contracting muscle, an enzyme is activated to split phosphocreatine (PCr). This releases the energy needed to reform ATP. If no other source of ATP resupply were available, PCr could probably maintain maximal muscle contractions for about 10 seconds.[15] But since other ATP sources kick in, PCr ends up the major source of energy for all events lasting up to about 1 minute (Table 12-1).

The main advantages of PCr is that it can be activated instantly and can replenish ATP at rates fast enough to meet the energy demands of the fastest and most powerful sports events, including jumping, lifting, throwing, and sprinting actions. The disadvantage of PCr is that there is not enough of it made and stored in the muscles to sustain a high rate of ATP resupply for more than a few minutes. Many attempts have been made over the years to improve the muscle ATP and PCr stores by dietary means, but none have been effective.[12]

TABLE 12-1

Energy systems for muscle cell use

System	When in Use	Example of an Exercise
ATP	At all times	All types
Phosphocreatine (PCr)	All exercise initially; extreme exercise thereafter	Shotput, jumping
Anaerobic glycolysis (carbohydrate)	High intensity exercise, especially lasting 30 seconds to 2 minutes	200-yard (200-meter) run for time
Aerobic glycolysis (carbohydrate)	Exercise lasting 2 minutes to 4 to 5 hours; the higher the intensity (such as running a 6-minute mile), the greater the use	Basketball, swimming, jogging
Aerobic fat use	Exercise lasting more than a few minutes; greater amounts are used at lower levels of exercise intensity	Long-distance running, long distance cycling; 70%-90% of fuel use in a brisk walk is fat
Aerobic protein use	Low levels during all exercise; moderate levels in endurance exercise, especially when carbohydrate fuel is lacking	Long-distance running

The fuel mix in exercise sustained over 1 hour or more is 60%-80% fat, 15%-30% carbohydrate, and up to 10% protein. As intensity increases, carbohydrate use climbs to about 40% and protein use to about 15%. Fat use falls accordingly.

Releasing the energy in carbohydrate begins with glycolysis

Carbohydrates are a valuable fuel for muscles. The most useful form of carbohydrate fuel is the simple sugar glucose. This is available to all cells from the bloodstream. The breakdown of liver glycogen (a storage form of glucose) helps maintain blood glucose levels. In muscles, breakdown of stored glycogen helps meet carbohydrate demand of that muscle.[16] In the catabolic pathway that breaks down glucose, the 6-carbon glucose splits into two 3-carbon compounds. The net energy produced equals two ATP. This is about 5% of the total number of ATP that can be made from one glucose.[21] But although this phase of glucose metabolism does not extract much energy from a single glucose molecule, a muscle cell can break down thousands of glucose molecules per second. Therefore this form of glucose metabolism resupplies ATP at a very high rate for a brief period.[15]

When glucose breaks down, the resulting 3-carbon compound follows either of two main routes. When oxygen supply in the muscle is limited (*anaerobic* conditions) and when the exercise is intense (e.g., running 400 meters or swimming 100 meters), the 3-carbon compound accumulates in the muscle and is converted to ***lactic acid.*** No further ATP is directly formed. This conversion of glucose to lactic acid is called anaerobic ***glycolysis*** (*glyco* means sugar and *lysis* means breakdown). Carbohydrate is the only fuel that can be used for this process.

If there is plenty of oxygen available in the muscle (***aerobic*** conditions) and the exercise activity is of moderate to low intensity (e.g., jogging or distance swimming), the bulk of the 3-carbon compound is shuttled to the ***mitochondria*** of the cell, where it is further metabolized into carbon dioxide and water. This is known as aerobic glycolysis because the breakdown of glucose takes place with the aid of oxygen. Aerobic glycolosis forms about 95% of the ATP made from glucose metabolism (Figure 12-2).[21]

Anaerobic • Not requiring oxygen.

Lactic Acid • A three-carbon acid formed during anaerobic cell metabolism; a partial breakdown of glucose; also called lactate.

Aerobic • Requiring oxygen.

Glycolysis • The pathway that results in the breakdown of glucose into two 3-carbon compounds.

Mitochondria • Structure inside most cells, including muscle cells. These are the main sites of energy production in a cell. Mitochondria also contain the pathway for burning fat for fuel, among other metabolic pathways.

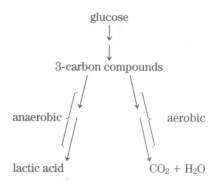

FIGURE 12-2
Carbohydrate, fat, and protein fuels can all supply ATP energy for a muscle cell.

Anaerobic glycolysis. The advantage of anaerobic glycolysis is that, other than PCr breakdown, it is the fastest way to resupply ATP. Anaerobic glycolysis provides most of the energy for events ranging from about 30 seconds to 2 minutes.[15] The two major disadvantages of anaerobic glycolysis are (1) the high rate of ATP production cannot be sustained for long events, and (2) the rapid accumulation of lactic acid greatly increases the acidity of the muscle. This acid inhibits the activities of key enzymes in the glycolysis pathway. That slows anaerobic ATP production and, in turn, causes fatigue.

For the most part, lactic acid accumulates in active muscle cells until it is released into the bloodstream. The liver picks up the lactic acid and resynthesizes it into glucose. Glucose then can reenter the bloodstream where it is available for cell uptake and breakdown. The heart also can use the lactic acid directly for its energy needs, as can less active muscle cells situated near active ones.[15]

Aerobic glycolysis. Aerobic glycolysis supplies ATP more slowly than does anaerobic glycolysis, but again more energy is released. Furthermore, the slower rate of aerobic energy supply can be sustained for hours. Accordingly, aerobic glycolysis makes a major energy contribution to sports events that last anywhere from 2 minutes to 4 or 5 hours (see Table 12-1).

Importance of glycogen versus blood glucose for carbohydrate fuel

It is important to note that muscle glycogen is the preferred fuel for both anaerobic glycolysis and for aerobic glycolysis in fairly intense muscular activities that last for less than about 2 hours. For these activities, the depletion of glycogen fuel in the muscle can cause fatigue. Diets high in carbohydrate can be used to build up muscle glycogen stores before athletic competition, thereby forestalling fatigue and improving endurance.[19] We discuss this technique in a later section.

As exercise duration increases beyond 20 to 30 minutes, blood glucose becomes increasingly important as a fuel for glycolysis. Use of glucose from the bloodstream can spare glycogen, saving it in the muscle for sudden bursts of effort that may be required, such as a sprint to the finish in a marathon race. Because it is important to maintain high concentrations of glucose in the bloodstream for prolonged exercise, many investigations have studied various types of carbohydrate feedings before and during exercise to maximize glucose supply. We will also discuss this issue in a later section.

CONCEPT CHECK

ATP is the main form of energy that cells use. Metabolic pathways use food energy to form ATP. Carbohydrate metabolism to form ATP begins as glucose becomes available from the bloodstream or from glycogen breakdown. In a muscle cell each glucose is broken down through a series of steps to yield either lactic acid or carbon dioxide (CO_2) plus water (H_2O). The process that occurs when glucose is broken down into carbon dioxide and water is called aerobic glycolysis, since oxygen is used. The conversion of glucose to lactic acid is called anaerobic glycolysis, since no oxygen is used. This latter process allows the cell to quickly reform ATP and supports the demand for energy during intense exercise.

Energy metabolism using fat

When fat stores in body tissues are broken down for energy, one triglyceride molecule first yields three fatty acids and a glycerol. The majority of the stored energy is found in the fatty acids. During physical activity, the fatty acids are released from various fat depots into the bloodstream and travel to the muscles, where they are taken into each cell and aerobically broken down to carbon dioxide and water.

The rate at which muscles use fatty acids is partly dependent on the concentration of fatty acids in the bloodstream. In other words, the more fatty acids that are released from fat stores into the bloodstream, the more fat will be used by the muscles. Recently, some athletes have attempted to raise their blood concentrations of fatty acids by consuming caffeinated beverages. This practice actually can increase fatty acid release from the fat depots and so can be helpful to some athletes (see the Nutrition Issue, p. 397).[22]

Fat is ultimately not a very useful fuel for intense, brief exercise, but it becomes a progressively more important energy source as duration of exercise increases, especially when exercise remains at a low or moderate (aerobic) rate (Figure 12-2). The reason for this is that some of the steps involved in fat breakdown simply cannot occur fast enough to meet the ATP demands of short duration, high intensity exercise. If fat were the only available fuel, we would be unable to exercise more intensely than a fast walk or jog. High-caliber sports events would be out of the question.

The advantage of fat fuel over other types is that it provides tremendous stores of energy in a relatively lightweight form. For a given weight of fuel, fat supplies more than twice as much energy as carbohydrate. For very lengthy activities, such as a triathalon, ultramarathon, manual labor in a foundry, or even sitting at a desk for 8 hours a day, fat supplies about 70% to 90% of the energy required. For short events, such as a 100-meter sprint or even a 1500-meter race, the contribution of fat used to resupply ATP is minimal. Keep in mind that the only fast-paced (anaerobic) fuel we eat is carbohydrate; slow and steady (aerobic) activity uses carbohydrate, fat, and protein energy sources (Figure 12-3).[15]

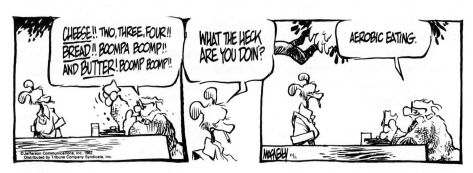

FIGURE 12-3
Shoe.

Does this mean we use protein to fuel activity?

Protein can be used for fueling muscles, but in most circumstances protein contributes only about 6% of the body's general energy needs.[18] This is also true for the typical energy needs of exercising muscles. However, proteins can contribute significantly to energy needs in endurance exercise, perhaps as much as 10% to 15%, especially as carbohydrate stores in the muscles are exhausted.[18] We easily eat enough to supply this amount of fuel.[11] Protein or amino acid supplements are not needed. Contrary to what many athletes believe, protein is used less for fuel in resistance types of exercise, such as weight lifting, than for endurance exercise, such as running. The primary fuels for weight lifting are phosphocreatine (PCr) and carbohydrate.

CONCEPT CHECK

Fat is a key aerobic fuel for muscle cells, especially at low exercise intensities. At rest muscles burn primarily fat for energy needs. On the other hand, little protein is used to fuel muscles. It supplies about 6% of energy needs, and at most 10% to 15% of energy needs during endurance events.

POWER FOOD: WHAT SHOULD AN ATHLETE EAT?

Athletic training and genetic makeup are two very important determinants of athletic performance. A good diet won't substitute for either, but as we have mentioned, diet can further enhance and maximize an athlete's potential. More importantly, a poor diet certainly can harm performance.[5]

How much food energy does an athlete need?

Athletes need varying amounts of food energy, depending on the athlete's body size and the type of training or competition being considered. A small person may need only 1700 kcalories daily to sustain normal daily activities without losing body weight. A large muscular man may need 3000 kcalories. These are only estimates and need to be individualized by trial and error for each athlete. Kcalories required for sports training or competition have to be added to energy needed for normal activities (see Table 12-2). An hour of bowling, for example, requires few kcalories in addition to those required to sustain normal daily living. On the other extreme, 12-hour endurance bicycle races over mountains can require an additional 4000 kcalories per day. Therefore some athletes may need as much as 7000 kcalories daily just to maintain body weight while training, whereas others may need 1700 kcalories or less.

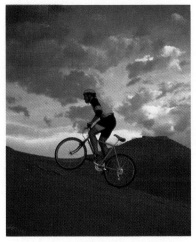

Carbohydrate and fat mostly fuel endurance exercise.

How can we determine whether an athlete is getting enough energy from food? The first step is to estimate the athlete's body fat percentage by measuring skinfold thickness, estimating bioelectrical impedance, or using the underwater weighing technique (see Chapter 11). Body fat should be in the desirable range—about 6% to 12% for most male athletes and 15% to 20% (but sometimes less) for most female athletes.[15] The next step is to monitor body-weight changes on a daily or weekly basis. If body weight starts to fall, food energy should be increased; if weight rises because of increases in body fat, the athlete should be encouraged to eat less.

If the body composition test shows that the athlete is too fat, the athlete should eat about 200 to 500 fewer kcalories per day until the desirable fat percentage is achieved while maintaining a regular exercise program. Reducing fat intake is the best nutrient-related approach. On the other hand, if the athlete needs to gain weight, an additional 200 to 500 kcalories per day will eventually lead to the needed weight gain. A mix of carbohydrate and fat is advised, coupled again with exercise to ensure the gain is mostly from lean tissue and not just added fat stores.

Rapid weight loss by dehydration. Wrestlers, boxers, boxers, judo players, and oarsmen often try to lose weight so that they can be certified to compete in a lower weight class. This helps them gain a mechanical advantage over an opponent of smaller stature. Most of the time, this weight is lost a few hours before stepping on the scale for weight certification. Athletes can lose up to 22 pounds (10 kilograms) of body water in 1 day by sitting in a sauna, exercising in a plastic sweat suit, and/or taking diuretic drugs that speed water loss from the kidneys. Losing as little as 3% of body weight by dehydration can sometimes adversely affect endurance performance.[2] A pattern of repeated weight loss and weight gain of more than 5% of body weight by dehydration carries some risk of kidney malfunction or heat illness. Dehydration also causes a reduction in blood volume, increases body temperature, and may result in heat cramps or heat exhaustion.

This habit of losing weight by dehydration is common in sports such as interscholastic and intercollegiate wrestling. Most competitors in wrestling face opponents who have gone through the same misery to gain an "advantage." If an athlete wishes to compete in a lower body-weight class and has enough extra fat stores, that athlete should begin a gradual, sustained reduction in food energy intake long before the competitive season starts. In so doing, the athlete will have a presumably healthier body composition (less fat) and can avoid the potentially harmful and certainly misery-creating effects of severe dehydration. An athlete who has no extra body fat should be discouraged from attempting to compete at a lower body-weight class. It is important for coaches and trainers to be aware of the decreased performance and serious side effects of severe dehydration.

TABLE 12-2

Approximate energy costs of various activities[1] for a 150-pound (68-kilogram) person

Activity	Kcal/Hour
Aerobics—heavy	544
Aerobics—light	204
Aerobics—medium	340
Backpacking	612
Basketball—vigorous	680
Bicycling (5.5 MPH)	204
Bowling	265
Calisthenics—heavy	544
Calisthenics—light	272
Canoeing (2.5 MPH)	224
Cleaning (female)	253
Cleaning (male)	236
Cooking	190
Cycling (13 MPH)	659
Dressing/showering	106
Driving	117
Eating (sitting)	93
Food shopping	245
Football—touch	476
Golf	244
Horseback trotting	346
Ice skating (10 MPH)	394
Jogging—medium	612
Jogging—slow	476
Lying—at ease	89
Racquetball—social	544
Roller skating	346
Running or jogging (10 MPH)	897
Skiing (10 MPH)	598
Sleeping	80
Swimming (.25 MPH)	299
Tennis	414
Volleyball	346
Walking (2.5 MPH)	204
Walking (3.75 MPH)	299
Water skiing	476
Weight lifting—heavy	612
Weight lifting—light	272
Window cleaning	240
Writing (sitting)	118

Source: Mosby Diet Simple, N-Squared Computing, Salem, Oregon, 97302

General principles for meeting nutrient needs in the training diet

Anyone who exercises regularly, including the dieter, needs to consume a diet that includes moderate to high amounts of carbohydrates.[4] This should be about 55% to 70% of total kcalories, rather than our typical 46%. Endurance athletes should meet the higher value. Fat intake should then fall from our typical 38% of total kcalories to 15% to 30%. Protein should make up the rest of the energy—about 10% to 15% of the total. This creates a plate with about two-thirds carbohydrate-rich foods and one-third protein-rich foods.[5]

All athletes should consume a variety of foods and adhere to the Guide to Daily Food Choices (see Chapter 2). Numerous selections of starches and fruits will help maintain adequate muscle glycogen stores and replace glycogen losses from the previous day.[7] Triathletes and marathon participants should consider eating close to 600 grams of carbohydrates a day, and even more if necessary, to (1) prevent chronic fatigue and (2) load the muscles and liver with

---

TABLE 12-3

Grams of carbohydrate in typical foods

Starchy vegetables, breads, and cereals—15 grams carbohydrate per serving
One serving:

½ cup dry breakfast cereals*	1 small baked potato
½ cup cooked breakfast cereals	½ bagel
½ cup cooked grits	½ English muffin
⅓ cup cooked rice	1 slice bread
½ cup cooked pasta	¾ ounce pretzels
¼ cup baked beans	6 saltine crackers
½ cup corn	2 four-inch-diameter pancakes
½ cup beans	2 taco shells

Vegetables—5 grams carbohydrate per serving
One serving:

½ cup cooked vegetables
1 cup raw vegetables
½ cup vegetable juice
Examples: carrots, green beans, broccoli, cauliflower, onions, spinach, tomatoes, vegetable juice

Fruits—15 grams carbohydrate per serving

One serving:

½ cup fresh fruit	12 cherries or grapes
½ cup fruit juice	½ grapefruit
¼ cup dried fruit	1 nectarine
1 small apple	1 orange
4 apricots	1 peach
½ banana	1-¼ cup watermelon

Milk—12 grams carbohydrate per serving
One serving:

1 cup milk
8 ounces plain lowfat yogurt

Sweets—15 grams carbohydrate per serving
One serving:

½ slice cake	½ cup ice cream
2 small cookies	¼ cup sherbet
3 ginger snaps	

---

*Note the carbohydrate contents of dry cereals vary widely. Check the label of the ones you choose and adjust serving size accordingly.

Modified from *Exchange Lists for Meal Planning* by the American Diabetes Association and American Dietetic Association, 1986, Chicago, American Dietetic Association.

glycogen. This practice is especially important when performing multiple training bouts in 1 day, such as swim practices, or heavy training on successive days, such as in cross-country running.[19] Table 12-3 can help plan a 600-gram carbohydrate intake. Table 12-4 provides an example of a high-carbohydrate diet. One does not have to give up any specific food. The diet focus just must turn to more of the best—high carbohydrate foods—and away from the rest—concentrated fat sources.

A further look at carbohydrate—carbohydrate loading

For athletes who compete in events lasting 90 to 120 minutes or longer or in shorter events repeated in a 24-hour period, it is often advantageous to undertake a *carbohydrate-loading* regimen to maximize muscle glycogen stores.[19] One possible regimen includes a gradual reduction or tapering of exercise intensity and duration coupled with a gradual increase in dietary carbohydrate

Carbohydrate-loading • A process in which a very high carbohydrate diet is consumed for 6 days before an athletic event in an attempt to increase muscle glycogen stores.

TABLE 12-4

A 600-gram carbohydrate diet

4000 kcalories:	
623 grams of carbohydrates	(61% of kcalories)*
139 grams of protein	(14% of kcalories)*
118 grams of fat	(26% of kcalories)*

Menu	Carbohydrate (grams)
Breakfast	
1 orange	14
2 cups oatmeal	50
1 cup skim milk	12
2 bran muffins	48
Snack	
³/₄ cup chopped dates	98
Lunch	
Lettuce salad:	
1 cup romaine lettuce	2
1 cup garbanzo beans	45
¹/₂ cup alfalfa sprouts	5.5
2 tablespoons French dressing	2
3 cups macaroni and cheese	80
1 cup apple juice	28
Snack	
2 slices whole-wheat toast	26
1 teaspoon margarine	—
2 tablespoons jam	14
Dinner	
2 ounces turkey breast (no skin)	—
2 cups mashed potatoes	74
1 cup peas and onions	23
1 banana	27
1 cup skim milk	12
Snack	
1 cup pasta with	33
2 teaspoons margarine and	—
2 tablespoons parmesan cheese	
1 cup cranberry juice	36
Total	628 grams

*A carbohydrate: protein: fat ratio of 60:15:25 is a good general goal when planning a diet to aid athletic performance.

as a percentage of energy intake. The procedure can begin with the athlete completing a hard workout lasting about 60 minutes about 6 days before competition. Workouts for the next 4 days should last about 40, 40, 20, and 20 minutes, respectively. Exercise intensities should be progressively reduced each day. On the final day before competition, the athlete should rest.

The dietary carbohydrate on the first 3 days of this regimen contributes 45% to 50% of energy intake (about 450 grams). This intake rises to 65% to 75% carbohydrate (about 600 grams) for the remaining 3 days before the competition. This carbohydrate-loading technique usually increases muscle glycogen storage by 50% to 85% over usual conditions, i.e., when a typical amount of carbohydrate is consumed (46% of kcalories). The greater carbohydrate stores then often result in improved athletic endurance.[19]

ANOTHER BITE	Appropriate Activities for Carbohydrate Loading	Inappropriate Activities for Carbohydrate Loading
	Marathons	Football games
	Long-distance swimming	10-kilometer runs
	Cross-country skiing	Downhill ski races
	30-kilometer runs	Walking and hiking
	Triathalons	Most swimming events
	Cycling time trials	Basketball games
	Long-distance canoe racing	Weight lifting
		Most track and field events
		Rowing events

A potential disadvantage of carbohydrate loading is that, along with the glycogen, some water is also stored in the muscles.[7] The water adds body weight and may cause muscle stiffness. For some people, this makes carbohydrate loading an unfeasible practice. Athletes considering carbohydrate loading should try it once during training (and well before an important event) to experience its effects on performance. They can then determine if it is worth the effort.

Sports nutritionists emphasize the difference between a high-carbohydrate meal and a high-carbohydrate/high-fat meal.[5] Before endurance events, such as marathons or triathalons, some athletes attempt carbohydrate loading by eating potato chips, French fries, banana cream pie, and pastries. These foods do contain carbohydrate, but they also contain a lot of fat. Better food choices are pasta, rice, potatoes, bread, and many breakfast cereals. Sports drinks appropriate for carbohydrate loading, such as GatorLode or Exceed High Carbohydrate Source, can also help. Eating a moderate amount of dietary fiber during the final day is a good precaution to reduce the chances of bloating and intestinal gas during the next day's event.

Muscle bulking diets

During muscle-building regimens, athletes should consume 1 to 1.5 grams of protein per kilogram (0.5 to 0.7 grams per pound) of body weight daily.[18] This range goes from slightly above to about double the protein RDA (0.8 grams per kilogram of desirable body weight). Anyone eating a variety of foods can easily meet the higher intake. For example, a 123-pound (53-kilogram) woman can consume close to her upper range of 80 grams of protein by eating 4 ounces of chicken (one chicken breast) and 3 ounces of beef (a small lean hamburger), and drinking 3 glasses of milk during a single day. And this does not even include the protein in the grains or vegetables she will also eat. A 180-pound (77-kilogram) man needs only to consume 6 ounces of chicken (a large chicken breast) and a 6-ounce can of tuna, and drink 3 glasses of milk during a day to obtain

Carbohydrate loading is safe for adolescents, but the activities this technique is useful for, like marathon runs, may not be. Physician approval should be sought for the latter.

close to his upper range of 115 grams of protein. Many athletes eat many more protein-rich foods as they meet their energy needs (see Table 12-3). Again, we see that protein supplements are not needed for athletes because their diets typically exceed even the most generous protein recommendation.

Athletes who either feel they must significantly limit their energy intake or are vegetarians should determine how much protein they eat; they should make sure it equals at least 1 gram per kilogram of desirable body weight. Skimping on protein is not a good idea.[5]

Vitamins and minerals

Athletes usually consume many kcalories, and so they tend to consume plenty of vitamins and minerals. The B-vitamins and minerals such as iron and copper are especially needed to support energy metabolism (Table 12-5). If a low-energy intake—less than 1200 kcalories—is needed, athletes should pay very close attention to their vitamin and mineral intake. A focus on nutrient-dense foods, such as lowfat milk, broccoli, tomatoes, oranges, strawberries, whole grains, lean beef, kidney beans, turkey, fish, and chicken is a good idea. Vitamin and mineral fortified foods (e.g., many breakfast cereals) also can be used. Vitamin and mineral intakes that greatly exceed the RDA are not needed. Note that vitamin and mineral supplements supply no known *ergogenic* (work-producing) benefit (see the Nutrition Issue on p. 397). They only benefit the body when a medically diagnosed deficiency exists![1]

Iron. Athletes, especially female and adolescent athletes, should focus special attention on iron intake. Iron losses in sweat, increased iron requirements for the enhanced red blood cell production associated with athletic fitness, foot-strike destruction of red blood cells (red cells are broken by trauma as they pass through the foot during exercise), and iron loss during menstruation deplete a woman's iron stores. If this iron is not replenished, iron-deficiency anemia and markedly impaired endurance performance can result.[12] Although true anemia (noted as a depressed blood hemoglobin concentration) is quite rare among athletes, it is a good idea, especially for adult women athletes, to have blood hemoglobin levels checked regularly and to monitor dietary iron intake. Vegetarian female athletes should be especially careful to watch iron status. If blood iron levels are consistently low, the use of iron supplements may be advisable. Iron supplements can improve athletic performance if the athlete is truly anemic, but they have no effect when the athlete simply has low blood levels of iron that have not resulted in anemia.

Calcium. Athletes, especially women who are attempting to lose weight by restricting their intake of dairy products, can have marginal or low dietary intakes of calcium. This practice does not contribute to optimum bone health. Of still greater concern are women athletes who have stopped menstruating as a result of arduous exercise training that has interfered with the normal secretion of the reproductive hormones. Disturbing reports show that female athletes who do not menstruate regularly have far less dense spinal bones—in other words, less calcium present—than both nonathletes and female athletes who menstruate regularly.[10]

Researchers have just begun to understand the importance of regular menstruation for the promotion of bone maintenance. Current studies imply that a woman runner who does not menstruate regularly may also have a higher risk for the development of a *stress fracture.* Female athletes whose menstrual cycles become irregular should consult a physician to ascertain the cause. Decreasing the level of training and/or increasing body weight often restores regular menstrual cycles. If irregular menstrual cycles persist, severe bone loss and osteoporosis may result. Extra calcium in the diet does not necessarily compensate for this loss of menstruation, but inadequate dietary calcium can make matters worse.

Ergogenic • Work-producing.

Stress Fracture • A fracture that occurs from repeated jarring of a bone. Common sites include bones of the foot.

Long distance runner Alberto Salazar experienced problems with sleeping and performance impairment until it was found to be related to his low iron intake and related iron-deficiency anemia.

Pre-event meal

A light meal (300 kcalories) should be eaten 2 to 4 hours before an endurance event to top off muscle and liver glycogen stores and prevent hunger during the event. Extra fluid intake is also advised. The foods in the overall meal should consist primarily of carbohydrate, contain little fat or dietary fiber, and include

TABLE 12-5

Vitamins and minerals: Function and usage with regard to exercise

Vitamins and Minerals	Exercise-related Function	Proposed Benefit to Performance	Effects of Supplementation in Excess of RDA/ESADDI
Thiamin	Carbohydrate metabolism	Enhances endurance performance	Does not enhance performance
Riboflavin	Energy metabolism	Enhances aerobic performance	Does not enhance performance
Niacin	Energy metabolism	Enhances energy metabolism	May impair performance by reducing fatty acid release
Vitamin B-6	Formation of hemoglobin	Enhances exercise performance	Does not enhance performance
Pantothenic acid	Energy metabolism	Enhances aerobic performance	Unclear research results to date
Vitamin B-12	Red blood cell development	Enhances endurance performance	Does not enhance performance
Folate	Cell synthesis; red blood cell formation		No studies available
Biotin	Fat and glycogen synthesis		No studies available
Vitamin C	Antioxidant	Prevents tissue damage; speeds repair	Well-controlled studies show no effect
Vitamin A	Antioxidant	Prevents tissue damage; speeds repair	Enhanced performance unlikely
Vitamin D	Bone mineral metabolism	Bone formation during muscle building	Does not affect work performance; may affect muscle building (one study), but needs likely do not exceed the RDA. Note excess intakes can be toxic
Vitamin E	Antioxidant	Prevents tissue damage; speeds repair	Does not enhance performance; may reduce exercise damage caused by breakdown in fat structure in cell membranes
Zinc	Carbohydrate, fat, and protein metabolism; tissue repair	Repair of exercise damage	Enhances some measures of muscle performance after 2 weeks (one study), but the dose was too high to be safely consumed on a regular basis (nine times the male RDA)
Copper	Red blood cell synthesis; energy metabolism	Enhances aerobic performance	Studies not available
Chromium	Carbohydrate metabolism; increases effects of insulin	Delays fatigue	Studies not available
Selenium	Antioxidant	Protects against exercise damage; delays fatigue	Studies not available
Iron	Oxygen transport and delivery	Reduces fatigue; enhances endurance	No effect on performance in nonanemic or non-iron-deficient subjects

From Clarkson PM: Vitamins and trace minerals. In Lamb DR and Williams M, editors: *Perspectives in exercise science and sports medicine*, vol 4, Ergogenics: Enhancement of exercise and sport performance, Indianapolis, 1991, Benchmark Press.

a moderate amount of protein.[5] Good choices are pasta, bagels, muffins, bread, and breakfast cereals with lowfat milk. Liquid meal replacement formulas also can be used. Fiber-rich foods should be consumed the previous day to help clear the bowels before the event, but not the night before. Foods that are fatty or fried, such as sausage, bacon, sauces, and gravies, should be avoided. A meal high in carbohydrate is quickly digested, promotes normal blood glucose levels, and avoids the need to dip right away into glycogen stores. If an athlete feels a pre-event meal harms performance, eating a high-carbohydrate diet the day and night before can help meet the same goal.

Consuming carbohydrate 15 to 45 minutes before competition was previously thought to adversely affect performance because it increases insulin release, and insulin causes blood glucose to fall. However, such feedings do not cause premature fatigue or decrease endurance for most people. In fact, recent studies show positive benefits of this type of pre-event feeding.[19] However, some athletes are extremely sensitive to an insulin surge. Thus athletes should experiment with pre-event carbohydrate feedings to see if their performance is adversely or positively affected.

Maximizing body fluids and energy stores during exercise

Athletes need enough water to maintain the body's ability to regulate its internal temperature and so keep itself cool.[2] Most energy released during metabolism appears immediately as heat. Unless this heat is quickly dissipated, heat cramps, heat exhaustion, or deadly heat stroke may ensue. As we noted in Chapter 10, sweat evaporating from the skin helps remove this heat from the body. Sweat rates during prolonged exercise range from 3 to 8 cups (750 to 2000 milliliters) per hour. To keep the body from becoming dehydrated, fluid intake during exercise, when possible, should be adequate to minimize body weight loss. However, most athletes find it very uncomfortable to replace more than about 75% to 80% of this sweat loss during exercise.

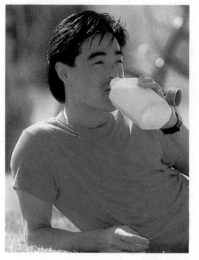

Attention to fluid consumption is one key for maintaining peak athletic performance.

By experimenting, athletes can determine how much fluid they require to maintain weight and how much fluid intake they can tolerate without experiencing stomach cramps. This determination will be most accurate if the athlete is weighed before and after a typical workout. For every 1 pound (½ kilogram) lost, 2 cups (0.5 liter) of water should be consumed during exercise or immediately afterward. For example, an athlete who loses 5 pounds during practice should drink 10 cups of water, that is, perhaps 7 to 8 cups during practice and 2 to 3 cups following practice.

Thirst is not a reliable indicator of fluid need.[11] By relying on thirst alone, an athlete might take 48 hours to replenish fluid loss. After several days of practice, the increasing fluid debt can begin to impair performance. By the time one feels thirsty, the person may have lost 3% of body weight through sweat.

A good rule of thumb is to drink beverages freely for up to 2 hours before an event. Don't worry about thirst. Then consume 1 to 2 cups (0.25 to 0.5 liters) of fluids (like water, diluted fruit juice, or sports drinks) about 15 minutes before a sports event. This is called hyperhydration. The extra fluid in the body will be ready to replace sweat losses as needed. Next, consume approximately 1 to 1.5 cups of fluid (preferably at refrigeration temperature on hot days to help cool the body) each 15 minutes for events that last longer than 30 minutes.[5] If the weather is hot and/or humid, even more fluids may be required. The athlete need not worry that gradual consumption of fluids will cause bloating or impair performance. But skipping fluids will almost certainly cause problems!

Carbohydrate intake during recovery from exercise

A large portion of the day's carbohydrate-rich foods should be consumed within 2 hours of a training exercise bout, and the sooner the better.[19] This period

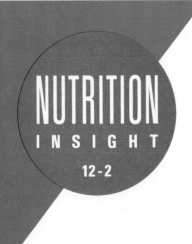

NUTRITION
I N S I G H T
12-2

SPORTS DRINKS: ARE THEY NECESSARY?

A question that often arises is whether to drink water or a sports-type carbohydrate-*electrolyte* drink, such as Bodyfuel, Exceed, Gatorade, or 10-K, during competition. For sports that require less than 30 minutes of exertion, replacing the water lost in sweat is the primary concern because losses of body carbohydrate stores and electrolytes (sodium, chloride, potassium, and other minerals) are not usually too great in such activities.[5] Electrolytes are lost in sweat, but the quantities lost in exercise of brief to moderate duration can be easily replaced later by consuming normal foods, such as orange juice, potatoes, or tomato juice.

Water is certainly cheaper than a sports drink. But sports-type drinks can taste better than water, which may make one drink more often—a clear benefit for fluid replenishment. In addition, the carbohydrate in these drinks quickly replaces carbohydrate used up during practice or competition. The sodium present also aids glucose absorption.

For endurance athletes—those whose sports demand exertion for longer than 30 minutes—the discussion of sports drinks becomes more critical.[2] Beverages for the endurance athlete must provide water for hydration, electrolytes to both enhance water absorption from the intestine and to help retain blood volume, and carbohydrate to provide energy. Beyond 60 to 90 minutes of exercise, electrolyte replacement becomes increasingly important.

Prolonged exercise results in large sweat losses, and some of the fluid for sweat comes from the bloodstream. If only water is used to replace the fluid losses in the blood, the concentration of essential electrolytes in the bloodstream may become too diluted. Small amounts of sodium and potassium are included in sports drinks to help maintain blood volume.

Including carbohydrates in sports drinks also has been found to delay fatigue in endurance exercise.[19] In exercise at intensities of a 3-hour marathon pace, ingesting carbohydrate improves endurance, presumably by either preventing great drops in blood glucose levels or by providing an outside source of glucose for muscle use.

The amount of carbohydrate recommended for consumption about 15 minutes before endurance exercise is 1 to 2 cups of a 10% to 20% solution of carbohydrate (10 to 20 grams of carbohydrate per 100 milliliters of water), such as GatorLode or Exceed High Carbohydrate Source. Once exercise begins, $1/2$ to 1 cup of a 5% to 8% carbohydrate solution (5 to 8 grams per 100 milliliters of fluid) should be consumed every 15 to 20 minutes. This is the carbohydrate concentration of typical sports drinks (check the label to be sure).

Some beverage labels mention *glucose polymers* (glucoses linked together in short chains). Solutions containing glucose polymers were initially thought to empty from the stomach faster than solutions containing glucose. We now know that there's little difference in stomach emptying times between sports drinks containing glucose polymers and those containing simple sugars such as glucose or sucrose. Furthermore, comparisons of drinks containing glucose polymers (more properly known as maltodextrins), glucose, or sucrose show that all of these carbohydrates have similar positive effects on exercise performance and physiological function as long as the concentrations of carbohydrate are in the 5% to 8% range. The exception to this rule is drinks whose only carbohydrate source is fructose. Fructose is absorbed from the intestine more slowly than glucose and often causes bloating or diarrhea. ●

Electrolytes • Compounds that break down into ions in water and, in turn, are able to conduct an electrical current. These include sodium, chloride, and potassium.

Glucose Polymer • Carbohydrate sources used in some sports drinks that consist of grouping of a few glucose molecules.

Alcohol and caffeine both have a dehydrating effect on the body, so fluids containing them should not be part of any hydration plan for exercise.

of time is when glycogen synthesis is the greatest. Athletes who are training hard can consume a simple sugar candy, sugared soft drink, fruit juice, or a sports-type carbohydrate supplement right after training as they attempt to reload their muscles with glycogen. At fast-food restaurants, the athlete can order extra crust on pizza, load up at the salad bar, and have extra rolls and muffins.

Fluid and electrolyte intake is also an essential component of the athlete's recovery diet. This helps reestablish normal levels of body fluids as quickly as possible. This is especially true if the athlete works out twice a day and if the environment is hot and humid.

ANOTHER BITE It cannot be emphasized enough that any nutrition strategies, including fluid replacement, should be tested during practice and trial runs. An athlete should never try a new food or beverage on the day of competition. Some food items or beverages may not be tolerated well, and the day of competition is not the time to find that out.

CONCEPT CHECK

All athletes would do well to plan a diet that follows the Guide to Daily Food Choices. High-carbohydrate foods should be emphasized, and these should dominate the pre-event meal. Additional protein intake above a usual American intake is not necessary. Nutrient supplements should be taken only to correct actual nutrient deficiencies. Fluid should be consumed as liberally as possible before, during, and after an event. A sports-type drink can be helpful for endurance athletes.

SUMMARY

- All energy available to humans comes from solar energy. ATP is the major form of energy used for cellular metabolism. Plants capture solar energy using photosynthesis. Human metabolic pathways are able to extract that energy from foodstuffs and convert it into ATP energy.

- In glycolysis, glucose is broken down into 3-carbon compounds, yielding some ATP. The 3-carbon compounds can then proceed to other aerobic pathways to form carbon dioxide (CO_2) and water (H_2O), or anaerobic pathways to form lactic acid.

- At low workloads, muscle cells mainly use fat for fuel. For intense exercise of short duration, muscles use phosphocreatine (PCr) for energy. For more sustained intense activity, muscle glycogen breaks down into lactic acid. For endurance exercise, fat and carbohydrate are used as fuels; carbohydrate is used increasingly as activity intensifies. Little protein is used to fuel muscles.

- Exercise is a vital part of a healthy lifestyle. Stretching exercises and aerobic stimulation of the heart constitute a good exercise plan. Physically active people show lower risks for premature heart disease, diabetes mellitus, and other common chronic diseases.

- Anyone who exercises regularly needs to consume a diet that is moderate to high in carbohydrates and that follows the suggestions of the Guide to Daily Food Choices. Weekend athletes should do the same, as the many health benefits experienced add to those from the exercise.

- Carbohydrate loading can double the usual stores of muscle glycogen. Participants in endurance events that last more than 2 hours benefit most from carbohydrate loading. This basically is a diet containing about 600 grams of carbohydrate for 3 to 4 days before the event.

- Athletes should consume enough fluid to both minimize loss of body weight and ultimately restore preexercise weight. A sports-type drink can be helpful for endurance athletes.

ARE YOU MEASURING UP TO THE NUMBERS?

In this chapter several key nutrients were discussed in relation to exercise performance. The following guidelines were mentioned (not only for athletes, but for those maintaining generally good fitness):

- eat a moderate to high amount of carbohydrates (55% or more of total kcalories)
- athletes should eat about of 1 gram of protein per kilogram of body weight
- consume the RDA for vitamins and minerals
- make sure iron and calcium intake is at RDA levels (especially in women)

Review the results of the dietary assessment you completed in Chapter 2. Remember that you assessed 1 day's food intake. Now answer the following questions (even if you are not an athlete):

1. What percentage of your kcalories came from carbohydrate? Was your intake 55% of your total kcalories or greater?

_____

2. Did you eat at least 0.8 grams of protein per kilogram of body weight? If you are an athlete, did you consume about 1 gram per kilogram of body weight?

_____

_____

3. Did you consume at least the RDA for all vitamins and minerals assessed, especially iron and calcium? Which ones were below the RDA?

_____

_____

_____

_____

_____

4. What can you do to improve your dietary intake to aid general fitness, and if you are an athlete, to promote maximal performance in your chosen event(s)?

_____

_____

_____

_____

REFERENCES

1. Aronsen VA: Vitamins and minerals as ergogenic aids, *The Physician and Sportsmedicine* 14:209, 1988.
2. Barr S, Costill D: Water: Can the endurance athlete get too much of a good thing? *Journal of the American Dietetics Association* 89:1629, 1989.
3. Blair SW and others: Physical fitness and all-cause mortality, *Journal of the American Medical Association* 26:2395,1989.
4. Burke L, Read R: Sports Nutrition: approaching the Nineties, *Sports Medicine* 8:80, 1989.
5. Clark N: *Nancy Clark's sports nutrition guidebook: eating to fuel your active lifestyle*, Champaign, Ill, 1990, Leisure Press.
6. Costill D: *Inside running: basics of sports physiology*, Indianapolis, Ind, 1985, Benchmark Press.
7. Costill D: Carbohydrates for exercise: Dietary demands for optimal performance, *International Journal of Sports Medicine* 9:1, 1988.
8. Hagen RD: Benefits of aerobic conditioning and diet for overweight adults, *Sports Medicine* 5:144, 1988.
9. Hallagan JB and others: Anabolic-androgenic steroid use by athletes, *The New England Journal of Medicine* 321:1042,1989.
10. Highet R: Athletic amenorrhea: An update on etiology,complications and management, *Sports Medicine* 7:82, 1989.
11. Hoffman CJ, Coleman E: An eating plan and update on recommended dietary practices for the endurance athlete, *Journal of the American Dietetic Association* 91:325, 1991.
12. Hultman E: Nutritional effects on work performance, *American Journal of Clinical Nutrition* 49:949, 1989.
13. Jacobson BH: Effect of amino acids on growth hormone release, *Physician and Sportsmedicine* 18(1):63, 1990.
14. Kavanagh T, Shephard RJ: Can regular sports participation slow the aging process? Data on Masters athletes, *Physician and Sportsmedicine* 18(6):94, 1990.
15. Lamb D: *Physiology of exercise: responses and adaptations*, New York, 1984, MacMillan Press.
16. Layzer RB: How muscles use fuel, *The New England Journal of Medicine* 324:411, 1991.
17. National Research Council, Committee on Diet and Health: *Diet and health*, Washington DC, 1989, National Academy Press.
18. Paul G: Dietary protein requirements of physically active individuals, *Sports Medicine* 8:154, 1989.
19. Sherman M, Lamb D: Nutrition and prolonged exercise. In Lamb D, Murray R, editors: *Perspectives in exercise science and sports medicine: prolonged exercise*, Indianapolis, Ind, 1988, Benchmark Press.
20. Shroyer JA: Getting tough on anabolic steroids: can we win the battle, *The Physician and Sportsmedicine* 18(2):106, 1990.
21. Stryer L: *Biochemistry*, ed 3, New York, 1988, WH Freeman.
22. Williams MH: Nutritional ergogenic aids and athletic performance, *Nutrition Today*, January/February, 1989, p 7.
23. Work JA: Are java junkies poor sports? *The Physician and Sportsmedicine* 19:83, 1991.

HOW MUCH HAVE I LEARNED?

What have you learned from Chapter 12? Here are 15 statements about nutrition and fitness. Read them to test your current knowledge. If you think the statement is true or mostly true, circle T. If you think the statement is false or mostly false, circle F. Use the scoring key at the end of the book to compute your total score. To review, take this test again later, and especially before tests.

1. T (F) A cell can directly use the energy stored in carbohydrate to fuel a muscle's energy demands. *must 1st convert to ATP energy*

2. T (F) Carbohydrates can be used for energy needs but fat cannot.

3. T (F) Carbohydrate metabolism does not require oxygen.

4. (T) F *(anaerobic) only initial stages. (aerobic) burning to H_2O & CO_2 does require O_2* Carbon dioxide is a by-product of energy metabolism.

5. T (F) Even when athletes are getting the RDA quantities of vitamins and minerals in the diet, it has been shown that supplements of vitamins and minerals will increase athletic performance.

6. T (F) There are really no disadvantages for an athlete who attempts to lose weight during the competitive season. *rapid wt. loss can weaken body - reduce muscle mass & glycogen storage*

7. T (F) It is particularly important for athletes to consume protein and amino acid supplements because it is hard for them to get enough protein from their diets. *athletes high kcal intake makes meeting protein needs easy.*

8. (T) F A large portion of carbohydrate food, like starches or fruits, should be consumed within 2 hours after an exercise bout to maximize glycogen synthesis because this is when glycogen synthesis is the greatest.

9. (T) F Sports-type drinks, like Gatorade, are not significantly better than water for fluid replacement for the everyday athlete. However, they may be advantageous for endurance athletes.

10. (T) F Caffeine use has improved athletic performance in some cases. *Can enhance fat use by muscles which can help performance in endurance events*

11. T (F) Your target heart rate for exercise is 80% to 95% of maximum heart rate. *60 - 85% promotes aerobic conditioning*

12. T (F) Warm-up exercises are not important to the week-end athlete.

13. T (F) Thirst is a good guide for fluid replacement after hard exercise. *better guide is wt. loss. for every pound lost drink 2 cups of water*

14. T (F) It is a good idea to eat lots of carbohydrate before a 100-meter dash. *Carbohydrate loading benefits exercise lasting longer than 1½ - 2 hrs*

15. (T) F Anabolic steroids are illegal ergogenic aids for athletes. *also - unsafe*

NUTRITION ISSUE

ERGOGENIC AIDS: SOME SUBSTANCES CAN ENHANCE ATHLETIC PERFORMANCE

Manipulating one's diet for better performance has a long history. As long as 30 years ago, American football players were encouraged on hot practice days to "toughen up" for competition by consuming salt tablets before and during practice and by not drinking water. Now it is recognized that this practice can be fatal. Today's athletes are also likely to experiment—bee pollen, seaweed, freeze-dried liver flakes, gelatin, ginseng, coenzyme Q10, creatine, amino acid supplements, and artichoke hearts are just some of the worthless substances known today as ergogenic aids.[22]

Still, modern-day athletes can benefit from recently documented scientific evidence that some dietary substances do have ergogenic properties. These include sufficient water, lots of carbohydrate, and a balanced and varied diet that follows the Guide to Daily Food Choices.[5] Amino acid supplements are not in the list. The average American eats plenty of protein, athletes included.

Clearly, it is not possible to change average athletes into champions simply by altering diets. This means nutrient supplements require careful evaluation. Use should be designed to meet a specific dietary weakness, such as a poor iron intake. These and other aids, whose benefit is often dubious and which nonetheless can pose health risks, must be given close scrutiny before use. The risk-benefit ratio of these ergogenic aids especially needs to be examined. Athletes must stay on guard against false promises.

Carnitine

The majority of the energy stored in the body for muscle use is found in fat. During physical activity, fatty acids are released into the bloodstream from the fat depots and travel to the muscles, where they are taken into each cell and aerobically broken down to carbon dioxide and water. These fatty acids must enter the cell's mitochondria before they can be broken down. The fatty acids are mostly transported from the fluid portion of the cell into the mitochondria using a transport system that contains a compound called **carnitine.** Athletes sometimes take carnitine pills hoping it will help them burn fat faster in exercise. But since our cells can make carnitine quite easily, carnitine supplements provide no reliable benefit.[22]

Bicarbonate loading

We have noted that muscles that contract vigorously during athletic performance produce lactic acid. Lactic acid buildup inhibits the activity of enzymes involved in energy metabolism and leads to early fatigue. In the 1930s, athletes attempted to counter lactic acid accumulation by ingesting small doses of **sodi-**

Carnitine • A compound used to shuttle fatty acids into the cell mitochondria. This allows for the fatty acids to be burned for energy.

Sodium Bicarbonate • An alkaline substance made of basically sodium and carbon dioxide ($NaHCO_3$).

Steroids • A group of hormones and related compounds that are derivatives of cholesterol.

Androgen • A general term for hormones that stimulate development in male sex organs and male characteristics, such as facial hair; for example, testosterone.

Growth Hormone • A pituitary hormone that produces body growth and release of fat from storage, among other effects.

um bicarbonate (a base). However, this failed to improve their athletic performances. On the other hand, more recent experiments using large doses of bicarbonate (30 milligrams per kilogram of body weight) demonstrate performance improvement. Athletes who consume large doses of bicarbonate 1 or 2 hours before exercise generally have improved strenuous performance lasting 2 to 10 minutes. About 20 minutes of warm-up typically precedes the event. The bicarbonate-loading apparently speeds the removal of lactic acid from contracting muscle cells. Unfortunate side effects of large doses of sodium bicarbonate are nausea and diarrhea, often at unpredictable times. For this reason, bicarbonate loading has so far not become popular with athletes.

Caffeine

Drinking three to four cups of coffee (4 to 5 milligrams of caffeine per kilogram of body weight) or using caffeine suppositories about 1 hour before an endurance competition (lasting more than 2 hours) enhances performance in some athletes. The effect is less apparent in athletes who have ample stores of glycogen. The reason for the overall effect is not well established: increased use of fatty acids for muscle fuel, psychological effects, or enhancement of glycolysis in muscle all deserve consideration. However, some athletes experience changes in heart rhythm, nausea, or lightheadedness that can actually impair performance.[23] Olympic officials view caffeine as a drug and do not condone its use. They consider a body level of caffeine exceeding the equivalent of five to six cups of coffee illegal.[22]

Anabolic steroids

Public attention focused on the use of anabolic *steroids* when Ben Johnson, winner of the gold medal for the 100-meter dash in the 1988 Olympic Games, was disqualified. Johnson acknowledged that he took anabolic steroids regularly as part of his training regimen. These steroids are used by athletes to enhance performance in a variety of sports but most commonly in strength sports, such as football, wrestling, weight lifting, and certain track-and-field events.[9] Steroids have also been used by swimmers and cyclists and are often used by male and female body builders and even nonathletic high school students in an attempt to "get big."

Steroids are synthetic versions of sex hormones that promote two types of effects: masculinization and growth promotion. Athletes have taken these drugs, often in doses 10 to 30 times normal *androgen* output, to increase muscle size, strength, and performance; no cardiovascular benefit has been found.[20]

Although they can increase muscle mass in some people, steroid use is unsafe and, in athletics, illegal. The consequences of steroid use also can occasionally be devastating. For example, steroids can cause growth plates in bones to close prematurely (thus limiting the adult height of a teenage athlete); produce bloody cysts in the liver; accelerate the development of heart disease; and cause high blood pressure, sterility, and many other detrimental physical effects. Psychological consequences vary from increasing aggressiveness, drug dependence, and mood swings to decreased sex drive, depression, and even roid-rage (violence attributed to steroid use).[9] Some football players consider the increased aggressiveness an additional benefit.

Athletes may begin to use steroids during high school, and perhaps as early as junior high school. Many serious athletes must make a hard choice—to not use steroids and face a large field of artificially endowed opponents or to use the drugs and risk side effects and legal sanctions (Table 12-6).

Growth hormone

There is too little scientific information available regarding the effects of *growth hormone* on muscle mass and strength to allow firm conclusions to be

TABLE 12-6

Suggestions for the athlete making choices about steroid use

1. Know the facts about steroids.
2. View your body as something to keep safe from harm and free from contamination.
3. Think about your plans for the future and your health.
4. Go for natural methods that allow you to look good and perform well.
5. Enjoy and appreciate your uniqueness; don't ever try to be somebody else.
6. When in doubt, check the recommendation out with somebody who really cares.
7. After considering all of the possible consequences, have the courage to make a good decision based on healthy practices.

From *American Family Physician* 41:1163, April, 1990.

Blood Doping • A technique by which an athlete's red blood cell count is increased. Blood is taken from the athlete. The red blood cells are concentrated and then later reintroduced into the athlete.

Diphosphoglycerate (DPG) • A compound in the red blood cell that is involved in oxygen release from hemoglobin.

made about this drug. However, it is known that the skin, tongue, and bones may grow abnormally under growth hormone stimulation. Abusing growth hormone may increase height if consumed at critical ages, but uncontrolled growth of the heart and other internal organs and even death are also potential consequences. All in all, use of growth hormone is dangerous—it requires careful monitoring by a physician. Arginine and ornithine supplements (basically amino acids), a new rage among body builders, are promoted as growth hormone boosters. Current evidence suggests that any increase in growth hormone after consuming amino acids is rather modest and probably of little physiological consequence.[13]

Blood doping

Injecting red blood cells into the bloodstream—known as **blood doping**—is a technique that may enhance aerobic capacity. In this procedure, an athlete donates at least 2 pints of blood at least 6 weeks before the event and freezes the cells while the body makes more blood to replace it. Then, 1 or 2 days before competition, the frozen red cells are thawed and reinfused into the veins; the added cells elevate the total red blood cell count and hemoglobin concentration above normal.

Studies of blood doping show that it is a means to improve endurance performance. Admissions by world-class athletes—including members of the victorious United States cycling team in the 1984 Olympics—that they used blood doping to reduce race times continue to stimulate questions about both sports ethics and how well the procedure actually works. Several studies confirm an aerobic benefit to the athlete as a result of blood doping, but the possible negative health consequences remain to be determined. It is also an illegal practice under Olympic guidelines.

Phosphate loading

Contrary to beliefs of many athletes and coaches, phosphate pills do not always improve performance or efficiency of heart function during endurance events. Some studies have suggested that loading phosphate for 4 days increased the levels of a metabolically important phosphate compound, **diphosphoglycerate (DPG)**, in red blood cells. These studies also showed that increased levels of DPG potentially improved the delivery of oxygen to muscles and reduced work by the heart during vigorous exercise. We now know that rigorously trained athletes already have high levels of DPG in their red blood cells. Thus although a single dose of phosphate can induce blood chemistry changes, it does not reliably improve the ability to perform endurance exercise, nor does it necessarily increase the efficiency of aerobic metabolism. ●

EATING DISORDERS

Most of us occasionally eat until we're stuffed and uncomfortable. Faced with savory and tempting foods, we find that we can't easily stop eating. Usually we forgive ourselves, vowing not to overeat the next time. Nevertheless, many of us have problems controlling our weight. Although creeping weight gain might eventually lead to medical problems, it is usually associated with simple overeating.

In stark contrast, the eating disorders we explore in this chapter involve severe distortions of the eating process. Dieting for a week on mostly grapefruit in order to fit into a bikini at Spring break does not amount to an eating disorder. Rather, the eating disorders we discuss can develop into life-threatening conditions. And what's most alarming about these disorders, anorexia nervosa and bulimia, is the increasing number of cases reported each year.

We live in a society where food is abundant, and although some of us regularly exercise, our lifestyles are fairly sedentary. Everyday we are bombarded with images of the "ideal" body. Television programs, billboard advertisements, magazine pictures, movies, and newspapers tell us that an ultra-slim body will bring happiness, love, and even success. Is happiness possible for those who aren't the perfect "10?" It is hard not to compare the media images with our own seemingly less-than-perfect bodies.

Some people are more receptive and vulnerable to these messages than others, because of both psychological and physical reasons. These people may be more likely to develop eating disorders. Moreover, the messages are not aimed at all people equally; they are overwhelmingly beamed at women, and women account for most cases of anorexia nervosa and bulimia. ●

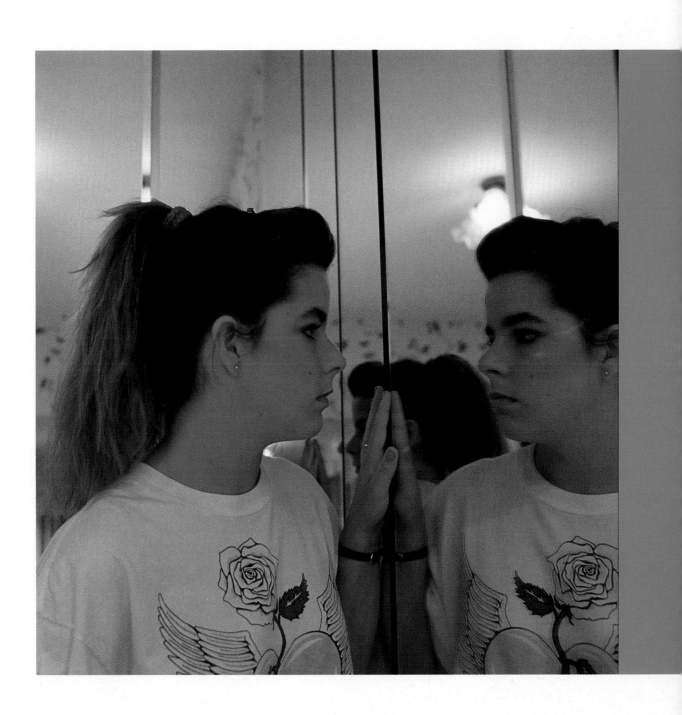

How Restrained Are You?

Circle the number of the answer that best completes the question.

1. How often do you diet?

0	never	3	often
1	rarely	4	always
2	sometimes		

2. What is the most weight (pounds) you have ever lost within 1 month?

0	0 to 4	3	15 to 19
1	5 to 9	4	20+
2	10 to 14		

3. What is the most weight (pounds) you have ever gained within 1 week?

0	0 to 1	3	3.1 to 5
1	1.1 to 2	4	5.1+
2	2.1 to 3		

4. In a typical week, how much does your weight (pounds) fluctuate?

0	0 to 1	3	3.1 to 5
1	1.1 to 2	4	5.11
2	1 to 3		

5. Would a weight fluctuation of 5 pounds affect the way you live your life?

0	not at all	2	moderately
1	slightly	3	very much

6. Do you eat sensibly in front of others and splurge alone?

0	never	2	often
1	rarely	3	always

7. Do you give too much time and thought to food?

0	never	2	often
1	rarely	3	always

8. Do you feel guilty after overeating?

0	never	2	often
1	rarely	3	always

9. How conscious are you of what you are eating?

0	not at all	2	moderately
1	slightly	3	extremely

10. How many pounds over your desired weight were you at your maximum weight?

0	0	3	11 to 20
1	1 to 5	4	21+
2	6 to 10		

Now add together all the numbers you circled. You could have a minimum score of 0 or a maximum of 35. Write your score in the blank here:_____

ASSESS YOURSELF

INTERPRETATION OF ASSESS YOURSELF

Pick out the appropriate category below based on your score:

0-15 Relatively unrestrained

16-23 Moderately restrained

24-35 Highly restrained

Often people with the eating disorder bulimia exhibit what is called *restraint*. This means that they regularly worry about what they are eating. They feel they are failures if they lapse even once and indulge on something that doesn't appear to help them control their weight. They try to eat "good" things like broccoli and avoid letting people see them eat "bad" things like candy bars. However, when they feel stressed or eat a "bad" thing it usually opens the floodgate for a secretive binge, hidden from everyone's sight.

When people are highly restrained, their self-denial sets them up for a pattern of binge eating in the future. The assessment you completed above encourages you to examine the degree of dietary restraint you practice in your life. If you fall into the moderately or highly restrained category, you might look at how you can change your beliefs about food and dieting to reduce your chances of struggling with binge eating.

This assessment is modified from Frankle RT, Mei-Uih Yang MU: The revised restraint scale in *Obesity and weight control*, Rockville, Md, 1988, Aspen Publications.

WE ALL NEED TO EAT

Eating—a completely instinctive behavior for animals—serves an extraordinary number of psychological, social, and cultural purposes for humans. As we mentioned in Chapter 1, eating practices may take on religious meanings; identify bonds among cultural, ethnic, and family groups; and be a means of expressing hostility and affection, prestige, and class values. Similarly, providing, preparing, and distributing food may be a means of expressing love or hatred, or even power in family relationships. Given these possibilities, it is not surprising that some eating behaviors take on unusual and strange rituals, progressing from (1) normal responses to hunger and satiety cues to (2) obsessive weight loss to (3) a full-blown eating disorder.

Food can represent much more than nutrients

From birth we link food with personal emotional experiences. An infant associates milk with security and warmth, and so the bottle or breast becomes a source of comfort as well as food. We are further exposed to the use of foods as rewards. Here are some typical statements heard at the dinner table:

"You can't play until you clean up your plate."

"I'll eat the broccoli if you let me watch TV."

"If you love me, you'll eat what I fixed for dinner."

On the surface, this practice appears harmless enough, but, eventually, both caregivers and children can build behavior patterns that use foods to achieve unstated goals. Food, then, can take on a much larger role. At the extreme—when food is regularly used as a tool of expression rather than simply as a source of nutrients—it can contribute to abnormal eating patterns. At worst, these patterns can lead to anorexia nervosa.

TWO COMMON TYPES OF EATING DISORDERS

Anorexia nervosa and *bulimia* (sometimes called bulimia nervosa) have been written about for centuries, at least as far back as the Middle Ages.

Anorexia Nervosa • An eating disorder involving a psychological loss of appetite and self-starvation, resulting in part from a distorted body image and various social pressures commonly associated with puberty.

Bulimia • An eating disorder in which large quantities of food are eaten at one time (binge eating) and then purged from the body by vomiting, use of laxatives, or other means.

Anorexia nervosa is characterized by extreme weight loss, poor and distorted body image, and an irrational, almost morbid, fear of obesity and weight gain. The term anorexia implies a loss of appetite; however, denying one's appetite more accurately describes anorectic behavior. By rough estimate, approximately 1 of every 100 girls (1%) between the ages of 12 and 18 years suffers from anorexia nervosa.[8] It occurs less commonly among adults. Few men are affected, partly because the ideal image for men is big and bulky. Men in weight control sports, such as wrestling or judo, may practice bulimia,[24] but poor self-esteem and other psychological problems don't seem to be the cause of this behavior. Most of these athletes vomit and dehydrate so that they can compete in lower weight classes. On the other hand, people with anorexia nervosa typically see themselves as fat even though they are extremely thin.

Bulimia means "ox hunger," or being as hungry as an ox.[10] It is characterized by episodes of binge eating followed by attempts to purge the food from the body, usually by vomiting, fasting, taking diuretics, or using laxatives. People with this disorder may be difficult to identify because they keep their binge-purge behaviors secret and their symptoms are not obvious. Researchers think that approximately 2% to 4% of adolescent and college-age women suffer from this disorder. A growing number of male athletes also report these practices, especially swimmers, wrestlers, and track participants. "Get thin and win" is a slogan heard around gyms.

The Diagnostic and Statistical Manual of Mental Disorders (3rd edition, revised) of the American Psychiatric Association lists specific criteria for diagnosing eating disorders (Figure 13-1).[18] People may exhibit some symptoms of an eating disorder but not sufficiently enough to enable a medical worker to diagnose it. People may also show characteristics of both anorexia nervosa and

Groups of people with long-standing histories of anorexia nervosa include models, ballet dancers, and gymnasts. Earning their living often depends on maintaining ultra-slim bodies.

CRITERIA FOR EATING DISORDER

Anorexia nervosa

A) Refusal to maintain body weight over a minimal normal weight for age and height, for example, weight loss leading to maintenance of body weight 15% below that expected; or failure to make expected weight gain during period of growth, leading to body weight 15% below that expected.

B) Intense fear of gaining weight or becoming fat, even though underweight.

C) Disturbance in the way in which one's body weight, size or shape is experienced. The person claims to "feel fat" even when emaciated, believes that one area of the body is "too fat" even when obviously underweight.

D) In females, absence of at least three consecutive menstrual cycles when otherwise expected to occur (primary or secondary amenorrhea). (A woman is considered to have amenorrhea if her periods occur only following hormone administration, such as estrogen.)

Bulimia nervosa

A) Recurrent episodes of binge eating (rapid consumption of a large amount of food in a discrete period of time).

B) A feeling of lack of control over eating behavior during the eating binges.

C) The person regularly engages in either self-induced vomiting, use of laxatives or diuretics, strict dieting or fasting, or vigorous exercise to prevent weight gain.

D) A minimum average of two binge eating episodes a week for at least 3 months.

E) Persistent overconcern with body shape and weight.

¹Source: *Diagnostic and Statistical Manual for Mental Disorders, DSM IIIR* (14).

FIGURE 13-1

Criteria for the diagnoses of anorexia nervosa and bulimia. Milder habits and symptoms that point in these directions are still troubling as they suggest the person is developing the ultimate disease patterns.

bulimia. The diseases overlap considerably (Figure 13-2). Studies suggest that 20% to 50% of women diagnosed as having anorexia nervosa eventually develop bulimic symptoms.[13]

Figure 13-3 lists some characteristics of people with anorexia nervosa and bulimia. Do you know someone who is at risk? If so, a professional diagnosis, coupled with professional help, is needed. The sooner help begins the better. The first step is to rule out other diseases, such as cancer, gastrointestinal disease, schizophrenia, and depression. If an eating disorder is diagnosed, the person should consider immediate treatment.[17] The best a friend can do is to lead the person to treatment. Professional help is often available at student health centers and student guidance/counselling facilities on college campuses. We need to be cautious of diagnosing eating disorders in friends and family members. A number of diagnostic criteria must be met before this is possible, and only a professional is equipped to do so.

There are no simple causes or solutions to eating disorders. They are rooted in multiple causes—biological, psychological, and social.[11] In the Nutrition Issue we review some sociological aspects of these disorders. From this perspective you might see how the disorders develop and why some people are more susceptible than others.

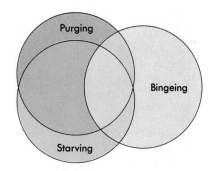

FIGURE 13-2
The overlap of eating disorders. A combination of binge eating, purging, and/or starving can be found in both anorexia nervosa and bulimia.

ARE YOU AT RISK FOR AN EATING DISORDER?

Characteristics of anorexia nervosa
- Rigid dieting causing dramatic weight loss
- False body perception—thinking "I'm too fat," even when emaciated; relentless pursuit of thinness
- Rituals involving food, excessive exercise, and other aspects of life
- Maintenance of rigid control in life-style; security found in control and order
- Feeling of panic after a small weight gain; intense fear of gaining weight
- Feelings of purity, power, and superiority through maintenance of strict discipline and self-denial
- Preoccupation with food, its preparation, and observing another person eat
- Helplessness in the presence of food
- Lack of menses after what should be the age of puberty

Characteristics of bulimia
- Secretive binge eating; never overeating in front of others
- Eating when depressed
- Bingeing followed by fasting, laxative abuse, self-induced vomiting, or excessive exercise
- Shame, embarrassment, deceit, and depression; low self-esteem and guilt (especially after a binge)
- Fluctuating weight resulting from alternate bingeing and fasting
- Loss of control; fear of not being able to stop eating
- Perfectionism, "people pleaser"; food is the only comfort/escape in an otherwise carefully controlled and regulated life
- Erosion of teeth, swollen glands

FIGURE 13-3
Some characteristics of eating disorders. This can be used as a tool for group discussion to help people discover their risks. Having some of these characteristics does not diagnose the disease but should cause a person to reflect on their eating habits and related concerns.

ANOREXIA NERVOSA

Anorexia nervosa evolves from a dangerous mental state to an extremely dangerous physical condition. People suffering from this disorder think they are fat and intensely fear obesity and weight gain. They lose much more weight than is healthy. Recent studies indicate that 3% to 8% of people with anorexia die prematurely—from suicide, heart ailments, and infections.[20] About half those who survive it recover within 6 years; the rest simply exist with the disease. The longer one suffers from anorexia nervosa, the poorer the chances for complete recovery. A young patient with a short episode and a cooperative family has a better outlook. Prompt and vigorous treatment with close follow-up improves the chances.[7, 23]

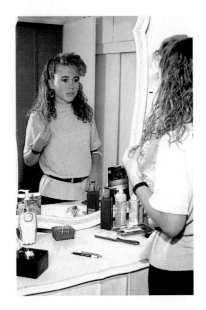

FIGURE 13-4
Self-image can be everchanging. For people with eating disorders, the difference between the real and desired body image may be too difficult to accept.

A person with anorexia nervosa may use the disorder to gain attention from the family, sometimes in hopes of holding the family together.

Anorexia may begin as a simple attempt to lose weight. A comment from a well-meaning friend or relative suggesting that the person seems to be gaining weight or is too fat may be all that is needed. The stress of having to maintain a certain weight to look attractive or competent on a job can set off a problem. Physical changes associated with puberty, the stress of leaving childhood, or losing a friend may also trigger extreme dieting (Figure 13-4). Leaving home for boarding school or college or starting a job can reinforce the desire to make oneself more "socially acceptable."

Adolescence is a period of turbulent sexual and social tensions. Teenagers seek—and are often expected—to establish separate and independent lives. While declaring independence they seek acceptance and support from peers and parents, and react intensely to how they think others perceive them.[7] At the same time, their bodies are changing, much of it beyond their control. Adolescents often lack appropriate coping mechanisms for the stresses of teen years. The attempt to take charge of their lives sometimes results in exercising extreme control over the body. At the same time, genetic factors also appear to increase the risk for anorexia nervosa: usually both identical twins—rather than only one—develop the disorder.[8]

Once dieting begins, a person developing anorexia nervosa does not stop. The results are long periods of semistarvation practiced rigidly, almost with a vengeance, in a relentless pursuit of thinness.[20] Anorexia may eventually lead to bingeing on large amounts of food in a short time, then purging. Purging occurs primarily through vomiting, but laxatives, diuretics, fasting, and exercise are also used. Thus a person with anorexia nervosa may exist in a state of semistarvation, or may alternate periods of starvation with periods of bingeing and purging.[3]

Once a person drops below 15% of normal body weight, there is great risk for lifelong suffering from anorexia nervosa. After falling 25% below normal body weight, a cure becomes very difficult, hospitalization is almost always necessary, and premature death is more likely.[20, 23]

Profile of a person with anorexia nervosa

A person with anorexia nervosa refuses to eat. This refusal is the hallmark of the disease, whether or not other practices, such as binge-purge cycles, appear. The person is usually a girl from the middle or upper socioeconomic class. Perhaps her mother also has distorted views of a desirable body shape and acceptable food habits. The girl is often described by parents and teachers as "the best little girl in the world." She is competitive and often obsessive.[3] Her parents set high standards for her. At home, she may not allow clutter in her bedroom. Physicians note that after a physical examination, she may fold her examination gown very carefully and clean up the examination room before leaving. Even though such behaviors may be apparent, it takes a skilled professional to tell the difference between anorexia nervosa and other common adolescent complaints, such as delayed puberty, fatigue, and depression.[7]

A common thread underlying many—but not all—cases of anorexia nervosa is conflict within the family structure, especially rooted in an overbearing mother.[19] When family expectations are always too high, resulting frustration leads to fighting. Overinvolvement, rigidity, overprotection, and denial also typically appear in the daily transactions of such families.[7] Often the eating disorder allows the person to exercise control over an otherwise powerless existence.

Early warning signs

A person developing anorexia nervosa will exhibit important warning signs. At first, dieting becomes the life focus.[17] The person may feel, "The only thing I am good at is dieting. I can't do anything else." This innocent beginning often leads

Many Americans feel that a thin body might make life perfect. This whirlwind hope especially appeals to young people. Quite vulnerable are young women who feel alienated from or suffocated by their parents. Parents may not consider a teenager mature enough to make decisions, for instance. She disagrees, and if the situation is very tense, may turn to purging or starving as a way to show her power. "You may try to control my life, but I can do anything I want with my body."

In the words of one young woman: "I couldn't get angry, because it would be like destroying someone else, like my mother. It felt like she would hate me forever. I got angry through anorexia nervosa. It was my last hope. It's my own body and this was my last ditch effort."

to very abnormal eating habits, such as cutting a pea in half before eating it. An anorectic woman may cook a large meal and watch others eat it while refusing to eat any herself. As the disease progresses, she narrows her own food choices considerably (Figure 13-5). For someone developing anorexia nervosa these practices say "I am in control." The anorectic person may be hungry but denies it. She is driven by the belief that good things will happen for her if she just becomes thin enough. It becomes a question of willpower.

Soon the anorectic person becomes irritable and hostile and begins to withdraw from family and friends. School performance generally crumbles. The person refuses to eat out with family and friends, thinking, "I won't be able to have the foods I want to eat," or "I won't be able to throw up afterward." The person also tends to be excessively critical of herself and others. Nothing is good enough. Because it cannot be perfect, life appears meaningless and hopeless. A sense of joylessness colors everything.

As stress increases in an anorectic person's life, sleep disturbances and depression are common. For a female these problems, coupled with lower and lower body weight and fat stores, cause menstrual periods to stop.[5] This may be the first sign of the disease a mother notices. Parents, teachers, friends, and coaches need to be aware of the early warning signs of anorexia nervosa. As we stated earlier, this disease is much easier to treat when caught at an early stage. If not treated right away, it quickly leads to self-destruction.

Ultimately, an anorectic person eats very little food; 300 to 600 kcalories daily is not unusual. In place of food the person may consume up to 20 cans of diet soft drinks each day.

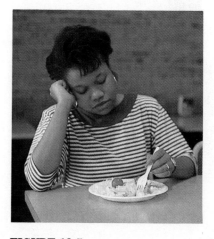

FIGURE 13-5
A serious distortion of eating behavior. When life reaches this stage, one needs professional help.

Physical signs and symptoms

Rooted in the emotional state of the victim, anorexia nervosa produces profound physical effects. A typical medical description reveals a reluctant young woman and a frantic family.[7] The anorectic person is often 20% to 40% below desirable body weight and appears to be skin and bones. This state of semistarvation disturbs many body systems as it forces the body to conserve as much energy as possible. Hormonal responses to semistarvation then cause an array of predictable effects:[5, 23]

- Lowered body temperature caused by loss of fat insulation.
- Slower basal metabolism caused by decreased synthesis of active thyroid hormone.
- Decreased heart rate as metabolism slows, leading to easy fatigue, easy fainting, and an overwhelming need for sleep.
- Iron-deficiency anemia from poor nutrient intake, which leads to further weakness.

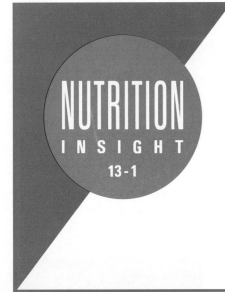

NUTRITION
I N S I G H T
13-1

ANOREXIA NERVOSA: A CASE STUDY

At fifteen Alma had been healthy and well-developed, had menstruated at age 12, was 5 feet 6 inches tall, and weighed 120 pounds. At that time her mother urged her to change to a school with a higher academic standing, a change she resisted; her father suggested that she should watch her weight, an idea that she took up with great eagerness, and she began a rigid diet. She lost rapidly and her menses ceased. That she could be thin gave her a sense of pride, power, and accomplishment. She also began a frantic exercise program, would swim by the mile, play tennis for hours, or do calisthenics to the point of exhaustion. Whatever low point her weight reached, Alma feared that she might become too fat if she regained as little as an ounce.

At age 20 when she came for a consultation with her physician, she looked like a walking skeleton; scantily dressed in shorts and a halter, with her legs sticking out like broomsticks, every rib showing, and her shoulder blades standing up like little wings. Alma insisted that she looked fine and that there was nothing wrong with being so skinny. ●

Lanugo • Downlike hair that appears after a person has lost much body fat through semistarvation. The hair stands erect and traps air, acting as insulation to the body to replace the insulation usually supplied by body fat.

- Rough, dry, scaly, and cold skin from a poor nutrient intake and anemia.
- Low white blood cell count caused by poor nutrient intake, especially protein and zinc. This condition increases the risk of infection, a cause of death in anorectic people.
- Loss of hair caused by a poor nutrient intake.
- Appearance of *lanugo,* downy hairs on the body that trap air, insulating against heat loss and in turn replacing some insulation lost with the fat layer.
- Constipation from semistarvation and laxative abuse.
- Low blood potassium because of a poor nutrient intake, possible vomiting, and the use of some types of diuretics. This increases the risk of heart rhythm disturbances, another leading cause of death in anorectic people.
- Loss of menstrual periods because of low body weight, low fat content, and the stress of the disease. Periods cease when body weight drops to around 100 pounds or less in many women. Accompanying hormonal changes cause a loss of bone mass and increase the risk of osteoporosis.
- Eventual loss of teeth caused by frequent vomiting. Loss of teeth and bone mass can be lasting signs of the disease, even if the other physical and mental problems are resolved.

A person with anorexia nervosa is psychologically and physically ill and needs help.

CONCEPT CHECK

Anorexia nervosa is an eating disorder characterized by semistarvation. It is found primarily—but not only—in adolescent girls, starting at or around puberty. An anorectic person dwindles essentially to "skin and bones," but often thinks she is fat. Semistarvation produces hormonal and other changes that lower body temperature, slow the heart rate, decrease immune response, stop menstrual periods, and contribute to hair loss. It is a very serious disease that often produces lifelong consequences. It can end with death.

Treatment of anorexia nervosa

Anorectic persons often sink into shells of isolation and fear. They deny that a problem exists. Frequently, friends and family members meet in a group with the person to confront the problem in a loving way. They present evidence of the problem and encourage entrance into treatment immediately. Treatment then requires a team of physicians, registered dietitians, psychologists, and other health professionals working together. An ideal setting is an eating disorders clinic in a medical center.[23]

Once the medical team has gained the cooperation of the anorectic person, they work together to restore a sense of balance, purpose, and future.[3] As we said, anorexia nervosa usually is rooted in psychological conflict. However, a person who has been barely existing in a state of semistarvation can not focus on much besides food.[23] A psychiatrist cannot counsel a starving person. Dreams and even morbid thoughts about food will interfere with therapy until sufficient weight is regained.

Nutrition therapy. The first goal of therapy then must be to have a person increase food intake. Weight gained must be enough to raise the metabolic rate to normal and to reverse as many physical signs of the disease as possible. Food intake is designed to first minimize or stop any further weight loss. Then the focus shifts to restoring regular food habits. After this is accomplished, the expectation can be switched to slow weight gain, from 1 to 4 pounds (0.5 to 2 kilograms) each week until weight exceeds 90% of preillness weight. Weight gain is not the sole goal of treatment but rather a prelude to fuller engagement in psychological issues.[19] The medical team should stress that patients will not be abandoned after they gain weight.[23]

One critical goal at early stages of treatment is to allow the person a feeling of control over life.[3] Only when the patient knows exactly what to expect can this be achieved. Unanticipated weight gain at this stage of treatment—even when caused by fluctuating menstrual fluids after periods resume—can easily set up a feeling of being completely out of control.

Experienced professional help is the key. An anorectic person may be on the verge of suicide and near starvation. Today suicide is the most common cause of death in these people.[20] In addition, anorectic people are often very clever and resistant. They may try to hide weight loss by wearing many layers of clothes, putting coins in their pockets, and drinking numerous glasses of water.

Psychological therapy. Once the physical problems are addressed, the therapist tries to determine how dieting became such a dominant force, knowing that it usually signals a deeper emotional illness.[17] To heal, the anorectic person must reject the sense of accomplishment associated with an emaciated body. If therapists can discover reasons for the disorder, they can develop strategies to restore normal weight and eating habits by resolving psychological conflicts.

A key aspect of psychological treatment is showing the person how to regain control of some facets of his or her life and how to cope with tough situations. As eating evolves into a normal routine, the person can turn to previously neglected activities.

Family therapy is important in treating anorexia nervosa.[3] It focuses on the role of the illness among family members, how individual family members react, and how their behavior might unknowingly contribute to the abnormal eating patterns. Therapy involves all family members relevant to the behavior problem. Frequently, a therapist finds family struggles at the heart of the problem. As the disorder resolves, the person has to relate to family members in new ways in order to gain the attention previously tied to the disease.[17] The family needs to help the young person ease into adulthood and to accept its responsibilities as well as its advantages.

Self-help groups for anorectic and bulimic persons, as well as their families and friends, represent nonthreatening first steps into treatment. People also can attend to get a sense of whether they really do have an eating disorder.

With professional help, many people with anorexia nervosa can again lead normal lives. They then do not have to depend on unusual eating habits to cope with daily problems. Although they may not be totally cured, they do recover a

Health professionals should measure and compare weight and height to standards—not merely rely on appearance—because our assessments of "thin" are distorted by the very thin models in advertisements.

These words are from a young woman on recovering from anorexia nervosa: "I have lost a specialness that I thought it gave me. I was different from everyone else. Now I know that I'm somebody who's overcome it, which not everybody does."[3]

sense of normalcy in their lives. There are no set answers or approaches; each case is different.[7] Medications are useful mainly when depression accompanies the disorder. Still, establishing a strong relationship with either a therapist or another supportive person is a key to recovery.[17] Once the anorectic person feels understood and accepted by another person, he or she can begin to build a sense of self and exercise some autonomy.[3]

CONCEPT CHECK

Treatment of anorexia nervosa first requires a person to be brought back from a semistarvation state. Once weight gain allows normal basal metabolism to be maintained, psychotherapy can begin to uncover the causes of the disease and to help the person develop skills needed to return to a healthy life. Family therapy is an important tool in treatment.

BULIMIA

One of your best friends may practice bulimia without your knowing it. The person may feel desperate, yet will go to great lengths to keep it secret. This eating disorder involves episodes of binge eating followed by attempts to purge the food. College-age students practice it most commonly.[22] Susceptible people may have both biological factors and lifestyle patterns that predispose them to becoming overweight. As teenagers, these people probably tried many weight-reduction diets. Now as young adults their fear of gaining weight is overwhelmed by periods of real hunger.

Bulimia was first characterized in 1979 in college students. Like people with anorexia nervosa, those with bulimia are usually female, successful, and perfectionists. But, they are usually at or slightly above a normal weight. Females with bulimia are more likely to be sexually active than those with anorexia nervosa. The person with bulimia may think of food constantly. The major difference from anorexia nervosa is actually that the bulimic person turns to food during a crisis or problem, not away from it. Also, unlike those with anorexia nervosa, people practicing bulimia know their behavior is abnormal.[17] These people often have very low self-esteem and are depressed. The world sees their competence, while inside they feel out of control, ashamed, and frustrated.

Bulimic people tend to be impulsive. It has been suggested that part of the problem may actually arise from an inability to control responses to impulse and desire.[12] Some studies have demonstrated that bulimic people tend to come from disengaged families, ones that are loosely organized. Roles for family members are not clearly defined. Too little protection is given for family members and rules are very loose. This is in contrast to anorectic people who come from engaged families where roles may be too well defined.

Pinpointing the number of people who practice bulimia is difficult if the strictest medical guidelines are followed. These guidelines specify that to be diagnosed as bulimic a person must vomit at least twice a week for 3 months. Approximately 2% to 4% of college-age women fit this description.[23] However, people with bulimia lead secret lives. There is really no way to tell just by looking that someone has this disorder. Estimates of cases come largely from self-report and may therefore be unreliable. The problem, especially of milder cases, may be much more widespread than we think.

Among sufferers of bulimia, binges often alternate with attempts to rigidly restrict food intake.[9] Elaborate "food rules" are common. One frequently encountered rule is to avoid eating sweets. Thus if even one cookie or donut is

Men, especially athletes, are increasingly likely targets of bulimia as they attempt to maintain a certain weight.[24]

consumed, the person may feel that he or she has broken a rule and must get rid of the objectionable food. Usually this leads to further overeating, both because it is easier to regurgitate a large amount of food than a small amount, and because "having blown it," a decision is made to "go all the way" and start over tomorrow.

Binge-purge cycles may be practiced daily, weekly, or at other intervals.[11] A special time is often set aside. Most binge eating occurs at night when other people are less likely to interrupt, and usually lasts from a half-hour to 2 hours. A binge can be triggered by a combination of stress, boredom, loneliness, and depression. It often follows a period of strict dieting, and so can be linked to intense hunger. The binge is not at all like normal eating and, once begun, seems to propel itself. The person loses control. Bulimic people often report that they do not taste or enjoy the food once the binge has started (Figure 13-6).

Foods chosen for a binge are usually convenience foods—cakes, cookies, pies, ice cream, donuts, and pastries. As much as 20,000 kcalories might be eaten in a binge.[11] Purging follows in hopes that no weight will be gained. But even when vomiting follows the binge very quickly, 20% to 33% of the kcalories taken in are still absorbed. Even more kcalories are absorbed when laxatives are used for purging. People are mistaken in thinking that there will be no caloric cost as long as they purge soon after a binge.

Since people beginning to practice bulimia often use their fingers to induce vomiting, bite marks around the knuckles are a characteristic sign of this disorder.[23] Therefore, it is important for physicians to routinely examine the hands of young people. Once the disease is established, however, a person often can vomit simply by contracting the abdominal muscles. Vomiting may also occur spontaneously.

People practicing bulimia are not proud of these behaviors. After a binge, they usually feel guilty and depressed. Over time they feel hopeless about their situations. Compulsive lying and drug abuse can further intensify these feelings. All this just makes things worse (Figure 13-7). If a person has just started a binge when somebody comes to visit, the response may be, "Get out of my house." The person distances herself from friends and family, becoming more preoccupied with bingeing and purging, an activity that takes up a lot of time.

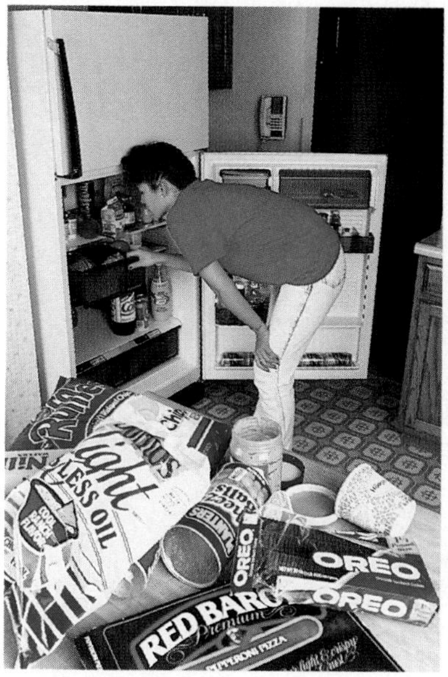

FIGURE 13-6

The binge-purge cycle. It can lead to a sense of helplessness.

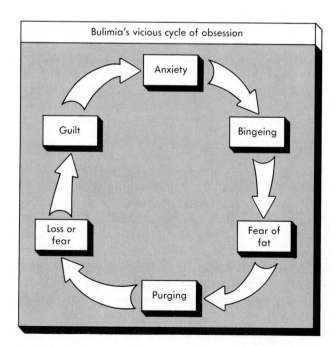

FIGURE 13-7

Bulimia's vicious cycle of obsession.

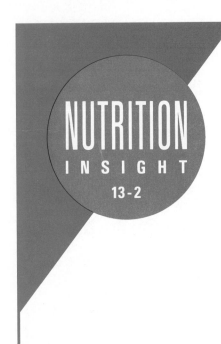

THOUGHTS OF A PERSON WITH BULIMIA

I am wide awake and immediately out of bed. I think back to the night before when I made a new list of what I wanted to get done and how I wanted to be. My husband is not far behind me on his way into the bathroom to get ready for work. Maybe I can sneak onto the scale to see what I weigh this morning before he notices me. I am already in my private world. I feel overjoyed when the scale says that I stayed the same weight as I was the night before, and I can feel that slightly hungry feeling. Maybe *it* will stop today; maybe today everything will change. What were the projects I was going to get done?

We eat the same breakfast, except that I take no butter on my toast, no cream in my coffee, and never take seconds (until Doug gets out the door). Today I am going to be really good and that means eating certain predetermined portions of food and not taking one more bite than I think I am allowed. I am very careful to see that I don't take more than Doug. I judge myself by his body. I can feel the tension building. I wish Doug would hurry up and leave so I can get going!

As soon as he shuts the door, I try to get involved with one of the myriad of responsibilities on my list. I hate them all! I just want to crawl into a hole. I don't want to do anything. I'd rather eat. I am alone; I am nervous; I am no good; I always do everything wrong anyway; I am not in control; I can't make it through the day; I know it. It has been the same for so long.

I remember the starchy cereal I ate for breakfast. I am into the bathroom and onto the scale. It measures the same, *but I don't want to stay the same!* I want to be thinner! I look in the mirror. I think my thighs are ugly and deformed looking. I see a lumpy, clumsy, pear-shaped wimp. There is always something wrong with what I see. I feel frustrated, trapped in this body, and I don't know what to do about it.

Health problems stemming from bulimia

Most health problems in bulimia arise from vomiting. While vomiting is the most effective way of purging, it is also the most physically destructive. Dental professionals are sometimes the first health professionals to notice signs of bulimia.[15] Repeated exposure to the acid in vomit demineralizes teeth. The person complains of painful teeth that are sensitive to heat, cold, and acids. Eventually, the teeth may severely decay, erode away from fillings, and finally fall out.

Blood potassium levels can drop significantly with regular vomiting or use of certain diuretics. This can disturb the heart's rhythm and even produce sudden death. Salivary glands may swell because of infection and irritation from the vomit. The person may even suffer from stomach ulcers and bleeding and tears in the esophagus. Constipation may result from frequent laxative use.[23]

Ipecac syrup, also used to induce vomiting, is poisonous to the heart, liver, and kidneys. It has caused accidental poisoning when taken repeatedly.

Treatment of bulimia

Therapy for bulimia, as for anorexia nervosa, requires a team approach. Treatment should last at least 15 to 20 weeks. Clinicians have yet to agree on the best method. Generally, psychotherapy aims primarily to help a person accept herself and to be less concerned with body weight (Figure 13-8).[17] Therapy focuses on correcting typical bulimic behaviors, such as the "all or none" thinking: if I'm not perfect, I'm a failure, so one slip-up—one cookie—justifies a binge. The person might be asked to role play a scientist testing assumptions and beliefs about food and weight. Patient and therapist together examine the validity of such beliefs. The premise for this therapy is that if abnormal attitudes and beliefs can be altered, normal eating will follow.[17] In addition, the therapist guides the person to establish behaviors that will mini-

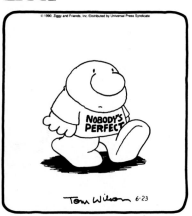

FIGURE 13-8

I float to the refrigerator knowing exactly what is there. I begin with last night's brownies. I always begin with the sweets. At first I try to make it look like nothing is missing, but my appetite is huge and I resolve to make another batch of brownies. I know there is half of a bag of cookies in the bathroom, thrown out the night before, and I polish them off immediately. I take some milk so my vomiting will be smoother. I like the full feeling I get after downing a big glass. I get out six pieces of bread and toast one side of each in the broiler, turn them over and load them with pats of butter, and put them under the broiler again until they are bubbling. I take all six pieces on a plate to the television and go back for a bowl of cereal and a banana to have along with them. Before the last piece of toast is finished, I am already preparing the next batch of six more pieces. Maybe another brownie or five, and a couple of large bowls full of ice cream, yogurt, or cottage cheese.

My stomach is stretched into a huge ball below my rib cage. I know I'll have to go into the bathroom soon, but I want to postpone it. I am in never-never land. I am waiting, feeling the pressure, pacing the floor in and out of the rooms. Time is passing. Time is passing. It is getting to be time.

I wander aimlessly through each of the rooms again, tidying, making the whole house neat and put back together. I finally make the turn into the bathroom. I brace my feet, pull my hair back and stick my finger down my throat, stroking twice, and get up a huge pile of food. Three times, four times, and another pile of food. I can see everything come back. I am so glad to see those brownies because they are *so* fattening. The rhythm of the emptying is broken and my head is beginning to hurt. I stand up feeling dizzy, empty, and weak. The whole episode has taken about an hour. ●

mize bingeing. Examples of these behaviors are eating regular meals and using alternate methods—other than food—to cope with stressful situations.[1] Group therapy is often useful. As in cases of anorexia nervosa, if a person enters treatment in a state of starvation, psychotherapy will be delayed.

One goal of therapy is to help a bulimic person accept as normal some depression and self-doubt. Therapists may prescribe antidepressant medications to combat some depression associated with bulimia. That often also works to reduce binge eating in early phases of treatment.

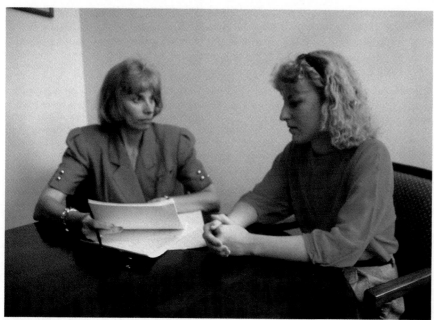

A person practicing bulimia should seek professional advice to help stop the process.

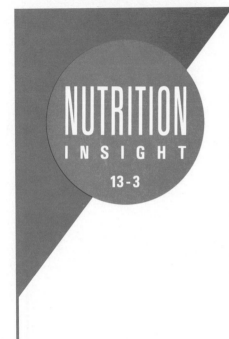

BARYOPHOBIA

Baryophobia, literally "the fear of becoming heavy," is a relatively new disorder. The term applies to children or young adults who grow slower and less than normal.[21] Decreased growth in a child usually reflects disease. If no hormonal or other abnormality can be found, the possibility of baryophobia should be investigated.

This disorder occurs when parents put their children on the same lowfat, high-carbohydrate diet that adults follow. Adults do this in an attempt to prevent their children from developing obesity or heart disease later in life. Today's parents or caregivers, themselves frequently harassed by weight problems, are determined to free their children from that ordeal. Well intended efforts to prevent obesity in their children can lead parents or caregivers to severely restrict their children's diets. The child doesn't get enough kcalories to maintain an adequate growth rate. In young adults, the low kcalorie diet may be self-imposed to avoid a perceived risk of obesity.

In these cases, counseling is needed. The caregivers and the young adult need to be informed of the nutrient requirements and weight gain patterns for the age group involved. The caregivers will learn that including some sweets and higher-fat foods in a young person's diet is appropriate (see Chapter 15). The diet can still minimize saturated fat, a more important focus in a diet designed to reduce the risk of heart disease. Supplying adequate kcalories and protein and other nutrients is the key to promoting growth—height and weight—in childhood and young adult years, and it can be done in a healthful manner. ●

Baryophobia • A disorder associated with a poor growth rate in a child because of parents underfeeding the child or young adult in an attempt to prevent development of obesity and heart disease.

Nutritional counseling can help correct misconceptions about food.[2] This entails teaching the person about bulimia and its consequences, focusing on its extreme means of weight control. In early stages it may be best for the person with bulimia to avoid eating binge foods or stepping on a scale. The primary goal, however, is to develop a normal eating pattern so that food choices become more mechanical. Some nutrition specialists achieve this goal by encouraging daily meal planning.

Nutritional counseling emphasizes setting up regular eating habits rather than stopping the bingeing and purging.[2] Usually a food diary is kept throughout treatment. This helps the person monitor food intake as well as feelings that accompany binge-purge cycles. Alternate coping strategies can then be tried. A therapist might use such information to identify events that seem to trigger binge episodes.

Once regular eating habits are established, the binge-purge cycle should stop by itself. The person should be discouraged from following strict food rules. Stressing the maintenance of healthful eating habits is a key to helping a person regain nutritional perspective.

Bulimia is a serious health problem. If not treated, grave medical complications can result. Since relapse is likely, therapy should be long term as we mentioned before.[17] People with bulimia can be very depressed and are at a high risk for suicide. For this reason they need professional help.

PREVENTING EATING DISORDERS

Parents, friends, and professionals working with young adults should consider the following advice for preventing eating disorders:

1. Discourage restrictive dieting, meal skipping, and fasting.
2. Provide information about normal changes that occur during puberty.
3. Correct misconceptions about nutrition, normal body weight, and approaches to weight loss.
4. Carefully phrase weight-related recommendations and comments.

Our society as a whole can benefit from a fresh focus on healthful food practices and a healthful outlook toward foods.

ANOTHER BITE

Aside from the references we list at the end of the chapter, sources to give you more insight into eating disorders include:

Hot line

Bulimia Anorexia Self Help/Behavior Adaptation Support and Healing (BASH) 1-800-762-3334—Available 24 hours, this is a treatment and research center for eating (anorexia, bulimia, overweight) and mood (depression, anxiety, phobias, panic attacks) disorders. It will provide assistance and information.

Books

Kano S: *Making peace with food,* Cottage Grove, Ore, 1985, Amity Publishing Company.

Vredevelt P, Whitman J: *Walking a thin line,* Portland, Ore, 1985, Multnomah Press.

Levenkron S: *Treating and overcoming anorexia nervosa,* New York, 1982, Charles Scribner's Son.

Newsletter

NAAS Quarterly Newsletter, 1925 Dublin Granville Rd., Columbus, Ohio 43229—Material is appropriate for professional and personal use. Ten back issues and "Overview of Eating Disorders" can be ordered for $10.00. A current subscription also is available through NAAS membership.

CONCEPT CHECK

Bulimia is characterized by episodes of binge eating followed by purging, usually by vomiting. Vomiting is very destructive to the body, often causing severe dental decay, stomach ulcers, irritation of the esophagus, and blood potassium imbalances. Treatment using nutrition counseling and psychotherapy attempts to restore normal eating habits, help the person correct distorted beliefs about diet and lifestyle, and find tools to cope with the stresses of life

SUMMARY

- The person with anorexia nervosa is usually a girl around the age of puberty who begins to diet but then finds it difficult to stop. She is generally a perfectionist and a high achiever, often described as the "best little girl in the world." Few cases are seen in men.

- Warning signs for anorexia nervosa include abnormal food habits, such as cutting a pea in half before eating it or cooking a large meal and watching others eat. Later, school performance crumbles, and the person often refuses to eat out with family and friends and develops a very critical and joyless nature.

- Physical effects of anorexia nervosa include decreases in body temperature and heart rate, iron-deficiency anemia, a low white blood cell count, hair loss, constipation, low blood potassium level, and the loss of menstrual periods. A person with anorexia nervosa is physically very ill.

- Treatment of anorexia nervosa includes increasing food intake to at least support basal metabolism and then to allow for gradual weight gain. Psychological counseling attempts to help the person establish regular food habits and to find means of coping with the life stresses that led to the disorder. Hospitalization may be necessary.

- Bulimia is characterized by bingeing on up to 20,000 kcalories at one sitting and then purging by vomiting, laxative use, exercise, or other means. Both men and women are at risk. Vomiting as a means of purging is especially destructive to the body; it can cause severe tooth decay, stomach ulcers, irritation of the esophagus, low blood potassium levels, and other problems. Bulimia poses a serious health problem and is associated with significant risk of suicide.

- Treatment of bulimia includes psychological as well as nutritional counseling. During treatment, the person learns to accept him/herself and to cope with problems in ways that do not involve food. Regular eating patterns are developed as the bulimic person begins to plan meals in an informed, healthy manner.

- Baryophobia describes a condition where children are underfed by parents in an attempt to limit risk of future disease, such as obesity or heart disease. Growth failure—weight and height gains—can result if nutrient intake is not increased to appropriate levels.

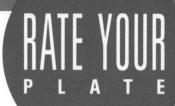

ASSESSING THE RISK OF HAVING AN EATING DISORDER

Figure 13-1 of this chapter lists the criteria for the eating disorders anorexia nervosa and bulimia. These criteria are repeated below. Put an "X" in the space before statements that describe your characteristics and lifestyle. Respond as honestly as possible.

_____ 1. You refuse to keep your body weight over a minimal normal weight for age and height.

_____ 2. You intensely fear gaining weight or becoming fat, even though you are underweight.

_____ 3. You feel fat even though you are quite thin.

_____ 4. If you are female, you have missed at least three consecutive menstrual cycles.

_____ 5. You have recurrent episodes of binge eating.

_____ 6. You feel out of control over eating behavior during the eating binges.

_____ 7. You regularly either self-induce vomiting, use laxatives or diuretics, diet strictly or fast, or vigorously exercise to prevent weight gain.

_____ 8. You engage in a minimum average of two binge eating episodes a week.

_____ 9. You have a persistent overconcern with body shape and weight.

Questions 1 through 4 pertain to anorexia nervosa and 5 through 9 to bulimia.

COMPLETE THIS ACTIVITY BY ANSWERING THE FOLLOWING QUESTIONS:

1. After having completed this checklist, do you feel that you might have an eating disorder or the potential to develop one?

_____

_____

2. Do you think some of your friends might have an eating disorder?

_____

_____

3. What counseling and education resources exist in your area or on your campus to help with a potential eating disorder?

_____

_____

_____

_____

_____

4. If a friend had an eating disorder, what do you think would be the best way to assist him or her in getting help?

_____

_____

_____

_____

If you would like more information you can contact the following national self-help groups:

American Anorexia/Bulimia Association, Inc.
418 East 76th Street
New York, New York 10021
212/734-1114

Anorexia Nervosa and Associated Disorders, Inc.
P.O. Box 271
Highland Park, IL 60035
312/831-3438

Anorexia Nervosa and Related Eating Disorders, Inc.
P.O. Box 5102
Eugene, OR 97405
503/344-1144

Bulimia, Anorexia Self Help
1027 Bellevue Avenue
St. Louis, MO 63117
314/567-4080

REFERENCES

1. Anonymous: Orderly dieting and disordered eating: a case report, *Nutrition Reviews* 49:16, 1991.
2. ADA Reports, Position of the American Dietetic Association: Nutrition intervention in the treatment of anorexia nervosa and bulimia nervosa, *Journal of The American Dietetic Association* 88:68, 1988.
3. Beresin EV and others: The process of recovering from anorexia nervosa, *Journal of The American Academy of Psychoanalysis* 17:103, 1989.
4. Collier SW and others: Assessment of attitudes about weight and dieting among college-aged individuals, *Journal of the American Dietetic Association* 90:276, 1990.
5. Comerci GD: Medical complications of anorexia nervosa and bulimia nervosa, *Medical Clinics of North America* 74:1293, 1990.
6. Feldman W and others: Culture versus biology: children's attitudes toward thinness and fatness, *Pediatrics* 81:190, 1988.
7. Field HL: Eating disorders, *Comprehensive Therapy* 15:3, 1989.
8. Goldbloom DS and others: Anorexia nervosa and bulimia nervosa, *Canadian Medical Association Journal* 140:1149, 1989.
9. Greene GW and others: Dietary intake and dieting practices of bulimic and non-bulimic female college students, *Journal of The American Dietetic Association* 90:576, 1990.
10. Health and Public Policy Committee, American College of Physicians: Eating disorder: anorexia nervosa and bulimia, *Nutrition Today* March/April, 1987, p 29.
11. Herzog D, Copeland P: Bulimia nervosa—psyche and satiety, *The New England Journal of Medicine* 319:716, 1988.
12. Kirkley BG, Burge JC: Dietary restriction in young women: issues and concerns, *Annals of Behavioral Medicine* 11:66, 1989.
13. Kreipe RE and others: Long-term outcome of adolescents with anorexia nervosa, *American Journal of Diseases of Children* 143:1322, 1989.
14. Mackenzie M: The pursuit of slenderness and addition to self-control: an anthropological interpretation of eating disorders. In Briggs GM, editor: *Nutrition update, 2,* New York, 1985, John Wyley & Sons.
15. Monehen R: Anorexia nervosa, bulimia, and the dental assistant, *Dental Assistant* July/August, 1989, p 19.
16. Morris A and others: The changing shape of female fashion models, *International Journal of Eating Disorders* 8:593, 1989.
17. Mynors-Wallis LM: The psychological treatment of eating disorders, *British Journal of Hospital Medicine* 41:470, 1989.
18. Nicholi AM, editor: *The new Harvard guide to psychiatry,* Cambridge, Mass, 1988, Harvard University Press.
19. Omizo SA: Anorexia nervosa: psychological considerations for nutritional counseling, *Journal of the American Dietetic Association* 88:49, 1988.
20. Patton G: The course of anorexia nervosa, *British Medical Journal* 299:139, 1989.
21. Pugliese MT and others: Fear of obesity: a cause of short stature and delayed puberty, *The New England Journal of Medicine* 309:513, 1983.
22. Schotte DE, Stunkard AJ: Bulimia versus bulimic behaviors on the college campus, *Journal of the American Medical Association* 258:1213, 1987.
23. Szmukler GI: Treatment of the eating disorders, *The Medical Journal of Australia* 151:583, 1989.
24. Thornton JS: Feast or famine: eating disorders in athletes, *The Physician and Sportsmedicine* 18:116, 1990.

HOW MUCH HAVE I LEARNED?

What have you learned from Chapter 13? Here are 15 statements about eating disorders. Read them to test your current knowledge. If you think the statement is true or mostly true, circle T. If you think the statement is false or mostly false, circle F. Use the scoring key at the end of the book to compute your total score. To review, take this test again later, and especially before tests.

1. **T F** Human societies deal irrationally with food.
2. **T F** Eating disorders are widespread in Western society.
3. **T F** People with anorexia nervosa have an intense fear of losing weight.
4. **T F** Bulimic people often induce vomiting to control their weight.
5. **T F** People with anorexia nervosa are often overachievers.
6. **T F** People with anorexia nervosa have a distorted view of their own bodies.
7. **T F** People with bulimia are aware that their eating patterns are abnormal.
8. **T F** People with bulimia are easy to identify because of their openness about their problem.
9. **T F** American society favors the lean and angular look.
10. **T F** The real problem underlying eating disorders is often how people feel about themselves.
11. **T F** People with eating disorders are often perfectionists.
12. **T F** Eating disorders are easier to treat at early stages of development.
13. **T F** Binge eating is characteristic of bulimia.
14. **T F** Treatment of bulimia emphasizes the immediate return to a strict diet.
15. **T F** Baryophobia is a new eating disorder found in children.

NUTRITION ISSUE

EATING DISORDERS: A SOCIOLOGICAL PERSPECTIVE

We evaluate ourselves in many ways. One way is based on body image. We identify our body with ourself and judge it as we think others see us, knowing that our appearance affects their opinions of us.

Early in life, we learn to recognize what "acceptable" and "unacceptable" body types look like. Of all attributes that constitute attractiveness, body weight is probably perceived as the most important, partly because it is an aspect we feel we can control somewhat.

Yet body weight is probably the aspect of image that dissatisfies us most. Fatness has been ranked as the most dreaded deviation from our cultural ideals of body image, the one most derided and shunned, even among schoolchildren.[6]

Women, in particular, are likely to diet because they have very strong feelings about what is an acceptable size and weight. In general, though, these women aren't technically obese. Rather, they diet to correct some perceived flaw or because they simply feel they should weigh less than they do now.

A Glamour magazine survey with 30,000 respondents indicated that 80% were ashamed of their bodies. This dissatisfaction focuses primarily on the desire for lower weight and smaller thighs, hips, buttocks, and waists, typical sites of greatest fat deposition in sexually mature women.[12]

Changing times

The "full-bodied" woman as a cultural ideal did not survive into the twentieth century. Over the course of this century, a woman's "ideal" body form has become thinner and thinner. Our passion for thinness may have its roots in the Victorian era, which specialized in denying "unpleasant" physical realities, such as appetite and sexual desire.[14] Flappers of the 1920s cemented a trend for thinness (Figure 13-9). Over the past 20 years, the ideal has gradually moved toward a thinner, more angular body shape. Female models for women's magazines have become taller, thinner, and more "tubular" in that bust and body circumferences have decreased compared to waist size.[16] At the same time, the population as a whole has gained weight. The same holds true for men in general: a lean, slightly muscular physique characterizes men in advertisements and movies.

Researchers have linked this preference for a lean body type to the recent surge in eating disorders. As the more full-figured woman (earth mother) is being replaced by the ultra-thin woman, our preoccupation with obesity and the number of people with eating disorders has increased. It appears that the cultural pressures toward thinness are stretching the physiological capabilities of many women and men. Given the natural variability in human basal metabolism, our easy access to food, and increasingly sedentary lifestyles, it is

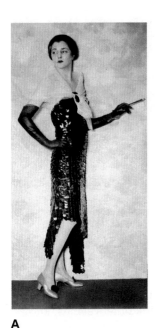

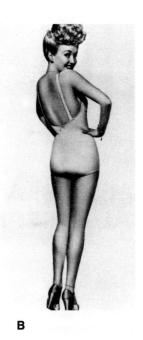

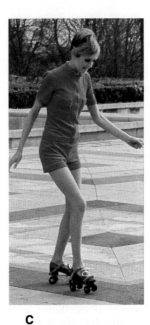

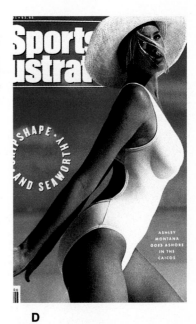

A　　　　　　　B　　　　　　　　　　　C　　　　　　　　　D

FIGURE 13-9

The changing views of desirable body weight. American society has imposed varying stereotypes for desirable body weight, especially for women. **A,** The svelte flapper of the 1920s. **B,** The "thin but curvaceous" look of the 1940s. **C,** Ultra-thin was in during the 1960s. **D,** Lean and well-toned physiques grace magazine covers of the 1980s and 1990s.

no surprise that some of us gain weight. People predisposed to eating disorders for either biological or emotional reasons may be nudged "over the edge" by this change in social values.

The pursuit of power

Today, society views obesity as a failure of control, willpower, competence, and productivity. At stake is social acceptance and even access to scarce resources, such as good jobs or an attractive spouse. Whether we like it or not, our appearance says a lot about us. The question implicit in our society's values is this: if a person cannot control himself enough to stay slim, can he supervise employees, organize the work day, and reliably bear heavy responsibilities?

Mixed messages

On top of the pressure for thinness, we receive mixed messages. Half the advertisements in women's magazines may be for diets, and the other half for tasty foods. Movie and television stars are almost always perfect physical specimens. Yet television advertisements encourage us to visit our local fast-food restaurant. There you can buy a hamburger, French fries, and milk shake, totaling about 1200 kcalories—about the amount of energy our daily basal metabolism uses—without even leaving the car.

New pressures

Divorce now ends about one-half of all marriages. This increases the stress on children and adolescents, who, like adults, may turn to food. Considering other prevalent stresses—alcoholism in the family, school and work pressures, and crowded urban conditions—many of us face family and social environments that encourage us to find a pressure release valve. That valve may be food.

Thin is in!

All in all, fat has lost favor in our society. Today's myth is that thin people are better than obese people—more competent, healthier, and more strong-willed.

Eating disorders are usually only a symptom of greater emotional trauma in a person's life. When psychiatrists are able to dig deeper, they find that eating disorders mask serious questions of self-worth, family struggles, and sometimes fears of puberty and the future.[10] The real illnesses are not the eating disorders—though they eventually contribute to poor health—but rather, the way people feel about themselves. And negative self-images are reinforced by current social values.

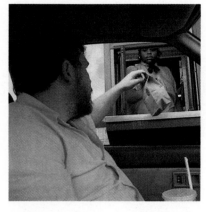

The easy availability of fast food has made weight control even harder for the average person.

By severely restricting calories for long periods of time, people with anorexia nervosa greatly compromise their nutritional status, impair their reproductive systems, retard growth, and put themselves at risk for osteoporosis and even death.[12] The harm produced by milder, shorter periods of diet restriction is not clear. Evidence, however, suggests that even moderate diet restriction, if continued, contributes to the risks for various anemias, pregnancy complications, low-birth-weight infants, and may reduce bone density and metabolic rate. As we mentioned, it can also impair growth in children and very young adolescents.[12] The percentage of adolescents and young adults who significantly restrict kcalories is not known. But at least two problems, iron-deficiency anemia and pregnancy complications, are significant problems in this age group.

cathy®   **by Cathy Guisewite**

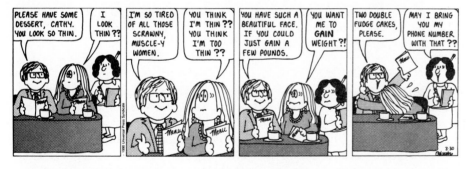

FIGURE 13-10

For women there are some glimmers of hope. Feminists are beginning to point out that true liberation means being free to find your natural weight. Women who combine careers and motherhood are saying that they have more important things to worry about; fashion leaders are tolerating more curves; exercise programs are encouraging walking, rather than jogging and working out to feel good. Writers, therapists, and some registered dietitians are working to help women accept and love their bodies.

What is the difference between people who can accept themselves—even with a few more pounds than the glamorous people have—and those who chronically diet and feel dissatisfied? Perhaps it is the willingness to recognize that satisfaction with appearance comes from within, not from what they see in the mirror or what someone else tells them (Figure 13-10). The challenge facing Americans today is achieving a healthy body weight without excessive dieting. This means adopting and maintaining sensible eating habits, a physically active lifestyle, and realistic and positive attitudes and emotions, while practicing creative ways to handle stress. ●

NUTRITION

A
FOCUS
ON
LIFE STAGES

PREGNANCY AND BREAST-FEEDING

Pregnancy can be a very special time for a couple. Along with the responsibility of shaping a child's health and personality comes the prospective exhilaration of watching the child develop and grow. Prospective parents often feel an overriding desire to produce a healthy baby, which opens them up to new nutrition and health information. The parents-to-be usually want to do everything possible to maximize their chances of having a healthy baby.

Producing a healthy baby is not just a matter of luck. True, some aspects of fetal and newborn health are beyond a parent's control. Still, conscious decisions about social, health, and nutritional factors significantly determine the baby's health and future.[16] What the parents do relates directly to the likelihood of having a healthy newborn. Let's examine the practices that help make a healthy baby a reality. ●

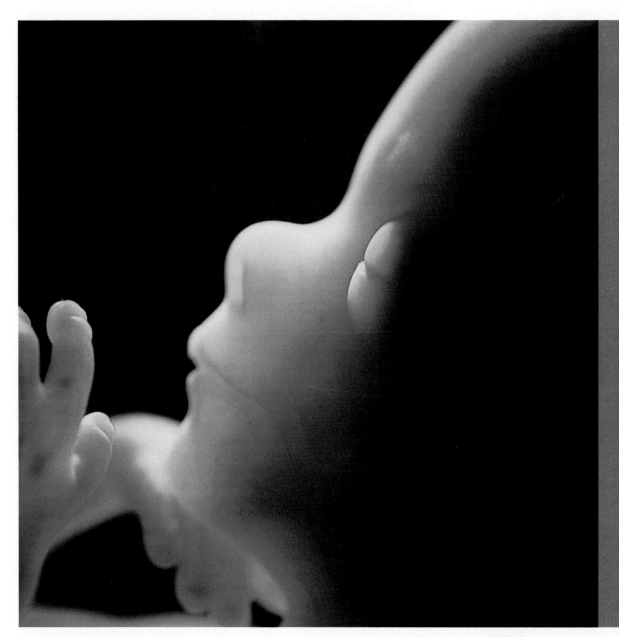

The fetus relies on the mother to supply the nutrients needed for growth and development.

To Breast-feed or Not to Breast-feed: That Is The Question

One important decision facing parents is whether to breast-feed or formula-feed their child. If you ever become a parent, you will want to participate in this decision. This assessment explores your feeding preference and reasons for it. Please answer the following questions.

PARENTAL/FAMILY INFLUENCE

1. As a baby, were you breast-fed or bottle-fed?

_____

2. Why did your parents choose that means of nourishing you? Ask them if you are not sure.

_____

_____

PERSONAL CHOICE

3. Which means do you prefer to use for your future children, breast-feeding or formula-feeding?

_____

REASONS

4. Why do you prefer one over the other?

_____

_____

_____

_____

5. To what degree will your parents' preference affect yours?

_____

_____

In this chapter we consider the benefits of breast-feeding. As you read about this issue, reconsider your answers to these questions.

ASSESS YOURSELF

PRENATAL GROWTH AND DEVELOPMENT

For 8 weeks after its conception, a human **embryo** develops from an **ovum** into a fetus. For another 30 weeks the incomplete fetus continues to develop. When its body is finally mature enough, the infant is born, about 38 weeks after it was conceived. Until birth, the mother nourishes it via a placenta, an organ that forms in her uterus to accommodate the growth and development of the fetus (Figure 14-1).

Women often do not suspect they are pregnant during the first few weeks. They may not even seek medical attention during the first **trimester.** Nevertheless, without fanfare, the embryo grows and develops daily. For that reason, a woman's health and nutritional habits are particularly important for several years before pregnancy. Note that a history of anorexia nervosa or bulimia does not set the stage for a healthy pregnancy. Some research suggests that an inadequate vitamin and mineral intake—especially of the vitamin folate—in the months before conceiving and during the first months of pregnancy may lead to birth defects.[15] Parents-to-be need to be aware of this kind of information.

Good nutrition practices then have a double significance—to the woman and her future fetus—during a woman's childbearing years. Other practices—such as smoking and using certain medications (even aspirin), illicit drugs (like cocaine), and alcohol—can harm a fetus during its development. Harmful effects can occur even before a woman realizes she is pregnant. On the other hand, once started, healthful habits can be carried into pregnancy, providing optimum health and nutrition from conception until birth.[16]

Embryo • The developing human life form from the second to eighth week after conception.

Ovum • The egg cell from which a fetus eventually develops if the egg is fertilized by a sperm cell.

Trimester • The normal pregnancy of 38 to 42 weeks is divided into three 13 to 14 week periods called trimesters.

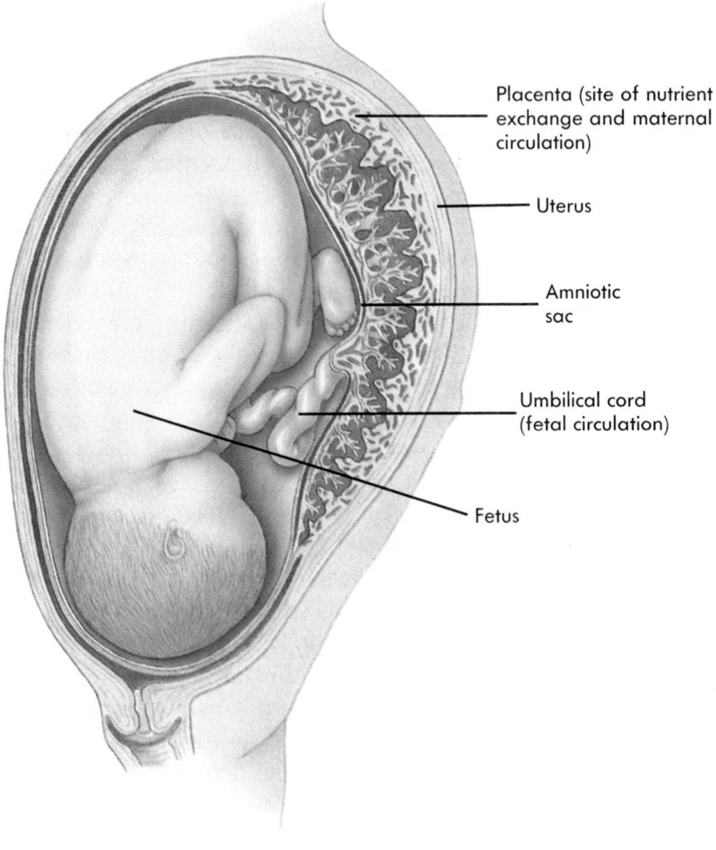

Placenta (site of nutrient exchange and maternal circulation)

Uterus

Amniotic sac

Umbilical cord (fetal circulation)

Fetus

FIGURE 14-1

The fetus in relationship to the placenta. The placenta is the organ through which nourishment flows to the fetus.

Miscarriage • Loss of pregnancy, also called spontaneous abortion, that occurs within 28 weeks of conception.

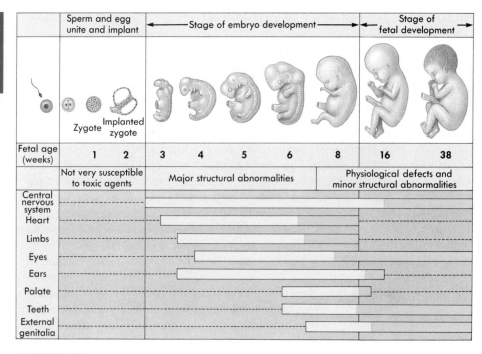

	Sperm and egg unite and implant		←——Stage of embryo development——→				Stage of fetal development ←——→	
	Zygote	Implanted zygote						
Fetal age (weeks)	1	2	3	4	5	6	8	16	38
	Not very susceptible to toxic agents		Major structural abnormalities				Physiological defects and minor structural abnormalities	
Central nervous system								
Heart								
Limbs								
Eyes								
Ears								
Palate								
Teeth								
External genitalia								

FIGURE 14-2

Vulnerable periods of development. The most serious damage from fetal exposure to toxins is likely to occur during the first 8 weeks after conception (yellow bars). As the chart shows, however, damage to vital parts of the body—including the eyes, brain, and genitals—also can occur during the last months of pregnancy (purple bars).

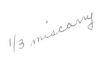

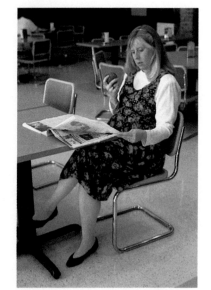

An expectant mother must be especially careful to eat foods that are healthy for both her and her unborn child.

Early growth—the first trimester

Embryo growth begins with a rapid increase in cell number. This type of growth also dominates fetal development. Newly formed cells then proceed to grow larger. Further growth and development combines increasing cell number and size.[22] At about 3 weeks, cells begin to form specialized organs and body parts. By the end of 13 weeks, the heart is complete and beating, most organs have formed, and the fetus can move (Figure 14-2).

Nutritional deficiencies and other insults to a fetus—for example, injuries caused by medications and other drugs, high doses of vitamin A, radiation, or trauma—can alter or arrest the progressing phase of development. The effects may last a lifetime. The most critical time for fetal development is during the first trimester. Most *miscarriages*—premature termination of a pregnancy—occur at this time. Currently, about one-third of all pregnancies miscarry, often so early that a woman does not realize she was indeed pregnant. Early miscarriages usually result from a genetic defect or fatal error in fetal development.

A woman must avoid substances that may harm the developing fetus, especially during the first trimester. This holds true for the time when a woman is trying to become pregnant. Note that she likely will not know of her pregnancy for at least a few weeks.[10] In addition, the fetus develops so rapidly during the first trimester that if an essential nutrient is not available, the fetus may be affected even before the deficiency appears in the mother. Though some women lose appetite and feel nausea during the first trimester, adequate nutrition is extremely important (Figure 14-3).

The second trimester

By the beginning of the second trimester, a fetus weighs about 1 ounce. Soon its movements can be detected by the mother. Arms, hands, fingers, legs, feet,

For Better or For Worse®   by Lynn Johnston

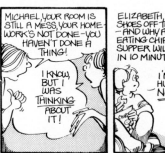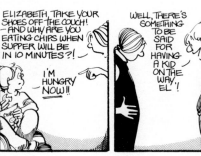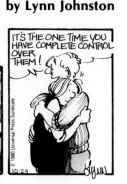

FIGURE 14-3

and toes are fully formed. The fetus has ears and begins to form tooth sockets in its jawbone. Organs continue to grow and mature, and with a stethoscope, physicians can detect the fetus' heart beat. Eventually, the fetus begins to look more like a baby (Figure 14-2). Most bones are distinctly evident throughout the body.

The third trimester

By the beginning of the third trimester, a fetus weighs about 2 to 3 pounds. After about 28 to 30 weeks of gestation, an infant born **prematurely** (before 37 weeks of gestation) has a good chance of survival if it is cared for in a nursery for high-risk newborns. However, the infant will not contain the mineral and fat stores normally accumulated during the last month of gestation. This and other medical problems, such as a poor ability for sucking and swallowing, complicate nutritional care for prematurely born infants.[22] More than one in ten infants in the United States are born prematurely.

At 9 months, the fetus weighs about 7 to 9 pounds (3 to 4 kilograms) and is about 20 inches (50 centimeters) long (Figure 14-4). A soft spot in the forehead (fontanel) indicates where the skull bones are growing together. The bones finally close after about 12 to 18 months.

What is a successful pregnancy?

Defining a successful pregnancy is difficult. No specific standards have been determined.[11] One dimension concerns protection of the mother's physical and emotional health. Two goals are commonly suggested for health of the infant: (1) a gestational period longer than 37 weeks and (2) a birth weight greater than 5.5 pounds (2500 grams). The longer the gestational age, the more time fetal lungs have to develop. Adequate lung development is critical for the infant's survival. By 37 weeks, fetal lungs are well developed, and other medical problems associated with premature birth occur less often.

Infants born after 37 weeks in the uterus that weigh less than 5.5 pounds are considered **small for gestational age (SGA)**.[22] About one in 14 infants is born SGA in the United States. These infants are more likely than normal-weight infants to have problems in regulating blood sugar and temperature and show reduced growth and development in the early weeks after birth.

In rating the success of a pregnancy, the newborn's quality of life must also be considered. This dimension involves the newborn's ability to grow, develop, learn, and eventually to reproduce. Parents should strive toward producing a baby who is born healthy, on time, and with the mental, physical, and physiological capabilities to take advantage of whatever life offers, while also protecting the mother's health.

431

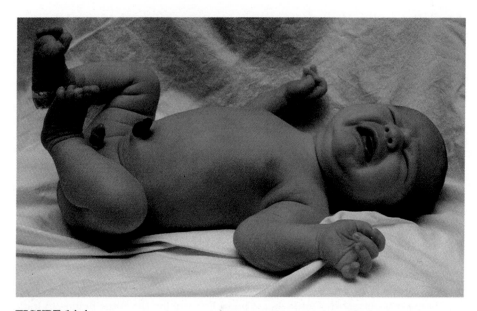

FIGURE 14-4
A healthy one-week-old baby. At birth the baby usually weighs about 7½ pounds and is 20 inches in length.

Nutrition is one key to a successful pregnancy.[16] Eating healthfully is vital during pregnancy to ensure the health of both the fetus and the mother. Fetal organs and body parts begin to develop very soon after conception. The first trimester (13 weeks) is an especially critical period when poor nutrition or drug use can result in birth defects.

CONCEPT CHECK

Infants born after 37 weeks of gestation and weighing more than 5.5 pounds (2.5 kilograms) have the fewest medical problems at birth. To help reduce infant and maternal medical problems or death, a mother should strive to carry her baby in the uterus for the entire 9 months and to have a large enough baby. Good nutrition and health practices aid in this goal. Limiting activities that increase the risk of having a premature or small-for-gestational-age (SGA) infant are also important.

MEETING INCREASED NUTRIENT NEEDS POSED BY PREGNANCY

Over the past century the medical community has changed nutritional advice for pregnant women. In the 1950s, doctors commonly recommended that women restrict weight gain to between 15 and 18 pounds. At times they also recommended severe kcalorie and sodium restrictions to keep the baby small, in hopes of easing labor and avoiding complications. Few of these practices were based on sound scientific information. We know now that many of these recommendations can actually harm the mother and fetus.

The first comprehensive scientific report about nutrition and pregnancy was issued in 1970 by The National Academy of Sciences and recently updated in 1990.[16] The document emphasizes an increase in nutritional requirements during pregnancy (not restrictions) and the importance of individually assessing and counseling mothers-to-be.

For Better or For Worse®   **by Lynn Johnston**

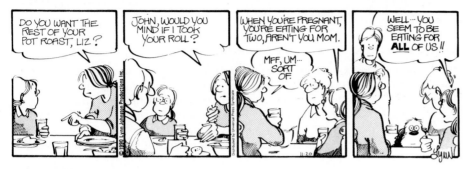

FIGURE 14-5

Increased energy needs

An average pregnancy requires about 80,000 extra kcalories: divided by 280 days, this averages approximately 300 extra kcalories daily.[22] Just 2 cups of lowfat milk and a piece of bread, for example, can provide this amount. The extra kcalories are mostly needed during the second and third trimesters of pregnancy. Though she may "eat for two," the pregnant woman must not double her normal kcalorie intake. She cannot afford a Big Mac for herself and another for the fetus (Figure 14-5). She will want to seek the best quality foods to create the best possible health for her child. Many vitamin and mineral needs increase, but the mother can meet those requirements by eating nutrient dense foods—ones that don't contribute many extra kcalories (Figure 14-6).

If a woman is active during pregnancy, she can add the extra kcalories she uses to the kcalorie allowance for pregnancy. Her greater body weight requires more energy for activity. Physicians strongly encourage women to continue most activities during pregnancy, except scuba diving, downhill skiing, weight lifting, and contact sports like hockey. Walking, cycling, swimming, and light

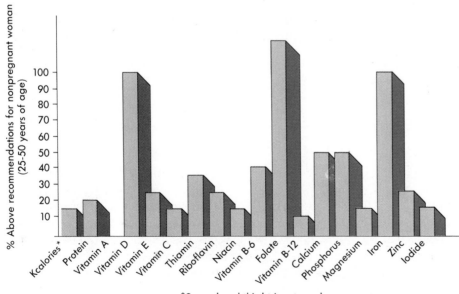

*Second and third trimester only

FIGURE 14-6
Changes in the 1989 RDA for pregnancy. During pregnancy, many nutrients are needed in greater amounts than at other times. These include vitamin D, folate, and iron. Note, however, that kcalorie needs do not change very much.

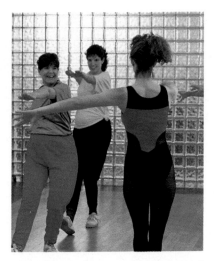

Moderate exercise can be performed throughout most stages of pregnancy.

aerobics are generally advised. However, many women find that they are quite inactive during the later months, partly because of their increased size, and so an extra 300 kcalories daily is usually enough.

 ANOTHER BITE

The American College of Obstetrics and Gynecology suggests the following guidelines for exercise during pregnancy:
1. Do not allow heart rate to exceed 130 beats/minute.
2. Avoid exercising in hot, humid weather.
3. Avoid contact and jarring sports.
4. Discontinue exercise that causes discomfort or overheating.
5. Drink plenty of liquids to avoid dehydration and overheating.
6. After about the fourth month, don't exercise while lying on your back.

Recommended weight gain

Adequate weight gain for a mother is one of the best predictors of pregnancy outcome. Her diet should allow for approximately 2 to 4 pounds (.9 to 1.8 kilograms) of weight gain during the first trimester, and then a subsequent weight gain of ¾ to 1 pound (0.5 kilogram) weekly during the second and third trimesters. Total weight gain goal normally averages about 25 to 35 pounds (11.5 to 16 kilograms).[19] Adolescents and black women, who often have smaller babies, are strongly advised to aim for the greater amount.[10]

For underweight women the goal increases to 28 to 40 pounds (12.5 to 18 kilograms). The goal decreases to 15 to 25 pounds (7 to 11.5 kilograms) for obese women. Figure 14-7 shows why the typical recommendation begins at 25 pounds. It accounts for the total weight of the baby (8 pounds), placenta (1 pound), amniotic fluid (2 pounds), the mother's increased breast tissue (3 pounds), increased blood supply (4 pounds), the increased fat (2 to 8 pounds), and increased muscle tissue (2 pounds) she needs to support pregnancy and lactation.

A weight gain of about 25 to 35 pounds has repeatedly been shown to yield optimum health for both mother and fetus.[2] This poundage especially reduces

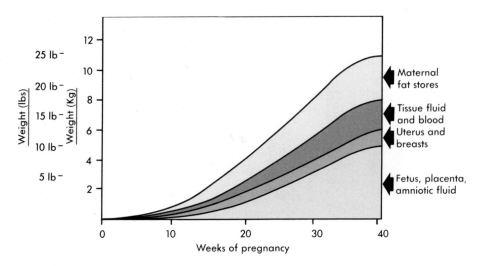

FIGURE 14-7

The components of weight gain in pregnancy. A weight gain of 25 to 35 pounds is recommended. Note the various components total about 25 pounds.

the risk for delivering an infant of **low birth weight** and should yield a birth weight of 8 to 9 pounds (3.5 to 4 kilograms). While some extra weight gain during pregnancy is usually not harmful, it can set the stage for creeping obesity during the childbearing years if the mother does not return to about her prepregnancy weight. This is especially true if the woman intends to have more than one child.[17]

Weight gain during pregnancy needs regular monitoring, especially in teenage years.[16] Infant birth weights improve if the mother's weight gain meets the above mentioned ranges. Keeping weekly records of a pregnant woman's weight gain can help assess how much to adjust her food intake (see Appendix N for an example of a weight gain chart). Weight gain is a key issue in prenatal care and a concern of many mothers (Figure 14-8). Inadequate weight gain can cause many problems. If a woman deviates from the desirable weight gain pattern, she should be warned of dangers.

cathy®   **by Cathy Guisewite**

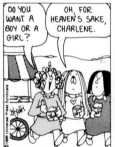
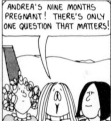
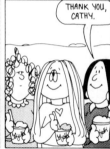
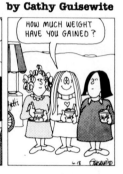

FIGURE 14-8
Weight gain in pregnancy is a concern of more than just the mother.

If a woman begins to gain too much weight during her pregnancy, she should not be encouraged to lose weight in order to get back on track. She should simply slow the increase in weight to parallel the rise on the prenatal weight gain chart. If a woman has not gained the desired weight by a given point in pregnancy, she shouldn't be encouraged to gain the needed weight rapidly. Instead, she should slowly gain a little more weight than the typical pattern in order to meet the goal by the end of pregnancy.

During pregnancy, women in America are more likely to gain excess weight and make poor food choices than to eat too few kcalories. The problem is more often how to limit weight gain so that they don't have many extra pounds to shed after pregnancy. Excessive weight gain increases risk for complications during pregnancy and encourages excess fetal growth, which makes birth trauma more likely. Loose, accommodating maternity clothes designed for comfort do not provide the usual feedback about weight gain, and fluid retention can likewise mask true weight gain during pregnancy. The woman and her physician should work together to monitor weight gain.

Increased protein and carbohydrate needs

The RDA for protein increases by 10 grams daily. A glass of milk alone contains 8 grams. Still, many nonpregnant women already eat the recommended 60 grams of protein per day. However, all women should check to make sure they are actually eating enough protein. Carbohydrate needs are at least 100 grams daily. This amount prevents ketosis, which can harm the fetus (see later section). Most women already consume almost twice this amount.

Increased vitamin needs

Vitamin needs generally increase, especially the need for vitamin D and folate (see Figure 14-6).

Vitamin D. The body increases its calcium metabolism during pregnancy to absorb and distribute extra calcium for forming fetal bones. The mother's need for vitamin D doubles to aid the calcium absorption. To provide it, pregnant women should get regular sunlight exposure. If exposure is impossible or insufficient, they can drink vitamin D–fortified milk to make up the difference. A quart (liter) suffices. Pregnant women can also consider a vitamin D supplement that contains 5 to 10 micrograms (200 to 400 IU). The typical prenatal supplement contains this extra amount of vitamin D.

Folate. The synthesis of DNA requires folate. This means that both fetal and maternal growth in pregnancy depends on an ample supply of folate. Red blood cell formation increases in pregnancy and that also requires folate. Serious anemia (the megaloblastic type; see Chapter 9) can result if folate intake is inadequate. The RDA doubles during pregnancy. As mentioned before, folate deficiency has been associated with birth defects.

Some women have difficulty consuming sufficient folate to satisfy their pregnancy needs. Recent studies show that some pregnant women consume only about the nonpregnant RDA. However, by choosing foods wisely—for example, folate-rich fruits and vegetables as outlined in the Guide to Daily Food Choices —a woman can meet her needs (Table 14-1). A prenatal vitamin supplement may be used to meet the RDA for folate, especially by women with histories of inadequate folate intake, frequent or multiple births, folate-related anemia, or use of medications that increase folate needs.[10] But normally, wise diet choices alone suffice.[16]

Increased mineral needs

Mineral needs generally increase during pregnancy, especially the need for iron, calcium, zinc, and fluoride (see Figure 14-6).

TABLE 14-1

A food plan for pregnancy and breast-feeding

Food group	Key nutrients supplied	Number of servings
Milk, yogurt, and cheese: 1 cup; 1½ ounces for cheese	Protein Riboflavin Calcium	3*
Meat, poultry, fish, dry beans, eggs, and nuts: 2-3 ounces meat; 1 cup beans; 2 eggs; ½ cup nuts	Protein Thiamin Vitamin B-6 Iron Zinc	3
Vegetables: ½ cup or ¾ cup raw	Vitamin A Vitamin C Folate Dietary Fiber	3 (to 5)
Fruits: 1 piece generally	Vitamin C Folate Dietary Fiber	2 (to 3)
Breads, cereals, rice, and pasta: 1 slice or ½ -¾ cup cooked	B-vitamins Iron Dietary Fiber	6 (to 11)

*Four servings if a teenager.

Iron. Extra iron (twice the RDA for nonpregnant women) is needed for hemoglobin synthesis during pregnancy by the mother and for providing iron stores to the fetus. The greatest need occurs mostly during the last two trimesters. A supplement is often needed to provide that much iron, especially if iron-fortified foods, such as breakfast cereals, are not eaten. Because iron supplements decrease appetite and can cause nausea and constipation, taking them along with food helps. Combining foods rich in vitamin C with an iron supplement increases iron absorption. Severe iron-deficiency anemia in pregnancy may lead to premature delivery, low birth weight, and increased risk for fetal death in the first weeks of life.

Calcium. Calcium is needed during pregnancy to promote adequate mineralization of the fetal skeleton and teeth. Most calcium is required during the third trimester, when skeletal bones are growing most and teeth are forming. However, extra calcium intake should start immediately. The RDA for calcium in pregnancy is the same as for women ages 11 to 24 years and one and a half times the RDA for women over age 24 years. The only practical food sources for calcium are the milk, yogurt, and cheese group and calcium-fortified orange juice. Calcium supplements are needed if these options are not possible.

Zinc. Zinc is a mineral important for supporting growth and development. The RDA increases 25% for pregnant women. The extra protein foods in the diet of a pregnant woman should supply this much zinc. A poor zinc status in pregnancy increases the risk for having a low-birth-weight infant.

Fluoride. Fluoride can improve fetal tooth development. Women should ask their dentists if extra fluoride is needed.

Is there an instinctive drive in pregnancy to eat more nutrients?

Extra needs in pregnancy for folate, iron, calcium, and zinc are the most difficult for women to satisfy. These, then, should be the focus of diet planning for pregnant women. Before we discuss diet planning, however, one important misconception about pregnancy needs to be dispelled. You may have heard that mothers instinctively know what to eat, and that their craving for pickles and ice cream is dictated by a natural desire to consume needed nutrients. These cravings are most common during the last two trimesters and could be related to hormonal changes in the mother. Still, it remains a puzzle why women devour clay, starch, ice, and other nonfood items during pregnancy.[9] Is this a natural drive or a learned behavior? We think the latter is true.

There may be a natural instinct to consume the right foods during pregnancy, but we are so far removed from surviving by instinct that relying on our desires is risky. Good nutritional counseling and the Guide to Daily Food Choices can focus food choices more reliably.

A FOOD PLAN FOR PREGNANCY

As stated earlier The Guide to Daily Food Choices provides a good diet approach during pregnancy (see Table 14-1). It includes three servings from the milk, yogurt, and cheese group (four servings for teens who are pregnant or breast-feeding); three servings from the meat, poultry, fish, dry beans, eggs, and nuts group; three to five servings from the vegetable group; two to three servings from the fruit group; and six to eleven servings from the breads, cereals, rice, and pasta group. More specifically, most of the servings from the milk, yogurt, and cheese group should be portions of lowfat milk, yogurt, or cheese. These supply needed protein, calcium, and riboflavin. Servings from the meat, poultry, fish, dry beans, eggs, and nuts group should include two animal sources and two vegetable sources. Besides protein, these provide some of the extra iron and zinc needed.

The servings of vegetables provide mostly vitamins and minerals. A good vitamin C source should be among the vegetable and fruit servings, as well as a

If a woman finds herself with no desire at all for pickles and ice cream or frijoles and hot fudge, there is no need to panic: about a third of pregnant women experience no strong food cravings.

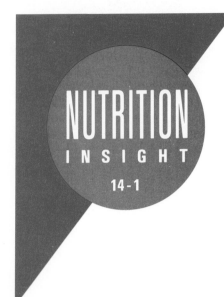

WHAT DO I REALLY HAVE TO GIVE UP WHEN I'M PREGNANT?

We have already mentioned that alcohol should not be consumed in pregnancy, and this suggestion is amplified in the Nutrition Issue on p. 458. We have also said that neither nutrient supplements nor any drug use—over the counter, prescription, or illicit—is advised without a doctor's approval. Light aerobics is allowed but hockey is not. Smoking should be stopped, and crash dieting is not recommended.

What else should be eliminated during pregnancy?

Caffeine

The potential danger of caffeine use during pregnancy has been debated for some time. Although evidence so far doesn't justify recommending abstinence during pregnancy, several recent studies have produced provocative findings. First, caffeine reduces iron absorption, a nutrient needed in high amounts during pregnancy. Second, moderate-to-heavy caffeine users have been found to have a significantly greater risk of spontaneous abortion during the late first and second trimesters than women who use less caffeine. Moderate caffeine use is defined as consuming at least 150 milligrams of caffeine daily, the equivalent of about 1½ cups of coffee. Another study concluded that the risk of low birth weight rose as the level of daily caffeine increased. The risk was more than four and a half times greater for women who consumed more than 300 milligrams of caffeine daily than for women who used no caffeine at all. Even though additional research is needed to confirm these observations, it seems justifiable at this point to advocate moderation in caffeine consumption during pregnancy.[7] This recommendation has wide support, especially to cut down to 2 cups or less of coffee daily. That is equivalent to four caffeine-containing soft drinks.

---

rich source of folate, such as orange juice or a green leafy vegetable. For the breads, cereals, rice, and pasta group, the servings should be whole grains or enriched grains. Recall that whole grains are good sources of dietary fiber. This basic diet plan can contain as little as 1800 kcalories and still meet the extra needs of pregnancy (Table 14-2).

When are prenatal vitamin and mineral supplements needed?

As outlined above, maternal dietary changes during pregnancy will enable the typical woman to meet all increased nutrient needs, except perhaps for iron. For most pregnancies, the National Academy of Sciences supports only the use of iron supplements.[16] However, physicians routinely prescribe a specially formulated prenatal supplement. They may do this because it is easier to prescribe supplements than to discuss diet changes. Also, some women are just not willing to improve their diets to meet their increased nutrient needs. The supplements typically include the critical nutrients for pregnancy—iron, folate, vitamin D, and calcium—and many others, as well (Appendix N).

There is no evidence that prenatal supplements cause problems, aside perhaps from the combined amounts of supplementary and dietary vitamin A (mainly during the first trimester). Under some conditions, such as poverty, teenage pregnancy, poor maternal diet, multiple fetuses, and vegetarianism, the necessity for use of supplements deserves a close look.[10]

The pregnant vegetarian

The vegetarian woman who becomes pregnant should not necessarily face special nutritional hurdles if she practices either lacto-ovo vegetarianism or lacto vegetarianism. Meeting iron needs is still the major problem. A total vegetari-

Pregnancy, in particular, is not a time to self-prescribe vitamin and mineral pills.

Food additives

Unfortunately, some pregnant women are frightened by rumors that various food additives cause abnormal fetal development. This fear is largely unjustified. True, we don't know the cause of most birth defects and, theoretically, some substances in the food supply could pose problems. But there is no solid proof of a connection between food additives and birth defects. Regulations currently enforced by FDA mandate that any company proposing to introduce a new additive into the U.S. food supply must prove its safety through a series of animal studies. The evidence must show that the additive causes neither cancer nor birth defects. Many additives that have been used in the American food supply for years are "generally recognized as safe" (see Chapter 17). Ongoing reevaluation of many of these substances has yielded little cause for concern.

Among the additives receiving much attention in the popular press is aspartame (NutraSweet and Equal). This sweetener has now replaced sugar and saccharin in many commercially manufactured products. Aspartame does not appear to adversely affect the fetus. Observations of human subjects have generated no data to suggest that aspartame use by pregnant women adversely affects the course and outcome of pregnancy. Some experts recommend only cautious use, if at all.[7] But it is hardly warranted to recommend that pregnant women abstain from using aspartame-sweetened products (see Chapter 6, reference no. 15).

There is still much mystery about why some babies develop abnormally or are delivered prematurely. At present, research suggests that pregnant women should meet their nutritional needs through sensible food choices, avoid alcohol, and use caffeine-containing foods and beverages judiciously. Above all, pregnant women in America should appreciate how lucky they are to have access to a superb food supply. They should delight in knowing that they can provide all the nutrition the fetus needs—except maybe iron—through wise food choices.

TABLE 14-2

A sample diet based on the minimum recommendations in Table 14-1

Breakfast
3/4 cup raisin bran
4 ounces orange juice
1/2 cup 1% milk

Snack
2 tablespoons peanut butter
1 slice whole-wheat toast
1/2 cup plain lowfat yogurt
1/2 cup strawberries

Lunch	**Dinner**
spinach salad with	3 ounces lean ham
2 tablespoons oil and vinegar dressing	1 cup navy beans
1/2 sliced tomato	1 cornbread muffin
2 slices whole-wheat toast	3/4 cup cooked broccoli
1 1/2 ounces of provalone cheese	1 teaspoon corn oil margarine
	iced tea or milk (the latter if a
Snack	teenager)
4 whole-wheat crackers	
1 cup 1% milk	

This diet meets the RDA for pregnancy and lactation for only 1800 kcalories (including 34 milligrams of iron).

an (vegan), on the other hand, must carefully plan a diet that includes sufficient protein, vitamin B-6, iron, calcium, zinc, and a vitamin B-12 supplement. The basic vegan diet listed in Chapter 8 should be supplemented in the grain group, as well as in the beans, nuts, and seeds group to supply more needed nutrients. Since iron and calcium are poorly absorbed from most plant foods, iron and calcium supplements are probably necessary. The levels provided by a typical prenatal supplement should suffice for iron needs but not for calcium needs.

CONCEPT CHECK

Women need an average of about 300 more kcalories daily during pregnancy, especially during their second and third trimesters. They should gain weight slowly and steadily. Women starting at normal weight should gain up to a total of 25 to 35 pounds. Protein, vitamin, and mineral needs all increase during pregnancy. Vitamin D, folate, iron, calcium, and zinc are nutrients of particular concern. A pregnant woman's diet should be varied and generally include more milk products than a nonpregnant woman's diet. Prenatal supplemental vitamins and minerals are commonly prescribed, but taking too many supplements, especially of vitamins A and D, can be hazardous to the fetus.

THE EFFECT OF NUTRITION ON THE SUCCESS OF PREGNANCY

Do we have evidence that all this attention to nutrition is worth the effort? Yes, the effort is justified. Extra nutrients and energy are used for the growth of the fetus as well as the changes made in the mother's body to accommodate the fetus. Her uterus and breasts grow, the placenta develops, her total blood volume increases, the heart and kidneys work harder, and stores of body fat increase. All these changes prepare a woman's body for birth and to produce milk. The nutrients needed for these support-system changes are added to the nutrient needs of both the growing fetus and the mother's own normal body functions.[22]

It is difficult to establish the specific harm to fetal development if a mother either gets too little energy and nutrients during pregnancy or has only minimal nutritional stores when pregnancy starts. A daily diet containing only 1000 kcalories has been shown to greatly retard fetal growth and development. Increased maternal and infant death rates recently seen in famine stricken areas of Africa add further evidence (see Chapter 18). For some nutrients, however, such as iron and calcium, the fetus may also use—and deplete—the mother's stores if she doesn't get enough in her diet.

The mother's body can adapt to the demands of pregnancy in a variety of ways; it may, for example, absorb more nutrients from foods. However, the success of this adaptation is unpredictable. Both environmental and nutritional factors, such as a mother's prepregnancy weight and weight gain during pregnancy, turn out to be much more important.[2] Figure 14-9 depicts many factors that influence the outcome of pregnancy.

Early research supports the importance of good nutrition in pregnancy

During World War II, parts of Russia and much of Holland were blockaded. Food supplies were quickly exhausted. The resulting undernutrition greatly affected birth weights of infants developing in second or third trimester. Birth defects also occurred more commonly, and the number of new pregnancies fell. After the blockades were lifted, birth weights, subsequent infant health, and the numbers of new pregnancies quickly returned to prewar statistics.[22]

At the same time, researchers working in Boston noticed that a good protein intake was associated with a greater success of pregnancy.[22] It appeared that

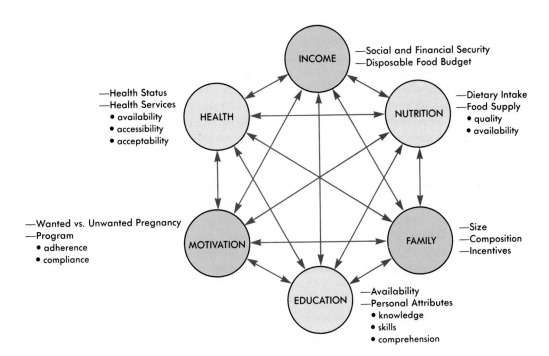

FIGURE 14-9
The seamless web of influences that can affect the outcome of pregnancy. Much more than luck goes into having a healthy baby at birth.

the mother's diet—not only during pregnancy but also preceding conception—affected the health of both mother and infant. Studies in Toronto then showed that dietary supplements and nutritional counseling improved the health of the pregnant mother and yielded a healthier baby. Complication rates also dwindled. In addition, researchers in Great Britain showed that height and social class could better predict the outcome of pregnancy than dietary intake during pregnancy.[5] Supporting this is a recent study of middle class black women in Chicago. Their risk of having low-birth-weight babies still exceeded that of middle class whites, possibly reflecting the effects of previous generations of poverty.[6] This finding again suggests that long-term nutritional intake may be critical to pregnancy outcome.

Laboratory animal studies have supported the importance of diet during pregnancy. Food deprivation during animal pregnancy led to smaller organ size in the offspring, even in the brain, which usually resists nutritional insults. In addition, placentas weighed less and fewer healthy offspring survived the first weeks of life.

Maternal and infant mortality—common consequences of poor nutrition

In the United States, approximately 12 of every 100,000 live births lead to the mother's death. Nine hundred and seventy infant deaths occur for each 100,000 live births. Compared with other industrial countries worldwide, the United States ranks 22nd—a poor showing. And for blacks in the United States, infant deaths are double that seen in whites or hispanics. Considerable efforts are being made to reduce both infant and maternal deaths. Good health care and nutritional practices are the keys to reducing these deaths.

Beyond nutrients

Many nutrition-related factors also affect the health of both the mother and the fetus (infant):[22]

Low socioeconomic status that leads to poverty, inadequate health care, poor health practices, lack of education, and unmarried status is associated with problems in pregnancy.[7] Currently in the United States about 25% of births are to unwed mothers.

Obesity leads to an increased rate of high blood pressure and diabetes mellitus during pregnancy.[8] Surgical and other complications during delivery likewise increase,[20] especially because the baby can be very large. These pregnancies require intense monitoring.

Poor, absent, or delayed prenatal care can allow maternal nutritional deficiencies to deprive a fetus of needed nutrients. The risk of fetal damage also increases in cases of chronic diseases, such as hypertension or diabetes mellitus. Without prenatal care, a woman is three times more likely to give birth to a low-birth-weight baby—one that will be 40 times more likely to die during the first 4 weeks of life than a normal-birth-weight infant. Ideally, prenatal care should start before conception.[16] Still, about 25% of women in the United States receive no prenatal care in the first trimester—again, a critical time to change habits.

Smoking, alcohol consumption, use of some medications, and illicit drug use in pregnancy all lead to harmful effects. The Nutrition Issue on p. 458 reviews one effect of alcohol—fetal alcohol syndrome. Smoking is linked to low infant birth weight. This occurs probably because the fetus can't get needed oxygen when nicotine constricts the arteries, cutting some of the blood supply.[22] Problem drugs include aspirin, hormone ointments, nose drops, rectal suppositories, weight-control pills, and medications that were prescribed for previous illnesses.

A recent survey of 36 hospitals throughout the United States found that overall 11% of women use illicit drugs during pregnancy. The actual range for individual hospitals was 0.4% to 27%. In 1989, research at a major hospital in Philadelphia revealed that 15% of 852 women tested had positive blood studies for cocaine or combinations of cocaine, marijuana, and narcotics. This percentage was equally distributed among private and medical-assistance patients. Clearly, this is not an issue for poor minorities alone: Infants in all socioeconomic and ethnic groups are adversely affected.

Fetal exposure to cocaine is of special concern. It has become more prevalent in recent years and has been linked to such problems as premature labor, small body and head size, physical malformations, and disturbed nervous system development.[13]

Pica is the practice of eating nonfood items, such as dirt, starch, ice, or clay, especially during pregnancy. Pica occurs more frequently among black women in the United States.[9] As we mentioned before, this practice probably results more from cultural influences than from a need for specific nutrients, like iron and zinc. Eating soil raises the risk of infections from parasites and can cause anemia as well as life-threatening blockages of the intestinal tract. Eating laundry starch should be discouraged because it contains toxic compounds. Eating ice can break teeth.

Prenatal ketosis is not desirable for the growing fetus. Ketone bodies are thought to be poorly used by the fetal brain. This suggests that they could slow fetal brain development. Researchers stress the need for a pregnant woman not to "crash" diet or fast for more than 12 hours. A pregnant woman can develop significant ketosis after only 20 hours of fasting. Eating about 100 grams of carbohydrate everyday prevents ketosis. We noted earlier even nonpregnant women usually eat twice this amount.

Inadequate weight gain, especially among underweight women, often produces infants of low birth weight (LBW).[2] Undernourished women often have borderline vitamin and mineral intakes. They should try to reach desired weight by the end of the first trimester. Most women can achieve that by consistently eating 300 more kcalories a day than usual. Overweight women who try to avoid weight gain during pregnancy may rob both themselves and their infants of essential nutrients. Also, to efficiently metabolize protein during pregnancy, enough kcalories from carbohydrate and fat are needed for energy needs.

In the United States, 7% to 10% of infants have a low birth weight, that is, they weigh less than 5.5 pounds (2.5 kilograms). Low-birth-weight infants are more susceptible to infections, illnesses, and disabilities and are more likely to die than normal weight infants. Premature birth, poor diet during pregnancy, some medical conditions in the mother, and the factors highlighted above influence an infant's birth weight. Reducing the number of low-birth-weight infants will help reduce infant deaths.

Education, an adequate diet, and early and consistent prenatal medical care maximize the chances of producing a healthy baby. The woman should be counseled to avoid x-ray exposure, smoking, vitamin A supplements, medicines, illicit drugs, and alcohol use. If diabetes mellitus is present or developing, it must be carefully controlled to minimize complications in the pregnancy.

Again, it is best to begin these examinations and counseling strategies before a woman becomes pregnant, but certainly they should begin early in pregnancy. Many potential problems that develop during pregnancy can be diagnosed and quickly treated medically.

Almost all women need prenatal nutritional counseling because nutrition needs are unique during pregnancy.[1] Food habits cannot be predicted from income, education, or lifestyle. While some women already have good nutritional habits, most can benefit from nutritional advice. All should be reminded of habits that may harm the growing fetus, such as severe dieting or fasting. By focusing on appropriate prenatal care, good nutritional intake, and proper health habits, as well as using common sense, parents give their fetus—and later infant—its best chance of thriving.

The U.S. government supports programs that aim to reduce infant mortality. Provision of high quality health care and foods helps alleviate the effects of poverty and poor education. An example of such a program is the Special Supplemental Food Program for Women, Infants, and Children (WIC). This program offers health assessments, counselling, and foods (or vouchers for foods) that supply high quality protein, calcium, iron, and vitamin C to pregnant women, infants, and children (to age 5 years) from low-income populations. The diets of pregnant women have improved markedly on this program, as has their likelihood of having a healthy baby.

Given close monitoring, women over the age of 35 have an excellent chance of producing healthy babies. Physicians once considered this a high-risk group. They now feel this age group has typical problems that are usually manageable.[18]

CONCEPT CHECK

Successful pregnancy depends in part on the mother's healthful diet. It must provide the nutrients necessary for body maintenance, building the new fetus, and development of the mother's physical support system in the uterus and breasts. A minimal nutrient intake can retard fetal development. Besides nutrient intake, other factors that contribute to poor pregnancy outcome are low socio-economic status; obesity; poor, absent, or delayed prenatal care; smoking; imprudent medicine use; alcohol consumption; illicit drug use; pica; teenage pregnancy; inadequate prenatal weight gain; and prenatal ketosis.

PHYSIOLOGICAL CHANGES CAN CAUSE DISCOMFORT IN PREGNANCY

During pregnancy, the fetus' needs for oxygen, nutrients, and excretion increase the burden on the mother's lungs, heart, and kidneys. Although a mother's digestive and metabolic systems work very efficiently, some discomfort accompanies the changes her body undergoes to accommodate the fetus.

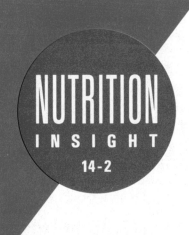

TEENAGE PREGNANCY

About half a million teenagers give birth to babies in the United States each year. Teenage pregnancy poses special health problems for both the mother and child. To accommodate their normal growth even when not pregnant, teenagers need an extraordinary nutrient supply. Women normally continue to grow taller for 2 years after they begin menstruating. Teen pregnancy adds the needs of the growing fetus to those of the growing mother. They both need considerable amounts of nutrients for their growing bodies.[14]

Teen diets—pregnant teens included—vary greatly in nutritional adequacy. Many teens have irregular eating habits, skip meals, snack on low-nutrient foods, and frequently diet. Many of them eat less than two-thirds of the RDA for many vitamins and minerals. Table 14-3 lists some of these problems.

TABLE 14-3

Nutrient-related risk factors in teenage pregnancy

- Low pregnancy weight gain
- Low prepregnancy weight for height (or other evidence of poor nutrition)
- Smoking
- Excessive prepregnancy weight for height
- Anemia

Other risk factors suggested by health histories
- Unhealthy lifestyle (i.e., use of drugs and alcohol)
- Unfavorable reproductive history
- Chronic diseases
- History of an eating disorder

Modified from ADA Reports: Position paper of the American Dietetic Association: Nutrition management of adolescent pregnancy, *Journal of The American Dietetic Association* 89:106, 1989.

Teenagers are more likely than most mothers to be underweight at the beginning of pregnancy and to gain less than 16 pounds during pregnancy. Consequently, teens frequently produce low-birth-weight infants.

The specific needs of the pregnant adolescent vary according to their own growth patterns, body build, and exercise habits. This makes it difficult to predict their nutrient needs. But health workers can evaluate the adequacy of their diet by checking for appropriate weight gain during pregnancy and appropriate food choices. To improve pregnancy outcomes and the health of pregnant teenagers, their eating practices should be routinely examined and they should be counseled concerning nutrition during their prenatal care.[1] They need information about the basic nutritional guidelines. They also need to be made aware of the risks they are taking if they smoke, drink alcohol, or use drugs not approved by their physician. ●

Heartburn, constipation, and hemorrhoids

Hormones produced by the placenta relax muscles in both the uterus and the intestinal tract. This often causes heartburn as stomach acid slips up into the esophagus (see Chapter 5).[22] When this occurs, the woman should avoid lying down after eating, eat less fat so that foods pass more quickly from the stomach into the small intestine, and avoid spicy foods she can't tolerate. She should also consume liquids between meals to decrease stomach volume and pressure.

Constipation often results as the intestinal muscles relax during pregnancy. It especially develops late in pregnancy as the fetus competes with the GI tract for space in the abdominal cavity. To offset these discomforts a woman should typically consume more water, dietary fiber, and dried fruits, and exercise. These practices can help avoid constipation and an often accompanying problem, hemorrhoids. Straining during defecation can lead to hemorrhoids, which are more likely to occur during pregnancy anyway because of other bodily changes.

Edema

Placental hormones cause various body tissues to retain fluid during pregnancy.[22] Blood volume also greatly expands during pregnancy. The extra fluid normally contributes some swelling (edema). There is no reason to severely restrict salt or use diuretics to limit mild edema. However, the edema may limit physical activity late in pregnancy and occasionally require the woman to elevate her feet to control the effects. Retaining fluid spells trouble only if hypertension and the appearance of protein in the urine accompany it. (We discuss this in a later section.)

Morning sickness

Women commonly feel nauseated during the early stages of pregnancy, which is possibly a reaction to pregnancy-related hormones circulating in the bloodstream.[22] Although known as "morning sickness," nausea may occur at any time and persist all day. It is often the first signal to a woman that she is pregnant. Some women partially control mild nausea by eating soda crackers or dry cereal before getting out of bed, cooking with open windows to dissipate nauseating smells, eating smaller, more frequent meals, and avoiding foods that increase nausea. Usually, nausea stops after the first trimester, but it can continue throughout the entire pregnancy. In cases of serious nausea, the preceding practices offer little relief. When appetite is severely reduced or vomiting persists, medical therapy is needed.

Anemia

To supply fetal needs, the mother's blood volume expands up to approximately 150% of normal. The red cell mass expands only 20% to 30% above normal and occurs more gradually. This leaves proportionately fewer red blood cells in a pregnant woman's bloodstream. The lower ratio of red blood cells to total blood volume is a condition known as ***physiological anemia***.[22] It is a normal response to pregnancy rather than the result of poor nutrient intake. If during pregnancy, however, iron stores and/or dietary iron intake is inadequate, any resulting iron-deficiency anemia requires medical evaluation.

Pregnancy-induced hypertension

Pregnancy-induced hypertension is a high-risk disorder. In its mild forms it is known as preeclampsia and in severe forms as eclampsia. The problem resolves once the pregnancy state ends. Early symptoms include a rise in blood pressure, excess protein in the urine, edema, changes in blood clotting, and nervous system disorders. Very severe effects, including convulsions, can occur in the second and third trimesters. Good nutrition, especially a good calcium intake, may prevent or lessen the symptoms.[3] Mild effects can be lessened by bedrest. If not controlled, eclampsia eventually damages the liver and kidneys, and mother and fetus may both die. Careful medical attention is needed.

• • •

Although pregnancy brings with it some physical discomforts for the mother, the inconvenience is temporary and many potential discomforts can be diffused through generally good eating and health habits. More than that, the good habits bring double benefits since they are the basis of good health for both mother and infant.

Physiological Anemia • The normal increase in plasma volume that dilutes the concentration of red blood cells, resulting in anemia; also called hemodilution.

Pregnancy-induced Hypertension • A serious disorder that can include high blood pressure, kidney failure, convulsions, and even death of the mother and fetus. Although exact cause is not known, good nutrition and prenatal care can prevent or limit its severity. Mild cases are known as preeclampsia; more severe cases are called eclampsia (formerly called toxemia).

Today, folate-related anemias do not often occur during pregnancy. Widespread use of prenatal supplements, which supply folate, is probably the major reason.

Let-down reflex • A reflex stimulated by infant suckling that causes the release (ejection) of milk from milk ducts in the mother's breasts.

Bottle-feeding a formula to an infant is also a nutritious choice. We discuss the how-to's in the next chapter.

CONCEPT CHECK

Heartburn, constipation, nausea, and vomiting from morning sickness, edema, and anemia are possible discomforts and complications of pregnancy. Changes in food habits can often ease these problems. Pregnancy-induced hypertension, with high blood pressure and kidney failure, can lead to severe complications, and if not treated, can lead to death of both the mother and fetus.

BREAST-FEEDING

Before the 1900s, if a mother didn't breast-feed, a "wet-nurse" was substituted. Formula-feeding was fraught with complications, primarily because people did not know the importance of sterilizing formulas against bacteria. Nor did people know much about the nutritional needs of infants. During the early 1900s, the technology of formulas and feeding improved. From the 1920s and especially in the 1940s when women worked in armament factories during World War II, more and more babies were fed formula. Throughout the 1950s and early 1960s, interest in breast-feeding further waned. In the 1970s, breast-feeding enjoyed a resurgence, which has since leveled off.

Recent statistics show that about 60% of white women nurse their babies in the hospital, and 25% of black women do so. The same approximate ratio of white to black women who breast-feed holds after four months. The women who choose to breast-feed usually find it an enjoyable and special time in their lives and in the relationship with their new babies.

Physiology of lactation

Almost all women can breast-feed their children.[12] Major problems are usually caused by a lack of information. Problems such as inverted nipples can be corrected during pregnancy. Breast size does not affect successful breast-feeding: the cells needed to produce milk are present. First-time mothers who plan to breast-feed should learn as much as they can about the process before delivering the baby. Interested women should learn the proper technique, as well as what problems to expect and how to respond to them. Familiarity with the process builds the confidence and knowledge necessary for success.

Producing human milk

During pregnancy, cells in the breast form milk-producing **lobules** (Figure 14-10). Hormones from the placenta stimulate these changes in the breast. After birth, the mother produces more **prolactin** hormone to maintain the changes in the breast, and therefore the ability to produce milk.[22] During pregnancy, breast weight increases by 1 to 2 pounds.

The hormone prolactin also stimulates the synthesis of milk. Suckling stimulates prolactin release. Milk synthesis then occurs as an infant nurses. The more the infant suckles, the more milk is produced. Milk production closely parallels infant demand.[12] In this way, even twins can be nursed. Demand is the driving force for milk production.

Most protein found in human milk is synthesized by breast tissue. Some proteins also enter the milk directly from the mother's bloodstream. These proteins include immune factors and enzymes. Fats in human milk come from the mother's diet, and some are also synthesized by breast tissue. The simple sugar galactose is synthesized in the breast, while glucose enters from the mother's bloodstream. Together these sugars form lactose, the main carbohydrate in human milk.

The let-down reflex

An important brain-breast connection—the **let-down reflex**—is necessary for breast-feeding (Figure 14-11).[22] The brain releases the hormone oxytocin to

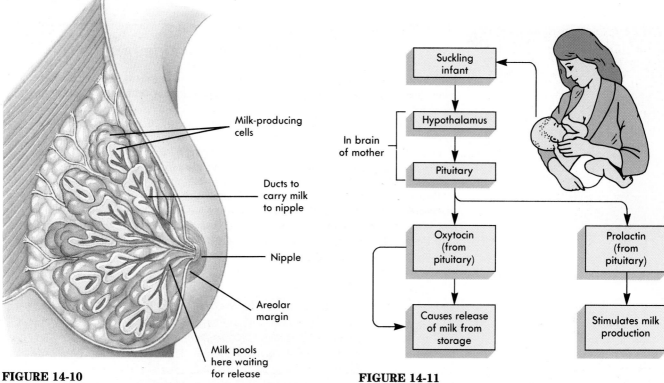

FIGURE 14-10

The breast automatically prepares itself for nourishing the infant. Many structures in the breast contribute to the production and release of human milk.

FIGURE 14-11

The let-down reflex. Suckling by the infant initiates hormonal changes that lead to milk production and the let-down reflex. This reflex releases the milk from storage cells in the breast.

allow the breast tissues to let down (release) the milk from storage sites. It travels to the nipple area. A tingling sensation signals the let-down reflex shortly before milk flow begins. If the let-down reflex doesn't operate, little milk is available to the infant. The infant then gets frustrated, and this can frustrate the mother.

The let-down reflex is easily inhibited by nervous tension, a lack of confidence, and fatigue. First-time mothers should be especially aware of the link between tension and a weak let-down reflex. They need to find a relaxed and supportive environment where they can breast-feed.

After a few weeks, the let-down reflex becomes almost automatic. The mother's response can be triggered just by thoughts about the baby or by seeing or hearing another baby. But at first, the reflex can be a bit bewildering. Because she cannot measure the amount of milk the infant takes in, a mother may fear that she is not adequately nourishing the baby. A good standard of comparison for a breast-fed baby is (1) it should have 6 or more wet diapers every day and show normal growth; (2) the stool should look like mustard (one to two stools every day is typical); and (3) the breast should soften during the feeding. If so, enough milk is being consumed.

The parents need not be concerned that breast-fed infants grow a bit more slowly after about 3 months of age than formula-fed infants. The infant's physician is the best judge of whether the rate of growth of the breast-fed infant is satisfactory. Growth will likely catch up to that of formula-fed babies by 2 years of age.[12]

It generally takes 2 to 3 weeks to fully establish a feeding routine. By then infant and mother should both feel comfortable, the milk supply should meet infant demand, and initial nipple soreness should have disappeared. Establishing the routine requires patience, but the rewards are great. The adjustments are easier if supplemental formula feedings are not introduced until breast-feeding is well-established. That occurs after about 2 to 3 months. However, providing water in a bottle during hot weather is fine.

Disposable diapers can absorb so much urine that it is difficult to judge when they are wet. A strip of paper towel laid inside a disposable diaper makes a good wetness indicator. Or, cloth diapers may be used for a day or two to assess whether nursing is supplying sufficient milk.

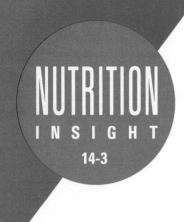

NUTRITION

I N S I G H T

14-3

THE MECHANICS OF BREAST-FEEDING

Each infant is unique and has a distinct personality that begins to form before birth. Some eagerly breast-feed the first time they get the chance; others may be disinterested for the first couple of days. A mother should expect the unexpected. She shouldn't be discouraged if her infant doesn't act like others she's seen. Her infant will soon become hungry and will breast-feed when ready.

In the hospital, a mother can begin breast-feeding by asking a nurse to help her. Nurses are experienced in helping women begin the process and can suggest various positions to try—traditional, football hold, or others (Figure 14-12).

To get started, a woman should take the dark area around the nipple, the **areola,** between two fingers so the infant can get a good hold. This is especially important with very large or full breasts. The mother should then rub the infant's cheek with the nipple. The infant will naturally "root" for the nipple and latch on. The mother may have to continue to hold on to the areola so that it won't block the infant's nose.

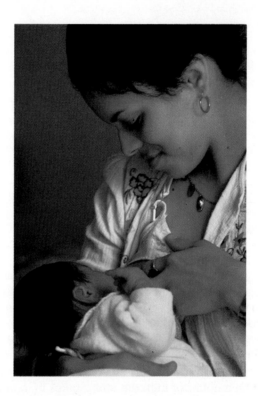

FIGURE 14-12
Breast-feeding fosters closeness between mother and infant. This is part of the process called bonding, which is part of the normal parent-child nurturing process. Bottle-feeding also allows for this.

It may take a few days for the mother and infant to get to know each other and to establish comfortable positions.[12] The mother should not be alarmed if after the first few days or weeks breast-feeding still does not feel totally natural. It takes time, especially with a first child.

A mother should begin by nursing about 5 minutes on each side every 1 to 2 hours and eventually increase nursing time to 10 or so minutes on each side spaced every 3 to 4 hours after about one week. Babies suck fairly vigorously when they are hungry and soften their suck as they get fuller. So it is a good idea to begin nursing on the breast on which the baby finished the previous feeding—it will feel heavier and fuller. It is important at the start for the mother not to allow the infant to use the breast as a pacifier. This can cause nipple soreness and much pain.

Babies cry for reasons other than hunger. The baby's only language is crying. If the baby is fussy less than 2 hours after the start of a feeding, caregivers should look for other causes for the crying before offering the breast. At times babies do nurse just for comfort, but they also have other needs. Some babies need to fuss (not hard crying) for several minutes before drifting off to sleep, even just after a feeding. At fairly predictable times because of growth spurts—about 10 days, 6 weeks, 3 months, and 4 to 6 months—the baby will suddenly fuss to nurse twice as often as usual for about 48 hours.[12] The more frequent emptying of the breasts will increase milk production, and then the baby will be getting more milk at each feeding and spread out the feedings again.

To get a baby's attention, a mother may try squirting a bit of milk into its mouth or perhaps change its diapers to wake it. To stop a session the mother can break an infant's suction by inserting a finger along the breast into the child's mouth. Merely pulling the infant off her breast could be quite painful. Then she should burp the baby and start on the other breast. To keep nursing enjoyable, the mother should try to reduce other stresses in life, eat a nutritious diet, and get plenty of sleep—at least 8 hours when possible.

Many babies need fairly frequent night-time feedings at first, which can fatigue the mother. The mother can lie down to nurse her baby but should not go to sleep, so as to reduce the risk of suffocation to the baby. The baby also must be positioned so that it cannot fall out of bed. A small blanket should be rolled up and placed against the baby's back to keep it on its side. In this position any spit-up milk can run out of the mouth.

When breast-feeding does not go perfectly

Problems may accompany nursing a baby. This is typical—there is no reason for panic. Breast-feeding is more a skill than an instinct—it takes practice.

Engorgement.   Engorgement of milk in the breast may occur when an infant isn't an established nurser. The breasts fill with milk, but the infant does not empty them. The woman should then express milk from the breast in order to reduce the size and resulting pain. It is probably best to buy an inexpensive (about $35) breast pump. Before pumping, the breasts can be stimulated with a towel soaked in warm water. The woman can also manually express milk by squeezing gently while moving her hands from the back to the front of the breast.[22]

Leakage.   Breasts may leak between feeding sessions, especially if a let-down reflex is stimulated. Pushing straight back to the chest wall on the nipple helps stop let-down. The mother can do this discreetly by folding her arms. Absorbent pads or a handkerchief can be worn to soak up any milk.

Nipple soreness.   If nipples become sore, using a pacifier can satisfy some of the infant's suckling needs. Allowing the nipples to air dry and using a lanolin cream should reduce tenderness in a couple of days. It is important to keep nursing sessions to 10 minutes per side and to use the sore side last until the soreness subsides.

Overall, the mother should expect that small problems will arise, but these can be easily dealt with. If the mother wants to continue to nurse, she should be able to do so.

When the baby is still hungry

When it appears an infant is not satisfied after 20 minutes of nursing, the mother should first attempt to breast-feed the infant more often, at least every 2½ to 4 hours. This will increase milk production and in turn probably satisfy the infant. In this way even twins can be nursed. Demand drives milk production. Foods other than breast milk or formula are rarely needed before 4 months of age. Recall that a breast-fed baby normally wets six to eight diapers a day and shows normal growth. ●

Areola • The circular dark area of skin at the center of the breast.

Colostrum • The first milk secreted during late pregnancy and the first few days after birth. This thick fluid is rich in immune factors and protein.

Meconium • The first stool passed after birth. It has a thick, mucuslike consistency.

Lactobacillus Bifidus Factor • A protective factor secreted in the colostrum that encourages growth of beneficial bacteria in the newborn's intestines.

Human milk is for humans

Human milk is composed of lactose, protein, fats, vitamins, minerals, and other constituents. It's composition differs from cow's milk. Unless altered, cow's milk should not be used in infant feeding for the first 6 to 12 months. The main protein in cow's milk forms a hard curd that is hard to digest unless it is first heat-treated. Infant kidneys are not mature enough to handle the high mineral content of the milk (see Chapter 15). For those reasons, many authorities advise against using cow's milk, unless processed into a baby formula, until the infant is at least 1 year old.

Colostrum. The first milk made by the human breast is **colostrum.** This type of milk is produced a few days before birth through the week or so after birth. It is yellowish and thick. Colostrum contains immune factors that protect the infant from some diseases. These immune factors compensate for the infant's immature immune system in its first few months of life.[12] They are one reason that breast-fed infants have fewer respiratory and intestinal infections than formula-fed infants.

Colostrum has potent laxative properties that help the baby pass **meconium,** a stool produced during fetal life. One compound in colostrum, the **Lactobacillus bifidus factor,** encourages the growth of beneficial *Lactobacillus bifidus* bacteria. These bacteria limit the growth of potentially toxic bacteria in the intestine, such as *Escherichia coli*, and promote the intestinal health of the breast-fed infant.

Mature milk. Human milk composition gradually changes until several days after delivery, when it achieves the normal composition of mature milk. Human milk looks very different from cow's milk. (Table 15-1 in the next chapter provides a direct comparison). Human milk is thin, almost watery in appearance, and often has a slight bluish tinge. Its nutritional qualities are impressive, especially the quality of protein.

Its main protein, lactalbumin, forms a soft, light curd in the infant's stomach, easing digestion.[22] The other proteins bind iron, reducing the growth of iron-requiring bacteria. Many of these types of bacteria cause diarrhea. Still other proteins offer the important immune protection already noted.

Human milk changes in fat composition during each feeding. The consistency of milk released initially (about 60% of the volume) resembles that of skim milk. The next amount (about 35% of the total volume) has a greater fat proportion, similar to whole milk. Finally the hindmilk (about 5% of the total), is essentially like cream, and is usually released 10 to 20 minutes into the feeding.[12] Babies need to nurse long enough to get the kcalories in the rich hindmilk in order to be satisfied between feedings and grow well.

A FOOD PLAN FOR WOMEN WHO BREAST-FEED

Nutrient needs for a breast-feeding mother change slightly—if at all—from those of the pregnant woman. Exceptions are decreases in folate and iron needs, and increases in kcalories (200), vitamin A, vitamin C, niacin, and zinc needs. However, the diet for breast-feeding women can be the same as that for pregnant women, except the woman should add an additional serving from the milk, yogurt, and cheese group if she is a teenager (see Table 14-1). It is important for the woman to drink fluids every time the baby nurses. A high fluid intake encourages ample milk production. If a woman restricts her kcalories too severely, the quantity of milk also decreases. This is not a time to crash diet.

Milk production requires approximately 800 kcalories everyday. The RDA for energy during lactation is an extra 500 kcalories daily above prepregnancy recommendations. The difference between kcalorie needs and intake should allow for gradual loss of the 3 to 5+ pounds of fat accumulated during pregnancy. This shows how practical the link is between pregnancy and breast-feeding.[4] If the mother continues to breast-feed beyond 4 to 6 months, or is physically active, she will need more kcalories.

ANOTHER BITE Most substances the mother ingests are secreted into the milk. For this reason, alcohol and caffeine intake should be limited or avoided, and all medications should be checked with a pediatrician. Some mothers believe that some foods, such as garlic and chocolate, flavor the breast milk and upset the infant. If a woman notices a connection between a food she eats and the infant's later fussiness, she could consider avoiding that food. However, she might want to experiment again with it later. Infants become fussy for many reasons, and the suspected ingredient may not be the cause.

CONCEPT CHECK

Recognition of the importance of breast-feeding has contributed to its greater popularity during the last 20 years. Almost all women have the ability to breast-feed. The hormone prolactin stimulates breast tissue to synthesize milk. Some components of human milk come directly from the mother's bloodstream. Infant suckling triggers a let-down reflex that releases the milk. The more an infant nurses, the more milk is synthesized. The nutrient composition of human milk is very different from that of cow's milk and changes as the infant matures. The first milk, colostrum, is rich in immune factors. The diet for breast-feeding is generally similar to that for pregnancy except for additional fluids, as well as an extra serving from the milk, yogurt, and cheese group for a teenage pregnancy.

MAKING THE DECISION TO BREAST-FEED
Advantages of breast-feeding

Human milk is tailored to meet infant nutrient needs for the first 4 to 6 months of life. The possible exceptions are fluoride, iron, and vitamin D. Infant supplements, given under the guidance of a pediatrician, can supply these. Regular sun exposure for the infant can supply needed vitamin D. Although formula feeding can satisfy the infant, mother, and the rest of the family (see Chapter 15), breast-feeding offers many physiological and practical advantages.

Fewer infections.   Breast-feeding reduces the general risk of infections to the infant. This is partially because of the immune bodies in human milk that an infant can use. As already mentioned, these reduce the risk of respiratory and intestinal infections. Breast-fed infants also have fewer ear infections because they do not sleep with a bottle in the mouth as bottle-fed infants often do. We strongly discourage allowing any infant to sleep with a bottle in its mouth. While an infant sleeps with a bottle in its mouth, milk pools there, backs up through the throat, and eventually settles in the ears, creating a growth media for bacteria. Infant ear infections are a common problem. By avoiding them parents can decrease discomfort for the infant and trips to the doctor and prevent possible hearing loss. Tooth decay because of night-time bottles is also likely (see Chapter 15).

Fewer allergies and intolerances.   Breast-feeding reduces the chances of allergies, especially in allergy-prone infants (see the Nutrition Issue on p. 490).[22] Cow's milk contains a number of potentially allergy-causing proteins that are missing from human milk. Infants tolerate human milk better than they do formulas. Formulas must sometimes be switched several times until caregivers find one the infant thrives on.

Convenience. Breast-feeding frees the mother from the time and expense involved in buying and preparing formula and washing bottles. Breast milk is ready to go and sterile. This allows the mother to spend more time with her baby. On the other hand, if the child is bottle-fed, the mother may be freed to do other things while others feed the baby. This trade-off needs to be considered.

Barriers to breast-feeding

A lack of role models, widespread misinformation, fear of appearing immodest, and working away from the children all serve as barriers to breast-feeding.

Misinformation. Probably the major barriers to breast-feeding are misinformation and lack of role models. If a woman is interested in breast-feeding, she should talk to women who have done it successfully. Experienced mothers can be an enormous help to the first-time mother. She should find a friend she can call on to ask questions. In almost every community, a group called La Leche League offers classes in breast-feeding and advises women who have problems with it.

Returning to an outside job. Working outside the home can complicate plans to breast-feed. One possibility after a month or two of breast-feeding is for the mother to regularly express and save her own milk. She can express milk using a breast pump or by hand into a sterile plastic bottle or nursing bag (used in a disposable bottle system). Saving breastmilk requires careful sanitation and rapid chilling.[12] It can be stored in the refrigerator for 1 day and be frozen for 1 month. There is a knack to learning how to express milk, but the freedom can be worth it. Then others can feed the mother's milk to the infant.

Some women can juggle both a job and breast-feeding, but others find it too cumbersome and decide instead to formula-feed. A compromise—balancing some breast-feedings, say early morning and night, with formula-feedings during the day—is possible. However, too many supplemental feedings decrease milk production.

> **ANOTHER BITE** A schedule of expressing milk and using supplemental formula-feedings is most successful if begun after 1 to 2 months of exclusive breast-feeding. After 2 months, the baby is well adapted to breast-feeding and probably feels enough emotional security and other benefits from nursing that it is willing to drink both ways.

The key months for breast-feeding are the first 2 to 3 months of an infant's life. A longer commitment is better. The American Academy of Pediatrics recommends it exclusively for the first 4 to 6 months, and as a supplement with solid food for the second 6 months of life. But the first few months are critically important ones. During that time human milk provides the antiinfective properties needed until the infant begins to synthesize its own immune factors in high concentrations.

Social reticence. Another barrier for some women is embarrassment when nursing a child in public. Our society historically has stressed modesty and frowned on baring breasts in public—even in so good a cause as nourishing babies. With appropriate clothing, it is possible to nurse quite discreetly.

When is breast-feeding not a good idea?

Mothers should not breast-feed their infants if they don't want to do so. There are distinct advantages to breast-feeding, but none so great that a woman who decides to bottle-feed should feel she is penalizing her infant.

Frozen human milk should not be thawed in a microwave. The heat can destroy immune factors present and create hot spots that can scald the infant's tongue.

Because human milk contains much phenylalanine, it often can not be fed to infants with the disease phenylketonuria. Infants with galactosemia can not have human milk because of the great amount of galactose in it (see Chapter 8). Mothers who take medications that pass into the milk and adversely affect the child also should not breast-feed. In addition, a woman who has a serious chronic disease, such as tuberculosis or hepatitis, or is being treated for cancer should not breast-feed.

What about environmental contaminants in human milk?

Some women wonder whether breast-feeding is safe. There is some legitimate concern over the levels of various environmental contaminants in human milk. But the benefits from human milk are very well established, and the risks from environmental contaminants are still largely theoretical. Thus it is probably best to operate with what we know works until sufficiently strong research data dissuade us.

A few measures a woman could take to counteract some known contaminants are (1) to avoid freshwater fish from polluted waters, (2) to carefully wash and peel fruits and vegetables, and (3) to remove the fatty edges of meat. In addition, a woman should not try to lose weight rapidly while nursing because contaminants stored in fat tissue then enter her bloodstream and, in turn, her milk. If a woman questions whether her milk is safe, especially if she has lived in an area known to have a high concentration of toxic wastes or environmental pollution, she should consult her local health department.

Can a premature infant be breast-fed?

There is no clear-cut answer to whether a woman can breast-feed a premature infant.[12] In some cases human milk is the most desirable form of nourishment. If so, it must usually be expressed from the breast and fed through a tube. This type of feeding demands great maternal dedication. Fortification of the milk with nutrients such as calcium, phosphorus, sodium, and protein is often needed to match an infant's rapid growth. In other cases, special feeding problems may prevent using human milk or necessitate supplementing it with formula. Sometimes even intravenous nutrition is the only option. Working as a team, the pediatrician, neonatal nurses, and registered dietitian guide the parents in this decision.

CONCEPT CHECK

Human milk provides most of an infant's nutritional needs for the first 6 months. Vitamin D, iron, and fluoride may be supplemented. The advantages of breast-feeding over formula-feeding include fewer intestinal, respiratory, and ear infections; fewer allergies and food intolerances; and convenience. Lack of role models, misinformation, and social reticence may dissuade a mother from breast-feeding. A combination of breast-feeding and formula-feeding is possible when a mother is regularly away from her infant. Breast-feeding is not desirable if a mother has certain diseases or must take medication potentially harmful to the infant. The premature infant, depending on its condition, may benefit from consuming human milk.

SUMMARY

- Adequate nutrition is vital during pregnancy to ensure the well-being of both the infant and the mother. Insults from poor nutrition and some medications can cause birth defects, especially if they occur in the first trimester. Growth retardation and altered development are possible if insults occur later in pregnancy.

- Infants born prematurely (before 37 weeks of gestation) or with low birth weight (less than 5.5 pounds or 2.5 kilograms) usually have more medical problems at birth than normal infants.

- Teenage pregnancy requires very careful prenatal and nutritional care. Complications are more common in these pregnancies because of the very high physiological demands and often poor social and economic support.

- Daily energy needs increase by an average of 300 kcalories during pregnancy. Weight gain should be gradual to a total of 25 to 35 pounds in a normal weight mother.

- Protein, vitamin, and mineral requirements increase during pregnancy. Three servings from the milk, yogurt, and cheese group (four if a teenager), in addition to the other recommendations of The Guide to Daily Food Choices, are recommended. Supplements of iron and folate, in particular, may be needed.

- Pregnancy-induced hypertension, heartburn, constipation, nausea, vomiting, edema, and anemia are all possible discomforts and complications of pregnancy. Nutritional therapy can often help minimize these problems.

- The popularity of breast-feeding has increased in the past 20 years. Almost all women have the ability to nurse their infants. The nutrient composition of human milk is very different from cow's milk. Colostrum, the first milk produced by humans, is very rich in immune factors. Mature milk is rich in important proteins.

- For the infant, advantages of breast-feeding over formula-feeding include fewer intestinal, respiratory, and ear infections; fewer allergies and food intolerances; and convenience. An infant can be adequately nourished with formula if the mother chooses not to breast-feed. Breast-feeding is not desirable if the mother has certain diseases or must take medication potentially harmful to the infant.

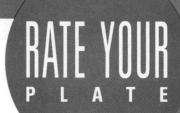

TARGETING NECESSARY NUTRIENTS FOR A PREGNANT WOMAN

In this chapter we mentioned that the nutrient needs hardest to meet during pregnancy are *folate, vitamin D, iron, calcium,* and *zinc.* Refer to Chapters 9 and 10 to find five foods rich in each nutrient. List them next to the appropriate heading below.

Nutrient	Foods			
	1		4	
Folate	2		5	
	3			
	1		4	
Vitamin D	2		5	
	3			
	1		4	
Iron	2		5	
	3			
	1		4	
Calcium	2		5	
	3			
	1		4	
Zinc	2		5	
	3			

Did you list any foods next to more than one nutrient? What are they?

_____

_____

Foods rich in more than one of these nutrients would be doubly useful and valuable. Those foods would be ones to focus on when pregnant.

Are there any reasons why it might be hard for a person to get the needed amount of these nutrients?

_____

_____

REFERENCES

1. ADA reports: Position of the American Dietetic Association: nutritional management of adolescent pregnancy, *Journal of the American Dietetic Association* 89:104, 1989.
2. Abrams B and others: Maternal weight gain and preterm delivery, *Obstetrics and Gynecology* 74:577, 1989.
3. Belizan JM and others: The relationship between calcium intake and pregnancy-induced hypertension: up-to-date evidence, *American Journal of Obstetrics and Gynecology* 158:898, 1988.
4. Brewer MM and others: Postpartum changes in maternal weight and body fat deposits in lactating vs nonlactating women, *American Journal of Clinical Nutrition* 49:259, 1989.
5. Carr-Hill R and others: Is birth weight determined genetically? *British Medical Journal* 295:687, 1987.
6. Collins JW, Jr, David RJ: The differential effect of traditional risk factors on infant birthweight among blacks and whites in Chicago, *American Journal of Public Health* 80:679, 1990.
7. Department of Health and Welfare: Canada's national guidelines on prenatal nutrition, *Nutrition Today* July/August, 1987, p 34.
8. Evans ER and others: Gestational diabetes, *American Family Physician* 36(6):119, 1987.
9. Horner RD and others: Pica practices of pregnant women, *Journal of the American Dietetic Association* 91:34, 1991.
10. Iannucci L: The perplexities of pregnancy, *FDA Consumer* November, 1990, p 17.
11. Jacobson HN: A healthy pregnancy, the struggle to define it, *Nutrition Today*, January/February, 1988, p 30.
12. Lawrence RA: *Breastfeeding*, ed 3, St. Louis, 1989, Mosby–Year Book.
13. Lipshultz SE and others: Cardiovascular abnormalities in infants prenatally exposed to cocaine, *Journal of Pediatrics* 118:44, 1991.
14. McGrew MC, Shore WB: The problem of teenage pregnancy, *The Journal of Family Practice* 32:17, 1991.
15. Milunsky A and others: Multivitamin/folic acid supplementation in early pregnancy reduces the prevalence of neural tube defects, *Journal of the American Medical Association* 262:2847, 1989.
16. National Academy of Sciences—Institute of Medicine: *Nutrition during pregnancy*, Washington DC, 1990, the academy.
17. Parham E and others: The association of pregnancy weight gain with the mother's postpartum weight, *Journal of The American Dietetic Association* 90:550, 1990.
18. Resnik R: The "elderly primigravida" in 1990, *The New England Journal of Medicine* 322:693, 1990.
19. Suitor CW: Perspectives on nutrition during pregnancy, *Journal of the American Dietetic Association* 91:96, 1991.
20. Thomson M, Hanley J: Factors predisposing to difficult labor in primiparas, *American Journal of Obstetrics and Gynecology* 158:1074, 1988.
21. Waterson EJ, Murray-Lyon IM: Preventing alcohol related birth damage: A review, *Social Science Medicine* 30:349, 1990.
22. Worthington-Roberts B and others: Nutrition in pregnancy and lactation, St. Louis, 1989, Mosby–Year Book

HOW MUCH HAVE I LEARNED?

What have you learned from Chapter 14? Here are 15 statements about pregnancy and breast-feeding. Read them to test your current knowledge. If you think the answer is true or mostly true, circle T. If you think the answer is false or mostly false, circle F. Use the scoring key at the end of the book to compute your total score. To review, take this test again later, and especially before tests.

1. (T) F — Infants weighing less than 5.5 pounds (2.5 kilograms) at birth are more likely to have medical problems.

2. T (F) — The most critical time for fetal development is during the last 13 weeks of pregnancy. *1st 13 wks when organs & body parts are forming greatest potential for birth defects*

3. (T) F — Nutritional factors are more important than genetic factors in determining birth weight. *avg. 300 kcal/day; kcal demands greatest during 2nd & 3rd trimester*

4. (T) F — A woman needs more kcalories when she is pregnant.

5. (T) F — Most women should gain about 25 to 35 pounds during pregnancy. *allows optimal fetal development & birth weight*

6. (T) F — Poor food choices in pregnancy are more common than low-kcalorie intakes. *gaining excessive weight from eating too many kcal can be a problem*

7. T (F) — Pregnant women know instinctively what to eat. *learning wise food choices / eating a healthful diet requires*

8. (T) F — Mineral needs increase during pregnancy. *especially iron, calcium & zinc; iron requirement usually necessitate taking iron supplements in addition to changing diet*

9. (T) F — Pregnancy can bring on a form of high blood pressure. *happens more frequently w/ poor nutrient intake - especially calcium*

10. (T) F — Breast-fed infants suffer fewer respiratory infections than formula-fed infants. *& intestinal infections*

11. (T) F — A major barrier to breast-feeding is often a lack of information. *most women can breastfeed - breast size & even feeding twins pose no special problems*

12. (T) F — Mothers who must take medications that pass into the milk should check with their doctor before breast-feeding. *many substances ingested by mom are secreted into milk*

13. (T) F — Through the placenta oxygen and nutrients transfer from the mother to the fetus. *and wastes - placenta is a specialized organ of pregnancy*

14. (T) F — Most miscarriages occur during the first trimester. *good nutrition & health habits should begin early, ideally b/4 pregnancy begins*

15. T (F) — Cow's milk can be substituted for human milk when an infant is 2 to 3 months old. *cow's milk too difficult to digest & fully metabolize until approx 6-12 months of age. infants kidneys aren't mature enough to handle high mineral content.*

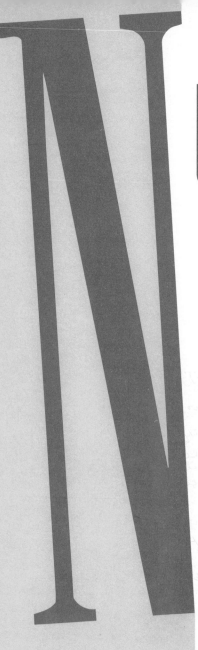

NUTRITION ISSUE

FETAL ALCOHOL SYNDROME

Although we know a great deal about diagnosing and treating some learning problems in children, many causes remain elusive. One particular question haunts many mothers: Did something happen while I was pregnant that created a learning disability for my child? This puzzle makes alcohol use during pregnancy a very important issue, especially since alcohol is the most common damaging substance fetuses are exposed to.

Scientists do not know if alcohol must be totally eliminated from the diet, but there is no question that large amounts of alcohol harm the fetus. Until a safe level can be established, it is recommended that women not drink alcohol at all during pregnancy. Women suffering from chronic alcoholism produce children with a recognizable pattern of malformations called *fetal alcohol syndrome (FAS).* [22] A diagnosis of FAS is based mainly on poor prenatal and infant growth, physical deformities (especially of facial features), and mental retardation (Figure 14-13). The infant is frequently irritable and proceeds to develop hyperactivity and short attention span. Poor eye-hand coordination is not uncommon.

The range of abnormalities varies from severe FAS to reduced birth weight, behavioral effects, growth retardation, and poor learning ability in infants of women who report only social drinking. The latter category is termed fetal alcohol effects (FAE).[22] Without the clue from the classic facial abnormalities to alert them to the condition's presence, parents may not suspect the presence of subtle defects caused by alcohol. Yet they may exist and can devastate learning potential. Annually, about 4000 to 7000 infants are born in the United States with FAS, and about 30,000 are born with FAE. This great number of alcohol-induced disorders and resulting mental retardation could be prevented.

Exactly how alcohol causes these defects is not known. Most likely, other factors, such as poor nutrition, cigarette smoking (nicotine intake), and other drug use, also contribute to the overall result. We further do not know how much alcohol it takes to produce the effects. Again, for this reason many authorities—including the U.S. Surgeon General and the American Medical Association—believe it is best for mothers-to-be to avoid alcohol altogether. Abstinence is especially important during the first trimester when key growth and development occur. Alcohol reaches the fetal blood at the same concentration as the mother's blood within 15 minutes of her drinking. However, the effect on the fetus may be up to ten times greater.

Just one bout of binge drinking can arrest and alter cell division occurring during a critical phase of fetal development. The fetus then may develop with an irreversible defect. Physical damage to the fetus results more from first-trimester drinking because tissues and organs are being developed; emotional

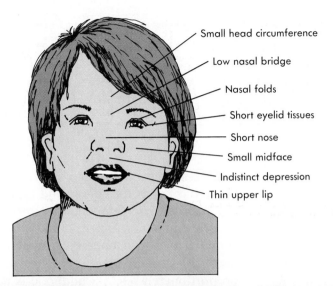

- Small head circumference
- Low nasal bridge
- Nasal folds
- Short eyelid tissues
- Short nose
- Small midface
- Indistinct depression
- Thin upper lip

Facial features that are characteristic of FAS.

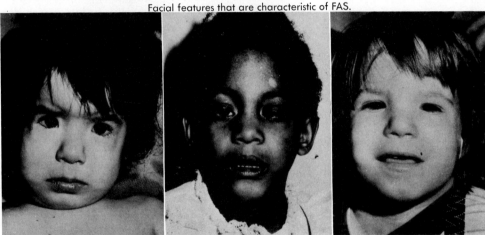

FIGURE 14-13

Fetal alcohol syndrome. Milder forms of alcohol-induced changes on the fetus (and so the infant) are known as fetal alcohol effects.

and learning problems stem more from third-trimester drinking because the brain is in a critical stage of development. And throughout the pregnancy, alcohol interferes with growth.[10]

Since alcohol has the capacity to adversely affect each stage of fetal development, the earlier in pregnancy that heavy drinking ceases, the greater the potential for improved outcome. The best course is to consider alcohol an indulgence that can be eliminated until after pregnancy.[21] Not only is it important for pregnant women to abstain from alcohol during pregnancy, but also when trying to conceive and anytime conception is possible. One step in the right direction is the new congressionally mandated warnings about drinking during pregnancy that appear on all alcoholic beverage containers. Recall that many women are not aware they are pregnant until 2 to 3 months after conception. Pregnancy lasts only 9 months. Parents may spend a lifetime caring for their needlessly handicapped offspring. ●

Fetal Alcohol Syndrome (FAS) • A group of physical and mental abnormalities in the infant that result from the mother consuming alcohol during pregnancy.

NUTRITION FROM INFANCY THROUGH ADOLESCENCE

As we grow through early years into adulthood, our needs for energy and nutrients change. Infants need huge amounts of energy, protein, vitamins, and minerals per pound of body weight to support their tremendous growth and development. As growth tapers, children need and eat proportionately less.[13] Childhood is regarded as a key time to establish healthy habits, including those related to food and physical activity.[14] The family is dominant over the child. Thus education designed to change the eating behaviors of children must be directed simultaneously at the main caregivers, as they usually determine what foods are purchased and how these are prepared.

Later, teenagers sprout quickly during another growth spurt, and they amaze their elders with the sheer amount of food they can put away. Often their eating habits and lifestyles encourage eating on the run.[20] Their typically hit-and-miss meal patterns challenge all meal planning that aims to meet their extra growth and nutrient needs. In exploring these stages of life we will look at the key role nutrients play, and how food habits can be tailored to met those needs. ●

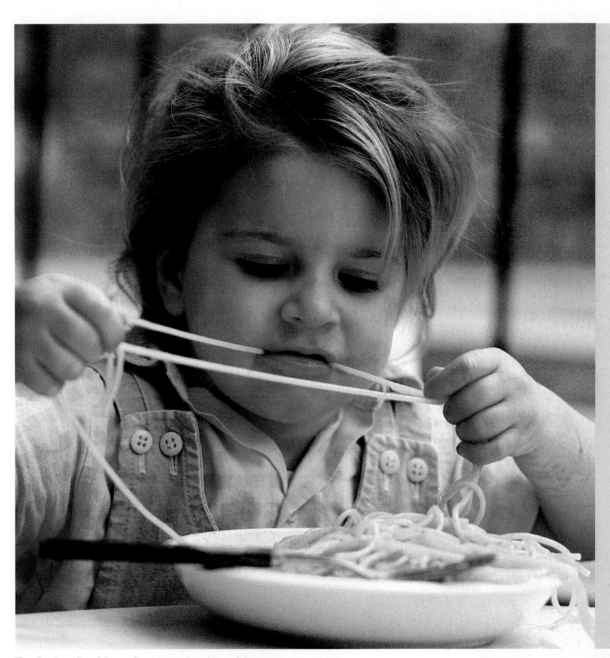

Exploring food is as fun as eating it at this stage.

Avoiding Table Wars

If you have children or have ever worked as a babysitter, you probably know how difficult it can be to get kids to eat on command. The problem doesn't go away—caregivers also worry later about the eating habits of their teenagers. During adolescence teenagers establish their own identities, and their busy lifestyles leave little time for structured eating.

How can household wars about eating be avoided? Listed below are some statements about children and adolescents and their eating habits. Which are true? Place a "T" in the blank to the left if you think the statement is true, or an "F" if false. If caregivers know the truths, they possibly can avoid table wars.

_F_ 1. Around 9 to 10 months of age, infants explore, test, and play with food. Unless they are disciplined to eat neatly and treat food seriously, they will be undisciplined eaters in the future.

_T_ 2. Expect babies to take only two or three bites of solid food at first meals.

_T_ 3. Infants enjoy bland foods much more than do adults.

_F_ 4. Infants should be encouraged to consume a lot of apple juice because it's rich in so many nutrients.

_F_ 5. Honey is a good sweetener for infants because it has a high nutrient content.

_T_ 6. Toddlers typically have less appetite than they had during the first year of life.

_F_ 7. You can normally expect children to avoid vegetables and whole grains.

_T_ 8. Adult modeling of good eating habits influences the children's behavior.

_T_ 9. A good policy is the one-bite rule, which asks children to take at least one bite of the foods presented to them.

_F_ 10. Children like foods with soft textures and strong flavors.

_F_ 11. Children should be made to eat three meals a day, rather than many small meals.

_T_ 12. Children often object to having foods mixed, as in stews and casseroles.

_F_ 13. Children should be forced to eat.

_F_ 14. Infants and children of all ages should eat lowfat diets to decrease their risk of future heart disease.

_T_ 15. Teenagers are more likely to try healthful foods when immediate positive outcomes are emphasized—such as their contributions to a better appearance and physique—as opposed to when potential future health hazards from a poor diet are stressed.

_T_ 16. Involving teenagers in cooking and purchasing food helps to promote good eating habits.

True: 2,3,6,8,9,12,15,16.
False: 1,4,5,7,10,11,13,14.

ASSESS YOURSELF

INFANT GROWTH AND PHYSIOLOGICAL DEVELOPMENT

During infancy a child's attitudes toward foods and the whole eating process begin to take shape. If parents and other caregivers practice good nutrition and are flexible, they can lead a child into lifelong beneficial food habits. Such an infant has a good chance of starting life with the nutrients needed to support brain and body growth spurts, and to develop a willingness to try new foods. However, these physical and psychological advantages alone do not guarantee that a child will thrive. Children additionally need specific attention focused on them; they need to grow in a stimulating environment, and they need a sense of security. Children hospitalized for growth failure tend to gain weight more quickly when tender loving care accompanies needed nutrients.

The growing infant

It seems that all babies do is eat and sleep. There is a good reason for this. An infant's birth weight doubles in the first 4 to 6 months and triples within the first year. Such rapid growth requires a lot of both nourishment and sleep. Beyond the first year growth is slower and steadier; it takes 5 more years to double the weight seen at 1 year. An infant also increases in length in the first year by 50% and then continues to gain height throughout preschool and teen years.[13] Height is essentially complete by age 19, though small increases may occur in the early 20s (Figure 15-1). Head size in proportion to total height shrinks from one fourth to one eighth during the climb from infancy to adulthood.

The human body needs a lot more food to support growth and development than to merely maintain itself once growth ceases. In some populations food is not regularly available. When nutrients are missing at critical phases of growth and development, growth slows and may even stop. From observations of Egyptian mummies we see that infants were about the same size in 300 B.C. as they are today. However, adult mummies are much smaller than adults today. Also, many suits of armor in museum collections of the Middle Ages are small

We will tend to use the term parents in this chapter, but we realize in America some infants and children are raised by other caregivers rather than their true biological parents.

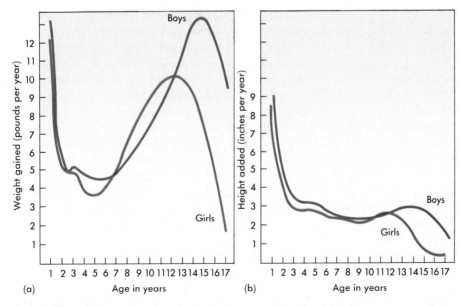

FIGURE 15-1

Growth rates. **A,** Average gains in weight for girls and boys. **B,** Average additions to height for girls and boys. The higher the line in any one year, the greater the amount of gain compared to other years. Note the great degree of length gained in infancy. Large gains in weight happen in infancy and at puberty.

In Utero • In the uterus; in other words, during pregnancy.

Weight primarily reflects current nutrient intake. Height is a measure of long-term nutrient intake.

Children under 2 to 3 years of age are measured with knees unflexed, lying on their backs, and so the term length is used rather than height.

in size. People of the past ate nutrient-poor diets that did not support the growth we typically experience today.

In Third World countries today, about half the children are short and underweight for their age. Poor nutrition—called undernutrition—is at the heart of the problem. This occurs to a lesser extent in America. The undernourished children are simply smaller versions of nutritionally fit children. In poorer countries, when breast-feeding ceases, children are often fed a high-carbohydrate, low-protein diet. This diet supports some growth but does not allow children to attain their genetic potential. To grow, children must consume adequate amounts of protein and other nutrients.

Infant development follows a pattern in which body water reduces from about 75% at birth to 60% at 1 year. This is also the proportion typical in adults. By 1 year of age an infant's body nitrogen content (and so, protein content) has increased from 2% of body weight at birth to 3%, indicating the infant has synthesized much new lean tissue.

The effect of undernutrition on growth

As with the fetus *in utero,* the long-term effects of nutritional problems in infancy and childhood depend on the severity, timing, and duration of the nutritional insult to cell processes.

Eating a poor diet as an infant hampers cell division that occurs at that stage. Getting an adequate diet later usually won't compensate for lost growth because high levels of key hormones are now missing from the bloodstream, though they were present during the critical time when cells should have divided. For example, a 15-year-old Central American girl who is 4 feet 8 inches tall cannot attain the adult height of a typical American simply by now eating better. Girls experience their peak rate of growth before the onset of the menses. Once the time for growth ceases (in women this is about 2 years after they start menstruating), a good nutrient intake will help maintain health and weight but will not make up for lost growth.

Assessing infant growth and development

Health professionals assess a child's increases in height and weight by comparing these with typical growth patterns recorded on charts.[13] The typical charts contain seven percentile divisions, which represent 90% of children (Figure 15-2). A percentile simply represents the rank of the person among 100 age-matched and gender-matched peers. Tony, for example, is at the ninetieth percentile height for age, meaning that of 100 boys of that age, he is shorter than ten and taller than 89. A child at the fiftieth percentile is considered average. Fifty children will be taller than this child; 49 will be shorter.

Individual growth charts are available for both males and females, for ages ranging from 0 to 36 months or 2 to 18 years (see Appendix O). Height for age, weight for age, and weight for height can be plotted. Infants and children should have their growth assessed during regular health checkups. It takes 1 to 3 years for an infant to establish its own genetic percentile. Once this figure is established, such as length- (height)-for-age, the child's measurement should then track along that percentile. If the child's growth does not keep up with its length-for-age percentile, a physician needs to investigate whether a medical or nutritional problem is impeding the predicted growth. Inappropriate weight gain—too little or too much—should also be investigated.

Infants born prematurely may catch up in growth in 2 to 3 years. This requires that the child jump up in the percentiles. If this occurs—especially in length-for-age—it is usually no cause for alarm. On the other hand, jumping percentiles in weight-for-height can be disturbing if the child approaches the eightieth to ninetieth percentiles. Generally a child at the ninetieth percentile

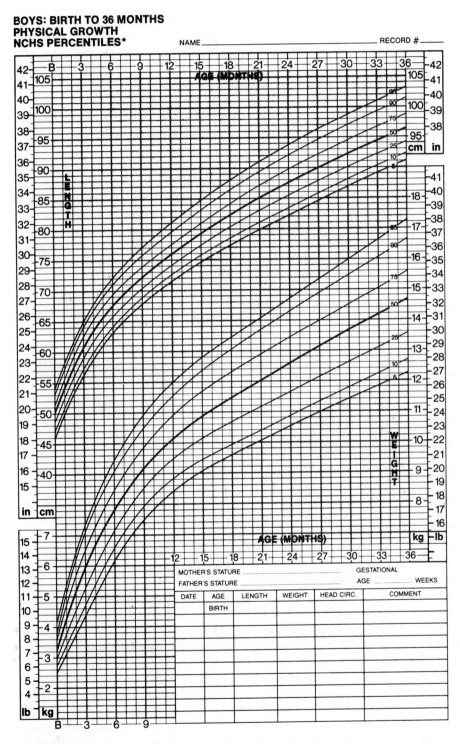

BOYS: BIRTH TO 36 MONTHS
PHYSICAL GROWTH
NCHS PERCENTILES*

NAME _____ RECORD # _____

FIGURE 15-2

Growth charts used to assess height (length) and weight in young boys. A certain weight and height (length) corresponds to a percentile value—which is a ranking of the person among 100 peers. See Appendix O for charts that apply to young girls and older children.

for weight-for-height is considered overweight. Above the ninety fifth percentile, the child is considered obese.

Brain growth

The brain grows faster at birth than at any other time of life. To accomodate the growth, an infant's head must be very large in proportion to the rest of the body. The rapid growth stops between 12 and 15 months of age. The rest of the body eventually grows to fit the head. In early physical checkups a health professional usually measures the head circumference as another means of assessing growth. How nutritional status affects brain development and intelligence quotient (IQ) is difficult to measure because we haven't figured out how to separate the effects of nature from nurture. However, studies from Central America suggest that IQ after age 5 years relates more closely to the amount of schooling a child receives than to nutritional intake during childhood.

Adipose (fat) tissue growth

Since 1970, researchers have speculated that overfeeding during infancy may increase fat tissue cell numbers. Today, we know that fat cells can also increase as adulthood obesity develops (see Chapter 11). Still, if kcalories are limited during infancy to keep down fat cell number, the growth of other organ systems may also be severely retarded. Special concern revolves especially around proper brain and nervous system development. In addition, most obese infants become normal-weight preschoolers. So it appears unwise to restrict an infant's diet, especially fat intake, to influence the growth of fat tissue.[9] About 40% of kcalories from fat is recommended. As mentioned earlier, without adequate nutrients, infants cannot eventually attain their potential adult height.

CONCEPT CHECK

Growth occurs rapidly during infancy: birth weight doubles in 4 to 6 months and triples within the first year. Lean tissue increases and the percentage of body water falls during infancy. Undernutrition can irreversibly inhibit growth and maturation. Infant and child growth is assessed by tracking body weight, height (or length), and head circumference over time. It is undesirable for infants to become obese, although no evidence strongly indicates that obese infants become obese adults.

Failure to thrive

Occasionally an infant does not grow much in the first few months. Physical problems that may contribute to retarded growth range from poor oral cavity development, infections, and heart irregularities to constant diarrhea associated with intestinal problems. However, more than half of the infants who fail to thrive have no apparent disease. Poor infant-parent interactions are the typical cause.[5] This stems from misinformation, no parent role model, or apathy about the child's welfare. Overall, the problems often arise from the parents' inexperience rather than intentional negligence.

Infants need cuddling, and they respond to voices and eye contact, especially at feeding times. New parents need to appreciate the importance of these practices to their infant's well-being. Some parents are also overcommitted to maintaining a lean child in hopes of preventing future obesity, as we discussed in Chapter 13. The result, even though well meaning, can be a child's failure to thrive.

When clinicians encounter an infant who is failing to thrive, they must first determine if the child is consuming enough energy. For infants, approximately 45 kcalories per pound (100 kcalories per kilogram) of body weight daily is adequate. For a breast-fed infant, the clinician needs to make sure that sufficient milk is being consumed. The child should be nursing about six to eight times a day for about 20 minutes a session and have six to eight wet diapers each day. The mother should consume adequate food and fluid (see Chapter 14). Children older than 2 years are less likely to fail to thrive because they can often get food for themselves. Younger children are limited to what the caregivers provide.

INFANT NUTRITIONAL NEEDS

An infant's nutrient needs vary as they grow, and these differ from adult needs in both amount and proportion (Figure 15-3). Initially, human milk or formula supplies needed nutrients. Solid foods are usually not needed until after 4 to 6 months.[13] Even after solid foods are added, the basis of an infant's diet for the first year is still human milk or formula.

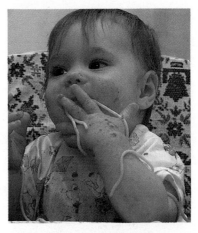

Early attempts at self-feeding provide exciting times for both infant and caregivers.

Energy

As mentioned earlier, infants need about 45 kcalories per pound of body weight daily (100 kcalories per kilogram) to supply them adequate energy. At 6 months of age this amounts to about 750 kcalories daily. Based on body weight, this amounts to two to four times more than adults need. Infants need an easy way to get these kcalories. Either human milk or formula is ideal for the first few months. Both are high in fat and supply about 650 kcalories per quart of fluid

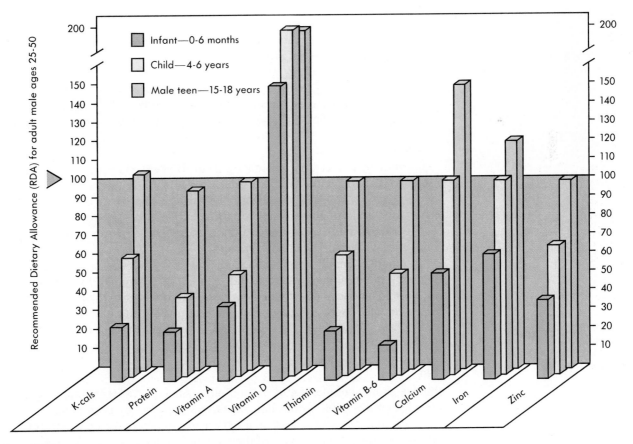

FIGURE 15-3

Compared to energy needs, infants need greater quantities of some nutrients than adults. This is illustrated by comparing the height of the kcals bar to all other bars for infants. The same comparison holds for children, but to a lesser extent.

TABLE 15-1

Composition of infant formulas per liter*

Milk or Formula	Kcalories	Protein (grams)	Fat (grams)	Carbohydrate (grams)	Minerals† (grams)
Human milk	750	11	45	70	2
Casein-based formulas					
Similac	680	15.5	36	72	3.3
Enfamil	670	15	38	69	3
SMA	670	15	36	72	2.5
Gerber	670	15	36	72	2.4
Cow's milk					
Whole	670	36	36	49	7
Skim	360	36	1	51	7
Soybean protein-based formulas					
ProSobee	670	20	36	68	4
Isomil	570	20	36	68	4
Nursoy	670	20	36	68	4
Predigested protein					
Nutramigen	670	19	26	90	1.1
Alimentum	670	19	38	70	1.2

*1 liter equals about 30 fluid ounces.
†Calcium, phosphorus, and other minerals

(700 kcalories per liter; Table 15-1). Later, human milk or formula, supplemented by solid foods, can provide even more energy.

The infant's high energy needs are primarily driven by its rapid growth and high metabolic rate. The high metabolic rate is caused in part by the ratio of the infant's great body surface to its weight. More body surface allows more heat loss from the skin; the body must use extra energy to replace that heat.

Protein

Daily protein needs vary in infancy from 0.7 to 1 gram of protein for each pound of body weight (1.6 to 2.2 grams per kilogram). About 40% of total protein intake should come from essential amino acids. Both of these goals are satisfied by either human milk or formula. Total protein intake should not exceed 20% of kcalorie needs. Excess nitrogen and minerals supplied by high-protein diets overtax an infant's kidneys.

In America, infant protein deficiency is unlikely, except in cases of mistaken feeding practices, such as overdiluting an infant's formula. Protein deficiency may also be induced by elimination diets used to detect food allergies. As foods are eliminated from the diets, infants may not be offered enough protein to compensate for the high protein sources no longer present (see the Nutrition Issue on p. 492, Food Allergies and Intolerances).

Fat

Infants should get about 40% of their energy from fat. More than 50% may lead to poor fat digestion. About half the energy supplied by both human milk and formula comes from fat. Essential fatty acids should make up 3% of total energy. Fats are an important part of the infant's diet because they are energy-dense and vital to the development of the nervous system. As a concentrated energy source, fat helps resolve the potential problem of the infant's high energy needs and small stomach capacity.

Vitamins of special interest

Vitamin K is routinely given (injected) to all infants at birth. This dose lasts until the infant's intestinal bacteria are established and begin to synthesize vitamin K. Formula-fed infants receive the rest of the vitamins they need from the formula. Breast-fed infants, especially dark-skinned ones, may require a vitamin D supplement if they are not exposed to much sunlight. (Sunlight hitting human skin activates synthesis of vitamin D; see Chapter 9.) The time needed in the sun is approximately 15 to 30 minutes daily on hands and face for white infants, and longer for dark-skinned babies. Breast-fed infants whose mothers are total vegetarians (vegans) should receive a vitamin B-12 supplement. Infants who drink goat's milk need a supplement of folate because the milk doesn't supply enough of it.

Minerals of special interest

The iron stores a child is born with are generally depleted by the time its birth weight doubles, in 4 to 6 months. To maintain a good iron status, the American Academy of Pediatrics recommends formula-fed infants be given an iron-fortified formula from birth. Breast-fed infants need solid foods to supply extra iron at about 6 months of age. The need for iron is a major consideration in deciding when to introduce solid foods. Some researchers recommend liquid iron supplements from birth or by 1 month of age for breast-fed infants.

Infants need adequate amounts of iodide and zinc to support growth. Human milk and formula adequately supply these needs when the infant's energy needs are met. In addition, fluoride supplements to aid tooth development may be needed for breast-fed infants. Fluoride supplements are also recommended for bottle-fed infants if the water supply used in home formula preparation does not contain fluoride. This applies to bottled water. Note that formula manufacturers use fluoride-free water in formula preparation. Parents should consult their dentist for advice on the need for flouride for the infant.

Water

An infant needs about 2 ounces of water per pound of body weight daily (about 150 milliliters per kilogram). Infants typically consume enough human milk or formula to supply this amount. In hot climates supplemental water may be necessary. And any conditions that pull water out of the body—diarrhea, vomiting, fever, too much sun, and allergies—often call for supplemental water. Infants are easily dehydrated, a condition that can have serious effects if not remedied. Dehydration can result in rapidly decreasing kidney function, and the infant may then require hospitalization for rehydration.

CONCEPT CHECK

When an infant does not grow properly, its failure to thrive may stem from physical problems or inappropriate feeding practices. Most nutrient needs in the first 6 months are met by human milk or formula. Breast-fed infants may need vitamin D, fluoride, and iron supplements, and formula-fed infants may need fluoride supplements. Infants usually get enough water in the human milk or formula they drink.

Formula-feeding for infants

We discussed breast-feeding in detail in Chapter 14. Let's now focus on formula-feeding. Recall that a major advantage of breast-feeding is provision of immune bodies that impart immune protection to the infant. That advantage is very important in the context of poverty and poor hygiene. It is less important in America, where high standards for water purity and cleanliness make formula feeding a safe alternative for infants.

Formula composition.   Infants cannot adequately tolerate cow's milk because of its high protein and mineral content. It must be altered. The altered forms, known as infant formulas, were first available commercially in 1931. Since 1980 they have been required to conform to strict guidelines for nutrient composition and quality set by federal law. Formulas generally contain lactose or sucrose for carbohydrate, heat-treated proteins from cow's milk, and vegetable oils for fat (Table 15-1). Soy protein-based formulas are available for infants who can't tolerate lactose. Formulas contain vitamins and minerals in amounts suggested by the guidelines of the American Academy of Pediatrics.

A variety of specialized formulas are available. Their compositions vary in energy content; types of protein, carbohydrate, and fat; and iron fortification.[13] These special formulas were developed in response to the special needs of some normal-term infants, premature infants, infants with allergies, infants with higher energy needs, and infants with special metabolic problems, such as phenylketonuria.

A severely malnourished 5-month-old infant was recently admitted to Arkansas Children's Hospital in Little Rock. Symptoms included heart failure, rickets, inflamed blood vessels, and possible nerve damage. According to the hospital, the baby girl had been fed nothing but Soy Moo since she was 3 days old. Soy Moo is a soy beverage sold in health food stores. This kind of soy beverage, sometimes improperly called soy milk should not be confused with soy-based infant formulas. Unlike true infant formulas, which are nutritionally complete and appropriate for infants, other soy beverages lack some nutrients infants need.[19]

Formula preparation.   In the 1950s, it was common to prepare a day's supply of bottles and then sterilize them in boiling water for about 30 minutes. Today, it is often more convenient to prepare bottles one at a time. All utensils should be washed before preparing the formula. Powdered formulas are measured into a bottle to which clean water is added (follow label directions). The formula is mixed and fed immediately to the infant. Either warm or cold water can be added, depending on preference. Most people preparing concentrated formula make up the whole can (13 ounces) and store it in the refrigerator in a clean, covered jar or pitcher until needed. Ready-to-feed formula is also available. This is poured into a bottle and fed immediately.

It is safe to refrigerate diluted formula for a day. However, formula left over from a feeding should be discarded because it will be contaminated by bacteria and enzymes in saliva. If well water is used, it should be boiled before making formula and should also be analyzed for excessive concentration of naturally occurring nitrates, which can lead to a severe form of anemia.

Because babies swallow a lot of air along with either formula or human milk, it is important to burp a baby after about 10 minutes of feeding, or 1 to 2 ounces (30 to 60 milliliters) from a bottle, and again at the end of feeding. Spitting up a bit of milk is normal at this time. Once fed, the child should be placed on its stomach with its head to one side. In this position the infant has the least chance of choking on any milk it spits up.

It is important to stop a bottle feeding when the infant indicates it is full. Pay attention to cues that signal the infant has had enough, such as turning its head away, inattention, falling asleep, and turning playful (Figure 15-4). Trust the

Formula for baby foods should not be heated in a microwave oven. Hot spots can develop that may burn the infant's mouth. Bottles are best warmed in a pot of water on the stove or under hot running water.

infant's appetite rather than a standardized serving recommendation, and allow the infant to refuse some milk in the bottle. It is difficult to tell how much milk a breast-fed baby gets. New mothers who breast feed often worry whether the baby has had enough milk. Again, watch for signs from the baby. After about 20 minutes, the baby has probably had enough.

SOLID FOODS

Development of feeding skills

By 6 to 7 months, the infant has learned to grab and transfer objects from one hand to the other (Table 15-2). About this time teeth begin to appear, and the infant begins to handle finger foods with some dexterity. Dry toast, sliced in fingers, offers hours of enjoyment.

By age 7 to 8 months the infant can push food around on a plate and play with a drinking cup. It can hold a bottle and self-feed a cracker or piece of toast.[13] In mastering these manipulations the infant develops self-confidence and self-esteem. It is important that parents be patient and support these early feeding attempts, even though they appear inefficient.

Around 10 months of age, the infant practices in earnest self-feeding finger foods and drinking from a cup. Feeding time is often very messy. Food is used as a means to explore the environment. By the infant's first birthday, its body has developed sufficiently to accommodate crawling, probably walking, and self-feeding. While attempts at feeding are still erratic, the developing child takes great pride in doing more things independently. As the child drinks from a cup more frequently, fewer bottle-feedings and/or breast-feedings are necessary. The added mobility of walking should naturally lead to gradual weaning from the bottle or breast.[13]

Introducing solid foods

The time to introduce solid foods into an infant's diet hinges on a few important factors:[13]

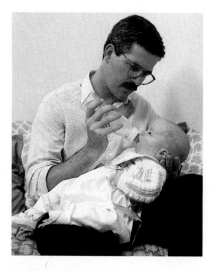

FIGURE 15-4
Careful attention during feeding allows the infant to signal the caregiver when the feeding should cease. Stopping the feeding before putting the infant to bed is important. This helps prevent nursing-bottle syndrome (described later) as the infant will not fall asleep with the bottle. Thus carbohydrate-laden fluid, which can lead to severe dental decay, will not pool in the oral cavity as the child sleeps.

TABLE 15-2

Feeding skills, as with other life skills, take time to develop

Age	Skills to Watch for
0-2 months	Can grasp a finger; crying is the only language
2-4 months	Thrashing movements common; these can interfere with feeding
4-5 months	Turns head to voices; begins eye-hand coordination
5-6 months	Sits erect when supported; crawling and finger-feeding begin
6-7 months	Transfers objects from hand to hand; chewing pattern (up and down) begins
7-8 months	Sits erect without support for a minute or so; reaches for, grabs, and closely inspects objects; can hold a bottle and self-feed a cookie
8-10 months	Makes efforts to stand; develops pincer grasp
10-11 months	Takes a few steps with support; mealtimes become more messy as food is something to be explored
11-12 months	Practices self-feeding in earnest; walking becomes more likely; develops likes and dislikes for foods; chewing is better developed; hands bottle to caregiver when finished
12-15 months	Becomes more skilled at walking and self-feeding; inquisitive toddlers explore everything, so household toxins must be safely stored out of reach
21-24 months	Vocabulary builds; food patterns become more individualized

This timeline is just an estimate. Infants vary. A pediatrician should be consulted if caregivers are concerned about an infant's developmental progress.

Nutritional need—As noted, iron stores are exhausted by about 6 months of age. Either solid foods or iron supplements are then needed to supply iron if the child is breast-fed or fed a formula not supplemented with iron. Iron, however, is not the only needed nutrient missing from human milk and unfortified formulas. Vitamin D and fluoride may also deserve attention. Still, adding solid foods is unnecessary for any nutrients other than iron before 4 to 6 months.

Physiological capabilities—Infants cannot actively digest starch before 3 months. As they age, their digestive capabilities increase. Kidney function likewise is quite limited until about 4 to 6 weeks of age. Until then, waste products from high levels of dietary protein or minerals are difficult to excrete.

Physical ability—Before 3 to 4 months, the infant practices tongue thrusting. Generally, the child quickly spits out any solid food put on the tongue. It takes about 4 to 6 months before an infant can sit up, turn the head away when full, and control tongue thrusting.

Preventing allergies—An infant's intestinal tract can readily absorb whole proteins from birth until 4 to 5 months of age. Early exposure to many types of proteins, particularly proteins in cow's milk may predispose a child to future allergies, including food allergies (see the Nutrition Issue on p. 492), as some types of these proteins may be absorbed intact. For this reason, it is best to minimize the number of different types of proteins in a child's diet during the first 3 months.

Keeping these considerations in mind—nutritional need, physiological and physical readiness, and allergy prevention—the American Academy of Pediatrics recommends that solid foods not be introduced until about 6 months of age (Table 15-3). In general, a child starting solid foods should weigh at least 13 pounds (6 kilograms) and should be drinking more than 32 ounces (1 liter) of formula daily or breast-feeding more than 8 to 10 times within 24 hours. This description applies to most 6-month-old infants.

Before 6 months, infants are not physically mature enough to consume much solid food. Attempts to push down solid foods have sometimes led to force-feeding with a feeder (a giant syringe) or to mixing infant cereal with milk and putting it in a bottle. Even if these are traditional alternatives in your family, there is no reason to carry on these practices. The inconvenience alone should make one consider whether all the effort is worth it. This practice is unnecessary nutritionally, tedious, and possibly dangerous for the infant because it increases the risk of allergies and choking or inhaling food when crying. Even so, many children are already eating solids by 2 months of age.[12]

Sometimes a rapidly growing infant—one who consumes more than 32 ounces (1 liter) of formula daily—needs solid foods at 4 months to meet high energy needs. However, most infants can easily wait until 6 months. By that age, the infant is ready for solid food and feeding is much easier.

A common reason offered for introducing solid foods early—before 4 to 6 months of age—is the belief that it helps the infant sleep through the night. However, many studies have shown that sleeping through the night is a developmental milestone for the infant. It has nothing to do with how much food it eats. Infants naturally begin sleeping through the night between the ages of 1 to 3 months. Girls reach this stage before boys. Filling them with cereal is not going to influence that process.

Which solid foods should be fed first?

Before 6 months of age, the first solid foods can be iron-fortified cereals. A good idea is to offer foods after some breast-feeding or formula-feeding to take the edge off hunger. This practice aids in early spoon-feeding. Rice cereal is the

TABLE 15-3

One approach for the introduction of semisolid foods and table foods in infancy

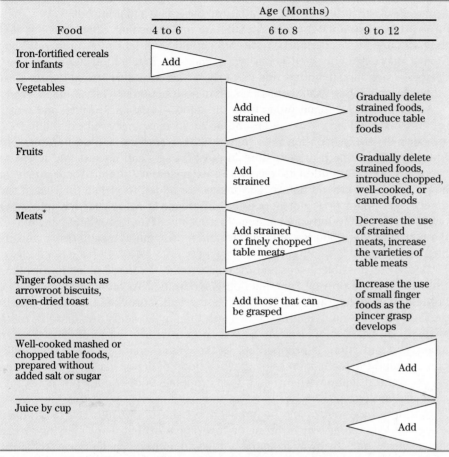

Food	Age (Months)		
	4 to 6	6 to 8	9 to 12
Iron-fortified cereals for infants	Add		
Vegetables		Add strained	Gradually delete strained foods, introduce table foods
Fruits		Add strained	Gradually delete strained foods, introduce chopped, well-cooked, or canned foods
Meats*		Add strained or finely chopped table meats	Decrease the use of strained meats, increase the varieties of table meats
Finger foods such as arrowroot biscuits, oven-dried toast		Add those that can be grasped	Increase the use of small finger foods as the pincer grasp develops
Well-cooked mashed or chopped table foods, prepared without added salt or sugar			Add
Juice by cup			Add

*These can be added first, if the infant begins solid foods at 4 to 6 months of age. At 1 year of age formula or human milk should also be replaced by cow's milk. Modified from Pipes PL: *Nutrition in infancy and childhood*, St. Louis, 1989, Mosby–Year Book.
The shape of the triangle indicates gradual addition or deletion of the food product.

best cereal to begin with because it is least likely to cause allergies. After the age of 6 months the first food is not such an important issue. Some pediatricians may recommend lean ground (strained) meats for more absorbable forms of iron. Although yogurt and cottage cheese are also well tolerated and their consistencies make them good candidates for early foods, they are not good sources of iron.

Once a new food has been fed for 7 days without ill effects, another food can be added to the infant's diet. At first, this can be another type of cereal, or perhaps a cooked and strained (blended) vegetable, meat, fruit, or egg yolk. Each feeding step builds on the last (Table 15-3).

Waiting 7 days between each new food is important because it can take that long for signs of an allergy to develop. Symptoms to look for are diarrhea, vomiting, a rash, or wheezing. If one or more of these symptoms appear, the suspected problem food should be avoided for several weeks and then reintroduced in a small quantity. If the problem continues, a doctor should be consulted. It is important not to introduce mixed foods until each component of the mixed food has been given separately. Otherwise, if an allergy or intolerance develops, it will not be easy to identify the offending food. Note that many babies outgrow food sensitivities in childhood (see the Nutrition Issue on p. 492).

Some foods that commonly cause an allergic response in infants are egg

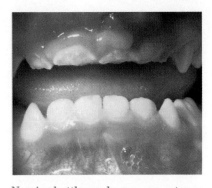

Nursing bottle syndrome—an extreme example of tooth decay. This child was probably often put to bed with a bottle. The upper teeth have decayed almost all the way to the gum line.

whites, chocolate, nuts, and cow's milk.[11] It is best not to introduce these foods early in infancy. However, the American Academy of Pediatrics accepts the use of cow's milk after the age of 6 months (up to about 24 ounces or about 0.75 liters daily), provided the child is consuming at least one-third of total energy from solid food. Still, it is best to wait until the infant's first birthday.

A variety of strained foods is available for infant feeding. Check this out next time you are in a supermarket. Parents should read labels on prepared baby food if they are concerned about sugar and salt. Single-food items are more desirable than mixed dinners and desserts, which are less nutrient-dense. Most brands have no added salt, but some fruit desserts contain a lot of added sugar.

As an alternative, plain foods from the table—vegetables, fruits, and meats (no seasoning added)—can be ground up in an inexpensive plastic baby food grinder/mill. Another option is to puree a larger amount of food in a blender, freeze it in ice-cube portions, store in plastic bags, and defrost and warm as needed. Careful attention to cleanliness is necessary. Infant foods made at home should be ground before seasonings are added to please the rest of the family. The infant does not notice the difference if salt, sugar, or spices are omitted. It is best to introduce infants to a variety of foods so that by the end of the first year the infant is consuming many foods—milk, meats, fruits, vegetables, and grains.

As early as possible, juices and formula should be offered in a cup. Drinking from a cup helps prevent "nursing bottle syndrome." As an infant plays with a bottle, the carbohydrate-rich fluid bathes the teeth, providing an ideal growth medium for bacteria. Bacteria on the teeth then make acids that dissolve tooth enamel. An infant should never be put to bed with a bottle or placed in an infant seat with a bottle propped up. As the child lies in bed, fluid (even milk) pools around the teeth, increasing the likelihood of dental caries. Again, infants need careful attention when being fed. Propping bottles does not constitute careful attention.

Getting a baby out of the bedtime-bottle habit is difficult. But determined caregivers can either wince through a few nights of their baby's crying or can slowly wean the baby away from the bottle with either a pacifier or water (for a week or so).

In the first attempts to introduce solid foods, just getting the food into the infant, instead of all over him, proves to be a challenge. The caregiver must proceed slowly. Initially, table foods supplement—rather than replace—formula or

Feeding toddlers is usually an interesting experience.

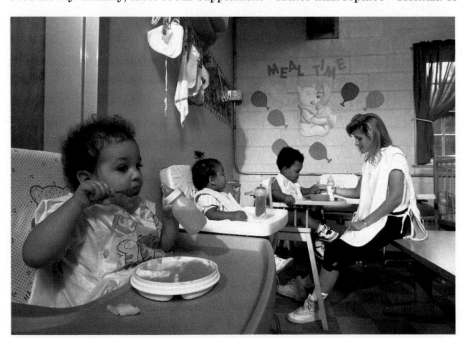

human milk. The infant controls the situation by signaling when he is hungry and when he has had enough to eat. Self-feeding skills require coordination and can develop only if the infant is allowed to practice and experiment. By 9 to 10 months, the infant's desire to explore, experience, and play with food can also hinder feeding. Caregivers need to relax and take this phase of infant development in stride. Sloppy, friendly mealtimes actually can make good memories.

To ease efforts in feeding solid foods, consider the following tips:

- Use a baby-sized spoon; a small spoon with a long handle is best.
- Hold the baby comfortably on the lap, as for breast-feeding or bottle-feeding, but a little more upright to ease swallowing. In this position, the baby expects food.
- Put a small dab of food on the spoon tip and gently place it on the baby's tongue.
- Convey a calm and casual approach to the baby. The baby needs time to get used to food.
- Expect the baby to take only two or three bites of the first meals. Anything more than that is real success.

By the end of the first year, finger-feeding becomes more efficient, drinking from a cup improves, and chewing is easier as more teeth erupt.[13] Still, experimentation and unpredictability are to be expected.

A summary of infant feeding recommendations

Breast-Fed Infants

- Breast-feed for 6 months or more
- Consider fluoride, iron, and vitamin D supplements
- Add iron-fortified cereal at about 6 months of age
- Provide a variety of basic, soft foods after 6 months of age

Formula-Fed Infants

- Use infant formula for at least 6 months, preferably an iron-fortified type
- Give fluoride supplement if water supply is not fluoridated
- Add iron-fortified cereal at about 6 months of age
- Provide a variety of basic, soft foods after 6 months

What not to feed an infant

Several foods and practices to avoid when feeding an infant are:

Honey and corn syrup—These products may contain spores of *Clostridium botulinum*. The spores can eventually develop into bacteria in the stomach and lead to a food poisoning known as botulism. This is often fatal in children under 1 year old (see Chapter 17).

Overly salty and overly sweet foods—Infants do not need a lot of sugar or salt added to their foods. They enjoy bland foods much more than do adults.[13]

Excessive formula or milk—more than 40 ounces (1.2 liters) of formula or 32 ounces (1 liter) of milk daily—Solid foods should play a greater role in satisfying an infant's increased appetite after 6 to 8 months. The switch needs to occur mainly because foods can contain much iron, whereas human milk, cow's milk, and low-iron formulas don't contain much. About 24 to 32 ounces (³/₄ to 1 liter) of human milk or formula daily is ideal after 6 months, with food supplying the rest of energy needs.

Foods that tend to cause choking—These foods include hot dogs (unless finely cut into sticks, not coin shapes), candy, whole nuts, grapes, coarsely cut meats, raw carrots, and popcorn. Hot dogs, grapes, chunks of meat, car-

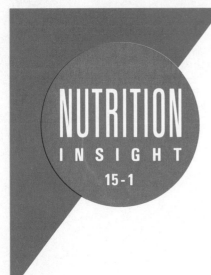

DIETARY GUIDELINES FOR INFANT FEEDING

In response to various controversies surrounding infant feeding, experts have written the following dietary guidelines for infants:[9]

- Build up to a variety of foods.
- Be sensitive to the baby's appetite to avoid overfeeding or underfeeding.
- Don't restrict fat and cholesterol too much.
- Don't overdo high-fiber foods.
- Sugar is fine in moderation.
- Sodium is fine in moderation.
- Babies need more iron per pound of body weight than do adults.

These guidelines have been accepted by the American Academy of Pediatrics and the American Dietetic Association. The recommendations in this chapter are also consistent with these guidelines. In essence, there is no evidence of positive effects of very restrictive diets during infancy, while their hazards are well documented. ●

rots, peanuts, popcorn and peanut butter cause the most choking deaths. Caregivers should discourage the practice of allowing younger children to gobble snack foods during playtime and should supervise all meals.

Lowfat or nonfat cow's milk—Beyond 2 years, children can use 2% or 1% fat milk because by then they are consuming enough solid foods to supply energy and fat needs. Before that age, the amount of lowfat milk needed for energy needs would supply too many minerals. That could overtax the kidneys. The lower fat intake might also harm nervous system development. The American Academy of Pediatrics strongly urges parents not to give children under the age of two reduced fat milk.

Excessive apple or pear juice—The simple carbohydrate sorbitol contained in these juices can lead to diarrhea because sorbitol is poorly absorbed. Diluting juices with an equal part of water is a good idea, but it should be begun early, before the infant becomes accustomed to full-strength juices.

CONCEPT CHECK

Infant formulas generally contain lactose or sucrose, heat-treated proteins from cow's milk, and vegetable oil. Formulas may or may not be fortified with iron. Sanitation is very important in preparing and storing formula. Solid food should not be added to an infant's diet until the child is both ready for and needs solid food, usually at about 6 months of age. The first solid food given can be iron-fortified infant cereals with very gradual additions of other foods; one at a time each week. Some foods to avoid giving infants in the first year include honey, lowfat cow's milk, overly salty or sweet foods, and foods that may cause choking.

NUTRITION-RELATED PROBLEMS IN INFANCY

Parents, other caregivers, and clinicians should be aware of a variety of potential problems related to infant nutrition.

Possible feeding problems

Feeding problems to watch out for in infancy include:
- Getting insufficient iron in the diet
- Excluding an entire food group of the Guide to Daily Food Choices from the diet during introduction and later regular use of solid foods

- Drinking raw milk from either cows or goats. This raw milk raises the possibility of viral and bacterial contamination (see Chapter 17). Goat's milk, as noted, is low in folate
- Not progressing from the bottle to a cup by 1 year of age
- Feeding from a bottle past 18 months of age
- Getting supplemental vitamins or minerals beyond 150% of an infant's or child's U.S. RDA.

All these problems require attention. Parents and other caregivers should consult with a physician.

Colic

The first time an infant has a lengthy, unexplained crying spell, most parents panic. Crying episodes that do not respond to typical remedies, such as feeding, holding, or diaper changes, are characteristic of infants who develop *colic*. Colic affects about 1 in 5 infants, so it is neither uncommon nor abnormal. Late afternoon and early evening can be the most difficult times. The infant may cry continuously. Nighttime sleeping is almost always disturbed by crying spells. Again, efforts to soothe a colicky infant—feeding, rocking, and holding—are usually ineffective overall. The only good news is that colic usually goes away after a few intense months.

Colic is thought to be caused by one of two reasons: (1) allergy-causing proteins in formula or human milk or (2) excess gas buildup in the gastrointestinal (GI) tract because of poor peristalsis.[4] Tucking the body into a ball is a common response to colic by the infant. Painful accumulation of gas in the GI tract may be the reason for this response. The crying is not usually related to feeding, but positioning a colicky baby upright during feeding allows him to more easily expel trapped air by burping. In addition, the infant should be burped regularly during feeding and fed for no longer than 30 minutes. The longer a child suckles at the bottle or breast, the more air he takes in.

Changing the infant's diet from a cow's milk protein-based formula to a predigested protein-formula sometimes helps in severe cases (Table 15-1).[4] A recent study suggests that it is helpful for the breast-feeding mother to avoid dairy products. In addition, the physician may prescribe medications to calm the child and reduce gas buildup. Overall, parents need the counsel and support of other adults to ease their distress during this trying period, which often lasts for the first 3 to 4 months.[21] Because it is so unnerving to feel powerless to calm an infant in pain, hearing from other parents who have experienced it is especially helpful.

Diarrhea

Diarrhea results from various causes in infancy, including bacterial and viral infections. In the United States, about 500 infants die each year of simple dehydration resulting from diarrhea. To prevent dehydration, infants with diarrhea should be given plenty of fluids—although not milk or full strength fruit juices. Specialized fluids, such as Pedialyte, are available. These contain glucose, sodium, potassium, chloride, and water. It is best to have a pediatrician's recommendations concerning fluid replacement.

Once diarrhea subsides, a bottle-fed infant may be switched to a soy-based, lactose-free formula for a few weeks. This allows time for the intestine to produce sufficient lactase enzyme to digest the large amount of lactose typically found in formulas. The breast-fed infant should continue at the breast throughout the duration.

Milk allergy

Over 25 proteins in milk can lead to allergies. Some of these are inactivated by heating (scalding) milk. However, some proteins are very heat stable. A "true"

Colic • Periodic crying in a healthy infant, apparently caused by gas buildup or allergies to proteins.

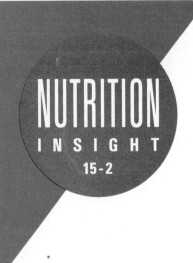

OBESITY IN THE GROWING YEARS

In America, 15% to 25% of children are overweight. About 15% of adolescents in America are obese (Figure 15-5).[7] In the short run, ridicule and embarrassment are the main problems accompanying obesity. Significant health problems associated with obesity usually first appear in adulthood. Unfortunately, about 40% of obese children and about 70% of obese adolescents become obese adults. The time to strike against obesity is in childhood because the chances are high that an obese school-age child will become an obese adult.

The easiest way to evaluate obesity in childhood is to plot weight-for-height on a growth chart. Children over the ninetieth percentile are considered overweight, and those over the ninety-fifth percentile are considered obese. Skinfold thickness can also be measured to assess obesity (see Chapter 11).

What causes childhood obesity?

Current research indicates that there are many potential causes for childhood obesity. Recall the nature versus nurture discussion in Chapter 11. Some infants are born with lower metabolic rates; they use energy more efficiently and, in turn, have an easier time saving kcalories for fat storage. Some infants are less active than others and so use fewer kcalories each day. Research shows a moderate relationship between the number of hours a child spends watching television and obesity. Obesity also tends to be hereditary. We can also expect further environmental influences, such as snacking, decreased physical activity, and high-fat/high-kcalorie food choices to contribute to childhood obesity.

Treating childhood obesity

A first approach to treating childhood obesity is assessing the child's activity level. If a child spends much free time in sedentary activities (such as watching television), more physical activities should be encouraged.[14] At the beginning of the week, a plan for a reasonable allotment of TV time and video games for each family member is needed. The TV generation now glues itself to the tube for an average of 22 hours a week. Activities to replace TV viewing and video games do not necessarily have to be competitive sports. Children should be given opportunities to enjoy

milk allergy is actually quite rare and develops in less than 1% of formula-fed infants.[13] However, infants may be switched to soy-based formulas in an attempt to decrease crying and spitting up. Just because a child thrives better on a soy-based formula does not mean he has a true milk allergy (see the Nutrition Issue on p. 492 to learn more about what causes allergies). If it is a true milk allergy, the soy formula is not likely to help in the long run. A special formula with predigested protein will be needed (see Table 15-1).

Iron-deficiency anemia

Iron-deficiency anemia typically occurs in infants who consume few solid foods and whose diets are dominated by cow's milk, which has little iron.[15] Iron stores are then quickly depleted by the daily demand for new red blood cells to be synthesized. To prevent iron-deficiency anemia, it is best to start an infant at about 6 months on iron-fortified cereals and meats and to limit formula to 16 to 25 ounces (500 to 750 milliliters) daily. The infant should also not consume cow's milk for the first year, and especially before 3 months of age, because cow's milk tends to cause intestinal bleeding. If anemia does develop, medicinal iron supplements are advised with a physician's guidance.

The premature infant

The premature infant is fed either human milk or a specially designed formula. As noted in Chapter 14, nutrients may be added to human milk to increase its

activities that they like, such as walking, cycling, swimming, and jazz dancing, and then encouraged to do these often. Getting the family together for a brisk walk after dinner, or finding an after-school sport the child enjoys are two good ideas.

Moderation in kcalorie intake is important, especially in limiting high-fat/high-kcalorie food choices and sugar-laden carbonated beverages. More nutrient-dense foods should be the primary focus. Resorting to a weight-loss diet is usually unnecessary. Changing habits should be the emphasis in the short run.[14] Children have an advantage over adults in losing weight—some stored kcalories can be used for growth. If weight gain can be moderated, height gains may soon catch up. This is one reason why treating obesity in childhood is so desirable. Further growth can contribute to success.

Sometimes weight loss is necessary if a child will still be obese after attaining ultimate adult height. Then weight loss should be gradual, perhaps 1/2 pound per week. The child should be closely watched to ensure that during this weight loss the rate of growth is normal. It is important that the child's kcalorie intake not be so low that gains in height diminish.

Behavior modification adds a third important component to treating childhood obesity. Children often need to find a new way to relate to foods, especially snack foods. An important family rule could be that children are allowed to eat only while sitting at the meal table. This could stop endless hours of snacking in front of the television. It might also help to put portions on plates rather than allow snacking to go on indefinitely, as often happens when children eat directly from a full box of crackers.

Parents play a key role in treating childhood obesity. After all, they select and bring the food home. Overweight children have greater long-term success controlling their weight if their parents provide early support for exercising and eating right. One goal is to keep healthy, nutrient-rich but kcalorie-light snacks on hand. The parents also must help a child turn his interest from eating toward other interests, such as sports, hobbies, and school. Any management plan for treating childhood obesity must involve the parents.

The self-esteem of a child is quite fragile. Obesity itself already affects the child's psyche. Humiliation does not work: it only makes the child feel worse. Support, admiration, and encouragement—these are offerings to be emphasized. ●

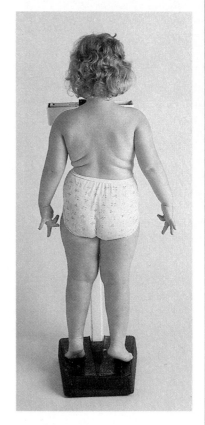

FIGURE 15-5
Childhood obesity. A female child like this one who is still obese after 5 years of age often faces a battle against obesity for the rest of her life.

protein, mineral, and energy content. The premature infant must be fed immediately because it has little fat or carbohydrate storage. Body composition of the full-term infant includes about 12% fat, while the composition of the very premature infant can include as little as 2% fat.

CONCEPT CHECK

Colic commonly is associated with GI tract discomfort. Switching to a formula with predigested proteins may help treat colic. It also may be helpful for breast-feeding mothers to avoid dairy products, under a physician's guidance. Diarrhea requires additional fluids to prevent dehydration. Allergy to milk proteins is rare and may require switching to a formula with predigested proteins. Introducing iron-containing solid foods at an appropriate time and avoiding early use of cow's milk can generally prevent iron-deficiency anemia in infancy.

CHILDHOOD

The rapid growth rate that characterizes infancy quickly tapers during the next few years. The average weight gain is only 5 pounds during the second year of life (Figure 15-1). As a toddler's growth rate tapers, eating behaviors change.[13] Feeding problems can stem from the decreasing appetite that characterizes preschool years. Adapting food choices to the slower growth rate and reduced

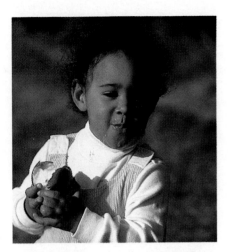

Childhood is the ideal time to begin to enjoy healthy foods.

hunger becomes a challenge. When the child consumes few foods, the nutrient density of each food choice is important. This is a good time to emphasize whole grains and vegetables without increasing fat intake. Choosing a whole-grained breakfast cereal with limited fat is an excellent choice. There is no need to decrease fat intake severely, but fatty food choices should not overwhelm more nutritious ones.

ANOTHER BITE Surprisingly, children eat what they are exposed to. Since learning to eat a variety of foods is a behavioral process, not intellectual, parents should expose children to different foods repeatedly. At this age, children can eat a well-rounded and healthy diet if one is served to them. If offered whole-grain breakfast cereals, whole-wheat bread, vegetables, salad, and fresh fruits regularly, young children accept most of these foods and eat them. Only a lack of imagination limits—and possibly deprives—a child's diet. If caregivers don't like a particular food, they should still offer it to the child.

The preschool years are the best time for a child to start a healthful pattern of living and eating, focusing on regular physical activity and nutritious foods. Self-esteem and successful eating are closely tied. Parents and other caregivers are role models: if they eat a variety of foods, the children will eat a variety of foods. A good policy is the one-bite rule: children should take at least one bite of the foods presented to them. For snacks, parents should decide the options. Children should then be allowed to choose; responsibility for food choice ideally should start early.[6,17]

In the early school years regular meals, especially breakfast, becomes an important focus. Some research suggests breakfast helps children learn better in the subsequent hours they spend in school.[10] The energy and nutrients consumed can stimulate attention, energy level, and motivation, yielding better test scores. Sports performance can be improved as well. This makes sense because depleted carbohydrate stores in the liver can be replenished at breakfast. Still, some researchers dispute the importance of breakfast in learning. They claim that it is the more motivated students who eat breakfast, rather than eating breakfast that motivates students. In our opinion it is a good idea to give breakfast to all students, especially to otherwise sluggish ones.

Breakfasts can be imaginative. Instead of conventional breakfast foods, caregivers can offer pizza, spaghetti, soups, yogurt with trail mix on top, chili, sandwiches, or shish kebab.

Most breakfast cereals today are fortified with vitamins and minerals. But if a child normally eats well-balanced meals the rest of the day, there is no need to get all the Recommended Dietary Allowances of vitamins and minerals at one sitting. So, cereals meeting the U.S. RDA offer no health advantage.

How to help a child choose nutritious foods

One way adults can encourage young children to eat nutritious, well-balanced meals is to serve new foods and repeat exposure to them. If a child observes adults and older children eating and enjoying a food, there is a good chance he will eventually accept it. The dinner hour is a good time for children to experience new foods and to develop their own likes and dislikes. Preschool children tend to be wary of new foods. If adults can be patient and persevere, children will build good food habits. Above all, the dinner table should not become a battle ground (Figure 15-6).

Perseverance with children is critical because it takes effort and commitment to guide them into liking a variety of foods. If left to their own devices, preschool children would find a few foods they like and eat them every day. But by constantly being introduced to new foods, children this age can expand their nutritional choices, develop an experimental approach, and learn to

FIGURE 15-6

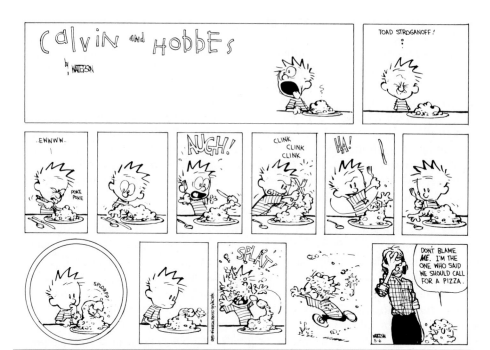

appreciate a variety of foods. It may take 10 to 15 exposures, but eventually most foods will be accepted. A positive outlook by the caregivers helps a lot.

Research shows that children like certain foods—especially those with crisp textures and mild flavors—and familiar foods.[22] Young children are especially sensitive to and reject hot-temperature foods.

Parents and other caregivers play a central role in teaching by example. Children more readily learn good table manners along with others who practice them. The harmony that comes from working at being polite creates a positive environment for learning good nutrition habits. Preschoolers eventually develop skill with spoons and forks and can even use dull knives. But finger foods are also a good idea. A goal should be to make mealtime a happy, social time. Share enjoyment of healthful foods. A regular family meal daily—whether breakfast, lunch, or dinner—is an appropriate setting for children to learn about healthy eating and to build good eating habits.

Childhood feeding problems

Tensions between parents, or between parents and children, often contribute to eating problems. Getting to the root of family problems and creating a more harmonious family atmosphere is an important part of resolving many childhood feeding problems. In addition, parents must often be educated as to what to expect of a preschool child and what goals to set. Given below are some typical problems, their causes, and suggestions for correcting them.

"My child won't eat as much or as regularly as he did as an infant."   This is to be expected. The growth rate slows after infancy, and a child does not need as much food. Parents must often be reminded that they shouldn't expect a 3-year-old to eat as voraciously as an infant or to eat adult-sized portions. Reducing serving size to two-thirds an adult's portion for servings from the Guide to Daily Food Choices is a good approach for young children age 2 years and older. Normal-weight children have a built-in feeding mechanism that adjusts hunger to regulate food intake at each stage of growth.[6] If a child is developing and growing normally and the caregiver is providing a variety of healthful foods, all can be confident the child isn't starving. One should avoid nagging, forcing, and bribing.

Appetite also varies with activity level and general health. An initial symptom of a sick child is poor appetite. Picky eating is also just another indication of a child's striving toward independence and its strong desire to establish routines. Asserting oneself about food preferences is a relatively easy way for the child to do this.

Parents should also be reminded that food likes and dislikes change rapidly in childhood and again are influenced by food temperature, appearance, texture, and taste. Sometimes children object to having foods mixed as in stews or casseroles, even if they normally like the ingredients separately.

Battling to get a child to eat more is rarely worth the effort.[17] Parents should present the food, eat some themselves, and let the child decide the serving size. In addition, they should recognize that this is an important age for children to explore the world around them. Even good eaters are sometimes more interested in exploring than in eating. There's room for occasional indulgences, a skipped meal or two, or once-in-a-while poor choices. It's eating and lifestyle habits over the course of a month and lifetime that matter.

"My child is always snacking, yet she never finishes her meal." Children have small stomachs. Offering them 6 or so small meals succeeds better than limiting them to three meals each day. Sticking to three meals a day offers no special nutritional advantages; it is just a social custom. Snacking is fine as long as good dental care is practiced. When we eat isn't nearly so important as what we eat. If nutritious snacks are readily available, these would be good to offer at midmorning or midafternoon when the child becomes hungry (Table 15-4). Fruits and vegetables (fresh, frozen, or juice) are always good snack accompaniments. Working parents should make sure their children are provided with nutritional snacks to tide them over until dinnertime.

When a child refuses to eat, it is best not to overreact.[17] Doing so may give the child the idea that eating is a means of getting attention or manipulating a scene. Most children do not starve themselves to any point approaching physical harm. When a child refuses to eat, have him sit at the table for a while, and if he still isn't interested in eating, remove the food and wait until the next scheduled meal or snack.

"My child never eats his vegetables." Everyone dislikes certain foods. Again, the one-bite policy can be encouraged, and guidelines can be set to discourage fussing over unfamiliar foods. Children eventually learn that they can eat foods they don't particularly like without first gagging, choking, and yelling "Oh gross!" It takes time for a child to become enthusiastic about a new food, but with continual exposure and a positive role model, chances are the child may even grow to like it.

Children cannot and should not be forced to eat. They need to develop independence and identities separate from their parents. In other words, children have to choose for themselves—a practice that should be encouraged. Hunger is still the best means for getting a child to eat. It may work to feed a child vegetables at the start of a meal, when he is hungriest. Offer new foods with familiar ones. A platter of raw or lightly cooked carrots, broccoli, green and red peppers, cabbage, and mushrooms eaten as a snack with friends can do a lot to remedy a vegetable problem. Nutritious dips sell vegetables to many children. Using heroes as role models may work. Vegetables may acquire more appeal when children help prepare them (Figure 15-7). A child about 4 or 5 years old can safely eat raw vegetables without fear of choking.

"How do I know if my child is eating healthfully?" The Guide to Daily Food Choices listed in Chapter 2 forms the basis for a healthy diet in children age 2 years and older. Again, serving size can increase to full adult portions as energy needs and appetite increase with age. A child who eats from the food groups and regularly gains height and weight is eating a good diet. Some nutrients that deserve special attention during childhood are calcium, iron, and vitamins A, B-6, and C.[16] These nutrients should be readily supplied if a child's diet includes choices from all the food groups—milk, yogurt, and cheese group; meat, poultry, fish, dry beans, eggs, and nuts group; fruit group; vegetable group; and breads, cereals, rice, and pasta group.

Caregivers can use snacks to fill in the foods missing from your meals. Fresh fruit, fruit or vegetable juices, ice milk or pudding, a sandwich or burrito, or a bowl of cereal are all good choices.

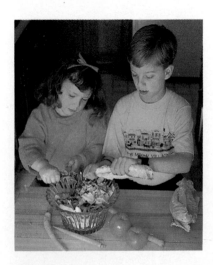

FIGURE 15-7
Parents can involve children in meal preparation. This can help children develop an interest in new foods.

TABLE 15-4

Serving nutritious snacks and beverages for school-age children

Snack suggestions:					
		Flour tortillas	Spread with refried beans or canned chili, sprinkle with grated cheese and broil; top with chili sauce	Popcorn	Serve plain or make three quarts and sprinkle with ¼ c grated cheese and ½ t garlic or onion salt
Fresh raw vegetables	Serve with a dip of cottage cheese or yogurt blended with dried buttermilk dressing	Ready-to-eat cereals	Use brands low in sugar and containing fiber. Serve with raisins.	Parfait	Make with yogurt, fruit and granola
Celery	Spread with peanut butter and sprinkle on raisins, shredded carrots or nuts finely chopped	Pita loaf	Place sliced meat, cheese, lettuce and tomato in open pocket	Gelatin	Add fruit or vegetable juice, vegetables, fruits, or cottage cheese
Bananas	Dip in sweetened yogurt or spread with peanut butter and roll in coconut, chopped nuts or granola	English muffins or pita bread	Top with spaghetti sauce, grated cheese and meats; broil or bake and cut in fourths	Frozen fruit cubes	Freeze pureed applesauce or fruit juice into cubes
Sliced apples or crackers	Serve with a dip of peanut butter, honey, nuts, raisins and coconut mixed together	Potato skins	Sprinkle with shredded cheese, broil and top with yogurt and bacon bits	Fruit fizz	Add club soda to juice instead of serving soft drinks
Bagels	Spread with cream cheese or peanut butter and top with chopped bananas, crushed pineapple or shredded carrots	Canned chili	Heat and top with onions, lettuce and tomato; use as dip for Italian or French bread, biscuits or corn bread	Fruit shake	Blend milk with fresh fruit (bananas, berries or a peach) and a dash of cinnamon or nutmeg
Quick bread or muffins	Make with carrots, zucchini, pumpkin, bananas, nuts, dates, raisins, lemons, squash, and berries	Kabobs	Make with any combination of the following: fruit, vegetables and sliced or cubed cooked meat (remove toothpicks before serving)	Yogurt frost	Combine fruit juice and yogurt; add fresh fruit if desired
				Hot chocolate	Make hot chocolate or cocoa with milk chocolate and a dash of cinnamon
				Seeds	Shelled sunflower seeds

From *A food guide for the first five years*, National Meat and Livestock Board, 444 North Michigan Avenue, Chicago, IL 60611.

Two-year-olds commonly prefer peculiar foods, and parents need not worry about this. A child may switch from one specific food focus (often called a jag) to another with equal intensity. If the caregiver continues to offer choices, the child will soon begin to eat a wider variety of foods again, and the specific food focus will disappear as suddenly as it appeared.

Major scientific groups, such as the American Dietetic Association and the American Society for Clinical Nutrition, believe that vitamin and mineral supplements are unnecessary for healthy children (see Chapter 3). It is better to emphasize good foods. However, a nutrient supplement at the RDA level may be needed when a child is ill, especially if the illness persists. Diets for children who eat totally vegetarian should especially focus on protein, vitamin B-12, iron, and zinc. Studies show that many parents offer children conservative amounts of vitamins, so toxicity is unlikely. Still, the practice of giving supplements is often unnecessary, especially given today's typically highly fortified breakfast cereals, which children often eat.

If current childhood feeding practices aim to follow the most healthful dietary plans, they should gradually shift away from high fat diets to diets containing more complex carbohydrates.[8] After 2 years of age, many authorities recommended eating patterns for children that contain no more than 30% of

School lunch menus follow federal guidelines in the United States. What is eaten is up to the student.

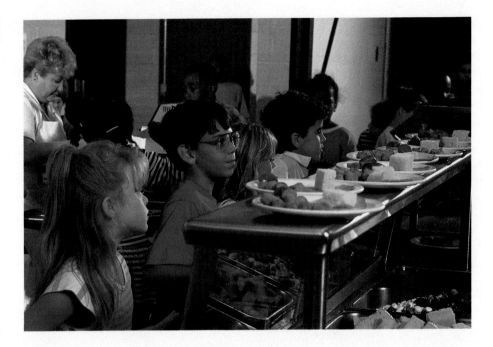

calories as fat and no more than 10% of calories as saturated fat. The Guide to Daily Food Choices, with its emphasis on starches, allows for such a pattern. Children are exposed to high-fat foods in fast-food restaurants. These foods are often sweet and high in salt as well. Caregivers can teach and model healthful ways to eat at fast-food restaurants by ordering from the salad bar. Children aren't born with a preference for high-fat foods; they develop this preference through repeated exposure.[22]

Many of us should consider a diet higher in carbohydrate and lower in fat. For children, the idea is not to force them to follow severely restricted diets, such as adults with weight or cholesterol problems might follow. Instead, children can simply limit the amount of high-fat, nutritionally empty foods they eat each day. Some easy diet changes to begin with are bagels instead of doughnuts, nonfat frozen yogurt instead of ice cream, lowfat milk instead of whole milk, fruit instead of crackers and cheese for snacks, and air-popped popcorn instead of chips.

Nutritional problems in childhood

The two most common nutritional problems in childhood are obesity, which we discuss in Nutrition Insight 15-2, and iron-deficiency anemia.

Iron-deficiency anemia

Childhood iron-deficiency anemia is most likely to appear in children between the ages of 6 and 24 months.[15] It can lead to poor stamina and decrease in learning ability because the oxygen supply to cells decreases. Less resistance to disease is also likely. Fortunately, the incidence of childhood anemia is decreasing. In 1970, about 12% of children ages 18 to 23 months were diagnosed as anemic in the United States. By 1984, the figure had dropped to 4%.[23] This decrease probably occurred because of the increased iron fortification of formulas and breakfast cereals that began in the early 1970s. In addition, the Special Supplemental Food Program for Women, Infants, and Children (WIC) sponsored by the federal government, also began in the early 1970s. This program emphasizes the importance of iron-fortified formulas and cereals and distributes them—along with nutrition education—to low-income parents of infants and preschool children considered to be at nutritional risk.

The best way to prevent iron-deficiency anemia in children is to regularly feed them foods that are adequate sources of iron.[15] Iron-fortified breakfast cereals and a few ounces of lean meat are convenient means of getting more iron into a child's diet. The high proportion of heme iron in many animal foods allows the iron to be more readily absorbed than iron from plant foods. Consuming a vitamin C source along with the less readily absorbed iron in plants and supplements will aid absorption (see Chapter 10).

Is childhood the time to start a diet designed to limit the risk for heart disease?

The American Academy of Pediatrics does not recommend lowfat diets (below 30% of total kcalories) for young children. It does recommend screening for blood cholesterol levels in children from families with histories of early heart disease and then treating children with high blood cholesterol levels with appropriate diet and drug therapy when needed.

Although there may be no reason to put children on lowfat diets, parents can introduce heart-healthy habits by limiting a child's exposure to saturated fats. Heart disease starts in childhood. Autopsies of young military men who died in Korea and Vietnam showed the early signs of plaque buildup in their blood vessels.[8] As we said before, it is best to encourage foods that have less overall fat and a higher proportion of monounsaturated and polyunsaturated fat. Moderation is the best strategy; very restrictive diets can be detrimental to overall growth. A child needs to consume adequate energy and to build good habits that can be practiced into the teen years.[8] One strategy to add to previous recommendations is to have children drink milk that is 2% or 1% fat after the age of 2 and to limit the intake of fatty meats, high-fat cheese, stick margarine, ice cream, and butter.

Are low-sodium diets appropriate for children?

Scientific data neither confirm nor refute the notion that eating less sodium will reduce the risk of future high blood pressure. Moderation in sodium consumption does help build good health habits for the future—especially if the person later develops hypertension and needs to eat even less sodium. If children become accustomed to less salt, they will be less inclined to eat very salty foods as adults.

CONCEPT CHECK

The rapid growth rate of an infant's first year slows during the toddler and preschool years (about ages 1 to 5). As a child's appetite decreases, adults need to serve nutrient-dense foods and allow the child to decide how much to eat. Snacking is fine if there is attention given to the selection of healthy foods and good dental hygiene. Vitamin and mineral supplements are usually not needed—a plan following the Guide to Daily Food Choices should meet nutrient needs. Children should have plenty of iron-rich foods available to prevent iron-deficiency anemia. Developing heart-healthy habits after age 2 years is good health insurance.

THE TEENAGE YEARS

Most girls begin a rapid growth spurt between the ages of 10 and 13 years, and most boys grow more between the ages of 12 and 15 years. Nearly every organ in the body grows during these periods of faster growth, which last about 3 years. Most noticeable are increases in height and weight and development of secondary sexual characteristics. Girls usually begin menstruating (reach menarche) during this growth spurt, and they grow very little—if at all—

beyond 2 years after menarche. Early maturing girls may begin their growth spurt as early as ages 7 to 8, while early maturing boys may begin growing by ages 9 to 10.

During the growth spurt, girls gain about 10 inches (25 centimeters) in height and boys gain about 12 inches (30 centimeters). Girls also tend to accumulate both lean and fat tissue, whereas boys tend to gain mostly lean tissue. This growth spurt provides about 42% to 51% of ultimate adult weight, and 15% to 25% of ultimate adult height (Figure 15-1).

Fortunately, as the growth spurt begins, teenagers begin to eat more. If teens choose nutritious food, they can take advantage of their increased hunger and easily satisfy their nutrient needs. As with other age groups, the Guide to Daily Food Choices provides the basis for meeting these nutrient needs (Table 15-5).

Nutritional problems of teens

We discussed anorexia nervosa and bulimia in Chapter 13. Other nutritional problems are more common during the teen years. A major concern is that many teenage girls stop drinking milk, and so they may not consume enough calcium to allow for maximum mineralization of bones through their early twenties. Many investigators are concerned that young women who do not drink milk are sowing the seeds for future osteoporosis. Again, 3 servings from the milk, yogurt, and cheese group per day are recommended. The RDA for calcium increases between ages 11 and 24 years from 800 to 1200 milligrams for both males and females. Only about 1 in 6 teenage girls consumes that much.

Another concern is iron deficiency. Iron-deficiency anemia sometimes appears in girls after they start menstruating and in boys during their growth spurt, especially if they are involved in athletics (see Chapter 12).[15] About 12% of teenagers have low iron stores. It is important that teenagers choose good food sources of iron, such as lean meats, whole grains, and enriched cereals. In addition, it is always a good idea to consume vitamin C with plant or supplemental sources of iron to increase iron absorption. Adolescent and teenage girls especially need to eat good sources of iron (or regularly consume an iron supplement), particularly those with heavy menstrual flows. Iron-deficiency anemia is not a desirable state for a teen. It can produce increased fatigue and decreased ability to concentrate and learn. School performance may suffer.

Another common problem during middle and late adolescence results from skipping meals. Busy schedules, part-time jobs, athletics, and social activities all may interfere with regular meal times. Breakfast is often skipped. Missing a meal may deprive a teen of sufficient kcalories and nutrients unless these can somehow be made up in snacks and other meals.

Another potential problem primarily involves boys during their growth spurt, when they are eating lots of foods. Because they expend a great deal of energy, boys often devour large amounts of saturated fat and cholesterol to meet their energy needs, especially if they regularly consume hamburgers, French fries, fried chicken, and milk shakes. The fats contribute to plaque buildup in the arteries, thus paving the way for early coronary heart disease. We believe it is prudent for boys to begin choosing heart-healthy foods, especially during the high energy intake years associated with the teen growth spurt.

Poor dietary habits formed during teenage years often continue into adulthood, giving rise to an increased risk of chronic diseases, such as heart disease, osteoporosis, and some types of cancer. Getting this message across to teenagers and their families is an important and challenging task for nutrition educators and health professionals.

A closer look at the diets of teenage girls

Teenagers are apt to adopt fad diets, eat away from home or miss meals completely, and snack a lot. Teenage girls, especially, are very concerned with

TABLE 15-5

Guide to Daily Food Choices for adolescents and teens[*]

	Include at Least this Many Servings Daily
Milk, yogurt, and cheese (preferably lowfat or nonfat)	3
Meats, poultry, fish, dry beans, eggs, and nuts	2-3
Vegetables	3-5
Fruits	2-4
Breads, cereals, rice, and pasta (preferably whole grain; otherwise enriched or fortified	6-11
Fats. oils. and sweets	Use sparingly

[*]Use serving sizes from adult Guide to Daily Food Choices.
Here we define "teen" as a person who has added height in the past year, and is at least 12 years old. This guide should be used through age 24 years.

weight gain, appearance, and acceptability. In an attempt to reach personal goals, they may eat dangerously little and stick to just a few items. If their limited food choices consist of French fries, soft drinks, and pastries, little room is left for foods that are good nutrient sources. It's not only calcium and iron that teenage girls need to be concerned about—they often don't get enough vitamin A, vitamin B-6, folate, vitamin C, and zinc as well.

Helping teens eat more nutritious foods

Teenagers face a variety of upheavals in their lives. They pursue their independence, experience identity crises, seek peer acceptance, and worry about physical appearance. Advertisers take advantage of this by pushing a vast array of products—candy, gum, soda pop, and snacks—targeted toward the teenage market. All these factors affect food choice.

Teens often do not think of the long-term benefits of good health.[20] They have a hard time relating today's actions to tomorrow's health outcomes. The future is far away. Many teenagers tend to think they can just change habits later; there is no hurry.

Overcoming the teenage mind set

One strategy for working with teenage boys is to stress the importance of nutrition for physical development—especially muscular development—and for fitness, vigor, and health. With teenage girls, one approach is to help them understand how to choose nutrient-dense foods that lead to better health while maintaining appropriate weight. It can be explained that beauty is based on the glow of health, something that sick people often do not have. For teenagers, it is better to focus on the many positive aspects of healthful foods they can reap right now than to talk about health hazards that may or may not happen at some later time if they eat less healthful food.[20]

Are teenage snacking practices harmful?

As with children, the major focus with snacks should be what one eats. Teens often obtain one-fourth to one-third of all their energy and major nutrients from

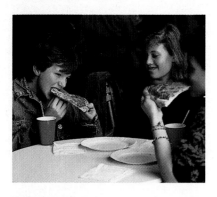

FIGURE 15-8
The teen years are noted for snacking. Still, nutritional problems associated with teenagers' eating fast food are caused more by food choice than the foods available.

snacks (Figure 15-8). Teenagers can obtain many nutrients from snacking. Even fast-food restaurants offer some good food choices. By choosing wisely and eating in moderation, teens can eat at fast-food restaurants and still consume a very good diet (see Nutrition Insight 3-1). Snacks and fast-food restaurants in and of themselves are not the problem; poor food choices are. Unfortunately, a recent Gallup poll has found just what you might expect—that teens snack mostly on potato chips, corn chips, cookies, candies, and ice cream.

CONCEPT CHECK

Another period of rapid growth occurs during the teen years. Girls generally start this earlier than boys. The Guide to Daily Food Choices should direct meal plans. Common nutritional problems in these years arise from poor food choices and include poor calcium intake in girls, iron-deficiency anemia, and sometimes excessive saturated fat intake. Because changes occur so rapidly during these years, and in so many areas—psychological, social, and physical—it may be difficult to stress the importance of nutrition to teenagers.

SUMMARY

- Growth is very rapid during infancy; birth weight doubles in 4 to 6 months, and length increases by 50% in the first year. An adequate diet, especially protein intake, is very important to support normal growth. Undernutrition can cause irreversible changes in growth and development. Growth in infants and children can be assessed by measuring body weight, height (or length), and head circumference over time.

- Nutrient needs in the first 6 months can be met by human milk or formula. Supplementary vitamin D and iron may be needed in the first 6 months for breast-fed infants, and all infants may need supplemental fluoride.

- Infant formulas generally contain lactose or sucrose, heat-treated proteins from cow's milk, and vegetable oil. Formulas may or may not be fortified with iron. Sanitation is very important when preparing and storing formula.

- Most infants do not need solid foods before about 6 months of age. Solid food should not be added to an infant's diet until the nutrients are needed; the GI tract can digest complex foods; the infant has the physical ability to control tongue thrusting; and the risk of developing food allergies decreases.

- The first solid food given should be iron-fortified infant cereals or ground meats. Other single foods can be added gradually, at the rate of about one each week. Some foods to avoid giving infants in the first year include honey, lowfat cow's milk, overly salty or sweet foods, or foods that may cause choking.

- Introducing iron-containing solid food at the appropriate time and not offering cow's milk until appropriate can generally prevent iron-deficiency anemia in late infancy.

- Obese children and adolescents are more likely to become obese adults and so incur greater health risks. Parents can provide healthy food choices, while children should control portion sizes. When controlled early, a problem of obesity may correct itself as the child continues to grow in height. Obese infants, on the other hand, do not necessarily go on to become obese children.

- A slower growth rate in preschool years underlines the importance of children eating nutrient-dense foods and reducing their food serving sizes. Choosing iron-rich foods, such as lean red meats, is important at this age. Portion sizes at meals of 1 tablespoon of each food for each year of life is a good rule of thumb. Teens and young adults particularly need adequate iron and calcium in the diet, especially girls.

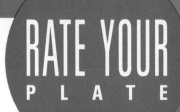

GETTING LITTLE BILLY TO EAT

Bill is 3 years old and his mother is worried about his eating habits. He absolutely refuses to eat vegetables, meat, and dinner in general. Some days he eats very little food. He wants to eat snacks most of time. His mother wants him to eat a formal lunch and dinner to make sure he gets all the nutrients he needs. Mealtime is a battle because Bill says that he isn't hungry, but his mother wants him to eat everything served on his plate. He drinks five to six glasses of whole milk per day because that is the one food he adores.

When his mother prepares dinner she makes plenty of vegetables, boiling them until they are soft, hoping this will appeal to Bill. Bill's dad waits to eat his vegetables last, regularly telling the family that he eats them only because he has to. He also regularly complains about how dinner has been prepared. Bill saves his vegetables until last and usually gags when his mother orders him to eat them. Billy has been known to sit at the dinner table for an hour until the war of wills ends. Bill's mother serves casseroles and stews regularly because these are her best dishes. Bill likes to eat breakfast cereal, fruit, and cheese and will regularly request these foods for snacks. However, his mother tries to deny his requests so he will have an appetite for dinner. Bill's mother comes to you and asks you what she should do to get Bill to eat.

ANALYSIS

1. Give six mistakes Bill's parents are making, contributing to Bill's poor eating habits.

_____

_____

_____

_____

_____

_____

2. Give six strategies they might try to promote good eating habits in Bill.

_____

_____

_____

_____

_____

_____

REFERENCES

1. Barrett S: Unproven allergies: an epidemic of nonsense, *Nutrition Today*, March/April, 1989, p 6.
2. Behrman RE and others: *Nelson Textbook of Pediatrics*, ed 13, Philadelphia, 1987, WB Saunders.
3. Butkus SN, Mahan LK: Food allergies: immunological reactions to food, *Journal of The American Dietetic Association* 86:601, 1986.
4. Colon AR, Dipalma JS: Colic, *American Family Physician* 40(6):122, 1989.
5. Fauson A, Wilson J: Family interactions surrounding feeding of infants with nonorganic failure to thrive, *Clinical Pediatrics* 26:518, 1987.
6. Forbes GB: Children and food: order amid chaos, *The New England Journal of Medicine* 324:262, 1991.
7. Gortmaker SL and others: Increasing pediatric obesity in the United States, *American Journal of Diseases of Children* 141:535, 1987.
8. Heald FP: Atherosclerosis during adolescence, *Medical Clinics of North America* 74:1321, 1990.
9. Johnson GH: *Dietary guidelines for infants*, Fremont, Mich, 1989, Gerber Products.
10. Lindeman AK, Clancy KL: Assessment of breakfast habits and social/emotional behavior of elementary school children, *Journal of Nutrition Education* 22:226, 1990.
11. Metcalfe DD: Diseases of food hypersensitivity, *The New England Journal of Medicine*, 321:255, 1989.
12. Parraga IM and others: Feeding patterns of urban black infants, *Journal of The American Dietetic Association* 88:796, 1988.
13. Pipes PL: *Nutrition in infancy and childhood*, St. Louis, 1989, Mosby–Year Book.
14. Rees JM: Management of obesity in adolescence, *Medical Clinics of North America* 74:1275, 1990.
15. Ritchey AK: Iron deficiency in children, *Postgraduate Medicine* 82:59, 1987.
16. Sanjur D and others: Dietary patterns and nutrient intake of toddlers from low-income families in Denver, Colorado, *Journal of the American Dietetic Association* 90:823, 1990.
17. Satter EM: Childhood eating disorders, *Journal of The American Dietetic Association* 86:357, 1986.
18. Snider, S: Acne, *FDA Consumer*, October, 1990, p 17.
19. Stehlin D: Feeding baby: nature and nurture, *FDA consumer* September, 1990, p 27.
20. Story M and others: Adolescent nutrition: self-perceived deficiencies and needs of practitioners working with youth, *Journal of The American Dietetic Association* 88:591, 1988.
21. Taubman B: Parental counseling compared with the elimination of cow's milk or soy milk protein for the treatment of infant colic syndrome: a randomized trial, *Pediatrics* 81:756, 1988.
22. Warwick ZS: Development of taste preferences: implications for nutrition and health, *Nutrition Today*, March/April, 1990, p 15.
23. Yip R: Declining prevalence of anemia among low-income children in the United States, *Journal of The American Medical Association* 258:1619, 1987.
24. Zeiger RS: Prevention of food allergy in infancy, *Annals of Allergy* 65:430, 1990.

HOW MUCH HAVE I LEARNED?

What have you learned from Chapter 15? Here are 15 statements about nutrition from infancy through adolescence. Read them to test your current knowledge. If you think the statement is true or mostly true, circle T. If you think the statement is false or mostly false, circle F. Use the scoring key at the end of the book to compute your total score. To review, take this test again later, and especially before tests.

1. T F   Consuming low-protein diets in childhood can greatly affect ultimate adult height.

2. T F   An infant's length increases by 50% in the first year.

3. T F   Brain growth is greatest during the teen years.

4. T F   Most obese infants become obese adults.

5. T F   Infants have lower energy needs per pound than do older children.

6. T F   An infant's diet should be very low in fat.

7. T F   Infants need solid food by 3 months of age.

8. T F   Infants enjoy blander foods than do adults.

9. T F   Colic may be caused by a gas buildup in the intestinal tract.

10. T F   Cow's milk fed during early infancy can cause allergies.

11. T F   Iron-deficiency anemia often occurs in infants whose diets consist mainly of cow's milk.

12. T F   It is nutritionally important to put children on a three-meals-per-day schedule.

13. T F   The two most common nutritional problems in childhood are obesity and anemia.

14. T F   Parents should carefully control the amount of food their children eat.

15. T F   Allergies can be avoided by limiting certain foods in the diet.

NUTRITION ISSUE

FOOD ALLERGIES AND INTOLERANCES

Adverse reactions to foods are commonly reported, in some cases approaching 8% to 33% of the population. They are reported more frequently by females. The most common ages for adverse food reactions are infancy and young adulthood. Allergic-related disease appears in about 0.3% to 7.5% of children. Types of reactions associated with food ingestion are:

Classical **allergy**—Itching, reddening skin, asthma, and a runny nose.
Gastrointestinal—Nausea, vomiting, diarrhea, intestinal gas, bloating, pain, constipation, and indigestion.
General—Headache, skin reactions, tension and fatigue, tremors, and psychological problems.

Allergic reaction symptoms vary with the location in the body as noted above. A generalized, all-systems reaction is called anaphylactic shock. This condition can be life-threatening.

About 90% of food allergies (also called hypersensitivities) are caused by milk, eggs, nuts (especially peanuts), corn, seafood, soy, and wheat. Other foods frequently identified with adverse reactions include alcoholic beverages, meat and meat products, vegetables, sugars, cereals, fish, fats and oils, fruits, chocolate, and cheese.[11] A family history of allergies greatly increases the risk.

Food allergies

A food allergy is caused by an immune response to a food substance. **Food sensitivity** is a term often used today to describe milder reactions. The word allergy specifies a disorder of the immune system. About 2% to 4% of food reactions in infants, children, and adults result from true allergies. Allergens are usually large proteins with specific sizes and configurations.

When an allergen enters an allergic-prone host for the first time, a specific immune reaction takes place, although it is not apparent. Subsequent exposures can then trigger various muscles to contract, increase permeability of blood vessels, and lead to nasal secretions, itching, and changes in dilation of the airways.[3]

Why do allergies occur?

A big question concerning food allergies is how intact food proteins can cross the natural barriers of the GI tract to interact with the immune system. Considering the thoroughness of the digestive system, it seems that these particles would break down into amino acids that the body could then metabolize with no adverse effects. Evidence now shows that large particles, however, can gain access to the immune system through gaps between intestinal cells. These large particles can eventually be transported via the bloodstream to various body sites where they can cause a reaction.

In a nonallergic person, immune factors synthesized by intestinal cells act as a natural barrier against absorption and transportation of large molecules. This protection doesn't seem to function efficiently for people with food allergies.

Testing for a food allergy

The first step in determining the presence of a food allergy is to record in detail a history of symptoms, time from ingestion to onset of symptoms, most recent reaction, quantity of food needed to produce a reaction, and the food suspected of causing a reaction. A family history of allergic disease can also help. The physician looks for signs of allergy, such as inflammation in the nasal cavity, skin diseases, and asthma. Skin testing can help pinpoint likely allergen suspects.

The next step usually is to eliminate from the diet all tested compounds that appear to cause allergic symptoms plus all other foods the person's history suggests may cause an allergy. If symptoms are still present, the person can restrict the diet even more severely or even use special formulas that are hypoallergenic. This type of elimination diet should eventually yield no symptoms.

After 2 to 4 weeks without symptoms, foods can be cautiously reintroduced, but not those thought to cause ***anaphylactic shock***. Foods should be tried in small quantities at first—$\frac{1}{2}$ to 1 teaspoon (2.5 to 5 milliliters). The amount is increased until the dose approximates usual intake. In this way allergenic substances can be identified if symptoms resume. In a clinical setting, this can be done using a double-blind approach where neither the patient nor the person scoring the results know whether the diet contains the potentially offending food (see Nutrition Issue 1). This is especially needed when a psychological component might complicate the reaction, or when symptoms are vague or ill-defined. Dried foods can be encapsulated and then given to the person.

Treatment of food allergies

Once potential allergens are identified, the best treatment is to avoid them, especially for people with zero tolerance. Cromolyn sodium, a prescription medication given as an inhalant, can limit the extent of an immune reaction in the lungs. An oral form of this that will lessen immune response in the intestine should be approved for use soon.

A major challenge for the clinician treating a person with a food allergy is to make sure that what remains in the diet can still provide essential nutrients. Children especially, with their small food intake, permit less leeway in removing offending foods that may contain numerous nutrients.

Allergy • An immune response that occurs when immune bodies (antibodies) react with a foreign substance (antigen).

Food Sensitivity • A mild reaction to a substance in a food that might be noticed as slight twitching or redness of the skin.

A bogus method used to test for food allergies is cytotoxic testing. Don't be taken in by this form of health fraud.[1]

ANOTHER BITE If an allergic-prone woman is pregnant or breast-feeding, she should avoid offending foods, like eggs and peanuts, because antigens can cross the placenta during pregnancy. Antigens will also be secreted in her milk. She should work with her doctor to make sure an adequate diet is still consumed. In addition when food allergies run in the family, women are advised to breast-feed their infants exclusively for 6 months. Formula-fed infants have a greater risk of developing allergies. Breast-feeding then should continue for as long as possible, preferably at least 1 year. Exclusive breast-feeding with delayed introduction of solid foods until 6 months of age has been shown to be an effective way to reduce development of allergies in infants.[24]

Prognosis • A forecast of a course of a disease.

Food Intolerance • An adverse reaction to food that does not involve the immune system.

The **prognosis** for food allergies that occur before 3 years of age is good. About 40% of children outgrow food allergies. Food allergies diagnosed after age 3 years are often more long-lived. Adults have reported reactions that still appear even 15 or more years after the first episode. Occasional reintroduction of foods can be tried every 6 months or so to see whether the allergy symptoms have decreased, but not before 1 year of age. If no symptoms appear, tolerance to the food has developed.

Food intolerances

In addition to food allergies, **food intolerances** also cause adverse food reactions. These do not involve the immune system, and so it is important to separate them from actual food allergies. Food intolerance also differs from allergies in that more of the offending food is required to produce symptoms. The treatments also differ. Food intolerances can be caused by:

- Substances, such as tomatoes or pineapples, that produce medicine-type activity.
- Toxic contaminants, such as bacterial toxins; synthetic compounds such as tartrazine (F, D, & C yellow no. 5); antibiotics; and insect parts (see Chapter 17).
- Deficiencies in digestive enzymes, such as lactase.
- Food poisoning caused by improper handling or cooking, as in *Clostridium botulinum* food poisoning, or viral and bacterial infections, as in *Salmonella* food poisoning.

All these conditions can lead to GI tract symptoms. In addition, anyone can expect to be sensitive to one or more of these causes of food intolerance—not only people with specific changes in their immune system.

Four other noteworthy food intolerances are induced by the presence of sulfites, monosodium glutamate (MSG), tartrazine, and tyramine in food. A sulfite reaction causes flushing, spasms of the airways, and a loss of blood pressure. Wine, dehydrated potatoes, dried fruits, gravy, soup mixes, and restaurant salad greens commonly are treated with sulfites. Evidence of reaction to MSG might be an increase in blood pressure, numbness, sweating, vomiting, headache, and facial pressure. A reaction to tartrazine includes spasm of the airways, itching, and reddening skin. MSG is commonly found in Chinese food and many processed foods, like soup. Tyramine can cause high blood pressure in people taking monoamine-oxidase inhibitor medications (for mental depression). Tyramines are commonly found in "aged" foods, such as cheeses and red wines.

The basic treatment for food intolerances is to avoid specific offending components. However, this usually does not require total elimination because people are generally not as sensitive to factors causing food intolerances as they would be to allergens. For instance, a slight amount of sulfites in a glass of wine may be tolerable, whereas a large dose from a chef's salad may cause a reaction. See Chapter 17 on food safety for more details about toxic reactions from foods.

How many children are sensitive to food additives?

In 1973, Dr. Benjamin Feingold suggested that food additives caused hyperactivity (now known as a part of the attention deficit disorder) in children. He theorized that because some children are allergic to aspirin-like compounds, and some food additives have aspirin-like structures, such children would also be allergic to certain food additives. Much research followed this proposal: generally, the research has not supported a strong or predictable association between the consumption of food additives and hyperactivity in children.

Today the incidence of attention deficit disorder with hyperactivity is seen in approximately 2% to 4% of school-age children; boys are affected four to six times more than girls. The initial identification of hyperactivity in children commonly occurs when they are 2 or 3 years of age as they enter nursery or elementary school. Teachers report that these students are uncontrollable, easily distracted, unable to sit still, act impulsively, bother other children, and, especially, intrude into other children's activities.

There are many pitfalls in studying any link to diet and hyperactive behavior. An additive-free diet is likely to be more nutrient-rich because it will contain more whole, less processed foods. So, it is difficult to know whether behavior changes in a hyperactive child on such a diet would result from eliminating additives or adding more nutrients. In addition, by giving the child a special diet and observing behavior, parents are giving that child more attention. The extra attention alone can decrease disruptive behavior.

The only definitive way to study this relationship is to use a double-blind protocol. A child would be given an additive-free food and then later a food full of additives. Neither the parents, the child, nor the researchers should know what is in the food. After the child has consumed the foods, the researchers score the child's behavior.

This procedure is much too cumbersome to be used in a school system or by a private pediatrician. Thus many suspected cases of food additive–linked hyperactivity are not tested in a definitive scientific manner. This is a real problem since some diets used for hyperactive children eliminate more than just food additives. Some popular approaches eliminate dietary essentials, such as milk, fruit, and some grain products. The more limited the diet, the greater the risk of nutrient deficiencies and poor growth.

If an additive-free diet follows the Guide to Daily Food Choices and actually improves a child's attention span and behavior, there is no reason not to employ it. About 5% to 10% of cases may be helped by this treatment.[2] Eliminating food colors from the diet has no harmful effect as such.

A physician should agree that special diet restrictions are worth trying. Even then, diet changes must be handled carefully. In addition, a child should not be singled out as different from his peers and shouldn't end up feeling deprived as a result of dietary restrictions. The child should not see his own behavior as more directed by diet than by how he feels. Parents who look for excuses for a child's behavior may often find it easier to blame inappropriate behavior on something concrete, like food.

Will anything actually help the hyperactive child? Time is a very important therapy; hyperactivity tends to decrease as a child matures. When hyperactivity contributes to a true attention deficit disorder syndrome, behavior therapies and stimulant medications (Ritalin, for example) can be used to treat the problem. The advice of a pediatrician skilled in this disease should be sought. ●

Chapter 6 discusses whether sugar causes hyperactivity or antisocial behavior.

NUTRITION FOR ADULT AND ELDERLY YEARS

Eating is one of our great pleasures. Guided by common sense and moderation, eating well is also a means to good health. Most of us want a long, productive life, free of illness. Yet, many people from early middle age onward suffer heart disease, strokes, diabetes mellitus, osteoporosis, or other chronic diseases. We can slow the development of and in some cases even prevent these diseases by pursuing a diet that works against them. This action is most profitable if we begin early and continue throughout adulthood. We serve ourselves best—as individuals and as a nation—by striving to be as free of disease as possible and to maintain vitality even in the last decade of life. This concept was first explored in Chapter 1. We will discuss it again in this chapter. We will also address the special nutrition needs of the elderly.

Keep in mind that present day-to-day health practices can significantly influence health during a person's elderly years. Many health problems that occur with age are not inevitable; they result from disease processes that influence physical health.[1] We have much to learn from healthy elderly people whose attention to health and physical activity—along with a little luck—keeps them active and vibrant while others are forced to watch from the sidelines. Successful aging is the goal. Age fast or slow—it is partly our choice. ●

CHAPTER

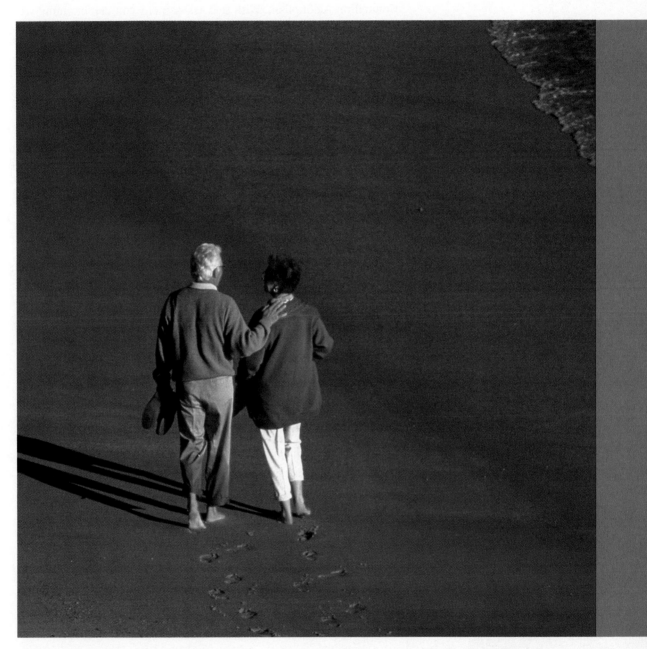

An active lifestyle continues to help maintain muscle mass and heart health in one's later years.

Could You or Someone You Know Have a Problem with Alcohol?

The Nutrition Issue on p. 525 discusses ethanol, commonly known as alcohol. Misuse of alcohol is one of our most preventable health problems. It is a prominent contributor to five of the ten leading causes of death in the United States. The social consequences of alcohol dependency include divorce, unemployment, and poverty. The following questionnaire was developed by the National Council on Alcoholism. With this assessment you can examine whether you or someone you know might need help. Answer the following questions by placing an "X" in the appropriate blank.

	Yes	No
1. Do you occasionally drink heavily after disappointment, a quarrel, or when someone gives you a hard time?	_____	_____
2. When you have trouble or feel under pressure, do you drink more heavily than usual?	_____	_____
3. Have you ever noticed that you're able to handle liquor better than you did when you first started drinking?	_____	_____
4. Do you ever wake up the morning after you've been drinking and discover that you can't remember part of the evening before, even though your friends tell you that you didn't pass out?	_____	_____
5. When drinking with other people, do you try to have a few extra drinks when others won't know it?	_____	_____
6. Are there certain occasions when you feel uncomfortable if alcohol isn't available?	_____	_____
7. Have you recently noticed that when you begin drinking, you're in more of a hurry to get the first drink than you used to be?	_____	_____
8. Do you sometimes feel a little guilty about your drinking?	_____	_____
9. Are you secretly irritated when your family or friends discuss your drinking?	_____	_____
10. Have you recently noticed an increase in the frequency of memory blackouts?	_____	_____
11. Do you often find that you wish to continue drinking after your friends say they've had enough?	_____	_____
12. Do you usually have a reason for the occasions when you drink heavily?	_____	_____
13. When you're sober, do you often regret things you have done or said while drinking?	_____	_____
14. Have you tried switching brands or following different plans for controlling your drinking?	_____	_____

ASSESS YOURSELF

	Yes	No
15. Have you often failed to keep promises you've made to yourself about controlling or cutting your drinking?	_____	_____
16. Have you ever tried to control your drinking by changing jobs or moving to a new location?	_____	_____
17. Do you try to avoid family or close friends while you're drinking?	_____	_____
18. Are you having an increasing number of financial and work problems?	_____	_____
19. Do more people seem to be treating you unfairly without good reason?	_____	_____
20. Do you eat very little or irregularly when you're drinking?	_____	_____
21. Do you sometimes have the "shakes" in the morning and find that it helps to have a little drink?	_____	_____
22. Have you recently noticed that you can't drink as much as you once did?	_____	_____
23. Do you sometimes stay drunk for several days at a time?	_____	_____
24. Do you sometimes feel very depressed and wonder whether life is worth living?	_____	_____
25. Sometimes after periods of drinking do you see or hear things that aren't there?	_____	_____
26. Do you get terribly frightened after you have been drinking heavily?	_____	_____

INTERPRETATION

These are all symptoms that may indicate alcoholism. "Yes" answers to several of the questions indicate the following stages of alcoholism:

Questions 1-8: Early Stage
Questions 9-21: Middle Stage
Questions 22-26: Final Stage

It is vital that people assess themselves honestly. If you or someone you know demonstrates some or a number of these symptoms, it is important that help be pursued. If there is even a question in your mind, go talk to a professional about it. Alcohol abuse is one of many problems adults face.

YOUR ADULT YEARS

People who practice healthy lifestyles and aim to prevent disease may or may not live longer. Heredity, accidents, and other things beyond our control influence longevity. However, health seekers often remain more active longer and spend less time immobilized. Many adults in America today have turned a healthful diet and moderate exercise regimen into lifetime pursuits in search of longevity.

A diet that optimizes long-term nutritional health emphasizes lowfat dairy products, lean meats and plant proteins, a variety of fruits and vegetables, and whole grain breads and cereals. The Guide to Daily Food Choices is a blueprint for this good diet.

To further refine food choices, recall also from Chapter 2 that Dietary Guidelines issued by USDA/DHHS encourage us to:

1. Eat a variety of foods.
2. Maintain healthy body weight.
3. Choose a diet low in fat, saturated fat, and cholesterol.
4. Choose a diet with plenty of vegetables, fruits, and grain products.
5. Use sugar only in moderation.
6. Use salt and sodium only in moderation.
7. If you drink alcoholic beverages, do so in moderation.

These guidelines provide a good general focus for diet planning. The practices recommended can accommodate many cultural dietary patterns. They are broad enough to allow you to include all the foods you enjoy in your eating plan—you may just have to eat some foods less frequently than others and/or in smaller portions, depending on your own health needs and preferences. Moderation—rather than elimination—is the overriding consideration.

Are adults following these diet recommendations?

In general, American adults are trying to follow the diet recommendations listed above. Since the mid-1950s we have consumed less saturated fat as more people substitute skim and lowfat milk for cream and whole milk. However, we eat more cheese, which is usually a concentrated form of saturated fat. Since 1963, we eat less butter, eggs, and animal fat and use more vegetable fats and oils and fish. These changes generally follow the recommendations to reduce the intake of saturated fat and instead emphasize unsaturated fat. Today, animal breeders are raising much leaner cows and hogs than in 1950. This helps us all. Our demand for chicken, a relatively lean source of animal protein, has also skyrocketed.

Other aspects of the average U.S. diet are more mixed. Nutritional surveys from the early 1980s (the most comprehensive to date) show that the major contributors of kcalories to the adult diet are:

- white bread, rolls, and crackers
- doughnuts, cakes, and cookies
- alcoholic beverages
- whole milk and beverages made with it
- hamburgers, cheeseburgers, and meatloaf

If the trend in diets were truly toward decreasing alcohol, sugar, and saturated fat and increasing fiber, the foods listed above could hardly appear at the top of the list. Our suggestions for improvement would stress lowfat milk; whole-wheat bread and whole-grain cereals; lean meat and tuna; peanuts and kidney beans; and oranges and broccoli. What would your list look like?

Your task, as an adult, is to pinpoint the lifestyle practices most likely to cause you illness and chronic disease and to change those specifically. Whether these changes include switching to bran cereal, rice, pasta, fish, chicken, asparagus, and bok choy and walking 2 miles every other day is up to you. These practices all provide a means to promote and maintain nutritional and

As stated in Chapter 1, a varied, balanced diet; maintaining a desirable body weight; performing regular exercise; minimizing tobacco use; and limiting (or adjusting to) stress are health practices we all should seriously consider.

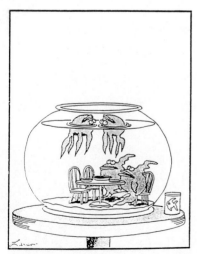

"Well the Parkers are dead. . . . You had to encourage them to take thirds, didn't you?"

FIGURE 16-1
The Far Side.

overall health. The overriding consideration should be quality and length of life and the impact dietary changes might have on them. Now is the time to design this plan (Figure 16-1). Learn more about your risk factors for chronic disease. Then review Chapter 3 for help in converting your plan into reality.

Life Span • The potential oldest age to which a person can survive.

Life Expectancy • The average length of life for a given group of people.

CONCEPT CHECK

The Dietary Guidelines form an effective framework for diet planning in adulthood. Additional recommendations for exercising regularly, not using tobacco products, and limiting stress can further maximize health potential. Surveys show that Americans are beginning to follow general health recommendations, but many goals still need more attention. Genetic background, medical conditions, and some lifestyle practices influence an individual's nutritional and health state. Individual nutrition and health plans should be developed by all of us.

NUTRITION IN THE ELDERLY YEARS

How long do your family members generally live? Of those who died early in adulthood, can you pinpoint some causes? Do you plan to live longer than your parents did or will? How long will that be? Some basic statistics can help you predict.

Life Span

Life span refers the maximum number of years humans live. As far as we know, this hasn't changed in recorded time. The longest human life documented to date is 116 years. In contrast, the domestic dog has a life span of 20 years, and a rat, 5 years.

Life expectancy

Life expectancy is the time an average person can expect to live. In 1988, life expectancy in America was 71 years for men and 78 years for women. Worldwide, the highest average age is 81 years for women in Switzerland and 75 years for men in Japan. Life expectancy hasn't always been this long; for primitive humans, it was about 30 to 35 years. It had increased to 49 years in Medieval England and remained so until the turn of this century in the United States. During the last 80 years, life expectancy for nearly all people has increased, mainly because of changes in the principal causes of death.

At the turn of this century, infectious diseases commonly caused death. Vaccines and antibiotics have tremendously lowered death from disease. The decline in infant and childhood deaths, coupled with better diets and health care, have allowed more people to age first into maturity and then into elderly years. Now the principal causes of death in Western societies are related to heart disease and cancer (Table 16-1).

In 1900, half of all whites died before reaching age 55. In 1940, half were still alive at age 68. Today, half are alive at ages exceeding 70 years. In the year 2035, about 20% of the population will be 65 years and older, twice as many as reach 65 years today (Figure 16-3). Among the older population, the 85+ years group is the fastest growing segment. Between 1986 and 2050, the population aged 85+ years is expected to increase from about 1% to more than 5% of the total U.S. population. This is the first time in history a society will need to deal with such a large elderly population.

The "graying" of America

The "graying" of America poses some problems. Today, while people older than age 65 account for 12% of the U.S. population, they account for more than 30% of all medications used, 40% of acute care hospital stays, and 50% of the federal health budget. Of the elderly, 85% have nutrition-related problems, such as

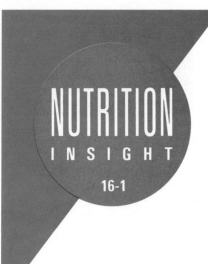

NUTRITION
I N S I G H T
16-1

A PRESCRIPTION FOR LONGEVITY?

Some of us live longer than others. Whole communities also show differences in longevity. In the United States, Seventh Day Adventist men live an average of 6 years longer than other men. They have unusually low death rates from heart disease and cancer. When we examine their lifestyles, we find that most do not smoke or drink alcoholic beverages, they eat less meat and more fruits, vegetables, and whole grains than average men. These and other health habits are clearly identified as factors influencing how quickly we age.[10]

A study of more than 6000 people in the San Francisco Bay area showed that those who followed seven simple health habits experienced a much lower death rate than those who did not. The long-lived group had the following habits: (1) They never smoked; (2) they moderated their alcohol consumption; (3) they ate breakfast regularly; (4) they didn't snack; (5) they slept 7 to 8 hours a night; (6) they exercised regularly; and (7) they maintained desirable body weight.

As we learned in the chapter on weight control, factors influencing weight, and hence longevity, appear to be related to nature as well as nurture. When researchers closely examine the genetic and lifestyle backgrounds of long-lived people, they surmise that vigorous physical activity, lowfat diets, and the prevention of excessive weight gain may be key factors of longevity.[14] Studies of families, and of twins in particular, also provide evidence for genetic control of human longevity. Identical twins tend to have very similar life spans and causes of death. Since identical twins have exactly the same genetic information, this argues strongly that longevity is at least partially because of hereditary.

What does animal research tell us about longevity?

Animal studies on longevity are quite extensive. By limiting kcalorie intake to about 60% of usual in rodents, life span can be increased by 35%[20] The same treatment results in at least 50% less incidence of cancer (see Chapter 9). Only kcalories should be limited; the diet is supplemented with vitamins and minerals. Some studies have shown that food restriction can be started late in life and still extend the life span of rats. Scientists have found similar results using low kcalorie diets in other species, including mice, hamsters, spiders, fish, and mollusks, and are optimistic that it may work in monkeys. A study of this possibility is currently underway. Many other hypotheses have been tested in animals, but none are as effective in extending life expectancy as kcalorie restriction.

There are many theories to explain how kcalorie restriction increases life expectancy in rodents. It may be that a greatly reduced caloric intake lowers the

FIGURE 16-3

Trend in age distribution of U.S. population (including Armed Forces overseas), 1900-2050. The United States has never had a population with so many elderly people as it will soon have.

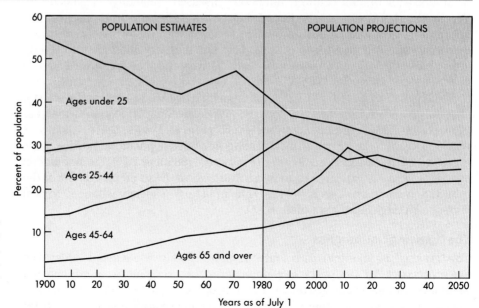

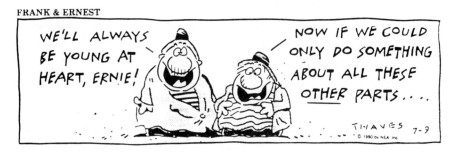

FIGURE 16-2

metabolic rate, which in turn reduces wear and tear on the body. Or the mechanism may involve the immune system. Fewer calories may mean a delay in the natural aging of the immune system, thereby postponing the onset of diseases more commonly associated with old age. Other theories focus on what happens to hormonal systems under conditions of severe caloric restriction. Less insulin release, for example, could reduce cell turnover—a factor associated with aging. The ability of cells to repair damaged DNA could also be affected by calories. It is likely that several of these mechanisms come into play when animals are underfed. Other reasons are also possible.[20]

The extended life expectancies gained from reduced feeding may actually be equal to the natural life span of animals in the wild. Perhaps what we see in the laboratory is an acceleration of the aging process caused by **ad libitum** (and so overfeeding) that is typically allowed for laboratory animals. Might well-fed western man again look to long-lived rural people for the fountain of youth?[10]

Pass the butter?

From the animal studies, we can infer that many mammalian species, and maybe humans, might live longer by restricting kcalories.[2] In every species studied so far, being thin has meant living longer. But, with humans the question is, are people willing to give up cheeseburgers and fries to have an unknown number of additional years of life? For most of us the deferred benefit of a longer, healthier life is overshadowed by the immediate pleasure of a hot fudge sundae. Clearly, we should consider striking a balance between immediate gratification and a pleasant long-term future (Figure 16-2). ●

Ad Libitum • At one's desire or pleasure.

heart problems, diabetes mellitus, hypertension, osteoporosis, and obesity (Table 16-2).

Postponing these chronic diseases for as long as possible will help control health care costs. The more independent, healthy years people live, the better life can be for them and the less they burden the health care system, which will increasingly have to scramble to accommodate a growing elderly population. Keep in mind that aging is not a disease, although the process of aging is still a mystery. It is difficult to design a model that predicts aging because so often disease speeds the process. But diseases that commonly accompany old age—osteoporosis and atherosclerosis, for example—are not an inevitable part of aging. Some people do die of old age, not as a direct result of disease.[9]

What actually is aging?

One view of aging describes it as processes of slow cell death beginning soon after fertilization. When we are young, aging is not apparent because the major metabolic activities are geared toward growth and maturation. We produce plenty of active cells to meet physiological needs. During late adolescence and

TABLE 16-1

Changes in the causes of death during this century in the United States

Chronic diseases, rather than the infectious diseases, are now the major "killers." AIDS is currently the eleventh leading cause of death.

	1900			**1989**	
Rank	**Percent Cause of Death**	**Mortality**	**Rank**	**Percent Cause of Death**	**Mortality**
1	Pneumonia and influenza	12	1	Heart disease	34
2	Tuberculosis	11	2	Cancer	23
3	Diarrhea and enteritis	8	3	Cerebrovascular disease (stroke)	7
4	Heart disease	8	4	Accidents	4
5	Cerebrovascular disease (stroke)	6	5	Pulmonary (lung) disease	4
6	Nephritis	5	6	Pneumonia and influenza	4
7	Accidents	4	7	Diabetes mellitus	2
8	Cancer	4	8	Suicide	1
9	Diphtheria	2	9	Liver disease and cirrhosis	1
10	Meningitis	2	10	Homicide and law enforcement	1

From National Center for Health Statistics: *Monthly vital statistics report*, August 30, 1990.

Reserve Capacity • The extent to which an organ can preserve essentially normal function, despite decreasing cell number or cell activity.

adulthood, the body's major task is to maintain cells. But, inevitably cells age and die. Eventually, as more cells die, the body cannot adjust to meet all physiological demands. Body functioning begins to decrease, but organs usually retain enough *reserve capacity* so that for a long time the body shows no outward disease. Although no symptoms appear, subclinical disease may develop, and if allowed to progress unchecked, organ function and then body function eventually deteriorate noticeably.[2]

The aging process is clearly illustrated by changes in the function of the enzyme lactase. For some people, lactase activity in the small intestine slows during childhood. Generally, however, clear symptoms of the deficiency—gas and bloating after milk consumption—do not appear until adulthood. Although lactase output decreases in these cases, perhaps from birth, enough enzyme is present to digest lactose until adulthood.

Cells age probably because of automatic cellular changes and environmental influences. Even in the most supportive of environments, cell structure and function inevitably change. Eventually, cells lose their ability to regenerate the internal parts they need, and they die. As more and more cells in an organ system die, organ function decreases. After age 14 months, human brain cells are

TABLE 16-2

Selected disease conditions associated with aging

	Rate of Occurrence Per 1000 Persons			
Chronic Condition	**Total**	**45-64 Years**	**65-74 Years**	**75+ Years**
Arthritis	131	280	460	508
Hypertension	124	265	408	395
Hearing impairments	91	149	261	381
Heart conditions	83	137	291	339
Visual impairments	35	46	72	136
Deformities or orthopedic impairments	121	175	191	198
Diabetes mellitus	26	55	98	92
Diverticula of intestines	8	15	36	45
Asthma	37	32	47	26

From the National Center for Health Statistics: *Vital and health statistics*, May 24, 1988.

Diabetes destroy can nephrons

continually lost, but we have enough reserve capacity to maintain mental function throughout life. **Kidney nephrons** are also continually lost. In some people this loss leads to eventual kidney failure, but most of us maintain sufficient kidney function. Again, in aging, there is first a reduction in reserve capacity. Only after that is exhausted does actual organ function noticeably decrease.

Theories on the causes of aging

Although the causes of aging remain a mystery, many hypotheses have been promoted to explain it:[9]

Errors crop up in copying the genetic blueprint (DNA)—Once enough errors in DNA copying accumulate, a cell can no longer synthesize the major proteins it needs to function, and therefore it dies.

Connective tissue stiffens—Collagen protein strands found mostly in connective tissues chemically bond to each other. The bonding decreases flexibility in key body components, altering organ function. Skin wrinkles and joints and arteries stiffen. The bonding may also restrict nutrients from entering cells.

Toxic products build-up—Breakdown products of fats may act as intracellular sludge, hampering normal metabolic processes by clogging cells. Brown spots on the skin are a sign of this process.

Electron-seeking compounds damage cell parts—Electron-seeking compounds can break down cell membranes and proteins. One way to prevent some damage from these compounds is to consume adequate—not excessive—vitamin E, vitamin C, selenium, and beta-carotene. In contrast, it's not so effective to consume cellular enzymes designed to break down the damaging compounds. The ingested enzymes are themselves broken down during digestion before they can act in the body. Despite that, some health food stores sell the enzyme superoxide dismutase, which is made by cells to destroy certain electron-seeking compounds.

Hormone function changes—The hormone dehydroepiandrosterone (DHEA), produced by adrenal glands (located near the kidneys), circulates at extremely high levels in young adults and falls sharply with age. This change has led to speculation that it may play a role in aging. Long-term effects of using products containing this hormone are unknown. FDA has not approved use of DHEA, so marketing it is illegal in the United States. A fall in growth hormone levels is also being investigated as a potentially treatable hormonal effect of aging. Replacing growth hormone has wide-ranging, unpredictable effects and it is very costly to obtain. The studies so far support the theory that growth hormone-related loss of lean body mass plays a role in aging.

The immune system loses some efficiency—The thymus gland (located in the upper chest) is a major component of the immune system. During adolescence the thymus gland reaches its maximum size and by age 50 it is barely visible. The immune system itself runs a somewhat parallel course. It is most efficient during childhood and young adulthood, but with advancing age, it is less able to recognize and counteract foreign substances, such as viruses, that enter the body. As we age then, the immune system's ability to detect and destroy developing cancer cells decreases. Some cancer cells then can take advantage of the opportunity to multiply wildly.

Autoimmunity develops—**Autoimmune** reactions occur when white blood cells and other immune bodies fail to distinguish between substances normally present in the body and invading foreign compounds. White blood cells and other immune bodies then begin to attack the body tissues in addition to foreign compounds. Many diseases, including some forms of diabetes mellitus and arthritis, involve this autoimmune response.

Death is programmed into the cell—Each human cell can divide only so

Kidney Nephrons • Unit of kidney cells that filters wastes from the bloodstream.

Autoimmune • Immune reactions against normal body cells; self against self.

As the number of possible cell divisions increases, so does life span. The Galapagos tortoise, whose cells divide about 140 times, has a life span of perhaps 200 years.

many times, about 50. Once this number of divisions occurs, the cell automatically succumbs.

Most likely, aging results from an interaction of these events and changes. Scientists point out that even very healthy people have a lower life expectancy if they are exposed to sufficient environmental stresses, such as radiation and certain chemical agents.[2] Because cell aging and diseases like cancer are aggravated by environmental factors, it makes good sense to avoid such risks as excess sunlight and hazardous chemicals. Again, as stressed at the outset, we have some say in how fast we age.

CONCEPT CHECK

While life span has not changed, life expectancy has increased dramatically over the past century. For many societies this means an increasing proportion of the population is, and will be, over 65 years of age. Sidestepping continually rising health care costs and maximizing satisfaction with life requires postponing chronic illness. Aging begins early in life and probably results from both automatic cellular changes and environmental influences. Some popular theories of aging suggest these possible causes: errors in DNA copying accumulate; connective tissue stiffens; fat by-products buildup; electron-seeking compounds break down cell parts; hormonal and immune systems don't function well; autoimmune responses damage the body. Proper diet and health habits can play a role in slowing some of these processes.

THE EFFECTS OF AGING ON THE NUTRITIONAL HEALTH OF THE ELDERLY

Elderly people vary more in health status among themselves than do any other age group. This means that chronological age is not so useful in predicting physical health status (physiological age) (Figure 16-4). Among people aged 65 and over, some are totally independent, healthy people, while others are frail and require almost total care. To predict the nutritional problems of an elderly person, it is necessary to know the extent of physiological change caused by aging (Figure 16-5) and whether the person shows early warning signs for long-term poor nutrition. As we examine how aging affects body systems and how these changes contribute to poor nutrition, we will suggest ways to lessen the risk in your life and parallel changes in diet to counteract problem conditions.

FIGURE 16-4

The declines in physiological function. Some decline seen in aging is inevitable. But overall the decline is especially evident in sedentary people.

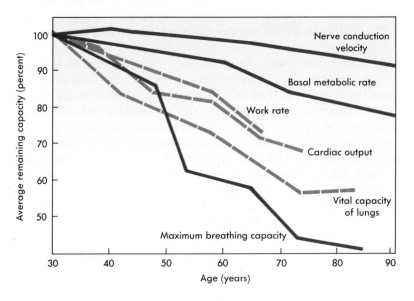

Taste and smell

Sensitivity to taste and smell often decreases with age.[2] Stronger seasonings may be required to make foods taste good. Food companies are carving a niche in the marketplace by capitalizing on this change; by using a variety of flavor enhancers they make foods tastier for the elderly. But for this group, a poor diet and possibly zinc deficiency can also contribute to a loss of taste. Therefore, a poor appetite should never be dismissed as a characteristic of old age. Many causes can be remedied.

Dental health

About 50% of people over age 50 years have lost all their teeth.[1] Attention to dental hygiene and dental care throughout life greatly lessens this risk. Gum disease also is common and encourages tooth loss. Replacement dentures enable some to chew normally, but many elderly people, especially men, have denture problems. A pureed diet is not necessarily the remedy.[4] Solving individual dietary needs requires identifying foods that need to be modified in consistency and can be eaten in a typical state. When people have problems chewing, nutrient-dense snacks like yogurt, bananas, and peanut butter can help. Sometimes just allowing extra time for swallowing and feeding encourages more eating.

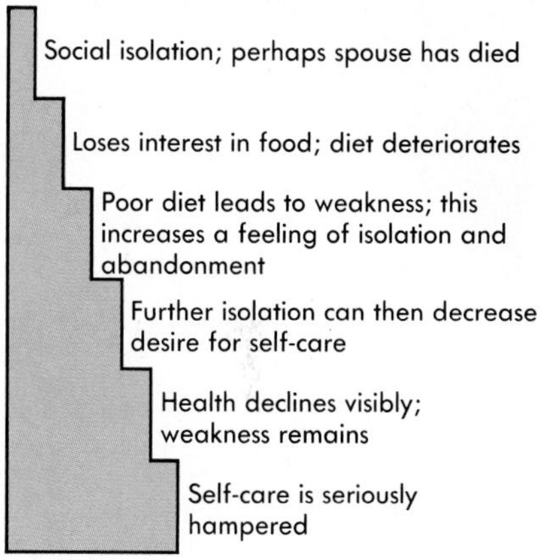

Thirst

Elderly people often partially lose their sense of thirst and in turn don't drink enough fluids. They are then more likely to become dehydrated, a condition that leads to confusion. It is important for them to consume enough fluids, and if necessary, they should be monitored to ensure they do so. About 8 cups of fluid daily is a good goal. An approximate fluid recommendation is the same as for younger adults, 1 milliliter per kcalorie burned.[2] This amount must be adjusted if diuretics are used or fluid is lost through other routes, such as from an **ostomy** (a surgically created opening in the body). Some important signs of dehydration, other than confusion, include dry lips, sunken eyes, increased body temperature, decreased blood pressure, constipation, decreased urine output, and nausea.

The intestinal tract

The main intestinal problem for the elderly is constipation[16] (see Chapter 5 for a review of this problem). To keep the intestinal tract performing efficiently, elderly people generally need to consume more dietary fiber than they may have in their youth, approximately 35 grams a day. They should also drink more fluid to move along masses that could form from high fiber intake. Exercise likewise helps keep things moving smoothly. Because medications can induce constipation, a physician should be consulted if constipation might be related to a medication. If mineral oil is taken as a laxative, it should always be used with caution—and not at mealtimes—because it binds fat-soluble vitamins and limits their absorption.

As we noted earlier, lactase production frequently slows with age. In the Nutrition Insight on p. 141 we list several options for people with lactose intolerance. The stomach slows its acid production as people age, usually limiting, in turn, the synthesis of intrinsic factor. These changes can contribute to poor absorption of vitamin B-12, and eventually, to pernicious anemia.

Less stomach acid may also hamper iron absorption. Other conditions that affect the body's iron status occur with regular use of aspirin, which frequently causes blood loss in the stomach, and use of antacids, which may bind iron. Ulcers and hemorrhoids can also cause blood loss (again, see Chapter 5 for a review). Careful attention to iron status is needed in these cases.

Ostomy • A surgically created short circuit in intestinal flow where the end point usually opens from the abdominal cavity rather than the anus, as in the case with a colostomy.

Social isolation; perhaps spouse has died

Loses interest in food; diet deteriorates

Poor diet leads to weakness; this increases a feeling of isolation and abandonment

Further isolation can then decrease desire for self-care

Health declines visibly; weakness remains

Self-care is seriously hampered

FIGURE 16-5
The descent of poor health in the elderly. This decline needs to be prevented whenever possible.

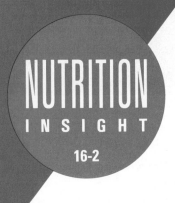

NUTRIENTS AND IMMUNITY

We have frequently mentioned the importance of good nutrition for immune function. Early humans were plagued by famine, infections, and death. Today, because of better nutrition, many of us avoid that cycle. In striving for good nutrition, however, it is easy to go too far. While a proper nutrient intake is needed to maintain immune function, excess quantities do not further boost immunity and can, in fact, decrease it. Let's review some major components of the immune system—the skin, intestinal cells, and white blood cells—and consider how nutrient intake affects each component (Figure 16-6).

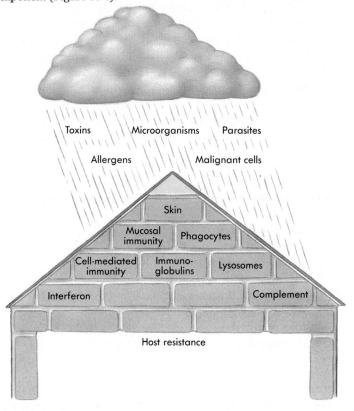

FIGURE 16-6

Host protective factors. The immune system has many arms—all are influenced by nutrient intake.

Skin

The skin forms an almost continuous barrier surrounding the body. Invading microbes have difficulty penetrating the skin. However, if the skin is split by lesions, bacteria can easily penetrate this barrier. Skin health is hampered by deficiencies of such nutrients as essential fatty acids, vitamin A, niacin, and zinc. Vitamin A deficiency also decreases gland secretions in the skin—necessary secretions that contain enzymes capable of killing bacteria. Bacterial eye infections in poorer countries are also often caused by vitamin A deficiency.

Intestinal cells

The cells of the intestines form an important barrier to invading microbes. Not only are the cells closely packed together, but also specialized cells that produce immune bodies are scattered throughout the intestinal tract. These immune bodies bind to the invading microbes, preventing them from entering the bloodstream. When both protein and vitamin A are deficient, the specialized cells produce fewer immune bodies.

For a person in a deficient nutritional state, the intestinal cells break down so that microbes more easily enter the body and cause infections. Two common results of undernutrition are diarrhea and bacterial infections of the bloodstream. To protect the health of the intestinal tract, an adequate nutrient intake is necessary—especially of protein, vitamin A, vitamin B-6, vitamin B-12, vitamin C, zinc, and other nutrients needed for intestinal cell synthesis and maintenance.

Opportunistic Infection
• An infection primarily seen in undernourished or otherwise weakened people.

White blood cells

Once a microbe enters the bloodstream, white blood cells move in to attack it. A variety of white blood cells participate in this response. These agents are notably less active in elderly years, partly because the thymus gland, which processes immune cells, shrinks after sexual maturity. One class of white blood cells matures in the thymus gland. As a group, together with specialized proteins, these cells make various immune bodies to bind, engulf, and digest microorganisms. In the process, they create a template (memory) that allows future recognition of the microbe. Recognition allows more rapid attacks in the future.

Undernutrition and immune function

Nutrient intake affects white blood cells and protein factors. Some white blood cells live only a few days. Their constant resynthesis requires a steady nutrient input. The immune system needs iron to produce an important killing factor that is used; it needs copper for the synthesis of a specific type of white blood cell; and it needs adequate amounts of vitamin C, protein, vitamin B-6, folate, and vitamin B-12 for general cell synthesis and, later, cell activity. Zinc and vitamin A are also needed for the overall growth and development of the immune cells.

One proof that nutrition is important to immune status is the body's response to microbes; microbes normally present in the body usually cause disease only in severely undernourished people. A good example is measles. Your parents probably have had this viral infection and survived. (You were probably vaccinated against measles.) However, many undernourished children who contract it die. Thus the presence of a virus or microbe in the body does not guarantee its triumph over the immune system. But if a person's health is already compromised through undernutrition, the chances of a destructive microbe winning are greater.

An infection that occurs primarily in undernourished people is called an ***opportunistic infection***. Opportunistic infections also are characteristic of acquired immune deficiency syndrome (AIDS), a disease where one class of white blood cells becomes severely depleted. A type of pneumonia that rarely occurs in people with normal immune function is often able to take hold in people with AIDS.

Immune function decreases with age. The effects are very similar to the changes that occur with undernutrition in the elderly. This means that elderly people need to be doubly sure that they meet their nutrient needs so that their immune systems will provide an effective defense against disease.

A note of caution

Many studies show that good nutritional status is associated with good immune status. However, other studies also show that an overabundance of certain nutrients can actually harm the immune system. Too much polyunsaturated fatty acids and vitamin E have been implicated in a decreased immune response in mice. Taking too much zinc (300 milligrams per day for 6 weeks) also appears to decrease immune function. This decrease may be partially caused by zinc interfering with copper absorption. The copper deficiency contributes to decreased synthesis of a specific class of white blood cells.

The message here is that eating a balanced diet will help us maintain the health of all components of our immune systems. Our bodies need this system to continuously defend us from harmful microbes in the environment. However, consuming more nutrients than needed is not going to boost the immune system to higher abilities. In fact, it can harm certain aspects of immune function. ●

Liver, gallbladder, and pancreas

With age, the liver functions less efficiently. When there is a history of significant alcohol consumption, fat buildup in the liver accounts for some decline. If cirrhosis develops, the liver functions even less efficiently (see the Nutrition Issue on p. 525). When liver function deteriorates it cannot efficiently detoxify many medications. The possibility for vitamin A toxicity in turn increases. Elderly people should be warned not to take excessive amounts of vitamin A, since toxic dosages can cause hair loss, malaise, headache, bone pain, liver dysfunction, and a decrease in white blood cell count.

The gallbladder also functions less efficiently as we age. Gallstones may dam up the fluids to be secreted through the gallbladder, causing them to pool and back up into the liver instead. Gallstones can also interfere with fat digestion by allowing less bile into the small intestine. A lowfat diet or even surgery may be necessary.

Although the digestive function of the pancreas may decline with age, the pancreas has a large reserve capacity. A sign of a failing pancreas is high blood glucose, which accumulates under several different conditions. Glucose may circulate in the bloodstream instead of being taken up by cells because the pancreas secretes less insulin or because cells resist insulin actions—especially adipose (fat) cells in obese people. Another cause can be insufficient chromium available in the body. Where appropriate, improved nutrient intake and weight loss can improve insulin action.

Kidney function

Incontinence—the inability to control the muscle responsible for retaining urine—afflicts up to 20% of the elderly living at home and 75% of those in nursing homes. The embarrassment of having to wear diapers causes many to avoid fluids (resulting in dehydration and constipation) and to become socially isolated.

Over time, the kidneys filter wastes more slowly as they lose nephrons (filters). As noted in Chapter 8, kidneys more often deteriorate in people who have regularly eaten excessive protein, and in some cases, excess kcalories (as inferred from studies on laboratory animals). The deterioration significantly decreases the kidneys' ability to excrete the products of protein breakdown. While an increased protein intake of 1 gram per kilogram of desirable body weight has been recommended for physically active elderly people,[12] that recommendation does not apply to people whose decreased kidney function causes urea—a main by-product of protein metabolism—to accumulate in the bloodstream.

Immune function

With age, the immune system often operates less efficiently. Consuming adequate protein and zinc helps maximize the health of the immune system. Recurrent sicknesses and poor wound healing are warning signs of deficient protein and zinc intake. Eating too little food in general or too few animal proteins is usually the reason. Older people often eliminate meat from their diet because it's too hard to chew. Recall that animal proteins are an excellent source of zinc. On the other hand, as we note in Nutrition Insight 16-2, overnutrition also appears to be equally harmful to the immune system. For example, obesity and excessive iron and zinc can suppress the immune system.

Lung function

Lung efficiency declines somewhat with age,[2] and is especially pronounced in elderly people who have smoked and continue to smoke tobacco products. Breathing becomes shallower and faster and more difficult as the number of lung air sacs decreases. Smoking often leads to emphysema and/or lung cancer. The decrease in lung efficiency contributes to a general downward spiral in body function; breathing difficulties limit physical activity and endurance and frequently discourage eating. These changes eventually cancel other efforts to maintain overall health.

Besides not smoking, exercise helps prevent lung problems. People need not lose their capacity to breathe deeply as long as sufficient aerobic exercise is part of their regular routine. Otherwise, merely walking can demand the "exertion" of a marathon pace.[7] Coupled with poor muscle tone and decreased muscle mass, movement becomes continually more difficult. What is the answer? Stay physically active throughout life.

Hearing and vision

Vision and hearing both decline as we age,[2] though hearing impairment occurs mainly in industrial societies with urban traffic, aircraft, loud music, and pile drivers. People differ as to when or if these losses become disabling. Vision and hearing losses can make food shopping difficult. Elderly people may be unable to drive or read food labels. They may also avoid social contacts as much as possible because they can't hear. Poor vision may make them afraid to walk for fear of falling. They may need assistance in shopping.

Decrease in lean tissue

Some muscle cells shrink and others are lost as muscles age; some muscles lose their ability to contract as they accumulate fat and collagen. Lifestyle greatly determines the rate of muscle mass deterioration. As you might predict, an active lifestyle tends to maintain muscle mass, whereas a very inactive one encourages its loss. Weight training has been shown to prevent muscle loss in elderly people.[7] Weight training exercises can also be used to help the elderly regain some muscle strength. But in one study, when older adults stopped the weight training program, any gains in muscle strength were quickly lost. This illustrates the importance of regular exercise throughout life.

Physical activity is also desirable for elderly people because it allows them to eat more food, thereby increasing their chances of consuming an adequate diet. Vitamin and mineral needs do not fall as we age, although food intake may. Another good practice is to decrease sugar and fat consumption in order to increase the diet's nutrient density. An elderly person may need to take a multivitamin and mineral supplement with a physician's guidance if they eat less than 1200 kcalories daily (see the Nutrition Issue on p. 91).

Increases in fat stores

As lean tissue decreases with age, the body often takes on more fat. Some researchers feel that some extra fat stores in the elderly may be fine.[2] Large population studies suggest that in otherwise healthy people, a little fat gain during the adult years does not pose health risks. The booklet accompanying the 1990 Dietary Guidelines allows ranges for healthy body weights at a given height to climb by 11 to 18 pounds once a person is over 35 years of age. The greater amounts are for taller people (Table 16-3). However, obesity is not desirable because it can raise blood pressure and blood glucose levels, as well as make it more difficult to walk and to care for oneself.

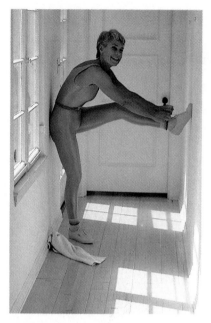
Age is no reason to stop exercising.

ANOTHER BITE In early adulthood and middle age, significant weight gain is a major problem. In the late elderly years, weight loss is more of a concern. Weight loss in elderly people often means increased risk of death. It may also indicate increased sickness and poor tolerance of medications. When assessing weight in elderly people, compare present weight with the previous year's weight.[8]

Cardiovascular health

The heart often pumps blood less efficiently in elderly people, usually because they have become less physically active. Poor heart conditioning allows fatty and connective tissues to infiltrate the heart's muscular wall. This decline in

Cardiac Output • The amount of blood pumped by the heart.

cardiac output is not inevitable with aging and does not occur among elderly people who remain physically active.

Heart attack and stroke—the major causes of death in all adults—are caused primarily by atherosclerosis and high blood pressure. As one ages, atherosclerotic plaque accumulates in the arteries, reducing their elasticity, constricting blood flow, and consequently, elevating blood pressure.

You already know the main way to limit the build up of atherosclerotic plaque—keep the serum cholesterol level below 200 milligrams per 100 milliliters. New evidence is even showing that strict diet control can cause some plaque to disappear.[13] Other studies use diet and medications or surgery to lower blood cholesterol levels, which, in turn, reduces the amount of plaque in the arteries supplying the heart. This suggests that a heart-healthy diet is more important during adult and elderly years than researchers previously thought.

High blood pressure—heavily implicated in both stroke and heart attack—can be lowered in most people by severe sodium restriction. A limit of 2 grams of sodium helps almost all people with hypertension, but that is a difficult diet to plan and follow. Alternatively, a mild sodium restriction (not to exceed 4 grams of sodium daily), while effective for salt-sensitive people, is not so helpful for those who are not sensitive. (The Nutrition Issue on p. 332 reviews the effects of other nutrients on blood pressure.)

We can do much to prevent heart attack and stroke just by eating nutritiously, walking briskly or exercising regularly, controlling blood pressure, and avoiding smoking.

Bone health

In Chapter 10 we discussed the decline in bone density associated with aging. Recall that bone loss in women occurs especially after menopause. Bone loss

TABLE 16-3

Suggested weights for adults

Height*	Weight in Pounds†	
	19 to 34 Years	35 Years and Over
5'0"	97-128‡	108-138
5'1"	101-132	111-143
5'2"	104-137	115-148
5'3"	107-141	119-152
5'4"	111-146	122-157
5'5"	114-150	126-162
5'6"	118-155	130-167
5'7"	121-160	134-172
5'8"	125-164	138-178
5'9"	129-169	142-183
5'10"	132-174	146-188
5'11"	136-179	151-194
6'0"	140-184	155-199
6'1"	144-189	159-205
6'2"	148-195	164-210
6'3"	152-200	168-216
6'4"	156-205	173-222
6'5"	160-211	177-228
6'6"	164-216	182-234

*Without shoes.
†Without clothes.
‡The higher weights in the ranges generally apply to men, who tend to have more muscle and bone; the lower weights more often apply to women, who have less muscle and bone.
From USDA/DHHS: *Dietary Guidelines for Americans,* 1990.

in men is slow and steady from middle age throughout the elderly years. For women, increasing calcium intake to 1500 milligrams per day can help maintain density in some types of bones, but it does not predictably prevent bone loss from the spine. Presently, only estrogen replacement therapy, active vitamin D hormone (calcitriol) therapy, and calcitonin therapy—administered with a physician's guidance—can claim that. From laboratory animal studies we infer that performing weight-bearing exercises also helps sustain bone.

If osteoporosis becomes very severe, it limits the ability of elderly people to exercise, shop, prepare food, and live normally.[17] They eat less and get fewer nutrients. There is additional concern that many elderly may suffer from hidden osteomalacia, a condition that occurs primarily when there is not enough sun exposure and possibly poor vitamin D synthesis in the skin.[6] When they can't get regular sun exposure—during the winter or when they are homebound—elderly people need a source for 10 micrograms (400 IU) of vitamin D per day. Either fortified milk products or a vitamin supplement can provide this amount.

OTHER FACTORS THAT INFLUENCE NUTRIENT NEEDS IN THE ELDERLY
Medications

Medications and old age often go together. Medications can improve health and quality of life, but some of them also profoundly affect nutrient needs in the elderly (Table 16-4). Forty-five percent of the elderly population regularly take multiple prescription drugs; many drugs affect appetite or absorption of nutrients.[15] Often, during later years people must take several medications for long periods of time. They should make sure to work with their physician and pharmacist to coordinate all medications taken.[1] Pharmacists can advise when to take drugs—with or between meals—for greatest effectiveness.[15]

Drug-related nutritional problems include (1) increased need for potassium when certain types of diuretics leach it out of the body and (2) changes in appetite caused by antidepressant agents or certain antibiotics. Blood loss from long-term use of aspirin or aspirin-like medications strains iron reserves and can lead to anemia.[15] We recommend that people who must take one or more medications for more than just a few weeks should closely watch their diets, eating nutrient-dense foods and possibly taking needed supplements to counteract effects of certain medications.

Depression and mental state

About 12% to 14% of elderly people experience significant depression. That, combined with isolation and loneliness as family and friends either die, move away, or become less mobile, frequently contributes to apathetic eating and weight loss in older people. People living alone do not necessarily make poor food choices, but they often eat fewer kcalories in part from skipping meals, especially men.[5] Depression can be a downward spiral where poor appetite produces weakness that leads to even poorer appetite. In the elderly, the resulting poor nutritional state can produce further mental confusion and increased isolation and loneliness[4,21] (Figure 16-5).

The role of nutrition in preserving mental function in the elderly remains unclear. Specific nutritional deficiencies of thiamin, niacin, vitamin B-6, and vitamin B-12, as well as excessive alcohol use, cause well-recognized central nervous system disorders. However, the subtle effects of eating minimal kcalories, leading to semistarvation, are often overlooked. In addition, as mentioned earlier, a poor fluid intake may lead to dehydration and, in turn, to confusion.[2]

We know mental illness can lead to a poor nutritional state, but the extent to which subtle nutritional deficiencies can lead to a poor mental state is not clear. It is important to prevent overt nutrient deficiencies, especially those

TABLE 16-4

Potential drug-nutrient interactions for some commonly used drugs

Drug	Use	Nutrient	Potential Side Effect
Alcohol	—	Thiamin, vitamin B-6, folate, and zinc	Poor absorption/poor utilization
Antacids (Maalox)	Reduce stomach acidity	Calcium, vitamin B-12 and iron	Decreased absorption due to altered gastrointestinal pH
Anticoagulants (coumadin)	Prevention of blood clots	Vitamin K	Poor utilization
Antihistamines (Benedryl)	Treatment of allergies and nausea; as local anesthetic	—	Weight gain
Beta-blocker (propanolol [Inderal])	Decrease hypertension	(Cholesterol)	Some can increase serum cholesterol levels
Aspirin	Anti-inflammatory, pain reduction	Iron	Anemia from blood loss
Cathartics (laxatives)	To induce bowel movement	Calcium, potassium	Poor absorption
Cholestyramine	Reducing blood cholesterol	Vitamins A, D, E, K	Poor absorption
Cimetidine (Tagamet)	Treatment of ulcers	Vitamin B-12	Poor absorption
Colchicine	Treatment of gout	Vitamin B-12, carotenes, and magnesium	Decreased absorption due to damaged intestinal mucosa
Corticosteroids (prednisone)	Anti-inflammatory	Zinc / Calcium	Poor absorption / Poor utilization
Furosemide (Lasix)	Potassium-wasting diuretic	Potassium and sodium	Increased loss
Isoniazid (INH)	Tuberculosis	Vitamin B-6	Poor utilization
Neomycin	Antibiotic	Fat, protein, sodium, potassium, calcium, iron, and vitamin B-12	Decreases pancreatic lipase, binds bile salts, and so interferes with absorption
MAO inhibitors (Parnate)	Antidepressant	(Tyramine in aged foods)	Hypertension caused by poor tyramine metabolism
Phenobarbital	Sedative; treatment of epilepsy	Vitamin D and folate	Reduced metabolism and utilization
Phenytoin (Dilantin)	Treatment of epilepsy	Vitamin D and folate	Reduced metabolism and utilization
Tricyclic antidepressants (Elavil)	Antidepressant	—	Weight gain due to appetite stimulation

Modified from Chernoff R: Aging and nutrition, *Nutrition Today* March/April, 1987, p 4.

mentioned above. Whether taking extra amounts of specific amino acids, such as tryptophan or tyrosine, and choline can increase synthesis of chemical messengers in the brain and therefore alter behavior is still unknown.

CONCEPT CHECK

Nutritional problems of the elderly often accompany chronic diseases and intensify as organ function decreases over time. As we age, our senses of taste, smell, thirst, hearing, and sight lose some sensitivity; our abilities to digest and absorb lose efficiency; our organs—liver, gallbladder, pancreas, kidneys, lungs, and heart—work less effectively; and our immune systems gradually lose capacity. In addition, muscle mass declines (largely because of inactivity), and bone mass gradually decreases. Diet changes and regular exercise can often help reduce the extent and impact of these typical results of aging.

DO THE RDA INCREASE IN THE ELDERLY YEARS?

Currently, the RDA for nutrients and kcalories includes one category for both men and women who are 51 years of age and older. Kcalorie recommendations assume an active lifestyle—a characteristic the RDA committee supports. Nutrient recommendations have largely been projected from studies of young adults. Scientists know very little about the nutrient needs of the elderly, especially for those over age 75 years.[2] Only during the last few years has much research focused on this question. Since the RDA applies only to healthy people, many elderly people—for example those with ulcers and heavy aspirin users—are not covered by the RDA. Indeed it is particularly tricky to evolve an RDA valid for most older people because many of them are ill and/or regularly take medications.

Recently, a noted research team suggested that the current RDA for healthy elderly people is probably too high for vitamin A; too low in protein (for the active elders), vitamins D, B-6, and B-12, and about right for the other nutrients.[18] In this case, the about right category may reflect either that studies suggest the RDA is adequate, or that we lack studies to make a more definitive statement. Still, a well-planned diet that follows the Guide to Daily Food Choices can meet all nutrient needs of the elderly (Table 16-5). Only when kcalorie intake is around 1500 or below should supplements be routinely advised.[11]

There is a concern that the RDA for calcium should be increased to help slow the acceleration of bone loss suffered by elderly women. Although taking extra calcium may affect only bone loss occurring in specific areas of the body, it is still better than doing nothing at all. Still, the focus on calcium is best directed to adolescents, who are building life-long supplies.

Elderly women need less iron because they no longer menstruate. However, chronic ulcers, hemorrhoids, and aspirin use may necessitate an increased iron intake.

Overall, nutrient needs for the elderly resemble those for younger adults, but individual modifications are necessary to compensate for specific diseases.

Planning a diet for the elderly

To supply energy needs for males 51 years of age and older, the recommendation is 2300 kcalories; for females, the recommendation is 1900 kcalories. Studies show that elderly men eat closer to 1600 to 1900 kcalories, while women eat about 1250 to 1550 kcalories.

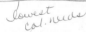
lowest cal. needs

TABLE 16-5

Sample diet of nutrient-dense food choices for the elderly that meets all RDA for 1600 kcalories

Breakfast	Lunch
1 cup Crispy Wheat 'n Raisins	Turkey sandwich
1 cup 1% milk	2 slices whole-wheat bread
1 orange	2 ounces roasted turkey
tea or coffee, if desired	breast
	mustard
	1 banana
	1 oatmeal raisin cookie
Dinner	1 cup 1% milk
Salad	
1 cup romaine lettuce	
½ cup tomatoes	
2 tablespoons Italian dressing	
¼ cup sunflower seeds	
4 ounces lean roast beef	
½ cup brown rice with au juis	
¾ cup carrot sticks	
1 oatmeal raisin cookie	

NOTE: This diet follows the Guide to Daily Food Choices discussed in Chapter 2.

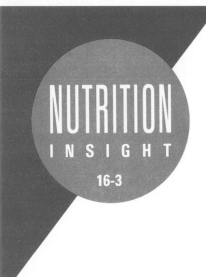

ALZHEIMER'S DISEASE

Alzheimer's Disease has become a dreaded possibility for many people approaching old age. Many of us have had first-hand experience as loved ones have been "lost" to this form of progressive *dementia*. Although it seems a disease of the times— with more and more people both in nursing homes or in families that devote more time to caring for these people—the disease has been around for quite awhile.

In 1907 Dr. Alois Alzheimer documented several cases of what seemed to be early senility. Typical symptoms of the disease included personality changes, unreasonable fears, outbursts, and general forgetfulness. Today, the disease Dr. Alzheimer first described affects about 3 to 4 million people in the United States— this includes about 25% of all people over age 85 and 50% of all people in nursing homes.[23]

More reports diagnosing Alzheimer's disease surface every day. Is this a disease of modern society or has it always been around but we didn't know how to diagnose it? Old age is often accompanied by a general decline in mental function. But what makes Alzheimer's disease different is that it can be diagnosed specifically by the presence of special protein deposits and tangled masses of nerves in the brain in areas linked to memory and thinking. However, this type of diagnosis can be done only at autopsy, and so it is difficult to know precisely how many cases of dementia in old age are actually the Alzheimer's type. Clinical assessments can be made, and as we know more about the typical course of the disease, these methods have become more reliable.[23]

Causes and physical effects

In general terms, Alzheimer's disease is best described as a progressive brain disorder marked by an inability to remember, reason, or understand what is going on. Age is the primary risk factor. Scientists propose causes including altered cell development, altered brain proteins, and unidentified blood-borne agents. Genetic predisposition is closely linked to a minor form that occurs at about age 40.[3] Aluminum is highly concentrated in abnormal protein accumulations in the brain, but the aluminum is more likely an effect than a cause of the disease. Whether there are other, as yet unknown, causes remains to be seen.

Alzheimer's is a progressive disease. Its course has been divided into three stages, although these can vary in duration and intensity with individuals. Generally it begins as (1) confusion, depression, anxiety, and short-term memory loss; (2) develops into long-term memory loss and problems in communication and perception; and (3) the individual with Alzheimer's disease may eventually become bedridden and completely dependent.[3] Death is frequently attributable to bacterial infection or pneumonia associated with accidental food inhalation.

Treatment

Today, treatment of Alzheimer's disease is usually limited to the use of antidepressants and other drugs that target related symptoms of the disease. Therapies cur-

Diet plans for the elderly should focus on nutrient density, especially on the nutrients vitamin D along with sun exposure, vitamins E, B-6, B-12, C, and thiamin, and the minerals iron, calcium, and zinc. A sample diet that meets all these needs appears in Table 16-5. Ideally, some protein should come from lean meats to help meet vitamin B-6 and zinc needs, two nutrients of special concern. Because physical activity simultaneously increases appetite and uses kcalories, it allows the exerciser to eat more. Taking in more nutrients in general then simplifies the planning of an adequate diet.

Fluid needs are 1 milliliter per kcalorie burned. A high-fiber diet can decrease

rently under investigation range from simple aspirin to overlapping doses of potent, synthetically produced brain chemicals.[22] But, in order to prevent a disease, we generally need to understand its causes. And unfortunately, we don't yet know as much as we need to about Alzheimer's disease.

Nutrition considerations

The main nutrition goal for people with this disease is a healthy diet that maintains body weight. Forgetfulness may lead to irregular eating habits with associated weight loss. Because one characteristic of Alzheimer's disease is the death of cells that secrete the brain chemical acetylcholine, scientists once thought that a diet that provided choline and the related compound lecithin might correct this deficit. However, studies have found this to have no effect on Alzheimer's patients.[23]

Abnormal food behaviors, such as gorging, are often seen early in the course of Alzheimer's disease. A craving for sweets may lead to a temporary weight gain that can be managed by offering lower kcalorie snacks and meals. At the other extreme there is often a partial or complete refusal to eat. Frequent, small meals and nutrient-dense snacks using favorite foods when possible may encourage more regular eating. People who are still leading reasonably independent lives may not be able to shop or to remember to eat meals. Congregate feeding programs and home-delivered meals may be helpful during the early stages of disease. Keep in mind that by the time the disease has been diagnosed, some people have already developed nutritional problems (see later section).

With the progression of the disease, there is more confusion and distractibility. At this stage, it is wise for others to oversee food planning and mealtimes. Measures should be taken to control distractions, such as television, radio, children, pets, and the telephone, that can disrupt a meal for someone with Alzheimer's disease. Others should monitor food temperatures because victims may ignore discomfort and burn themselves. Tough, crunchy foods that may easily cause choking should be avoided. For those still capable of self-feeding, assistance devices should be used when appropriate: roller-rocker knives, bowls, plate guards, a damp washcloth under the plate to prevent skidding, cups with tops, flexible straws, and large bibs. These are available at medical supply houses. As people with Alzheimer's disease become less able to manage eating by themselves, it becomes more of a challenge to those trying to feed them. They may hold food in the mouth, forget how to eat or to swallow, spit out food, and play with and then refuse food.[3]

All of us need to pay attention to dietary recommendations to promote and maintain health. People with Alzheimer's disease may not be able to do this on their own. In later stages of this disease, people may not be tuned in to their own needs. The responsibility for providing good nutrition will ultimately fall to family, health care providers, and nursing home staff.

The fastest-growing segment of the population is made up of people 85 and older. Thus in the future Alzheimer's disease could have devastating consequences for America's already strained health-care system. The disease also takes an immense emotional toll on its victims and their family members[3] (Figure 16-7). ●

Dementia • General loss or decrease in mental function.

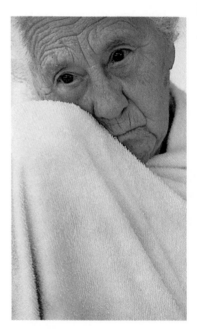

FIGURE 16-7
Alzheimer's disease. One in ten people over age 65 may have Alzheimer's disease. This ratio poses dire implications for public health in the future.

constipation, but fiber intake should be slowly increased to about 35 grams, making sure a glass of water (or other fluid) accompanies each dose of fiber.

Singles of all ages face logistical problems with foods: purchasing, preparing, storing, and using foods with minimal waste are challenges. Economy packages of meats and vegetables are normally too large to be useful for a single person. Many singles live in small dwellings, some without kitchens and freezers. Gearing a diet to accommodate a limited budget, limited facilities, and a single appetite requires special considerations.

Following are some practical suggestions for diet planning for singles:

- If you own a freezer, cook large amounts, divide into portions, and freeze.

- Buy only what you can use; small containers may be expensive, but letting food spoil also is costly.
- Ask the grocer to break open a family-sized package of wrapped meat or fresh vegetables.
- Buy only several pieces of a fruit—perhaps a ripe one, a medium-ripe one, and an unripe one—so that the fruit can be eaten over a period of several days.
- Keep a box of dry milk handy to add a nutritious punch to recipes for baked goods and whatever other foods for which this addition is acceptable.

Regularly taking vitamin and mineral supplements can be expensive—an important consideration for people on fixed, and possibly inadequate, incomes. Too much of some supplements can lead to toxicity. Between about 35% and 70% of elderly people regularly take supplements, some at potentially toxic levels. If supplements are necessary, the elderly person should then work closely with a physician to determine which nutrients to include and the least amounts that are necessary.

Feeding sick, infirm, and/or mentally confused people is time-consuming and demanding work that requires special training. Friends, relatives, and health personnel should look for poor nutrient intake in all the elderly, even in those who live in nursing home settings. Note that about 5% of the elderly live in nursing homes. The figure jumps to about 20% for those over age 85. Research projects that 43% of adults now age 65 will spend some time in a nursing home. Family members have a unique opportunity to make sure nutrient needs of the elderly are met by looking for weight maintenance based on regular healthy meal patterns. If problems arise in instituting a healthful diet, registered dietitians can offer professional and personalized advice.

From surveys it appears that the majority of elderly people like most vegeta-

---

TABLE 16-6

Guidelines for promoting healthful eating in later years

- Eat regularly; small frequent meals may be best.
- Find out which convenience foods and labor-saving devices can be of help.
- Try new foods, new seasonings, and new ways of preparing foods. Don't just use convenience foods and canned goods.
- Keep some easy-to-prepare foods on hand for times when tired.
- Add nonfat dry milk to recipes for baked goods and other appropriate foods to boost nutrition value.
- Have a treat occasionally, perhaps an expensive cut of meat or a favorite fresh fruit.
- Eat in a well-lit or sunny area; serve meals attractively; use foods with different flavors, colors, shapes, and textures.
- Arrange things so food preparation and clean-up are easier.
- Eat with friends, relatives, or at a senior center when possible.
- Share cooking responsibilities with a neighbor.
- Use community resources for help in shopping and other daily care needs.
- Stay physically active.
- If possible, take a walk before eating to stimulate appetite.
- When necessary, chop, grind, or blend hard-to-chew foods. Softer, protein-rich foods can be substituted for meat when poor dental function limits normal food intake.
- If eating movements are limited, cut the food ahead of time, use utensils with deep sides or handles, and obtain more specialized utensils if needed.

bles, despite misconceptions that older people do not like broccoli because it forms gas or tomatoes because they contain too much acid. By the time we reach adulthood, our eating habits reflect regional tastes, social class, ethnic group, and life experiences. There is no generic food list for the elderly.[4]

Overall, good nutrition benefits the elderly in many ways. It delays some disease progression; improves management of some existing diseases; hastens recovery from many illnesses; can increase mental, physical, and social well-being; and often decreases the need for and length of hospitalization. Overall, a good nutritional intake should be a vital part of the health maintenance program for elderly people. A variety of strategies can promote healthful eating in the elderly years (Table 16-6). These should focus on presenting nutritious, tasty foods in a pleasant, friendly environment.

COMMUNITY NUTRITION SERVICES FOR THE ELDERLY

Health care advice and services for the elderly can come from clinics, private practitioners, hospitals, and health maintenance organizations. Home health care agencies, adult day-care programs, adult overnight-care programs, and *hospice* centers (for the terminally ill) can supply day-to-day care.

Hospice • Hospital care that emphasizes comfort and dignity in death.

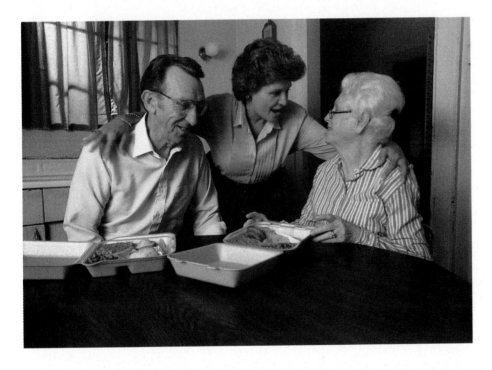

The home-delivered meals program represents a gift of nutrition and caring by a community to its elderly citizens.

Nutrition programs for those age 60 and over offer congregate meal programs, which provide lunch at a central location, and home-delivered meals (often known as Meals-On-Wheels if sponsored by local private or public agencies). Federal commodity distribution is available in some areas of the United States to low income elderly people. Food stamps can also aid the elderly who live below the poverty level. Food cooperatives and a variety of clubs and social organizations provide additional aid to the elderly. The congregate meal programs and home-delivered meals are funded partially by the U.S. government under Title III of the Older Americans Act (Figure 16-8) and through volunteer community efforts.

The U.S. government sets specific standards for home-served meals and for those served in congregate feeding centers. The meals are designed to provide one-third of the RDA. The basic meal pattern is 3 ounces of meat or meat alternative, 2.5 cups of fruit or vegetable, 1 slice of bread or alternative, 1 teaspoon

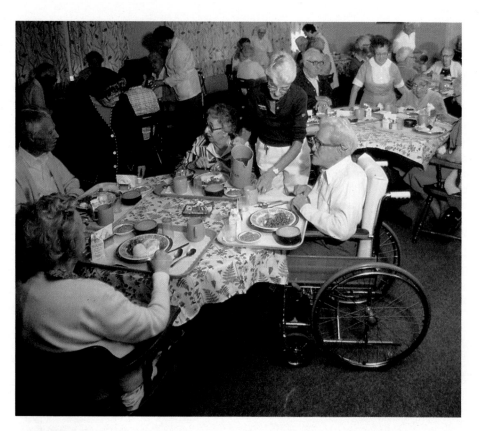

FIGURE 16-8
Congregate meals for the elderly. Sites in many communities in the United States provide nutritious meals and an opportunity to socialize for elderly people.

of butter or margarine, 1 cup of milk, and ½ cup of dessert. Foods rich in vitamin A and vitamin C are emphasized. The social aspect often improves an elderly person's appetite and general outlook.

Many eligible elderly are missing meals and are poorly nourished simply because they don't know of available programs. Irregular meal patterns and weight loss, often because of difficulties in preparing foods, are warning signs that this may be the case. An effort should be made to identify and inform these people of community services.

The ideal is to remain healthy and to live independently for as long as possible without becoming socially isolated. Personal living situations can greatly determine whether an elderly person is well-nourished. For some, just getting to the store or having to carry groceries may be a major problem. Relatives and friends can be a real help. Special transportation arrangements may also be available through a local transit company or taxi service.

Studies have found that congregate meal programs can positively influence the nutritional status of otherwise homebound people. Still, congregate meal programs provide at most one meal a day, and usually not every day of the week. So if people come to depend on them exclusively, they eat too few meals. The problem with home-delivered meals is that they may never be eaten, and if not eaten on delivery and left at room temperature, they may become unsafe to eat later. Thus these programs help the elderly, but even more help still is needed.

CONCEPT CHECK

Specific nutrient requirements for the elderly are only now being extensively studied. Diet plans for the elderly should be modified for decreased physical abilities, presence of drug-nutrient interactions, possible depression, and economic constraints. Particular attention should be paid to sun exposure and intake of the vitamins D, E, B-6, B-12, C, and thiamin, as well as the minerals iron, calcium, and zinc. A nutrient-dense diet helps to meet these needs. In the United States many nutrition services, such as congregate and home delivered meals are available to help the elderly population obtain a healthy diet.

SUMMARY

- A goal for all of us should be to delay symptoms of and disabilities from chronic diseases for as many years as possible. Good nutritional habits—especially following the Guide to Daily Food Choices and Dietary Guidelines—play a role in this process.

- A basic plan for health promotion and disease prevention includes eating a proper diet, exercising regularly, abstaining from smoking, limiting alcohol intake, and limiting stress.

- The 1990 Dietary Guidelines for Americans recommend that individuals eat a variety of foods; maintain desirable weight; choose a diet low in fat, saturated fat, and cholesterol; choose a diet rich in vegetables, fruits, and grains; use salt and sugar in moderation; and, drink alcoholic beverages in moderation for those who do so. Genetic background, medical conditions, and other lifestyle practices influence a person's optimal diet.

- While life span has not changed, life expectancy has increased dramatically over the past century. For societies this means an increasing proportion of the population is over 65 years of age. As health care costs rise, the goal of delaying disease becomes even more important for all of us.

- Aging begins before birth. Cell aging probably results from automatic cellular changes and environmental influences, such as DNA damage. Add to this list damage caused by electron-seeking compounds, hormonal changes, and alterations in the immune system as possible causes.

- Nutritional problems of the elderly are related to the presence of chronic diseases and to the normal decreases in organ function that occur with time. These include loss of teeth, lessened sensitivity in the senses of taste and smell, changes in gastrointestinal tract function, and deterioration in heart and bone health. Although disease affects nutritional state, the reverse is also true. Immune function is adversely affected by undernutrition, setting the stage for infection.

- Alzheimer's disease is a progressive and irreversible brain disorder. Its causes are unknown. It differs from other types of senile dementia in that the brain tissue accumulates protein plaques and tangled nerves (observable by autopsy). Nutritional health for people in advanced stages of disease is often complicated by special feeding problems.

- Specific nutrient needs for the elderly are only now being studied extensively. Diet plans should be based on a nutrient-dense approach and individualized for present health problems, decreased physical abilities, presence of drug-nutrient interactions, possible depression, and economic constraints. Specific nutrients, such as vitamins D, E, B-6, C, B-12, and thiamin, as well as the minerals iron, zinc and calcium, often deserve special attention in diet planning.

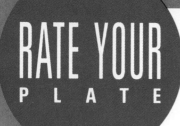

RATE YOUR PLATE

Most people, during their lifetimes, usually eat meals with families or loved ones. As elderly people reach even older ages, many of them are faced with living and eating alone. In a study of the diets of 4400 older Americans, one man of every five living alone and over age 55 was eating poorly. One of four women between ages 55 and 64 years was following a low-quality diet. These poor diets can contribute to deterioration of mental and physical health. Consider the following example of the living situation of an elderly person:

Neal, a 70-year-old man, lives alone in a house in a local suburban area. He lost his wife 1 year ago. He doesn't have many friends; his wife was his primary confidant. His neighbors across the street and adjacent are friendly, and Neal used to help them with yard projects in his spare time. Neal's health has been good, but he has trouble with his teeth recently. His diet has been poor, and in the last 3 months his physical and mental vigor has deteriorated. He has been slowly lapsing into a depression and so keeps the shades drawn and rarely leaves his house. Neal keeps very little food in the house because his wife did most of the cooking and shopping and he just isn't that interested in food.

If you were one of Neal's relatives and learned of Neal's situation, what six things could you do or suggest to help improve his nutritional status and mental outlook? Look back into the chapter to get some ideas.

1. _____

_____

2. _____

_____

_____

3. _____

_____

4. _____

_____

5. _____

_____

6. _____

_____

REFERENCES

1. The American Dietetic Association: Nutrition, aging, and the continuum of health care: technical support paper, *Journal of the American Dietetic Association* 87:345, 1987.
2. Chernoff R: Aging and nutrition, *Nutrition Today*, March/April, 1987, p 4.
3. Claggett MS: Nutritional factors relevant to Alzheimer's disease, *Journal of the American Dietetic Association* 89:392, 1989.
4. Davies L: Practical nutrition for the elderly, *Nutrition Reviews* 46:83, 1988.
5. Davis MA and others: Living arrangements and dietary quality of older US adults, *Journal of the American Dietetic Association* 90:1667, 1990.
6. Delvin EE: Vitamin D nutritional status and related biochemical indices in autonomous elderly population, *American Journal of Clinical Nutrition* 48:373, 1988.
7. Fiatarone MA and others: High-intensity strength training in nonagenarians, *Journal of the American Medical Association* 263:3029, 1990.
8. Fischer J, Johnson MA: Low body weight and weight loss in the aged, *Journal of the American Dietetic Association* 90:1697, 1990.
9. Goldstein S and others: Biologic theories of aging, *American Family Physician* 40(3):195, 1989.
10. Leaf A: The aging process: lessons from observations in man, *Nutrition Reviews* 46:40, 1988.
11. McIntosh WA and others: The relationship between beliefs about nutrition and dietary practices of the elderly, *Journal of American Dietetic Association* 90:671, 1990.
12. Munro HN and others: Nutritional requirements of the elderly, *Annual Reviews of Nutrition* 7:23, 1987.
13. Ornish D: Can lifestyle changes reverse coronary heart disease? *Lancet* 336:129, 1990.
14. Paffenbarger RS and others: Physical activity, all-cause mortality, and longevity of college alumni, *The New England Journal of Medicine* 314:605, 1986.
15. Roe DA: Therapeutic affects of drug-nutrient interactions in the elderly, *Journal of the American Dietetic Association* 85:174, 1985.
16. Shamburek RD, JT Farrar: Disorders of the digestive system in the elderly, *The New England Journal of Medicine* 322:438, 1990.
17. Stehlin D: Women and nutrition, *FDA Consumer* January/February, 1991, p 11.
18. Suter BM, Russell RM: Vitamin requirements of the elderly, *American Journal of Clinical Nutrition* 45:501, 1987.
19. U.S. Preventive Service Task Force: Screening for alcohol and other drug abuse, *American Family Physician* 40(1):137, 1989.
20. Walford RL and others: Dietary restriction and aging: historical phases, mechanisms and current directions, *Journal of Nutrition* 117:1650, 1987.
21. Walker D, Beauchene RE: The relationship of loneliness, social isolation, and physical health to dietary adequacy of independently living elderly, *Journal of the American Dietetics Association* 91:300, 1991.
22. Warshaw GA: New perspectives in the management of Alzheimer's disease, *American Family Physician* 42(5):41S, 1990.
23. Weiss R: Toward a future with memory, *Science News* 137:120, 1990.
24. Wilson JD and others: *Harrison's principles of internal medicine*, New York, 1991, McGraw-Hill.

HOW MUCH HAVE I LEARNED?

What have you learned from Chapter 16? Here are 15 statements about nutrition for the older adult. Read them to test your current knowledge. If you think the answer is true or mostly true, circle T. If you think the answer is false or mostly false, circle F. Use the scoring key at the end of the book to compute your total score. To review, take this test again later, and especially before tests.

1. **T** **F** The maximum age at which people die has increased dramatically.

2. **T** **F** Elderly adults should exercise regularly to try to slow loss of muscle mass.

3. **T** **F** Medications taken by the elderly can cause nutritional problems.

4. **T** **F** People over age 65 years account for more than half the health care costs in the United States.

5. **T** **F** Optimal diets can stop the aging process.

6. **T** **F** The senses of taste and smell usually increase with age.

7. **T** **F** Older people often lose their desire for liquids.

8. **T** **F** Vitamin B-12 absorption often decreases in elderly people.

9. **T** **F** The most frequently occurring intestinal problem in the elderly is constipation.

10. **T** **F** An excessive intake of vitamin A supplements in the elderly can cause bone pain and hair loss.

11. **T** **F** Poor wound healing should alert a clinician to examine the protein, zinc, and vitamin C intakes of an elderly person.

12. **T** **F** An active lifestyle tends to maintain muscle mass.

13. **T** **F** People over 65 years of age are quite similar in physical capabilities.

14. **T** **F** Cirrhosis of the liver can result from a practice of drinking seven beers a day.

15. **T** **F** Zinc enhances the immune system and can be safely taken in high doses by the elderly.

ETHANOL—ITS METABOLISM AND POTENTIAL TO INFLUENCE HEALTH

Alcoholism is an important issue for all adults to carefully examine. From early adulthood through elderly years, alcohol's ability to tear away at nutritional and overall health is enormous.

Alcohol absorption and action

After someone swallows an alcoholic beverage, their blood level of alcohol rises rapidly. Alcohol, also known as ethanol, is readily absorbed into the blood from all levels of the gastrointestinal tract. You've probably been warned—with good reason—not to drink on an empty stomach. Alcohol absorption depends partly on the rate of stomach emptying. Food, particularly fat, slows the stomach's emptying rate and stimulates secretions. These dilute the alcohol and slow its absorption into the bloodstream.

Some alcohol is metabolized in the cells lining the stomach, especially in men. Most of the remaining alcohol is metabolized in the liver.[24] About 10% of the ethanol in the body is directly eliminated by diffusion through the kidneys or lungs.

Alcohol affects the brain more than any other organ. Acting as a sedative, alcohol tends to relieve the drinker's anxiety, slur speech, reduce coordination in walking, impair judgment, and encourage uninhibited behavior. Because it lowers inhibitions, alcohol appears to act as a stimulant, but in fact it is a powerful depressant to the body. As William Shakespeare wrote: "It stirs up desire, but takes away the performance." Because it cuts off secretion of the body's antidiuretic hormone, alcohol increases urination (see Chapter 10). It also causes the blood vessels to dilate, releasing body heat.

Metabolism

A social drinker who weighs 150 pounds and has normal liver function metabolizes about 7 to 14 grams (the equivalent of ½ to 1 beer) of alcohol per hour (100 to 200 milligrams of alcohol per kilogram of body weight per hour). If a person drinks slightly less alcohol each hour than the amount that can be metabolized by the liver, the blood alcohol content remains low. In that case, a person can drink large amounts of alcohol over long periods of time without becoming noticeably intoxicated. When the rate of alcohol consumption exceeds the liver's metabolic capacity, the blood alcohol content rises and symptoms of intoxication appear (Table 16-7).

When a man and woman of similar size drink the same amount of alcohol, the woman retains more alcohol in her bloodstream; women cannot metabolize as much alcohol in their stomach cells. They have lower levels of the key alcohol-metabolizing enzyme, alcohol dehydrogenase. Women are also much quick-

TABLE 16-7

Blood alcohol levels and symptoms

Level (mg/dl)	Sporadic Drinker	Chronic Drinker
50 (party level)	Congenial euphoria; decreased tension	No observable effect
75	Gregarious	Often no effect
100 (0.1%)	Uncoordinated; legally drunk (as in drunk driving) in most states; a level of 0.08% is legal drunkenness in some stricter locations	Minimal signs
125-150	Unrestrained behavior; episodic dyscontrol; legally drunk at 0.15% in all states	Pleasurable euphoria or beginning of incoordination
200-250	Alertness lost; lethargic	Effort required to maintain emotional and motor control
300-350	Stupor to coma	Drowsy and slow
>500	Some will die	Coma

Modified from Wyngaarder JB and Smith LH: *Cecil textbook of medicine*, Philadelphia 1988, WB Saunders.

While the liver is metabolizing alcohol, it cannot rapidly metabolize medications, such as sedatives. Consequently, high amounts of alcohol mixed with some sedatives may cause a person to lapse into coma and die.

er to develop alcohol-related ailments, such as cirrhosis of the liver, than are men with the same drinking history.

When a person drinks a lot of alcohol, alcohol dehydrogenase in the liver cannot break it all down. For this and other reasons, another liver enzyme system begins to metabolize alcohol. The liver usually uses the same system to metabolize medications and other "foreign" compounds. Once the extra system is activated, alcohol tolerance increases since the rate of alcohol metabolism increases.[19]

Alcohol and overall health

About 32% of all Americans have three drinks or less each week, 22% have two drinks or less a day. Only 11% have more than two drinks a day. Although the public health impact of alcohol abuse is still being calculated, in and of itself, misuse of alcohol is one of the most preventable health problems in the United States. Drinking alcohol excessively contributes significantly to 5 of the 10 leading causes of death in the United States—certain forms of cancer, cirrhosis of the liver, motor vehicle and other accidents, suicides, and homicides.[19] Tobacco reacts with alcohol in a way that reinforces its effects in causing esophageal and oral cancer. In addition, excessive alcohol drinking increases the risk of some types of heart disease, high blood pressure (especially in blacks), nerve diseases, nutritional deficiencies (discussed later), damage to a pregnant woman's fetus, and many other disorders. A major cause of lasting mental retardation that begins in infancy is fetal exposure to alcohol (see Chapter 14).

Social consequences of dependence on alcohol include divorce, unemployment, and poverty. An estimated 27 million American children are more likely to develop abnormally in psychosocial skills and relationships because their parents abuse alcohol.[19]

For the above reasons, alcohol should be used cautiously and in moderation, if at all. Drinking even small amounts of alcohol can lead to dependence on it. Approximately 10% of those who drink alcoholic beverages in the United States are alcoholics. As many as 18 million Americans are estimated to have alcohol problems. Of these, 41% (7.2 million) are alcohol abusers, drinkers who experienced at least one severe or moderately severe consequence of alcohol abuse, such as job loss, arrest, or illness, in the previous year.

The people who drink the most alcohol are those in the 20- to 40-year age group. The practice often begins earlier. In a 1985 survey, 66% of the high school seniors interviewed reported that they had consumed alcohol in the past month and 5% described themselves as daily drinkers.

Studies of adoptees raised by nonalcoholic adoptive parents indicate a genetic component in alcoholism. On reaching adulthood, the biological children of alcoholic parents have a four-fold greater incidence of alcoholism than biological children of nonalcoholic parents, even where the adopting families had similar patterns of alcohol consumption. Other studies question a strong genetic component to the disorder.

Cirrhosis

Long-term alcohol use causes fatty liver, alcoholic hepatitis, and cirrhosis. Cirrhosis is a chronic and usually relentlessly progressive disease characterized by fatty infiltration of the liver. Eventually the fat chokes off the blood supply, depriving the liver cells of oxygen and nutrients. Liver cells then die and are replaced by connective (scar) tissue. This scarring process is what we call cirrhosis.[24] In America, most cases of liver cirrhosis are caused by alcohol consumption. Cirrhosis develops in 12% to 31% of cases of alcoholism. In addition to the amount and duration of alcohol consumption, genetic factors and individual differences determine the body's response to alcohol.

No specific amount of alcohol consumption guarantees cirrhosis of the liver. Rather, some people are very susceptible to its effects, others are not. One observable pattern is that cirrhosis commonly results from a 15-year consumption of approximately 80 grams of alcohol per day (Table 16-8). This is equivalent to 7 beers per day. Some evidence suggests the dose may be effective when it's as low as 40 grams a day for men and 20 grams a day for women. Early

TABLE 16-8

Caloric, carbohydrate, and alcohol content of alcoholic beverages

Beverage	Amount (ounces)	Alcohol (grams)	Carbohydrate (grams)	Energy (kcalories)
Beer				
Regular	12	13	14	150
Light	12	10	6	90
Extra light	12	8	3	70
Near	12	2	12	60
Distilled				
Gin, rum, vodka, whiskey	1.5	15	—	105
Brandy, cognac	1.0	11	—	75
Wine				
Red	4	12	1	85
Dry white	4	11	0.5	80
Sweet	4	12	5	103
Sherry	2	9	1.5	75
Port, muscatel	2	7	7	95
Vermouth, sweet	3	12	14	141
Vermouth, dry	3	13	4	105
Manhattan	3	21	2	165
Martini	3	19	1	140
Old-fashioned	3	21	1	180

From Guthrie HA: *Introductory nutrition*, ed 7, St Louis, 1989, Mosby–Year Book.

stages of alcoholic liver injury are reversible, while advanced stages usually are not. The only known prevention for alcoholic cirrhosis is to limit consumption of alcohol.

A poor nutritional status makes the liver more vulnerable to toxic substances by depleting supplies of antioxidants, such as vitamin E and vitamin C. A nutritious diet can help prevent some complications associated with alcoholism, but usually alcoholism wreaks serious destruction on the body with or without an adequate diet. Laboratory animal studies clearly show that even when one consumes a nutritious diet, alcoholism can lead to cirrhosis of the liver.

Alcohol and nutrition

Nutritional problems in a person with alcoholism result from deficiencies of a variety of nutrients:

Vitamin A deficiency may be caused by a poor diet, an inability of the liver to produce retinol-binding protein, or poor zinc status, which reduces retinol-binding protein synthesis. In addition, the chemical-detoxifying systems in the liver induced by chronic alcohol consumption may hasten the degradation of vitamin A in the liver.

Thiamin deficiency can be caused by decreased thiamin absorption or decreased liver synthesis of the active thiamin coenzyme. People with alcoholism often exhibit nervous system problems similar to those seen in a thiamin deficiency.[24]

Niacin deficiency and resulting pellagra can be caused by a poor diet.

Vitamin B-6 deficiency is one of the most common deficiencies of alcoholism, probably stemming from a poor dietary intake of the vitamin and increased breakdown of the vitamin B-6 coenzyme.

Folate deficiency can be caused by a poor diet and poor nutrient absorption. This, along with vitamin B-6 deficiency, are the two most common vitamin deficiencies of alcoholism.[24]

Vitamin D deficiency is usually caused by the liver's decreased capacity to convert vitamin D into the final usable form. Alcohol also may encourage bone cell dysfunction that diminishes bone formation and reduces bone mineralization. This can lead to osteoporosis.

Vitamin C deficiency may result primarily from a decrease in dietary intake or from altered liver metabolism, or both.

Vitamin K deficiency probably occurs because less of it is synthesized in intestinal bacteria, less is consumed, and less is absorbed.

General recommendations for drinking alcohol

The Surgeon General's Office recommends that to reduce the risk of chronic disease, people should (1) drink alcohol only in moderation (no more than two drinks a day), if at all; (2) avoid drinking any alcohol before or while driving, operating machinery, taking medications, or engaging in any other activity requiring judgment; and (3) avoid drinking alcohol while pregnant.

The National Academy of Science's report on *Diet and Health* also does not recommend alcohol consumption. For those who do drink alcoholic beverages, the committee recommends limiting consumption to the equivalent of less than 1 ounce of pure alcohol in a single day. This is the equivalent of two cans of beer, two small glasses of wine, or two average cocktails. Again, pregnant women should avoid alcoholic beverages altogether.

Do you have a problem with alcohol?

Asking a person about the quantity and frequency of alcohol consumption is an important means of detecting abuse and dependence. The following questionnaire (CAGE) is popular for use in routine health care:[19]

CAGE Questionnaire to Screen for Alcohol Abuse

C: Have you ever felt you ought to *Cut* down on drinking?

A: Have people *Annoyed* you by criticizing your drinking?

G: Have you ever felt bad or *Guilty* about your drinking?

E: Have you ever had a drink first thing in the morning to steady your nerves or get rid of a hangover (*Eye-opener*)?

Another key point to question is tolerance. Does it take more to make you inebriated than it did in the past? More than one positive response suggests an alcohol problem.

Treatment

Once a diagnosis of alcohol abuse or dependence is established, a physician should arrange appropriate treatment and counseling for the patient and family. The drinker must confront the immediate problem of how to stop the drinking. Total abstinence must be the primary goal.[24] For people with alcoholism, there is no such thing as controlled drinking. A problem drinker cannot return safely to social drinking. The person should enter an Alcoholics Anonymous (AA) program, or one similar, and the spouse should join Al-Anon. Success is usually proportionate to participation in AA, other social agencies, religious counseling, and other resources. About 2 years of treatment should be expected.

Current research does not support the generally negative public opinion about the prognosis for alcoholism. In most industrial alcoholism treatment programs, where workers are socially stable and—because of the risk to jobs and pensions—well motivated, recovery rates run at the 70% to 80% level. This remarkably high cure rate is probably accounted for by early detection. Once a person moves from problem drinking to an advanced stage of alcoholism, success rates seldom exceed 40% to 50%. Early identification and intervention remain the most important steps in the treatment of alcoholism. ●

The medical deterrent drug disulfiram (Antabuse) can be of critical importance in helping the alcoholic to make the essential decision to stop drinking. An early step in alcohol metabolism is blocked by the action of this drug. As a result, a highly toxic alcohol by-product accumulates in the blood, producing prostrating nausea, vomiting, diffuse flushing, and a shocklike reaction when alcohol is consumed.

NUTRITION

BEYOND THE NUTRIENTS THEMSELVES

FOOD SAFETY

At the turn of the century, conditions in Chicago's meat-packing industry were sickening. Moldy, spoiled meat was commonly doused with borax to cover up the smell and glycerine was added to make it look fresh. Upton Sinclair outraged the American public with his first-hand account of these deplorable conditions in *The Jungle.* In 1906, increasing public pressure forced the passage of the first Food and Drug Act in the United States. Federal inspection then safeguarded the public from worm-infested and diseased meat and generally improved food preparation standards. Indeed, today we have come a long way.

Still, food poisoning warnings pop up everywhere.[18] Attention has turned to more contemporary food safety concerns, such as microbial and chemical contamination. If you take to heart every scary headline about pesticides, food additives, and bacterial contamination, you will find yourself eating precious few foods. On one hand, we are told to eat more fruits, vegetables, fish, and poultry; on the other hand, we are warned that these foods may contain dangerous substances. So, we still must ask, "How safe is our food?"

Scientists and health authorities agree that Americans enjoy one of the safest, most wholesome food supplies in the world.[23] Over the past 50 years tremendous progress has been made in food safety. Despite the progress, a health risk from microbes and chemicals is still found in foods. This chapter focuses on these hazards—how real they are and how we can minimize them. ●

CHAPTER

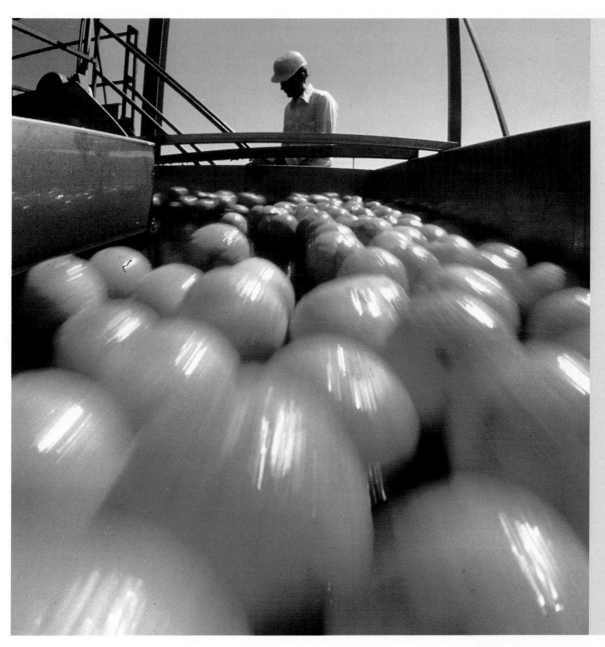

Food processing, in this case oranges, is necessary if we are to continue to enjoy a rich and varied diet year round.

Test Your Food Safety Knowledge

Take this quiz to see how aware you are about the safety of some basic foods. Place a check in the appropriate column, depending on if you think the item is safe or risky to eat.

	Safe	Risky
1. Hot dogs that have been stored unopened in the refrigerator for over 7 days?	_____	_____
2. A bruised or moldy piece of fruit?	_____	_____
3. Frozen ham that was thawed on the counter?	_____	_____
4. An opened jar of mayonnaise that has been in the refrigerator for 6 months?	_____	_____
5. A foil-covered baked potato left out on the counter since the night before?	_____	_____
6. Meat loaf that's pink in the middle after cooking?	_____	_____
7. Raw ground beef that turns brown after 1 to 2 days of refrigeration?	_____	_____
8. An uncooked potato with a greenish cast, eaten with the peel left on?	_____	_____
9. Lettuce moistened by poultry drippings in a grocery bag?	_____	_____
10. Steak that was thawed in the refrigerator and then refrozen with some ice crystals still present?	_____	_____
11. Cooked shrimp that was never deveined?	_____	_____
12. Mustard or ketchup with a black, crusty ring around the rim of the jar?	_____	_____
13. Moldy or shriveled peanuts?	_____	_____

Now that you've completed this assessment, check your answers below.

SAFE: 1,2,4,7,10,11,12
RISKY: 3,5,6,8,9,13

Explanations of the safety or risk of these foods can be found in this chapter. It may have been hard for you to answer these questions. Many people don't know much about proper food preservation, handling, and cooking to avoid significant illness.

Modified from What do you know about food safety? *Tufts University Diet and Nutrition Letter* 3(11):7-8, 1986.

ASSESS YOURSELF

SETTING THE STAGE

The greatest health risk from food is contamination from bacteria and, to a lesser extent, from molds, fungi, yeasts, and viruses. These microbes can all cause food poisoning.[14] But even though microbial contamination is the cause of most food poisoning incidents,[19] Americans seem more concerned about health risks from chemicals in foods. Fully 75% of consumers surveyed in a recent Gallup poll said that pesticide contamination was a major concern to them. In the long run there is some merit to this concern. But on a day-to-day basis, according to the Centers for Disease Control in Atlanta, Georgia, only 2% of all cases of food-borne illness in the United States is caused by food additives.

We will first discuss food poisoning, because it is by far the more important issue for our day-to-day health. Then we will cover the use and safety of food additives.

FOOD POISONING

About one-third to one-half of all diarrhea cases in America—upward of 20 million each year—are induced by food-borne organisms.[9] It is estimated that diarrhea caused by food poisoning hits about one of every ten to thirty-five Americans each year at a cost to the economy of $1 billion to $10 billion. For most of us, the typical result—a brief yet distressing episode of diarrhea, such as traveler's diarrhea—presents no real health risk. But for many, it can be more serious. Some people, especially children, the elderly, people with alcoholism or with underlying health problems, such as cancer or acquired immune deficiency syndrome (AIDS), can suffer greatly from illnesses caused by food-borne microbes. Some bouts of food poisoning are lengthy and lead to food allergies, seizures, blood poisoning (from toxins or microbes in the bloodstream), or other illnesses.

Part of the responsibility for preventing food-borne illness lies with each one of us, for 30% of all such illness results from unsafe handling of food at home.[9] Usually you can't tell by taste, smell, or sight that a particular food contains harmful microbes. So you might not even be aware that food poisoning was the cause of your distress. But, in fact, the last case of stomach or intestinal "flu" you had may have been caused by something you ate. The symptoms of both disorders are often the same: diarrhea, vomiting, fever, and weakness.

Why is food poisoning so common?

The risk of having food poisoning is common, partly because the food industry tries to increase the shelf life of products. Longer shelf life at room temperatures allows more time for bacteria in foods to multiply. Some bacteria grow even at refrigeration temperatures. Partially cooked—and some fully cooked—products pose a special risk because refrigerated storage may only slow—not prevent—bacterial growth. FDA is especially concerned about this problem.

Food poisoning risk is even increasing as we rely more heavily on centralized kitchens outside the home to prepare our foods. Supermarkets have become major food processors over the past decade and now offer a variety of prepared foods from specialty meat shops, salad bars, and bakeries. With so many two-income families, people are looking for convenient, easy-to-prepare nutritious foods. Supermarkets offer entrees that can be served immediately or reheated. The foods are usually prepared in central kitchens or processing plants and shipped to individual stores. If a food product is contaminated in the central kitchen or processing plant, patrons of stores over a wide area can suffer food poisoning. A malfunction in a dairy plant in 1985 resulted in 16,284 confirmed cases of *Salmonella* bacteria infections and at least two deaths from contaminated milk.[23]

Still another cause of increased food-poisoning incidents in America is

TABLE 17-1

Organisms that cause foodborne illness: their source, symptoms, and prevention

Organism	Source of Illness	Symptoms	Prevention Methods
Bacteria			
Staphylococcus aureus	Live in nasal passages and in cuts on skin. Toxin is produced when food contaminated by bacteria is left for extended time at room temperature. Meats, poultry, egg products, tuna, potato, and macaroni salads, and cream-filled pastries are likely targets.	Onset: 2-6 hours after eating. Diarrhea, vomiting, nausea, and abdominal cramps. Mimics flu. Lasts 24-48 hours. Rarely fatal.	• Sanitary food-handling practices • Prompt and proper refrigeration of foods • Keep cuts on skin covered
Salmonella	Found in raw meats, poultry, eggs, fish, milk, and products made with these items. Multiplies rapidly at room temperature. The bacteria themselves are toxic.	Onset: 5-72 hours after eating. Nausea, fever, headache, abdominal cramps, diarrhea, and vomiting. Can be fatal in infants, the elderly, and the sick.	• Handling food in a sanitary manner • Thorough cooking of foods • Prompt and proper refrigeration of foods • Watch cross-contamination
Clostridium perfringens	Widespread in environment. Generally found in meat and poultry dishes. Multiply rapidly when foods are left for extended time at room temperature. The bacteria themselves are toxic.	Onset: 8-24 hours after eating (usually 12 hours). Abdominal pain and diarrhea. Symptoms last a day or less, usually mild. Can be more serious in older or already ill people.	• Sanitary handling of foods, especially meat and meat dishes, gravies, and leftovers • Thorough cooking and reheating of foods • Prompt and proper refrigeration
Clostridium botulinum	Widespread in the environment. However, bacteria produce toxin only in low-acid, anaerobic (oxygen-free) environments, such as in cans of green beans, mushrooms, spinach, olives, and beef. Honey may carry spores.	Onset: 12-36 hours after eating. Symptoms include double vision, inability to swallow, speech difficulty, and progressive paralysis of the respiratory system. OBTAIN MEDICAL HELP IMMEDIATELY. BOTULISM CAN BE FATAL.	• Using proper methods for canning low acid foods • Avoiding commercial cans of low acid foods that have leaky seals or are bent, bulging, or broken • Toxin can be destroyed after can or jar is opened by boiling contents hard for 20 minutes, but discard if suspect toxin is present because of off-odors
Campylobacter jejuni	Found on poultry and beef and can contaminate meat and milk. Chief food sources are raw poultry and meat and unpasteurized milk.	Onset: 3-5 days after eating, or longer. Diarrhea, abdominal cramping, fever, and sometimes bloody stools. Lasts 2-7 days.	• Thorough cooking of foods • Handling food in a sanitary manner • Avoiding unpasteurized milk
Listeria monocytogenes	Found in soft cheeses and unpasteurized milk. Resists acid, heat, salt, and nitrate well.	Onset: 4-21 days. Fever, headache, vomiting, and sometimes even more severe symptoms. May be fatal.	• Thorough cooking of foods • Handling food in a sanitary manner • Avoiding unpasteurized milk

TABLE 17-1 cont'd

Organisms that cause foodborne illness: their source, symptoms, and prevention

Organism	Source of Illness	Symptoms	Prevention Methods
Bacteria			
Yersinia enterocolitica	Common in nature; carried in food and water. They multiply rapidly at both room and refrigerator temperatures. Generally found in raw vegetables, meats, water, and unpasteurized milk.	Onset: 2-3 days after eating. Fever, headache, nausea, diarrhea, and general malaise. Mimics flu and appendicitis. An important cause of intestinal distress in children.	• Thorough cooking of foods • Sanitizing cutting instruments and cutting boards before preparing foods that are eaten raw • Avoidance of unpasteurized milk and unchlorinated water.
Viruses			
Hepatitis A virus	Chief food sources: shellfish harvested from contaminated areas and foods that are handled a lot during preparation and then eaten raw (such as vegetables).	Onset: 30 days. Jaundice, fatigue. May cause liver damage and death.	• Sanitary handling of foods • Use of pure drinking water • Adequate sewage disposal • Adequate cooking of foods
Parasites			
Trichinella spiralis	Found in pork and wild game.	Onset: weeks-months. Muscle weakness, fluid retention in face, fever, flu-like symptoms.	• Thoroughly cooking pork and wild game
Anisakis	Found in raw fish.	Onset: 12 hours. Stomach infection, severe stomach pain.	• Thoroughly cooking fish.
Tapeworms	Found in raw beef, pork, and fish.	Abdominal discomfort, diarrhea.	• Thoroughly cooking all animal products
Mycotoxins			
A group of toxic compounds produced by molds, such as aflatoxin.	Produced in foods that are relatively high in moisture. Chief food sources: beans and grains that have been stored in a moist place.	May cause liver and/or kidney disease.	• Checking foods for visible mold and discarding those that are contaminated. • Proper storage of susceptible foods.

greater consumption of ready-to-eat foods imported from foreign countries. In the past, food imports were mostly raw products processed here under strict sanitation standards. Now, however, we import more processed foods, such as cheese from France and seafood from Asia, some of which are contaminated.

Finally, more cases of food-borne disease are reported now because we are more aware of the role of various players in the process. Every decade the list of microorganisms suspected of causing food poisoning expands (Table 17-1).[17] And besides serving as a good growth medium for some microorganisms, we now know food simply transmits many others as well.

Food preservation—past, present, and future

For centuries, salt, sugar, smoke, fermentation, and drying have been used to preserve food. Most preserving methods work on the principle of decreasing free water—the amount of water not bound to other components in the food.

Salts and sugar decrease free water by binding to it. The process of drying drives off free water. Bacteria need abundant stores of water to grow; yeasts and molds can grow with less water, but some is still necessary.

Decreasing the water content of some rather high-moisture foods, however, would cause them to lose essential characteristics. To preserve such foods—cucumber pickles, sauerkraut, milk (yogurt), wine—fermentation has been a traditional alternative. Selected bacteria are used to ferment or pickle foods. The fermenting bacteria make acids and alcohol, which minimize the growth of other microbes. The acid produced is especially helpful in preventing the growth of the deadly bacterium *Clostridium botulinum.*

Today, we can add ***pasteurization,*** sterilization, refrigeration, freezing, ***irradiation,*** canning, and chemical preservatives to the list of food preservation techniques. A new method for food preservation—***aseptic processing***—simultaneously sterilizes the food and package separately before the food enters the package. Liquid foods, such as fruit juices, are especially easy to process in this manner. With aseptic packaging, boxes of sterile milk and juices can remain on supermarket shelves, free of microbial growth, for many years.

Food poisoning: when undesirable microbes alter foods

In 1871, an Italian scientist named Selmi proposed that food poisoning was caused by ptomaines, breakdown residues of proteins produced during bacterial spoilage of food. Although people still refer to ptomaine poisoning, this idea has been rejected for a long time because ptomaines are not so poisonous as was once assumed. Today, we know that specific toxin-producing bacteria and other microbes cause food poisoning. These organisms cause health problems either **directly,** by invading the intestinal wall, or **indirectly,** by producing a toxin in the food that later harms us.

Salmonella organisms in contaminated food deliver a direct hit to the intestine, causing ***food-borne infections.*** The *Staphylococcus* bacterium produces a toxin, which in turn causes a ***food-borne intoxication.*** Many different types of bacteria cause food poisoning, such as *Bacillus, Campylobacter, Clostridium, Escherichia coli, Listeria monocytogenes, Vibrio, Yersinia pestis, Salmonella, and Staphylococcus.*[17] Because each teaspoon of soil contains about two billion bacteria, we are constantly at risk for food poisoning. Luckily, only a small number of all bacteria actually pose a threat. Determining which microbe has caused a food-poisoning incident entails identifying the clinical features of the poisoning, the incubation period for symptoms, and the food source (Table 17-1).

General rules for preventing food poisoning

You can greatly reduce the risk of food poisoning by following some very important rules:

- Wash your hands thoroughly with hot, soapy water before handling food. Always wash your hands after handling raw meat, fish, poultry, or eggs.
- When grocery shopping, select frozen foods and perishables, such as meat, poultry, or fish, last. Always put these products in separate plastic bags so that drippings don't contaminate other foods in the shopping cart. Then, don't let groceries sit in a warm car; this allows bacteria to grow. Refrigerate or freeze food promptly.
- Don't buy or use food from containers that leak, bulge, or are severely dented. Don't buy or use food from jars that are cracked or have loose or bulging lids. Don't taste or use food that has a foul odor or that spurt liquid when opened. The deadly *Clostridium botulinum* toxin is probably present.
- Wash thoroughly all counters, cutting boards, dishes, and other equipment in hot soapy water, and rinse. Do this both before and after coming

---

**Pasteurization • ** The process of heating food products to kill pathogenic microorganisms; one method heats milk at 161° F for at least 20 seconds.

**Irradiation • ** A process whereby radiation energy is applied to foods, creating compounds (ions) within the food that destroy cell membranes, break down DNA, link proteins together, limit enzyme activity, and alter a variety of other proteins and cell functions that can lead to food spoilage.

**Aseptic Processing • ** A method by which both food and container are simultaneously sterilized; it allows manufacturers to produce boxes of milk that can be stored at room temperature. Variations of this process are also known as ultra high temperature (UHT) packaging.

**Food-borne Infection • ** Food poisoning that is caused directly by bacteria or other microbes in food.

**Food-borne Intoxication • ** Food poisoning that is caused by toxins produced by bacteria or other microbes in food.

Unless properly treated and stored, even dried fruits can support the growth of molds.

in contact with raw meat, fish, poultry, and eggs, to rid *Salmonella* present.

- Wash fresh fruit and vegetables carefully to remove dirt.
- If possible, cut foods to be eaten raw on a clean, plastic cutting board reserved for that purpose. If the same board must be used for both meat and other foods, cut the items to be eaten raw before cutting any potentially contaminated items, such as meat.
- Cook animal foods thoroughly. Internal temperature for beef should reach 160° F or 71° C; for poultry 180° F or 82° C; for fish and pork 170° F or 77° C; and for eggs the yolk should at least be semisolid and the white hard. A good general precaution is to eat no raw animal products. This includes any use of raw or undercooked eggs (cooked to less than 160° F or 71° C).[2] Many people are poisoned each year by eating raw seafood (Figure 17-1). Undercooked pork can allow infection by the parasite that causes trichinosis. The U.S. Department of Agriculture (USDA) will answer questions on safe preparation and use of animal products by phone (1-800-535-4555).
- Once a food is cooked, cool it rapidly (to 40° F or 4° C) within 2 to 4 hours if it is not to be eaten immediately. Greater surface area allows quicker cooling, so separate foods into several pans. Don't recontaminate cooked food through contact with raw meat or juices that might be on your hands, cutting boards, or dirty utensils.
- Reheat leftovers to 165° F (74° C) and reheat gravy to a rolling boil to kill potential *Clostridium perfringens* bacteria present.[15] Stopping at an acceptable eating temperature is not good enough.
- Keep hot foods hot and cold foods cold. Avoid time and temperature abuses. Store food below 40° F (4° C) or above 140° F (60° C) (Figure 17-2). Food poisoning microbes thrive in more moderate temperatures (60° to 90° F or 16° to 32° C). Observe timelines for safe food storage (see Appendix P). This is important because some food-poisoning microbes can grow in the refrigerator. Do not leave cooked or refrigerated foods, such as meat and salads, at room temperature for more than 2 hours because this allows microbes to grow and to cause food poisoning.
- Insulate perishable items if fresh-prepared food is taken on a picnic or other outing, or even if it is a long drive home from the store. Pack cold food in a cooler with plenty of ice. A cooler without ice can be used to keep hot food warmer.
- Avoid coughing and sneezing over foods, even when you are healthy. Cover cuts on hands. This helps stop *Staphylococcus aureus* from entering your food.
- Make sure the refrigerator stays below 40° F (4° C). Generally keep it as cold as possible without freezing the milk or lettuce.
- Cook stuffing separately from poultry (or wash the bird thoroughly, stuff it immediately before cooking, and then transfer the stuffing to a clean bowl immediately after cooking). Make sure the stuffing reaches a temperature of 165°F (74° C). *Salmonella* is the major concern with poultry.
- Consume only pasteurized milk and pasteurized cheese. This is especially important for pregnant women because very toxic bacteria and viruses that thrive in unpasteurized milk can harm the fetus.
- Completely remove moldy portions of food or don't eat the food. When in doubt, throw the food out. Mold growth is prevented by properly storing foods at cold temperatures and using the foods within a reasonable length of time (again see Appendix P).

Microbes that cause food poisoning commonly enter food through cross-contamination (usually from improper food handling) and grow because they are maintained at temperatures favorable to them.[1] Many foods contain prob-

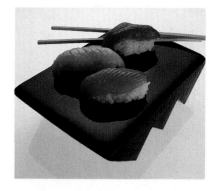

FIGURE 17-1

Sushi, like all raw animal food dishes, is a high-risk choice. Animal foods should be cooked thoroughly before eating.

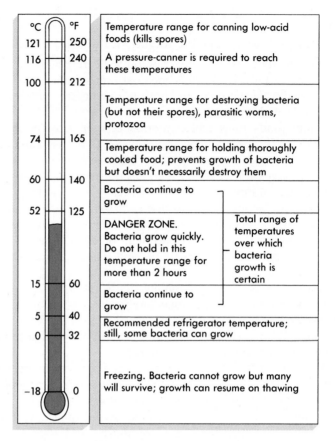

FIGURE 17-2

Effects of temperature on microbes that cause food-borne illness. (Modified from Temperature Guide to Food Safety: *Food and home notes*, Washington, 1977, USDA.)

lem microbes. Most food poisoning incidents could be eliminated through sanitary food-handling procedures and appropriate storage.

Watch for safe food handling techniques when you eat out. Check that foods in a salad bar are iced; custard and pudding pies are chilled; hot foods served on a hot food bar are hot; and vending machines are checked regularly, especially those with sandwiches and milk. Foods stored and served in dormitories should be properly handled.

Several practices can reduce the risk of bacteria surviving during microwave cooking:

- **Cover food with glass or ceramic when possible. The trapped steam helps decrease evaporation and heats the surface.**
- **Stir the product occasionally to avoid cold spots. Then allow microwaved food to stand, covered, after cooking is completed. The heat concentrated inside the food will radiate outward, helping to cook the exterior and equalize the temperature throughout.**
- **Thaw meats in the refrigerator. If thawed in the microwave, use the oven's defrost setting. Note that ice crystals in frozen foods are not heated well by the microwave oven and can create cold spots that later cook more slowly.**

Treatment for food poisoning

If you suffer some food poisoning, you can offset the effects of diarrhea by drinking a lot of fluids. Bedrest speeds recovery, and aspirin can ease the aches and pains. A fever of 102° F (39° C) or greater, blood in the stool, or dehydration from frequent vomiting or diarrhea (a sign of dehydration is dizziness when standing) deserves a physician's evaluation, especially if symptoms persist for more than 2 or 3 days. To prevent further contamination, wash your hands thoroughly and avoid handling food until the diarrhea disappears. In cases of suspected botulism, consult a physician immediately because an antitoxin may be available to speed recovery.

The USDA specifies three particular situations in which it is vital for consumers to report food poisoning incidents to the local health department:

- if the food in question was eaten at a large gathering.
- if the item came from a restaurant, delicatessen, sidewalk vendor, or a kitchen that serves large numbers of people.
- if the suspected food was a commercial product, such as a canned good or a frozen, packaged item.

CONCEPT CHECK

Bacteria and the toxins they produce cause most food poisoning. Traditionally, several methods were commonly used to prevent the growth of microorganisms in food: sugar or salt was added to bind water, or the foods were pickled, smoked, or dried before storage. Today, we have additional food processing methods, such as pasteurization, sterilization, canning, and irradiation. Also, food handling practices, including cleanliness, storage of foods at proper temperatures, and thorough cooking of foods help prevent contamination. All raw animal products and any cooked food must be treated with special care to reduce their potential as food poisoners. Symptoms of food poisoning resemble those associated with stomach or intestinal "flu": diarrhea, vomiting, abdominal bloating, and headache. Treatment in mild cases generally requires only bed rest and extra fluids. On the whole, we have a safe, sanitary food supply and many of the public's food safety problems can be avoided if we use caution in food preparation.

A CLOSER LOOK AT MICROBES THAT CAUSE FOOD POISONING

We noted that finding a food-poisoning agent requires some detective skills. Determining the agent depends on knowing the food source, the incubation time for symptoms, the types of symptoms, and the duration of illness associated with an outbreak. Let's look at the characteristics of the major problem microbes individually.

Staphylococcus aureus (S. aureus)

The organism *Staphylococcus aureus (S. aureus)* causes 20% to 40% of food poisoning cases each year. This microbe produces toxins in food that, once ingested, cause nausea, vomiting, diarrhea, headaches, and abdominal cramps. Symptoms usually develop within 2 to 6 hours of eating the contaminated food. The person rarely dies from this type of food poisoning, but also develops no immunity against future attacks. Bed rest and fluids are generally the only treatment. Recovery takes place usually within 2 to 3 days.

S. aureus bacteria live mainly in the nasal passages and in skin sores. These microbes enter food when people sneeze and cough over food or handle food while they have open skin sores. Once present in significant numbers in a food, *S. aureus* can make enough toxin to cause human illness in about 4 hours if the food temperature stays near 100° F (38° C). The toxin is undetectable by flavor, odor, and appearance, and can even withstand prolonged cooking.

Common foods associated with *S. aureus* food poisoning are custard, ham, egg salad, cheese, seafood, cream-filled pastries, and milk. Whipped cream standing at room temperature for hours is a typical source. Keeping these and other foods above 140° F (60° C) or below 40° F (4° C) prevents both the bacterium's growth and further toxin production. To eliminate the spread of this microbe, it is important to work with clean hands, working surfaces, and utensils; direct coughs and sneezes away from food; and cover skin cuts on hands and arms when handling food.

Salmonella food poisoning

Many varieties of *Salmonella* bacteria cause food poisoning. All 2000 types of *Salmonella* can be killed by normal cooking. Yet, they are responsible for almost 60% of food poisoning incidents. These bacteria are commonly found in animal and human feces and enter food via infected water, contaminated cutting boards, contaminated meat products, cracked eggs, and actual bits of feces in food. Ingesting the live bacteria causes the problem. FDA calculates that *Salmonella* food poisoning costs more than $10 billion a year in medical care and lost work time in the United States.

Symptoms of *Salmonella* food poisoning are the same as those of *S. aureus* food poisoning but can take longer to develop, from 5 to 72 hours. Again, bed rest and fluids are the only treatment, and recovery usually occurs within 2 to 3 days. Fatalities are rare. *Salmonella* food poisoning occurs most frequently from consuming eggs, chicken, meat, meat products, custard made with infected eggs, raw milk, and inadequately refrigerated and reheated leftovers. Raw chicken is often contaminated, and undercooked food poses a special risk. Again, thorough cooking kills *Salmonella* bacteria.

To be safe, eggs should be boiled in water for 7 minutes, poached for 5 minutes (hard), or fried for 3 minutes on each side until the yolk is at least semisolid and the white is firm. Raw eggs should *not* be used in salads, sauces, eggnogs, or milkshakes.[2] Hollandaise sauce, often warmed at low heat, is especially prey to *Salmonella*, as are eggs in uncooked homemade ice cream and mayonnaise. Recent research indicates that *Salmonella* can even be found in intact eggs—as well as cracked ones—especially if the egg has been left at room temperature for a few hours.[4] This is a major concern for FDA and currently the focus of much research.

Most outbreaks of *Salmonella* food poisoning can be traced to improper food handling. Picnics pose a special challenge because food is frequently held for hours at a dangerous temperature (between 40° F to 140° F or 4° C to 60° C) (Figure 17-3). It takes only about 8 hours for *Salmonella* bacteria to multiply sufficiently to cause illness. Observing the temperature precautions for *S. aureus* organisms also prevents *Salmonella* bacteria growth.

Salmonella food poisoning is likely caused by cross-contamination of foods. To avoid outbreaks, keep hands and utensils clean when preparing foods and scrub a plastic cutting board with a chlorinated cleanser after contact with raw meat or poultry. Avoid wooden cutting boards; they pose a special risk because food and juices lodged in cracks make them difficult to sanitize. Store foods at temperatures either hot or cold enough to prevent bacterial growth. Do not allow susceptible foods to stand for more than 2 hours at room temperature. Marinate meat and seafood in the refrigerator. Finally, thaw foods in the refrigerator, in a microwave oven, or under a stream of cold water—not on the kitchen counter.

Clostridium perfringens (C. perfringens)

The bacterium *C. perfringens*, another major cause of food poisoning, lives throughout the environment, especially in soil, the intestines of farm animals and humans, and in sewage. It is called the "cafeteria germ" because most foodborne outbreaks by this organism are associated with the food service industry or with events where large quantities of food are prepared and served.[15] Symptoms of an infection resemble those of *Salmonella* food poisoning, but the victim usually doesn't vomit. Symptoms occur within 8 to 24 hours of consuming enough live bacteria. Again, bed rest and fluids are the only treatment, and recovery usually occurs within a day or so.

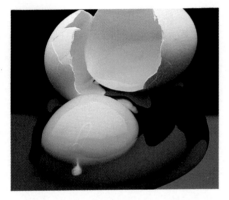

Eggs carry a high risk for *Salmonella* food poisoning unless cooked until the white is hard and the yoke is no longer running.

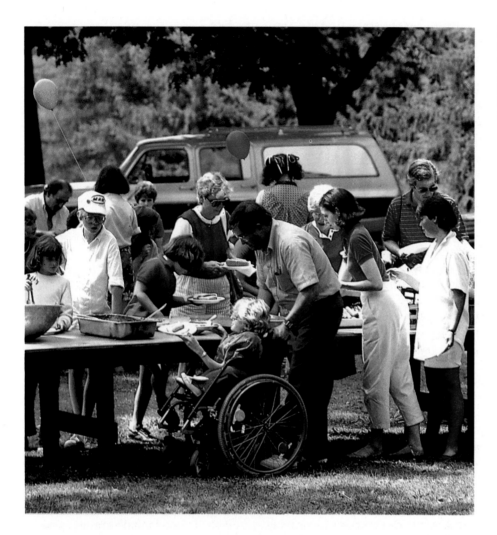

FIGURE 17-3
Outdoor events demand special preventive measures. Many cases of food poisoning happen at events like this family picnic. This is because foods may be out in the warm air for hours at a time.

C. perfringens thrives in an oxygen-free environment. It forms heat-resistant spores that germinate and transform into bacteria at temperatures between 70° F and 120° F (21° C to 49° C). The bacteria then can quickly multiply to disease-causing levels. Foods stored in deep serving dishes are especially fertile media for growth of this bacteria because the centers are isolated from air and stay warm.

C. perfringens organisms are often found in cooked beef, turkey, gravy, dressing, stews, and casseroles.[15] The best insurance against promoting their growth is to maintain proper holding temperatures and to divide large leftover portions into smaller ones. The more surface exposed to air, the less oxygen-deprived the centers will be. Be especially careful to cook meats completely and cool them rapidly in small containers. Thoroughly reheat leftover meat to 165° F (74° C) before serving. Always bring leftover gravy to a rolling boil. Refrigerate cold cuts and sliced meats at 40° F or 4° C, and serve them cold.

Clostridium botulinum (C. botulinum)

The *C. botulinum* bacteria can cause botulism, a food poisoning that can be fatal. This microbe comes from soil and may exist as a bacterium or spore in all foods. As they multiply in food, the bacteria release a deadly toxin. The death rate for botulism is about 60% and is related to the amount of toxin consumed. Although botulism receives much public attention, few cases are reported each year in the United States.

Symptoms of botulism appear within 12 to 36 hours of ingesting contaminated food. The toxin blocks nerve function, causing vomiting, abdominal pain, double vision, dizziness, and acute respiratory failure. If the person survives, recovery occurs within 10 days. Normally, bed rest is the only therapy. With quick diagnosis, treatment with an antiserum is possible. Still, ultimate recovery may be slow.

Since *C. botulinum* grows only in the absence of air, it thrives primarily in canned food, especially improperly home-canned, low-acid foods, such as string beans, corn, mushrooms, beets, and asparagus. Recently, other foods with oxygen-deprived centers, such as potato salad, sauteed onions, stew, and chopped garlic have caused botulism. Cured meats also pose a risk for botulism; however, the nitrates and vitamin C used to preserve commercial products strongly inhibit bacterial growth.

Home canned foods are a common source of botulism. While the canning process may kill all bacteria and the heat may drive out all oxygen, spores of *C. botulinum* can still survive if the heating is insufficient. When the can or jar cools, the spores germinate into bacteria that produce the toxin. Commercial canning factories are less likely to allow this to happen.

Always check all cans carefully. Look for rust on the seams, holes, and swollen sides or tops. Make sure the can sucks in air when opened and the liquid inside is clear, not milky, and does not smell bad. If there are any signs of spoilage, return the can to the store or to the nearest public health department. Whatever you do, *do not taste the food. One string bean can contain enough toxin to kill you.*

The bacteria discussed above are the key offenders. However, the list of problem microbes—bacteria, fungi, molds, parasites, and viruses—as we noted earlier, is much longer.[14,17] Molds growing on foods can produce toxins that have a wide range of effects when consumed. Aflatoxins are produced by a mold that often grows on peanuts, corn, wheat, and oil seeds, such as cottonseed. Although aflatoxins cause cancer in animals, FDA allows them at acceptable levels because they are considered unavoidable contaminants.

Parasites are another food-poisoning agent. Most of us know to thoroughly cook pork. This kills a small parasitic worm, *Trichinella spiralis*, which can be live in raw or undercooked pork and causes the disease trichinosis (Figure 17-4). Symptoms can take weeks or months to develop and include muscle weakness, fever, and fluid retention in the face. Equally harmful is the parasitic worm, *Anisakis*, found in its early growth stages in some raw fish.[11] People who eat the popular Japanese dishes made of raw fish, sushi or sashimi, are particularly vulnerable to this type of food poisoning. Symptoms usually occur within 12 hours of consumption and can include serious stomach pain if the young parasites penetrate the stomach lining. Thoroughly cooking fish or freezing it for at least 72 hours are reliable methods for eliminating the threat of Anisakis disease.

Viruses, such as the hepatitis A, can also be transmitted in food. Symptoms include intestinal problems, weakness, fatigue, jaundice, and sometimes even development of serious liver disease requiring hospitalization. Since symptoms can take a month to show up, pinpointing the cause can be difficult. Unsanitary food handling in restaurants and raw seafood are the usual culprits.

Recently, researchers have noted botulism poisoning caused by spores (as opposed to bacteria) that enter the body. Infants between 2 and 6 months of age are at special risk, as are people with poor stomach acid production. Bacteria spores then germinate in the stomach and produce toxin. For this reason, honey—which can contain the *C. botulinum* spores—should not be given to infants under 1 year.

THE FAR SIDE   By GARY LARSON

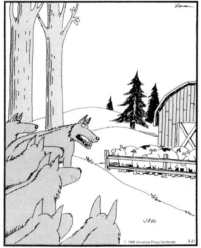

"I say we do it . . . and trichinosis be damned!"

FIGURE 17-4

CONCEPT CHECK

To prevent food poisoning from *Staphylococcus aureus* organisms, cover cuts on hands and avoid sneezing on foods. To avoid *Salmonella* food poisoning, work with clean hands and utensils and separate raw meats, especially poultry products, from other foods. Thoroughly cook meat and poultry products to destroy any *Salmonella* present. To avoid poisoning from *Clostridium perfringens,* rapidly cool leftover foods and thoroughly reheat them. To avoid botulism from

Clostridium botulinum, carefully examine canned foods and don't allow cooked foods to stand for more than 2 hours at room temperature. For other less frequent causes of food poisoning, carefully handle raw animal products so that their juices do not contaminate other foods; thoroughly cook all foods, especially fish and other seafood; and consume only pasteurized dairy products.

Intentional Food Additive •
Additives knowingly (directly) incorporated into food products by manufacturers.

Incidental Food Additives •
Additives that gain access to food products indirectly from environmental contamination of food ingredients or during the manufacturing process.

FOOD ADDITIVES

Food additives are used to maintain or increase a food's nutritional value, preserve freshness, enhance flavor or appearance, or aid in processing and/or preparation. Appendix Q provides a comprehensive list of food additives and their purposes in foods.

Do we need food additives?

Limiting food spoilage accounts for the bulk of additive use. Food additives, such as potassium sorbate, are used to maintain the safety and acceptability of foods by retarding the growth of problem microbes implicated in food poisoning.[20]

Additives are also used to combat some enzymes that lead to undesirable changes in color and flavor in foods, but do not cause anything so serious as food poisoning. This second type of food spoilage occurs when enzymes in a food react to oxygen; for example, when apple and peach slices darken or turn rust color as they are exposed to air. Antioxidants are a type of preservative that retards the action of oxygen-requiring enzymes on food surfaces. These preservatives are not necessarily novel chemicals. They include vitamin E, vitamin C, and a variety of sulfites.

ANOTHER BITE

When buying products, especially perishables, check the product date for safety. Four types of dates are commonly used. The pack date is the day the product was manufactured. The pull or sell date indicates the last date the product should be sold. It allows some time for storing food at home before eating. Check the expiration date of foods stored at home because that is the last date the food can safely be consumed. Last, baked goods may have a freshness date, indicating that the product may safely be eaten for a short time after the date but may not taste the same.

Without the use of some food additives, it would be impossible to safely produce massive quantities of foods and distribute them nationwide or worldwide, as is now done. Despite consumer concerns about the safety of food additives, many have been extensively studied and proven safe when FDA guidelines for their use are followed.[8]

Intentional versus incidental food additives

Food additives are classified into two types: those that are ***intentionally*** (directly) added to foods and those that have ***incidentally*** (indirectly) entered foods. Both types of additives are regulated by FDA. Currently, more than 2800 different substances are intentionally added to foods. As many as 10,000 other substances enter foods incidentally. This includes substances that may reasonably be expected to enter food through surface contact with processing equipment or packaging materials.

Today, sugar, salt, corn syrup, and citric acid still constitute 98% of all additives by weight.

The GRAS list

In 1958, all food additives used in the United States and considered safe at that time were put on a **generally recognized as safe (GRAS)** list.[23] Congress established the GRAS list because it felt manufacturers did not need to prove the safety of substances that were already generally regarded as safe by knowledgeable scientists. As is still the case, FDA was assigned responsibility for proving that a substance did not belong on the GRAS list. Since 1958, some substances on the list have been reviewed. A few, such as cyclamates, failed the review process and were removed from the list. Recently the additive red dye #3 was banned because it is linked to cancer. Many chemicals on the GRAS list have not yet been rigorously tested, primarily because of expense. These chemicals have received a low priority for testing mostly because they have long histories of use without evidence of harm and/or because their chemical structures do not suggest they are potential health hazards.

Are synthetic chemicals always bad?

Nothing about a natural product makes it inherently safer than a synthetic (man-made) product.[18] Many synthetic products are simply laboratory copies of chemicals that also occur in nature (see the discussion in Chapter 18 on biotechnology for some examples). And although humans contribute some toxins to foods, such as synthetic pesticides and industrial chemicals, nature's poisons are often even more potent and prevalent. Dr. Bruce Ames, a noted cancer researcher, suggests that we ingest at least 10,000 times more (by weight) natural toxins produced by plants than we do man-made pesticide residues. This comparison doesn't make man-made chemicals any less toxic, but it does lend perspective.

Consider the familiar food additive baking powder, which is used to make the batter rise in cakes, pancakes, and other quick breads. When manufacturers list potassium acid tartrate, sodium aluminum phosphate, or monocalcium phosphate on cake mix labels, they are referring to baking powder by its chemical names. Baking soda could be listed by its proper name, sodium bicarbonate, just as ordinary table salt could be called sodium chloride. The question should not be whether a food additive, such as salt, is a chemical, but rather whether the chemical additive is safe to use.

Vitamin E is often added to food to prevent rancidity of fats. This chemical is safe when used within certain limits. However, high doses have been associated with health problems (see Chapter 9). Thus even well-known chemicals we are comfortable using can be toxic in some circumstances and at some concentrations.

Testing food additives for safety

Food additives are tested under FDA scrutiny for safety on at least two animal species, usually rats and mice (Figure 17-5). Scientists determine the highest dose of the additive that produces **no observable effects** in the animals. High doses are needed to reduce the cost and length of the tests. Still, these doses are proportionately much higher than humans are ever exposed to. The maximum dosage level is then divided by at least 100 to establish a margin of safety for human use.[18] The rationale for reducing the no observable effect level by a 100-fold margin is that we assume humans are at least 10 times more sensitive to food additives than laboratory animals and that any one person might be ten times more sensitive than another.[23] This very broad margin essentially ensures that the food additive in question will cause no deleterious health effects in humans. Other terms used to express this margin of safety concept are tolerance, allowable level, and acceptable levels.

One important exception applies to the schema for testing intentional food additives: if an additive is shown to cause cancer, even though caused by very

Odyssey © L. Taha 1988

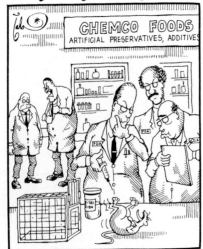

Darn it! He knows the FDA is here. He's faking it.

FIGURE 17-5

high doses, no margin of safety is allowed. The food additive cannot be used because it would violate the **Delaney clause** in the 1958 Food Additive Amendments. This clause prohibits intentionally adding to foods a compound that was introduced after 1958 and causes cancer.[23] Evidence for cancer could come from either laboratory animal or human studies.

Recently, the value of animal cancer tests has been questioned. Research suggests that when rats are fed massive doses of chemicals, as they typically are in the tests, it may be the dose itself, rather than the chemical action, that causes cancer. The scientific community is currently debating which is the best method to test additives to evaluate cancer risk in humans.[6] The question boils down to how to test chemicals efficiently and how to apply data obtained from laboratory animals to humans. Nevertheless, we are left with our current approach until a better method is established.[18]

Incidental food additives are another matter altogether. FDA cannot simply ban various industrial chemicals and mold toxins from foods, even though some types can cause cancer. These products are not purposely added to foods—they are present whether we like it or not. FDA sets an acceptable level for these substances. Basically, it establishes a cancer safety margin of one million, which means that a substance can be added to foods only if the product that results does not contribute to more than one cancer case during the lifetimes of one million people.[18]

Obtaining approval for a new food additive

Today, before a new substance can be added to foods, FDA must approve its use. Besides rigorously testing an additive to establish its safety margins, manufacturers must give FDA information that: (1) identifies the new additive, (2) gives its chemical composition, (3) states how it is manufactured, and (4) specifies laboratory methods used to measure its presence in the food supply at levels of intended use.

Manufacturers also must offer proof that the additive will accomplish its intended purpose in a food, that it is safe, and that the level present is no higher than needed. Additives cannot be used to hide defective food ingredients, such as rancid oils, deceive customers, or replace good manufacturing practices. A manufacturer must establish that the ingredient is necessary for producing a specific food product.

Common food additives

A list of food additive categories appears in Table 17-3. Let's look at some of the major categories to understand exactly why food additives are used and to learn more about the specific substances that are used as food additives.[20]

Acidic or alkaline agents.   Acids, such as calcium lactate, have many uses in foods. As flavor enhancing agents, they impart a tart taste to soft drinks, sherbets, and cheese spreads, for example. As preservatives, they inhibit microbial growth. As antioxidants, they prevent discoloration and rancidity. They also adjust acid and base balance. Adding acids during food processing increases the margin of safety from botulism in naturally low-acid vegetables, such as beets.

Alkaline products, such as sodium hydroxide, can alter the texture and flavor of foods, including chocolate. In processing, alkaline products are sometimes used to produce a milder flavor by neutralizing the acids produced during fermentation.

Anticaking agents.   By absorbing moisture, compounds such as calcium silicate, ammonium citrate, magnesium stearate, and silicon dioxide keep table salt, baking powder, powdered sugar, and other powdered food products free-flowing. These chemicals prevent the caking and lumping that would make powdered or crystalline products hard to use.

Delaney Clause • This clause to the 1958 Food Additives Amendment of the Pure Food and Drug Act in the United States prevents the intentional (direct) addition to foods of a compound introduced after that date, which has been shown to cause cancer in animals or man.

Note that the margin of safety for some vitamins and trace minerals is much lower than for additives. In a few cases, five to ten times our needs for a nutrient can be toxic. So food additives are subjected to much stricter limits than are essential nutrients, such as copper and vitamin D.

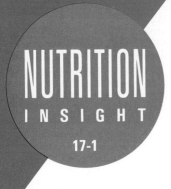

PROTECTING THE U.S. FOOD SUPPLY

A variety of federal, state, and local agencies in the United States monitor food safety. The history of the food laws they enforce is listed in Table 17-2. Some of the agencies involved are:

- *The U.S. Department of Agriculture (USDA).* This agency enforces standards for wholesomeness and quality of grains and produce, meat, poultry, milk, and eggs produced in the United States. Its activities include inspection of production plants and of grains, fruits, vegetables, meat, poultry, and dairy products.[23] USDA also routinely monitors animal foods for antibiotics.

TABLE 17-2

Key U.S. Food Laws[6]

1906: **Pure Food and Drug Act**—This most importantly defined adulterated foods: those foods containing "any added poisons or other added deleterious ingredient which may render such article injurious to health."

1938: **Federal Food, Drug, and Cosmetic Act**—This provided for exemptions and safe tolerances for substances that, although not desirable in foods, were either necessary in production or unavoidable.

1958: **Food Additives Amendment (and the Color Additives Amendment of 1960)**—These made it necessary for manufacturers to demonstrate the safety of a new food additive before approval by FDA. The 1958 act also included the Delaney clause: "no additive shall be deemed to be safe if it is found to produce cancer when ingested by man or animals, or if it is found after tests which are appropriate for the evaluation of the safety of the food additives to induce cancer in man or animals."

- *Bureau of Alcohol, Tobacco, and Firearms.* This agency is responsible for enforcing laws that cover the production, distribution, and labeling of most alcoholic beverages.
- *Environmental Protection Agency (EPA).* This agency regulates pesticides. EPA must approve all pesticides before they are sold in the United States. It determines the safety of new pesticide products and sets allowable limits for pesticide residue in foods. This limit is not necessarily set at the maximum safe level of a pesticide in a food; EPA sets limits no higher than needed for a product's intended use. These levels are then enforced by FDA.[1] EPA also establishes water quality standards, including those for drinking water.
- *Food and Drug Administration (FDA).* This agency is responsible for ensuring the safety and wholesomeness of all foods sold in interstate commerce (except for meat and poultry, which are primarily under USDA jurisdiction). Follow their actions by reading *FDA Consumer.* FDA also sets standards for specific foods and enforces federal regulations for labeling, food and color additives, food sanitation, and the safety of foods. The agency inspects food plants, imported food products, and mills that make feeds containing medications or nutritional supplements for animals destined for human consumption.

  FDA acts primarily when the public health is endangered or when proper medical care is being discouraged. It regulates products, not people. FDA cannot control what people say, just what is on the label and how a product is promoted. FDA gives low priority to simple economic deception by products.

  To monitor foods for contaminants, FDA routinely samples items that are of dietary importance, such as produce. Foods suspected of containing illegal residues receive a more intensive evaluation. An important part of FDA's safety sampling is a "market basket" study of foods that typify the American diet.[7] Four times a year, identical purchases of 234 foods, including pro-

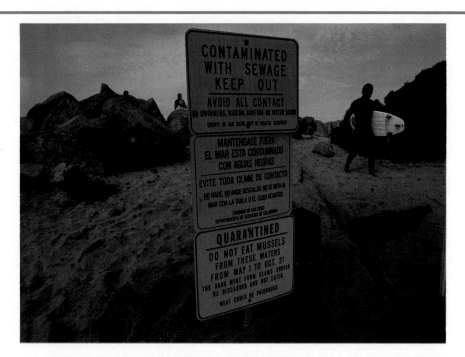

FIGURE 17-6
Purchase seafood from reputable suppliers. They must be able to guarantee the food has been legally harvested.

cessed foods, are analyzed for pesticide residues, radioactive elements, toxic metals, and other undesirable substances. Imported foods with illegal residues can be refused entry into the country by FDA.[21]

ANOTHER BITE Traditionally, FDA does not regularly inspect food-processing plants. It relies instead on its "Good Manufacturers Procedures" plan that food processors and manufacturers are expected to follow. FDA inspectors may visit a specific food processing establishment only infrequently. The agency relies on consumer complaints to alert it to potential dangers—then it researches these in greater detail.

- *National Marine Fishery Service.* This agency is part of the Department of Commerce. It is responsible for seafood quality and other aspects of fisheries management. Its inspection program for fish products is voluntary, not mandatory.[1] This is probably one reason why one-fourth of all food poisoning incidents in the United States involve fish, according to the Centers for Disease Control in Atlanta (Figure 17-6). FDA does inspect seafood processing plants and spotchecks imported fish and seafood.
- *State and local government.* States inspect restaurants, retail food establishments, dairies, grain mills, and other food-related establishments within their borders (Figure 17-7). States have the primary responsibility for milk safety. FDA provides guidelines to state and local governments for regulating dairy products and restaurants.
- *Foreign Governments.* Governments of at least 40 nations are now partners with the United States in ensuring food safety through agreements that cover 24 food products, including shellfish. International cooperation in food inspection and regulatory standards is expanding.

The limited budgets of government enforcement agencies at all levels may limit the number and thoroughness of inspections. So individuals must assume some responsibility for these protective activities themselves. We must remain alert in cases of apparent abuse and contact the appropriate government agency. ●

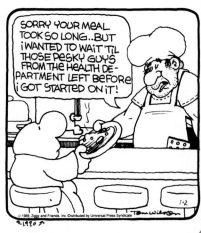

FIGURE 17-7

TABLE 17-3

Food additive categories

Anticaking	Formulation aids: carriers, binders, fillers, plasticizers	Processing aids: clarifying, clouding, catalyst, floculants, filter aids, crystallization inhibitors
Antimicrobial		
Antioxidants		
Color, and adjuncts	Fumigants	
Conditioners	Humectants	
Curing and pickling	Leavening	Propellants
Dough strengtheners	Lubricants and release agents	Sequestrants
Drying agents		Solvents and vehicles
Emulsifiers	Nonnutritive sweeteners	Stabilizers and thickeners
Enzymes	Nutritive sweeteners	
Firming agents	Oxidizing and reducing pH control	Surface active agents
Flavor enhancers		Surface-finishing agents
Flavoring agents		Synergists
Flour treating		Texturizers

See Appendix Q for examples of compounds that fall within these categories.
From Hegarty V: *Decisions in nutrition*, St. Louis, 1988, Mosby–Year Book.

Antioxidants. These preservatives help delay food discoloration from oxygen exposure, such as occurs when potatoes are diced. They also help keep fats from turning rancid. Two widely used antioxidants are BHA (butylated hydroxyanisole) and BHT (butylated hydroxytoluene). Vitamin E and related compounds also serve as antioxidants.

Sulfites also are widely used as antioxidants in foods. Sulfites are actually a group of sulfur-based chemicals—sulfur dioxide, gas, sodium and potassium bisulfite, and sodium and potassium meta bisulfite. After ingesting sulfites, people who are very sensitive to them may have difficulty breathing, wheeze, vomit, have hives, diarrhea, abdominal pain, cramps, and dizziness. FDA now limits the use of sulfites on raw fruits and vegetables—an action directed mainly at salad bars. Potatoes are not covered by that regulation.[10] FDA also requires manufacturers to declare the presence of sulfites on labels of packaged foods containing at least 10 parts per million of sulfites. Labels on wine bottles often list a sulfite warning.

Colors. Color additives do not improve nutritional qualities, but they can make foods more eye appealing. Food colorings can not be used to deceive consumers, for example, by covering blemishes, or to conceal inferiority, or to mislead people in any way. Although colorings are arguably unnecessary additives, manufacturers have satisfied FDA that color is "necessary" for the production of certain foods.

Controversy has surrounded the use of some food colors. Currently, the safety of using tartrazine (FD&C yellow No. 5) is disputed. It has caused allergic symptoms, such as hives, itching, and nasal discharge in sensitive individuals, especially in people allergic to aspirin. Although few Americans are sensitive to tartrazine, FDA requires manufacturers to list FD&C yellow No. 5 on labels of food products containing it. Some red dyes have also raised alarms, and some have been banned.[6]

Emulsifiers. These products, by distributing and suspending fat in water, improve the uniformity, smoothness, and body of foods, such as bakery goods, ice cream, and candies. In mayonnaise, for example, egg yolks act as emulsifiers in holding together the oil and the acids, such as vinegar or lemon juice. Lecithin, derived from soybeans, acts as an emulsifier in chocolate and margarine. Monoglycerides and diglycerides, found also as by-products of fat digestion, are used as emulsifiers in cake mixes.

Fat replacements. Fat replacements, such as Paselli SA2, Dur-Low, and Sta-Slim 143, are being produced for commercial use. These carbohydrate-based products add to another major player—Simplesse—discussed in Chapter 7.

Flavors and flavoring agents.   Naturally occurring and artificial agents can impart more flavor to foods. These agents include extracts from spices and herbs, as well as man-made agents. You probably have recognized flavors of some spices and of liquid derivatives of onion, garlic, cloves, and peppermint in foods. To meet the demand of industry, manufacturers have developed synthetic flavors that not only taste like natural flavors, but also have the advantage of stability. Often artificial flavors, such as butter or banana flavors, have the same chemical composition that makes up part of the natural flavor.

Flavor enhancers.   These substances—monosodium glutamate (MSG), for example—help bring out the natural flavors of foods. Some people are sensitive to MSG and experience flushing, chest pain, facial pressure, dizziness, sweating, rapid heart rate, nausea, vomiting, and high blood pressure after exposure. Because MSG is often used in Chinese food, reactions have been called Chinese restaurant syndrome. The onset of symptoms occurs about 10 to 20 minutes after ingestion and may last from 2 to 3 hours. People who find themselves sensitive to MSG should avoid it.

Humectants.   These chemicals, such as glycerol, propylene glycol, and sorbitol, are added to foods to help retain proper moisture, fresh flavor, and texture. They are often used in candies, shredded coconut, and marshmallows.

Leavening Agents.   Air and steam can be used to create a light texture in breads and cakes; however, carbon dioxide bubbles are much more reliable for this purpose. Common leavening agents that produce carbon dioxide gas include yeast, baking powder, and baking soda. Baking soda needs to react with acids to generate carbon dioxide. Baking powder can be used in either acid or alkaline conditions.

Maturing and bleaching agents.   Compounds such as bromates, peroxides, and ammonium chloride hasten the natural aging and whitening processes of milled flour. This shortens the delay in using flour in baked products. Otherwise, freshly milled flour lacks the qualities necessary to make a stable, elastic dough, and otherwise requires several months to be useful in baking.

Nutrient supplements.   Vitamin and mineral supplements are added to foods to improve their nutritional quality. Sometimes they replace nutrients lost in processing, as occurs when enriching flour. Vitamin A is added to margarine and to some forms of milk. Vitamin D is added to some dairy products. Potassium iodide is added to salt, and calcium to some flours. Breakfast cereals often contain a variety of added nutrients.

Preservatives.   There are many types of preservatives. Some inhibit microbial growth, others function as antioxidants or sequestrants (discussed below). Sodium benzoate, sorbic acid, and calcium propionate are common preservatives. Sorbic acid is a potent inhibitor of molds and fungal growth. Calcium propionate, a natural part of some cheeses, inhibits mold growth.

Nitrates—and the related form, nitrites—are used as preservatives, especially to prevent growth of *Clostridium botulinum*. Sodium and potassium nitrates and nitrites are used to preserve meats, such as bacon, ham, salami, and hot dogs. Nitrates and nitrites have been used for centuries—in conjunction with salt—to preserve meat. An added effect of nitrates is their reaction with myoglobin pigments in meat to form a bright pink color. This gives the characteristic appearance to ham, hot dogs, and other cured meats.

Nitrate consumption from both cured foods and natural vegetables has been associated with the synthesis of nitrosamines in the stomach. Nitrosamines are potent cancer-causing agents, particularly for the stomach and esophagus. Actual risk appears to be low, however, except for people who secrete little stomach acid (some elderly people, for example). FDA also feels that consumers take for granted a margin of microbial safety gained from nitrite use in cured meats. People often serve these meats cold or at least underheated. Consequently government agencies have chosen not to ban nitrate or nitrite

Infants are more sensitive to MSG because they have not yet developed a complete blood-brain barrier. This means they cannot fully exclude such substances as MSG from the brain.

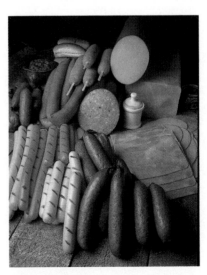

Cured meats rely on nitrates/nitrites for their pink color.

Sequestrants • Compounds that bind free metal ions; by so doing, they reduce the ability of ions to cause rancidity in foods containing fat.

use in foods, but rather to change manufacturing practices to lower amounts of preformed nitrosamines.

 If nitrates and nitrites form chemical substances that can cause cancer, why aren't they banned by the Delaney clause? In the United States, the USDA regulates the use of chemicals in meats. The laws which govern USDA functions are separate from the 1938 Federal Food, Drug, and Cosmetic Act. Because of this, the Delaney clause, an amendment to the 1938 law, does not apply to USDA actions. Currently, USDA sees no clear threat to public safety from the regulated use of nitrates and nitrites in meats, and so no action has been taken.

The addition of vitamin C to cured meats, such as bacon, is one way to reduce the amount of nitrosamines formed in foods. This is a common practice today. Other antioxidants, such as vitamin E, also inhibit synthesis of nitrosamines.

Most nitrites and nitrates in the U.S. food supply occur naturally in foods, primarily in vegetables and baked goods. About one-third of nitrites and one-seventh of nitrates in our food supply are added in manufacturing.

Alternative sweeteners. Currently, saccharin and acesulfame (Sunette) are the only nonnutritive sweeteners used in foods. Since aspartame (Nutrasweet) yields energy, it is considered a nutritive sweetener (see Chapter 6). Saccharin is carcinogenic to rats when administered over two generations. The cancers are found primarily in the bladder. However, population studies of humans have not found an increased risk of developing bladder cancer from exposure to saccharin. Congress has prevented FDA from banning saccharin through 1992, but a warning label must accompany any use. Because Congress has exempted saccharin, the Delaney clause can't be applied to it.

Stabilizers and thickeners. These additives impart a smooth texture and uniform color and flavor to candies, ice creams, and other frozen deserts, chocolate milk, and artificially sweetened beverages. Commonly used substances are pectins, vegetable gums (such as guar gum and carrageenan), gelatins, and agars. They work by absorbing water. Without stabilizers and thickeners, ice crystals form in ice cream and other frozen desserts, and particles of chocolate separate from chocolate milk. Stabilizers are also used to prevent evaporation and deterioration of flavorings used in cakes, puddings, and gelatin mixes.

Sequestrants. These compounds include EDTA and citric acid. They bind many free chemical ions, and by doing so, reduce the ability of ions to cause rancidity in products containing fat.

In general, if you consume a variety of foods in moderation, the chances of food additives jeopardizing your health are minimal. Pay attention to your body. If you suspect an intolerance or sensitivity, consult your physician for further evaluation. Remember that, in the short run, you are more likely to suffer from either poor food handling practices that allow bacteria to grow in food or from consuming raw animal foods than from eating additives. Excess kcalories, saturated fat, and other potential "problem" nutrients pose the greatest long-term risk.

 Look at the ingredients listed on a typical box of flavored gelatin dessert. Besides the expected sugar and gelatin, there is a long list of vitamins and minerals, adipic acid, disodium phosphate, fumaric acid, artificial color, and artificial flavor. You may wonder whether this is a smart food choice. If you are bewildered or concerned about all the additives generally creeping into your diet, you can easily avoid most of them by emphasizing unprocessed whole foods. However, no evidence shows that this will necessarily make you healthier. It amounts to a personal decision. Do you have faith that FDA and food manufacturers are adequately protecting your health and welfare, or do you want to take more personal control by minimizing your intake of compounds not naturally found in foods? Choose the path that seems best to you. If you prepare your own dinner tonight, make a point of reading each label to discover more about what you are eating.

CONCEPT CHECK

Food additives are used to reduce spoilage caused by microbial growth, oxygen, some chemical ions and other compounds. Additives are also used by food manufacturers to improve flavor and color, leaven, provide nutritional fortification, thicken, and emulsify food components. Additives are classified as intentional (direct)—those purposefully added to foods—and incidental (indirect)—those that end up in foods through environmental contamination or manufacturing practices. Additives in foods are limited to at most 1/100 of the highest amount that causes no observable effect when consumed by animals. The Delaney clause further limits intentionally adding to foods most cancer-causing compounds introduced after 1958 under FDA jurisdiction. Carcinogens that incidentally enter foods have maximum levels set for them. These are monitored primarily by FDA.

NATURALLY OCCURRING TOXINS IN FOODS

Foods contain a variety of naturally occurring toxic substances. Following are some of the more important examples:[13]

Mushrooms—some species are poisonous.

Safrole—found in sassafras, mace, and nutmeg; causes cancer.

Solanine—found in potato shoots and green spots on potato skins; inhibits nervous system action.

Aflatoxin—found on moldy grains and peanuts; causes cancer. FDA rigorously inspects peanut butter to ensure that it's safe for consumption.

Avidin—found in raw egg whites; binds biotin, preventing its absorption. Cooking inactivates avidin.

Goitrogens—found in raw rutabagas, turnips, brussels sprouts, broccoli, kale, and soybeans; inhibit thyroid hormone metabolism. Cooking destroys them.

Thiaminase—found in raw clams and mussels; it destroys the vitamin thiamin. Cooking inactivates thiaminase.

Glycyrrhizic acid—found in pure licorice extracts; causes hypertension.

Tetrodotoxin—found in puffer fish; causes respiratory paralysis.

Protease inhibitor—found in raw soybeans; inhibits digestive enzymes.

Saponins—found in alfalfa sprouts; destroy red blood cell membranes.

Tannins—found in tea; bind calcium and iron.

Oxalic acid—found in spinach; binds calcium.

Herbal teas—containing senna or comfrey; can cause diarrhea and liver damage.

Nitrates—found in spinach, lettuce, and beets; can be converted into the carcinogen nitrosamine.

Browning products—found in toasted grains; can cause genetic (DNA) changes.

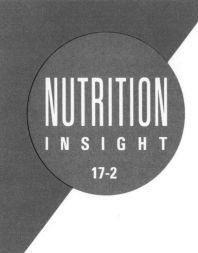

NUTRITION
I N S I G H T
17-2

ENVIRONMENTAL CONTAMINANTS IN FOOD

A variety of environmental contaminants may be found in foods. We mention some of the more important ones here:

Lead. Ingesting this metal can cause anemia, kidney disease, and damage to the nervous system. Because it has a high atomic weight, it is a "heavy" metal. Many heavy metals are toxic at low doses. Lead toxicity is especially a problem for children and causes poor learning ability.[12] It is important not to store food in a can with a lead solder joint after the can has been opened. Contact with air speeds degradation of the solder joint and the release of lead into the food product. This is especially important for acidic food products, such as tomatoes. Many cans today are lead free if used for acidic products, such as soft drinks.

Never store acidic products, such as fruit juice, sauerkraut, or pickled vegetables, in galvanized, tin, or other metal containers, except stainless steel. This includes opened tin cans. Acid can dissolve the metal, and lead will then leach into the food product. Lead can also leak out of solder joints in copper pipes, so let tap water run a minute or more before drinking it or cooking with it, especially first thing in the morning.

Lead can enter the food supply via leaded crystal and pottery glazes. Lead is no longer used in glazes on commercially produced dishes in the United States because of this hazard. However, there is no way to ensure the safety of homemade or imported pottery items. It is important not to use antiques or collectibles—this includes any leaded glass—for food or beverage storage because of the potential lead contamination.

Dioxin. This is an abbreviated name for a complex chemical defoliant. Dioxin is believed to cause cancer and other harmful effects in animals, even in small doses.[5] For Americans, major food sources of dioxin are bottom-feeding fish from the Great Lakes—an area with a great deal of industrial activity and chemical production. Dioxin is primarily a problem for people who frequently consume fish caught locally. People who eat commercial fish normally eat a variety, and even people who stick to one type of fish do not usually have a problem because fish in interstate commerce generally come from different waters, only a few of which may contain dioxin.

Dioxin has also been detected in some paper products. Levels in milk cartons and coffee filters have currently been reduced to the point that they are so low they cannot be distinguished from "background" dioxin levels typically found in foods.

Mercury. FDA first limited mercury, another heavy metal, in foods in 1969 after 120 people in Japan became ill from eating fish contaminated with high amounts. Birth defects in offspring of some of those people were also blamed on the mercury poisoning. The fish most often contaminated was swordfish. Currently, swordfish shipments are automatically detained until they are shown to meet mercury standards. For freshwater fish in America, it is best to eat the younger, and hence smaller, fish. These have had less time to accumulate mercury than larger, older fish.

Urethane in alcoholic beverages. This chemical forms during fermentation of alcoholic beverages. If the fermented product is heated, as in the production of sherry and bourbon, urethane levels increase even more. Although urethane causes cancer in animals, it is unclear whether it causes cancer in humans. FDA research on urethane in food products is now a high priority.

Polychlorinated biphenyls (PCBs). These chemicals were widely used for years in a variety of industrial products, but because they are linked to liver tumors and reproductive problems in animals, they are no longer produced. FDA has banned their use in machinery associated with food and animal feed and has established limits for PCBs in susceptible foods and in paper used for food-packaging material.

The most significant food source of PCB residues is fish, primarily freshwater fish, such as Coho and Chinook salmon from the Great Lakes and bottom-feeding freshwater species from waters in other industrial areas. A key point in fish consumption is variety and moderation when local sources have the potential for contamination. ●

People have coexisted for centuries with these naturally occurring toxins, learning to avoid some of them. Farmers know potatoes must be stored in the dark so that solanine won't be synthesized. Grain elevator operators check grain deliveries under ultraviolet light for the presence of aflatoxins. And we have naturally limited our consumption of other toxins and developed cooking and food preparation methods to limit their potency. Some are toxic only in doses higher than people ordinarily consume. For example, the amount of saponins in alfalfa sprouts eaten on a sandwich or salad daily will not harm you. Nevertheless, it is important to understand that some potentially harmful chemicals in foods occur naturally.

Overall, the best practice is to emphasize variety and moderation in selecting foods. You can avoid many food contaminants by consuming unprocessed foods. A general program to minimize exposure to naturally occurring and environmental toxins also includes: (1) learning which foods pose risks; (2) thoroughly rinsing and scrubbing fruits and vegetables; (3) removing outer leaves of leafy vegetables; (4) eating smaller, rather than the larger, species of fresh water game fish (toxins accumulate more over the longer lifetime of the larger fish); (5) trimming fat and skin from meat, poultry, and fish; and (6) discarding any fat that is rendered from meat or fish during cooking. This practice helps because many food contaminants dissolve in fat.

SUMMARY

- Bacteria and other microbes in foods are the agents most likely to cause food poisoning. To guard against food poisoning in the past, people used salt, sugar, smoke, fermentation, and drying to preserve foods. Today, we also recognize the importance of proper cooking and of keeping hot foods hot and cold foods cold. Pasteurization has also greatly improved the safety of dairy products.

- Cross-contamination commonly causes food poisoning. It occurs when bacteria on raw animal products reach other foods that can support bacterial growth. Because of the risk of cross-contamination, no food should be kept at room temperature for more than 2 hours if it has come in contact with raw animal products and can support bacterial growth.

- Treatment for food poisoning usually requires drinking a lot of fluids, avoiding food handling while diarrhea is present, thorough hand washing, and bed rest.

- The major causes of food poisoning today are the bacteria *Salmonella, Staphylococcus aureus,* and *Clostridium perfringens.* To protect against these agents of food poisoning, cover cuts on the hands, do not sneeze on foods, avoid contact between raw meat or poultry products and other food products, and rapidly cool and then thoroughly reheat leftovers. Thorough cooking of foods and the use of pasteurized dairy products further protects against other problem microbes. Viruses, molds, and parasites also account for many cases of food poisoning. Again, taking care to select, handle, and cook foods properly can prevent problems.

- Food additives are used primarily to extend shelf life by preventing microbial growth and destruction of food components by oxygen, certain chemical ions, and other substances. Food additives are classed as those intentionally added to foods and those that incidentally end up in foods. An additive to a food is limited by FDA to at most 1/100 of the greatest amount that causes no observable effects in animals. In most cases, the Delaney clause bans use of any intentional food additive introduced after 1958 in the United States if it causes cancer.

- Antioxidants, such as vitamin E and sulfites, prevent oxygen and enzyme destruction of food products. Emulsifiers suspend fat in water, improving the uniformity, smoothness, and body of foods, such as ice cream. Common preservatives include sodium benzoate and sorbic acid, which prevent bacterial growth. Sequestrants bind free chemical ions, preventing them from causing fats to become rancid.

- Toxic substances occur naturally in a variety of foods, such as green potatoes, moldy grains, raw soybeans, and raw egg whites. Cooking foods limits their toxic effects. Over the centuries, people have purposely avoided some of these foods, such as moldy grains and the green parts of potatoes.

- A variety of environmental contaminants can be found in food. Because most of them dissolve in fat, trimming fat from meats and discarding fat that is rendered during cooking of meats, fish, and poultry are good steps to minimize exposure. In addition, it is helpful to wash fruits and vegetables thoroughly and to discard the outer leaves of leafy vegetables.

CAN YOU CHOOSE THE IMPROPER FOOD SAFETY PRACTICES?

In this chapter you learned the following facts:

- One-third to one-half of all diarrhea cases in America are induced by food-borne organisms.
- Diarrhea caused by food poisoning hits about one of every ten to thirty-five Americans per year.

Carefully preparing foods to prevent food-borne illness can minimize its occurrence for most of us. Read the excerpt below and pick out the food safety violations that could contribute to food poisoning.

John Noseguard, a local health department inspector, gives the following account of his visit to a local diner:

Workers at the Morningside Diner try hard to give good service and provide tasty, satisfying food. As I walked through the kitchen I noticed that each food handler washed his/her hands thoroughly with hot, soapy water before handling the food, especially after handling raw meat, fish, poultry, or eggs. Before preparing raw foods they also thoroughly wash the cutting boards, dishes, and other equipment. As they use their cutting boards, after cutting food, they wipe them with a damp rag and use them again to cut more food.

When preparing fresh fruits and vegetables, they wash them but are careful to leave a little dirt on them for fear of washing important nutrients from the outside. The cooks generally cook meats to an internal temperature of 180° F (82° C). However, for pork, to preserve the flavor, it is cooked to an internal temperature of 140° F (60° C). Some cooked foods, which are to be served later, are cooled to 40° F (4° C) within 2 hours, and foods like beef stew are cooled in shallow pans.

To save the customer money, the management of the diner uses canned foods, even when the cans are dented. Often these can be purchased at lower prices. When leftovers are reheated, they are raised to an internal temperature of 150° F (66° C) and served. Food handlers take great care to remove moldy portions of food. The cooks prepare stuffing separately from the poultry. The temperature of their refrigerators were approximately 55° F (13° C).

1. Below, list the violations of food safety practices that could contribute to food poisoning.

_____

_____

_____

2. If you were writing a report describing ways the Morningside Diner could correct these practices, what would you say?

_____

_____

_____

REFERENCES

1. American Dietetic Association. Food and water safety, *Journal of the American Dietetic Association* 90:111, 1990.

2. Anonymous: Eggs-ercise care, *FDA Consumer*, December, 1988, p 3.

3. Blair D: Uncertainties in pesticide risk estimation and consumer concern, *Nutrition Today*, November/December, 1989, p 13.

4. Blumenthal D: From the chicken to the egg, *FDA Consumer*, April, 1990, p 7.

5. Blumenthal D: Deciding about dioxins, *FDA Consumer*, February, 1990, p 10.

6. Blumenthal D: Red Dye No. 3 and other colorful controversies, *FDA Consumer*, May, 1990, p 18.

7. Farley D: Setting safe limits on pesticide residues, *FDA Consumer*, October, 1988, p 8.

8. Fennema OR: Food additives—an unending controversy, *American Journal of Clinical Nutrition* 46:201, 1987.

9. Hecht A: Preventing food-borne illness, *FDA Consumer*, January/February, 1991, p 18.

10. Leikos CW: An order of fries—hold the sulfites, *FDA Consumer*, March, 1988, p 10.

11. McKerrow JH, Sakanari J: Anisakiasis: revenge of the sushi parasite, *The New England Journal of Medicine* 319:1228, 1988.

12. Needleman HL and others: The long-term effects of exposure to low doses of lead in childhood, *The New England Journal of Medicine* 322:83, 1990.

13. Newberne PM: Naturally occurring food-borne toxicants. In Schills ME, Young VR, editors: *Modern nutrition in health and disease*, Philadelphia, 1988, Lea & Febiger.

14. Nightingale SL: Foodborne disease: an increasing problem, *American Family Physician* 35(3):353, 1987.

15. Peterson LR and others: A large *Clostridium perfringens* foodborne outbreak with an unusual attack rate pattern, *American Journal of Epidemiology* 127:605, 1988.

16. Rogan A, Glaros G: Food irradiation: the process and implications for dietitians, *Journal of the American Dietetic Association* 88:833, 1988.

17. Ryser ET, Marth EH: New food-borne pathogens of public health significance, *Journal of the American Dietetic Association* 89:948, 1989.

18. Segal M: Determining risk—is it worth the worry? *FDA Consumer*, June, 1990, p 7.

19. Segal M: Invisible villains—tiny microbes, our biggest food hazard, *FDA Consumer*, July/August, 1988, p 9.

20. Senti FR: Food additives and contaminants. In Schills ME, Young VR, editors: *Modern nutrition in health and disease*, Philadelphia, 1988, Lea & Febiger.

21. Snider S: FDA insures quality of imports, *FDA Consumer*, March, 1991, p 13.

22. Thonney PR, Bisogni CA: Residues of agricultural chemicals on fruits and vegetables, *Nutrition Today*, November/December, 1989, p 6.

23. Young FE: Weighing food safety risks, *FDA Consumer*, September, 1989, p 8.

HOW MUCH HAVE I LEARNED?

What have you learned from Chapter 17? Here are 15 statements about food safety. Read them to test your current knowledge. If you think the answer is true or mostly true, circle T. If you think the answer is false or mostly false, circle F. Use the scoring key at the end of the book to compute your total score. To review, take this test again later, and especially before tests.

1. **T F** In America, as many as one of every ten people may suffer a bout of diarrhea from food poisoning each year.

2. **T F** You can usually tell from a food's taste, odor, or appearance if that food poses a risk for food poisoning.

3. **T F** Imported food does not pose a risk for food poisoning because of careful inspection on entry into this country.

4. **T F** Synthetic (man-made) chemicals are necessarily more harmful than those that occur in nature.

5. **T F** Exposure to oxygen causes some foods to spoil.

6. **T F** Food can be preserved by reducing its water content.

7. **T F** Most kinds of bacteria can cause food poisoning.

8. **T F** Most food-poisoning microbes thrive on temperatures between 40° F and 140° F (4° C and 60° C).

9. **T F** Symptoms of food poisoning resemble stomach or intestinal "flu" symptoms.

10. **T F** Food-poisoning victims receive some immunity against future attacks.

11. **T F** Chickens are a common source of *Salmonella* food poisoning.

12. **T F** Botulism is the deadliest form of food poisoning, and the bacteria that cause it are present in soil.

13. **T F** *Clostridium botulinum,* the bacterium that causes botulism, grows only in the absence of air.

14. **T F** Eating raw fish can cause serious health problems.

15. **T F** Alcoholic beverages are free of toxic compounds.

NUTRITION ISSUE

PESTICIDES IN FOODS

Pesticides used in food production produce both good and unwanted effects. Most health authorities feel the benefits outweigh the risks. Pesticides help ensure an adequate food supply, make foods available at reasonable cost, and help ensure safety of the food supply. Alternatively, sentiment is growing nationwide that pesticides pose significant an avoidable health risks. Consumers have come to assume that man-made is dangerous and "organic" is safe. But such is not always the case. Some researchers believe this sentiment is grounded in fear and fueled by unbalanced reports. Other researchers say concern about pesticides is valid and overdue.[3]

The public is struggling to make sense of conflicting information. Most concern about pesticide residues in foods focuses on chronic rather than acute toxicity since the amounts of residues, if present at all, are extremely small. These low concentrations found in foods are not known to produce adverse effects in the short-term, although the high levels that occasionally result from accidents or misuse have done so. For humans, pesticides pose a danger mainly in their cumulative effects.[3] Hence, their threats to health are difficult to determine. However, growing evidence, including the problems of contamination of underground water supplies,[1] indicates that we would be better off as a nation if we reduced our use of pesticides.

 Alar in apples illustrates the public's problem with conflicting information. Apple growers have routinely sprayed Alar on trees to control ripening. We now know that one component of Alar changes into a potential carcinogen when heated, as it is when apples are processed into juice. Manufacturers and apple growers have now moved quickly to eliminate the use of Alar. Still, as some school systems were taking apples off menus, the U.S. Environmental Protection Agency (EPA) stated that it is unlikely that a person would be harmed from eating apples containing Alar. The agency felt it was safer to eat apples while Alar was being phased out than it was to drive a car or live on mostly hamburgers and candy bars. Furthermore, FDA analysis of 683 samples between 1981 and March 1989 turned up no apples with amounts of Alar that even approached EPA's safe limits.[23]

What is a pesticide?

Federal law defines a pesticide as any substance or mixture of substances intended to prevent, destroy, repel, or mitigate any pest.[22] Their built-in toxic properties lead to the possibility that other nontarget organisms, including humans, might also be harmed. The term pesticide tends to be used as a gener-

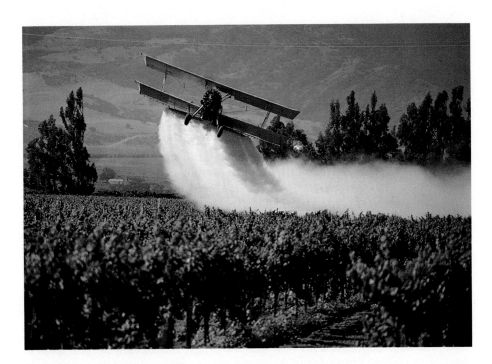

FIGURE 17-8
Pesticide use poses a risk versus benefit question. Each side has points we need to consider.

ic reference to many types of products, including insecticides, herbicides, fungicides, and rodenticides. A pesticide product may be chemical or bacterial, natural or man-made. For agriculture, the EPA allows about 10,000 pesticide uses, involving some 300 active ingredients.[22] Pesticide use in general substantially contributes to the chemical load applied intentionally to the earth's surface. About 2.6 billion pounds of pesticides are used each year in the United States, 60% of which is applied to agricultural crops (Figure 17-8).[3]

Once a pesticide is applied, it can turn up in a number of unintended and unwanted places. It may be carried in the air and dust by wind currents, remain in soil attached to soil particles, be taken up by organisms in the soil, decompose to other compounds, be taken up by plant roots, or enter aquatic habitats. Each is a route to the food chain; some are more direct than others.

Why use pesticides?

In the United States alone, pests destroy nearly $20 billion of food crops yearly, despite extensive pesticide use. The primary reason for using pesticides is economic—use of agricultural chemicals increases production and lowers the cost of food, at least in the short run. It decreases erosion by eliminating cultivation otherwise needed to get rid of weeds. Unless pesticides are applied, farming must depend much more on crop rotations to limit damage from pests. Government subsidies in the United States that encourage planting the same crops year after year discourage crop rotation, and so stimulate pesticide use. (See the discussion on sustainable agriculture in Chapter 18. Crop rotation is a key feature of that farming technology.)

Consumer demands have also changed over the years. At one time we would not think twice about buying an apple with a worm hole; we simply took it home, cut out the wormy part, and ate the apple. Today, consumers find worm holes less acceptable, and so farmers rely more and more on pesticides to produce cosmetically attractive fruits and vegetables.[18] On the practical side, pesticides can protect against rotting and decay of fresh fruits and vegetables. This is helpful since our food distribution system does not usually permit consumer purchase within hours of harvest. Also, food grown without pesticides can contain naturally occurring organisms that produce carcinogens at levels far above current standards for pesticide residues. For example, fungicides help prevent the potent carcinogen aflatoxin (caused by growth of a mold) from forming on some crops. So while some pesticides may improve the appearance of food products, others help keep some foods fresher and safer to eat.

Regulating pesticides

Currently, a newly proposed pesticide is exhaustively tested, perhaps over 10 years or more, before it can be used. EPA must decide both that the pesticide causes no unreasonable adverse effects to man and the environment, and that benefits outweigh the risks of using it. However, there is concern about older chemicals registered before 1970, when less stringent testing conditions were permitted.[3,22] EPA is now asking chemical companies to retest the old compounds using more rigorous tests. But inadequate funding at EPA has hampered the review of older pesticides. The slow pace for this retesting has angered the critics of pesticide use. When weighing whether to approve or cancel a pesticide, EPA considers how much more it would cost the farmer to use an alternative pesticide or process and whether cancellation would decrease productivity.[23] After determining the dollar cost to the farmer, EPA then looks at costs to processors and consumers as well.

Once approved for use, at least a 100-fold margin of safety is a standard requirement to minimize health effects other than cancer (such as kidney damage or birth defects).[7] These tolerances (limits) set the safety standard at 100 times less than the highest dose at which the pesticide causes no ill effects in animals—or lower. If the pesticide causes cancer, its use must not incur more than one cancer case in one million people. And, if the pesticide causes cancer and its level in finished foods is higher than that allowed for use on crops, its use is banned by the Delaney clause.[3]

How safe are pesticides?

A person's risk of poisoning from exposure to pesticides through food depends on the how potent the chemical poison is, how concentrated it is in the food, how much and how frequently it's eaten, and the person's resistance or susceptibility to the substance. Pesticide use is clearly associated with impure water quality. Accumulating information also links pesticide use to increased cancer rates in farm communities. For U.S. rural counties, the incidence of lymph, genital, and digestive tract cancers increases with higher-than-average herbicide use.[3] Respiratory cancer cases increase with greater insecticide use. In tests using laboratory animals, scientists have found that some of the chemicals present in pesticide residues cause birth defects, sterility, tumors, organ damage, and injury to the central nervous system. Some pesticides persist in the environment for years.

Still, an article published in the April 1987 issue of *Science* magazine and authored by Dr. Bruce Ames stated that cancer risk from pesticide residues was hundreds of times less than the risk of eating such common foods as peanut butter, brown mustard, and basil. Plants manufacture their own toxic substances to defend themselves against insects, birds, and grazing animals (including humans). When plants are stressed or damaged, they produce even more of these toxins. Because of this, many foods contain naturally occurring chemicals considered toxic, even carcinogenic. Other scientists argue that if natural carcinogens in large numbers are already in the food supply, then we should reduce the number of added carcinogens whenever possible. In other words, we should do what we can to help the problem.

The mere presence of a pesticide in food or water at any concentration frightens some people. But, the levels of pesticide residues found in foods are almost always well below the tolerance levels that have been set to meet safety concerns.[7] High and obviously hazardous concentrations are very rare, usually as the result of spills or improper uses. But the major challenge for scientists and regulators goes beyond detecting and measuring pesticide residues; it is rather a question of what, if any, biological significance they have.[22]

If EPA suspects any pesticide poses an imminent hazard to health, the agency can immediately stop its use.[23]

The risks of pesticides to children

Any discussions of pesticides and associated health risks need to focus attention on children. Children face a higher risk from pesticides than adults for several reasons.[3]

1. Their exposure is greater; children eat more food in proportion to their body weight than do adults.
2. Children consume more foods that are potential sources of pesticide residues, than do adults. They eat more fruit, for example.
3. Exposure at an early age carries a greater risk than exposure later in life; residues accumulate to toxic levels over a longer period. Also cancer has more time to develop.
4. Physiological susceptibility to the effects of carcinogens and neurotoxins in pesticides may be greater; the cells in children are dividing rapidly and the enzyme systems that detoxify chemicals are not fully developed.

Until recent years, EPA did not consider these factors in risk calculations. EPA now looks at age-level consumption data for approval of new pesticides. Although children are at greater risk from pesticides, the magnitude of that risk and how best to calculate it are open to debate.

Testing levels of pesticides in foods

FDA tests thousands of raw products a year for pesticide residues and consistently finds 96% to 98% free of illegal residues.[7] (A pesticide is considered illegal in this case if it is not approved for use on the crop in question or if the amount used exceeds the allowed levels.) Residues sometimes appear on the wrong crops or in excess amounts because of contamination from nearby farms via wind or water. Still, actual crop residues are usually considerably lower than the legal limits because worst-case scenarios of crop treatment and residue level are used to set the limits. When a problem is identified, FDA takes steps to make sure it's corrected and that the tainted food in question never reaches the consumer. However, of 600 pesticides available on international markets, many are not even detected by any of FDA's multiresidue tests.[3] This has raised concern by pesticide critics with regards to imported foods. Better tests that detect single residues are less frequently used because of cost.

Personal action

We often take risks in our own lives, but we prefer to have a choice in the matter after weighing the pros and cons. For instance, we can choose not to immunize a child, but we do so with the understanding that the child might get sick. It is a personal risk that we choose to take. One can also choose to risk cancer from smoking or to avoid that risk. But in regards to pesticides in produce, someone else is deciding what is acceptable and what is not.[23] Our only choice is whether to buy or avoid pesticide-containing foods. And, in reality it is almost impossible to avoid pesticides entirely because even organic produce often contains traces of pesticides, probably cross-contaminated from nearby farms.

Short-term studies of the effects of pesticides on laboratory animals cannot pinpoint long-term cancer risks precisely. But it should be clearly understood that the presence of minute traces of an environmental chemicals in food does not mean that any adverse effect will result from consumption of that food. FDA feels the hazards are comparatively low and, in the short run, are less than the hazards of food poisoning created in our own kitchens.[7] We can't avoid the risks entirely, but we can limit pesticide exposure by carefully washing vegetables and fruits and following the other advice on p. 555.

In the future, we can encourage farmers to use fewer pesticides to protect our foods and water supplies (see Chapter 18), and we will have to settle for produce that isn't perfect in appearance. Are you concerned enough about pesticides on food to change your shopping habits and take more political action? ●

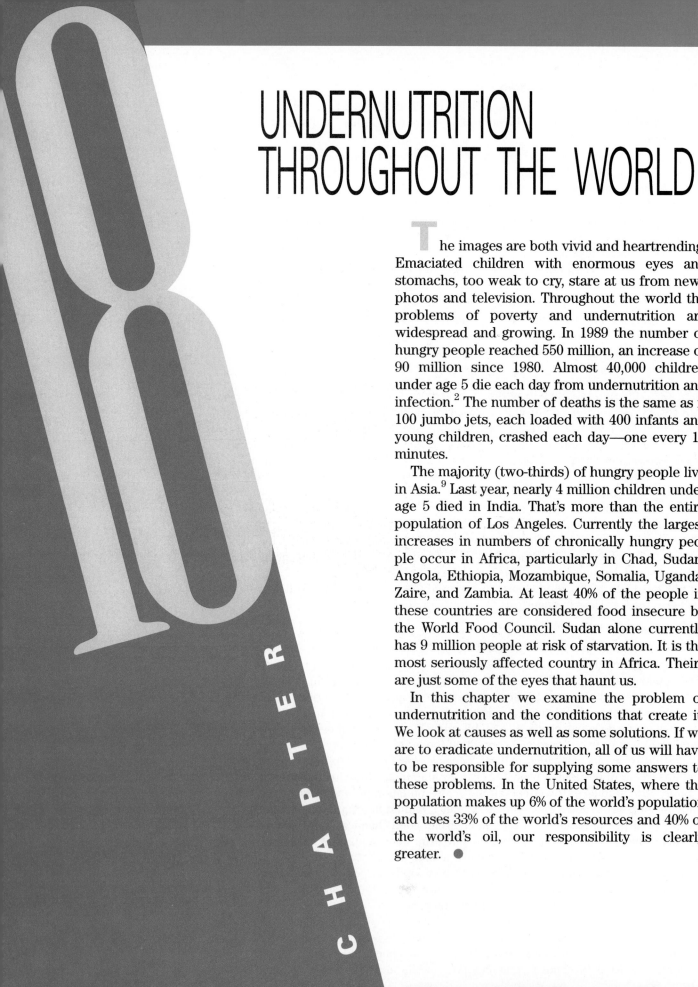

UNDERNUTRITION THROUGHOUT THE WORLD

The images are both vivid and heartrending. Emaciated children with enormous eyes and stomachs, too weak to cry, stare at us from news photos and television. Throughout the world the problems of poverty and undernutrition are widespread and growing. In 1989 the number of hungry people reached 550 million, an increase of 90 million since 1980. Almost 40,000 children under age 5 die each day from undernutrition and infection.[2] The number of deaths is the same as if 100 jumbo jets, each loaded with 400 infants and young children, crashed each day—one every 14 minutes.

The majority (two-thirds) of hungry people live in Asia.[9] Last year, nearly 4 million children under age 5 died in India. That's more than the entire population of Los Angeles. Currently the largest increases in numbers of chronically hungry people occur in Africa, particularly in Chad, Sudan, Angola, Ethiopia, Mozambique, Somalia, Uganda, Zaire, and Zambia. At least 40% of the people in these countries are considered food insecure by the World Food Council. Sudan alone currently has 9 million people at risk of starvation. It is the most seriously affected country in Africa. Theirs are just some of the eyes that haunt us.

In this chapter we examine the problem of undernutrition and the conditions that create it. We look at causes as well as some solutions. If we are to eradicate undernutrition, all of us will have to be responsible for supplying some answers to these problems. In the United States, where the population makes up 6% of the world's population and uses 33% of the world's resources and 40% of the world's oil, our responsibility is clearly greater. ●

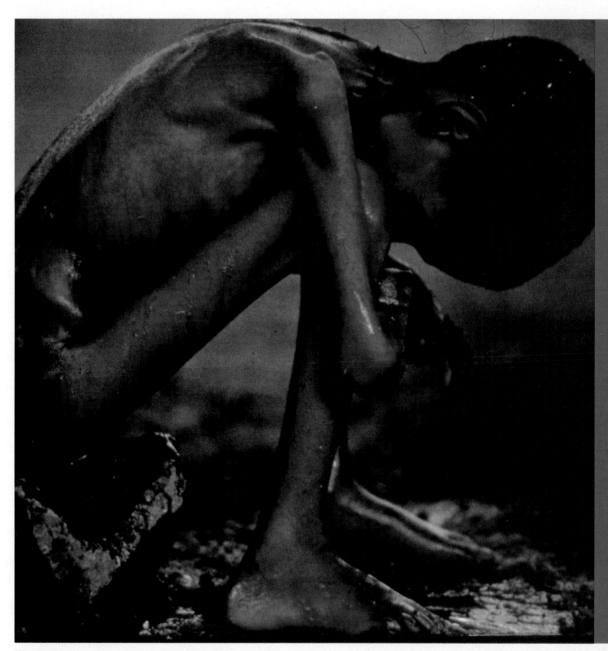

The tragedy of poverty, undernutrition, and illness. How can you help this child?

Broadening A Narrow Vision

Many people in the United States are unaware of the magnitude of undernutrition in the world, as well as in this country itself. Reading this chapter will open your eyes to the nutritional state of the world's peoples. You will discover what you can do to help correct the problem. But before you read this chapter, think about the following questions and provide the best answers you can:

1. Who is most likely to experience undernutrition in the United States?

_____

_____

_____

2. What are the major causes of undernutrition in the United States?

_____

_____

_____

3. What are the major causes of undernutrition in the developing countries of the world?

_____

_____

_____

_____

4. To what degree are you concerned about undernutrition in the United States and the world?

_____

_____

These questions were designed to get you think about the issues addressed in this chapter. As you read this chapter, these and other questions will be answered.

ASSESS YOURSELF

WORLD HUNGER CONTINUES TO PLAGUE MANKIND

In November 1974, the United Nations World Food Conference proclaimed the bold objective "that within a decade no child will go to bed hungry, that no family will fear for its next day's bread, and that no human being's future and capacities will be stunted by malnutrition." Not only does this promise remain unfulfilled, 17 years later hunger is a daily experience for one in eight people.[2]

The famines that occurred in Ethiopia in the 1980s called special attention to the problem of undernutrition in the developing world. The plight of millions of starving people consolidated widespread public support for immediate aid for the victims of famine. The acute crisis that existed has eased in some areas; starvation is less in the public eye as a world concern. However, as we just noted, the problem of undernutrition in developing nations is ongoing. And it is one that requires political and technological solutions.

UNDERNUTRITION AND POVERTY

Let's begin our look at these problems by first defining some key words:

Hunger is the physiological state that results when not enough food is eaten to meet energy needs. It also describes an uneasiness, discomfort, weakness, or pain caused by lack of food. If hunger is not attended to, the resulting medical and social costs from undernutrition are high—infant prematurity and mental retardation, inadequate growth and development in childhood that contribute to poor school performance, decreased work output in adulthood, and chronic disease (Table 18-1).[1] Symptoms of chronic hunger can be found not only in the developing world, but also in many people living at or below the poverty level in America.[3]

The primary cause of chronic hunger is poverty. Unemployment and under-employment, homelessness, drug addiction, functional illiteracy, marital breakups leading to single parent families (often headed by a woman who has limited earning potential), wage discrimination, poor health, inadequate governmental programs, and war/civil strife all contribute to this poverty. In devel-

---

TABLE 18-1

The Realities of Undernutrition

- There are 550 million hungry people in the world. About 730 million people are chronically undernourished with respect to iron, zinc, and iodide.
- Each year, 15 to 20 million people die of hunger-related causes, including diseases brought on by lowered resistance caused by undernutrition. Of every four of these, three are children.
- 17 million children died last year from preventable diseases—one every 2 seconds, 40,000 a day. At least 250,000 children are permanently blinded each year simply through lack of vitamin A.
- Women in poor countries average up to four times more births than women in the U.S.
- Every day, the world produces about 3000 kcal/day for each person, well above the average need of 2300 kcal.
- A person born in the rich world will consume 30 times as much food as a person born in the Third World.
- Poor women in Third World countries face a 300 fold increased risk of death in pregnancy compared to women in the U.S.
- Almost half the world's people earn less than $200 a year—many use 80% to 90% of that income to obtain food.
- Of the nearly 5.3 billion people on earth, more than 1.2 billion drink contaminated water.
- In many poor countries, life expectancy of the population is one-half to two-thirds of that in the United States.
- 1.8 billion people in the world are without proper sanitation facilities.
- Poor countries have two-thirds of the 8 to 10 million AIDS cases worldwide.

Malnutrition • Failing health that results from a long-standing dietary intake that either fails to meet or greatly exceeds nutritional needs.

oping nations the problems stemming from poverty, a lack of resources, and inadequacy of governmental programs are intensified.

Malnutrition is a condition of impaired development or function caused by a long-term deficiency, excess, or imbalance of kcalories and/or nutrients. The occurrence of specific diseases of malnutrition depends mostly on the food/population ratio.[19] When food supplies are low and the population is large, undernutrition leading to nutritional deficiency diseases, such as xeroph-

TABLE 18-2

Nutrient deficiency diseases commonly seen in states of undernutrition in the world.

Disease and Key nutrient involved	Typical result	Some natural sources for the nutrient
Xerophthalmia		
Vitamin A	Blindness, poor growth, increased infections	Liver, sweet potatoes, spinach, greens, carrots, cantaloupe, apricots, mangos, papayas
Rickets		
Vitamin D	Weakened bones, bow legs, fractures	Fish oils, (sun exposure)
Beriberi		
Thiamin	Nerve degeneration, poor muscle coordination, heart problems	Sunflower seeds, pork, whole grains, dried beans
Ariboflavinosis		
Riboflavin	Inflammation of face and oral cavity	Milk, mushrooms, spinach, liver
Pellagra		
Niacin	Diarrhea, skin inflammation, mental deterioration	Mushrooms, bran, tuna, chicken, beef, peanuts, whole grains
Scurvy		
Vitamin C	Poor wound healing, bleeding skin and gums	Citrus fruits, strawberries, broccoli, mangos, papaya
Iron-deficiency anemia		
Iron	Poor work output, poor growth, increased health risk in pregnancy	Meats, spinach, seafood, peas, bran, whole grains
Goiter		
Iodide	Enlarged thyroid gland, poor growth in infancy and childhood, possible mental retardation	Saltwater fish, seaweed

Note that often two or more nutrition deficiency diseases are found simultaneously in an undernourished person in the Third World. This discussion of individual nutrients makes it easier to see the important role of each nutrient.

thalmia (eye problems caused by a poor vitamin A intake), is common. However, when the food supply is ample or overabundant, poor food choices coupled with an excessive intake can lead to nutrition-related chronic diseases, such as certain forms of diabetes mellitus. Note, however, pockets of undernutrition among the poor may still be found in food abundant areas, such as the United States.

Genetics plays an important role in both forms of malnutrition. Not every child in Thailand who eats mainly rice develops *protein-energy malnutrition* (see Chapter 8); similarly, not every adult in New York City who consumes a high-fat, high-kcalorie diet suffers a heart attack.[19] Genetics influences the development of these diseases.

Undernutrition, referred to many times in this book, is the malnutrition that results from an inadequate intake, absorption, or use of the nutrients or kcalories needed for optimal growth, development, and body function. The earliest response to undernutrition is a reduction in activity. This allows the individual to preserve energy for growth and other vital functions. With persistent undernutrition, the second response is a reduced rate of weight gain or poor weight maintenance. Later, in children, the rate of growth in height is reduced.

Undernutrition is the most common form of malnutrition among the poor in both developing and developed countries. It is also the primary cause of specific nutrient deficiencies that in turn can result in muscle wasting, blindness (from xerophthalmia), scurvy, pellagra, beriberi, anemia, rickets, goiter, and a host of other effects (Table 18-2). For example, more than 250,000 children develop blindness from xerophthalmia each year. About half of all women in the Third World suffer from anemia caused by iron deficiency and malaria. Of the 5.3 billion people in the world, at least half a billion suffer some form of undernutrition.[2] Death and disease from infections, particularly those causing acute and prolonged diarrhea or acute lower respiratory disease, are dramatically increased when the infections are superimposed on a state of chronic undernutrition.

Protein-energy malnutrition (PEM) is a form of undernutrition caused by an extremely deficient intake of kcalories and/or protein. The typically dramatic results of protein-energy malnutrition—kwashiorkor and marasmus—were covered in Chapter 8. We will concentrate in this chapter on the more subtle effects of a chronic lack of food.

CONSEQUENCES OF UNDERNUTRITION—A CLOSER LOOK

Prolonged undernutrition is detrimental to health at any time throughout life, but consequences are more critical during some periods of growth and throughout the elderly years.

The critical periods

The human organism is particularly susceptible to the effects of undernutrition during periods of rapid growth, especially pregnancy, infancy, and childhood.

Pregnancy. The period of greatest health risk from undernutrition is during pregnancy. A pregnant woman needs extra nutrients to meet her own needs as well as those of her developing fetus. If the mother's nutrient intake is inadequate during pregnancy, her own health can be seriously jeopardized.[13] Stores of maternal nutrients may be depleted to provide for the baby. Maternal iron-deficiency anemia is one possible consequence. Pregnancy-induced hypertension (preeclampsia), a life-threatening condition involving rapid weight gain from fluid retention and a sharp increase in blood pressure, is also thought to be influenced by inadequate prenatal nutrition.

In Africa, women give birth, on average, to more than six live babies. Coupled with chronic undernutrition, this high birthrate creates a one in 20 lifetime risk of dying from pregnancy-related causes for women. In contrast,

Undernutrition • Failing health that results from a long-standing dietary intake that does not meet nutritional needs.

Protein-Energy Malnutrition (PEM) • This results when a person regularly consumes insufficient amounts of kcalories and protein. The deficiency eventually results in body wasting and an increased susceptibility to infections.

Gestation • The time between conception and birth of the infant.

American women face a risk of one in about 6000 from pregnancy-related causes. No other social indicator—literacy, life expectancy, and infant morality included—shows a wider gap between the developing world and the industrialized world.

Fetal and infant stages. The greatest risk from undernutrition during pregnancy actually is borne by the fetus. A growing fetus requires a diet rich in protein, vitamins, and minerals as it develops. When these needs are not met, the infant is often born before 37 weeks of **gestation** —about 40 weeks of gestation is ideal. Results of prematurity include poor lung function and a weakened immune response. These conditions lessen health and make death more likely. Long-term problems in growth and development can result if the infant does survive. At the extreme, low-birth-weight babies, 2500 grams or less (about 5.5 pounds or less), face 30 to 40 times the normal risk of dying before the age of 1 year, primarily because of their poor lung development. When low birth weight is accompanied by other physical abnormalities, medical intervention can cost $100,000 or more. When severe retardation occurs, the lifetime cost of care can be over $2 million.

In the United States, low birth weight accounts for more than half of all infant deaths and for 75% of deaths of babies under 1 month of age.[3] Worldwide, more than half of infant deaths stem from low birth weight.

Childhood. The rapid growth years of early childhood comprise another period of high risk from undernutrition. Because the human brain grows most rapidly from conception through early childhood, the brain and central nervous system are particularly vulnerable. After the preschool years, brain growth and development slows dramatically until maturity, when it stops. Nutritional deprivation, especially in early infancy, can lead to permanent brain impairment. Beyond early childhood, learning may be jeopardized by a deprived environment, but the basic size and structure of the brain are set.[3]

In general, poor children experience more nutritional deprivation and overall illness and are more severely affected by these effects than are other children. For example, iron-deficiency anemia, indicated by the presence of an abnormally low concentration of hemoglobin in the blood, is much more common among poor children than nonpoor children. This deficiency can lead to reduced stamina and learning problems. Undernutrition in childhood also can weaken resistance to infection, as immune function decreases when nutrients such as protein and zinc are very low in a diet.[4] Poorly nourished youngsters are then at risk for more frequent colds, ear infections, and other infectious diseases. Note that nearly half of all black children in the United States live in poverty.

Symptoms of undernutrition in children are not always obvious. Visitors to developing countries may not notice undernutrition in children—children who appear to be 3 or 4 years old actually may be 8 or 9 years old. Failure of children to grow is a common result of undernutrition and a warning sign that more extreme effects may follow. In a recent survey of 76 developing countries, stunting was seen in more than one-third of children aged 2 to 5 years old.[2]

We also need to consider one more group at risk for undernutrition—the elderly and the chronically ill. These people often require nutrient-dense foods, the amount depending on each person's state of health and level of activity. Because many have fixed incomes and significant medical costs, food is often a low priority item. In addition, the elderly and the chronically ill are often unable to take care of all their own needs, are sometimes isolated, and are more apt to be depressed—all important factors that can influence food intake .

General effects of semistarvation

The results of undernutrition from semistarvation in their initial stages are often so mild that physical symptoms are absent, and blood tests typically do not detect the slight changes in metabolism. Even in the absence of clinical symptoms, however, undernourishment may affect reproductive capacity, resistance to or recovery from disease, activity and work output, and attitudes and behavior. Recall from Chapter 2 that as tissues continue to be depleted of nutrients, blood tests eventually detect biochemical changes, such as a drop in blood hemoglobin concentration. Physical symptoms, such as body weakness, become apparent with further depletion. Finally, the full-blown symptoms of the predominating deficiency become obvious enough to be recognized, such as edema associated with a protein deficiency.

In general, the occurrence of severe deficiency in a few people in a population represents the tip of the iceberg. This usually means that a much greater number have milder degrees of undernutrition. As we have noted, mild nutrient deficiencies, though perhaps not life threatening, can in certain critical combinations still cause very important practical difficulties in health, as well as in life in general. These should not, therefore, be dismissed as trivial, especially in the developing world.[4] It is becoming clear that combined deficiencies of certain vitamins, iron, and zinc, although less severe than those causing overt physical symptoms, can seriously reduce work performance. *Marginal* deficiencies of iodide, iron and zinc are known to affect hundreds of millions of people worldwide.

Detailed experiments studying the effects of chronic undernutrition were performed by Dr. Ansel Keys in the 1940s. He maintained 32 men on a diet averaging about 1600 kcalories daily for 6 months. During this time the men lost an average of 24% of their body weight. After about 3 months, the subjects complained of tiredness, muscle soreness, irritability, and hunger pains. They showed a loss of ambition, poor self-discipline, and poor concentration. They were often moody and depressed. Their ability to laugh heartily and sneeze was reduced, and they became intolerant to heat. Decreases in heart rate and muscle tone were also noted.

These cumulative stresses of undernutrition, then, eventually caused emotional instability and an overall apathetic frame of mind. Persistent hunger made it difficult for the subjects to pursue cultural interests, perform manual activities, and study. This in turn produced a frustrating discrepancy between their desire and ability to pursue activities. When they were permitted to eat normally again, even after 12 weeks of rehabilitation, the desire for more food and a feeling of tiredness continued for the subjects. By 20 weeks they had largely, but not fully, recovered—full recovery required about 33 weeks.

These same responses can be expected from undernutrition wherever it appears in the world. This state diminishes the ability of people, communities, and even whole countries to perform at peak levels of physical and mental capacity, robbing people and nations of human resources. Furthermore, the effects of undernutrition in poor countries are even greater than that seen by Dr. Keys because his subjects had adequate vitamin and mineral intakes. In addition, the populations in poorer countries must also contend with recurrent infections, poor sanitary conditions, extreme weather conditions, and regular exposure to very infectious diseases. Their greater nutrient requirements—especially iron—to combat rampant parasite and other infections compounds the problem further. As mentioned before, iron and zinc deficiency both can lead to poor immune function and so increase the risk of disease caused by infections, such as diarrhea, pneumonia, and dysentery.

As we mentioned earlier, a common consequence of undernutrition both in the United States and worldwide is an increased rate of infant mortality. The United States infant mortality rate is currently twenty-second worldwide, the

Marginal • Noticeable, but not severe.

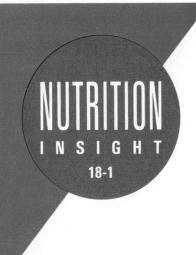

UNDERNUTRITION INFLUENCES THE POTENTIAL TO LEARN

The influence of nutrition on normal growth and development has long been observed, and tragic consequences of severe undernutrition on the structure and function of the brain of the growing child have been amply documented. The first two to three years of life are a critical period of brain development, during which it grows in spurts. Most of the brain's nerve cells stop dividing by the time of birth. The brain grows after birth by forming connections, or *synapses,* between the nerve cell, and developing structures necessary for normal conduction of nervous impulses.

Since the brain is capable of growing so rapidly only during this critical period, brain size and structure are highly susceptible to the complications of undernutrition in early childhood. Seriously undernourished children have smaller heads and lower brain weights than their well-nourished counterparts, a condition that unfortunately remains irreversible. Thus growth deficits among the poor worldwide suggest that children are losing out on physical, social, and cognitive activities necessary for optimal development.

Public health workers in the United States have noted an increase in cases of stunted growth, anemia, and abnormal weight in poor children. These children need more nutrients to grow and develop properly.[3] Studies indicate that hunger, even such as that following a morning fast, can inhibit the ability of children to perform their best in school, even if they are not undernourished.

The most common nutritional deficiency in American children is iron deficiency. Physical activity and the capacity for work are reduced by iron deficiency. Iron's influence on growth and learning has also been well documented.[12] Infants and preschool and school-age children who are iron deficient show slower growth and less progress in mental development, attention span, learning skills, and in educational achievement test scores.

Cognitive growth (intelligence), however, is not the only aspect of normal growth affected by iron deficiency. Mental development in children is also dependent on interaction with the larger world. A child's active exploration of his physical and social environment is a prerequisite for normal development. If a young child is deprived of adequate kcalories and/or nutrients, like iron, to meet his or her energy needs, he soon spends minimal energy on activities not directly related to survival. As a result, the child becomes apathetic and listless, and reduces time spent in play, social interaction, and exploring the environment. If such inactivity is prolonged, normal mental development will be impaired. Neglect or abuse by parents adds to the problem.

These effects of undernutrition may be substantially diminished by vigorous nutritional rehabilitation, especially when combined with appropriate social stimulation. However, some studies indicate that particular nutrient deficiencies and their affects may not be totally reversible. ●

Synapse • Spaces between nerve cells. One nerve cell stimulates other nearby cells, including other nerve cells, by releasing chemicals that cross the synapse. These chemicals are what excites neighboring cells.

second worst showing for any industrialized nation.[2] Scandinavia, Western European nations, such as England, France and Germany, and Asian nations, such as Japan, all have lower infant mortality rates. The United States' position has declined from a rank of sixth in infant mortality rates in the 1950s to its current position. The black infant mortality rate in the United States is 18.4 per 1000 live births, a figure comparable to that of developing countries. The rate for white Americans is 9.4 per 1000. Additional data for poor whites in the United States suggest that this black to white ratio reflects the impact of economic and social circumstances, rather than any biological difference between racial groups.

CONCEPT CHECK

Hunger is the uneasiness and pain that results when insufficient food is eaten to meet energy needs. Chronic hunger leads to undernutrition and, in turn, to growth failure for children and weakness in adults. Risk of infection increases and nutrient deficiency diseases also result. The primary cause of undernutrition is poverty. The critical periods when undernutrition most adversely influences health are pregnancy, infancy, and childhood. The effects in infancy are quite dramatic, as evidenced by infant mortality rates about twice that of healthy populations.

UNDERNUTRITION IN UNITED STATES—HOW WIDESPREAD IS IT?

At least 32 million Americans live at or near the poverty level—currently estimated at about $12,700 annually for a family of four. More than two-thirds of these people live in metropolitan areas. These poor include nearly a quarter of all children. About two-thirds—18 to 20 million—of these Americans experience chronic hunger; 7 to 8 million are children.[3] These citizens eat enough to prevent overt starvation, so undernutrition in the United States presents itself quite differently from that in the developing world. Kwashiorkor and marasmus, evident in the pictures of Ethiopian children in the mid 1980s, rarely occur. Instead, undernutrition in the United States tends to take the form of silent undernutrition, a term coined by the World Health Organization. It is reflected in the young child whose weight is several pounds below the low end of the normal range on a growth chart.[3] The untrained eye may not recognize the condition or simply see the child as skinny. The trained professional will recognize that the child's size reflects growth failure.

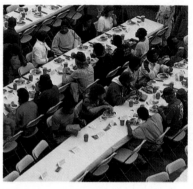

500 Christmas meals provided by volunteers in Los Angeles.

Poor Americans often face difficult choices: whether to buy groceries for the family or pay this month's rent; whether to have dental work done or pay the current utility bill; or whether to replace clothes the children have outgrown or pay for transportation to apply for a job. Food is one of the few flexible items in a poor person's budget. Rents are fixed, utility costs aren't negotiable, the price of medical care and prescription drugs can't be bargained down, and bus drivers won't accept less than the going rate to transport riders. But a person can always eat less. The short term consequences may be less dramatic than having the utilities shut off. The long-term cumulative effects, however, are disturbing.

In sheer numbers, as well as in severity of health risks posed, undernutrition in the United States is a troubling problem. Its existence is all the more disturbing since the threat of undernutrition for most Americans was virtually eliminated in the 1970s.[3] The fact that major pockets of undernutrition were conquered and then reemerged and spread rapidly in the 1980s suggests that the roots of undernutrition are mainly political and socioeconomic, rather than technical. Resources are available for feeding all Americans. In the developing world, far more factors complicate this problem, as we will discuss later.

ANOTHER BITE

The presence of undernutrition in the United States raises a broad question for our society at large; where can people in such situations turn when their own resources fail? The responsibility for helping those in need could lie with the federal government, state government, local government, religious groups, charitable organizations, or perhaps with the individuals themselves. All can be part of the solution.

Undernutrition in the United States is not a new problem

The problem of undernutrition in the United States actually began soon after the Pilgrims landed. Studies in the 1930s during the Depression documented both undernutrition and the existence of widespread pellagra (niacin deficiency) and rickets (vitamin D deficiency). In response, the government opened soup kitchens and began distributing food commodities.[14] Congress organized school lunch programs in 1946 after testimony by the United States Surgeon General that 70% of the men who had poor nutrition during the Depression era (10 to 12 years earlier) were being rejected for physical reasons by the draft.

In the 1950s, it was assumed that all Americans had enough to eat. Nevertheless, occasional reports of undernutrition surfaced, mostly among the chronic poor: migrant workers, Native Americans, southern blacks, unemployed minorities, and some elderly people.

After observing extensive hunger and poverty during his presidential campaign, John F. Kennedy in the 1960s revitalized the food stamp program, a program begun two decades earlier, and expanded commodity distribution programs.[3] The program for low income people, still in effect, allows recipients to use food stamps like cash to purchase food and seeds—but not tobacco, cleaning items, alcoholic beverages, or nonedible products—at stores authorized to accept them (Table 18-3).

The school breakfast program won passage in 1965 as politicians began to see firsthand the number of children coming to school hungry. Both school lunch and breakfast programs still enable low-income students to receive meals at reduced cost or no cost if certain income guidelines are met. In the same year Congress funded group noon-time (called congregate) meals and home-delivered meals for all senior citizens over 60 years of age.[14] Both are still active programs serving the elderly.

Political and social awareness of hunger and undernutrition in the late 1960s was spurred on by the book *Hunger USA* and a resulting television documentary, *Hunger in America*, shown in May 1968. The film graphically demonstrated that hunger existed in all areas and ethnic groups in the United States.[14] The response was dramatic. Between 1969 and 1971, some already large federal food programs were expanded, and others were newly created.[3] The Food Stamp program served only 2 million people in 1968, but by 1971 it was serving 11 million citizens. Today it serves more than 19 million people. The School Lunch program, which served only 2 million poor children before 1970, was serving 8 million children by 1971. In 1990 about 12 million children had the cost of their lunch fully-subsidized or partly-subsidized by the program. The School Breakfast program, which was still only a pilot program for children living in poverty areas, became nationally available by 1975.

In the early 1970s the Special Supplemental Feeding Program for Women, Infants, and Children (WIC) was authorized. This program provides food vouchers and nutrition education to low-income pregnant and lactating women and their young children. WIC has been repeatedly shown to be cost effective, especially in reducing the numbers of premature, low-birth-weight babies.[14] WIC is also credited for the widespread drop in iron-deficiency anemia seen in children in the last decade. The current federal budget shortfalls have over the last few years threaten both the scope and existence of this program. This raises a yearly struggle for support of the program. "Of all the dumb ways of saving money, not feeding pregnant women and kids is the dumbest," says Dr. Jean Mayer, one of the world's leading experts on nutrition.

Undernutrition in United States—a reevaluation

In 1977, a team of physicians resurveyed areas of undernutrition studied 10 years earlier. They found that the degree of poverty in regions like Appalachia and the slums of big cities had not changed. If anything, poverty was often

TABLE 18-3

Some federally subsidized programs that supply food for Americans

Program	Eligibility	Description
Food Stamps	Low income	Coupons are given to purchase food at grocery stores, the amount based on size of household and income
Emergency Food System	Low income	Food stamps issued on 24-hour notice for one month while eligibility for further use of the program can be investigated
Commodity Supplemental Food Program	Certain low income populations, such as pregnant women and young children	USDA surplus foods are distributed by county agencies
Special Supplemental Feeding Program for Women, Infants, and Children (WIC)	Low income pregnant/lactating, infant, child less than 5 years old at nutritional risk	Coupons are given to purchase milk, cheese, fruit juice, cereal, infant formula, and other specific food items at grocery stores
School Lunch	Low income	Free or reduced price lunch distributed by the school; meal follows USDA pattern based on the Guide to Daily Food Choices; cost for the child depends on family income.In schools without a lunch program, special milk programs may be available.
School Breakfast	Low income	Free or reduced price breakfast distributed by the school. Meal follows USDA pattern. Cost for the child depends on family income.
Child Care Food Program	Child enrolled in organized child care program; income guidelines are the same as School Lunch Program	Reimbursement given for meals supplied to children at the site. Meals must follow USDA guidelines based on the Guide to Daily Food Choices
Congregate Meals for the Elderly	Age 60 or over (no income guidelines)	Free noon meal is furnished at a site; meal follows specific pattern based on $1/3$ of the RDA
Home-delivered Meals	Age 60 or over, homebound	Noon meal is delivered at no cost or for a fee, depending on income; at least 5 days a week. Sometimes other meals for later consumption are delivered at the same time; private organizations who sponsor these problems often refer to them as Meals on Wheels

worse than in 1967. Yet undernutrition had essentially disappeared as a social phenomenon.[3] As a population, Americans had more food resources available to them. The large federal food programs—Food Stamps, the School Lunch and School Breakfast programs, and WIC—contributed to this difference. Politicians had responded to the demands of the American people by directing federal resources toward a massive human problem, and the effort succeeded.[3] Certainly some Americans still fell through the cracks, but a food "safety net" was catching many whose needs had not been met before.

The 1980s

The first official recognition in 1982 that widespread hunger reappeared in the United States came from the a conference of mayors. While the news media had been reporting the appearance of soup kitchens and breadlines in the nation's cities since the beginning of the decade, the mayors identified growing hunger as a national problem.[3]

Why was there a sudden increase in hungry people in the United States? First, unemployment in the United States rose from 6.2% in early 1980 to 10.8% in 1983. Although the rate has since fallen to about 6% to 7%, more Americans are unemployed today than were unemployed in 1980. Second, in every year but 1 since 1976, the scope of the Food Stamp program has been narrowed and eligibility tightened, so that participants lost $7 to $10 billion worth of foods in the period from 1982 to 1985. In 1981, the School Lunch program was reduced by one-third. In addition, during that time funding levels for the senior citizen meals programs lagged far behind the increases in food and operating costs, as well as behind the increasing numbers in this age group.[1]

In a 1985 report, *Hunger in America: The Growing Epidemic*, a group of physicians associated the reappearance of widespread hunger in the United States with government policies and budget cutbacks.[3] Other contemporary reports pointed out that for the majority of food programs, at least half the clients were families with children—those most at risk from undernutrition.

Although cuts in the Food Stamp and school meal programs were made in the early 1980s, attempts to cut WIC were not successful. A bipartisan coalition in Congress protected WIC against proposed funding reductions. This coalition maintained and even increased WIC participation in the mid 1980s in the face of annual efforts to cut funds. This points to the political nature of the problems we discuss in the United States. Who went hungry depended very heavily on political decisions.

Congress acts again

During 1986 and 1987, concern over undernutrition and associated adverse health outcomes began to take hold in Washington. Congressional leaders became more concerned. Four hundred million dollars were then added back to the Food Stamp and school meals programs, and Congress increased funding for WIC.[14] These changes, however, while signaling a growing awareness of undernutrition, still fall far short of the amount needed to end the problem. For instance, the need for WIC services still greatly outstrips resources allocated to the program. This forces children to be disenrolled from the program, as currently pregnant women and infants are given the highest priority. As a nation, the United States is not as well off nutritionally as in the late 1970s, but much better off today than in 1985.

Poverty is also at the heart of the current problem

The root cause of hunger and undernutrition in the United States continues to be poverty. In 1988, there were more than 32 million Americans living at or below the poverty threshold. Recent increases were fueled by the unequal distribution of wealth in the 1980s. From 1980 to 1989, the richest 20% of American families received a 33% increase in after-tax income. The richest 5% of families received a 51% increase.[14] Meanwhile, the poorest 20% of families netted a 0.5% decrease in after-tax income. Of the 13 million jobs created between 1980 and 1985, most were in the service sector, such as fast-food restaurants. These usually offer low pay. If both parents have such full-time, low-paying jobs, the family may still operate at or below the poverty level, again currently $12,700 for a family of four. Thus not only have the impoverished in the United States had to exist with less federal assistance, they have also netted a dwindling amount of the national family income.

HOMELESSNESS IN THE UNITED STATES

The economics of poverty and undernutrition have recently changed in one more very important way. Homelessness is much more evident now than in 1980. Estimates of the number of homeless vary widely, ranging from 350,000 to 3 million.[2] Homelessness exists partly because the cost of housing has substantially increased and partly because federal support for subsidized housing was cut dramatically during the 1980s. In 1969, the average American spent about 33% of his or her income on housing. People at or below the poverty line spent about 50% for housing. In 1989 half of all poor renter households paid at least 70% of their income in rent and utilities.[14] Many families below the poverty line pay 80%. When so much is spent for shelter, almost every other expense is pushed aside, including enough food for children. The larger the family, the less money left to feed each child. Other important causes of homelessness include release of the mentally ill from mental institutions in the 1980's, unemployment, substance abuse, and personal crises.

The stereotypical image of a homeless person is someone out of step with society who might refuse to work. However, each year, as more and more typical Americans find themselves on the streets, we are having to rethink this stereotype.[11] In Columbus, Ohio during 1989, of the 10,562 people who used structures funded by the Community Shelter Board over a 9-month period, 47% had at least a high school diploma, 22% were employed, 17% had recently been employed, and 18% were children; the total included 513 families. In an affluent California community (Contra Costa County) in 1989, investigators found 48% of emergency food recipients were members of families with children; only 2% were transients; and 45% of adult emergency food recipients were employed in low-paying jobs or had recently lost a job. Many emergency food recipients were disabled (16% of survey respondents), raising dependent children alone (27%), or were children themselves (33%).

FOOD AND SHELTER FOR ALL AMERICANS

The reasons for both homelessness and undernutrition in America are many. Blaming the victims obscures the real issues. These problems increased dramatically in the 1980s, linked to political and economic factors. Opponents of federal nutrition programs raise the issue of cost, often citing the federal deficit as a reason for limiting spending and stating much money is wasted by bureaucrats and drug-addicted recipients. This argument in our opinion does not outweigh the even greater need to meet the nutritional and housing needs of American citizens. The approximately 1.2 trillion dollar budget of the United States, 26% of which goes for defense spending, allows for many choices.

Undernutrition especially is a condition that need not exist. Nutrition pro-

The availability of cooking facilities is an additional important variable related to nutrient intake of the poor. In the absence of cooking facilities, people may buy expensive foods that require no preparation. These typically are processed snack foods, which provide kcalories but often limited nutrients.

Infrastructure • The basic framework of a system or organization. For a society, this includes roads, bridges, telephones, and other basic technologies.

Geometric Ratio • A group of numbers where the division of each number by the one to the left of it yields the same answer.

Arithmetic Ratio • A group of numbers where the difference between each number is the same.

grams and community intervention, if used fully and effectively, could go a long way toward meeting the food needs of those at highest risk.[14] More employment opportunities could then help solidify the improvements. The near elimination of large-scale undernutrition in the United States in the 1970s demonstrates that this national problem can be solved. Until the economy can accept all of us, a federal food safety net is important.

Private emergency food network systems also are important, but not sufficient to meet all food needs in the United States. Private donations often taper off during economic hardship in a given geographic area. In addition, much of what is donated is limited in nutritional value. Of necessity, processed and canned grocery items predominate, rather than protein-rich foods or perishable items, such as fresh produce and milk. During recent years, an extensive network of private agencies to feed the hungry has emerged.[3] There are numerous food banks around the United States in the Second Harvest system. These food banks distribute corporate surplus to thousands of soup kitchens and food pantries operating out of church basements and social service agencies. Yet despite this extraordinary effort, a huge gap remains between federal aid and human need. There is no escaping the fact that federal assistance is the most effective way to help poor Americans get adequate nutrition. When federal assistance is a priority, undernutrition can be beaten.

CONCEPT CHECK

Hunger and undernutrition in the United States were recognized by political leaders in the 1960s. In response, federally subsidized food programs, such as food stamps, school lunch, and congregate meals for the elderly, were started or received substantially increased funding. This federal response greatly reduced undernutrition in the United States; but the number of at-risk people increased in the 1980s as funding for these programs was reduced, and an economic recession took place. Since 1985 some funding has been restored, but elimination of undernutrition remains a challenge for the United States.

UNDERNUTRITION IN THE THIRD WORLD

Undernutrition in the Third World is also tied to poverty, so any true solution must address this problem. However, the countries that are considered to be Third World nations—that are neither industrialized nor have a planned economy as seen in the Soviet Union—have a multitude of problems so complex and interrelated that they cannot be treated separately. Programs that have proven immensely helpful in the United States would only be a starting point in the Third World. Solutions have to consider major obstacles, such as:

- extreme imbalances in the food/population ratio in different regions of a country
- the rapid depletion of natural resources
- cultural attitudes towards certain foods
- poor *infrastructure* especially poor housing, sanitation and storage facilities, education, communications, and transportation systems
- war and civil unrest
- mounting external debt

Let's examine each problem individually. In this context, Figure 18-1 depicts key factors relating to an individual's food intake.

THE FOOD/POPULATION RATIO

Whether the earth can yield enough food for all people has been a long-standing question. As early as 1798, the English clergyman and political economist,

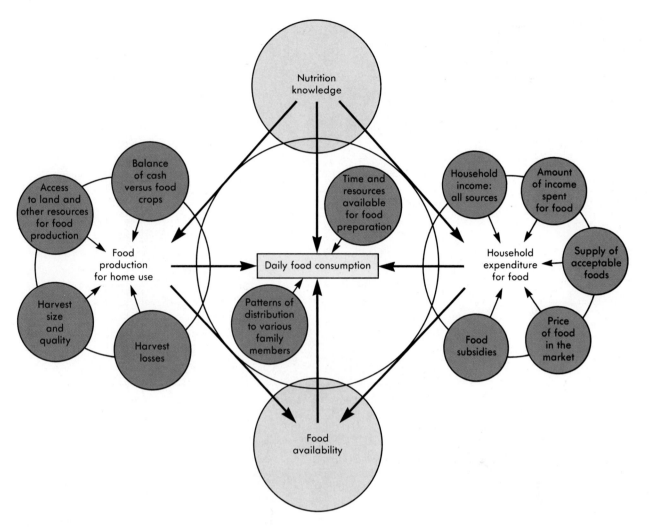

FIGURE 18-1
The many factors affecting household food consumption.

Thomas Malthus, proposed a rather pessimistic view of the prospects for humans. He said that given the passion between the sexes (which he felt was something to be counseled against) the population would always increase in a **_geometric ratio_**—2, 4, 8, 16, 32 and so on. Meanwhile, at best, the food supply would increase only **_arithmetically_**—2, 4, 6, 8, 10 and so on. This prediction means that while the food/population ratio might begin at 2/2, eventually population will grow to 32 while food supplies will only increase to feed 10.[19]

Malthus felt that in the likely absence of sexual restraint, the growing population would be subject to recurring checks imposed by widespread starvation, war, or natural catastrophe brought on by disease. His proposals became the object of intense controversy in England and elsewhere, often meeting vigorous opposition. Eminent scientists in Britain pointed out that scientific advances in agriculture would greatly increase food production. In fact, that has been true. Nevertheless, the population explosion is just that.[8] Malthus was correct in his prediction of geometric growth in the world population. So far this growth has not been slowed significantly by either natural checks or recent human interventions, such as birth control (Figure 18-2).

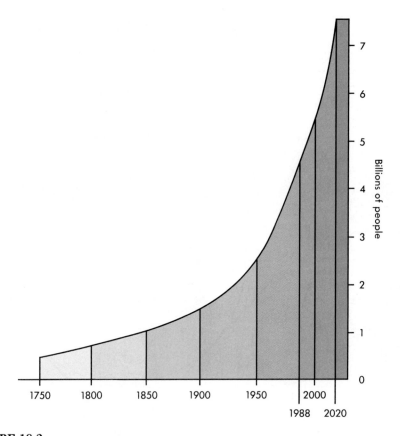

FIGURE 18-2
World population trends since 1750.
Adapted from Ehrlich PR and Ehrlich AH: Population, plenty and poverty, *National Geographic*, December, 1988, p 913.

Birth control programs have been effective in developed countries, but have been relatively ineffective in developing countries that could really profit from them. Whereas women in the United States average 1.9 live births each, women in Rwanda (in eastern Africa) average 8.5 live births each (Figure 18-3).

At this time, there are about 5.3 billion persons in the world. About three-quarters live in developing Third World countries. Many experts believe that the global supply of food would provide adequate nutrition for all 5.3 billion of us, about 3000 kcalories each. But food supplies are not distributed equally among consumers.[22] Gross disparities exist between developed and developing countries, among the rich and poor within countries, and even within families. In some instances, women and children get less to eat than men, and sometimes girl children get less than boy children.[13]

As well, food supply and population trends within the developing world itself are clearly different. Latin America and Asia both have had declining population growth rates since 1970, and their share of the world population will have risen only marginally between 1950 and 2025. On the other hand, the population in Africa will have more than doubled to 19% of the world population over the same 75-year period.

Economists estimate that world food production will continue to increase more rapidly than the world population in the near future, allowing the food/population ratio to increase through the year 2000. In the short run then, the primary problem appears not to be food production, but distribution and use, especially in poverty-stricken areas of the developing nations.[9]

Eventually, though, it is likely that food production will begin to lag behind population growth. And we are currently drifting in that direction, especially

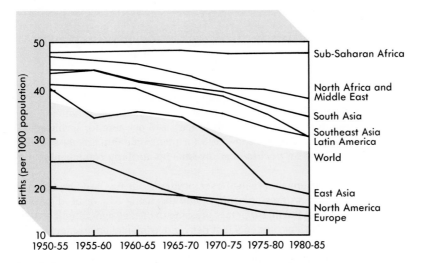

FIGURE 18-3

Birth rates in regions throughout the world. Rates have declined since the end of World War II. The only exception to this trend is in sub-Saharan Africa. As a result, Africa may account for nearly one-quarter of the world's population by the late twenty-first century.

when one examines worldwide grain reserves.[2] Most good farmland in the world is already in use, and because of poor farming practices or competing land-use demands, the number of farmable acres worldwide decreases annually. For many reasons, sustainable world food output—that which does *not* deplete the earth's resources—is now running well behind food consumption. This suggests that food production in less-developed countries will barely keep up with population growth, and will soon lag behind.[20] That in turn will reduce the reserves needed to both combat and help stave off undernutrition, particularly widespread starvation, in poor countries.

A renewed focus on population control

While efforts on the supply side of the food/population ratio are essential, some, but not all scientists in this area of research feel there is no substitute for reducing the demand side.[8] They argue that the survival of our civilization depends on limiting reproduction.

For millions of years, maximizing reproduction has been a measure of biological success. Because disease and difficult living conditions often claimed young lives, producing many offspring by couples was one strategy for carrying on the family. These conditions still hold in Third World countries and constitute as well a key method for providing support in old age. More children also means more helpers to farm, hunt, and prepare food. Traditionally, poorer people bear more children—unlike what you might predict.

Now, in an evolutionary blink of the eye—mere decades—poor people in developing nations are being asked to change their entire attitude toward having children. It is a difficult undertaking. In 1888, 1.5 billion people inhabited the earth. Now the population exceeds 5.3 billion and is growing fast—by some 90 million in 1988 alone. Currently the population increases by three people every second, or about a quarter of a million people every day. In essence the world must accommodate a new population roughly equivalent to that of the United States and Canada every 3 years!

Even though the overall rate of growth has begun to decline, most popula-

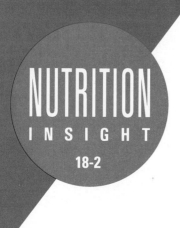

NUTRITION INSIGHT 18-2

PROTECTING THE ENVIRONMENT WITH LOW INPUT SUSTAINABLE AGRICULTURE

The central focus of agricultural science and policy for the last 50 years has been high crop yield. The central question that high yield agriculture poses today is: Can it be sustained, given its cost to the farmer and its impact on the environment?

Today a midwestern corn farmer spends at least $46 per acre for fertilizer, $17 per acre for pesticides, $17 for seeds, and $18 for fuel. Some farmers are spending as much as $35,000 a year on **herbicides.** Investments for farm equipment can be substantial as well.

Given the recent consumer uprisings over pesticides in food and water, incidents of farmer and farm worker poisonings, and the rising cost of production, a growing and broad base of public support is pressing to change agricultural production systems, particularly those systems that deliver detrimental environmental and public health side effects.

Low input sustainable agriculture (LISA) seeks to reduce use of purchased inputs (chemicals, machinery, etc.), while maintaining or increasing yields and farm profits.[6] The overall objective is to reduce costs, environmental and health hazards, and natural resource degradation. Sustainable agriculture offers a system of farm production that relies chiefly on working with nature, rather than trying to conquer it. The biological and stewardship techniques employed have already demonstrated adequate agricultural returns, without locking farmers into an expensive and environmentally damaging array of new farm inputs. Pesticides, fertilizers, water, and soil erosion are all receiving special attention. The LISA concept is gaining support both in the United States and Third World countries as water and soil conservation are needs that exist worldwide.

Reduction in pesticide use

LISA is especially effective in offering solutions to the problems of pesticides in the environment and in food. In the United States there is a growing market for meat and other agricultural products that are free of pesticide residues, as well as free of added growth hormones and antibiotics. Farmers can grow crops profitably on a commercial scale using technologies that substantially reduce the need for pesticides. Rather than resorting to herbicide exclusively to knock out weeds, farmers can combine timely cultivation with variations in planting dates and seeding rates to produce thicker canopies at the right time to shade out weeds. LISA is also reintroducing crop rotations—a traditional farming practice that provides effective pest control with sufficient economic returns. In many instances commercial pesticides are still the best, most cost-effective, or only means for growing a successful crop. But, LISA techniques can substantially reduce use of chemical pesticides.

Export of agrichemicals made in the United States to Third World countries is a time bomb in the area of worker safety. Virtually all chemical use in those countries is by hand application. Many of the extremely toxic materials, such as methyl parathion, are virtually impossible to apply safely by hand under tropical conditions. Sooner or later, political, if not moral pressure will force an industry response to this very real problem.

Reducing fertilizer use

Today, the conventional emphasis on maximum yields relies on heavy additions of fertilizers. The LISA farm community is seeking soil nutrient management practices that focus instead on long-term soil health rather than short-term yields. This in turn allows for maximum economic return, use of the soil's internal capacity for regeneration, and minimization of damage to ground and surface water. Crop rotation is an important tool in this effort.

Lessening water and soil erosion

Although not widely recognized at this time, recent growth in world food output has been achieved in part by practicing unsustainable methods such as plowing highly erodible land and depleting water tables through over-irrigation. In Africa, a land area twice the size of New Jersey is turned into unproductive desert each year because of soil erosion (Figure 18-4).[8] The erosion is caused by over-grazing livestock, destructive farming techniques, and destroying mature rain forests. Soil erosion is also a problem in the United States. LISA can help slow this erosion.

Many of Africa's cash crops damage the land, draining the soil of vital nutrients. Then, when the land has been used up, farmers move on to other areas, leaving behind desolated land ripe for soil erosion. In the short run, farmers can over-plow and over-pump with impressive results, but in doing so they are using up the natural resources on which long-term productivity depends.

Nearly all available irrigation water worldwide is currently used, and groundwater supplies are becoming depleted at rapid rates in many regions. China, which has more than 20% of the world's irrigated land, is plagued with a growing scarcity of fresh water. Third World countries often over-concentrate poultry, swine, and milk production around metropolitan areas, in turn polluting and over-drawing ground water.

A world view

The Food and Agriculture Organization (FAO) of the United Nations works on this principle: "The fight to ensure that all people have enough nutritious food to eat is worthy of our greatest efforts, but it must be fought with the full recognition that it cannot be won unless agricultural, fisheries, and forestry production returns to the earth as much—or more—than it takes." These words suggest we need to take immediate steps to protect an already fragile environment from further deterioration if the world is to feed a population of 6 billion by the year 2000. LISA is one alternative for the future. ●

Herbicide ● A compound that reduces the growth and reproduction of plants.

Low Input Sustainable Agriculture (LISA) ● A form of farming that attempts to limit use of purchased inputs, such as manufactured fertilizers and pesticides. Use of manure and crop rotation are typical substitute inputs.

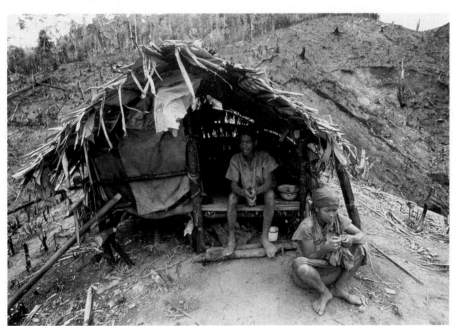

FIGURE 18-4

The need for LISA exists worldwide. Losing ground in their effort to grow rice, farmers in Madagascar survey erosion on hills cleared of rain forest. Farming further depletes the soil, and in turn new land must be cleared. Slash-and-burn farming destroys 50 acres of rain forest an hour worldwide.

tion experts believe population size will still pass 8 billion during the next 50 years. The poorest countries are increasing the most, further straining their ability to cope. A 1988 United Nations World Food Council report concluded that earlier progress in fighting undernutrition and poverty has either come to a halt or was being reversed in many parts of the world. This is particularly evident in Africa. The pressure of more people to feed will intensify the problems.

Attempts to stem the human tide

Attempts to implement family-planning programs in Third World nations have been met with only partial success. Some small countries, such as Singapore, Taiwan, Thailand, Columbia, Costa Rica, and several Caribbean countries have achieved substantial reductions in their birthrates. Larger countries, including India and Mexico, are struggling.[8]

China has explicitly recognized that it is already overpopulated. It has the world's most stringent family-planning program; the government allows only one child per urban couple—two at most in rural areas. Penalties for having extra children include restricted housing and employment opportunities. China's program, though successful by world standards, has encountered opposition. A new policy that allows families to earn private income, while very successful in increasing food production, has unexpectedly created an incentive to have more children to help earn the income.[8] The overall result has been a recent surge in the birthrate, which has been countered by new efforts to impose restraints.

In the final analysis, successful birth control programs have to recognize that only when people have enough to eat and are financially secure will they feel safe having fewer children. By providing the poor with a livelihood that allows access to food, shelter, health care, and enough money to support themselves in old age, experts believe more couples will then *choose* to have fewer children.

Promoting breast-feeding is important to family health. It helps naturally space births farther apart. Solely breast-feeding an infant lessens ovulations in women, and so fertilization, for an average of about 6 months (though it cannot be relied on totally as a form of birth control). When childbirths are more widely spaced, the health of mother and infant are aided, and fewer total births occur. In addition, in Third World Countries breast-feeding cuts infant mortality by providing some of the mother's immune factors for the infant, while also lessening the risk from water-borne diseases. Exclusive breast-feeding in early infancy improves the chances of infant survival, compared with a combination of breast and bottle-feeding. Other nutritional benefits will be discussed later.

In 1960, families in South Korea averaged six children each. Economic policies coupled with a strong family-planning program transformed South Korea from a struggling country to an economic success. Today, Korean families average slightly fewer than two children each and the population will soon stabilize.[8] However, nations do not have to wait to become industrialized before launching population control programs. Indonesia, South Korea, and Thailand took great economic strides and at the same time controlled population growth. Still, to date, population stabilization—as in Western countries—has mainly been accompanied by relative wealth and security.

In addition to economics, another unavoidable roadblock to family-planning programs lies with ancient cultural, religious, and traditional beliefs. In subSaharan Africa, being childless not only carries an aura of evil for the woman, but also marks the end of a line of descent. The Yoruba believe, for example, that a childless woman has made a pact with evil spirits before her own birth to kill her children and, devoid of descendants, will return to join these evil spirits in some other worldly sphere. These women are almost as afraid of being rendered functionally infertile by the death of all their children as they are of bearing none.[5] Thus female sterilization and even contraception are widely feared. Even women with four or five children fear, not unreasonably, that all the children may suddenly die.

In India, a rigid class structure that leaves those in the lower classes destitute and poor encourages these families to have more children for many of the economic reasons discussed above. Also, Moslem religious practices typically promote a large, abundant family as a sign of prosperity and health.

Malthus' gloomy mathematical prediction may soon become fact. If we cannot find ways of humanely controlling population growth, nature may solve the problem by killing off large portions of humanity in the ways Malthus predicted.[8] Only the future will tell.

Green Revolution • A time during the 1960s when there was much emphasis in improving strains and cultivation practices of cereal grains, such as rice, wheat, and corn.

Ecosystem • A community in nature that includes plant and animals and the environment associated with them.

CONCEPT CHECK

Currently, world food production is sufficient to meet the energy needs of the world's population. Undernutrition exists, despite adequate food resources, because of poverty, politics, and unequal distribution. In addition, projected population growth may soon overwhelm food production. Limiting population growth, especially in Third World countries where birth rates are high, is a challenging priority encouraged by some scientists.

THE DECLINING STATE OF AGRICULTURAL RESOURCES

Population control has become more critical lately as we quickly deplete, and in some cases exhaust, the earth's resources. The productive capacity of agriculture is approaching its limits worldwide. As we mentioned, food production, especially in parts of the Third World, is being undermined by environmentally-unsustainable farming methods.[22]

The term *green revolution* describes a phenomenon starting in the 1960s where a dramatic rise in crop yields in some countries, such as the Philippines, India, and Mexico, was made possible because of increased use of fertilizers and the development of superior crops through careful plant breeding. Many of the green revolution technologies have now achieved most of their potential. One example is that rice yield has not increased significantly since the release of superior varieties in 1966. Wheat is another example. India more than tripled its wheat harvest between 1965 and 1983, a period when high-yielding crop strains were introduced. Since then, its grain output has not increased. Future gains in productivity may be much harder to accomplish because of the need to farm less productive soils.[2] Until the introduction of yet another superior wheat or rice strain, developing countries will not benefit greatly from recent, more modest breakthroughs in biotechnology (see the Nutrition Issue on p. 596).[17,22]

Areas of the world that remain uncultivated or ungrazed are mostly of poor quality: rocky, steep, infertile, too dry, too wet, or inaccessible.[8] Much of this land is also invaluable for providing humans crucial *ecosystem* benefits. This is particularly true for humid tropical areas, such as the Amazon basin rain forests, which significantly influence the earth's climate, notably through oxygen production. Some nations, such as Brazil, can still expand onto land that will sustain cultivation, but such countries are in the distinct minority. And even then, this expansion in Brazil comes at the expense of further rain forest devastation. The overwhelming experience over the last few decades has been overextension of agriculture onto erodible land, followed by predictable degradation, erosion, and abandonment.

The prospects of obtaining substantially more food from the oceans are also poor. Since the early 1970s, the world fish catch per person has been declining. Clearly, we can exploit the earth's resources only so far—world population likely cannot continue to expand as it does today without potentially invoking serious famine and death.

ATTITUDES TOWARD CERTAIN FOODS

Culture affects food use just as it does family size. In India, for example, the Hindu reverence for cattle has multiplied some already significant nutrition problems. These sacred cows consume food rather than provide it; the wandering cows also considerably damage vegetation that could otherwise feed humans. Although the cows provide milk, there is no effort to improve milk production through selective breeding practices.

In certain areas of India, a child may not be fed milk curds because of a superstitious belief that these inhibit growth or bananas because they supposedly cause convulsions. These are obstacles, but not roadblocks to good nutrition. Given enough food resources, a healthful diet that allows for individual food taboos and prejudices is possible.

THE EFFECTS OF POOR INFRASTRUCTURE ON HEALTH: SHELTER AND SANITATION IN THE THIRD WORLD

When people die from undernutrition in Third World countries, other influences almost always contribute, such as inadequate shelter and sanitation. Poor sanitation raises the risk for infection, as does undernutrition. Together these represent a lethal combination (Figure 18-5). More than one billion people today occupy inadequate and deteriorating shelter with poor conditions. The future looks even worse. By the year 2000, Mexico City will house more than 26 million people, with Sao Paulo, Calcutta, and Bombay not far behind.[8] Many of the 15 million child deaths each year in developing countries (half of them in chil-

Note that in the United States many of us shun potential foods like horse-meat, insects, textured soy protein, and algae.

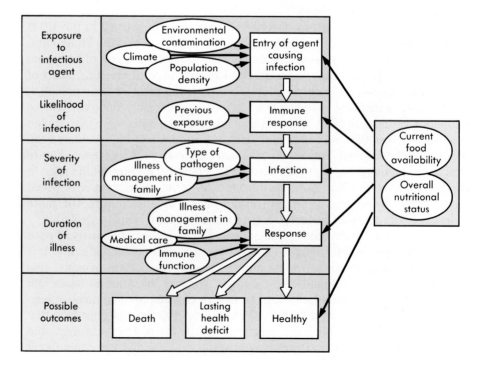

FIGURE 18-5

Nutrition and infection. The ultimate effect of an infection depends in part on the nutritional state of the person, as well as on many environmental influences.

dren under 5 years old) could be prevented if standards of environmental hygiene were improved.

Urban populations of some developing countries are currently growing at an annual rate of 5% to 7%. This urban explosion is the result of both high birth rates and continuing migration of people to the cities from the countryside. People come to the cities to find employment and resources the countryside can no longer provide. It is estimated that by the year 2000 about half of the world's population will live in cities and towns. Such a skewed population distribution will result in further impoverishment.

In Third World countries, the poor make up most of the urban population, and their needs for housing and community services often outstrip available governmental resources. Most of these urban poor live in over-crowded, self-made shelters that are only partially served by public utilities and lack a safe and adequate water supply. The shanty towns and ghettos of the Third World provide surroundings that are often worse than the rural areas the people left behind (Figure 18-6). And because the people now need cash to purchase food, they find themselves with diets that are even more meager than the home-grown rural fare.[13] To make matters worse, makeshift shelters often lack facilities to protect food from spoilage or from the ravages of insects and rodents. In some developing countries food losses can amount to as much as 30% to 40% of the perishable foods.[13]

A move from rural to urban life takes its greatest toll on infants and children. Infants are often weaned early from the breast, partly because the mother seeks employment and partly because she may be trying to emulate the image of sophisticated, formula-using women promoted in advertisements. Unfortunately, infant formulas are relatively expensive, and so poor parents may use too little to meet the baby's needs, or they may over-dilute the mixture. Since the water supply may not be safe, the prepared formula is also likely to be grossly contaminated with bacteria. In many nations, bottle-fed infants contract far more illnesses and are as much as 25 times more likely to die in childhood than those who are exclusively breast-fed for the first 6 months of life. On the other hand, breast milk is generally much more hygienic, readily available, nutritionally sound, and again provides infants with some immune factors. In spite of this grim fact, major corporations continue to market infant formulas in these regions heavily.

In Brazil migrants displaced by multinational land developers have flooded from the north and northeast into Rio de Janeiro and Sao Paulo, attracted by the prospect of jobs. There they have built shanty towns next to apartment towers and affluent suburbs, but the jobs do not materialize and the desperate poverty begets more poverty.

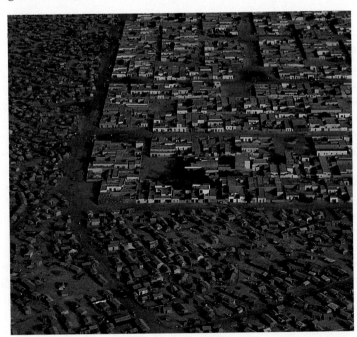

FIGURE 18-6
Urban centers in Africa can bear little resemblance to western experiences.

Overall, the most important single activity that can be undertaken for the health of people, wherever they live, is the provision of a safe and convenient water supply. The World Health Organization (WHO) estimates that 1.2 billion people, about one-fifth of all people, are without a safe and adequate water supply in 1990.

Poor sanitation, another example of inadequate infrastructure in the Third World, creates a further critical public health problem. It is common to see human feces, rotting garbage, and associated insect and rodent infestations in Third World cities. Human urine and feces is a potent source of disease organisms, and ends up as one of the most dangerous substances with which people can come into contact. In some developing countries, diarrheal diseases account for as many as one-third of all deaths in children under 5 years of age. WHO estimates that even with progress in housing, 1.8 billion people in the world are still without proper sanitation in 1990.

To this already unbalanced equation, add the threat of sickness from Acquired Immune Deficiency Syndrome (AIDS). Developing countries now have two-thirds of the world's 8 million to 10 million human immunodeficiency virus (HIV) infections, and could have 80% of the 15 million to 20 million infections expected by the year 2000.[2] Even more than 3 million people in the Western Hemisphere will be infected with the AIDS virus by the mid 1990s.

Still, the continent hardest hit by AIDS is Africa. The pattern for transmission of HIV is different in most of Africa than in industrialized nations. Reuse of hypodermic needles, infected blood supplies, transfer of the virus to the infant at birth, and prostitution all contribute to the spread of HIV in Africa.

The economic impact as more become ill from AIDS will be enormous. In an already undernourished population, the long-term effects may be similar to a prolonged war.

CONCEPT CHECK

Poor housing conditions, impure water, and inadequate sanitation worldwide increase the risk for infection and disease. Infection then combines with undernutrition to further compromise health status. A healthy diet, clean drinking water, and sanitary handling of human waste all contribute to health—these should be the rights of every human being.

WAR AND CIVIL UNREST

The president of Mali recently stated "Only by translating our sense of common destiny into action will we be able to resolve the paradox of currently spending $1000 billion each year in the production of lethal weapons, while only a fraction of that sum would make our planet a land of prosperity for millions of people who today suffer from illness, hunger, thirst and ignorance."

Worldwide military spending has doubled over the past 20 years to more than $1000 billion yearly. The amount spent on weapons every minute could feed 2000 undernourished children for a year. The Third World's share of the global arms budget increased from 9% to 16% from 1977 to 1987, draining resources that could be used to combat poverty and hunger. Although Africa has been ravaged by economic decay and famines for years, military spending in Africa more than doubled in the 1970s and held firm in the early 1980s.[2]

In the worst of cases, civil disruptions and war contribute in large measure to massive undernutrition.[15] War-related famine affects at least 20 million people in southern and northeastern Africa. In southern Sudan, 3 to 4 million men, women, and children were starving in 1991 because civil war has prevented them from planting their fields and restocking their herds. Even when food might be available, political divisions may well impede distribution to the point that undernutrition will continue to be the lot of many people for years into the future. In addition, aid programs aimed at the poor, especially during emergencies, have been undermined by poor administration, corruption, and political influence. In the 1970s, the problem of undernutrition was perceived as a technical one—how to produce enough food for the growing world population. Today, the problem is largely a political one—how to achieve cooperation among and within nations.

EXTERNAL DEBT

At a recent meeting of the United Nations, many developing countries asserted that they were on the verge of economic collapse and felt that a major contributing factor was the $1.3 trillion external debt they collectively owed. Latin American debt represents 45% of the region's gross regional output of goods and services. Nearly 40% of total export earnings are spent in paying off this debt. One option is for Latin American nations to form a comprehensive plan aimed at renegotiating the external debt on more realistic terms. The current debt of the United States limits its ability to correct this problem (and to help its own poor as well).

Many African nations carry large debt burdens. Still, they need to import—and pay for—machinery, concrete, trucks, and consumer goods. To make up the difference between export income and import expenses, countries have been forced to borrow billions of dollars from international banks. While the African debts are much smaller in absolute terms than the debts of Brazil, Argentina, and Mexico, for example, the actual burden is greater when national incomes and export earnings are considered. Nearly half the money African nations earn from exports goes to paying off the continent's multi-billion dollar debt. As a result, African nations have had to impose austerity programs. The effects of wage cuts and the increased prices for food and consumer goods can push many of these poor nations over the edge into widespread undernutrition.

SOLUTIONS TO UNDERNUTRITION IN THE THIRD WORLD

As you have probably guessed, eliminating undernutrition in the Third World will be complicated. In the 1980s it was a common practice for the more abundant nations of the world to supply famished areas with direct food aid. Though highly publicized and praised at the time, direct food aid is not a long-term solution.[21] While reducing the number of deaths from famine, it can also reduce incentives for local production by driving down local prices. In addition, the affected countries may have little or no means of transporting the food to those who need it most. Furthermore, the donated foods may meet with little cultural acceptance.

In the short run, there is no choice—aid must be given because people are starving. Still, improving the infrastructure for poor people, especially rural people, needs to be the long-term focus. This is because the most significant factor affecting undernutrition of people in impoverished areas of the world is their reliance on outside sources for basic needs. Their dependence makes them constantly vulnerable.

Recall that in the last 20 years world food supplies have grown faster than population. Thus the increase in undernutrition during this time period is caused by an increase in the number of people cut off from their fair share of this supply. Millions of farmers are losing access to resources they need in order to be self-reliant. And the number of households with insufficient means to support themselves is growing. In response, careful small-scale, regional development is needed. There is a growing realization that the rural landless will flock to the overcrowded cities unless economic opportunities can be created for them.

Poor people in less developed countries benefit from access to the land to help maintain food security.

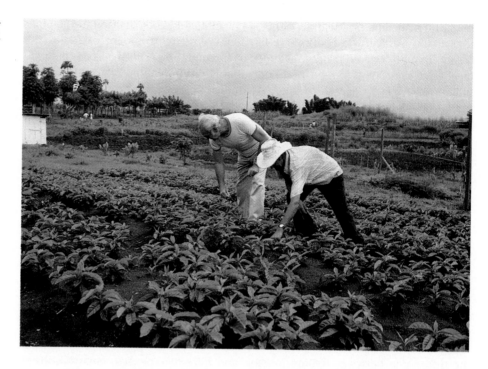

Small-scale rural enterprises and off-farm activities would ensure that poor people in rural areas who have no access to land or other assets can acquire entitlement to food. Such enterprises can be run by the people who stand to benefit, either as individuals or as members of small groups, using very limited capital. A prerequisite would be access to credit, appropriate technologies, a market, and ability to transport the product to that market. Households that presently have land could be helped in different ways so that they would be able to feed themselves.

For the most part, the problem is one of helping people produce much of their own needs and directing them to resources and employment opportunities. Experience has shown that credit—along with training, food storage facilities, and marketing—allows rural people to participate in development to their benefit and the benefit of their families and communities. Suitable technologies for processing, preserving, marketing, and distributing nutritious local staples need to be encouraged so small farmers—men and women—can flourish.

Land ownership brings many advantages, particularly available food.[15] But if food resources instead become concentrated in the hands of a few, as often happens in unequal land ownership, these won't be equally distributed unless efficient transportation systems are in place. Inequitable distribution then proves a very difficult problem to resolve.

Raising the economic status of impoverished people by employing them turns out to be as important as expanding the food supply. If an increase in food supply is achieved without an accompanying rise in employment, then there may be no long-term change in the number of undernourished people. It is possible to see food prices fall with increased mechanization, use of fertilizers, and other modern technologies. But these very same advances also can displace people from jobs. When this happens, the food that is produced will still be out of reach for those who need it most.

A shipment of high-technology tractors, for example, might put local laborers out of work. Rice might be planted more efficiently using farm machinery, but using human power eventually leaves more humans with the resources to buy food. Success in reducing undernutrition in the Third World must occur by employing more poor people more productively on available land or by providing other jobs. From a Third World point of view, it is of little consequence that these jobs are technologically primitive by Western standards.

It is also prudent to assume that the developing world will have to rely largely on its own resources to finance development, especially in light of the current budget deficit in the United States. It is even more essential then to make full use of human resources available in the developing world itself. The right choice for production ends up depending on the relative need to employ people and the numbers of people available to do the work.

Over-emphasizing **cash crops**, such as coffee, tea, rubber, and cocoa—as some developing countries have done, especially Latin American ones—is not likely to solve the nutritional problems of poor people. Cash crops are usually grown at the expense of food crops, on the assumption that money earned from the cash crops will be used to purchase enough food for the families of the workers. However, this is not always the case.[13] Food can be bought, but it may not be enough and it would be more expensive. In such a situation, poorer families are at greater risk than others since the money earned from cash crops is often not enough to meet other basic family needs, let alone their food needs. As with poor families in the United States, buying quality foods often takes second priority, resulting in nutritional deprivation.

The battle against world undernutrition then is twofold: to supply nutrients to the undernourished and to reduce the number of people in danger of undernutrition. The second part of this battle is a very real one. Many delegates to a recent Food and Agriculture Organization of the United Nations (FAO) conference stressed the need for strategies that could supply food to vulnerable households, subsidize basic commodities purchased by the poor, and raise the employment and income-generating capacity of the poor.

Today, one-third of the earth's population does not receive enough food to maintain an active working life, though enough grain is still produced to supply 3000 kcalories daily for every man, woman, and child on the planet. More than half of it is grown in the Third World. The economic loss from undernutrition is staggering, and the amount of human pain and suffering is incalculable. With all the international relief efforts, government assistance, and private organizations combined, we are still operating in the Dark Ages in our battle against undernutrition (Figure 18-7).

Cash Crop • Crops grown by countries with specific intent to export in order to gain the ability to purchase goods from other countries, rather than to feed the country's citizens. Examples are coffee, tea, cocoa, and bananas.

FIGURE 18-7

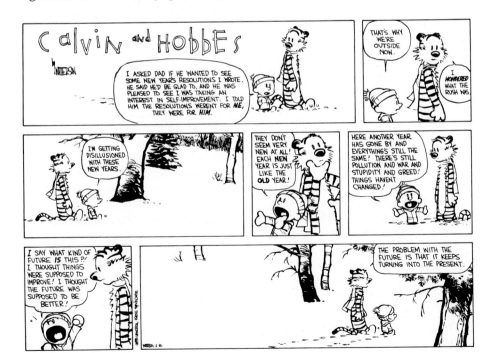

CONCEPT CHECK

War, civil strife, and external debt contribute to the difficulty of ending undernutrition in many Third World countries. Overall, the solution seems to lie in providing sufficient employment so that people can purchase the food their family needs and/or providing access to land and other food production resources. Programs must be sensitive to regional conditions to ensure that new technologies introduced don't intensify existing problems for the poorest people. Simple approaches are appropriate if people using them are left with the resources needed to feed their families.

SUMMARY

- Poverty is a common thread wherever people suffer from undernutrition. Malnutrition can occur when the food supply is either scarce or abundant. The resulting deficiency conditions or degenerative diseases are influenced by genetic makeup.

- Undernutrition is the most common form of malnutrition in developing countries. It results from inadequate intake, absorption, or use of nutrients or kcalories. Many deficiency conditions then appear and infectious diseases thrive because the immune system cannot function properly.

- The greatest risk of undernutrition occurs during critical periods of growth and development: pregnancy, infancy, and childhood. Low birth weight is a leading cause of infant deaths worldwide. Many developmental problems are caused by nutritional deprivation during critical periods of brain growth.

- Undernutrition diminishes both physical and mental capabilities. In poor countries, this is worsened by recurrent infections, poor sanitary conditions, extreme weather, inadequate shelter, and exposure to diseases.

- In the United States, famine has been nonexistent since the 1930s, but undernutrition is present. Soup kitchens, food stamps, school lunch and breakfast programs, and the Supplemental Feeding Program for Women, Infants, and Children (WIC) have focused on improving the nutritional health of poor and at-risk people. These programs have proven effective in reducing undernutrition when adequately funded.

- Multiple factors contribute to the problem of undernutrition in Third World countries. In densely populated countries, food resources may be inadequate and the means for distributing food may be poor. Farming methods often encourage erosion, which deprives the soil of valuable nutrients, thus defeating future efforts to grow food. Poor water availability hampers food production. Naturally occurring devastation from droughts, excessive rainfall, fire, crop infestation and human causes, such as urbanization, civil unrest, war, debt, and poor sanitation, all contribute to the major problem of undernutrition.

- Any proposed solutions to the problem of world undernutrition must consider the interaction of multiple factors, many of which are thoroughly embedded in cultural traditions. Family planning efforts, for example, may not succeed until life expectancy can be raised. Through education, efforts should be made to improve farming methods, encourage breast-feeding, and improve sanitation and hygiene. Direct food aid is only a short-term solution. In what may appear to be a step backward, a focus on subsistence-level farming, away from the specialization of cash crops, is needed in order to increase the economic status of people reliant on traditional rain-fed agriculture. This is one way to gain meaningful employment and purchasing power for vast numbers of the rural poor.

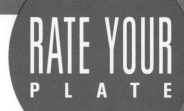

FIGHTING WORLD UNDERNUTRITION ON A PERSONAL LEVEL

The following are suggested activities for doing something about world and domestic undernutrition. Like any change in behavior, don't try to do too many things at once. Try one or two of them, representing your personal stand against this gigantic problem.

1. Go on a 1- or 2-day fast. Keep a diary of how you feel physically and emotionally through the day. At the end of the fasting period record what you learned about being without food. NOTE: *If you have a medical problem that demands regular consumption of food, like diabetes mellitus, or you are pregnant—do not choose this activity.*

2. Fast one meal per day for a month (e.g., lunch). Save an amount of money equivalent to the amount you would spend eating this meal out (e.g., $4.00). Donate the money to a voluntary agency that does anti-hunger work, such as those listed below:

Bread For the World
6411 Chillum Pl. NW
Washington, D.C. 20012

Oxfam America
115 Broadway
Boston, MA 02116

Seeds
222 East Lake Dr.
Decatur, GA 30030

Food Research and Action Center
1319 F St. NW Suite 500
Washington, D.C. 20004

Lutheran World Relief
390 Park Ave. S
New York, NY 10016

Save the Children Federation
P.O. Box 970
Westport, CT 06881

The Hunger Project
2015 Steiner St.
San Francisco, CA 94115

Institute for Food and
Development Policy
1885 Mission St.
San Francisco, CA 94103

Interreligious Taskforce
on U.S. Food Policy
110 Maryland Ave. NE
Washington, D.C. 20002

Catholic Relief Services
209 W Fayette St.
Baltimore, MD 21201

CARE
660 First Ave.
New York, NY 10016

3. Write a letter to one of your senators or congressperson asking what they are doing about ending domestic and world undernutrition.

4. Volunteer at a local soup kitchen or homeless shelter for a time limited period (1 month).

5. Call your local social service agency and ask what services are available locally to deal with hunger and undernutrition in the community. Then ask about how to donate money or volunteer your services.

6. Sponsor a child in a foreign country with monthly financial aid for food and clothing. To do this you can write:

World Vision International
Box O
Pasadena, CA 91109

7. Contribute to World Food Day activities each October 16th.
8. Organize students on your campus. At Miami University in Oxford, Ohio, two students saw the successful culmination of a year-long effort to provide food for the homeless in the suburban Cincinnati area by distributing excess food from the university's dining halls. Let us know about your efforts!

REFERENCES

1. American Dietetic Association: Position of The American Dietetic Association: domestic hunger and inadequate access to food, *Journal of The American Dietetic Association* 90:1437, 1990.
2. Bread for the World Institute: *Hunger 1990*, Washington DC, 1990, the institute.
3. Brown JL, Allen D: Hunger in America, *Annual Reviews of Public Health* 9:503, 1988.
4. Buzina R and others: Workshop on functional significance of mild-to-moderate malnutrition, *American Journal of Clinical Nutrition* 50:172, 1989.
5. Caldwell JC, Caldwell P: High fertility in sub-Saharan Africa, *Scientific American* May, 1990, p 118.
6. Chabot BF: Sustainable agriculture is model for extension, *Community Nutrition Institute News* March 8, 1990, p 4.
7. Council on scientific affairs: Biotechnology and the American agricultural industry, *Journal of the American Medical Association* 265:1429, 1991.
8. Ehrlich PR, Ehrlich AH: Population, plenty, and poverty, *National Geographic*, December, 1988, p 913.
9. Helmuth JW: World hunger amidst plenty, *USA Today*, March, 1989, p 48.
10. Keusch GT: Vitamin A supplements—too good not to be true, *The New England Journal of Medicine* 323:985, 1990.
11. Lenhart NM and others: Demographic profile and nutrient intake assessment of individuals using emergency food programs, *Journal of The American Dietetic Association* 89:1269, 1989.
12. Latham MC and others: Improvements in growth following iron supplementation in young Kenyan school children, *Nutrition* 6:159, 1990.
13. Marangu L: Food crisis in Africa, *Canadian Home Economics Journal* 39:144, 1989.
14. Mayer J: Nutritional problems in the United States: Then and now two decades later, *Nutrition Today*, January/February, 1990, p 17.
15. Mellor JW, Gavian, S: Famine: causes, prevention, and relief, *Science* 235:539, 1987.
16. Meyers AF: Undernutrition, hunger, and learning in children, *Nutrition News* 52(2):1, 1989.
17. Miller HI, Ackerman SJ: Perspective on food biotechnology, *FDA Consumer*, March, 1990, p 6.
18. NIH technology assessment conference statement on bovine somatotropin, *Journal of the American Medical Association* 265:1423, 1991.
19. Olson RE: World food production and problems in human nutrition, *Nutrition Today*, January/February, 1989, p 18.
20. Saran R: Food and the environment, *Food Policy*, February, 1990, p 76.
21. Singer HW: The African food crisis and the role of food aid, *Food Policy*, August, 1989, p 196.
22. Stokes B: Crowds, food and gloom, *National Journal*, September 16, 1989, p 2263.

HOW MUCH HAVE I LEARNED?

What have you learned from reading Chapter 18? Here are 15 statements about undernutrition in the world. Read them to test your current knowledge. If you think the statement is true or mostly true, circle T. If you think the statement is false or mostly false, circle F. Use the scoring key at the end of the book to compute your total score. To review, take this test again later, and especially before tests.

1. **T F** Hunger is the physiological state that results when not enough food is eaten.

2. **T F** The primary cause of undernutrition is poverty.

3. **T F** Diabetes mellitus is more common when food supplies are low.

4. **T F** Undernutrition is the most common form of malnutrition among the poor.

5. **T F** The risk of dying from pregnancy-related causes highlights the gap between the developing and industrialized countries.

6. **T F** The greatest risk from poor nutrition during pregnancy is borne by the infant.

7. **T F** 9-year-old children suffering from undernutrition can look like 4-year-old children.

8. **T F** Marginal deficiencies of iron affect few people worldwide.

9. **T F** Years of undernutrition can be overcome in several weeks on a high-protein, high-carbohydrate diet.

10. **T F** Compared with other industrialized countries, the United States has one of the lowest infant mortality rates in the world.

11. **T F** Homelessness in the United States is much more evident today as compared with 1980.

12. **T F** The world's population is rapidly outstripping the global food supply.

13. **T F** Traditionally, poorer people bear more children.

14. **T F** In Third World countries, the urban population consists mostly of the poor.

15. **T F** Wherever they live, a key factor for the health of people is a safe water supply.

BIOTECHNOLOGY AS AN ANSWER TO FOOD SHORTAGES?

The human ability to manipulate nature has enabled us to improve the production and yield of many important foods. Traditional **biotechnology** is almost as old as agriculture. The first farmer to selectively improve his stock by breeding the best bull with the best cows was implementing biotechnology in a simple sense. The first baker who used yeast to make bread rise was likewise using biotechnology to produce an improved product.[17]

By the 1930s, biotechnology made it possible to selectively breed better plant hybrids; as a result corn production in the United States quickly doubled. Through similar methods, agricultural wheat was crossed with wild grasses in order to acquire more desirable properties, such as greater yield, increased resistance to mildew and bacterial diseases, and tolerance to salt or adverse climatic conditions.

Another type of biotechnology uses hormones rather than breeding. In the last decade Canadian salmon have been treated with a hormone that allows them to mature three times faster than normal—without changing the fish in any other way. Overall, then, biotechnology is the use of living things—plants, animals, bacteria—to manufacture products.[17]

The new biotechnology

The *new biotechnology* that is part of agriculture today includes a number of methods that directly modify products. It differs from traditional methods because it directly changes some of the genetic material (DNA) of organisms to improve characteristics. No longer is cross-breeding plants or animals the only tool. The new process, called **genetic engineering,** was developed mostly in the 1970s. It now covers a wide range of cell and subcell techniques for synthesizing and then placing genetic material in organisms.[7] This allows access to a wider gene pool, and it permits faster and more accurate production of new and more useful microbial, plant, and animal species. Traditional breeding has been hit or miss. But biotechnology is precise—scientists select the traits they want and genetically engineer or introduce the gene that produces the desired trait into animals.[17] However, it is important to note that genetic engineering does not replace conventional breeding practices; both work together.

Currently, genetic engineering at the farm level has led to new types of seeds, availability of new growth hormones, and application of microbial inoculants to stop pests and frost damage. Biotechnology is also being used to develop drought-tolerant crops, as well as for methods to better detect the food-poisoning bacteria *Listeria* and other food-borne microbes. Plants are being engineered to grow without chemical pesticides, and new forms of potatoes can last without preservatives. To our eyes and palates, these first benefits of

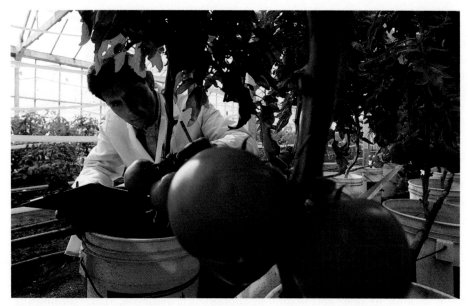

Much traditional biotechnology has gone into the tomato we enjoy today.

Biotechnology • Use of advanced scientific techniques to alter and ideally improve characteristics of plants, animals, and other forms of life.

Genetic Engineering • Alteration of genetic material in plants or animals with the intent of improving growth, disease resistance, or other characteristics.

the new biotechnology may seem only subtly different, but the ultimate benefits could be substantial.

Questions surround the use of the new biotechnology. Take, for instance, research on a new tomato that is genetically engineered to allow it to stay firm longer. Is it still a tomato? It looks the same, feels the same, tastes the same, and even has the identical nutritional value as that of the original product. The only change researchers have made is to counteract the action of a single gene in the DNA that makes tomatoes rot rapidly. The reversal of just one gene out of 10,000 is the only change needed to make the *biotech* tomato significantly different from the standard garden variety.

Still, ultimately the question remains—how many properties can be changed in a plant, animal, or bacteria before it becomes something else? A tomato altered in only one specific way still seems to be a tomato, but does it remain one if it is improved in 10 or 20 ways? When traditional methods crossed a tangerine with a grapefruit, the new genetic structure was clearly something else, now commonly known as a tangelo.

Is the new biotechnology safe?

New biotechnology continues to develop under protest. Although genetically modified organisms offer the possibility of reducing environmentally detrimental activities, such as the use of chemical pesticides, critics point out past mistakes of releasing foreign agents, such as insects and plants, into areas with no natural predators. While the risks may appear to be momentarily negligible, they may be cumulative, and so, dangerous in the long run.

Public opinion has long been turning against processes perceived as harmful to the environment, such as producing unnatural products. Since food reserves are high in the United States, Canada, and Europe, increasing food production has been questioned. The prime example of skepticism concerning unnatural products is Western Europe's ban of the growth hormone previously used in beef production there.[17] They felt the increase in meat supply was not worth the perceived risks posed by the product. In the United States, FDA has recently approved the first genetically engineered food product for humans, an enzyme called renin, traditionally used in making cheese. What will its political fate be?

Other potentially beneficial applications of the new biotechnology are currently being studied by both scientists and concerned consumer groups. Bovine somatotropin (BST), a hormone produced by cattle, has been known since the 1930s to increase milk production when injected into dairy cattle. Today an identical BST produced through genetic engineering can be used to greatly increase milk yield 10% to 25%.[18] Porcine somatotropin (PST), also produced by genetic engineering, increases swine growth. Because these are proteins, any BST or PST in the milk or meat produced would be digested and, therefore, inactivated when eaten. People even produce their own form of somatotropin, but it is structured considerably different.

Since cows produce BST naturally, it has always been present in their milk. Treating the animals with the proposed higher levels of BST won't increase the level of hormone occurring naturally in the milk, nor will it alter the milk's nutrient composition.

While FDA has yet to approve release of BST for routine use, the agency has determined that the milk and meat from treated animals is safe for humans.[18] Still, the public appears to oppose it, and European Economic Community has banned its use. Again, with milk surpluses in the United States and Europe, there is little to help garner public support. Furthermore, dairy farmers in Wisconsin, as well as other dairy producing regions, are generally opposed to the introduction of the hormone because they fear negative consumer reaction will cause lower milk consumption. The industry is also concerned that a sharp increase in milk output would adversely affect prices and, in turn, harm thousand of small dairy farms facing an already precarious economic situation.

Will the new biotechnology help reduce Third World undernutrition?

Whether genetically engineered applications will help reduce Third World undernutrition remains to be seen. Unless price cuts parallel the increased production, landowners and suppliers of biotechnology will capture the benefits of biotechnology, and so its rewards will most likely remain unshared. This principle needs to be emphasized; the person who couldn't afford a tangelo yesterday probably won't be able to afford one tomorrow. The same can be said for improved tomatoes. And as with most innovations, the more successful farmers, often those with larger farms, will adopt the new biotechnology first. Because of this, the present trend to fewer, larger farms will continue in the Third World—a trend that is counterproductive in addressing the most pressing undernutrition issues there. Furthermore, biotechnology does not promise dramatic gains in grain production—the primary food resource in the world.

For the Third World, the focus needs to be on providing people with resources to produce and/or purchase their own food rather than on simply growing more food. Biotechnology is merely a useful tool, not a panacea, to the complex scourge of world undernutrition. ●

APPENDIXES

A Food Composition Tables
B Clinical Measures and Physical Evidence of Nutritional Status
C Nutrient Recommendations for Canadians
D Dietary Intake Assessment
E U.S. Recommended Daily Allowances and Reference Daily Intakes
F The Exchange System
G Exchange System Lists
H The Cell—Primary Site for Metabolism
I National Cholesterol Education Program for Adults—Dietary Advice
J Important Chemical Structures in Nutrition
K Determination of Frame Size
L Caffeine Content of Foods
M Energy Cost of Various Activities
N An Example of Prenatal Vitamin/Mineral Supplements and Prenatal Weight Gain Chart
O Infant and Child Growth Charts
P Safe Food Storage
Q Common Food Additives
R Sources of Nutrition Information
S Evaluation of Protein Quality

APPENDIX A
FOOD COMPOSITION TABLES

Nutritive Components for Baby Foods

Food Name	Serving Portion	WT. Gm	KCAL Kc	PROT Gm	CARB Gm	FAT Gm	CHOL Mg	SAFA Gm	MUFA Gm	PUFA Gm	SOD Mg
BABY-TEETHING BISCUITS	1.000 ITEM	11.000	43.000	1.200	8.400	0.500	—	—	—	—	40.000
BABY-MIXED CEREAL/MILK	1.000 SERVING	28.400	32.000	1.300	4.500	1.000	—	—	—	—	13.000
BABY-OATMEAL CEREAL/MILK	1.000 SERVING	28.400	33.000	1.400	4.300	1.200	—	—	—	—	13.000
BABY-RICE CEREAL/MILK	1.000 SERVING	28.400	33.000	1.100	4.700	1.000	—	—	—	—	13.000
BABY-BEEF LASAGNA	1.000 SERVING	28.400	22.000	1.200	2.800	0.600	—	—	—	—	129
BABY-BEEF STEW	1.000 SERVING	28.400	14.000	1.400	1.500	0.300	3.550	0.160	0.120	0.010	98.000
BABY-MIXED VEGETABLES	1.000 SERVING	28.400	11.000	0.300	2.700	0.000	—	—	—	—	2.000
BABY-TURKEY & RICE	1.000 SERVING	28.400	14.000	0.500	2.100	0.400	2.840	0.120	0.150	0.040	5.000
BABY-VEAL & VEGETABLES	1.000 SERVING	28.400	20.000	1.700	1.700	0.800	—	—	—	—	7.000
BABY-APPLE BLUEBERRY	1.000 SERVING	28.400	17.000	0.100	4.600	0.100	0.000	—	—	—	0.000
BABY-APPLESAUCE	1.000 SERVING	28.400	12.000	0.100	3.100	0.000	0.000	0.000	0.000	0.000	1.000
BABY-PEACHES	1.000 SERVING	28.400	20.000	0.100	5.400	0.000	0.000	0.000	0.000	0.000	2.000
BABY-PEARS	1.000 SERVING	28.400	12.000	0.100	3.100	0.000	0.000	0.000	0.000	0.000	1.000
BABY-APPLE JUICE	1.000 FL OZ	31.000	14.000	0.000	3.600	0.000	0.000	0.000	0.000	0.000	1.000
BABY-APPLE PEACH JUICE	1.000 FL OZ	31.000	13.000	0.000	3.200	0.000	0.000	0.000	0.000	0.000	—
BABY-ORANGE JUICE	1.000 FL OZ	31.000	14.000	0.200	3.200	0.100	—	—	—	—	0.000
BABY-BEEF	1.000 SERVING	28.400	30.000	3.900	0.000	1.500	—	0.730	0.620	0.060	23.000
BABY-CHICKEN	1.000 SERVING	28.400	37.000	3.900	0.000	2.200	—	0.580	1.010	0.540	13.000
BABY-EGG YOLKS	1.000 SERVING	28.400	58.000	2.800	0.300	4.900	223	1.470	—	—	11.000
BABY-HAM	1.000 SERVING	28.400	32.000	3.900	0.000	1.600	—	0.550	0.780	0.220	12.000
BABY-LAMB	1.000 SERVING	28.400	29.000	4.000	0.000	1.300	—	0.660	0.530	0.060	18.000
BABY LIVER	1.000 SERVING	28.400	29.999	4.100	0.400	1.100	52.000	0.390	0.220	0.020	21.000
BABY-PORK	1.000 SERVING	28.400	35.000	4.000	0.000	2.000	—	0.680	1.020	0.220	12.000
BABY-TURKEY	1.000 SERVING	28.400	32.000	4.000	0.000	1.700	—	0.540	0.620	0.410	16.000
BABY-BEANS-GREEN	1.000 SERVING	28.400	7.000	0.400	1.700	0.000	0.000	0.000	0.000	0.000	1.000
BABY-COOKIE-ARROWROOT	1.000 ITEM	6.000	24.000	0.400	4.300	0.900	—	0.200	0.520	0.020	22.000
BABY-GARDEN VEGETABLES	1.000 SERVING	28.400	11.000	0.700	1.900	0.100	—	—	—	—	10.000
BABY-PEAS	1.000 SERVING	28.400	11.000	1.000	2.300	0.100	—	—	—	—	1.000
BABY-SQUASH	1.000 SERVING	28.400	7.000	0.200	1.600	0.100	—	—	—	—	1.000
BABY-SWEET POTATOES	1.000 SERVING	28.400	16.000	0.300	3.700	0.000	—	0.000	0.000	0.000	6.000
BABY-PRETZELS	1.000 ITEM	6.000	24.000	0.700	4.900	0.100	—	—	—	—	16.000
BABY-ZWIEBACK	1.000 PIECE	7.000	30.000	0.700	5.200	0.700	1.460	0.280	0.240	0.050	16.000
BABY-CEREAL & EGG YOLKS	1.000 SERVING	28.400	15.000	0.500	2.000	0.500	18.000	0.170	0.220	0.040	9.000
BABY-APPLE BETTY	1.000 SERVING	28.400	20.000	0.100	5.600	0.000	—	—	—	—	3.000
BABY-BEEF & EGG NOODLES	1.000 SERVING	28.400	15.000	0.600	2.000	0.500	—	—	—	—	8.000
BABY-BEANS-GREEN-BUTTERED	1.000 SERVING	28.400	9.000	0.300	1.900	0.200	—	—	—	—	1.000
BABY-BEETS	1.000 SERVING	28.400	10.000	0.400	2.200	0.000	0.000	0.000	0.000	0.000	24.000
BABY-CORN-CREAMED	1.000 SERVING	28.400	16.000	0.400	4.000	0.100	—	—	—	—	12.000
BABY-PEAS-CREAMED	1.000 SERVING	28.400	15.000	0.600	2.500	0.500	—	—	—	—	4.000
BABY-SPINACH-CREAMED	1.000 SERVING	28.400	11.000	0.700	1.600	0.400	—	—	—	—	14.000

Key to Abbreviations

KCAL, kcalories	**POT,** potassium	**V-B6,** vitamin-B6
PROT, protein	**MAG,** magnesium	**FOL,** folate
CARB, carbohydrate	**IRON,** iron	**V-B12,** vitamin-B12
FAT, fat	**ZINC,** zinc	**CALC,** calcium
CHOL, cholesterol	**V-A,** vitamin A	**PHOS,** phosphorus
SAFA, saturated fat	**V-C,** vitamin C	**SEL,** selenium
MUFA, monounsaturated fat	**THIA,** thiamin	**FIBD,** dietary fiber
PUFA, polyunsaturated fat	**RIBO,** riboflavin	**V-ET,** vitamin ET
SOD, sodium	**NIAC,** niacin	

OT Mg	MAG Mg	IRON Mg	ZINC Mg	V-A RE	V-C Mg	THIA Mg	RIBO Mg	NIAC Mg	V-B6 Mg	FOL Ug	V-B12 Ug	CALC Mg	PHOS Mg	SEL Mg	FIBD Gm	V-ET mg
35.000	4.000	0.390	0.102	1	1.000	0.026	0.059	0.476	0.012	—	0.008	29.000	18.000	—	—	—
56.000	8.000	2.960	0.202	6	0.300	0.122	0.165	1.640	0.019	3.200	—	62.000	40.000	—	0.000	0.045
58.000	10.000	3.440	0.262	6	0.400	0.143	0.160	1.700	0.017	2.800	—	62.000	45.000	0.001	—	0.054
54.000	13.000	3.460	0.182	6	0.300	0.132	0.142	1.480	0.032	2.300	—	68.000	50.000	0.001	0.000	0.074
35.000	3.000	0.250	0.198	100	0.500	0.020	0.025	0.384	0.020	—	—	5.000	11.000	—	—	0.062
40.000	3.000	0.200	0.247	95	0.900	0.004	0.018	0.372	0.021	—	—	3.000	12.000	0.003	0.340	0.062
34.000	—	0.090	—	77	0.800	0.004	0.009	0.142	—	2.300	—	6.000	—	0.000	—	0.128
12.000	—	0.070	—	27	0.300	0.001	0.006	0.087	0.009	0.900	—	6.000	6.000	—	0.000	0.062
43.000	2.000	0.170	0.284	21	0.500	0.006	0.021	0.457	0.024	—	0.128	3.000	15.000	—	—	0.062
20.000	—	0.060	—	1	7.900	0.005	0.010	0.034	0.010	1.000	—	1.000	2.000	0.000	—	0.165
20.000	1.000	0.060	0.007	0	10.900	0.003	0.008	0.017	0.009	0.500	—	1.000	2.000	0.000	—	0.165
46.000	2.000	0.070	0.024	5	8.900	0.003	0.009	0.173	0.004	1.100	—	2.000	3.000	0.000	—	0.165
37.000	2.000	0.070	0.021	1	7.000	0.004	0.008	0.054	0.002	1.000	—	2.000	3.000	0.000	—	0.165
28.000	1.000	0.180	0.009	1	18.000	0.002	0.005	0.026	0.009	0.000	—	1.000	2.000	0.000	—	0.180
30.000	1.000	0.170	0.008	2	18.100	0.002	0.003	0.066	0.007	0.400	—	1.000	1.000	0.000	—	0.180
57.000	3.000	0.050	0.017	2	19.400	0.014	0.009	0.074	0.017	8.200	—	4.000	3.000	0.000	—	0.180
62.000	5.000	0.420	0.696	16	0.600	0.003	0.040	0.808	0.040	1.600	0.403	2.000	24.000	0.003	0.000	0.111
40.000	4.000	0.400	0.343	11	0.500	0.004	0.043	0.923	0.057	2.900	—	18.000	27.000	0.003	0.000	0.111
22.000	2.000	0.780	0.543	107	0.400	0.020	0.075	0.007	0.045	26.100	0.437	22.000	81.000	0.005	0.000	0.170
58.000	4.000	0.290	0.637	3	0.600	0.039	0.044	0.746	0.071	0.600	—	2.000	23.000	0.003	0.000	0.111
58.000	4.000	0.420	0.781	7	0.300	0.005	0.057	0.829	0.043	0.600	0.621	2.000	27.000	0.004	0.000	0.111
64.000	4.000	1.500	0.844	3247	5.500	0.014	0.514	2.360	0.097	95.700	0.612	1.000	58.000	0.007	0.000	0.111
63.000	3.000	0.280	0.644	3	0.500	0.041	0.058	0.643	0.058	0.500	0.281	1.000	27.000	0.004	0.000	0.111
65.000	4.000	0.340	0.519	48	0.600	0.005	0.059	1.040	0.051	3.200	0.284	7.000	36.000	0.003	0.000	0.111
45.000	7.000	0.210	0.058	13	1.500	0.007	0.024	0.098	0.011	9.800	—	11.000	6.000	0.000	—	0.128
9.000	1.000	0.180	0.032	—	0.300	0.030	0.026	0.344	0.002	—	0.004	2.000	7.000	—	0.000	0.014
48.000	6.000	0.240	0.074	172	1.600	0.017	0.020	0.221	0.028	11.400	—	8.000	8.000	0.000	—	0.128
32.000	4.000	0.270	0.099	16	1.900	0.023	0.017	0.289	0.020	7.400	—	6.000	12.000	0.000	—	0.128
51.000	3.000	0.080	0.040	57	2.200	0.003	0.016	0.100	0.018	4.400	—	7.000	4.000	0.000	—	0.128
75.000	4.000	0.100	0.058	183	2.800	0.008	0.009	0.101	0.026	2.800	—	4.000	7.000	0.000	—	0.128
8.000	2.000	0.230	0.047	0	0.200	0.028	0.021	0.214	0.005	—	—	1.000	7.000	—	0.000	0.009
21.000	1.000	0.040	0.038	0	0.400	0.015	0.017	0.092	0.006	—	—	1.000	4.000	—	0.000	—
11.000	1.000	0.130	0.081	11	0.200	0.003	0.012	0.014	0.006	0.900	0.020	7.000	11.000	—	0.000	0.071
14.000	—	0.050	—	0	9.800	0.004	0.010	0.013	—	0.100	—	5.000	—	—	0.000	0.065
13.000	2.000	0.120	0.106	31	0.300	0.010	0.012	0.205	0.014	1.400	0.026	3.000	8.000	0.003	—	0.062
45.000	—	0.360	—	13	2.300	0.005	0.030	0.096	—	8.100	—	18.000	—	0.170	—	0.128
52.000	4.000	0.090	0.034	1	0.700	0.003	0.012	0.037	0.007	8.700	—	4.000	4.000	—	—	0.128
26.000	2.000	0.080	0.054	2	0.600	0.004	0.013	0.145	0.012	3.200	0.005	6.000	9.000	—	—	0.128
25.000	—	0.160	0.110	2	0.500	0.025	0.016	0.230	0.013	6.400	0.023	4.000	9.000	—	—	0.128
54.000	16.000	0.180	0.088	118	2.500	0.004	0.029	0.061	0.021	17.200	—	25.000	15.000	—	—	0.128

Nutritive Components for Beverages

Food Name	Serving Portion	WT. Gm	KCAL Kc	PROT Gm	CARB Gm	FAT Gm	CHOL Mg	SAFA Gm	MUFA Gm	PUFA Gm	SOD Mg
CARN INST BREAK-CHOC-ENV	1.000 ITEM	36.000	130	7.000	23.000	1.000	—	—	—	—	136
CHOC BEV DRINK-NO MILK-DRY	1.000 SERVING	28.000	97.700	0.924	25.300	0.868	0.000	0.513	0.283	0.025	58.800
BEER-REGULAR	1.000 FL OZ	29.700	12.000	0.100	1.100	0.000	0.000	0.000	0.000	0.000	2.000
WHIS/GIN/RUM/VOD-80 PROOF	1.000 FL OZ	27.800	64.000	0.000	0.000	0.000	0.000	0.000	0.000	0.000	0.000
WHIS/GIN/RUM/VOD-86 PROOF	1.000 FL OZ	27.800	69.000	0.000	0.000	0.000	0.000	0.000	0.000	0.000	0.000
WHIS/GIN/RUM/VOD-90 PROOF	1.000 FL OZ	27.700	73.000	0.000	0.000	0.000	0.000	0.000	0.000	0.000	1.000
WINE-DESSERT	1.000 FL OZ	30.000	46.000	0.100	3.500	0.000	0.000	0.000	0.000	0.000	3.000
WINE-RED-TABLE	1.000 FL OZ	29.500	21.000	0.100	0.500	0.000	0.000	0.000	0.000	0.000	19.000
CLUB SODA	1.000 FL OZ	29.600	0.000	0.000	0.000	0.000	0.000	0.000	0.000	0.000	6.000
COFFEE-BREWED	1.000 FL OZ	30.000	1.000	0.000	0.100	0.000	0.000	0.000	0.000	0.000	1.000
COFFEE-INSTANT-PREPARED	1.000 FL OZ	30.300	0.610	0.000	0.121	0.000	0.000	0.000	0.000	0.000	0.910
TEA-BREWED	1.000 FL 0Z	29.600	0.000	0.000	0.100	0.000	0.000	0.000	0.000	0.000	1.000
TEA-INSTANT-PREP-UNSWEET	1.000 CUP	237	2.000	0.100	0.400	0.000	0.000	0.000	0.000	0.000	8.000
TEA-INSTANT-PREP-SWEETENED	1.000 CUP	259	87.000	0.100	22.100	0.100	0.000	0.008	0.003	0.021	—
CORDIALS/LIQUEUR-54-PROOF	1.000 FL OZ	34.000	97.000	—	11.500	0.000	—	0.000	0.000	0.000	1.000
BRANDY/COGNAC-PONY	1.000 ITEM	30.000	73.000	—	—	—	—	—	—	—	—
CIDER-FERMENTED	1.000 FL OZ	30.000	11.800	—	0.300	—	—	—	—	—	0.000
WHIS/GIN/RUM/VOD-94 PROOF	1.000 FL OZ	27.800	76.500	0.000	0.000	0.000	0.000	0.000	0.000	0.000	0.000
WHIS/GIN/RUM/VOD-100 PROOF	1.000 FL OZ	27.800	82.000	0.000	0.000	0.000	0.000	0.000	0.000	0.000	0.000
CHAMPAGNE-DOMESTIC-GLASS	1.000 ITEM	120	84.000	0.200	3.000	—	—	—	—	—	—
WINE-VERMOUTH-DRY-GLASS	1.000 ITEM	100	105	0.000	1.000	0.000	0.000	0.000	0.000	0.000	4.000
WINE-VERMOUTH-SWEET-GLASS	1.000 ITEM	100	167	0.000	12.000	0.000	0.000	0.000	0.000	0.000	—
BEER-LIGHT	1.000 FL OZ	29.500	8.000	0.100	0.400	0.000	0.000	0.000	0.000	0.000	1.000
CREAM SODA	1.000 FL OZ	30.900	16.000	0.000	4.100	0.000	0.000	0.000	0.000	0.000	4.000
PERRIER-MINERAL WATER	1.000 CUP	237	0.000	0.000	0.000	0.000	0.000	0.000	0.000	0.000	3.000
OVALTINE-CHOC-PREP/MILK	1.000 CUP	265	227	9.530	29.200	8.790	—	—	—	—	228
COFFEE SUBSTITUTE-PREPARED	1.000 FL OZ	30.300	1.520	0.030	0.192	0.000	0.000	0.000	0.000	0.000	1.210
POSTUM-INST GRAIN BEV-DRY	1.000 SERVING	28.400	103	1.930	24.100	0.028	0.000	0.000	0.000	0.000	28.400
TANG-INST DRINK-ORANGE-DRY	1.000 SERVING	28.400	104	0.000	26.100	0.000	0.000	0.000	0.000	0.000	12.800
WINE-WHITE-TABLE	1.000 FL OZ	29.500	20.000	0.000	0.200	0.000	0.000	0.000	0.000	0.000	18.000
WINE COOLER-WHITE WINE/7UP	1.000 SERVING	102	54.900	0.050	5.720	0.000	0.000	0.000	0.000	0.000	7.480
WATER	1.000 CUP	237	0.000	0.000	0.000	0.000	0.000	0.000	0.000	0.000	7.000
LEMON LIME SODA-7UP	1.000 FL OZ	30.700	12.000	0.000	3.200	0.000	0.000	0.000	0.000	0.000	3.000
TEA-HERB-BREWED	1.000 FL OZ	29.600	1.000	0.000	0.100	0.000	0.000	0.000	0.000	0.000	0.000
GATORADE-THIRST QUENCHER	1.000 FL OZ	30.100	7.000	0.000	1.900	0.000	0.000	0.000	0.000	0.000	12.000
TONIC WATER-QUININE SODA	1.000 FL OZ	30.500	10.000	0.000	2.700	0.000	0.000	0.000	0.000	0.000	1.000
WINE-ROSE-TABLE	1.000 FL OZ	29.500	21.000	0.000	0.400	0.000	0.000	0.000	0.000	0.000	1.000

Nutritive Components for Breads

Food Name	Serving Portion	WT. Gm	KCAL Kc	PROT Gm	CARB Gm	FAT Gm	CHOL Mg	SAFA Gm	MUFA Gm	PUFA Gm	SOD Mg
BAGEL-EGG	1.000 ITEM	55.000	163	6.020	30.900	1.410	8.000	0.500	—		198
BAGEL-WATER	1.000 ITEM	55.000	163	6.020	30.900	1.410	—	0.200	—		198
BISCUITS-PREPARED/MIX	1.000 ITEM	28.000	93.200	2.070	13.600	3.320	—	0.600	—		262
BREADCRUMBS-DRY-GRATED	1.000 CUP	100	390	13.000	73.000	5.000	0.000	1.000	—		736
BREAD-CRACKED WHEAT	1.000 SLICE	25.000	65.500	2.320	12.500	0.868	0.000	0.100	—		108
BREAD-FRENCH-ENRICHED	1.000 SLICE	35.000	98.000	3.330	17.700	1.360	0.000	0.200	—		193
BREAD-RAISIN-ENRICHED	1.000 SLICE	25.000	69.500	2.050	13.200	0.990	—	0.200	—		94.000
BREAD-RYE-AMERICAN-LIGHT	1.000 SLICE	25.000	65.500	2.120	12.000	0.913	0.000	0.000	0.000	0.000	174
BREAD-PUMPERNICKEL	1.000 SLICE	32.000	81.600	2.930	15.400	1.100	0.000	0.100	—		173
BREAD-WHITE-FIRM	1.000 SLICE	23.000	61.400	1.900	11.200	0.902	0.000	0.200	—		118
BREAD-WHITE-FIRM-TOASTED	1.000 SLICE	20.000	65.000	2.000	12.000	1.000	0.000	0.200	—		117
BREAD-WHOLE WHEAT-FIRM	1.000 SLICE	25.000	61.300	2.410	11.300	1.090	0.000	0.100	—		159
BREAD-WHEAT-FIRM-TOASTED	1.000 SLICE	21.000	59.000	2.310	10.900	1.050	—	0.100	—		153
CORNMEAL-DEGERM-ENR-COOKED	1.000 CUP	240	120	3.000	26.000	0.000	0.000	0.000	0.000	0.000	264
MUFFIN-BLUEBERRY-HOME REC	1.000 ITEM	40.000	110	3.000	17.000	4.000	21.000	1.100	—		252

A

T Mg	MAG Mg	IRON Mg	ZINC Mg	V-A RE	V-C Mg	THIA Mg	RIBO Mg	NIAC Mg	V-B6 Mg	FOL Ug	V-B12 Ug	CALC Mg	PHOS Mg	SEL Mg	FIBD Gm	V-ET mg
422	80.000	4.500	3.000	525	27.000	0.300	0.070	5.000	0.400	0.000	0.600	100	150	—	—	—
165	27.400	0.879	0.434	0.568	0.196	0.010	0.041	0.143	0.003	—	0.000	10.400	35.800	—	—	0.056
7.000	2.000	0.010	0.000	0	0.000	0.002	0.008	0.135	0.015	1.800	0.010	1.000	4.000	—	—	—
1.000	0.000	0.030	0.020	0	0.000	0.002	0.000	0.000	0.000	0.000	0.000	0.000	1.000	0.000	0.000	0.000
1.000	0.000	0.010	0.010	0	0.000	0.002	0.000	0.014	0.000	0.000	0.000	0.000	2.000	0.000	0.000	0.000
0.000	0.000	0.000	0.000	0	0.000	0.000	0.000	0.000	0.000	0.000	0.000	0.000	0.000	0.000	0.000	0.000
3.000	3.000	0.070	0.020	0	0.000	0.005	0.005	0.064	0.000	0.100	0.000	2.000	3.000	—	0.000	—
0.700	4.000	0.130	0.030	0	0.000	0.001	0.008	0.024	0.010	0.600	0.000	2.000	4.000	—	0.000	—
0.000	0.000	—	0.030	0	0.000	0.000	0.000	0.000	0.000	0.000	0.000	1.000	0.000	—	0.000	—
3.000	2.000	0.120	0.000	0	0.000	0.000	0.000	0.066	0.000	0.000	0.000	1.000	0.000	0.000	0.000	—
7.900	1.210	0.015	0.009	0	0.000	0.000	0.000	0.088	0.000	0.000	0.000	0.910	0.910	0.000	0.000	0.000
1.000	1.000	0.010	0.010	0	0.000	0.000	0.004	0.000	0.000	1.500	0.000	0.000	0.000	0.000	0.000	—
7.000	5.000	0.040	0.080	0	0.000	0.000	0.005	0.088	0.005	0.700	0.000	5.000	3.000	0.000	0.000	—
0.000	5.000	0.050	0.080	0	0.000	0.000	0.047	0.093	—	9.600	0.000	6.000	3.000	0.000	—	—
1.000	0.000	0.020	0.020	—	0.000	—	—	—	—	—	—	0.000	0.000	—	—	—
—	—	—	—	—	—	—	—	—	—	—	—	—	—	—	—	—
—	—	—	—	—	—	—	—	—	—	—	—	—	—	—	—	—
0.000	0.000	0.010	0.010	0	0.000	0.002	0.001	0.004	0.000	0.000	0.000	0.000	1.000	—	0.000	—
9.000	0.000	0.010	0.010	0	0.000	0.002	0.001	0.004	0.000	0.000	0.000	0.000	1.000	—	0.000	—
5.000	—	—	—	—	—	0.010	0.010	0.200	—	—	—	8.000	—	0.005	0.000	—
															0.000	
5.000	1.000	0.010	0.010	0	0.000	0.003	0.009	0.116	0.010	1.200	0.000	1.000	4.000	0.000	—	—
0.000	0.000	0.020	0.022	0	0.000	0.000	0.000	0.000	0.000	0.000	0.000	2.000	0.000	—	0.000	—
0.000	1.000	0.000	0.000	0	0.000	0.000	0.000	0.000	0.000	0.000	0.000	32.000	0.000	—	0.000	—
600	52.000	4.770	1.130	700	29.000	0.630	0.970	12.700	0.766	29.000	0.871	392	302	—	—	—
7.270	1.210	0.018	0.009	0	—		0.000	0.065	—	—	0.000	0.910	2.120	—	0.000	—
896	—	1.870	—	0	0.000	0.165	0.076	6.760	—	—	—	76.700	189	—	0.000	—
9.900	—	0.028	—	535	107	0.000	0.000	0.000	—	—	—	71.000	75.800	—	—	—
3.300	3.000	0.090	0.020	0	0.000	0.001	0.001	0.020	0.004	0.100	0.000	3.000	4.000	—	0.000	—
1.000	5.000	0.193	0.063	—	—	0.002	0.003	0.043	0.007	0.100	0.000	6.110	6.950	—	—	—
1.000	2.000	0.010	0.060	0	0.000	0.000	0.000	0.000	0.000	0.000	0.000	5.000	0.000	—	0.000	—
9.000	0.000	0.020	0.020	0	0.000	0.000	0.000	0.005	0.000	0.000	0.000	1.000	0.000	—	0.000	0.000
3.000	0.000	0.020	0.010	0	0.000	0.003	0.001	0.000	0.000	0.200	0.000	1.000	0.000	—	0.000	0.000
3.000	0.000	0.020	0.010	0	0.000	0.002	0.000	0.000	0.000	0.000	0.000	0.000	3.000	—	0.000	0.000
9.000	0.000	—	—	0	0.000	0.000	0.000	0.000	0.000	0.000	0.000	0.000	0.000	—	0.000	0.000
9.000	3.000	0.110	0.020	0	0.000	0.001	0.005	0.022	0.007	0.300	0.000	2.000	4.000	—	0.000	—

T Mg	MAG Mg	IRON Mg	ZINC Mg	V-A RE	V-C Mg	THIA Mg	RIBO Mg	NIAC Mg	V-B6 Mg	FOL Ug	V-B12 Ug	CALC Mg	PHOS Mg	SEL Mg	FIBD Gm	V-ET mg
0.700	11.000	1.460	0.286	23.5	0.000	0.209	0.160	1.940	0.024	13.200	0.052	23.100	36.900	—	0.506	—
0.700	11.000	1.460	0.286	0	0.000	0.209	0.160	1.940	0.024	13.200	0.000	23.100	36.900	—	0.506	—
0.000	6.720	0.574	0.176	37	0.000	0.120	0.106	0.840	0.013	1.680	0.045	58.200	128	—	—	—
152	32.000	3.600	—	0	0.000	0.350	0.350	4.800	—	—	—	122	141	0.020	—	—
300	8.750	0.665	—	0	0.000	0.095	0.095	0.840	0.023	—	0.000	16.300	31.800	0.011	1.000	0.025
100	7.000	1.080	0.221	0	0.000	0.161	0.123	1.400	0.019	13.000	0.000	38.500	28.400	0.010	0.546	0.042
000	6.250	0.775	0.155	0	0.000	0.083	0.155	1.020	0.009	8.750	0.000	25.500	22.500	—	0.550	—
000	6.000	0.680	0.318	0	0.000	0.103	0.080	0.828	0.023	9.750	0.000	20.000	36.300	0.007	1.650	—
139	21.800	0.877	0.365	0	0.000	0.109	0.166	1.060	0.049	—	0.000	22.700	69.800	0.014	1.160	—
.800	4.830	0.653	0.143	0	0.000	0.108	0.071	0.863	0.008	8.050	0.000	29.000	24.800	0.006	0.621	0.028
000	4.800	0.600	0.142	0	0.000	0.070	0.060	0.800	0.008	8.000	0.000	22.000	23.000	0.006	0.540	0.024
000	23.300	0.855	0.420	0	0.000	0.088	0.053	0.958	0.047	13.800	0.000	18.000	65.000	0.011	2.830	0.030
400	22.50	0.823	0.403	0	0.000	0.067	0.050	0.920	0.045	13.200	0.000	17.200	63.000	0.011	2.380	0.025
000	16.800	1.000	—	98.4	0.000	0.140	0.100	1.200	0.600	57.600	0.000	2.000	34.000	0.006	0.700	0.192
000	10.000	0.600	—	18	0.000	0.090	0.100	0.700	—	—	—	34.000	53.000	—	—	—

Continued.

A

Nutritive Components for Breads—cont'd.

Food Name	Serving Portion	WT. Gm	KCAL Kc	PROT Gm	CARB Gm	FAT Gm	CHOL Mg	SAFA Gm	MUFA Gm	PUFA Gm	SOD Mg
MUFFIN-BRAN-HOME REC	1.000 ITEM	40.000	112	2.960	16.700	5.080	21.000	1.200	—	—	168
MUFFIN-CORN-HOME REC	1.000 ITEM	40.000	125	3.000	19.000	4.000	21.000	1.200	—	—	192
MUFFIN-PLAIN-HOME REC	1.000 ITEM	40.000	120	3.000	17.000	4.000	21.000	1.000	—	—	176
ROLL-BROWN & SERVE-ENR	1.000 ITEM	26.000	85.000	2.000	14.000	2.000	—	0.400	—	—	144
ROLL-HAMBURGER/HOTDOG	1.000 ITEM	40.000	114	3.430	20.100	2.090	—	0.500	—	—	241
ROLL-HARD-ENRICHED	1.000 ITEM	50.000	155	5.000	30.000	2.000	—	0.400	—	—	312
ROLL-SUBMARINE/HOAGIE-ENR	1.000 ITEM	135	390	12.000	75.000	4.000	0.000	0.900	—	—	761
MUFFIN-ENGLISH-PLAIN	1.000 ITEM	56.000	133	4.430	25.700	1.090	—	—	—	—	358
MUFFIN-ENGLISH-PLAIN-TOAST	1.000 ITEM	53.000	154	5.130	29.800	1.260	—	—	—	—	414
BREAD-CORN-HOME REC	1.000 SLICE	45.000	108	2.210	15.600	3.940	0.000	—	—	—	126
BREAD-MIXED GRAIN	1.000 SLICE	25.000	64.300	2.490	11.700	0.930	0.000	—	—	—	103
BREAD-WHOLE WHEAT-HOME REC	1.000 SLICE	25.000	66.500	2.250	11.600	1.610	0.000	—	—	—	89.000
BREAD-PITA	1.000 ITEM	38.000	105	3.950	20.600	0.570	—	—	—	—	215
ROLL-WHOLE WHEAT-HOMEMADE	1.000 ITEM	35.000	90.000	3.500	18.300	1.000	—	—	—	0.000	197
CROISSANT-ROLL-SARA LEE	1.000 ITEM	26.000	109	2.300	11.200	6.100	—	—	—	—	140
MUFFIN-SOY	1.000 ITEM	40.000	119	3.900	16.700	4.400	—	—	—	0.400	—
BREAD STICK-VIENNA TYPE	1.000 ITEM	35.000	106	3.300	20.300	1.100	—	—	—	—	548

Nutritive Components for Breakfast Cereals

Food Name	Serving Portion	WT. Gm	KCAL Kc	PROT Gm	CARB Gm	FAT Gm	CHOL Mg	SAFA Gm	MUFA Gm	PUFA Gm	SOD Mg
CEREAL-CORN GRITS-ENRICHED	1.000 CUP	242	146	3.500	31.400	0.500	0.000	0.000	0.000	0.000	0.000
CEREAL-FARINA-COOK-ENR	1.000 CUP	233	116	3.400	24.600	0.200	0.000	0.000	0.000	0.000	1.000
CEREAL-WHEAT-ROLLED-COOKED	1.000 CUP	240	180	5.000	41.000	1.000	0.000	—	—	—	535
CEREAL-WHEAT-WHOLE MEAL	1.000 CUP	245	110	4.000	23.000	1.000	0.000	—	—	—	535
CEREAL-FROST FLAKE-KELLOGG	1.000 CUP	35.000	133	1.800	31.700	0.100	0.000	0.000	0.000	0.000	284
CEREAL-CORN-SHREDDED-SUGAR	1.000 CUP	25.000	95.000	2.000	22.000	0.000	0.000	—	—	—	247
CEREAL-OATS-PUFFED-SUGAR	1.000 CUP	25.000	100	3.000	19.000	1.000	0.000	—	—	—	294
CEREAL-RICE-PUFFED-PLAIN	1.000 CUP	14.000	56.000	0.900	12.600	0.100	0.000	0.000	0.000	0.000	0.000
CEREAL-RICE-PUFFED-SUGAR	1.000 CUP	28.000	115	1.000	26.000	0.000	0.000	—	—	—	21.000
CEREAL-WHEAT FLAKES-SUGAR	1.000 CUP	30.000	105	3.000	24.000	0.000	0.000	—	—	—	368
CEREAL-WHEAT-PUFFED-PLAIN	1.000 CUP	12.000	44.000	1.800	9.500	0.100	0.000	—	—	—	0.480
CEREAL-WHEAT-PUFFED-SUGAR	1.000 CUP	38.000	140	3.000	33.000	0.000	0.000	—	—	—	57.000
CEREAL-WHEAT-SHRED-BISCUIT	1.000 ITEM	23.600	83.000	2.600	18.800	0.300	0.000	0.000	0.000	0.000	0.472
CEREAL-WHEAT GERM-TOASTED	1.000 CUP	113	431	32.900	56.100	12.100	0.000	2.090	1.750	7.330	4.000
CEREAL-CREAM/WHEAT-PACKET	1.000 ITEM	150	132	2.500	28.900	0.400	0.000	0.000	0.000	0.000	241
CEREAL-OATMEAL-INST-PACKET	1.000 ITEM	177	104	4.400	18.100	1.700	0.000	—	—	—	286
CEREAL-RALSTON-COOKED	1.000 CUP	253	134	5.500	28.200	0.800	0.000	0.000	0.000	0.000	4.000
CEREAL-ALL BRAN	1.000 CUP	85.200	212	12.200	63.400	1.530	0.000	—	—	—	961
CEREAL-ALPHA BITS	1.000 CUP	28.400	111	2.200	24.600	0.600	—	—	—	—	219
CEREAL-BRAN BUDS	1.000 CUP	85.200	220	11.800	64.800	2.040	—	—	—	—	523
CEREAL-BRAN CHEX	1.000 CUP	49.000	156	5.100	39.000	1.400	0.000	—	—	—	455
CEREAL-C.W. POST-PLAIN	1.000 CUP	97.000	432	8.700	69.400	15.200	0.000	11.300	1.720	1.420	167
CEREAL-CHEERIOS	1.000 CUP	22.700	88.800	3.420	15.700	1.450	0.000	0.270	0.515	0.597	246
CEREAL-CORN BRAN	1.000 CUP	36.000	124	2.500	30.400	1.300	0.000	—	—	—	310
CEREAL-CORN CHEX	1.000 CUP	28.400	111	2.000	24.900	0.100	—	—	—	—	271
CEREAL-CORN FLAKES-KELLOGG	1.000 CUP	22.700	88.300	1.840	19.500	0.068	0.000	0.000	0.000	0.000	281
CEREAL-CRACKLIN BRAN	1.000 CUP	60.000	229	5.500	41.100	8.800	0.000	—	—	—	487
CEREAL-CRISPY RICE	1.000 CUP	28.000	111	1.800	24.800	0.100	0.000	0.000	0.000	0.000	205
CEREAL-FORTIFIED OAT FLAKE	1.000 CUP	48.000	177	9.000	34.700	0.700	0.000	0.000	0.000	0.000	429
CEREAL-BRAN FLAKES-KELLOGG	1.000 CUP	39.000	127	4.900	30.500	0.700	0.000	0.000	0.000	0.000	363
CEREAL-FROSTED MINI WHEATS	1.000 ITEM	7.100	25.500	0.731	5.860	0.071	0.000	0.000	0.000	0.000	2.060
CEREAL-GRANOLA-HOMEMADE	1.000 CUP	122	595	15.000	67.300	33.100	0.000	5.840	9.370	17.200	12.000
CEREAL-GRAPE NUTS	1.000 CUP	114	407	13.300	93.500	0.456	0.000	0.000	0.000	0.000	792
CEREAL-GRAPE NUTS FLAKES	1.000 CUP	32.500	116	3.480	26.600	0.358	0.000	0.000	0.000	0.000	250

T Mg	MAG Mg	IRON Mg	ZINC Mg	V-A RE	V-C Mg	THIA Mg	RIBO Mg	NIAC Mg	V-B6 Mg	FOL Ug	V-B12 Ug	CALC Mg	PHOS Mg	SEL Mg	FIBD Gm	V-ET mg
.800	35.200	1.260	1.080	40	2.480	0.100	0.112	1.260	0.111	16.800	0.092	53.600	111	—	2.520	—
.000	18.400	0.700	—	25	0.000	0.100	0.100	0.700	—	—	—	42.000	68.000	—	—	—
.000	10.800	0.600	—	8	0.000	0.090	0.120	0.900	—	—	—	42.000	60.000	—	—	—
.000	5.460	0.800	0.190	0	0.000	0.100	0.060	0.900	0.016	9.880	—	20.000	23.000	0.008	—	0.203
.800	7.600	1.190	0.248	0	0.000	0.196	0.132	1.580	0.014	14.800	—	53.600	32.800	0.012	—	0.016
.000	11.500	1.200	0.300	0	0.000	0.200	0.120	1.700	0.018	29.500	0.000	24.000	46.000	0.015	—	0.020
122	—	3.000	—	0	0.000	0.540	0.320	4.500	0.047	—	—	58.000	115	0.041	—	0.054
314	10.600	1.580	0.403	0	0.000	0.258	0.179	2.100	0.022	17.900	0.000	90.700	62.700	0.015	—	—
364	12.200	1.830	0.466	0	0.000	0.239	0.207	2.430	0.026	20.700	0.000	105	72.600	0.015	—	—
.300	8.100	0.671	0.212	7.25	0.000	0.081	0.081	0.675	0.032	4.500	0.077	48.600	43.700	—	—	—
.500	12.300	0.815	0.300	0	0.000	0.098	0.095	1.040	0.026	16.300	0.000	26.000	53.000	0.011	1.000	0.025
.000	23.300	0.670	0.562	10.8	0.000	0.068	0.038	0.798	0.050	12.300	0.027	19.800	63.300	0.011	2.830	0.025
.800	—	0.916	—	0	0.000	0.171	0.076	1.400	—	—	—	30.800	38.000	—	0.357	—
102	40.000	0.800	—	0	0.000	0.120	0.050	1.100	—	—	—	34.000	98.000	0.016	—	0.035
.000	7.000	1.040	—	8.2	0.000	0.280	0.100	1.200	—	—	—	12.000	32.000	—	—	—
—	52.000	0.900	—	40	0.000	0.080	0.100	0.500	—	—	—	35.000	56.000	—	—	—
.000	—	0.300	—	0	0.000	0.020	0.030	0.300	—	—	—	16.000	31.000	—	—	—

T Mg	MAG Mg	IRON Mg	ZINC Mg	V-A RE	V-C Mg	THIA Mg	RIBO Mg	NIAC Mg	V-B6 Mg	FOL Ug	V-B12 Ug	CALC Mg	PHOS Mg	SEL Mg	FIBD Gm	V-ET mg
.000	11.000	1.560	0.170	—	—	0.240	0.150	1.960	0.058	1.000	—	1.000	29.000	—	0.600	0.290
.000	4.000	1.170	0.160	—	—	0.190	0.120	1.280	0.023	6.000	—	4.000	28.000	—	0.400	—
202	52.800	1.700	1.150	0	0.000	0.170	0.070	2.200	—	26.400	—	19.000	182	—	—	2.540
118	53.900	1.200	1.180	0	0.000	0.150	0.050	1.500	—	27.000	—	17.000	127	—	—	2.6
.000	3.000	2.200	0.050	463	19.000	0.500	0.500	6.200	0.600	124	—	1.000	26.000	—	2.200	—
—	3.500	0.600	0.088	0	13.000	0.330	0.050	4.400	0.450	88.300	1.330	1.000	10.000	0.002	—	0.090
—	28.000	4.000	0.693	275	13.000	0.330	0.380	4.400	0.450	5.500	1.330	44.000	102	0.006	0.125	1.168
.000	3.000	0.150	0.140	0	0.000	0.020	0.010	0.420	0.011	3.000	—	1.000	14.000	0.001	0.100	0.094
.000	7.560	0.000	1.480	300	15.000	0.000	0.000	0.000	0.504	98.800	1.480	3.000	14.000	0.002	0.200	0.188
.000	32.700	4.800	0.669	330	16.000	0.400	0.450	5.300	0.540	9.000	1.590	12.000	83.000	0.003	2.000	0.126
.000	17.000	0.570	0.280	0	0.000	0.020	0.030	1.300	0.020	4.000	—	3.000	43.000	—	0.400	0.080
.000	22.800	0.000	2.010	0	20.000	0.500	0.570	6.700	0.684	134	2.010	7.000	52.000	—	0.400	—
.000	40.000	0.740	0.590	0	0.000	0.070	0.060	1.080	0.060	12.000	—	10.000	86.000	—	2.200	0.085
1070	362	10.300	18.800	50	7.000	1.890	0.930	6.310	1.110	398	—	50.000	1294	—	7.800	15.9
.000	9.000	8.100	0.230	1250	—	0.400	0.200	5.000	0.500	100	—	40.000	20.000	—	—	—
100	—	6.320	—	455	—	0.530	0.290	5.490	0.742	150	—	163	133	—	1.620	1.060
153	59.000	1.640	1.420	0	—	0.200	0.180	2.050	0.114	18.000	0.109	14.000	148	—	4.200	—
1051	318	13.500	11.200	1125	45.200	1.110	1.280	15.000	1.530	301	—	69.000	794	0.025	25.500	1.270
110	17.000	1.800	1.500	375	—	0.400	0.400	5.000	0.500	100	1.500	8.000	51.000	—	0.300	—
1425	271	13.500	11.200	1125	45.200	1.110	1.280	15.000	1.530	301	—	57.100	740	0.025	23.600	0.903
394	126	7.800	2.140	11	26.000	0.600	0.260	8.600	0.900	173	2.600	29.000	327	0.010	7.900	—
198	67.000	15.400	1.640	1284	—	1.300	1.500	17.100	1.700	342	5.100	47.000	224	—	2.200	—
.000	31.300	3.610	0.629	300	12.000	0.295	0.341	4.000	0.409	4.990	1.200	38.800	107	0.010	0.863	—
.000	18.000	12.200	4.000	7.56	—	0.380	0.700	10.900	0.858	232	1.390	41.000	52.000	0.002	6.840	—
.000	4.000	1.800	0.100	14	15.000	0.400	0.070	5.000	0.500	100	1.500	3.000	11.000	0.002	0.500	—
.900	2.720	1.430	0.064	300	12.000	0.295	0.341	4.000	0.409	80.100	—	0.681	14.300	0.001	0.250	0.023
355	116	3.800	3.200	794	32.000	0.800	0.900	10.600	1.100	212	—	40.000	241	0.010	9.100	—
.000	12.000	0.700	0.460	0	1.000	0.100	0.000	2.000	0.044	3.000	0.082	5.000	31.000	0.004	1.000	—
343	58.000	13.700	1.500	636	—	0.600	0.700	8.400	0.900	169	2.500	68.000	176	0.010	1.200	—
248	71.000	11.200	5.100	516	—	0.500	0.600	6.900	0.700	138	2.100	19.000	192	0.004	5.500	0.164
.200	55.800	0.447	0.376	94	3.760	0.092	0.107	1.250	0.128	25.100	—	2.340	18.500	—	0.540	0.026
612	141	4.840	4.470	10	1.000	0.730	0.310	2.140	0.428	99.000	—	76.000	494	0.040	4.360	—
381	76.300	4.950	2.510	1500	—	1.480	1.710	20.100	2.050	402	6.040	43.300	286	0.034	5.470	—
113	35.800	5.170	0.650	430	—	0.423	0.488	5.720	0.585	115	1.720	13.000	96.900	0.010	2.080	0.137

Continued.

A

Nutritive Components for Breakfast Cereals—cont'd.

Food Name	Serving Portion	WT. Gm	KCAL Kc	PROT Gm	CARB Gm	FAT Gm	CHOL Mg	SAFA Gm	MUFA Gm	PUFA Gm	SOD Mg
CEREAL-HEARTLAND NATURAL	1.000 CUP	115	499	11.600	78.600	17.700	0.000	—	—	—	294
CEREAL-HONEY NUT CHEERIOS	1.000 CUP	33.000	125	3.600	26.500	0.800	0.000	0.130	0.310	0.300	299
CEREAL-HONEY BRAN	1.000 CUP	35.000	119	3.100	28.600	0.700		0.000	0.000	0.000	202
CEREAL-LIFE-PLAIN/CINNAMON	1.000 CUP	44.000	162	8.100	31.500	0.800	0.000	0.000	0.000	0.000	229
CEREAL-LUCKY CHARMS	1.000 CUP	32.000	125	2.900	26.100	1.200	0.000	0.220	0.430	0.490	227
CEREAL-GRANOLA-NATURE VAL	1.000 CUP	113	503	11.500	75.500	19.600	0.000	13.000	2.930	2.750	232
CEREAL-NUTRI GRAIN-BARLEY	1.000 CUP	41.000	153	4.500	33.900	0.300	0.000	0.000	0.000	0.000	277
CEREAL-NUTRI GRAIN-CORN	1.000 CUP	42.000	160	3.400	35.500	1.000	0.000	—	—	—	276
CEREAL-NUTRI GRAIN-RYE	1.000 CUP	40.000	144	3.500	33.900	0.300	0.000	0.000	0.000	0.000	272
CEREAL-NUTRI GRAIN-WHEAT	1.000 CUP	44.000	158	3.800	37.200	0.500	0.000	0.000	0.000	0.000	299
CEREAL-100% BRAN	1.000 CUP	66.000	178	8.300	48.100	3.300	0.000	0.590	0.570	1.870	457
CEREAL-PRODUCT 19	1.000 CUP	33.000	126	3.200	27.400	0.200	0.000	0.000	0.000	0.000	378
CEREAL-RAISIN BRAN-KELLOGG	1.000 CUP	49.200	154	5.300	37.100	0.984	0.000	—	—	—	359
CEREAL-RICE CHEX	1.000 CUP	25.200	99.500	1.340	22.500	0.101	0.000	0.000	0.000	0.000	211
CEREAL-RICE KRISPIES	1.000 CUP	28.400	112	1.900	24.800	0.200	0.000	0.000	0.000	0.000	340
CEREAL-SPECIAL K	1.000 CUP	21.300	83.100	4.200	16.000	0.085	0.000	0.000	0.000	0.000	199
CEREAL-SUGAR CORN POPS	1.000 CUP	28.400	108	1.400	25.600	0.100	0.000	0.000	0.000	0.000	103
CEREAL-SUGAR SMACKS	1.000 CUP	37.900	141	2.650	33.000	0.720	0.000	0.000	0.000	0.000	100
CEREAL-TEAM	1.000 CUP	42.000	164	2.700	36.000	0.700	0.000	0.000	0.000	0.000	259
CEREAL-TOASTIES	1.000 CUP	22.700	87.800	1.840	19.500	0.045	0.000	0.000	0.000	0.000	238
CEREAL-TOTAL	1.000 CUP	33.000	116	3.300	26.000	0.700	0.000	0.100	0.070	0.340	409
CEREAL-TRIX	1.000 CUP	28.000	108	1.500	24.900	0.400	0.000	0.000	0.000	0.000	179
CEREAL-WHEAT CHEX	1.000 CUP	46.000	169	4.500	37.800	1.100	0.000	—	—	—	308
CEREAL-WHEAT GERM-SUGAR	1.000 CUP	113	426	24.700	68.700	9.100	0.000	1.570	1.320	5.500	3.000
CEREAL-WHEATIES	1.000 CUP	29.000	101	2.800	23.100	0.500	0.000	0.070	0.050	0.240	363
CEREAL-CREAM/WHEAT-REG-HOT	1.000 CUP	251	134	3.800	27.700	0.500	0.000	0.000	0.000	0.000	2.000
CEREAL-CREAM/WHEAT-INSTANT	1.000 CUP	241	152	4.400	31.600	0.600	0.000	0.000	0.000	0.000	6.000
CEREAL-MALT O MEAL-COOK	1.000 CUP	240	122	3.500	25.800	0.300	0.000	0.000	0.000	0.000	2.000
CEREAL-MAYPO-COOK-HOT	1.000 CUP	240	170	5.800	31.800	2.400	0.000	—	—	—	9.000
CEREAL-ROMAN MEAL-COOKED	1.000 CUP	241	147	6.600	33.000	1.000	0.000	—	—	—	3.000
CEREAL-WHEATENA-COOKED	1.000 CUP	243	135	5.000	28.700	1.100	0.000	—	—	—	5.000
CEREAL-WHOLE WHEAT NATURAL	1.000 CUP	242	151	4.900	33.200	0.900	0.000	—	—	—	1.000
CEREAL-OATMEAL-RAW	1.000 CUP	81.000	311	13.000	54.200	5.100	—	0.940	1.800	2.080	3.000

Nutritive Components for Combination Foods

Food Name	Serving Portion	WT.Gm.	KCAL Kc	PROT Gm	CARB Gm	FAT Gm	CHOL Mg	SAFA Gm	MUFA Gm	PUFA Gm	SOD Mg
BEEF-RAVIOLIOS-CANNED	1.000 SERVING	28.400	27.500	1.140	4.260	0.568	—	—	—	—	131
SALAD-THREE BEAN-DEL MONTE	1.000 SERVING	28.400	22.400	0.710	5.060	0.056	0.000	0.000	0.000	0.000	101
SALAD-TUNA	1.000 CUP	205	350	30.000	7.000	22.000	68.000	4.300	—	—	434
BEEF-POTPIE-HOME RECIPE	1.000 SLICE	210	515	21.000	39.000	30.000	44.000	7.900	12.900	7.400	596
CHILI CON CARNE/BEANS-CAN	1.000 CUP	255	340	19.000	31.000	16.000	38.000	7.500	7.200	1.000	1354
MACARONI & CHEESE-ENR-CAN	1.000 CUP	240	230	9.000	26.000	10.000	42.000	4.200	—	—	729
MACARONI & CHEESE-ENR-HOME	1.000 CUP	200	430	17.000	40.000	22.000	42.000	8.900	—	—	1086
SPAGHETTI/TOM/CHE-HOME REC	1.000 CUP	250	260	9.000	37.000	9.000	4.000	2.000	—	—	955
SPAGHETTI/TOM/CHE-CAN	1.000 CUP	250	190	6.000	39.000	2.000	4.000	0.500	—	—	955
SPAGHETTI/TOM/MEAT-HOME	1.000 CUP	248	330	19.000	39.000	12.000	75.000	3.300	—	—	1009
SPAGHETTI/TOM/MEAT-CAN	1.000 CUP	250	260	12.000	29.000	10.000	39.000	2.200	—	—	1220
SALAD-POTATO	1.000 CUP	250	358	6.700	27.900	20.500	171	3.570	6.200	9.300	1323
SALAD-FRUIT-CAN/JUICE	1.000 CUP	249	125	1.280	32.500	0.060	0.000	0.010	0.012	0.027	13.000
SALAD-COLESLAW	1.000 TBSP	8.000	6.000	0.100	0.990	0.210	1.000	0.031	0.057	0.108	2.000
TACO	1.000 ITEM	81.000	187	10.600	12.700	10.400	21.100	—	—	—	456
PIZZA-PEPPERONI-BAKED	1.000 SLICE	120	306	13.000	36.700	11.500	—	—	—	—	817
SAND-BAC/LET/TOM/MAYO	1.000 ITEM	148	282	6.800	28.800	15.600	—	—	—	—	—
SANDWICH-CLUB	1.000 ITEM	315	590	35.600	41.700	20.800	—	—	—	—	—
SALAD-MACARONI	1.000 SERVING	28.400	50.700	0.700	5.300	3.000	—	—	—	—	148

T Mg	MAG Mg	IRON Mg	ZINC Mg	V-A RE	V-C Mg	THIA Mg	RIBO Mg	NIAC Mg	V-B6 Mg	FOL Ug	V-B12 Ug	CALC Mg	PHOS Mg	SEL Mg	FIBD Gm	V-ET mg
385	147	4.330	3.040	—	—	0.360	0.160	1.610	—	64.000	—	75.000	416	—	5.400	—
115	39.000	5.200	0.870	437	17.000	0.400	0.500	5.800	0.600	—	1.700	23.000	122	—	1.300	—
151	46.000	5.600	0.900	463	19.000	0.500	0.500	6.200	0.600	23.000	1.900	16.000	132	—	3.900	—
197	14.000	11.600	1.450	—	—	0.950	1.000	11.600	—	37.000	—	154	238	—	1.400	—
6.000	27.000	5.100	0.560	424	17.000	0.400	0.500	5.600	0.600	—	1.700	36.000	88.000	—	0.600	—
389	116	3.780	2.190	—	—	0.390	0.190	0.830	—	85.000	—	71.000	354	0.037	4.200	—
108	32.000	1.450	5.400	543	22.000	0.500	0.600	7.200	0.700	145	2.200	11.000	126	0.027	2.400	—
8.000	27.000	0.890	5.500	556	22.000	0.500	0.600	7.400	0.800	148	2.200	1.000	120	0.003	2.600	0.042
2.000	31.000	1.130	5.300	530	21.000	0.500	0.600	7.000	0.700	141	2.100	8.000	104	—	2.560	0.040
120	34.000	1.240	5.800	583	23.000	0.600	0.700	7.700	0.800	155	2.300	12.000	164	0.007	2.800	0.044
824	312	8.120	5.740	0	63.000	1.600	1.800	20.900	2.100	—	6.300	46.000	801	0.020	19.500	—
4.000	12.000	21.000	0.500	1748	70.000	1.700	2.000	23.300	2.300	466	7.000	4.000	47.000	—	0.400	—
256	63.500	6.000	5.020	500	—	0.492	0.590	6.690	0.689	133	2.020	17.200	183	0.005	5.310	—
9.200	6.300	1.590	0.348	1.85	13.400	0.328	—	4.440	0.454	89.000	1.340	3.530	24.700	0.004	0.151	0.010
0.000	10.000	1.800	0.480	375	15.000	0.400	0.400	5.000	0.500	100	—	4.000	34.000	0.004	0.100	0.011
6.800	11.700	3.390	2.810	280	11.300	0.277	0.320	3.750	0.383	75.200	—	6.180	41.300	—	0.170	—
7.000	2.000	1.800	1.500	375	15.000	0.400	0.400	5.000	0.500	100	—	1.000	28.000	—	0.200	0.026
6.100	18.200	2.390	0.379	500	20.100	0.493	0.569	6.670	0.682	134	—	4.170	41.300	—	0.531	—
4.000	19.000	2.570	0.580	556	22.000	0.500	0.600	7.400	0.800	—	2.200	6.000	65.000	0.007	0.400	—
6.300	3.410	0.597	0.066	300	—	0.295	0.341	4.000	0.409	80.100	1.200	0.908	10.000	—	0.386	—
123	37.000	21.000	0.780	1748	70.000	1.700	2.000	23.300	2.300	466	7.000	56.000	137	—	2.400	—
6.000	6.000	4.500	0.130	371	15.000	0.400	0.400	4.900	0.500	—	1.500	6.000	19.000	—	0.100	—
174	58.000	7.300	1.230	—	24.000	0.600	0.170	8.100	0.800	162	2.400	18.000	182	—	3.400	0.193
803	272	7.710	14.100	0	—	1.410	0.700	4.730	0.829	298	—	38.000	971	—	5.700	—
108	32.000	4.600	0.650	384	15.000	0.400	0.400	5.100	0.500	0.000	1.500	44.000	100	0.003	2.000	0.122
3.000	10.000	10.300	0.330	0	—	0.200	0.100	1.500	—	9.000	—	51.000	42.000	—	—	—
8.000	14.000	12.000	0.410	0	—	0.200	0.100	1.800	—	11.000	—	59.000	43.000	—	—	—
—	—	9.500	0.170	0	—	0.400	0.300	5.900	0.019	6.000	—	5.000	23.000	—	0.600	—
211	51.000	8.400	1.490	702	28.000	0.700	0.800	9.400	0.900	9.000	2.800	125	248	—	1.200	—
302	109	2.120	1.780	0	—	0.240	0.120	3.080	0.113	24.000	—	30.000	215	—	—	—
187	49.000	1.360	1.680	0	—	0.020	0.050	1.340	0.046	17.000	—	11.000	146	0.058	2.600	—
171	54.000	1.500	1.160	0	—	0.170	0.120	2.150	—	26.000	—	17.000	167	0.058	2.700	2.570
284	120	3.410	2.480	8.2	—	0.590	0.110	0.630	0.097	26.000	—	42.000	384	—	4.600	0.203

T Mg	MAG Mg	IRON Mg	ZINC Mg	V-A RE	V-C Mg	THIA Mg	RIBO Mg	NIAC Mg	V-B6 Mg	FOL Ug	V-B12 Ug	CALC Mg	PHOS Mg	SEL Mg	FIBD Gm	V-ET mg
5.700	—	0.312	—	50	0.426	0.026	0.023	0.398	—	—	—	4.540	—	—	0.230	0.045
3.300	6.250	0.284	0.093	8	0.852	0.014	0.014	0.085	—	—	—	9.660	16.200	—	—	—
—	—	2.700	—	118	2.000	0.080	0.230	10.300	—	—	—	41.000	291	—	1.030	0.000
334	—	3.800	—	344	6.000	0.300	0.300	5.500	—	—	—	29.000	149	—	—	1.180
594	—	4.300	—	30	—	0.080	0.180	3.300	0.263	—	—	82.000	321	—	5.000	—
139	—	1.000	—	52	0.000	0.120	0.240	1.000	—	—	—	199	182	—	1.440	0.384
240	52.000	1.800	—	172	0.000	0.200	0.400	1.800	—	—	—	362	322	—	1.200	0.320
408	—	2.300	—	216	13.000	0.250	0.180	2.300	—	—	—	80.000	135	—	2.500	—
303	28.000	2.800	—	186	10.000	0.350	0.280	4.500	—	—	—	40.000	88.000	—	2.500	—
665	—	3.700	—	—	22.000	0.025	0.300	4.000	—	—	—	124	236	—	2.730	—
245	28.000	3.300	—	200	5.000	0.150	0.180	2.300	—	—	—	53.000	113	—	2.750	—
635	39.000	1.630	0.780	82.5	24.900	0.193	0.150	2.230	0.353	16.800	0.385	48.000	130	—	5.250	—
288	21.000	0.620	0.360	149	8.300	0.027	0.035	0.886	—	—	0.000	28.000	36.000	0.001	1.640	—
4.000	1.000	0.050	0.020	6.56	2.600	0.005	0.005	0.022	0.010	2.100	0.002	4.000	3.000	—	—	—
263	36.500	1.150	1.560	147	0.810	0.089	0.065	1.410	0.122	11.300	0.405	109	134	—	—	—
216	—	2.520	—	54	2.400	0.324	0.288	5.150	0.096	78.000	0.360	196	—	—	2.160	—
—	—	1.500	—	174	13.000	0.160	0.140	1.600	—	—	—	53.000	89.000	—	—	—
—	—	4.300	—	350	27.000	0.380	0.410	10.200	—	—	—	103	394	—	—	—
4.000	—														0.290	—

Continued.

Nutritive Components for Combination Foods—cont'd.

Food Name	Serving Portion	WT.Gm.	KCAL Kc	PROT Gm	CARB Gm	FAT Gm	CHOL Mg	SAFA Gm	MUFA Gm	PUFA Gm	SOD Mg
SALAD-CARROT-RAISIN-HOME	1.000 CUP	268	306	3.800	55.800	11.600	—	—	—	—	—
SALAD-MANDARIN ORANGE GEL	1.000 SERVING	28.400	22.700	0.400	5.700	0.000	—	0.000	0.000	0.000	14.000
SALAD-CHICKEN	1.000 CUP	205	502	26.000	17.400	36.200	—	—	—	—	1395
CHILI WITH BEANS-CANNED	1.000 CUP	255	286	14.600	30.400	14.000	43.000	6.000	5.950	0.923	1330
SALAD-GREEN SALAD-TOSSED	1.000 SERVING	130	25.000	1.310	5.190	0.291	0.000	0.040	0.027	0.136	12.800
MEAT LOAF-CELERY/ONIONS	1.000 SERVING	87.600	213	15.800	5.230	13.900	107	5.290	5.900	0.613	103
SALAD-CHEF SALAD-HAM/CHEES	1.000 SERVING	200	196	13.400	7.420	12.700	46.000	6.980	4.090	0.739	567
PIZZA-CHEESE-BAKED	1.000 SLICE	120	290	14.600	39.100	8.640	56.400	3.400	2.400	1.000	698
BEEF & VEGETABLE STEW	1.000 CUP	245	220	16.000	15.000	11.000	72.000	4.900	4.500	0.500	1006
RICE-SPANISH-HOME RECIPE	1.000 CUP	245	213	4.400	40.700	4.200	—	—	—	—	774

Nutritive Components for Dairy Products

Food Name	Serving Portion	WT. Gm	KCAL Kc	PROT Gm	CARB Gm	FAT Gm	CHOL Mg	SAFA Gm	MUFA Gm	PUFA Gm	SOD Mg
CHEESE-BLUE	1.000 PIECE	28.000	100	6.070	0.660	8.150	21.000	5.300	2.210	0.230	396
CHEESE-CAMEMBERT-WEDGE	1.000 ITEM	38.000	114	7.520	0.180	9.220	27.000	5.800	2.670	0.280	320
CHEESE-CHEDDAR-SHREDDED	1.000 CUP	113	455	28.100	1.450	37.500	119	23.800	10.600	1.060	701
CHEESE-COTTAGE-4%-LAR CURD	1.000 CUP	225	232	28.100	6.030	10.100	33.800	6.410	2.880	0.315	911
CHEESE-CREAM	1.000 SERVING	28.000	99.000	2.140	0.750	9.890	31.000	6.230	2.790	0.360	84.000
CHEESE-MOZZARELLA-SKIM MILK	1.000 PIECE	28.000	72.000	6.880	0.780	4.510	16.000	2.870	1.280	0.130	132
CHEESE-PARMESAN-GRATED	1.000 CUP	100	456	41.600	3.740	30.000	79.000	19.100	8.730	0.660	1862
CHEESE-PROVOLONE	1.000 PIECE	28.000	100	7.250	0.610	7.550	20.000	4.840	2.100	0.220	248
CHEESE-RICOTTA-SKIM MILK	1.000 CUP	246	340	28.000	12.600	19.500	76.000	12.100	5.690	0.640	307
CHEESE-ROMAN0	1.000 PIECE	28.000	110	9.020	1.030	7.640	29.000	—	—	—	340
CHEESE-SWISS	1.000 PIECE	28.000	107	8.060	0.960	7.780	26.000	5.040	2.060	0.280	74.000
CHEESE-AMERICAN-PROCESSED	1.000 PIECE	28.000	106	6.280	0.450	8.860	27.000	5.580	2.540	0.280	406
CHEESE-SWISS-PROCESSED	1.000 PIECE	28.000	95.000	7.010	0.600	7.090	24.000	4.550	2.000	0.180	388
CHEESE FOOD-AMERICAN-PROC	1.000 SERVING	28.000	93.000	5.560	2.070	6.970	18.000	4.380	2.040	0.200	337
CHEESE SPREAD-PROCESSED	1.000 SERVING	28.000	82.000	4.650	2.480	6.020	16.000	3.780	1.760	0.180	381
CREAM-HALF & HALF-FLUID	1.000 CUP	242	315	7.160	10.400	27.800	89.000	17.300	8.040	1.030	98.000
CREAM-COFFEE-TABLE-LIGHT	1.000 CUP	240	469	6.480	8.780	46.300	159	28.900	13.400	1.720	95.000
CREAM-WHIPPING-HEAVY	1.000 CUP	238	821	4.880	6.640	88.100	326	54.800	25.400	3.270	89.000
CREAM-WHIP-PRESSURIZED	1.000 CUP	60.000	154	1.920	7.490	13.300	46.000	8.300	3.850	0.500	78.000
CREAM-SOUR-CULTURED	1.000 CUP	230	493	7.270	9.820	48.200	102	30.000	13.900	1.790	123
CREAM-WHIP-IMIT-FROZ	1.000 CUP	75.000	239	0.940	17.300	19.000	0.000	16.300	1.210	0.390	19.000
CREAM-WHIP-IMIT-PRESSURIZE	1.000 CUP	70.000	184	0.690	11.300	15.600	0.000	13.200	1.350	0.170	43.000
MILK-WHOLE-3.3% FAT-FLUID	1.000 CUP	244	150	8.030	11.400	8.150	33.000	5.070	2.350	0.300	120
MILK-2% FAT-LOWFAT-FLUID	1.000 CUP	244	121	8.120	11.700	4.680	18.000	2.920	1.350	0.170	122
MILK-2%-MILK SOLIDS ADDED	1.000 CUP	245	125	8.530	12.200	4.700	18.000	2.450	1.360	0.180	128
MILK-1%-FAT-LOWFAT-FLUID	1.000 CUP	244	102	8.030	11.700	2.590	10.000	1.610	0.750	0.100	123
MILK-BUTTERMILK-FLUID	1.000 CUP	245	99.000	8.110	11.700	2.160	9.000	1.340	0.620	0.080	257
MILK-EVAPORATED-WHOLE-CAN	1.000 CUP	252	338	17.200	25.300	19.100	73.100	11.600	5.900	0.605	267
MILK-EVAPORATED-SKIM-CAN	1.000 CUP	255	199	19.300	28.900	0.510	10.200	0.309	0.158	0.016	293
MILK-CONDENSED-SWEET-CAN	1.000 CUP	306	982	24.200	166	26.600	104	16.800	7.430	1.030	389
MILK-CHOCOLATE-WHOLE	1.000 CUP	250	208	7.920	25.900	8.480	30.000	5.260	2.480	0.310	149
MILK-EGGNOG-COMMERCIAL	1.000 CUP	254	342	9.680	34.400	19.000	149	11.300	5.670	0.860	138
MILKSHAKE-CHOCOLATE-THICK	1.000 ITEM	300	356	9.150	63.500	8.100	32.000	5.040	2.340	0.300	333
MILKSHAKE-VANILLA-THICK	1.000 ITEM	313	350	12.100	55.600	9.480	37.000	5.900	2.740	0.350	299
YOGURT-FRUIT FLAVOR-LOWFAT	1.000 CUP	227	231	9.920	43.200	2.450	10.000	1.580	0.670	0.070	133
YOGURT-PLAIN-LOWFAT	1.000 CUP	227	144	11.900	16.000	3.520	14.000	2.270	0.970	0.100	159
YOGURT-PLAIN-NONFAT	1.000 CUP	227	127	13.000	17.400	0.410	4.000	0.264	0.112	0.012	174
YOGURT-PLAIN-WHOLE	1.000 CUP	227	139	7.880	10.600	7.380	29.000	4.760	2.030	0.210	105
CHEESE-FETA	1.000 SERVING	28.000	75.000	4.030	1.160	6.030	25.000	4.240	1.310	0.170	316
CHEESE-GOUDA	1.000 PIECE	28.000	101	7.070	0.630	7.780	32.000	4.990	2.200	0.190	232
CHEESE-LIMBURGER	1.000 PIECE	28.000	93.000	5.680	0.140	7.720	26.000	4.750	2.440	0.140	227
CHEESE-MONTEREY	1.000 PIECE	28.000	106	6.940	0.190	8.580	—	—	—	—	152

T Mg	MAG Mg	IRON Mg	ZINC Mg	V-A RE	V-C Mg	THIA Mg	RIBO Mg	NIAC Mg	V-B6 Mg	FOL Ug	V-B12 Ug	CALC Mg	PHOS Mg	SEL Mg	FIBD Gm	V-ET mg
—	—	3.000	—	1100	12.000	0.160	0.160	1.000	—	—	—	96.000	130	—	—	—
000	—	—	—	—	—	—	—	—	—	—	—	—	—	—	0.000	—
521	—	—	—	—	—	—	—	—	—	—	—	—	—	—	—	—
932	115	8.750	5.100	86.7	4.300	0.122	0.268	0.913	0.337	—	0.030	119	393	—	—	—
279	14.000	0.885	0.211	235	18.600	0.074	0.069	0.632	0.069	61.200	0.000	30.700	31.100	0.001	2.110	0.483
182	13.600	1.910	3.080	12.3	0.725	0.052	0.148	3.160	0.162	10.900	1.520	22.800	112	0.001	0.110	0.068
415	28.400	1.170	1.730	740	24.000	0.337	0.240	2.210	0.206	46.000	0.474	227	251	0.019	2.390	0.719
230	31.200	1.610	1.670	74	2.400	0.336	0.288	4.210	0.120	55.200	0.480	220	216	—	1.900	—
613	—	2.900	—	480	17.000	0.150	0.170	4.700	—	—	0.002	29.000	184	—	3.190	0.515
566	—	1.500	—	162	37.000	0.100	0.070	1.700	—	—	—	34.000	96.000	—	—	—

T Mg	MAG Mg	IRON Mg	ZINC Mg	V-A RE	V-C Mg	THIA Mg	RIBO Mg	NIAC Mg	V-B6 Mg	FOL Ug	V-B12 Ug	CALC Mg	PHOS Mg	SEL Mg	FIBD Gm	V-ET mg
000	7.000	0.090	0.750	61.2	0.000	0.008	0.108	0.288	0.047	10.000	0.345	150	110	0.006	0.000	0.179
000	8.000	0.120	0.900	105	0.000	0.011	0.185	0.239	0.086	24.000	0.492	147	132	0.008	0.000	0.243
111	31.000	0.770	3.510	359	0.000	0.031	0.424	0.090	0.084	21.000	0.935	815	579	0.018	0.000	0.723
189	11.300	0.315	0.833	110	0.000	0.047	0.367	0.284	0.151	27.000	1.400	135	297	0.052	0.000	1.440
000	2.000	0.340	0.150	122	0.000	0.005	0.056	0.029	0.013	4.000	0.120	23.000	30.000	0.001	0.000	0.181
000	7.000	0.060	0.780	49.8	0.000	0.005	0.086	0.030	0.020	2.000	0.232	183	131	0.003	0.000	0.179
107	51.000	0.950	3.190	211	0.000	0.045	0.386	0.315	0.105	8.000	—	1376	807	0.024	0.000	0.640
000	8.000	0.150	0.920	69.4	0.000	0.005	0.091	0.044	0.021	3.000	0.415	214	141	—	0.000	0.179
308	36.000	1.080	3.300	319	0.000	0.052	0.455	0.192	0.049	—	0.716	669	449	—	0.000	1.570
—	—	—	—	48.6	0.000	—	0.105	0.022	—	2.000	—	302	215	—	0.000	0.179
000	10.100	0.050	1.110	72.1	0.000	0.006	0.103	0.026	0.024	2.000	0.475	272	171	0.003	0.000	0.179
000	6.000	0.110	0.850	103	0.000	0.008	0.100	0.020	0.020	2.000	0.197	174	211	0.003	0.000	0.179
000	8.000	0.170	1.020	68.8	0.000	0.004	0.078	0.011	0.010	—	0.348	219	216	0.003	0.000	0.179
000	9.000	0.240	0.850	77.8	0.000	0.008	0.125	0.040	—	—	0.317	163	130	0.006	0.000	0.179
000	8.000	0.090	0.730	67	0.000	0.014	0.122	0.037	0.033	2.000	0.113	159	202	0.006	0.000	0.179
314	25.000	0.170	1.230	315	2.080	0.085	0.361	0.189	0.094	6.000	0.796	254	230	0.001	0.000	—
292	21.000	0.100	0.650	519	1.820	0.077	0.355	0.137	0.077	6.000	0.528	231	192	0.001	0.000	—
179	17.000	0.070	0.550	1051	1.380	0.052	0.262	0.093	0.062	9.000	0.428	154	149	—	0.000	—
000	6.000	0.030	0.220	165	0.000	0.022	0.039	0.042	0.025	—	0.175	61.000	54.000	—	0.000	—
331	26.000	0.140	0.620	546	1.980	0.081	0.343	0.154	0.037	25.000	0.690	268	195	—	0.000	—
000	1.000	0.090	0.020	194	0.000	0.000	0.000	0.000	0.000	0.000	0.000	5.000	6.000	—	0.000	—
000	1.000	0.010	0.010	99.4	0.000	0.000	0.000	0.000	0.000	0.000	0.000	4.000	13.000	—	0.000	—
370	33.000	0.120	0.930	92.2	2.290	0.093	0.395	0.205	0.102	12.000	0.871	291	228	0.003	0.000	0.146
377	33.000	0.120	0.950	150	2.320	0.095	0.403	0.210	0.105	12.000	0.888	297	232	0.003	0.000	0.146
397	35.000	0.120	0.980	150	2.450	0.098	0.424	0.220	0.110	13.000	0.936	313	245	0.003	0.000	0.147
381	34.000	0.120	0.950	150	2.370	0.095	0.407	0.212	0.105	12.000	0.898	300	235	0.003	0.000	0.146
371	27.000	0.120	1.030	24.3	2.400	0.083	0.377	0.142	0.083	—	0.537	285	219	0.003	0.000	—
764	60.500	0.479	1.940	184	4.740	0.118	0.796	0.489	0.126	20.200	0.411	658	509	0.003	0.000	—
847	68.900	0.740	2.300	300	3.160	0.115	0.788	0.444	0.140	23.000	0.609	740	497	0.003	0.000	—
136	78.000	0.580	2.880	302	7.960	0.275	1.270	0.643	0.156	34.000	1.360	868	775	0.003	0.000	—
417	33.000	0.600	1.020	90.7	2.280	0.092	0.405	0.313	0.100	12.000	0.835	280	251	0.003	0.300	0.225
420	47.000	0.510	1.170	268	3.810	0.086	0.483	0.267	0.127	2.000	1.140	330	278	0.003	0.000	—
672	48.000	0.930	1.440	77.5	0.000	0.141	0.666	0.372	0.075	15.000	0.945	396	378	0.005	0.900	—
572	37.000	0.310	1.220	107	0.000	0.094	0.610	0.457	0.131	21.000	1.630	457	361	0.005	0.200	—
442	33.000	0.160	1.680	31.2	1.500	0.084	0.404	0.216	0.091	21.000	1.060	345	271	—	0.800	—
531	40.000	0.180	2.020	45	1.820	0.100	0.486	0.259	0.111	25.000	1.280	415	326	—	0.000	—
579	43.000	0.200	2.200	4.8	1.980	0.109	0.531	0.281	0.120	28.000	1.390	452	355	—	0.000	—
351	26.000	0.110	1.340	83.8	1.200	0.066	0.322	0.170	0.073	17.000	0.844	274	215	—	0.000	—
000	5.000	0.180	0.820	36.3	0.000	—	—	—	—	—	—	140	96.000	—	0.000	0.179
000	8.000	0.070	1.110	55	0.000	0.009	0.095	0.018	0.023	6.000	—	198	155	—	0.000	0.179
000	6.000	0.040	0.600	109	0.000	0.023	0.143	0.045	0.024	16.000	0.295	141	111	—	0.000	0.179
000	8.000	0.200	0.850	80.8	0.000	—	0.111	—	—	—	—	212	126	—	0.000	0.179

Continued.

A

Nutritive Components for Dairy Products—cont'd.

Food Name	Serving Portion	WT. Gm	KCAL Kc	PROT Gm	CARB Gm	FAT Gm	CHOL Mg	SAFA Gm	MUFA Gm	PUFA Gm	SOD Mg
CHEESE-ROQUEFORT	1.000 SERVING	28.000	105	6.110	0.570	8.690	26.000	5.460	2.400	0.370	513
CREAM-SOUR-HALF & HALF	1.000 TBSP	15.000	20.000	0.440	0.640	1.800	6.000	1.120	0.520	0.070	6.000
CREAM-SOUR-IMITATION	1.000 SERVING	28.000	59.000	0.680	1.880	5.530	0.000	5.040	0.170	0.020	29.000
MILK-WHOLE-LOW SODIUM	1.000 CUP	244	149	7.560	10.900	8.440	33.000	5.260	2.440	0.310	6.000
HOT COCOA-PREP/MILK-HOME	1.000 CUP	250	218	9.100	25.800	9.050	33.000	5.610	2.650	0.330	123
MILK-HUMAN-WHOLE-MATURE	1.000 CUP	246	171	2.530	17.000	10.800	34.000	4.940	4.080	1.220	42.000

Nutritive Components for Desserts

Food Name	Serving Portion	WT. Gm	KCAL Kc	PROT Gm	CARB Gm	FAT Gm	CHOL Mg	SAFA Gm	MUFA Gm	PUFA Gm	SOD Mg
ICE CREAM-VAN-HARD-10% FAT	1.000 CUP	133	269	4.800	31.700	14.300	59.000	8.920	—	—	116
ICE CREAM-VAN-SOFT SERVE	1.000 CUP	173	377	7.040	38.300	22.500	153	13.500	—	—	153
ICE MILK-VAN-SOFT-2.6% FAT	1.000 CUP	175	223	8.030	38.400	4.620	13.000	2.880	—	—	163
SHERBET-ORANGE-2% FAT	1.000 CUP	193	270	2.160	58.700	3.820	14.000	2.380	—	—	88.000
CUSTARD-BAKED	1.000 CUP	265	305	14.000	29.000	15.000	278	6.800	—	—	209
PUDD-TAPIOCA CREAM-HOME	1.000 CUP	165	220	8.000	28.000	8.000	80.000	4.100	—	—	257
PUDD-CHOC-COOKED-MIX/MILK	1.000 CUP	260	320	9.000	59.000	8.000	32.000	4.300	—	—	335
PUDD-CHOC-INST-MIX/MILK	1.000 CUP	260	325	8.000	63.000	7.000	28.000	3.600	—	—	322
CAKE-ANGELFOOD-MIX/PREP	1.000 SLICE	53.000	142	4.200	31.500	0.122	0.000	—	—	—	142
CUPCAKE/CHOCOLATE ICING	1.000 ITEM	36.000	130	2.000	21.000	5.000	15.000	2.000	1.700	0.700	120
CAKE-GINGERBREAD-MIX/PREP	1.000 SLICE	63.000	175	2.000	32.000	4.000	1.000	1.100	—	—	90.000
CAKE-YELLOW/ICING-HOME REC	1.000 SLICE	69.000	268	2.900	40.300	11.400	36.000	3.000	3.000	1.400	191
CAKE-FRUIT-DARK-HOME REC	1.000 SLICE	15.000	55.000	1.000	9.000	2.000	73.000	0.500	—	—	23.000
CAKE-SHEET-NO ICING-HOME	1.000 SLICE	86.000	315	4.000	48.000	12.000	1.000	3.300	—	—	382
CAKE-POUND-HOME RECIPE	1.000 SLICE	33.000	160	2.000	16.000	10.000	68.000	5.900	3.000	0.600	58.000
CAKE-SPONGE-HOME RECIPE	1.000 SLICE	66.000	188	4.820	35.700	3.140	162	1.100	—	—	164
COOKIE-CHOCOLATE CHIP-MIX	1.000 ITEM	10.500	50.000	0.500	6.960	2.420	5.520	0.700	0.900	0.600	37.800
COOKIE-CHOC CHIP-HOME REC	1.000 ITEM	10.000	46.300	0.500	6.410	2.680	5.250	0.600	1.150	0.800	20.600
COOKIE-MACAROON	1.000 ITEM	19.000	90.000	1.000	12.500	4.500	0.000	—	—	—	6.000
COOKIE-OATMEAL/RAISIN-MIX	1.000 ITEM	13.000	61.500	0.732	8.930	2.600	0.000	0.500	—	—	37.100
COOKIE-SANDWICH-CHOC/VAN	1.000 ITEM	10.000	50.000	0.500	7.000	2.250	0.000	0.550	—	—	63.000
COOKIE-VANILLA WAFER	1.000 ITEM	4.000	18.500	0.200	3.000	0.600	2.500	0.100	0.200	0.100	10.000
DANISH PASTRY-PLAIN	1.000 ITEM	65.000	250	4.060	29.100	13.600	0.000	4.700	—	—	249
DOUGHNUTS-CAKE-PLAIN	1.000 ITEM	25.000	104	1.280	12.200	5.770	10.000	1.200	1.200	2.000	139
DOUGHNUTS-YEAST-GLAZED	1.000 ITEM	50.000	205	3.000	22.000	11.200	13.000	3.000	5.800	3.300	117
PIE-APPLE-HOME REC	1.000 SLICE	135	323	2.750	49.100	13.600	0.000	3.900	—	—	207
PIE-BANANA CREAM-HOME REC	1.000 SLICE	130	285	6.000	40.000	12.000	40.000	3.800	—	—	252
PIE-CHERRY-HOME REC	1.000 SLICE	135	350	4.000	52.000	15.000	0.000	4.000	—	—	410
PIE-CUSTARD-HOME REC	1.000 SLICE	130	285	8.000	30.000	14.000	—	4.800	—	—	373
PIE-LEMON MERINGUE-HOME	1.000 SLICE	120	300	3.860	47.300	11.200	0.000	3.700	—	—	223
PIE-MINCE-HOME REC	1.000 SLICE	135	365	3.000	56.000	16.000	0.000	4.000	—	—	604
PIE-PEACH-HOME REC	1.000 SLICE	135	345	3.000	52.000	14.000	0.000	3.500	—	—	361
PIE-PECAN-HOME REC	1.000 SLICE	118	495	6.000	61.000	27.000	0.000	4.000	—	—	260
PIE-PUMPKIN-HOME REC	1.000 SLICE	130	275	5.000	32.000	15.000	0.000	5.400	—	—	278
PIECRUST-MIX/PREP-BAKED	1.000 ITEM	160	743	10.000	70.500	40.500	0.000	11.400	—	—	1300
GRANOLA BAR	1.000 ITEM	24.000	109	2.350	16.000	4.230	—	—	—	—	66.700
COOKIE-SUGAR-MIX	1.000 ITEM	20.000	98.800	0.908	13.100	4.790	—	—	—	—	109
CAKE-CHEESECAKE-COMMERCIAL	1.000 SLICE	85.000	257	4.610	24.300	16.300	—	—	—	—	189
ICE CREAM SUNDAE-HOT FUDGE	1.000 ITEM	165	312	7.260	46.500	10.900	18.200	—	—	—	177
TURNOVER-APPLE	1.000 SERVING	28.400	85.200	0.738	10.500	4.710	1.420	—	—	—	109
COOKIE-PEANUT BUTTER-MIX	1.000 ITEM	10.000	50.000	0.800	5.870	2.640	—	—	—	—	56.600
PUDD-RICE/RAISINS	1.000 CUP	265	387	9.500	70.800	8.200	—	—	—	—	188
TWINKIE-HOSTESS	1.000 ITEM	42.000	143	1.250	25.600	4.200	21.000	—	—	—	189

T Mg	MAG Mg	IRON Mg	ZINC Mg	V-A RE	V-C Mg	THIA Mg	RIBO Mg	NIAC Mg	V-B6 Mg	FOL Ug	V-B12 Ug	CALC Mg	PHOS Mg	SEL Mg	FIBD Gm	V-ET mg
.000	8.000	0.160	0.590	89.2	0.000	0.011	0.166	0.208	0.035	14.000	0.182	188	111	—	0.000	0.179
.000	2.000	0.010	0.080	20.4	0.130	0.005	0.022	0.010	0.002	2.000	0.045	16.000	14.000	—	0.000	—
.000	—	—	—	0	0.000	0.000	0.000	0.000	0.000	0.000	0.000	1.000	13.000	—	0.000	—
617	12.000	—	—	95.2	—	0.049	0.256	0.105	0.083	—	0.876	246	209	0.003	0.000	0.146
480	56.000	0.780	1.220	95.5	2.400	0.102	0.435	0.365	0.107	12.000	0.870	298	270	—	0.300	—
126	8.000	0.070	0.420	178	12.300	0.034	0.089	0.435	0.027	13.000	0.111	79.000	34.000	0.004	0.000	2.160

T Mg	MAG Mg	IRON Mg	ZINC Mg	V-A RE	V-C Mg	THIA Mg	RIBO Mg	NIAC Mg	V-B6 Mg	FOL Ug	V-B12 Ug	CALC Mg	PHOS Mg	SEL Mg	FIBD Gm	V-ET mg
257	18.000	0.120	1.410	133	0.700	0.052	0.329	0.134	0.061	3.000	0.625	176	134	0.002	0.000	0.180
338	25.000	0.430	1.990	199	0.920	0.080	0.448	0.178	0.095	9.000	0.996	236	199	0.003	0.000	0.104
412	29.000	0.280	0.860	44	1.170	0.117	0.541	0.184	0.133	5.000	1.370	274	202	0.003	0.000	—
198	15.000	0.310	1.330	39	3.860	0.033	0.089	0.131	0.025	14.000	0.158	103	74.000	—	0.000	—
387	—	1.100	—	87	1.000	0.110	0.500	0.300	—	—	—	297	310	0.003	—	—
223	—	0.700	—	60	2.000	0.070	0.300	0.200	—	—	—	173	180	—	0.000	—
354	—	0.800	—	68	2.000	0.050	0.390	0.300	—	—	—	265	247	—	0.000	—
335	—	1.300	—	68	2.000	0.080	0.390	0.300	—	—	—	374	237	—	0.000	—
.900	5.830	0.451	0.106	0	0.000	0.064	0.122	0.594	0.007	4.770	0.015	50.000	63.000	0.003	0.000	1.430
.000	—	0.400	—	12	0.000	0.050	0.060	0.400	—	—	—	47.000	71.000	0.003	—	0.050
173	14.000	0.900	0.284	0	0.000	0.090	0.110	0.800	0.048	5.000	0.066	57.000	63.000	0.004	0.000	—
.500	13.100	0.787	0.338	9.5	0.000	0.076	0.097	0.656	0.023	5.520	0.123	57.300	60.700	0.004	—	1.860
.000	—	0.400	—	3.6	0.000	0.020	0.020	0.200	—	—	—	11.000	17.000	0.001	—	—
.000	12.000	0.900	0.301	30	0.000	0.130	0.150	1.100	0.024	6.020	0.087	55.000	88.000	0.006	—	2.310
.000	—	0.500	—	16	0.000	0.050	0.060	0.400	—	1.980	—	6.000	24.000	0.002	0.080	0.888
.400	7.260	1.110	0.799	25	0.000	0.092	0.132	0.726	0.037	14.500	0.332	25.100	65.300	0.004	0.000	1.780
.500	2.520	0.228	0.053	6.09	0.000	0.014	0.022	0.195	0.002	0.945	—	2.940	7.460	0.001	0.040	0.280
.500	3.500	0.249	0.044	1	0.000	0.015	0.015	0.146	0.002	0.900	0.010	3.300	8.400	0.001	0.080	0.267
.000	—	0.150	—	0	0.000	0.010	0.030	0.100	—	—	—	5.000	16.000	0.001	—	0.507
.600	3.640	0.285	0.085	2.08	0.000	0.022	0.021	0.241	0.006	1.560	—	4.420	14.400	0.001	—	0.347
.750	5.100	0.175	0.086	0	0.000	0.015	0.025	0.175	0.004	0.300	0.000	2.500	24.000	0.001	—	0.257
.900	0.680	0.060	—	1	0.000	0.010	0.009	0.080	—	—	—	1.600	2.500	0.000	0.010	0.103
.500	9.750	1.200	0.546	11	0.000	0.156	0.150	1.470	—	—	—	68.900	66.300	—	—	—
.300	5.750	0.365	0.128	2.2	0.000	0.060	0.050	0.428	0.009	2.000	—	11.000	55.000	—	0.090	0.180
.000	9.500	0.600	—	5	0.000	0.100	0.100	0.800	—	11.000	—	16.000	33.000	—	0.300	0.360
115	10.800	1.220	0.230	5.1	2.000	0.149	0.108	1.240	0.035	6.750	0.000	12.200	31.100	0.015	—	2.150
264	—	1.000	—	66	1.000	0.110	0.220	1.000	—	—	—	86.000	107	0.015	—	—
142	9.450	0.900	—	118	0.000	0.160	0.120	1.400	—	—	0.000	19.000	34.000	0.015	—	2.150
178	—	1.200	—	60	0.000	0.110	0.270	0.800	—	—	—	125	147	0.015	0.000	2.070
.800	7.200	0.900	0.336	33.4	3.660	0.096	0.120	0.720	0.029	10.800	0.191	15.600	48.000	0.013	0.000	1.910
240	24.300	1.900	—	0	1.000	0.140	0.120	1.400	—	—	—	38.000	51.000	0.015	—	2.150
.000	9.450	1.200	—	198	4.000	0.150	0.140	2.000	—	—	0.000	14.000	39.000	0.015	—	2.150
145	—	3.700	—	40	0.000	0.260	0.140	1.000	—	—	—	55.000	122	0.012	—	—
208	16.900	1.000	—	320	0.000	0.110	0.180	1.000	—	—	—	66.000	90.000	0.015	—	2.070
500	—	3.050	—	0	0.000	0.535	0.395	4.950	—	—	—	65.500	136	—	—	0.784
200	—	0.763	—	—	—	0.067	0.026	—	—	—	0.000	14.400	66.500	—	—	—
600	1.600	0.386	0.054	2.96	0.000	0.036	0.024	0.466	0.011	1.800	—	20.800	37.800	0.001	—	0.514
300	8.500	0.408	0.357	43	4.250	0.026	0.111	0.391	0.054	15.300	0.421	47.600	74.800	—	—	—
413	34.700	0.611	0.990	46.2	3.300	0.066	0.314	1.120	0.132	9.900	0.660	216	238	—	—	0.693
900	2.560	0.312	0.054	2.28	0.284	0.028	0.020	0.332	0.011	1.140	0.028	3.980	11.400	—	—	0.452
400	3.900	0.190	0.750	3.04	0.000	0.019	0.016	0.381	0.008	2.400	—	11.500	23.500	—	—	0.257
469	—	1.100	—	35	0.000	0.080	0.370	0.500	—	—	—	260	249	—	—	—
	—	0.545	—	8.1	0.000	0.055	0.060	0.500	—	—	—	19.000	—	—	—	—

A

Nutritive Components for Eggs

Food Name	Serving Portion	WT. Gm	KCAL Kc	PROT Gm	CARB Gm	FAT Gm	CHOL Mg	SAFA Gm	MUFA Gm	PUFA Gm	SOD Mg
EGG-WHOLE-RAW-LARGE	1.000 ITEM	50.000	79.000	6.070	0.600	5.580	274	1.670	2.230	0.720	69.000
EGG-WHITE-RAW-LARGE	1.000 ITEM	33.000	16.000	3.350	0.410	0.000	0.000	0.000	0.000	0.000	50.000
EGG-YOLK-RAW-LARGE	1.000 ITEM	17.000	63.000	2.790	0.040	5.600	272	1.680	2.240	0.730	8.000
EGG-HARD-LARGE-NO SHELL	1.000 ITEM	50.000	79.000	6.070	0.600	5.580	274	1.670	2.230	0.720	69.000
EGG-POACHED-WHOLE-LARGE	1.000 ITEM	50.000	79.000	6.040	0.600	5.550	273	1.670	2.220	0.720	146
EGG-SUBSTITUTE-LIQUID	1.000 CUP	251	211	30.100	1.610	8.310	3.000	1.660	2.250	4.020	444

Nutritive Components for Fast Foods

Food Name	Serving Portion	WT. Gm	KCAL Kc	PROT Gm	CARB Gm	FAT Gm	CHOL Mg	SAFA Gm	MUFA Gm	PUFA Gm	SOD Mg
MCDONALDS-BIG MAC HAMBURGER	1.000 ITEM	204	563	26.000	41.000	33.000	86.000	—	—	—	1010
MCDONALDS-CHEESEBURGER	1.000 ITEM	115	307	15.000	30.000	14.000	37.000	—	—	—	767
MCDONALDS-HAMBURGER	1.000 ITEM	102	255	12.000	30.000	10.000	25.000	—	—	—	520
MCDONALDS-QP HAMBURGER	1.000 ITEM	166	424	24.000	33.000	22.000	67.000	—	—	—	735
MCDONALDS-QP HAMBURGER W/CH	1.000 ITEM	194	524	30.000	32.000	31.000	96.000	—	—	—	1236
MCDONALDS-FILET O FISH	1.000 ITEM	139	432	14.000	37.000	25.000	47.000	—	—	—	781
MCDONALDS-EGG MCMUFFIN	1.000 ITEM	138	327	19.000	31.000	15.000	229	—	—	—	885
TACO BELL-BEAN BURRITO	1.000 ITEM	166	343	11.000	48.000	12.000	—	—	—	—	272
TACO BELL-BEEF BURRITO	1.000 ITEM	184	466	30.000	37.000	21.000	—	—	—	—	327
TACO BELL-BEEFY TOSTADA	1.000 ITEM	184	291	19.000	21.000	15.000	—	—	—	—	138
TACO BELL-TACO-REGULAR	1.000 ITEM	83.000	186	15.000	14.000	8.000	—	—	—	—	79.000
TACO BELL-TOSTADA-REGULAR	1.000 ITEM	138	179	9.000	25.000	6.000	—	—	—	—	101
TACO BELL-BURRITO SUPREME	1.000 ITEM	225	457	21.000	43.000	22.000	—	—	—	—	367
WENDYS-SINGLE HAMBURGER	1.000 ITEM	200	470	26.000	34.000	26.000	70.000	—	—	—	774
WENDYS-DOUBLE HAMBURGER	1.000 ITEM	285	670	44.000	34.000	40.000	125	—	—	—	980
WENDYS-TRIPLE HAMBURGER	1.000 ITEM	360	850	65.000	33.000	51.000	205	—	—	—	1217
DAIRY QUEEN-CONE-REGULAR	1.000 ITEM	142	230	6.000	35.000	7.000	20.000	—	—	—	—
DAIRY QUEEN-DIP CONE-REG	1.000 ITEM	156	300	7.000	40.000	13.000	20.000	—	—	—	20.000
DAIRY QUEEN-SUNDAE-REGULAR	1.000 ITEM	177	290	6.000	51.000	7.000	20.000	—	—	—	20.000
DAIRY QUEEN-MALT-REGULAR	1.000 ITEM	418	600	15.000	89.000	20.000	50.000	—	—	—	—
DAIRY QUEEN-FLOAT	1.000 ITEM	397	330	6.000	59.000	8.000	20.000	—	—	—	—
DAIRY QUEEN-BANANA SPLIT	1.000 ITEM	383	540	10.000	91.000	15.000	30.000	—	—	—	—
JACK/BOX-JUMBO JACK HAMBUR	1.000 ITEM	246	551	28.000	45.000	29.000	80.000	—	—	—	1134
JACK/BOX-JUMBO JACK/CHEESE	1.000 ITEM	272	628	32.000	45.000	35.000	110	—	—	—	1666
JACK/BOX-ONION RINGS-BAG	1.000 ITEM	85.000	351	5.000	32.000	23.000	24.000	—	—	—	318
BURGER KING-WHOP HAMBURGER	1.000 ITEM	261	630	26.000	50.000	36.000	—	—	—	—	990
ARTHUR TREACHER-CHICK SAND	1.000 ITEM	156	413	16.200	44.000	19.200	—	—	—	6.700	708
CHURCHS CHICK-WHITE MEAT	1.000 ITEM	100	327	21.000	10.000	23.000	—	—	—	—	498
JACK/BOX-BREAK JACK SAND	1.000 ITEM	121	301	18.000	28.000	13.000	182	—	—	—	1037
JACK/BOX-MOBY JACK	1.000 ITEM	141	455	17.000	38.000	26.000	56.000	—	—	—	837

Nutritive Components for Fats and Oils

Food Name	Serving Portion	WT. Gm	KCAL Kc	PROT Gm	CARB Gm	FAT Gm	CHOL Mg	SAFA Gm	MUFA Gm	PUFA Gm	SOD Mg
BUTTER-REGULAR-TABLESPOON	1.000 TBSP	14.000	100	0.119	0.008	11.400	30.700	7.070	3.280	0.421	116
BUTTER-WHIPPED-TABLESPOON	1.000 TBSP	9.000	64.500	0.077	0.005	7.300	19.700	4.540	2.110	0.271	74.300
SHORTENING-VEGETABLE-SOY	1.000 CUP	205	1812	0.000	0.000	205	0.000	51.200	89.000	52.200	—
MARGARINE-DIET-MAZOLA	1.000 TBSP	14.000	50.000	0.000	0.000	5.700	0.000	1.000	2.100	2.600	130
MARGARINE-VEG SPRAY-MAZOLA	1.000 SERVING	0.720	6.000	0.000	0.000	0.720	0.000	0.080	0.170	0.400	0.000
MARGARINE-REG-HARD-STICK	1.000 ITEM	113	815	1.000	1.000	91.300	0.000	17.900	40.600	28.800	1.070
VEGETABLE OIL-CORN	1.000 CUP	218	1927	0.000	0.000	218	0.000	27.700	52.700	128	0.000
VEGETABLE OIL-OLIVE	1.000 CUP	216	1909	0.000	0.000	216	0.000	30.700	159	18.200	0.080

OT Mg	MAG Mg	IRON Mg	ZINC Mg	V-A RE	V-C Mg	THIA Mg	RIBO Mg	NIAC Mg	V-B6 Mg	FOL Ug	V-B12 Ug	CALC Mg	PHOS Mg	SEL Mg	FIBD Gm	V-ET mg
65.000	6.000	1.040	0.720	95.2	0.000	0.044	0.150	0.031	0.060	32.000	0.773	28.000	90.000	0.012	0.000	0.350
45.000	3.000	0.010	0.010	0	0.000	0.002	0.094	0.029	0.001	5.000	0.021	4.000	4.000	0.002	0.000	—
45.000	3.000	0.950	0.580	97	0.000	0.043	0.074	0.012	0.053	26.000	0.647	26.000	86.000	0.003	0.000	0.349
65.000	6.000	1.040	0.720	84	0.000	0.037	0.143	0.030	0.057	24.000	0.657	28.000	90.000	—	0.000	0.350
65.000	6.000	1.040	0.720	95.2	0.000	0.035	0.127	0.026	0.051	24.000	0.616	28.000	90.000	—	0.000	0.350
828	—	5.270	3.260	542	0.000	0.276	0.753	0.276	—	—	0.748	133	304	—	0.000	—

OT Mg	MAG Mg	IRON Mg	ZINC Mg	V-A RE	V-C Mg	THIA Mg	RIBO Mg	NIAC Mg	V-B6 Mg	FOL Ug	V-B12 Ug	CALC Mg	PHOS Mg	SEL Mg	FIBD Gm	V-ET mg
237	38.000	4.000	4.700	106	2.200	0.390	0.370	6.500	0.270	21.000	1.800	157	314	—	—	—
156	23.000	2.400	2.600	118	2.000	0.250	0.230	3.800	0.120	21.000	0.910	132	205	—	—	0.530
142	19.000	2.300	2.100	45.6	1.700	0.250	0.180	4.000	0.120	17.000	0.810	51.000	126	—	—	0.428
322	37.000	4.100	5.100	67	1.700	0.320	0.280	6.500	0.270	23.000	1.880	63.000	249	—	—	—
341	41.000	4.300	5.700	211	2.700	0.310	0.370	7.400	0.230	23.000	2.150	219	382	—	—	—
150	27.000	1.700	0.900	43.8	1.400	0.260	0.200	2.600	0.100	20.000	0.820	93.000	229	—	1.110	—
168	26.000	2.900	1.900	150	1.400	0.470	0.440	3.800	0.210	29.000	0.750	226	322	—	—	—
235	78.000	2.800	1.400	240	15.200	0.370	0.220	2.200	—	—	—	98.000	173	—	—	—
320	—	4.600	—	41.7	15.200	0.300	0.390	7.000	—	—	—	83.000	288	—	—	—
277	—	3.400	—	383	12.700	0.160	0.270	3.300	—	—	—	208	265	—	—	—
143	40.700	2.500	2.200	257	0.200	0.090	0.160	2.900	—	—	—	120	175	—	—	—
172	—	2.300	—	187	9.700	0.180	0.150	0.800	—	—	—	191	186	—	—	—
350	—	3.800	—	216	16.000	0.330	0.350	4.700	—	—	—	121	245	—	—	—
—	—	5.300	4.800	93.4	0.600	0.240	0.360	5.800	—	—	—	84.000	239	—	—	—
—	—	8.200	8.400	30.6	1.500	0.430	0.540	10.600	—	—	—	138	364	—	—	—
—	—	10.700	13.500	47.4	2.000	0.470	0.680	14.700	—	—	—	104	525	—	—	—
—	—	0.000	—	87.4	0.000	0.090	0.260	0.000	—	—	0.600	200	150	—	—	—
—	—	0.400	—	90.1	0.000	0.090	0.340	0.000	—	—	0.600	200	150	—	—	—
—	—	1.100	—	74.5	0.000	0.060	0.260	0.000	—	—	0.600	200	150	—	—	—
—	—	3.600	—	225	3.600	0.120	0.600	0.800	—	—	1.800	500	400	—	—	—
—	—	0.000	—	30	0.000	0.120	0.170	0.000	—	—	0.600	200	200	—	—	—
—	—	1.800	—	225	18.000	0.600	0.600	0.800	—	—	0.900	350	250	—	—	—
492	44.000	4.500	4.200	73.9	3.700	0.470	0.340	11.600	0.300	—	2.680	134	261	—	—	—
499	49.000	4.600	4.800	220	4.900	0.520	0.380	11.300	0.310	—	3.050	273	411	—	—	—
109	16.000	1.400	0.400	2.4	1.200	0.240	0.120	3.100	0.070	—	0.260	26.000	69.000	—	—	0.587
520	—	6.000	—	192	13.000	0.020	0.030	5.200	—	—	—	37.000	—	—	—	—
279	27.000	1.700	—	36.9	19.000	0.170	0.240	8.100	—	—	—	59.000	147	—	—	—
186	—	1.000	—	48	1.000	0.100	0.180	7.200	—	—	—	94.000	—	—	—	—
190	24.000	2.500	1.800	133	3.000	0.410	0.470	5.100	0.140	—	1.100	177	310	—	—	—
246	30.000	1.700	1.100	72.1	1.000	0.300	0.210	4.500	0.120	—	1.100	167	263	—	—	—

OT Mg	MAG Mg	IRON Mg	ZINC Mg	V-A RE	V-C Mg	THIA Mg	RIBO Mg	NIAC Mg	V-B6 Mg	FOL Ug	V-B12 Ug	CALC Mg	PHOS Mg	SEL Mg	FIBD Gm	V-ET mg
3.640	0.280	0.022	0.007	105	0.000	0.001	0.005	0.006	0.000	0.420	—	3.360	3.220	—	0.000	0.221
2.340	0.180	0.014	0.005	67.9	0.000	0.000	0.003	0.004	0.000	0.270	—	2.160	2.070	—	0.000	0.142
—	—	—	—	—	—	—	—	—	—	—	—	—	—	—	0.000	27.900
—	—	0.000	—	130	0.000	0.000	0.000	0.000	—	—	—	0.000	—	—	0.000	0.112
—	—	0.000	—	0	0.000	0.000	0.000	0.000	—	—	—	0.000	0.000	—	0.000	—
48.100	2.950	0.070	—	338	0.181	0.011	0.042	0.026	0.010	1.340	0.108	33.900	26.000	—	0.000	13.200
0.000	0.000	0.000	0.000	0	0.000	0.000	0.000	0.000	0.000	0.000	0.000	0.000	0.000	—	0.000	31.100
0.000	0.020	0.830	0.130	0	0.000	0.000	0.000	0.000	0.000	0.000	0.000	0.380	2.630	—	0.000	25.700

Continued.

A

Nutritive Components for Fats and Oils—cont'd.

Food Name	Serving Portion	WT. Gm	KCAL Kc	PROT Gm	CARB Gm	FAT Gm	CHOL Mg	SAFA Gm	MUFA Gm	PUFA Gm	SOD Mg
SAL DRESS-BLUE CHEESE	1.000 TBSP	15.300	77.100	0.700	1.100	8.000	9.000	1.500	1.900	4.300	167
SAL DRESS-BLUE CHE-LOW CAL	1.000 TBSP	16.000	10.000	0.000	1.000	1.000	4.000	0.500	—	—	177
SAL DRESS-FRENCH	1.000 TBSP	15.600	67.000	0.100	2.700	6.400	1.950	1.500	1.200	3.400	214
SAL DRESS-FRENCH-LOW CAL	1.000 TBSP	16.300	21.900	0.000	3.500	0.900	1.000	0.100	0.200	0.500	128
SAL DRESS-ITALIAN	1.000 TBSP	14.700	68.700	0.000	1.500	7.100	0.000	1.000	1.700	4.100	116
SAL DRESS-ITALIAN-LOW CAL	1.000 TBSP	15.000	15.800	0.000	0.700	1.500	1.000	0.200	0.300	0.900	118
SAL DRESS-MAYONNAISE TYPE	1.000 TBSP	14.700	57.300	0.000	3.500	4.900	4.000	0.700	1.300	2.600	104
SAL DRESS-MAYO-LOW CAL	1.000 TBSP	16.000	20.000	0.000	2.000	2.000	2.000	0.400	—	—	44.000
SAUCE-TARTAR-REGULAR	1.000 TBSP	14.000	75.000	0.000	1.000	8.000	9.000	1.500	—	—	98.000
SAL DRESS-THOUSAND ISLAND	1.000 TBSP	15.600	58.900	0.000	2.400	5.600	4.900	0.900	1.300	3.100	109
SAL DRESS-THOU ISL-LOW CAL	1.000 TBSP	15.300	24.300	0.100	2.500	1.600	2.000	0.200	0.400	1.000	153
ANIMAL FAT-COOKING-CHICKEN	1.000 TBSP	12.800	115	0.000	0.000	12.800	11.000	3.800	5.700	2.700	—
MARGARINE-CORN-REG-HARD	1.000 TSP	4.700	33.800	0.000	0.000	3.800	0.000	0.600	2.200	0.800	44.300
MARGARINE-CORN-REG-SOFT	1.000 TSP	4.700	33.700	0.000	0.000	3.800	0.000	0.700	1.500	1.500	50.700
MAYONNAISE-IMITATION-SOY	1.000 TBSP	15.000	34.700	0.000	2.400	2.900	4.000	0.500	0.700	1.600	74.600
SAL DRESS-RUSSIAN-LOW CAL	1.000 TBSP	16.300	23.100	0.100	4.500	0.700	1.000	0.100	0.200	0.400	141
SAL DRESS-RUSSIAN	1.000 TBSP	15.300	76.000	0.200	1.600	7.800	0.000	1.100	1.800	4.500	133
SAL DRESS-VINEGAR/OIL-HOME	1.000 TBSP	15.600	71.800	0.000	0.400	8.000	0.000	1.500	2.400	3.900	0.100
SANDWICH SPREAD-COMMERCIAL	1.000 TBSP	15.300	59.500	0.100	3.400	5.200	12.000	0.800	1.100	3.100	—
MAYONNAISE-LIGHT-LOW CAL	1.000 TBSP	14.000	40.000	0.000	1.000	4.000	5.000	—	—	—	—
MIRACLE WHIP-LIGHT-LOW CAL	1.000 TBSP	14.000	45.000	0.000	2.000	4.000	5.000	—	—	—	95.000
SAL DRESS-CAESAR	1.000 TBSP	15.000	70.000	0.000	1.000	7.000	—	—	—	—	—
SAL DRESS-RANCH STYLE	1.000 TBSP	15.000	54.000	0.400	0.600	5.700	—	—	—	—	97.000

Nutritive Components for Fish

Food Name	Serving Portion	WT. Gm	KCAL Kc	PROT Gm	CARB Gm	FAT Gm	CHOL Mg	SAFA Gm	MUFA Gm	PUFA Gm	SOD Mg
FISH-BLUEFISH-BAKED/BUTTER	1.000 ITEM	155	246	40.600	0.000	8.100	108	—	—	—	161
FISH-CLAMS-RAW-MEAT ONLY	1.000 SERVING	85.000	63.000	10.900	2.180	0.830	29.000	0.080	0.068	0.240	47.000
FISH-CLAM-CAN-SOLID/LIQUID	1.000 SERVING	28.400	15.000	2.330	0.667	0.333	17.700	0.067	—	—	14.700
FISH-CRAB MEAT-KING-CAN	1.000 CUP	135	135	24.000	1.000	3.200	135	0.600	0.600	2.000	675
FISH-STICK-BREAD-FROZ-COOK	1.000 ITEM	28.000	76.000	4.380	6.650	3.420	31.000	0.882	1.420	0.886	163
FISH-PERCH-BREADED-FRIED	1.000 PIECE	85.000	195	16.000	6.000	11.000	32.000	2.700	—	—	128
FISH-OYSTERS-RAW-MEAT ONLY	1.000 CUP	248	170	17.500	9.700	6.140	136	1.570	0.620	1.830	277
FISH-SALMON-PINK-CAN	1.000 SERVING	85.000	118	16.800	0.000	5.140	—	1.310	1.540	1.740	471
FISH-SARDINES-CAN/OIL	1.000 ITEM	12.000	25.000	2.960	0.000	1.380	17.000	0.184	0.465	0.618	60.500
FISH-SHAD-BAKE/MARG/BACON	1.000 SERVING	100	201	23.200	0.000	11.300	69.400	—	—	—	79.000
FISH-SHRIMP-MEAT-CAN	1.000 CUP	128	154	29.600	1.320	2.510	222	0.477	0.375	0.966	216
FISH-SHRIMP-FRENCH FRIED	1.000 SERVING	85.000	206	18.200	9.750	10.400	150	1.770	—	—	292
FISH-TUNA-CAN/OIL-DRAINED	1.000 SERVING	85.000	169	24.800	0.000	6.980	15.000	1.300	2.510	2.450	301
FISH-TUNA-WHITE-CAN/WATER	1.000 SERVING	85.000	116	22.700	0.000	2.090	35.000	0.556	0.551	0.780	333
FISH-TUNA-DIET-LOW SODIUM	1.000 SERVING	28.400	35.500	7.670	0.011	0.540	9.940	—	—	0.199	11.400
FISH-TUNA-LIGHT-CAN/WATER	1.000 SERVING	85.000	111	25.100	0.000	0.430	—	0.136	0.122	0.111	303
FISH-ANCHOVY-FILLET-CAN	1.000 ITEM	4.000	8.400	1.160	0.000	0.388	—	0.088	0.151	0.102	147
FISH-COD-COOKED-DRY HEAT	1.000 PIECE	180	189	41.100	0.000	1.550	99.000	0.302	0.223	0.526	141
FISH-CRAB CAKE	1.000 ITEM	60.000	93.000	12.100	0.290	4.510	90.000	0.890	1.690	1.360	198
FISH-CRAB-STEAMED-PIECES	1.000 CUP	155	150	30.000	0.000	2.390	82.200	0.206	0.287	0.831	1662
FISH-SOLE/FLOUNDER-BAKED	1.000 SERVING	127	148	30.700	0.000	1.940	86.000	0.461	0.392	0.523	133
FISH-HADDOCK-COOK-DRY HEAT	1.000 SERVING	85.000	95.000	20.600	0.000	0.790	63.000	0.142	0.128	0.263	74.000
FISH-MACKEREL-ATLANTIC-CAN	1.000 CUP	190	296	44.000	0.000	12.000	150	3.390	5.160	0.165	720
FISH-ROCKFISH-CKD-DRY HEAT	1.000 SERVING	100	121	24.000	0.000	2.010	44.000	0.474	0.447	0.594	77.000
FISH-ROE-RAW-EGGS	1.000 SERVING	28.400	39.000	6.250	0.420	1.800	105	0.408	0.465	0.744	—
FISH-SALMON-SMOKED	1.000 SERVING	100	117	18.300	0.000	4.320	23.000	0.929	2.020	0.995	784
FISH-SCALLOPS-STEAMED	1.000 SERVING	28.400	31.800	6.590	0.511	0.398	15.100	—	—	—	75.200
FISH-SWORDFISH-BROIL/MARG	1.000 SERVING	100	174	28.000	0.000	6.000	4.000	—	—	—	25.000
FISH-TROUT-BROOK-COOKED	1.000 SERVING	100	196	23.500	0.400	11.200	—	—	—	—	78.800

OT Mg	MAG Mg	IRON Mg	ZINC Mg	V-A RE	V-C Mg	THIA Mg	RIBO Mg	NIAC Mg	V-B6 Mg	FOL Ug	V-B12 Ug	CALC Mg	PHOS Mg	SEL Mg	FIBD Gm	V-ET mg
6.120	—	0.000	—	9.5	0.300	0.000	0.020	0.000	—	—	—	12.400	11.300	—	0.050	—
5.000	—	0.000	—	9	0.000	0.000	0.010	0.000	—	—	—	10.000	8.000	—	0.000	—
12.300	—	0.100	0.010	3.12	—	—	—	—	—	—	—	1.700	2.200	—	0.000	—
13.000	—	0.100	0.030	0	—	—	—	—	—	—	—	2.000	2.000	—	0.090	—
2.000	—	0.000	0.020	3.53	—	0.000	0.000	0.000	—	—	—	1.000	1.000	—	0.050	—
2.000	—	0.000	—	0	—	0.000	0.000	0.000	—	—	—	0.000	1.000	—	0.090	—
1.000	0.290	0.000	—	9.6	—	0.000	0.000	0.000	—	—	—	2.000	4.000	—	0.000	—
1.000	—	0.000	—	12	—	0.000	0.000	0.000	—	—	—	3.000	4.000	—	0.000	—
11.000	—	0.100	—	3	0.000	0.000	0.000	0.000	—	—	—	3.000	4.000	—	—	—
18.000	—	0.100	0.020	14.8	0.000	0.000	0.000	0.000	—	—	—	2.000	3.000	—	0.600	—
17.000	—	0.100	—	0	0.000	0.000	0.000	0.000	—	—	—	2.000	3.000	—	0.300	—
—	—	—	—	47	—	—	—	—	—	—	—	—	—	—	0.000	—
1.990	0.120	—	—	47	0.008	0.000	0.002	0.001	0.000	0.060	0.004	1.410	1.080	—	0.000	0.606
1.770	0.110	—	—	0	0.007	0.000	0.002	0.001	0.000	0.050	0.004	1.250	0.950	—	0.000	0.500
—	—	—	0.020	2.61	—	—	—	—	—	—	—	—	—	—	0.000	3.110
26.000	—	0.100	—	31.80	—	—	—	—	—	—	—	3.000	6.000	—	0.200	—
24.000	—	0.100	0.070	0	1.000	0.010	0.010	0.100	—	—	—	3.000	6.000	—	0.000	—
1.200	—	—	—	—	—	—	—	—	—	—	—	—	—	—	0.000	—
—	—	—	—	—	—	—	—	—	—	—	—	—	—	—	—	—
—	—	—	—	—	—	—	—	—	—	—	—	—	—	—	0.000	2.900
—	—	—	—	—	—	—	—	—	—	—	—	—	—	—	—	—
—	—	—	—	—	—	—	—	—	—	—	—	—	—	—	—	—
—	—	—	—	—	—	—	—	—	—	—	—	—	—	—	0.000	—

OT Mg	MAG Mg	IRON Mg	ZINC Mg	V-A RE	V-C Mg	THIA Mg	RIBO Mg	NIAC Mg	V-B6 Mg	FOL Ug	V-B12 Ug	CALC Mg	PHOS Mg	SEL Mg	FIBD Gm	V-ET mg
—	43.300	1.100	—	24	—	0.170	0.160	2.900	—	—	1.640	44.600	445	0.047	0.000	—
267	8.000	11.900	1.160	76.5	—	—	0.181	1.500	—	—	42.000	39.000	144	0.016	0.000	0.209
89.700	—	1.170	0.347	—	—	0.003	0.030	0.300	—	—	5.400	15.700	38.700	0.046	0.000	0.629
149	29.000	1.100	5.830	—	—	0.110	0.110	2.600	—	—	13.500	61.000	246	0.072	0.000	1.650
3.000	7.000	0.210	0.190	8.8	—	0.036	0.050	0.596	0.017	5.100	0.503	6.000	51.000	0.003	0.300	—
242	—	1.100	—	—	—	0.100	0.100	1.600	—	—	0.850	28.000	192	0.020	0.050	1.060
568	135	16.600	226	223	—	0.340	0.412	3.250	0.124	24.600	47.500	111	344	0.156	0.000	2.040
277	29.000	0.720	0.780	14.5	0.000	0.020	0.158	5.560	0.255	13.100	5.850	—	279	0.045	0.000	1.150
7.500	4.500	0.350	0.155	8.04	—	0.010	0.027	0.630	0.020	1.400	1.070	46.000	59.000	—	0.000	—
377	—	0.600	—	9.01	—	0.130	0.260	8.600	—	—	—	24.000	313	—	0.000	2.000
269	53.000	3.500	1.610	23	—	0.035	0.047	3.530	0.142	2.300	1.440	75.000	299	0.041	0.000	3.640
191	34.000	1.070	1.170	47.6	—	0.110	0.116	2.610	0.083	6.900	1.590	57.000	185	0.027	0.480	0.807
176	26.000	1.180	0.770	19.6	—	0.032	—	—	0.094	4.500	—	11.000	265	—	0.000	1.420
241	—	0.510	—	20.4	—	0.003	0.039	4.930	—	3.500	—	—	—	—	0.000	—
3.800	9.090	0.341	0.142	6.91	—	0.009	0.014	3.520	0.105	0.000	0.398	1.420	62.500	0.033	0.000	—
267	25.000	2.720	0.370	19.6	—	—	—	—	0.321	4.000	—	10.000	158	—	0.000	—
1.800	2.800	0.186	0.098	0.84	—	0.003	0.015	0.796	0.008	—	0.035	9.200	10.000	0.002	0.000	0.012
440	76.000	0.880	1.040	25.2	1.800	0.158	0.142	4.520	0.509	—	1.890	25.000	248	—	—	—
195	20.000	0.650	2.460	48.6	—	—	—	—	—	—	3.560	63.000	128	—	0.028	—
406	52.700	1.180	11.800	14	—	0.082	0.085	2.080	—	—	—	91.500	434	0.076	0.000	—
436	74.000	0.430	0.800	14.4	—	0.102	0.145	2.770	0.305	—	3.190	23.000	368	—	0.000	—
339	43.000	1.140	0.410	16.2	—	0.034	0.038	3.940	0.294	—	1.180	36.000	205	0.025	0.000	0.510
369	70.000	3.880	1.940	247	1.700	0.076	0.403	11.700	0.399	10.200	13.200	458	572	0.089	0.000	—
520	34.000	0.530	0.530	66	0.870	0.044	0.084	3.920	—	—	—	12.000	228	0.039	0.000	—
—	—	0.170	—	22.4	3.980	0.028	0.216	0.398	—	—	—	4.250	98.100	—	0.000	—
175	18.000	0.850	0.310	26	—	0.023	0.101	4.720	0.278	1.900	3.260	11.000	164	0.061	0.000	—
135	—	0.852	—	—	—	—	—	—	—	—	—	32.700	96.000	0.015	0.000	—
—	—	1.300	—	616	—	0.040	0.050	10.900	—	—	—	27.000	275	0.047	0.000	—
—	35.000	1.100	—	95.8	1.000	0.120	0.060	2.500	—	—	—	218	272	—	0.000	—

Continued.

A

Nutritive Components for Fish—cont'd.

Food Name	Serving Portion	WT. Gm	KCAL Kc	PROT Gm	CARB Gm	FAT Gm	CHOL Mg	SAFA Gm	MUFA Gm	PUFA Gm	SOD Mg
FISH-WHITEFISH-BAKE/STUFF	1.000 SERVING	100	215	15.200	5.800	14.000	—	—	—	—	195
FISH-WHITE PERCH-FRI-FILET	1.000 ITEM	65.000	108	12.500	0.000	5.300	0.000	—	—	—	—
FISH-CARP-COOKED-DRY HEAT	1.000 SERVING	85.000	138	19.400	0.000	6.100	72.000	1.180	2.540	1.560	54.000
FISH-CATFISH-FRIED-BREADED	1.000 SERVING	85.000	194	15.400	6.830	11.300	69.000	2.800	4.770	2.830	238
FISH-FLATFISH-CKD-DRY HEAT	1.000 SERVING	85.000	99.000	20.500	0.000	1.300	58.000	0.309	0.263	0.350	89.000
FISH-GROUPER-CKD-DRY HEAT	1.000 SERVING	85.000	100	21.100	0.000	1.110	40.000	0.254	0.228	0.343	45.000
FISH-MACKEREL-CKD-DRY HEAT	1.000 SERVING	85.000	223	20.300	0.000	15.100	64.000	3.550	5.960	3.660	71.000
FISH-OCEAN PERCH-CKD-DRY	1.000 SERVING	85.000	103	20.300	0.000	1.780	46.000	0.266	0.681	0.465	82.000
FISH-PERCH-COOKED-DRY HEAT	1.000 SERVING	85.000	99.000	21.100	0.000	1.000	98.000	0.201	0.166	0.401	67.000
FISH-POLLOCK-CKD-DRY HEAT	1.000 SERVING	85.000	96.000	20.000	0.000	0.950	82.000	0.196	0.148	0.445	98.000
FISH-POMPANO-CKD-DRY HEAT	1.000 SERVING	85.000	179	20.100	0.000	10.300	54.000	3.820	2.820	1.240	65.000
FISH-SALMON-CKD-MOIST HEAT	1.000 SERVING	85.000	157	23.300	0.000	6.400	42.000	1.190	2.220	1.870	50.000
FISH-SEA BASS-CKD-DRY HEAT	1.000 SERVING	85.000	105	20.100	0.000	2.180	45.000	0.557	0.462	0.810	74.000
FISH-SMELT-COOKED-DRY HEAT	1.000 SERVING	85.000	106	19.200	0.000	2.640	76.000	0.492	0.699	0.965	65.000
FISH-RED SNAPPER-CKD-DRY	1.000 SERVING	85.000	109	22.400	0.000	1.460	40.000	0.310	0.274	0.500	48.000
FISH-SURIMI	1.000 SERVING	85.000	84.000	12.900	5.820	0.770	25.000	—	—	—	122
FISH-POLLOCK-ATLANTIC-RAW	1.000 SERVING	85.000	78.000	16.500	0.000	0.830	60.000	0.115	0.095	0.411	73.000
FISH-SWORDFISH-COOKED-DRY	1.000 SERVING	85.000	132	21.600	0.000	4.370	43.000	1.200	1.680	1.010	98.000
FISH-TROUT-RAINBOW-CKD-DRY	1.000 SERVING	85.000	129	22.400	0.000	3.660	62.000	0.707	1.130	1.310	29.000
FISH-TUNA-YELLOWFIN-RAW	1.000 SERVING	85.000	92.000	19.900	0.000	0.810	38.000	0.200	0.131	0.241	31.000
FISH-WHITING-CKD-DRY HEAT	1.000 SERVING	85.000	98.000	20.000	0.000	1.430	71.000	0.269	0.309	0.456	113
FISH-CRAB-IMITATION-SURIMI	1.000 SERVING	85.000	87.000	10.200	8.690	1.110	17.000	—	—	—	715
FISH-CRAYFISH-CKD-MOIST	1.000 SERVING	85.000	97.000	20.300	0.000	1.150	151	0.197	0.320	0.281	58.000
FISH-LOBSTER-CKD-MOIST	1.000 CUP	145	142	29.700	1.860	0.860	104	0.155	0.232	0.132	551
FISH-SHRIMP-CKD-MOIST HEAT	1.000 SERVING	85.000	84.000	17.800	0.000	0.920	166	0.246	0.167	0.374	190
FISH-CLAMS-BREADED-FRIED	1.000 SERVING	85.000	171	12.100	8.780	9.480	52.000	2.280	3.860	2.440	309
FISH-CLAMS-CKD-MOIST HEAT	1.000 SERVING	85.000	126	21.700	4.360	1.650	57.000	0.160	0.146	0.469	95.000
FISH-MUSSEL-BLUE-CKD-MOIST	1.000 SERVING	85.000	147	20.200	6.280	3.810	48.000	0.723	0.862	1.030	313
FISH-OYSTER-EASTERN-CANNED	1.000 CUP	248	170	17.500	9.700	6.140	136	1.570	0.620	1.830	277
FISH-OYSTER-EAST-CKD-MOIST	1.000 SERVING	85.000	117	12.000	6.650	4.210	93.000	1.070	0.425	1.260	190
FISH-OYSTERS-PACIFIC-RAW	1.000 SERVING	85.000	69.000	8.030	4.210	1.960	—	0.434	0.304	0.760	90.000
FISH-SQUID-COOKED-FRIED	1.000 SERVING	85.000	149	15.300	6.620	6.360	221	1.600	2.340	1.820	260
FISH-HALIBUT-BROILED-DRY	1.000 SERVING	85.000	119	22.700	0.000	2.490	35.000	0.354	0.822	0.799	59.000

Nutritive Components for Frozen Dinners

Food Name	Serving Portion	WT. Gm	KCAL Kc	PROT Gm	CARB Gm	FAT Gm	CHOL Mg	SAFA Gm	MUFA Gm	PUFA Gm	SOD Mg
FISH DIVAN-LEAN CUISINE	1.000 ITEM	351	270	31.000	6.000	10.000	85.000	—	—	—	780
FETTUCINI ALFREDO-STOUFFER	1.000 ITEM	142	270	8.000	19.000	18.000	—	—	—	—	1195
TURKEY PIE-STOUFFER	1.000 ITEM	284	460	20.000	35.000	26.000	—	—	—	—	1735
MEATBALLS/NOODLES-STOUFFER	1.000 ITEM	312	475	25.000	33.000	27.000	—	—	—	—	1620
BEEF/GREEN PEPPERS-STOUF	1.000 ITEM	220	225	10.000	18.000	11.000	—	—	—	—	960
LASAGNA-STOUFFER	1.000 ITEM	298	385	28.000	36.000	14.000	—	—	—	—	1200
MEATLOAF-FROZ DIN-BANQUET	1.000 ITEM	312	412	20.900	29.000	23.700	—	—	—	—	1991
HAM-FROZ DIN-BANQUET	1.000 ITEM	284	369	16.800	47.700	12.200	—	—	—	—	1590
SALISBURY STEAK DIN-BANQ	1.000 ITEM	312	390	18.100	24.000	24.600	—	—	—	—	2059
CAKE-STRAWBERRY SHORTCAKE	1.000 SERVING	175	344	4.800	61.200	8.900	—	—	—	—	—
FROZ YOGURT-FRUIT VARIETY	1.000 CUP	226	216	7.000	41.800	2.000	—	—	—	—	—
CHICKEN KIEV-LE MENU	1.000 ITEM	234	500	21.000	35.000	30.000	—	—	—	—	745
VEGETABLE LASAGNE-LE MENU	1.000 ITEM	312	400	15.000	30.000	24.000	—	—	—	—	1135
BEEF SIRLOIN TIPS-LE MENU	1.000 ITEM	326	390	32.000	24.000	18.000	—	—	—	—	1100
CHICKEN PARMIGIANA-LE MENU	1.000 ITEM	326	400	27.000	27.000	20.000	—	—	—	—	895
MANICOTTI-CHEESE-LE MENU	1.000 ITEM	241	310	18.000	29.000	13.000	—	—	—	—	840
SOLE-LIGHT-VAN DE KAMP'S	1.000 ITEM	142	293	16.000	17.000	18.000	—	—	—	—	412
MEXICAN DINNER-SWANSON	1.000 ITEM	454	590	20.000	64.000	29.000	—	—	—	—	1865
BEEF DINNER-SWANSON	1.000 ITEM	326	320	25.000	34.000	9.000	—	—	—	—	1085

POT Mg	MAG Mg	IRON Mg	ZINC Mg	V-A RE	V-C Mg	THIA Mg	RIBO Mg	NIAC Mg	V-B6 Mg	FOL Ug	V-B12 Ug	CALC Mg	PHOS Mg	SEL Mg	FIBD Gm	V-ET mg
291	—	0.500	—	601	0.000	0.110	0.110	2.300	—	—	—	—	246	—	—	—
—	—	0.700	—	0	0.000	0.040	0.050	2.700	—	—	—	9.000	113	0.016	0.000	0.813
363	32.000	1.350	1.620	7.65	1.400	—	—	—	0.186	—	1.250	44.000	452	—	0.000	—
289	23.000	1.220	0.730	6.8	0.000	0.062	0.113	1.940	—	—	—	37.000	183	—	0.800	—
292	50.000	0.280	0.530	9.35	—	0.068	0.097	1.850	0.204	—	2.130	16.000	246	—	0.000	—
403	32.000	0.960	0.430	42.5	—	0.069	0.005	0.324	—	—	0.588	18.000	121	—	0.000	—
341	83.000	1.330	0.800	45.9	0.300	0.135	0.350	5.820	0.391	—	16.200	13.000	236	—	0.000	—
298	33.000	1.000	0.520	11.9	—	—	0.114	2.070	—	—	0.981	117	235	—	0.000	—
293	33.000	0.980	1.210	8.5	—	—	—	—	—	—	—	87.000	218	—	0.000	—
329	—	0.240	0.510	19.6	—	0.063	0.065	1.400	0.059	3.000	3.570	5.000	—	—	0.000	—
541	27.000	0.570	0.590	30.6	—	—	—	—	—	—	—	36.000	290	—	0.000	—
454	—	0.760	0.440	15.3	0.900	—	—	—	—	—	—	—	—	—	0.000	—
279	45.000	0.320	0.440	54.4	—	—	—	—	—	—	—	11.000	211	—	0.000	—
316	33.000	0.980	1.800	14.5	—	—	0.124	1.500	—	—	3.370	65.000	251	—	0.000	—
444	31.000	0.200	0.370	29.8	—	0.045	0.003	0.294	—	—	—	34.000	171	—	0.000	—
95.000	—	0.220	—	17	—	0.017	0.018	0.187	—	—	—	7.000	—	—	0.000	—
302	57.000	0.390	0.400	9.01	—	0.040	0.157	2.780	0.244	—	2.710	51.000	188	—	0.000	—
314	29.000	0.880	1.250	34.9	0.900	0.037	0.099	10.000	0.324	—	1.720	5.000	287	—	0.000	—
539	33.000	2.070	1.180	18.7	3.100	0.072	0.191	—	—	—	—	73.000	272	—	0.000	—
—	—	0.620	0.450	15.3	—	0.369	0.040	8.330	—	—	—	14.000	163	—	0.000	—
369	23.000	0.360	0.450	28.9	—	0.058	0.051	1.420	0.153	12.800	2.210	53.000	242	—	0.000	—
77.000	—	0.330	—	17	—	0.027	0.023	0.153	—	—	—	11.000	—	—	0.000	—
298	27.000	2.670	1.420	18.7	2.800	—	0.065	2.500	—	—	2.940	26.000	280	—	0.000	—
510	51.000	0.570	4.230	7.38	—	0.010	0.096	1.550	0.112	16.100	4.510	88.000	268	—	0.000	—
154	29.000	2.620	1.330	56.1	—	0.026	0.027	2.200	0.108	2.900	1.270	33.000	116	—	0.000	—
277	12.000	11.800	1.240	76.5	—	—	0.207	1.750	—	—	34.200	54.000	160	—	0.320	—
534	16.000	23.800	2.320	145	—	—	0.362	2.850	—	—	84.100	78.000	287	—	0.000	—
228	32.000	5.710	2.270	77.4	—	—	—	—	—	—	—	28.000	242	—	0.000	—
568	135	16.600	226	223	—	—	0.412	3.090	0.236	22.100	47.500	111	344	—	0.000	—
389	92.000	11.400	155	145	—	—	0.282	2.210	0.081	15.200	32.500	76.000	236	—	0.000	—
143	19.000	4.340	14.100	68.9	—	0.057	0.198	1.710	—	—	—	7.000	138	—	0.000	0.723
237	33.000	0.860	1.480	9.35	3.500	0.048	0.389	2.120	0.049	—	1.040	33.000	213	—	0.300	—
490	91.000	0.910	0.450	45.9	—	0.059	0.077	6.060	0.337	—	1.160	51.000	242	—	0.000	—

POT Mg	MAG Mg	IRON Mg	ZINC Mg	V-A RE	V-C Mg	THIA Mg	RIBO Mg	NIAC Mg	V-B6 Mg	FOL Ug	V-B12 Ug	CALC Mg	PHOS Mg	SEL Mg	FIBD Gm	V-ET mg
850	—	—	—	—	—	—	—	—	—	—	—	—	—	—	—	—
240	—	—	—	—	—	—	—	—	—	—	—	—	—	—	—	—
270	—	—	—	—	—	—	—	—	—	—	—	—	—	—	—	—
395	—	—	—	—	—	—	—	—	—	—	—	—	—	—	—	—
420	—	2.330	—	136	0.000	0.078	0.155	3.880	—	—	—	0.000	—	—	—	—
580	—	3.150	—	248	0.000	0.210	0.420	4.200	—	—	—	410	—	—	—	—
468	—	4.300	—	427	8.000	0.160	0.220	4.200	—	—	—	84.000	243	—	—	—
125	—	2.500	—	1311	57.000	0.570	0.230	3.400	—	—	—	151	278	—	—	—
387	—	3.500	—	791	7.000	0.160	0.190	3.600	—	—	—	90.000	206	—	—	—
—	—	2.000	—	86	89.000	0.170	0.210	1.300	—	—	—	73.000	84.000	—	—	—
—	24.000	0.000	—	0	0.000	0.010	0.260	0.000	—	—	—	200	200	—	—	—
—	—	—	—	—	—	—	—	—	—	—	—	—	—	—	—	—
—	—	—	—	—	—	—	—	—	—	—	—	—	—	—	—	—
—	—	—	—	—	—	—	—	—	—	—	—	—	—	—	—	—
—	—	—	—	—	—	—	—	—	—	—	—	—	—	—	—	—

Continued.

Nutritive Components for Frozen Dinners—cont'd.

Food Name	Serving Portion	WT. Gm	KCAL Kc	PROT Gm	CARB Gm	FAT Gm	CHOL Mg	SAFA Gm	MUFA Gm	PUFA Gm	SOD Mg
TURKEY DINNER-SWANSON	1.000 ITEM	326	340	20.000	42.000	10.000	—	—	—	—	1295
CHICKEN DINNER-SWANSON	1.000 ITEM	326	660	26.000	64.000	33.000	—	—	—	—	1610
EGG ROLL-BEEF/SHRIMP-FROZ	1.000 ITEM	12.000	27.000	0.900	3.500	1.000	—	—	—	—	80.500
FISH & CHIPS-VAN DE KAMPS	1.000 ITEM	224	500	16.000	45.000	30.000	—	—	—	—	551
CHICKEN CACCIATORE-STOUF	1.000 ITEM	319	310	25.000	29.000	11.000	—	—	—	—	1135
VEAL PARMIGIANA-FROZ DIN	1.000 ITEM	213	296	24.000	17.000	14.000	—	—	—	—	973
CABBAGE ROLL/TOM SAUC-HORM	1.000 SERVING	28.4000	23.000	1.100	3.200	0.700	3.000	0.281	0.226	0.043	127

Nutritive Components for Fruits

Food Name	Serving Portion	WT. Gm	KCAL Kc	PROT Gm	CARB Gm	FAT Gm	CHOL Mg	SAFA Gm	MUFA Gm	PUFA Gm	SOD Mg
APPLES-RAW-UNPEELED	1.000 ITEM	138	81.000	0.270	21.100	0.490	0.000	0.080	0.021	0.145	1.000
APPLE JUICE-CANNED/BOTTLED	1.000 CUP	248	116	0.150	29.000	0.280	0.000	0.047	0.012	0.082	7.000
APPLESAUCE-CAN-SWEETENED	1.000 CUP	255	194	0.470	50.800	0.470	0.000	0.077	0.018	0.138	8.000
APPLESAUCE-CAN-UNSWEETENED	1.000 CUP	244	106	0.400	27.600	0.120	0.000	0.020	0.005	0.034	5.000
APRICOT-RAW-WITHOUT PIT	1.000 ITEM	35.300	16.900	0.494	3.930	0.138	0.000	0.010	0.060	0.027	0.353
APRICOTS-DRIED-UNCOOKED	1.000 CUP	130	310	4.750	80.300	0.600	0.000	0.042	0.260	0.117	13.000
APRICOTS-DRIED-COOKED-UNSW	1.000 CUP	250	211	3.240	54.800	0.410	0.000	0.028	0.178	0.080	9.000
AVOCADO-RAW-CALIFORNIA	1.000 ITEM	173	306	3.640	12.000	30.000	0.000	4.480	19.400	3.530	21.000
BANANAS-RAW-PEELED	1.000 ITEM	114	105	1.180	26.700	0.550	0.000	0.211	0.047	0.101	1.000
BLACKBERRIES-RAW	1.000 CUP	144	74.000	1.040	18.400	0.560	0.000	0.000	0.000	0.000	0.000
BLUEBERRIES-RAW	1.000 CUP	145	82.000	0.970	20.500	0.550	0.000	0.000	0.000	0.000	9.000
CHERRIES-SWEET-RAW	1.000 ITEM	6.800	4.900	0.082	1.130	0.065	0.000	0.015	0.018	0.020	0.000
CRANBERRY SAUCE-CAN-SWEET	1.000 CUP	277	419	0.550	108	0.420	0.000	—	—	—	80.000
DATES-NATURAL-DRIED-CHOP	1.000 CUP	178	489	3.500	131	0.800	0.000	—	—	—	5.000
GRAPEFRUIT-RAW-PINK & RED	1.000 ITEM	246	74.000	1.360	18.500	0.240	0.000	0.034	0.032	0.060	0.000
GRAPEFRUIT-RAW-WHITE	1.000 ITEM	236	78.000	1.620	19.800	0.240	0.000	0.034	0.030	0.056	0.000
GRAPEFRUIT JUICE-RAW	1.000 CUP	247	96.000	1.240	22.700	0.250	0.000	0.035	0.032	0.059	2.000
GRAPEFRUIT JUICE-CAN-UNSW	1.000 CUP	247	93.000	1.290	22.100	0.240	0.000	0.032	0.032	0.057	3.000
GRAPEFRUIT JUICE-CAN-SWEET	1.000 CUP	250	116	1.450	27.800	0.230	0.000	0.030	0.030	0.053	4.000
GRAPEFRUIT JUICE-FROZ-DILU	1.000 CUP	247	102	1.370	24.000	0.330	0.000	0.047	0.044	0.079	2.000
GRAPE JUICE-CAN & BOTTLE	1.000 CUP	253	155	1.410	37.900	0.190	0.000	0.063	0.008	0.056	7.000
GRAPE JUICE-FROZ-DILUTED	1.000 CUP	250	128	0.470	31.900	0.230	0.000	0.073	0.010	0.065	5.000
GRAPE DRINK-CANNED	1.000 CUP	250	135	0.000	35.000	0.000	0.000	—	—	—	2.000
LEMONS-RAW-PEELED	1.000 ITEM	58.000	17.000	0.640	5.410	0.170	0.000	0.023	0.006	0.052	1.000
LEMON JUICE-RAW	1.000 CUP	244	60.000	0.920	21.100	0.000	0.000	0.000	0.000	0.000	2.000
LEMON JUICE-CAN & BOTTLE	1.000 CUP	244	52.000	0.980	15.800	0.700	0.000	0.093	0.027	0.207	50.000
LEMONADE-FROZ-DILUTED	1.000 CUP	248	105	0.000	28.000	0.000	0.000	0.000	0.000	0.000	0.000
LIME JUICE-RAW	1.000 CUP	246	66.000	1.080	22.200	0.250	0.000	0.027	0.025	0.066	2.000
LIME JUICE-CAN & BOTTLE	1.000 CUP	246	51.000	0.610	16.500	0.570	0.000	0.064	0.054	0.157	39.000
MELONS-CANTALOUPE-RAW	1.000 CUP	160	57.000	1.400	13.400	0.440	0.000	0.000	0.000	0.000	14.000
MELONS-HONEYDEW-RAW	1.000 CUP	170	60.000	0.770	15.600	0.170	0.000	0.000	0.000	0.000	17.000
ORANGES-RAW-ALL VARIETIES	1.000 ITEM	131	62.000	1.230	15.400	0.160	0.000	0.020	0.030	0.033	0.000
ORANGE JUICE-RAW	1.000 CUP	248	111	1.740	25.800	0.500	0.000	0.060	0.089	0.099	2.000
ORANGE JUICE-CAN	1.000 CUP	249	104	1.460	24.500	0.360	0.000	0.045	0.062	0.085	6.000
ORANGE JUICE-FROZ-DILUTED	1.000 CUP	249	112	1.680	26.800	0.140	0.000	0.017	0.025	0.030	2.000
PAPAYAS-RAW	1.000 CUP	140	54.000	0.860	13.700	0.200	0.000	0.060	0.053	0.043	4.000
PEACHES-RAW-WHOLE	1.000 ITEM	87.000	37.000	0.610	9.650	0.080	0.000	0.009	0.030	0.039	0.000
PEACHES-RAW-SLICED	1.000 CUP	170	73.000	1.190	18.900	0.160	0.000	0.017	0.058	0.077	1.000
PEACHES-CAN/WATER PACK	1.000 CUP	244	58.000	1.070	14.900	0.140	0.000	0.015	0.051	0.068	8.000
PEACHES-DRIED-UNCOOKED	1.000 CUP	160	383	5.770	98.100	1.220	0.000	0.131	0.445	0.587	12.000
PEACHES-DRIED-COOKED-UNSW	1.000 CUP	258	198	2.990	50.800	0.630	0.000	0.067	0.230	0.304	6.000
PEACHES-FROZ-SLICED-SWEET	1.000 CUP	250	235	1.560	59.900	0.330	0.000	0.035	0.120	0.160	16.000
PEARS-RAW-BARTLETT-UNPEELED	1.000 ITEM	166	98.000	0.650	25.100	0.660	0.000	0.037	0.139	0.156	1.000
PINEAPPLE-RAW-DICED	1.000 CUP	155	77.000	0.600	19.200	0.660	0.000	0.050	0.074	0.226	1.000
PINEAPPLE JUICE-CAN	1.000 CUP	250	139	0.800	34.400	0.200	0.000	0.013	0.023	0.070	2.000

POT Mg	MAG Mg	IRON Mg	ZINC Mg	V-A RE	V-C Mg	THIA Mg	RIBO Mg	NIAC Mg	V-B6 Mg	FOL Ug	V-B12 Ug	CALC Mg	PHOS Mg	SEL Mg	FIBD Gm	V-ET mg
—	—	—	—	—	—	—	—	—	—	—	—	—	—	—	—	—
—	—	—	—	—	—	—	—	—	—	—	—	—	—	—	—	—
—	—	—	—	—	—	—	—	—	—	—	—	—	—	—	0.120	—
—	—	—	—	—	—	—	—	—	—	—	—	—	—	—	—	—
300	—	—	—	—	—	—	—	—	—	—	—	—	—	—	—	—
466	—	2.300	—	123	6.400	0.300	0.380	6.800	—	—	—	97.000	—	—	—	—
87.000	4.000	0.250	0.190	—	0.180	0.760	0.020	0.290	0.030	2.900	0.100	5.900	15.700	—	—	—

POT Mg	MAG Mg	IRON Mg	ZINC Mg	V-A RE	V-C Mg	THIA Mg	RIBO Mg	NIAC Mg	V-B6 Mg	FOL Ug	V-B12 Ug	CALC Mg	PHOS Mg	SEL Mg	FIBD Gm	V-ET mg
159	6.000	0.250	0.050	7.4	7.800	0.023	0.019	0.106	0.066	3.900	0.000	10.000	10.000	0.001	3.200	0.814
296	8.000	0.920	0.070	0.2	2.300	0.052	0.042	0.248	0.074	0.200	0.000	16.000	18.000	0.002	0.520	0.025
156	7.000	0.890	0.100	2.8	4.400	0.033	0.071	0.479	0.066	1.500	0.000	9.000	17.000	0.001	4.340	0.230
183	7.000	0.290	0.060	7	2.900	0.032	0.061	0.459	0.063	1.400	0.000	7.000	18.000	0.001	4.150	0.220
104	2.820	0.191	0.092	92.2	3.530	0.011	0.014	0.212	0.019	3.040	0.000	4.940	6.710	—	0.670	0.314
1791	61.000	6.110	0.970	941	3.100	0.010	0.196	3.900	0.203	13.400	0.000	59.000	152	—	10.500	—
1222	42.000	4.170	0.660	591	3.900	0.015	0.075	2.360	0.285	0.000	0.000	40.000	104	—	6.700	—
1097	70.000	2.040	0.730	106	13.700	0.187	0.211	3.320	0.484	113	0.000	19.000	73.000	—	6.130	3.660
451	33.000	0.350	0.190	9.2	10.300	0.051	0.114	0.616	0.659	21.800	0.000	7.000	22.000	0.001	2.650	0.308
282	29.000	0.830	0.390	23.7	30.200	0.043	0.058	0.576	0.084	18.000	0.000	46.000	30.000	0.001	8.930	5.040
129	7.000	0.240	0.160	14.5	18.900	0.070	0.073	0.521	0.052	9.300	0.000	9.000	15.000	0.001	3.920	—
15.200	0.800	0.026	0.004	1.46	0.480	0.003	0.004	0.027	0.002	0.286	0.000	1.000	1.300	0.000	0.100	0.009
71.000	8.000	0.610	0.140	5.5	5.500	0.042	0.058	0.277	0.039	—	0.000	10.000	16.000	0.001	3.200	—
1161	63.000	2.050	0.520	8.9	0.000	0.160	0.178	3.920	0.342	22.400	0.000	58.000	70.000	—	15.500	—
312	20.000	0.300	0.180	63.7	91.000	0.098	0.050	0.492	0.104	23.200	0.000	36.000	22.000	0.001	3.200	0.615
350	22.000	0.070	0.160	2.4	78.600	0.088	0.048	0.634	0.102	23.600	0.000	28.000	18.000	0.001	2.500	0.590
400	30.000	0.490	0.130	2.47	93.900	0.099	0.049	0.494	—	51.200	0.000	22.000	37.000	0.001	0.500	0.098
378	24.000	0.500	0.210	1.8	72.000	0.104	0.049	0.571	0.049	25.600	0.000	18.000	27.000	0.001	0.000	0.099
405	24.000	0.890	0.150	0	67.300	0.100	0.058	0.798	0.050	25.900	0.000	20.000	27.000	0.001	0.000	0.100
337	26.000	0.340	0.130	2.2	83.400	0.101	0.054	0.536	0.109	8.900	0.000	19.000	34.000	0.001	0.000	0.099
334	24.000	0.600	0.130	2	0.200	0.066	0.094	0.663	0.164	6.580	0.000	22.000	27.000	0.001	0.000	—
53.000	11.000	0.260	0.100	1.9	59.700	0.038	0.065	0.310	0.105	3.100	0.000	9.000	11.000	0.001	0.000	—
88.000	—	0.300	—	2.02	0.000	0.030	0.030	0.300	—	—	—	8.000	10.000	0.001	0.000	—
80.000	—	0.350	0.040	1.7	30.700	0.023	0.012	0.058	0.046	6.200	0.000	15.000	9.000	0.001	0.580	—
303	16.000	0.080	0.120	4.9	112	0.073	0.024	0.244	0.124	31.500	0.000	18.000	14.000	0.001	0.732	—
248	20.000	0.310	0.150	3.7	60.400	0.100	0.022	0.481	0.105	24.600	0.000	26.000	21.000	0.001	0.732	—
40.000	—	0.100	—	1	17.000	0.010	0.020	0.200	—	12.000	—	2.000	3.000	0.001	—	—
268	14.000	0.080	0.150	2.5	72.100	0.049	0.025	0.246	0.106	—	0.000	22.000	18.000	—	0.000	—
185	16.000	0.560	0.150	4	15.700	0.081	0.007	0.401	0.066	19.500	0.000	30.000	24.000	0.001	0.000	—
494	17.000	0.340	0.250	516	67.500	0.058	0.034	0.918	0.184	27.300	0.000	17.000	27.000	0.001	1.400	0.224
461	12.000	0.120	—	6.8	42.100	0.131	0.031	1.020	0.100	—	0.000	10.000	17.000	0.001	1.530	0.238
237	13.000	0.130	0.090	26.9	69.700	0.114	0.052	0.369	0.079	39.700	0.000	52.000	18.000	0.002	2.620	0.314
496	27.000	0.500	0.130	49.6	124	0.223	0.074	0.992	0.099	136	0.000	27.000	42.000	0.001	1.980	0.099
436	27.000	1.100	0.170	43.7	85.700	0.149	0.070	0.782	0.219	136	0.000	21.000	36.000	0.001	0.260	0.100
474	24.000	0.240	0.130	19.4	96.900	0.197	0.045	0.503	0.110	109	0.000	22.000	40.000	0.001	0.700	0.100
359	14.000	0.140	0.100	282	86.500	0.038	0.045	0.473	0.027	—	0.000	33.000	7.000	0.001	1.270	—
171	6.000	0.100	0.120	46.5	5.700	0.015	0.036	0.861	0.016	3.000	0.000	5.000	11.000	0.001	2.000	0.087
334	11.000	0.190	0.230	91	11.200	0.029	0.070	1.680	0.031	5.800	0.000	9.000	21.000	0.001	3.910	0.170
241	12.000	0.770	0.220	130	7.000	0.020	0.046	1.270	0.046	8.200	0.000	6.000	25.000	0.001	1.080	—
1594	67.000	6.500	0.920	346	7.700	0.003	0.339	7.000	0.107	10.600	0.000	45.000	191	0.001	14.000	—
825	35.000	3.370	0.470	50.8	9.500	0.013	0.054	3.920	0.098	0.200	0.000	23.000	99.000	0.001	6.700	—
325	12.000	0.930	0.130	70.9	235	0.033	0.088	1.630	0.045	—	0.000	6.000	28.000	0.001	—	—
208	9.000	0.410	0.200	3.3	6.600	0.033	0.066	0.166	0.030	12.100	0.000	19.000	18.000	0.001	4.650	0.820
175	21.000	0.570	0.120	3.5	23.900	0.143	0.056	0.651	0.135	16.400	0.000	11.000	11.000	0.001	2.390	0.155
334	34.000	0.650	0.290	1.2	26.700	0.138	0.055	0.643	0.240	57.800	0.000	42.000	20.000	0.002	0.250	—

Continued.

A

Nutritive Components for Fruits—cont'd.

Food Name	Serving Portion	WT. Gm	KCAL Kc	PROT Gm	CARB Gm	FAT Gm	CHOL Mg	SAFA Gm	MUFA Gm	PUFA Gm	SOD Mg
PLUMS-RAW-PRUNE TYPE	1.000 ITEM	28.000	20.000	0.000	6.000	0.000	0.000	0.000	0.000	0.000	0.000
PRUNES-DRIED-UNCOOKED	1.000 CUP	161	385	4.200	101	0.830	0.000	0.066	0.547	0.180	6.000
PRUNE JUICE-CAN & BOTTLE	1.000 CUP	256	181	1.550	44.700	0.080	0.000	0.008	0.054	0.018	11.000
RAISINS-SEEDLESS	1.000 CUP	145	434	4.670	115	0.670	0.000	0.218	0.026	0.196	17.000
RAISINS-SEEDLESS-PACKET	1.000 ITEM	14.000	42.000	0.451	11.100	0.064	0.000	0.021	0.003	0.019	1.680
RASPBERRIES-RAW	1.000 CUP	123	61.000	1.110	14.200	0.680	0.000	0.023	0.065	0.385	0.000
RHUBARB-RAW-COOKED-SUGAR	1.000 CUP	270	380	1.000	97.000	0.000	0.000	0.000	—	—	5.000
STRAWBERRIES-RAW-WHOLE	1.000 CUP	149	45.000	0.910	10.500	0.550	0.000	0.030	0.077	0.277	2.000
TANGERINES-RAW-PEELED	1.000 ITEM	84.000	37.000	0.530	9.400	0.160	0.000	0.018	0.029	0.031	1.000
WATERMELON-RAW	1.000 CUP	160	50.000	0.990	11.500	0.680	0.000	0.000	0.000	0.000	3.000
APPLES-RAW-PEELED-BOILED	1.000 CUP	171	91.000	0.450	23.300	0.610	0.000	0.099	0.024	0.178	1.000
APPLE JUICE-FROZEN-DILUTED	1.000 CUP	239	111	0.340	27.600	0.250	0.000	0.043	0.005	0.074	17.000
APRICOTS-CAN/JUICE	1.000 CUP	248	119	1.560	30.600	0.090	0.000	0.007	0.042	0.017	9.000
BLACKBERRIES-FROZEN-UNSW	1.000 CUP	151	97.000	1.780	23.700	0.650	0.000	—	—	—	2.000
BLUEBERRIES-FROZEN-UNSWEET	1.000 CUP	155	78.000	0.650	18.900	0.990	0.000	—	—	—	1.000
BOYSENBERRIES-FROZEN-UNSW	1.000 CUP	132	66.000	1.460	16.100	0.350	0.000	—	—	—	2.000
FIGS-DRIED-UNCOOKED	1.000 CUP	199	508	6.060	130	2.320	0.000	0.466	0.513	1.110	22.000
FRUIT COCKTAIL-CAN/JUICE	1.000 CUP	248	113	1.130	29.400	0.030	0.000	0.005	0.007	0.015	9.000
KIWIFRUIT-RAW	1.000 ITEM	76.000	46.000	0.750	11.300	0.340	0.000	0.000	0.000	0.000	4.000
LIMES-RAW	1.000 ITEM	67.000	20.000	0.470	7.060	0.130	0.000	0.015	0.013	0.037	1.000
MELONS-CASABA-RAW	1.000 CUP	170	45.000	1.530	10.500	0.170	0.000	0.000	0.000	0.000	20.000
NECTARINES-RAW	1.000 ITEM	136	67.000	1.280	16.000	0.620	0.000	—	—	—	0.000
PAPAYA NECTAR-CAN	1.000 CUP	250	142	0.430	36.300	0.380	0.000	0.118	0.103	0.088	14.000
PEARS-CAN/JUICE	1.000 CUP	248	123	0.850	32.100	0.160	0.000	0.010	0.035	0.037	10.000
PINEAPPLE-CAN/JUICE	1.000 CUP	250	150	1.040	39.200	0.210	0.000	0.015	0.025	0.073	4.000
PINEAPPLE JUICE-FROZ-DILU	1.000 CUP	250	129	1.000	31.900	0.080	0.000	0.005	0.008	0.025	3.000
POMEGRANATES-RAW	1.000 ITEM	154	104	1.470	26.400	0.460	0.000	—	—	—	5.000
STRAWBERRIES-FROZ-UNSWEET	1.000 CUP	149	52.000	0.630	13.600	0.160	0.000	0.009	0.022	0.080	3.000
CRANAPPLE JUICE-CAN	1.000 CUP	253	180	0.177	45.900	0.127	0.000	—	—	—	17.700
FRUIT PUNCH DRINK-CAN	1.000 FL OZ	31.000	14.000	0.000	3.700	0.000	0.000	0.000	0.000	0.000	7.000
FRUIT ROLL UP-CHERRY	1.000 ITEM	14.400	50.000	0.000	12.000	1.000	—	—	—	—	5.000

Nutritive Components for Grains

Food Name	Serving Portion	WT. Gm	KCAL Kc	PROT Gm	CARB Gm	FAT Gm	CHOL Mg	SAFA Gm	MUFA Gm	PUFA Gm	SOD Mg
CRACKERS-GRAHAM-PLAIN	1.000 ITEM	7.000	27.500	0.500	5.000	0.500	0.000	0.100	0.250	0.150	33.000
CRACKERS-RYE WAFERS	1.000 ITEM	6.500	22.500	1.000	5.000	0.000	0.000	—	—	—	57.000
CRACKERS-SALTINES	1.000 ITEM	2.750	12.500	0.250	2.000	0.250	0.750	0.100	0.100	0.050	36.800
MACARONI-COOKED-FIRM-HOT	1.000 CUP	130	190	7.000	39.000	1.000	0.000	—	—	—	1.000
NOODLES-EGG-ENR-COOKED	1.000 CUP	160	200	7.000	37.000	2.000	50.000	—	—	—	3.000
PANCAKES-BUCKWHEAT-MIX	1.000 ITEM	27.000	55.000	2.000	6.000	2.000	20.000	0.800	—	—	160
PANCAKES-PLAIN-HOME RECIPE	1.000 ITEM	27.000	60.000	2.000	9.000	2.000	20.000	0.500	—	—	160
PANCAKES-PLAIN-MIX	1.000 ITEM	27.000	58.900	1.850	19.000	2.170	20.000	0.700	—	—	160
POPCORN-POPPED-PLAIN	1.000 CUP	6.000	25.000	1.000	5.000	0.000	0.000	0.000	0.000	0.000	0.000
POPCORN-POPPED-SUGAR COAT	1.000 CUP	35.000	135	2.000	30.000	1.000	0.000	0.500	—	—	0.000
PRETZEL-THIN STICK	1.000 ITEM	0.300	1.190	0.028	0.242	0.011	0.000	—	—	—	4.830
RICE-WHITE-INSTANT-HOT	1.000 CUP	165	180	4.000	40.000	0.000	0.000	0.000	—	—	13.000
RICE-WHITE-LONG GRAIN-COOK	1.000 CUP	205	225	4.000	50.000	0.000	0.000	0.000	0.000	0.000	6.000
RICE-WHITE-PARBOIL-COOKED	1.000 CUP	175	185	4.000	41.000	0.000	0.000	0.000	0.000	0.000	4.000
SPAGHETTI-COOK-TENDER-HOT	1.000 CUP	140	155	5.000	32.000	1.000	0.000	—	—	—	1.000
WAFFLES-ENR-HOME RECIPE	1.000 ITEM	75.000	245	6.930	25.700	12.600	45.000	2.300	—	—	445
FLOUR-WHEAT-ENR-SIFTED	1.000 CUP	115	420	12.000	88.000	1.000	0.000	0.200	—	—	2.000
BISQUICK MIX-DRY	1.000 CUP	112	480	8.000	76.000	16.000	—	—	—	—	1400
TORTILLA CHIPS-DORITOS	1.000 SERVING	28.000	139	2.000	18.600	6.600	0.000	1.430	3.190	1.770	180
CRACKERS-TRISCUITS	1.000 ITEM	4.500	21.000	0.400	3.100	0.750	—	—	—	—	—
CRACKERS-WHEAT THINS	1.000 ITEM	1.800	9.000	0.125	1.250	0.350	—	—	—	—	—

OT Mg	MAG Mg	IRON Mg	ZINC Mg	V-A RE	V-C Mg	THIA Mg	RIBO Mg	NIAC Mg	V-B6 Mg	FOL Ug	V-B12 Ug	CALC Mg	PHOS Mg	SEL Mg	FIBD Gm	V-ET mg
48.000	1.960	0.100	0.028	8	1.000	0.010	0.010	0.100	0.023	0.616	0.000	3.000	5.000	0.000	0.588	0.196
1200	73.000	3.990	0.850	320	5.400	0.130	0.261	3.160	0.425	5.900	0.000	82.000	127	0.001	11.000	—
706	36.000	3.030	0.520	0.9	10.600	0.041	0.179	2.010	—	1.000	0.000	30.000	64.000	0.001	0.100	—
1089	48.000	3.020	0.380	1.1	4.800	0.226	0.128	1.190	0.361	4.800	0.000	71.000	140	0.001	12.600	1.020
105	4.620	0.291	0.039	0.112	0.462	0.022	0.012	0.115	0.035	0.462	0.000	6.860	13.600	0.000	1.220	0.098
187	22.000	0.700	0.570	16	30.800	0.037	0.111	1.110	0.070	6.000	0.000	27.000	15.000	0.001	5.500	0.369
548	32.400	1.600	0.216	22	16.000	0.050	0.140	0.800	0.054	14.300	0.000	211	41.000	0.001	5.400	0.540
247	16.000	0.570	0.190	4.1	84.500	0.030	0.098	0.343	0.088	26.400	0.000	21.000	28.000	0.001	3.200	0.179
132	10.000	0.090	—	77.3	25.900	0.088	0.018	0.134	0.056	17.100	0.000	12.000	8.000	0.001	1.680	—
186	17.000	0.280	0.110	58.5	15.400	0.128	0.032	0.320	0.230	3.400	0.000	13.000	14.000	0.001	0.300	—
150	5.000	0.320	0.070	7.5	0.300	0.027	0.021	0.162	0.075	1.000	0.000	8.000	13.000	0.001	4.100	0.086
301	12.000	0.610	0.090	—	1.400	0.001	0.036	0.091	0.079	0.700	0.000	14.000	16.000	0.002	0.000	0.024
409	24.000	0.740	0.270	420	12.200	0.045	0.047	0.853	—	—	0.000	30.000	50.000	0.001	2.810	2.210
211	33.000	1.210	0.370	17.2	4.700	0.044	0.069	1.820	0.092	51.300	0.000	44.000	46.000	0.001	7.550	—
83.000	8.000	0.280	0.110	12.6	3.800	0.050	0.057	0.806	0.091	10.400	0.000	12.000	18.000	0.001	4.940	—
183	21.000	1.120	0.290	8.9	4.100	0.070	0.049	1.010	0.074	83.600	0.000	36.000	36.000	0.001	5.150	—
1418	118	4.450	1.000	26.4	1.700	0.141	0.175	1.380	0.446	15.000	0.000	286	136	—	14.000	—
235	17.000	0.530	0.210	75.7	6.800	0.030	0.040	0.999	—	—	0.000	20.000	34.000	0.001	1.510	—
252	23.000	0.310	—	13.3	74.500	0.015	0.038	0.380	—	—	0.000	20.000	31.000	—	2.900	—
68.000	—	0.400	0.070	0.7	19.500	0.020	0.013	0.134	—	5.500	0.000	22.000	12.000	0.001	—	—
357	14.000	0.680	—	5.1	27.200	0.102	0.034	0.680	—	—	0.000	9.000	12.000	0.001	2.000	0.238
288	11.000	0.210	0.120	100	7.300	0.023	0.056	1.350	0.034	5.100	0.000	6.000	22.000	0.001	2.990	—
78.000	8.000	0.860	0.380	27.7	7.500	0.015	0.010	0.375	0.023	5.200	0.000	24.000	1.000	0.001	0.125	—
238	17.000	0.710	0.220	1.4	4.000	0.027	0.027	0.496	—	—	0.000	21.000	29.000	0.001	4.710	—
304	35.000	0.700	0.240	9.5	23.800	0.238	0.048	0.710	—	—	0.000	34.000	16.000	0.002	1.880	0.250
340	23.000	0.750	0.290	2.5	30.000	0.175	0.050	0.500	0.185	—	0.000	28.000	20.000	0.002	0.300	—
399	—	0.460	—	0	9.400	0.046	0.046	0.462	0.162	—	0.000	5.000	12.000	0.001	1.100	—
220	16.000	1.120	0.190	6.6	61.400	0.033	0.055	0.688	0.042	25.000	0.000	23.000	20.000	0.001	3.900	0.313
70.800	5.060	0.304	0.455	0	81.000	0.025	0.051	0.152	—	—	—	12.700	5.060	0.001	0.000	—
8.000	1.000	0.060	0.040	1.2	9.200	0.007	0.007	0.007	0.000	0.400	0.000	2.000	0.000	0.000	0.000	—
45.000	—	—	—	—	—	—	—	—	—	—	—	—	—	—	—	—

OT Mg	MAG Mg	IRON Mg	ZINC Mg	V-A RE	V-C Mg	THIA Mg	RIBO Mg	NIAC Mg	V-B6 Mg	FOL Ug	V-B12 Ug	CALC Mg	PHOS Mg	SEL Mg	FIBD Gm	V-ET mg
27.500	3.570	0.250	0.053	0	0.000	0.010	0.040	0.250	0.006	0.910	0.000	3.000	10.500	0.001	0.200	0.026
39.000	—	0.250	—	0	0.000	0.020	0.015	0.100	—	—	—	3.500	25.000	0.001	0.866	0.024
3.250	0.770	0.125	0.017	0	0.000	0.125	0.013	0.100	0.001	0.495	0.000	0.500	2.500	0.004	0.039	0.010
103	26.000	1.400	0.700	0	0.000	0.230	0.130	1.800	0.083	15.600	0.000	14.000	85.000	0.032	1.040	0.026
70.000	43.200	1.400	—	11	0.000	0.220	0.130	1.900	0.141	19.200	0.000	16.000	94.000	0.094	1.440	—
66.000	5.130	0.400	0.192	12	0.000	0.040	0.050	0.200	0.057	2.970	0.355	59.000	91.000	0.002	—	—
33.000	5.130	0.400	0.192	6	0.000	0.060	0.070	0.500	0.057	2.970	0.355	27.000	38.000	0.002	—	—
43.200	5.130	0.265	0.192	7.66	0.000	0.038	0.059	0.254	0.057	2.970	0.355	35.600	70.700	0.003	—	—
—	—	0.200	0.500	—	0.000	—	0.010	0.100	0.012	—	0.000	1.000	17.000	0.001	0.400	—
—	—	0.500	—	—	0.000	—	0.020	0.400	—	—	—	2.000	47.000	0.007	—	—
0.303	0.072	0.006	0.003	0	0.000	0.001	0.001	0.013	0.000	0.048	0.000	0.078	0.273	—	—	0.000
—	13.200	1.300	0.700	0	0.000	0.210	0.000	1.700	0.056	16.500	0.000	5.000	31.000	0.033	1.710	0.182
57.000	16.400	1.800	0.700	0	0.000	0.230	0.020	2.100	0.871	22.600	0.000	21.000	57.000	0.041	2.130	0.226
75.000	—	1.400	0.700	0	0.000	0.190	0.020	2.100	0.744	19.300	0.000	33.000	100	0.035	1.820	0.193
85.000	23.800	1.300	0.700	0	0.000	0.200	0.110	1.500	0.090	16.800	0.000	11.000	70.000	0.085	0.980	0.084
129	16.500	1.480	0.653	28	0.000	0.180	0.240	1.460	0.054	14.300	0.365	154	135	—	—	—
109	28.800	3.300	0.800	0	0.000	0.740	0.460	6.100	0.069	24.200	0.000	18.000	100	0.005	3.230	0.046
—	—	—	—	—	—	—	—	—	—	—	—	—	—	—	—	0.302
51.000	21.000	0.500	0.240	—	0.000	0.030	0.030	0.040	0.100	4.000	0.000	30.000	59.000	—	1.850	—
—	—	—	—	—	0.000	—	—	—	—	—	—	—	—	0.001	—	0.017
—	—	—	—	5.2	—	—	—	—	—	—	—	—	—	0.000	—	0.007

Continued.

A

Nutritive Components for Grains—cont'd.

Food Name	Serving Portion	WT. Gm	KCAL Kc	PROT Gm	CARB Gm	FAT Gm	CHOL Mg	SAFA Gm	MUFA Gm	PUFA Gm	SOD Mg
CROUTONS-HERB SEASONED	1.000 CUP	30.000	100	4.290	20.000	0.000	—	0.000	0.000	0.000	372
TORTILLA-FLOUR	1.000 ITEM	30.000	95.000	2.500	17.300	1.800	—	—	—	—	—
CRACKERS-CHEESE	1.000 ITEM	1.000	5.380	0.091	0.520	0.327	—	0.090	—	—	12.000
CRACKERS-GRAHAM-SUG/HONEY	1.000 ITEM	7.000	30.100	0.519	5.400	0.732	—	0.300	—	—	32.900
FRENCH TOAST-HOME RECIPE	1.000 SLICE	65.000	153	5.670	17.200	6.730	—	—	—	—	257
CORN CHIPS	1.000 SERVING	28.400	155	1.700	16.900	9.140	0.000	1.500	3.390	4.250	164
TACO SHELLS	1.000 ITEM	11.000	49.800	0.967	7.240	2.150	—	—	—	—	—
TORTILLA-CORN	1.000 ITEM	30.000	67.200	2.150	12.800	1.140	—	—	—	—	53.400
WAFFLES-FROZEN	1.000 ITEM	37.000	103	2.150	15.900	3.520	—	—	—	—	256
CRACKERS-RY KRISP-NATURAL	1.000 ITEM	2.100	7.500	0.250	1.670	0.033	0.000	—	—	—	18.500
CRACKERS-ANIMAL	1.000 ITEM	1.900	8.670	0.127	1.470	0.200	—	—	—	—	7.530
CRACKERS-CHEDDAR SNACKS	1.000 ITEM	1.600	7.220	0.144	1.110	0.261	—	—	—	—	14.300
RICE-BROWN-UNCLE BEN'S	1.000 CUP	146	220	5.000	46.400	1.820	0.000	—	—	—	2.400
SHAKE'N BAKE	1.000 SERVING	28.400	116	2.440	17.700	4.260	—	—	—	—	984
CRACKERS-RITZ	1.000 ITEM	3.330	18.000	0.233	2.130	0.967	—	—	—	—	32.300
STUFFING-MIX-DRY FORM	1.000 CUP	30.000	111	3.900	21.700	1.100	—	—	—	—	399
STUFFING-MIX-PREPARED	1.000 CUP	140	501	9.100	49.800	30.500	—	—	—	—	1254
RICE CAKE-REGULAR	1.000 ITEM	9.310	35.000	0.700	7.600	0.280	—	—	—	—	10.800
NOODLES-RAMEN-ORIENTAL	1.000 CUP	227	207	5.900	30.700	8.600	—	—	—	—	829

Nutritive Components for Meats

Food Name	Serving Portion	WT. Gm	KCAL Kc	PROT Gm	CARB Gm	FAT Gm	CHOL Mg	SAFA Gm	MUFA Gm	PUFA Gm	SOD Mg
BACON-PORK-BROILED/FRIED	1.000 SLICE	6.300	36.300	1.930	0.036	3.120	5.330	1.100	1.500	0.367	101
ROAST BEEF-RIB-LEAN/FAT	1.000 SLICE	85.000	308	18.300	0.000	25.500	73.000	10.800	11.400	0.900	52.000
ROAST BEEF-RIB-LEAN	1.000 SLICE	51.000	122	13.900	0.000	7.030	41.300	2.960	3.060	0.209	37.700
STEAK-SIRLOIN-LEAN/FAT	1.000 ITEM	85.000	271	22.700	0.000	19.400	77.000	8.070	8.670	0.770	52.000
STEAK-SIRLOIN-LEAN-BROILED	1.000 ITEM	56.000	133	17.000	0.000	6.630	50.000	2.710	2.920	0.280	37.000
STEAK-ROUND-LEAN/FAT	1.000 SERVING	85.000	179	26.200	0.000	7.490	72.000	2.800	3.080	0.330	51.000
CORNED BEEF HASH-CANNED	1.000 CUP	220	400	19.000	24.000	25.000	50.000	11.900	—	—	1188
LAMB-CHOP-LEAN/FAT-BROILED	1.000 ITEM	89.000	360	18.000	0.000	32.000	86.000	14.800	6.800	1.000	62.000
LAMB-CHOP/RIB-LEAN-BROILED	1.000 ITEM	57.000	120	16.000	0.000	6.000	56.000	2.500	2.150	0.336	39.000
LAMB-LEG-LEAN/FAT-ROASTED	1.000 SLICE	85.000	235	22.000	0.000	16.000	82.000	7.300	—	—	59.000
BEEF-LIVER-FRIED/MARG	1.000 SLICE	85.000	184	22.700	6.680	6.800	410	2.400	1.460	1.530	90.000
HAM-REG-ROASTED-PORK	1.000 CUP	140	249	31.700	0.000	12.600	83.000	4.360	6.220	1.980	2100
HAM-REG-LUNCH MEAT-11% FAT	1.000 SLICE	28.400	52.000	4.980	0.880	3.000	16.000	0.960	1.400	0.340	373
PORK-CHOP-LEAN/FAT-BROILED	1.000 ITEM	82.000	284	19.300	0.000	22.300	77.000	8.060	10.200	2.530	54.000
PORK-CHOP-LEAN-BROILED	1.000 ITEM	66.000	169	18.400	0.000	10.100	63.000	3.480	4.530	1.230	49.000
PORK-LOIN-LEAN/FAT-ROAST	1.000 ITEM	88.000	268	22.400	0.000	19.100	80.000	6.920	8.760	2.180	56.000
PORK-LOIN-LEAN-ROASTED	1.000 SLICE	72.000	180	21.400	0.000	9.810	68.000	3.380	4.410	1.190	52.000
PORK-TENDERLOIN-LEAN-ROAST	1.000 SERVING	28.400	47.000	8.160	0.000	1.360	26.300	0.470	0.613	0.163	19.000
BOLOGNA-PORK	1.000 SLICE	23.000	57.000	3.520	0.170	4.570	14.000	1.580	2.250	0.490	272
BRAUNSCHWEIGER-SAUS-PORK	1.000 SLICE	18.000	65.000	2.430	0.560	5.780	28.000	1.960	2.680	0.670	206
SAUSAGE-PATTY-PORK-COOKED	1.000 ITEM	27.000	100	5.310	0.280	8.410	22.000	2.920	3.750	1.030	349
DEVILED HAM-CANNED	1.000 TBSP	13.000	45.000	2.000	0.000	4.000	10.000	1.500	—	—	160
FRANKFURTER-HOT DOG-NO BUN	1.000 ITEM	57.000	183	6.430	1.460	16.600	29.000	6.130	7.790	1.560	639
SAUSAGE-LINK-PORK-COOKED	1.000 ITEM	13.000	48.000	2.550	0.130	4.050	11.000	1.400	1.810	0.500	168
SALAMI-DRY OR HARD-PORK	1.000 SLICE	10.000	41.000	2.260	0.160	3.370	8.000	1.190	1.600	0.370	226
SALAMI-COOKED-BEEF	1.000 SLICE	23.000	58.000	3.380	0.570	4.620	14.000	1.940	2.140	0.200	266
ITALIAN SAUSAGE-PORK-LINK	1.000 ITEM	67.000	217	13.400	1.010	17.200	52.000	6.050	8.010	2.200	618
CANADIAN BACON-PORT-GRILL	1.000 SLICE	23.300	43.000	5.640	0.315	1.960	13.500	0.660	0.940	0.185	360
LIVERWURST/LIVER SAUS-PORK	1.000 SLICE	18.000	59.000	2.540	0.400	5.140	28.000	1.910	2.400	0.470	215
POLISH SAUSAGE-PORK	1.000 ITEM	227	740	32.000	3.700	65.200	159	23.400	30.600	6.990	1989
KIELBASA-PORK/BEEF	1.000 SLICE	26.000	81.000	3.450	0.560	7.060	17.000	2.580	3.360	0.800	280
KNOCKWURST-PORK/BEEF-LINK	1.000 ITEM	68.000	209	8.080	1.200	18.900	39.000	6.940	8.710	1.980	687
MORTADELLA-PORK/BEEF	1.000 SLICE	15.000	47.000	2.460	0.460	3.810	8.000	1.430	1.710	0.470	187

OT Mg	MAG Mg	IRON Mg	ZINC Mg	V-A RE	V-C Mg	THIA Mg	RIBO Mg	NIAC Mg	V-B6 Mg	FOL Ug	V-B12 Ug	CALC Mg	PHOS Mg	SEL Mg	FIBD Gm	V-ET mg
38.600	11.400	1.540	0.300	0	—	0.129	0.200	1.720	0.000	0.000	—	—	—	—	—	—
—	7.000	1.100	—	0.2	0.000	0.010	0.080	1.000	—	—	—	46.000	25.000	—	—	—
1.860	0.220	0.035	0.010	—	0.000	0.004	0.004	0.082	—	—	—	1.050	2.100	0.000	0.025	0.003
11.700	2.310	0.183	0.053	0	0.000	0.024	0.019	0.218	0.006	0.910	0.000	2.660	8.260	0.001	0.200	0.026
85.800	11.700	1.340	0.553	22.2	0.000	0.124	0.163	1.010	0.038	17.600	0.291	72.200	84.500	—	—	—
43.300	21.900	0.376	0.435	—	—	0.048	0.026	0.554	0.054	—	0.000	37.100	54.600	—	1.660	—
—	11.400	0.286	0.142	—	—	0.032	0.017	0.189	—	—	0.000	15.600	25.400	—	—	—
52.200	19.500	0.570	0.426	—	0.000	0.048	0.030	0.384	0.091	5.700	0.000	42.000	54.900	—	1.090	—
77.700	7.770	1.800	0.303	95	0.000	0.167	0.200	1.930	0.098	0.740	—	30.000	141	—	—	—
10.200	2.500	0.092	0.057	—	—	0.006	0.005	0.033	0.007	0.833	—	0.833	6.830	0.001	0.280	0.008
1.670	0.267	0.059	0.009	0	0.000	0.005	0.009	0.073	0.000	0.200	0.001	0.200	1.200	0.000	0.027	0.007
2.170	0.278	0.068	0.012	0.18	0.000	0.009	0.007	0.067	0.001	0.222	0.009	1.220	1.890	0.001	—	0.006
172	—	0.900	—	—	0.000	0.180	0.040	4.200	—	—	—	16.000	222	0.057	4.820	0.993
56.800	—	0.710	—	62	0.284	0.162	0.184	2.190	—	—	—	13.900	43.500	—	—	—
2.670	—	0.100	—	—	—	0.013	0.013	0.100	—	—	—	5.000	8.000	—	—	0.012
52.000	—	1.000	—	0	0.000	0.070	0.080	1.000	—	—	—	37.000	57.000	—	—	—
126	—	2.200	—	91	0.000	0.130	0.170	2.100	—	—	—	92.000	136	—	—	—
27.200	—	—	—	—	—	—	—	—	—	—	—	—	—	—	—	—
—	—	—	—	—	—	—	—	—	—	—	—	—	—	—	2.040	—

OT Mg	MAG Mg	IRON Mg	ZINC Mg	V-A RE	V-C Mg	THIA Mg	RIBO Mg	NIAC Mg	V-B6 Mg	FOL Ug	V-B12 Ug	CALC Mg	PHOS Mg	SEL Mg	FIBD Gm	V-ET mg
30.700	1.670	0.103	0.206	0	2.130	0.044	0.018	0.464	0.017	0.333	0.110	0.667	21.300	0.002	0.000	0.033
257	17.000	1.770	4.270	0	0.000	0.065	0.146	2.650	0.250	5.000	2.370	10.000	140	0.020	0.000	0.119
192	12.800	1.330	3.540	0	0.000	0.042	0.107	2.100	0.153	4.080	1.490	5.100	109	0.012	0.000	0.092
297	23.000	2.490	4.730	15	0.000	0.092	0.218	3.210	0.330	7.000	2.220	9.000	180	0.029	0.000	0.111
226	17.900	1.880	3.650	3	0.000	0.071	0.165	2.400	0.252	5.600	1.600	6.160	137	0.019	0.000	0.073
365	26.000	2.390	4.590	0	0.000	0.097	0.221	4.980	0.460	10.000	2.080	5.000	203	0.029	0.000	0.111
440	—	4.400	—	—	—	0.020	0.200	4.600	—	—	—	29.000	147	—	0.000	0.066
200	15.100	1.000	3.500	0	—	0.110	0.190	4.100	0.245	2.670	1.800	8.000	139	0.016	0.000	0.142
174	12.500	1.100	2.480	0	—	0.090	0.150	3.400	0.157	1.710	1.230	6.000	121	0.010	0.000	0.091
241	17.000	1.400	3.500	—	—	0.130	0.230	4.700	0.234	2.550	1.830	9.000	177	0.015	0.000	0.043
309	20.000	5.340	4.630	9216	19.400	0.179	3.520	12.300	1.220	187	95.000	9.000	392	0.042	0.000	0.536
573	30.000	1.880	3.460	0	31.700	1.020	0.462	8.610	0.430	—	0.980	12.000	393	0.066	0.000	0.392
94.000	5.000	0.280	0.610	0	8.000	0.244	0.071	1.490	0.100	1.000	0.240	2.000	70.000	0.013	0.000	—
287	20.000	0.660	2.010	2.1	0.200	0.690	0.294	4.320	0.310	4.000	0.810	5.000	193	0.014	0.000	0.131
276	19.000	0.610	1.930	1.5	0.200	0.641	0.278	3.930	0.300	4.000	0.710	5.000	184	0.011	0.000	0.106
284	17.000	0.870	1.800	2.1	0.300	0.727	0.210	4.440	0.350	1.000	0.530	5.000	173	0.028	0.000	0.139
271	16.000	0.820	1.710	1.8	0.300	0.681	0.196	4.090	0.340	0.000	0.450	4.000	164	0.023	0.000	0.114
152	7.000	0.437	0.850	0.601	0.100	0.266	0.111	1.330	0.120	1.670	0.157	2.330	81.700	0.009	0.000	0.113
65.000	3.000	0.180	0.470	0	8.100	0.120	0.036	0.897	0.060	1.000	0.210	3.000	32.000	0.003	0.000	0.014
36.000	2.000	1.680	0.510	759	2.000	0.045	0.275	1.510	0.060	—	3.620	2.000	30.000	0.002	0.000	0.063
97.000	5.000	0.340	0.680	0	0.000	0.200	0.069	1.220	0.090	—	0.470	9.000	50.000	0.003	0.000	0.043
—	1.690	0.300	0.238	0	—	0.020	0.010	0.200	0.042	—	0.091	1.000	12.000	0.002	0.000	—
95.000	6.000	0.660	1.050	0	15.000	0.113	0.068	1.500	0.080	2.000	0.740	6.000	49.000	0.013	0.000	0.080
47.000	2.000	0.160	0.330	0	0.000	0.096	0.033	0.587	0.040	—	0.220	4.000	24.000	0.004	0.000	0.021
—	2.000	0.130	0.420	0	—	0.093	0.033	0.560	0.060	—	0.280	1.000	23.000	0.002	0.000	0.011
52.000	3.000	0.460	0.490	0	3.000	0.029	0.059	0.785	0.050	0.000	1.110	2.000	23.000	0.004	0.000	0.025
204	12.000	1.010	1.590	0	1.300	0.417	0.156	2.790	0.220	—	0.870	16.000	114	0.022	0.000	0.107
90.500	5.000	0.190	0.395	0	5.000	0.192	0.046	1.610	0.105	1.000	0.180	2.500	69.000	0.003	0.000	—
—	—	1.150	—	—	—	0.049	0.185	—	0.030	5.000	2.420	5.000	41.000	0.003	0.000	0.063
538	31.800	3.270	4.380	0	2.270	1.140	0.336	7.820	0.431	—	2.220	27.200	309	0.066	0.000	0.363
70.000	4.000	0.380	0.520	0	6.000	0.059	0.056	0.749	0.050	—	0.420	11.000	38.000	0.004	0.000	0.042
136	8.000	0.620	1.130	0	18.000	0.233	0.095	1.860	0.110	—	0.800	7.000	67.000	0.010	0.000	—
24.000	2.000	0.210	0.320	0	4.000	0.018	0.023	0.401	0.019	—	0.220	3.000	15.000	0.002	—	0.024

Continued.

A

Nutritive Components for Meats—cont'd.

Food Name	Serving Portion	WT. Gm	KCAL Kc	PROT Gm	CARB Gm	FAT Gm	CHOL Mg	SAFA Gm	MUFA Gm	PUFA Gm	SOD Mg
POT ROAST-ARM-BEEF-COOKED	1.000 SLICE	100	231	33.000	0.000	9.980	101	3.790	4.350	0.400	66.000
STEAK-RIB-COOKED	1.000 ITEM	100	225	28.000	0.000	11.600	80.000	4.930	5.100	0.350	69.000
BACON BITS	1.000 TBSP	6.000	26.600	1.920	1.720	1.550	0.000	—	—	—	165
SPARERIBS-PORK-BRAISED	1.000 SERVING	28.400	113	8.230	0.000	8.580	34.300	3.330	4.010	0.997	26.300
HAMBURGER-GROUND-REG-BAKED	1.000 SERVING	85.000	244	19.600	0.000	17.800	74.000	6.990	7.790	0.660	51.000
HAMBURGER-GROUND-REG-FRIED	1.000 SERVING	85.000	260	20.300	0.000	19.200	75.000	7.530	8.390	0.710	71.000

Food Name	Serving Portion	WT. Gm	KCAL Kc	PROT Gm	CARB Gm	FAT Gm	CHOL Mg	SAFA Gm	MUFA Gm	PUFA Gm	SOD Mg
PICKLE/HOT DOG RELISH	1.000 SERVING	28.400	35.000	0.000	8.000	0.000	0.000	0.000	0.000	0.000	200
PICKLE/HAMBURGER RELISH	1.000 SERVING	28.400	30.000	0.000	7.000	0.000	0.000	0.000	0.000	0.000	325
VINEGAR-CIDER	1.000 TBSP	15.000	0.000	0.000	1.000	0.000	0.000	0.000	0.000	0.000	0.125
YEAST-BAKER-DRY-ACT-PACKET	1.000 SERVING	7.000	20.000	3.000	3.000	0.000	0.000	0.000	0.000	0.000	1.000
YEAST-BREWERS-DRY	1.000 TBSP	8.000	25.000	3.000	3.000	0.000	0.000	—	—	—	9.000
BAKING POWDER-HOME USE	1.000 TSP	3.000	5.000	0.000	1.000	0.000	0.000	0.000	0.000	0.000	339
BAKING POWDER-LOW SODIUM	1.000 TSP	4.300	5.000	0.000	2.000	0.000	0.000	0.000	0.000	0.000	0.000
GELATIN-DRY-ENVELOPE	1.000 ITEM	7.000	25.000	6.000	0.000	0.000	0.000	0.000	0.000	0.000	8.000
GELATIN DESSERT-PREP	1.000 CUP	240	140	4.000	34.000	0.000	0.000	0.000	0.000	0.000	0.000
OLIVES-GREEN-PICKLED-CAN	1.000 ITEM	4.000	3.750	0.100	0.100	0.500	0.000	0.050	0.350	0.035	80.800
OLIVES-MISSION-RIPE-CAN	1.000 ITEM	3.000	5.000	0.100	0.100	0.667	0.000	0.067	0.410	0.034	19.200
PICKLE-DILL-CUCUMBER-MED	1.000 ITEM	65.000	5.000	0.000	1.000	0.000	0.000	0.000	0.000	0.000	928
PICKLE-FRESH PACK-CUCUMBER	1.000 ITEM	7.500	5.000	0.000	1.500	0.000	0.000	0.000	0.000	0.000	50.000
PICKLE-SWEET/GHERKIN-SMALL	1.000 ITEM	15.000	20.000	0.000	5.000	0.000	0.000	0.000	0.000	0.000	128
PICKLE-RELISH-SWEET	1.000 TBSP	15.000	20.000	0.000	5.000	0.000	0.000	0.000	0.000	0.000	124
POPSICLE	1.000 ITEM	95.000	70.000	0.000	18.000	0.000	0.000	0.000	0.000	0.000	0.000
CHILI POWDER	1.000 TSP	2.600	8.000	0.320	1.420	0.440	0.000	—	—	—	26.000
CINNAMON-GROUND	1.000 TSP	2.300	6.000	0.090	1.840	0.070	0.000	0.010	0.010	0.010	1.000
OREGANO-GROUND	1.000 TSP	1.500	5.000	0.170	0.970	0.150	0.000	0.040	0.010	0.080	0.225
PAPRIKA	1.000 TSP	2.100	6.000	0.310	1.170	0.270	0.000	0.040	0.030	0.170	1.000
PARSLEY-DRIED	1.000 TSP	0.300	1.000	0.070	0.150	0.010	0.000	—	—	—	1.000
PEPPER-BLACK	1.000 TSP	2.100	5.000	0.230	1.360	0.070	0.000	0.020	0.020	0.020	1.000
SALT-TABLE SALT	1.000 TSP	5.000	0.000	0.000	0.000	0.000	0.000	0.000	0.000	0.000	1955
BAKING SODA	1.000 TSP	3.000	0.000	0.000	0.000	0.000	0.000	0.000	0.000	0.000	821
JELLO-GEL-SUGAR FREE-PREP	1.000 CUP	240	16.000	2.000	0.000	0.000	0.000	0.000	0.000	0.000	120
GEL-D ZERTA-LOW CAL-PREP	1.000 CUP	240	16.000	4.000	0.000	0.000	0.000	0.000	0.000	0.000	—
CHEWING GUM-WRIGLEYS	1.000 ITEM	3.000	10.000	0.000	2.300	—	0.000	—	—	—	0.000
VINEGAR-DISTILLED	1.000 CUP	240	29.000	0.000	12.000	0.000	—	0.000	0.000	0.000	2.000
CHEWING GUM-CANDY COATED	1.000 ITEM	1.700	5.000	—	1.600	—	—	—	—	—	—

Food Name	Serving Portion	WT. Gm	KCAL Kc	PROT Gm	CARB Gm	FAT Gm	CHOL Mg	SAFA Gm	MUFA Gm	PUFA Gm	SOD Mg
NUTS-ALMOND-SHELLED-SLIVER	1.000 CUP	115	677	22.900	23.500	60.000	0.000	5.690	39.000	12.600	12.700
NUTS-BRAZIL-DRIED-SHELLED	1.000 CUP	140	919	20.100	17.900	92.700	0.000	22.600	32.200	33.800	2.000
NUTS-COCONUT-DRI-FLAKE-CAN	1.000 CUP	77.000	341	2.580	31.500	24.400	0.000	21.600	1.040	0.267	15.000
NUTS-FILBERT/HAZEL-DRI-CHOP	1.000 CUP	115	727	15.000	17.600	72.000	0.000	5.300	56.500	6.900	3.000
NUTS-PEANUTS-OIL ROASTED	1.000 CUP	145	840	38.800	26.700	71.300	0.000	9.900	35.500	22.600	22.000
PEANUT BUTTER-SMOOTH TYPE	1.000 TBSP	16.000	95.000	4.560	2.530	8.180	0.000	1.360	3.950	2.460	75.000
NUTS-PECANS-DRIED-HALVES	1.000 CUP	108	721	8.370	19.700	73.100	0.000	5.850	45.500	18.100	1.000
NUTS-WALNUT-BLACK-DRI-CHOP	1.000 CUP	125	759	30.400	15.100	70.700	0.000	4.540	15.900	46.900	2.000
NUTS-WALNUT-PERSIAN/ENGLISH	1.000 CUP	120	770	17.200	22.000	74.200	0.000	6.700	17.000	47.000	12.000
ALFALFA SEEDS-SPROUTED-RAW	1.000 CUP	33.000	10.000	1.320	1.250	0.230	0.000	0.023	0.018	0.135	2.000

POT Mg	MAG Mg	IRON Mg	ZINC Mg	V-A RE	V-C Mg	THIA Mg	RIBO Mg	NIAC Mg	V-B6 Mg	FOL Ug	V-B12 Ug	CALC Mg	PHOS Mg	SEL Mg	FIBD Gm	V-ET mg
289	24.000	3.790	8.660	0	0.000	0.081	0.289	3.720	0.330	11.000	3.400	9.000	268	0.006	0.000	0.140
394	27.000	2.570	6.990	0	0.000	0.105	0.216	4.800	0.400	8.000	3.320	13.000	208	0.006	0.000	0.092
—	—	0.300		0	0.180	0.025	0.018	0.138	—	—		8.400	18.100			
90.700	7.000	0.527	1.300	0.901	—	0.116	0.108	1.550	0.100	1.330	0.307	13.300	74.000	0.005	0.000	0.045
188	13.000	2.050	4.160	0	0.000	0.026	0.136	4.040	0.200	7.000	1.990	8.000	117	—	0.000	0.375
255	17.000	2.080	4.310	0	0.000	0.026	0.170	4.960	0.200	8.000	2.300	10.000	145	—	0.000	0.315

POT Mg	MAG Mg	IRON Mg	ZINC Mg	V-A RE	V-C Mg	THIA Mg	RIBO Mg	NIAC Mg	V-B6 Mg	FOL Ug	V-B12 Ug	CALC Mg	PHOS Mg	SEL Mg	FIBD Gm	V-ET mg
—	—	0.189	—	—	—	—	—	—	—	—	—	5.600	3.700	0.000		
—	—	0.189	—	—	—	—	—	—	—	—	—	5.670	3.780	0.000		
15.000	—	0.100	0.020	—	—	—	—	—	0.000	—	—	1.000	1.000	—	0.000	
140	3.780	1.100	—	0	0.000	0.160	0.380	2.600	0.140	286	0.000	3.000	90.000	0.000	—	0.006
152	18.400	1.400	—	0	0.000	1.250	0.340	3.000	0.200	313	0.000	17.000	140	0.000	—	—
5.000	—	—	—	0	0.000	0.000	0.000	0.000	—	—	—	58.000	87.000	0.000	0.000	—
471	—	—	—	0	0.000	0.000	0.000	0.000	—	—	—	207	314	0.000	0.000	—
180	—	0.400	—	—	4.000	0.000	0.000	0.000	0.000	—	—	0.000	0.000	—	0.000	—
—	—	—	—	—	—	—	—	—	—	—	—	—	—	—	0.000	
1.750	—	0.050	—	1	—	—	—	—	—	0.040	0.000	2.000	0.500	0.000	0.080	—
0.667	—	0.033	0.010	1	—	0.000	0.000	—	0.000	0.033	0.000	3.000	0.333	0.000	0.060	—
130	7.800	0.700	0.176	7	4.000	0.000	0.010	0.000	0.005	0.650	0.000	17.000	14.000	0.000	—	—
—	—	0.150	0.020	1	0.500	0.000	0.000	0.000	0.001	0.075	0.000	2.500	2.000	0.000	—	—
—	0.150	0.200	0.020	1	1.000	0.000	0.000	0.000	0.001	0.150	0.000	2.000	2.000	0.000	—	—
—	—	0.100	0.010	—	—	—	—	—	—	—	—	3.000	2.000	0.000	—	—
—	—	0.000	—	0	0.000	0.000	0.000	0.000	—	—	—	0.000	—	—	—	—
50.000	4.000	0.370	0.070	908	1.670	0.009	0.021	0.205	—	—	0.000	7.000	8.000	0.001	—	—
11.000	1.000	0.880	0.050	6.000	0.650	0.002	0.003	0.030	—	—	0.000	28.000	1.000	0.001	—	—
25.000	4.000	0.660	0.070	104	—	0.005	—	0.093	—	—	0.000	24.000	3.000	—	—	—
49.000	4.000	0.500	0.080	1273	1.490	0.014	0.037	0.322	—	—	0.000	4.000	7.000	0.000	—	—
11.000	1.000	0.290	0.010	70.000	0.370	0.001	0.004	0.024	0.003	—	0.000	4.000	1.000	—	—	—
26.000	4.000	0.610	0.030	4.000	—	0.002	0.005	0.024	—	—	0.000	9.000	4.000	0.000	0.500	—
0.300	0.000	0.000	—	0.000	0.000	0.000	0.000	0.000	0.000	0.000	0.000	14.000	2.000	—	—	0.000
—	—	—	—	0	0.000	0.000	0.000	0.000	0.000	0.000	0.000	—	—	—	0.000	
—	—	—	—	—	—	—	—	—	—	—	—	—	—	—	0.000	
—	—	—	—	—	—	—	—	—	—	—	—	—	—	—	0.000	
0.000	0.000	0.000	0.000	0	0.000	0.000	0.000	0.000	0.000	0.000	0.000	3.000	0.000	—	—	—
36.000	0.000													0.074	—	—
—	—	—	—	—	0.000	0.000	0.000	0.000								

POT Mg	MAG Mg	IRON Mg	ZINC Mg	V-A RE	V-C Mg	THIA Mg	RIBO Mg	NIAC Mg	V-B6 Mg	FOL Ug	V-B12 Ug	CALC Mg	PHOS Mg	SEL Mg	FIBD Gm	V-ET mg
842	340	4.210	3.360	0	0.690	0.243	0.896	3.870	0.130	67.500	0.000	306	598	0.005	10.700	27.600
840	315	4.760	6.420	—	1.000	1.400	0.171	2.270	0.351	5.600	0.000	246	840	0.144	10.800	8.970
249	38.000	1.420	1.230	0	0.000	0.023	0.015	0.235	—	—	0.000	11.000	79.000	—	4.400	0.539
512	328	3.760	2.760	7.7	1.200	0.575	0.127	1.300	0.704	82.600	0.000	216	359	0.002	9.770	27.300
1020	273	2.780	9.600	0	0.000	0.425	0.146	21.500	0.576	153	0.000	125	733	0.055	11.100	9.990
110	28.000	0.290	0.470	—	0.000	0.024	0.017	2.150	0.062	13.100	0.000	5.000	60.000	0.002	1.400	1.120
423	138	2.300	5.910	13.8	2.100	0.916	0.138	0.958	0.203	42.300	0.000	39.000	314	0.003	8.300	3.350
655	252	3.840	4.280	37	—	0.271	0.136	0.863	—	—	—	72.000	580	0.024	11.800	1.050
602	203	2.930	3.280	14.8	3.900	0.458	0.178	1.250	0.670	79.200	0.000	113	380	0.023	—	3.140
26.000	9.000	0.320	0.300	511.000	2.700	0.025	0.042	0.159	0.011	12.200	0.000	10.000	23.000	—	0.726	—

Continued

A

Nutritive Components for Nuts and Seeds—cont'd.

Food Name	Serving Portion	WT. Gm	KCAL Kc	PROT Gm	CARB Gm	FAT Gm	CHOL Mg	SAFA Gm	MUFA Gm	PUFA Gm	SOD Mg
NUTS-CASHEWS-DRY ROASTED	1.000 CUP	137	787	21.000	44.800	63.500	0.000	12.500	37.400	10.700	21.000
NUTS-CHESTNUTS-ROASTED	1.000 SERVING	28.400	68.000	1.270	14.900	0.340	0.000	0.050	0.176	0.087	1.000
NUTS-COCONUT-DRIED-SHRED	1.000 CUP	93.000	466	2.680	44.300	33.000	0.000	29.300	1.400	0.361	244
NUTS-COCONUT CREAM-RAW	1.000 CUP	240	792	8.700	16.000	83.200	0.000	73.800	3.540	0.910	10.000
NUTS-MACADAMIA-DRIED	1.000 CUP	134	940	11.100	18.400	98.800	0.000	14.800	77.900	1.700	6.000
NUTS-MIXED-DRY ROASTED	1.000 CUP	137	814	23.700	34.700	70.500	0.000	9.450	43.000	14.800	16.000
NUTS-MIXED-OIL ROASTED	1.000 CUP	142	876	23.800	30.400	80.000	0.000	12.400	45.000	18.900	16.000
NUTS-PEANUTS-SPANISH-DRIED	1.000 CUP	146	827	37.500	23.600	71.800	0.000	9.960	35.600	22.700	23.000
NUTS-PECANS-OIL ROASTED	1.000 CUP	110	754	7.650	17.700	78.300	0.000	6.270	48.800	19.400	1.000
NUTS-PISTACHIO-DRIED	1.000 CUP	128	739	26.300	31.800	61.900	0.000	7.840	41.800	9.360	7.000
NUTS-PISTACHIO-DRY ROASTED	1.000 CUP	128	776	19.100	35.200	67.600	0.000	8.560	45.600	10.200	8.000
SEEDS-PUMPKIN/SQUASH-ROAST	1.000 CUP	64.000	285	11.900	34.400	12.400	0.000	2.350	3.860	5.660	12.000
SEEDS-SESAME-ROASTED-WHOLE	1.000 SERVING	28.400	161	4.820	7.310	13.600	0.000	1.910	5.150	5.980	3.000
SEEDS-SUNFLOWER-OIL ROAST	1.000 CUP	135	830	28.800	19.900	77.600	0.000	8.130	14.800	51.200	4.000
PEANUT BUTTER-LOW SODIUM	1.000 TBSP	16.000	95.000	5.000	2.500	8.500	0.000	—	—	—	5.000
NUTS-PEANUTS-OIL-SALTED	1.000 CUP	145	841	38.800	26.800	71.300	0.000	9.930	35.500	22.600	626
PEANUT BUTTER-CHUNK STYLE	1.000 CUP	258	1520	62.000	55.700	129	0.000	24.700	60.800	37.000	1255
PEANUT BUTTER-OLD FASHION	1.000 TBSP	16.000	95.000	4.200	2.700	8.100	0.000	1.500	—	2.700	75.000

Nutritive Components for Poultry

Food Name	Serving Portion	WT. Gm	KCAL Kc	PROT Gm	CARB Gm	FAT Gm	CHOL Mg	SAFA Gm	MUFA Gm	PUFA Gm	SOD Mg
CHICKEN-BREAST-FRIED FLOUR	1.000 ITEM	196	436	62.400	3.220	17.400	176	4.800	6.860	3.840	150
CHICKEN-DRUMSTICK-FRIED	1.000 ITEM	49.000	120	13.200	0.800	6.720	44.000	1.790	2.660	1.580	44.000
CHICKEN-BREAST-FRI/BATTER	1.000 ITEM	280	728	69.600	25.200	36.900	238	9.860	15.300	8.620	770
CHICKEN A LA KING-HOME REC	1.000 CUP	245	470	27.000	12.000	34.000	186	12.900	13.400	6.200	759
CHICKEN CHOW MEIN-CANNED	1.000 CUP	250	95.000	7.000	18.000	0.000	98.000	0.000	0.000	0.000	722
CHICKEN POTPIE-BAKED-HOME	1.000 SLICE	232	545	23.000	42.000	31.000	72.000	11.000	13.500	5.500	593
TURKEY-DARK MEAT-NO SKIN	1.000 CUP	140	262	40.000	0.000	10.100	119	3.400	2.290	3.030	110
TURKEY-LIGHT-NO SKIN-ROAST	1.000 CUP	140	219	41.900	0.000	4.500	97.000	1.440	0.790	1.200	89.000
TURKEY-LIGHT/DARK-NO SKIN	1.000 CUP	140	238	41.000	0.000	6.950	107	2.290	1.450	2.000	99.000
TURK-BREAST-NO SKIN-ROAST	1.000 ITEM	612	826	184	0.000	4.500	510	1.440	0.780	1.200	318
CHICKEN-GIBLETS-FRI/FLOUR	1.000 CUP	145	402	47.200	6.310	19.500	647	5.500	6.410	4.900	164
CHICKEN-GIBLETS-SIMMERED	1.000 CUP	145	228	37.500	1.370	6.920	570	2.160	1.730	1.560	85.000
CHICKEN-LIVER-SIMMERED	1.000 CUP	140	219	34.100	1.230	7.630	883	2.580	1.880	1.250	71.000
CHICKEN-BREAST-ROASTED	1.000 ITEM	196	386	58.400	0.000	15.300	166	4.300	5.940	3.260	138
CHICKEN-BREAST-STEWED	1.000 ITEM	220	404	60.300	0.000	16.300	166	4.580	6.380	3.480	136
CHICKEN-BREAST-N0 SKIN-FRI	1.000 ITEM	172	322	57.500	0.880	8.100	156	2.220	2.960	1.840	136
CHICK-BREAST-NO SKIN-ROAST	1.000 ITEM	172	284	53.400	0.000	6.140	146	1.740	2.140	1.320	126
CHICKEN-LEG-ROASTED	1.000 ITEM	114	265	29.600	0.000	15.400	105	4.240	5.970	3.420	99.000
CHICKEN-LEG-NO SKIN-ROAST	1.000 ITEM	95.000	182	25.700	0.000	8.010	89.000	2.180	2.900	1.870	87.000
CHICKEN-LEG-NO SKIN-STEWED	1.000 ITEM	101	187	26.500	0.000	8.140	90.000	2.220	2.950	1.900	78.000
CHICKEN-THIGH-FRIED/FLOUR	1.000 ITEM	62.000	162	16.600	1.970	9.290	60.000	2.540	3.640	2.110	55.000
CHICK-THIGH-NO SKIN-ROAST	1.000 ITEM	52.000	109	13.500	0.000	5.660	49.000	1.570	2.160	1.290	46.000
CHICKEN-WING-FRIED/FLOUR	1.000 ITEM	32.000	103	8.360	0.760	7.090	26.000	1.940	2.840	1.580	25.000
CHICKEN-WING-ROASTED	1.000 ITEM	34.000	99.000	9.130	0.000	6.620	29.000	1.850	2.600	1.410	28.000
CHICKEN-WING-STEWED	1.000 ITEM	40.000	100	9.110	0.000	6.730	28.000	1.880	2.640	1.430	27.000
DUCK-FLESH & SKIN-ROASTED	1.000 ITEM	764	2574	145	0.000	217	640	73.900	98.600	27.900	454
DUCK-NO SKIN-ROASTED	1.000 ITEM	442	890	104	0.000	49.500	396	18.400	16.400	6.300	286
CHICKEN-FRANKFURTER	1.000 ITEM	45.000	116	5.820	3.060	8.760	45.000	2.490	3.810	1.820	617
CHICKEN-LIVER PATE-CAN	1.000 TBSP	13.000	26.000	1.750	0.850	1.700	—	—	—	—	—
CHICKEN ROLL-LIGHT	1.000 SLICE	28.400	45.000	5.540	0.695	2.090	14.000	0.575	0.840	0.455	166
CHICKEN SPREAD-CANNED	1.000 TBSP	13.000	25.000	2.000	0.700	1.520	—	—	—	—	—
TURK HAM-CURED THIGH MEAT	1.000 SLICE	28.400	36.500	5.370	0.105	1.440	—	0.485	0.325	0.430	283
TURKEY LOAF-BREAST	1.000 SERVING	28.400	31.200	6.380	0.000	0.447	11.500	0.137	0.127	0.078	406
TURKEY PASTRAMI	1.000 SLICE	28.400	40.000	5.210	0.470	2.060	—	1.030	0.580	0.450	297
TURKEY ROLL-LIGHT	1.000 SERVING	28.400	42.000	5.300	0.150	2.050	12.000	0.570	0.710	0.490	139
STEAK-CHICKEN FRIED	1.000 ITEM	100	389	17.900	12.300	30.000	—	—	—	—	815

OT Mg	MAG Mg	IRON Mg	ZINC Mg	V-A RE	V-C Mg	THIA Mg	RIBO Mg	NIAC Mg	V-B6 Mg	FOL Ug	V-B12 Ug	CALC Mg	PHOS Mg	SEL Mg	FIBD Gm	V-ET mg
774	356	8.220	7.670	0	0.000	0.274	0.274	1.920	0.351	94.800	0.000	62.000	671	0.007	10.000	0.781
135	26.000	0.430	0.260	1.000	—	0.043	0.026	0.426	—	—	0.000	5.000	29.000	0.002	2.190	0.142
313	47.000	1.780	1.690	0	0.600	0.029	0.019	0.441	—	—	0.000	14.000	99.000	0.016	3.900	0.651
781	—	5.470	2.300	0	6.700	0.072	0.000	2.140	—	—	0.000	26.000	293	—	—	—
493	155	3.230	2.290	0	—	0.469	0.147	2.870	—	—	0.000	94.000	183	0.007	12.400	—
817	308	5.070	5.210	2.1	0.600	0.274	0.274	6.440	0.406	69.000	0.000	96.000	596	0.007	11.600	—
825	333	4.560	7.220	2.8	0.700	0.707	0.315	7.190	0.341	118	0.000	153	659	0.007	10.900	—
1047	262	4.710	4.780	0	0.000	0.969	0.191	20.700	0.432	147	0.000	85.000	560	0.007	13.600	11.400
395	142	2.330	6.050	—	—	—	—	—	—	—	0.000	37.000	324	0.006	8.470	1.360
1399	203	8.670	1.710	29.9	—	1.050	0.223	1.380	—	74.200	0.000	173	644	0.007	9.900	6.670
1242	166	4.060	1.740	30.7	—	0.541	0.315	1.800	—	—	0.000	90.000	609	0.007	9.900	6.670
588	168	2.120	6.590	3.84	—	—	—	—	—	—	0.000	35.000	59.000	—	—	—
135	101	4.190	2.030	0.284	—	—	—	—	—	—	0.000	281	181	—	5.320	—
652	171	9.050	7.040	6.75	1.900	0.432	0.378	5.580	—	316	0.000	76.000	1538	—	—	66.800
—	—	—	—	—	—	—	—	—	—	—	—	—	—	0.002	1.700	1.120
1020	273	2.780	9.600	0	0.000	0.425	0.146	21.500	0.577	153	0.000	125	733	0.055	11.200	10.100
1928	409	4.900	7.170	0	0.000	0.323	0.289	35.300	1.160	237	0.000	105	817	—	9.800	0.969
110	30.000	0.300	0.500	—	—	0.010	0.010	2.300	—	—	—	5.000	60.000	—	—	0.960

OT Mg	MAG Mg	IRON Mg	ZINC Mg	V-A RE	V-C Mg	THIA Mg	RIBO Mg	NIAC Mg	V-B6 Mg	FOL Ug	V-B12 Ug	CALC Mg	PHOS Mg	SEL Mg	FIBD Gm	V-ET mg
506	58.000	2.340	2.140	29.4	0.000	0.160	0.256	26.900	1.140	8.000	0.680	32.000	456	0.021	—	0.686
112	11.000	0.660	1.420	12.3	0.000	0.040	0.110	2.960	0.170	4.000	0.160	6.000	86.000	0.005	—	0.172
564	68.000	3.500	2.660	56.5	0.000	0.322	0.408	29.500	1.200	16.000	0.820	56.000	516	0.030	—	0.980
404	—	2.500	—	226	12.000	0.100	0.420	5.400	—	—	—	127	358	—	—	0.931
418	—	1.300	—	30	13.000	0.050	0.100	1.000	—	—	—	45.000	85.000	—	—	0.000
343	—	3.000	—	618	5.000	0.340	0.310	5.500	—	—	—	70.000	232	—	—	0.882
406	34.000	3.270	6.250	0	0.000	0.088	0.347	5.110	0.500	13.000	0.520	45.000	286	—	0.000	0.896
426	39.000	1.880	2.850	0	0.000	0.085	0.181	9.570	0.750	8.000	0.520	27.000	307	—	0.000	0.126
418	37.000	2.490	4.340	0	0.000	0.087	0.255	7.620	0.640	10.000	0.520	35.000	298	—	0.000	0.896
1784	178	9.360	10.600	0	0.000	0.264	0.802	45.900	3.420	38.000	2.360	76.000	1370	—	0.000	0.551
478	37.000	15.000	9.090	5195	12.700	0.141	2.210	15.900	0.880	550	19.300	26.000	414	0.025	—	—
229	30.000	9.340	6.630	3234	11.600	0.126	1.380	5.950	0.490	545	14.700	18.000	331	0.025	0.000	—
196	29.000	11.900	6.070	6886	22.200	0.214	2.450	6.230	0.820	1077	27.100	20.000	437	0.099	0.000	—
480	54.000	2.080	2.000	54.7	0.000	0.130	0.234	24.900	1.080	6.000	0.640	28.000	420	0.053	0.000	0.686
390	48.000	2.020	2.120	54.1	0.000	0.090	0.254	17.200	0.640	6.000	0.460	28.000	344	0.053	0.000	0.770
474	54.000	1.960	1.860	12	0.000	0.136	0.216	25.400	1.100	8.000	0.620	28.000	424	0.031	0.000	0.602
440	50.000	1.780	1.720	10.8	0.000	0.120	0.196	23.600	1.020	6.000	0.580	26.000	392	0.046	0.000	0.602
256	26.000	1.520	2.960	46.2	0.000	0.078	0.243	7.060	0.370	8.000	0.350	14.000	199	0.016	10.000	0.399
230	23.000	1.240	2.710	18	0.000	0.071	0.220	6.000	0.350	8.000	0.310	12.000	174	0.013	0.000	0.333
192	21.000	1.410	2.810	18	0.000	0.060	0.218	4.850	0.220	8.000	0.230	11.000	151	0.013	0.000	0.354
147	15.000	0.930	1.560	18.3	0.000	0.058	0.151	4.310	0.210	5.000	0.190	8.000	116	0.011	0.040	0.217
124	12.000	0.680	1.340	10.2	0.000	0.038	0.120	3.390	0.180	4.000	0.160	6.000	95.000	0.021	0.000	0.182
57.000	6.000	0.400	0.560	12	0.000	0.019	0.044	2.140	0.130	1.000	0.090	5.000	48.000	0.006	0.000	0.112
62.000	7.000	0.430	0.620	16.2	0.000	0.014	0.044	2.260	0.140	1.000	0.100	5.000	51.000	0.006	0.000	0.119
56.000	6.000	0.450	0.650	15.9	0.000	0.016	0.041	1.850	0.090	1.000	0.070	5.000	48.000	0.006	0.000	0.140
1560	124	20.600	14.200	483	0.000	1.330	2.060	36.900	1.400	50.000	2.260	86.000	1190	—	0.000	—
1114	88.000	11.900	11.500	103	0.000	1.150	2.080	22.500	1.100	44.000	1.760	52.000	898	—	0.000	—
—	—	0.900	—	17.1	—	0.030	0.052	1.390	—	—	—	43.000	—	0.010	—	—
—	—	1.190	—	28.2	1.300	0.007	0.182	0.977	—	—	—	1.000	—	—	—	0.036
54.500	5.000	0.275	0.205	6.82	—	0.019	0.037	1.500	—	—	—	12.000	44.500	—	—	—
—	—	0.300	—	3.25	—	0.001	0.015	0.357	—	—	—	16.000	—	—	—	0.036
92.000	—	0.785	—	0	—	0.015	0.070	1.000	—	—	—	2.500	54.000	—	—	—
78.800	5.670	0.113	0.318	0	0.000	0.011	0.030	2.360	0.100	—	0.572	2.000	64.800	—	0.000	—
73.500	4.000	0.470	0.610	0	—	0.016	0.071	1.000	—	—	—	2.500	56.500	—	—	—
71.000	5.000	0.360	0.440	0	—	0.025	0.064	1.990	—	—	—	11.000	52.000	—	—	—
126	—	2.300	—	26.000	—	0.110	0.140	2.700	—	—	—	11.000	110	—	—	0.130

Nutritive Components for Sauces and Dips

Food Name	Serving Portion	WT. Gm	KCAL Kc	PROT Gm	CARB Gm	FAT Gm	CHOL Mg	SAFA Gm	MUFA Gm	PUFA Gm	SOD Mg
SAUCE-HEINZ 57	1.000 TBSP	15.000	15.000	0.400	2.700	0.200	0.000	0.000	0.000	0.000	265
SAUCE-CHILI-BOTTLED	1.000 TBSP	15.000	16.000	0.400	3.700	0.000	0.000	0.000	0.000	0.000	201
DIP-GUACAMOLE-KRAFT	1.000 TBSP	15.000	25.000	0.500	1.500	2.000	0.000	—	—	—	108
DIP-FRENCH ONION-KRAFT	1.000 TBSP	15.000	30.000	0.500	1.500	2.000	0.000	—	—	—	120
SAUCE-TACO-CANNED	1.000 FL OZ	16.000	11.000	0.400	2.200	0.700	0.000	—	—	—	128
SAUCE-SALSA/CHILIES-CANNED	1.000 FL OZ	16.000	10.000	0.400	2.000	0.700	0.000	0.000	0.000	0.000	111
SAUCE-PICANTE-CANNED	1.000 FL OZ	16.000	9.000	0.300	1.900	0.500	0.000	0.000	0.000	0.000	218
SAUCE-BARBECUE	1.000 CUP	250	188	4.500	32.000	4.500	0.000	0.670	1.940	1.710	2032
MUSTARD-YELLOW-PREPARED	1.000 TSP	5.000	5.000	0.100	0.100	0.100	0.000	0.000	0.000	0.000	65.000
SAUCE-MARINARA-CANNED	1.000 CUP	250	171	4.000	25.500	8.380	0.000	1.200	4.280	2.300	1572
SAUCE-TOMATO-CAN-SALT ADD	1.000 CUP	245	74.000	3.250	17.600	0.410	0.000	0.059	0.061	0.164	1481
SAUCE-TOMATO-SPANISH-CAN	1.000 CUP	244	80.000	3.520	17.700	0.640	0.000	0.092	0.098	0.264	1152
SAUCE-SPAGHETTI-CANNED	1.000 CUP	249	272	4.530	39.700	11.900	0.000	1.700	6.070	3.250	1236
SAUCE-SOUR CREAM-MIX/MILK	1.000 CUP	314	509	19.100	45.400	30.300	91.000	16.100	9.880	2.760	1007
SAUCE-TERIYAKI-BOTTLED	1.000 TBSP	18.000	15.000	1.070	2.870	0.000	0.000	0.000	0.000	0.000	690
HORSERADISH-PREPARED	1.000 TBSP	15.000	6.000	0.200	1.400	0.000	0.000	0.000	0.000	0.000	165
SAUCE-WORCESTERSHIRE	1.000 TBSP	15.000	12.000	0.300	2.700	0.000	—	0.000	0.000	0.000	147
SAUCE-TABASCO	1.000 TSP	5.000	0.000	0.100	0.100	0.000	—	0.000	0.000	0.000	22.000
MUSTARD-BROWN-PREPARED	1.000 CUP	250	228	14.800	13.300	15.800	—	—	—	—	3268
SAUCE-TOMATO-CAN-LOW SOD	1.000 CUP	226	90.000	4.000	18.000	0.000	—	0.000	0.000	0.000	65.000
SAUCE-BEARNAISE-MIX/MILK	1.000 CUP	255	701	8.320	17.500	68.200	189	41.800	19.900	3.030	1265
SAUCE-CHEESE-MIX/MILK	1.000 CUP	279	307	16.000	23.200	17.100	53.000	9.320	5.310	1.580	1566
SAUCE-CURRY-MIX/MILK	1.000 CUP	272	270	10.700	25.700	14.700	35.000	6.050	5.160	2.760	1276
SAUCE-MUSHROOM-MIX/MILK	1.000 CUP	267	228	11.300	23.800	10.300	34.000	5.400	3.270	1.100	1533
SAUCE-SWEET/SOUR-MIX/PREP	1.000 CUP	313	294	0.760	72.700	0.080	0.000	0.010	0.020	0.040	779
SAUCE-SOY	1.000 TBSP	18.000	11.000	1.560	1.500	0.000	0.000	0.000	0.000	0.000	1029
GRAVY-BEEF-CANNED	1.000 CUP	233	124	8.730	11.200	5.490	7.000	2.750	2.300	2.210	117
GRAVY-CHICKEN-CANNED	1.000 CUP	238	189	4.590	12.900	13.600	5.000	3.360	6.080	3.580	1375
GRAVY-TURKEY-CANNED	1.000 CUP	238	122	6.200	12.200	5.010	5.000	1.480	2.150	1.170	—

Nutritive Components for Soups

Food Name	Serving Portion	WT. Gm	KCAL Kc	PROT Gm	CARB Gm	FAT Gm	CHOL Mg	SAFA Gm	MUFA Gm	PUFA Gm	SOD Mg
SOUP-CREAM/CHICK-CAN-MILK	1.000 CUP	248	191	7.460	15.000	11.500	27.000	4.630	4.450	1.640	1046
SOUP-CREAM/MUSHROOM-MILK	1.000 CUP	248	203	6.050	15.000	13.600	20.000	5.120	2.980	4.610	1076
SOUP-TOMATO-CAN-MILK	1.000 CUP	248	160	6.090	22.300	6.010	17.000	2.910	1.600	1.110	932
SOUP-BEAN/BACON-CAN-WATER	1.000 CUP	253	173	7.890	22.800	5.940	3.000	1.530	2.180	1.820	952
SOUP-BEEF BROTH-CAN-READY	1.000 CUP	240	16.000	2.740	0.100	0.530	0.605	0.260	0.100	0.020	782
SOUP-CLAM-MANHATTAN-WATER	1.000 CUP	244	78.000	4.180	12.200	2.310	2.000	0.440	0.410	1.320	1808
SOUP-MINESTRONE-CAN-WATER	1.000 CUP	241	83.000	4.260	11.200	2.510	2.000	0.540	0.690	1.110	911
SOUP-PEA-SPLIT-CAN-WATER	1.000 CUP	253	189	10.300	28.000	4.400	8.000	1.760	1.800	0.630	1008
SOUP-TOMATO-CAN-WATER	1.000 CUP	244	86.000	2.060	16.600	1.920	0.000	0.360	0.430	0.960	872
SOUP-VEGETABLE BEEF-CAN	1.000 CUP	245	79.000	5.580	10.200	1.900	5.000	0.850	0.800	0.110	957
SOUP-VEGETARIAN-CAN-WATER	1.000 CUP	241	72.000	2.100	12.000	1.930	0.000	0.290	0.830	0.730	823
SOUP-BEEF BROTH-DEHY-CUBED	1.000 ITEM	4.000	6.000	0.620	0.580	0.140	0.144	0.070	0.060	0.010	864
SOUP-ONION-DEHY-PACKET	1.000 SERVING	39.000	115	4.520	20.900	2.330	2.000	0.540	1.360	0.270	3493
SOUP-CREAM/CELERY-CAN-MILK	1.000 CUP	248	165	5.690	14.500	9.680	32.000	3.950	2.470	2.650	1010
SOUP-CHEESE-CAN-MILK	1.000 CUP	251	230	9.450	16.200	14.600	48.000	9.120	4.100	0.440	1020
SOUP-CHICK BROTH-CAN/WATER	1.000 CUP	244	39.000	4.930	0.930	1.390	1.000	0.410	0.630	0.290	776
SOUP-CHICKEN NOODLE-CAN	1.000 CUP	241	75.000	4.040	9.350	2.450	7.000	0.650	1.110	0.550	1107
SOUP-CLAM-NEW ENGLAND-MILK	1.000 CUP	248	163	9.460	16.600	6.600	22.000	2.950	2.260	1.080	992
SOUP-CREAM/POTATO-CAN-MILK	1.000 CUP	248	148	5.780	17.200	6.450	22.000	3.760	1.730	0.560	1060
SOUP-BLACK BEAN-CAN-WATER	1.000 CUP	247	116	5.640	19.800	1.510	0.000	0.400	0.540	0.470	1198
SOUP-BEEF-CHUNKY-CAN	1.000 CUP	240	171	11.700	19.600	5.140	14.000	2.550	2.140	0.200	867
SOUP-CHICKEN-CHUNKY-CAN	1.000 CUP	251	178	12.700	17.300	6.630	30.000	1.980	2.970	1.390	887
SOUP-CHICKEN/RICE-CAN	1.000 CUP	240	127	12.300	13.000	3.190	12.000	0.950	1.430	0.670	888

T Mg	MAG Mg	IRON Mg	ZINC Mg	V-A RE	V-C Mg	THIA Mg	RIBO Mg	NIAC Mg	V-B6 Mg	FOL Ug	V-B12 Ug	CALC Mg	PHOS Mg	SEL Mg	FIBD Gm	V-ET mg
—	—	—	—	—	—	—	—	—	—	—	—	—	—	0.000	—	—
5.000	—	0.100	—	21	2.000	0.010	0.010	0.200	—	—	—	3.000	8.000	0.000	—	—
—	—	—	—	—	—	—	—	—	—	—	—	—	—	—	—	—
8.000	—	0.300	—	4.4	6.200	0.020	0.010	0.270	—	—	—	5.900	9.800	—	—	—
7.000	—	0.280	—	39	9.100	0.020	0.010	0.290	—	—	—	4.200	9.300	—	—	—
7.000	—	0.250	—	23	8.800	0.020	0.010	0.220	—	—	—	3.800	8.000	—	—	—
435	—	2.250	—	218	17.500	0.075	0.050	2.250	0.188	—	0.000	48.000	50.000	—	2.300	—
7.000	2.000	0.100	—	—	—	—	—	—	—	—	—	4.000	4.000	0.000	0.060	0.088
1061	59.000	2.000	0.670	240	31.900	0.113	0.148	3.980	—	—	0.000	44.000	88.000	—	—	—
908	46.000	1.880	0.600	240	32.100	0.162	0.142	2.820	—	—	0.000	34.000	78.000	—	—	—
—	—	8.500	—	242	21.000	0.180	0.152	3.150	—	—	0.000	40.000	—	—	—	—
957	60.000	1.620	0.530	306	27.900	0.137	0.147	3.750	—	—	0.000	70.000	90.000	—	—	—
733	—	0.610	1.370	144	—	—	0.704	0.556	—	—	—	546	—	—	—	—
4.000	11.000	0.310	0.018	0	0.000	0.005	0.013	0.229	0.018	3.600	0.000	4.000	28.000	—	—	—
4.000	—	0.100	—	—	—	—	—	—	—	—	—	9.000	5.000	—	—	—
120	—	0.900	—	5.1	27.000	0.000	0.030	0.000	—	—	—	15.000	9.000	—	—	—
3.000	—	—	—	—	—	0.000	0.010	0.000	—	—	—	—	—	—	—	—
325	—	4.500	—	—	—	—	—	—	—	—	—	310	335	—	—	4.380
—	—	—	—	—	—	—	—	—	—	—	—	—	—	0.002	—	—
—	—	—	—	757	—	—	—	—	—	—	—	—	—	—	0.090	—
554	47.000	0.270	0.972	117	2.300	0.148	0.564	0.318	—	—	—	570	437	—	0.100	—
—	—	—	—	40.8	—	—	—	—	—	—	—	485	280	—	0.900	—
—	—	—	—	93.5	—	—	—	—	—	—	—	—	—	—	0.500	—
6.000	—	1.620	0.091	0	—	—	0.097	—	—	—	0.000	41.000	—	—	—	—
4.000	8.000	0.490	0.036	0	0.000	0.009	0.023	0.605	0.031	1.900	0.000	3.000	38.000	—	—	—
189	—	1.630	2.330	0	0.000	0.074	0.084	1.540	0.023	—	0.230	14.000	70.000	—	—	—
260	—	1.120	1.910	264	0.000	0.041	0.103	1.060	0.024	—	—	48.000	69.000	—	—	—
—	—	1.670	—	0	0.000	0.048	0.191	3.100	—	—	0.000	10.000	—	—	—	—

T Mg	MAG Mg	IRON Mg	ZINC Mg	V-A RE	V-C Mg	THIA Mg	RIBO Mg	NIAC Mg	V-B6 Mg	FOL Ug	V-B12 Ug	CALC Mg	PHOS Mg	SEL Mg	FIBD Gm	V-ET mg
273	18.000	0.670	0.675	94	1.300	0.074	0.258	0.923	0.067	7.700	—	180	152	0.008	0.500	—
270	20.000	0.590	0.640	38	2.300	0.077	0.280	0.913	0.064	—	—	178	156	0.008	—	—
450	23.000	1.820	0.290	108	67.700	0.134	0.248	1.520	0.164	20.900	0.440	159	148	0.008	0.800	—
403	44.000	2.050	1.030	89	1.600	0.089	0.033	0.567	0.040	31.900	—	81.000	132	0.008	3.200	—
130	—	0.410	—	0	0.000	0.005	0.050	1.870	—	—	—	15.000	31.000	0.008	0.000	—
262	10.000	1.890	0.927	96	3.200	0.063	0.049	1.340	0.083	9.500	2.190	34.000	57.000	0.008	—	—
312	7.000	0.920	0.735	234	1.100	0.053	0.043	0.942	0.099	16.100	0.000	34.000	56.000	0.008	1.900	—
399	48.000	2.280	1.320	44	1.400	0.147	0.076	1.480	0.068	2.500	0.000	22.000	213	0.008	—	—
263	8.000	1.760	0.244	69	66.500	0.088	0.051	1.420	0.112	14.700	0.000	13.000	34.000	0.008	0.900	—
173	6.000	1.110	1.550	189	2.400	0.037	0.049	1.030	0.076	10.600	0.310	17.000	40.000	0.008	0.980	—
209	7.000	1.080	0.460	300	1.400	0.053	0.046	0.916	0.055	10.600	0.000	21.000	35.000	0.008	1.210	—
5.000	2.000	0.080	0.008	0.54	—	0.007	0.009	0.119	—	—	—	—	8.000	0.000	—	—
260	25.000	0.580	0.231	1	0.900	0.111	0.238	1.990	—	6.300	—	55.000	126	0.000	2.200	—
309	22.000	0.690	0.196	68	1.400	0.074	0.248	0.436	0.064	8.500	—	186	151	0.008	0.770	—
340	20.000	0.810	0.688	147	1.200	0.063	0.334	0.502	0.078	—	0.440	288	250	0.008	—	—
210	2.000	0.510	0.249	0	0.000	0.010	0.071	3.350	0.024	—	0.240	9.000	73.000	0.008	0.000	—
5.000	5.000	0.780	0.395	72	0.200	0.053	0.060	1.390	0.027	2.200	—	17.000	36.000	0.008	—	—
300	23.000	1.480	0.799	40	3.500	0.067	0.236	1.030	0.126	9.700	10.300	187	157	0.008	—	—
323	17.000	0.540	0.675	67	1.100	0.082	0.236	0.642	0.089	9.200	—	166	160	0.008	—	—
273	42.000	2.160	1.410	49	0.800	0.077	0.054	0.534	0.094	24.700	0.020	45.000	107	0.008	—	—
336	—	2.320	2.640	261	7.000	0.058	0.151	2.710	0.132	13.400	0.610	31.000	120	0.008	—	—
176	—	1.730	1.000	130	1.300	0.085	0.173	4.420	0.050	4.600	0.250	24.000	113	0.008	—	—
—	—	1.870	—	586	3.800	0.024	0.098	4.100	—	3.800	—	35.000	—	0.008	—	—

Continued.

A

Nutritive Components for Soups—cont'd.

Food Name	Serving Portion	WT. Gm	KCAL Kc	PROT Gm	CARB Gm	FAT Gm	CHOL Mg	SAFA Gm	MUFA Gm	PUFA Gm	SOD Mg
SOUP-ONION-CAN-WATER	1.000 CUP	241	57.000	3.750	8.180	1.740	0.000	0.260	0.750	0.650	1053
SOUP-PEA-GREEN-CAN-WATER	1.000 CUP	250	164	8.590	26.500	2.940	0.000	1.410	1.000	0.380	987
SOUP-TOMATO RICE-CAN-WATER	1.000 CUP	247	120	2.110	21.900	2.720	2.000	0.520	0.600	1.350	815
SOUP-TURKEY-CHUNKY-CAN	1.000 CUP	236	136	10.200	14.100	4.410	9.000	1.220	1.780	1.080	923
SOUP-TURKEY NOODLE-CAN	1.000 CUP	244	69.000	3.900	8.630	1.990	5.000	0.560	0.810	0.490	815
SOUP-TURKEY VEGETABLE-CAN	1.000 CUP	241	74.000	3.090	8.640	3.020	2.000	0.900	1.330	0.670	905

Nutritive Components for Sugars and Sweets

Food Name	Serving Portion	WT. Gm	KCAL Kc	PROT Gm	CARB Gm	FAT Gm	CHOL Mg	SAFA Gm	MUFA Gm	PUFA Gm	SOD Mg
SUGAR-WHITE-POWDER-SIFTED	1.000 CUP	100	385	0.000	100	0.000	0.000	0 .000	0.000	0.000	0.830
CANDY-MILK-CHOC/PEANUTS	1.000 SERVING	28.000	154	4.000	12.600	10.800	—	—	—	—	19.000
CANDY-MILK-CHOC/ALMONDS	1.000 SERVING	28.000	151	2.600	14.500	10.100	—	—	—	—	23.000
SUGAR-SWEET & LOW-PACKET	1.000 ITEM	1.000	4.000	—	0.900	—	—	—	—	—	4.000
SUGAR-EQUAL-PACKET	1.000 ITEM	1.000	4.000	0.000	1.000	0.000	—	0.000	0.000	0.000	0.000
CANDY-LIFE SAVERS	1.000 ITEM	2.000	7.800	0.000	1.940	0.020	—	0.000	—	—	0.600
CANDY-M & M'S-PACKAGE	1.000 ITEM	45.000	220	3.000	31.000	10.000	—	—	—	—	—
CANDY-SNICKERS BAR	1.000 ITEM	57.000	270	6.000	33.000	13.000	—	—	—	—	—
CANDY-MILKY WAY BAR	1.000 ITEM	60.000	260	3.000	43.000	9.000	—	—	—	—	—
CANDY-KIT KAT BAR	1.000 ITEM	43.000	210	3.000	25.000	11.000	—	—	—	—	38.000
CANDY-BIT O HONEY	1.000 SERVING	28.000	121	0.900	21.200	3.600	—	—	—	—	—
CANDY-ALMOND JOY	1.000 SERVING	28.000	151	1.700	18.500	7.800	—	—	—	—	—
CANDY-JELLY BEANS	1.000 ITEM	2.800	6.600	0.000	1.670	0.000	—	0.000	0.000	0.000	0.300
CANDY-PEANUT BRITTLE	1.000 SERVING	28.000	123	2.400	20.400	4.400	—	—	—	—	9.000
CANDY-PEANUT BUTTER CUP	1.000 PIECE	17.000	92.000	2.200	8.700	5.350	2.500	3.000	—	—	54.500
CANDY-LOLLIPOP	1.000 ITEM	28.000	108	0.000	28.000	0.000	0.000	0.000	0.000	0.000	—
ICING-CAKE-WHITE-BOILED	1.000 CUP	94.000	295	1.000	75.000	0.000	0.000	0.000	0.000	0.000	134
ICING-CAKE-WHITE/COCO-BOIL	1.000 CUP	166	605	3.000	124	13.000	0.000	11.000	—	—	195
ICING-CAKE-CHOC-MIX/PREP	1.000 CUP	275	1035	9.000	185	38.000	0.000	23.400	—	—	882
ICING-CAKE-FUDGE-MIX/WATER	1.000 CUP	245	830	7.000	183	16.000	0.000	5.100	—	—	568
ICING-CAKE-WHITE-UNCOOKED	1.000 CUP	319	1200	2.000	260	21.000	0.000	12.700	—	—	156
CANDY-CARAMELS-PLAIN/CHOC	1.000 SERVING	28.000	115	1.000	22.000	3.000	0.000	1.600	—	—	74.000
CANDY-MILK CHOCOLATE-PLAIN	1.000 SERVING	28.000	145	2.000	16.000	9.000	0.000	5.500	—	—	28.000
CANDY-CHOCOLATE-SEMISWEET	1.000 CUP	170	860	7.000	97.000	61.000	0.000	36.200	—	—	3.000
CANDY-CHOC COATED PEANUTS	1.000 SERVING	28.000	160	5.000	11.000	12.000	0.000	4.000	—	—	16.000
CANDY-FONDANT-UNCOATED	1.000 SERVING	28.000	105	0.000	25.000	1.000	0.000	0.100	—	—	60.000
CANDY-FUDGE-CHOC-PLAIN	1.000 SERVING	28.000	115	1.000	21.000	3.000	0.000	1.300	—	—	54.000
CANDY-GUM DROPS	1.000 SERVING	28.000	100	0.000	25.000	0.000	25.000	0.000	0.000	0.000	10.000
CANDY-HARD	1.000 SERVING	28.000	110	0.000	28.000	0.000	0.000	0.000	0.000	0.000	9.000
MARSHMALLOWS	1.000 SERVING	28.000	90.000	1.000	23.000	0.000	0.000	0.000	0.000	0.000	11.000
HONEY-STRAINED/EXTRACTED	1.000 TBSP	21.000	65.000	0.000	17.000	0.000	0.000	0.000	0.000	0.000	1.000
JAMS/PRESERVES-REGULAR	1.000 TBSP	20.000	55.000	0.000	14.000	0.000	0.000	0.000	0.000	0.000	2.000
MOLASSES-CANE-LIGHT	1.000 TBSP	20.000	50.000	0.000	13.000	—	0.000	—	—	—	3.000
MOLASSES-CANE-BLACKSTRAP	1.000 TBSP	20.000	45.000	0.000	11.000	—	0.000	—	—	—	18.000
SUGAR-BROWN-PRESSED DOWN	1.000 CUP	220	820	0.000	212	0.000	0.000	0.000	0.000	0.000	66.000
SUGAR-WHITE-GRANULATED	1.000 TBSP	12.000	45.000	0.000	12.000	0.000	0.000	0.000	0.000	0.000	0.120

...T Mg	MAG Mg	IRON Mg	ZINC Mg	V-A RE	V-C Mg	THIA Mg	RIBO Mg	NIAC Mg	V-B6 Mg	FOL Ug	V-B12 Ug	CALC Mg	PHOS Mg	SEL Mg	FIBD Gm	V-ET mg
9.000	2.000	0.670	0.612	0	1.200	0.034	0.024	0.600	0.048	15.200	0.000	26.000	11.000	0.008	—	—
190	39.000	1.950	1.710	20	1.700	0.108	0.068	1.240	0.053	1.800	0.000	27.000	124	0.008	—	—
330	5.000	0.790	0.514	76	14.800	0.062	0.049	1.060	0.077	—	0.000	23.000	33.000	0.008	1.700	—
361	—	1.910	2.120	716	6.400	0.035	0.106	3.590	0.307	11.100	2.120	50.000	104	0.008	2.500	—
5.000	5.000	0.940	0.583	29	0.200	0.073	0.063	1.400	0.037	—	—	12.000	48.000	0.008	0.700	—
175	4.000	0.760	0.612	244	0.000	0.029	0.039	1.010	0.048	—	0.170	17.000	40.000	0.008	0.964	—

...T Mg	MAG Mg	IRON Mg	ZINC Mg	V-A RE	V-C Mg	THIA Mg	RIBO Mg	NIAC Mg	V-B6 Mg	FOL Ug	V-B12 Ug	CALC Mg	PHOS Mg	SEL Mg	FIBD Gm	V-ET mg
3.000	—	0.100	—	0	0.000	0.000	0.000	0.000	—	—	—	0.000	0.000	0.001	0.000	—
138	—	0.400	—	15	0.000	0.070	0.070	1.400	—	—	—	49.000	83.000	0.001	—	0.308
125	—	0.500	—	21	0.000	0.020	0.120	0.200	—	—	—	65.000	77.000	0.001	—	0.308
3.000	—	—	—	—	—	—	—	—	—	—	—	—	—	0.000	—	—
0.000	0.000	0.000	0.000	0	0.000	0.000	0.000	0.000	0.000	0.000	0.000	0.000	0.000	0.000	—	—
0.000	—	0.040	—	0	0.000	0.000	0.000	0.000	—	—	—	0.400	0.200	0.000	0.000	—
—	—	—	—	—	—	—	—	—	—	—	—	—	—	0.002	—	0.495
—	—	—	—	—	—	—	—	—	—	—	—	—	—	0.002	—	0.627
—	—	—	—	—	—	—	—	—	—	—	—	—	—	0.002	—	0.660
129	19.000	0.560	0.430	9	—	0.030	0.110	0.100	—	—	—	65.000	78.000	0.002	—	0.301
—	—	0.250	—	—	—	0.000	0.130	1.400	—	—	—	13.000	—	0.001	—	0.048
—	—	—	—	—	—	—	—	—	—	—	—	—	—	0.001	—	0.308
0.000	—	0.030	—	0	0.000	0.000	—	—	—	—	—	0.300	0.100	0.000	0.000	—
3.000	—	0.560	—	2.4	0.000	0.020	0.010	1.300	—	—	—	11.000	35.000	0.001	—	—
8.000	14.500	0.240	0.240	1	—	0.050	0.030	0.800	—	—	—	14.500	41.000	0.001	—	0.187
—	—	0.000	—	0	0.000	0.000	0.000	0.000	—	—	—	0.000	0.000	0.001	0.000	—
7.000	—	0.000	—	0	0.000	0.000	0.030	0.000	—	—	—	2.000	2.000	0.001	0.000	—
277	—	0.800	—	0	0.000	0.020	0.070	0.300	—	—	—	10.000	50.000	0.002	—	—
536	—	3.300	—	174	1.000	0.060	0.280	0.600	—	—	—	165	305	0.003	—	—
238	—	2.700	—	0	0.000	0.050	0.200	0.700	—	—	—	96.000	218	0.003	—	—
7.000	—	0.000	—	258	0.000	0.000	0.060	0.000	—	—	—	48.000	38.000	0.003	0.000	—
4.000	1.000	0.400	—	0	0.000	0.010	0.050	0.100	—	—	—	42.000	35.000	0.001	—	0.048
109	16.000	0.300	—	24	0.000	0.020	0.100	0.100	—	1.960	—	65.000	65.000	0.001	—	0.196
553	—	4.400	—	9	0.000	0.020	0.140	0.900	—	—	—	51.000	255	0.006	—	1.190
143	—	0.400	—	0	0.000	0.100	0.050	2.100	—	—	—	33.000	84.000	0.001	—	0.196
1.000	—	0.300	—	0	0.000	0.000	0.000	0.000	—	—	—	4.000	2.000	0.001	0.000	—
2.000	12.600	0.300	—	0	0.000	0.010	0.030	0.100	—	—	—	22.000	24.000	0.001	—	0.196
1.000	—	0.100	—	0	0.000	0.000	0.000	0.000	—	—	—	2.000	0.000	0.001	0.000	—
1.000	—	0.500	—	0	0.000	0.000	0.000	0.000	—	—	—	6.000	2.000	0.001	0.000	0.048
2.000	—	0.500	0.010	0	0.000	0.000	0.000	0.000	—	—	—	5.000	2.000	0.000	0.000	—
1.000	0.630	0.100	0.020	0	0.000	0.000	0.010	0.100	0.004	—	0.000	1.000	1.000	0.001	0.060	—
8.000	—	0.200	—	0	0.000	0.000	0.010	0.000	0.004	1.600	0.000	4.000	2.000	0.000	—	0.018
183	—	0.900	—	—	—	0.010	0.010	0.000	0.040	—	0.000	33.000	9.000	0.026	0.000	0.082
585	—	3.200	—	—	—	0.020	0.040	0.400	0.040	—	0.000	137	17.000	0.026	0.000	0.082
757	—	7.500	—	0	0.000	0.020	0.070	0.400	—	—	—	187	42.000	0.003	0.000	—
0.000	—	0.000	0.006	0	0.000	0.000	0.000	0.000	—	—	—	0.000	0.000	0.000	0.000	—

Nutritive Components for Vegetables

Food Name	Serving Portion	WT. Gm	KCAL Kc	PROT Gm	CARB Gm	FAT Gm	CHOL Mg	SAFA Gm	MUFA Gm	PUFA Gm	SOD Mg
V-8 VEG JUICE-LOW SODIUM	1.000 CUP	243	51.000	0.000	9.720	0.000	0.000	0.000	0.000	0.000	58.300
TOMATO JUICE-LOW SODIUM	1.000 CUP	244	42.000	1.860	10.300	0.140	0.000	0.010	0.022	0.058	24.400
BEANS-NAVY PEA-DRY-COOKED	1.000 CUP	190	225	15.000	40.000	1.000	0.000	—	—	—	13.000
BEANS/PORK/FRANKFURTER-CAN	1.000 CUP	257	366	17.300	39.600	16.900	15.000	6.050	7.270	2.150	1105
BEANS/PORK/TOM SAUCE-CAN	1.000 CUP	253	247	13.000	49.000	2.600	17.000	1.000	1.120	0.331	1113
BEANS/PORK/SWEET SAUCE-CAN	1.000 CUP	253	282	13.400	53.100	3.690	17.000	1.420	1.600	0.473	849
BEANS-RED KIDNEY-CAN	1.000 CUP	255	230	15.000	42.000	1.000	0.000	—	—	—	833
PEAS-SPLIT-DRY-COOKED	1.000 CUP	200	230	16.000	42.000	1.000	0.000	—	—	—	8.000
POTATO-HASHED BROWN-FROZ	1.000 CUP	156	340	4.920	43.800	17.900	—	7.010	8.010	2.070	54.000
POTATO-MASHED-MILK/BUTTER	1.000 CUP	210	222	3.950	35.100	8.870	4.000	2.170	3.720	2.540	619
POTATO-MASHED-DEHY-PREP	1.000 CUP	210	166	4.200	27.500	4.620	4.000	1.430	1.350	1.330	491
POTATO CHIPS-SALT ADDED	1.000 ITEM	2.000	10.500	0.128	1.040	0.708	0.000	0.181	0.125	0.360	9.400
RADISHES-RAW	1.000 ITEM	4.500	0.700	0.027	0.161	0.024	0.000	0.001	0.001	0.002	1.100
SAUERKRAUT-CANNED	1.000 CUP	236	44.000	2.150	10.100	0.330	0.000	0.083	0.031	0.144	1561
SPINACH-RAW-CHOPPED	1.000 CUP	56.000	12.000	1.600	1.960	0.200	0.000	0.032	0.006	0.082	44.000
SPINACH-RAW-BOIL-DRAIN	1.000 CUP	180	41.000	5.350	6.750	0.470	0.000	0.076	0.013	0.194	126
SPINACH-FROZ-BOIL-CHOPPED	1.000 CUP	205	57.400	6.440	10.900	0.431	0.000	0.068	0.012	0.176	176
SQUASH-SUMMER-BOIL-SLICED	1.000 CUP	180	36.000	1.630	7.760	0.560	0.000	0.115	0.041	0.236	2.000
SQUASH-WINTER-BAKE-MASH	1.000 CUP	205	79.000	1.810	17.900	1.290	0.000	0.267	0.096	0.543	3.000
SWEET POTATO-BAKE-PEEL	1.000 ITEM	114	118	1.960	27.700	0.130	0.000	0.027	0.005	0.056	12.000
SWEET POTATO-BOIL-MASHED	1.000 CUP	328	344	5.400	79.600	0.970	0.000	0.210	0.036	0.433	42.000
SWEET POTATO-CANDIED	1.000 PIECE	105	144	0.910	29.300	3.410	0.000	1.420	0.658	0.154	73.000
SWEET POTATO-CAN-MASHED	1.000 CUP	255	258	5.050	59.200	0.510	0.000	0.110	0.020	0.227	191
TOMATO-RAW-RED-RIPE	1.000 ITEM	135	24.000	1.090	5.340	0.260	0.000	0.037	0.039	0.107	10.000
TOMATO-RED-CAN-WHOLE	1.000 CUP	240	47.000	2.240	10.300	0.590	0.000	0.084	0.089	0.238	390
TOMATO CATSUP	1.000 TBSP	15.000	15.000	0.000	4.000	0.000	0.000	0.000	0.000	0.000	156
TOMATO JUICE-CAN	1.000 CUP	244	42.000	1.860	10.300	0.140	0.000	0.020	0.022	0.058	882
TOMATO POWDER	1.000 SERVING	28.400	85.800	3.670	21.200	0.125	0.000	0.018	0.019	0.050	38.100
VEGETABLES-MIXED-FROZ-BOIL	1.000 CUP	182	108	5.220	23.800	0.280	0.000	0.056	0.018	0.132	64.000
SQUASH-HUBBARD-BOIL-MASH	1.000 CUP	236	70.000	3.500	15.200	0.880	0.000	0.179	0.066	0.368	12.000
SQUASH-BUTTERNUT-BAKED	1.000 CUP	205	83.000	1.840	21.500	0.180	0.000	0.039	0.014	0.078	7.000
SQUASH-ACORN-BAKED	1.000 CUP	205	115	2.290	29.900	0.290	0.000	0.059	0.021	0.121	9.000
LETTUCE-ROMAINE-RAW-SHRED	1.000 CUP	56.000	8.000	0.900	1.320	0.120	0.000	0.014	0.004	0.060	4.000
SOYBEAN-DRY-COOKED	1.000 CUP	180	234	19.800	19.400	10.300	—	—	—	—	4.000
TOFU-SOYBEAN CURD	1.000 PIECE	120	86.000	9.400	2.900	5.000	0.000	—	—	—	8.000
BEANS-GARBANZO-CAN	1.000 SERVING	28.400	27.800	1.310	4.660	0.511	0.000	—	—	—	113
TOMATO-CAN-LOW SODIUM-DIET	1.000 CUP	240	47.000	2.240	10.300	0.590	0.000	0.084	0.089	0.238	31.200
SPINACH-CAN-SOLIDS/LIQUIDS	1.000 CUP	234	44.000	4.930	6.840	0.870	0.000	0.140	0.023	0.363	747
TOMATO PASTE-CAN-SALT ADD	1.000 CUP	262	220	9.900	49.300	2.330	0.000	0.332	0.351	0.948	2070
ARTICHOKES-BOIL-DRAIN	1.000 ITEM	120	53.000	2.760	12.400	0.200	0.000	0.048	0.006	0.086	79.000
BEANS-LIMA-CAN	1.000 CUP	248	186	11.300	34.400	0.740	0.000	0.168	0.043	0.358	618
BEANS-PINTO-FROZ-BOIL	1.000 SERVING	28.400	46.000	2.640	8.770	0.135	0.000	0.017	0.010	0.078	—
BEANS-SHELLIE-CAN	1.000 CUP	245	75.000	4.300	15.200	0.470	0.000	0.056	0.034	0.270	819
CHIVES-RAW-CHOPPED	1.000 TBSP	3.000	1.000	0.080	0.110	0.020	0.000	0.003	0.003	0.007	0.000
TOMATO PASTE-CAN-LOW SOD	1.000 CUP	262	220	9.900	49.300	2.330	0.000	0.332	0.351	0.948	172
TOMATO PUREE-CAN-LOW SOD	1.000 CUP	250	102	4.180	25.100	0.290	0.000	0.040	0.043	0.118	49.000
VEGETABLE JUICE-CAN	1.000 CUP	242	44.000	1.520	11.000	0.220	0.000	0.032	0.034	0.092	884
BEANS-REFRIED BEANS	1.000 CUP	253	270	15.800	46.800	2.700	—	1.040	—	—	1071
MIS0-FERMENTED SOYBEANS	1.000 CUP	275	565	32.500	76.900	16.700	0.000	2.420	3.690	9.430	10030
TOMATO PUREE-CAN-SALT ADD	1.000 CUP	250	102	4.180	25.100	0.290	0.000	0.040	0.043	0.118	998
BEANS-BAKED BEANS-CANNED	1.000 CUP	254	235	12.200	52.100	1.140	0.000	0.295	0.099	0.493	1008
EGGPLANT-BOILED-DRAINED	1.000 CUP	96.000	27.000	0.800	6.370	0.220	0.000	0.042	0.019	0.089	3.000
GARLIC-RAW-CLOVE	1.000 ITEM	3.000	4.000	0.190	0.990	0.020	0.000	0.003	0.000	0.007	1.000
LEEKS-BOIL-DRAIN	1.000 ITEM	124	38.000	1.010	9.450	0.250	0.000	0.033	0.004	0.138	13.000
MUSHROOMS-BOIL-DRAIN	1.000 ITEM	12.000	3.000	0.260	0.620	0.060	0.000	0.007	0.001	0.022	0.000
MUSHROOMS-CAN-DRAIN	1.000 ITEM	12.000	3.000	0.220	0.600	0.040	0.000	0.005	0.001	0.014	—
ONION RINGS-FROZ-PREP-HEAT	1.000 ITEM	10.000	40.700	0.534	3.820	2.670	0.000	0.858	1.090	0.511	37.500
PEPPERS-JALAPENO-CAN-CHOP	1.000 CUP	136	33.000	1.090	6.660	0.820	0.000	0.084	0.046	0.445	1990
POTATO SKIN-BAKED	1.000 ITEM	58.000	115	2.490	26.700	0.060	0.000	0.015	0.001	0.025	12.000
POTATO-AU GRATIN-HOME REC	1.000 CUP	245	322	12.400	27.600	18.600	58.000	11.600	5.270	0.676	1060
POTATO-HASH BROWN-PREP-RAW	1.000 CUP	156	326	3.770	33.300	21.700	—	8.480	9.690	2.500	38.000

T Mg	MAG Mg	IRON Mg	ZINC Mg	V-A RE	V-C Mg	THIA Mg	RIBO Mg	NIAC Mg	V-B6 Mg	FOL Ug	V-B12 Ug	CALC Mg	PHOS Mg	SEL Mg	FIBD Gm	V-ET mg
571	—	1.460	—	437	53.000	0.049	0.073	1.940	—	—	—	38.900	—	0.001	2.700	—
536	28.000	1.420	0.360	137	44.600	0.114	0.076	1.640	0.270	48.400	0.000	20.000	46.000	0.001	2.800	0.537
790	—	5.100	1.800	0	0.000	0.270	0.130	1.300	1.060	66.500	0.000	95.000	281	—	9.310	0.646
604	71.000	4.450	4.790	38.6	5.900	0.149	0.144	2.320	0.118	77.100	0.870	123	267	—	12.800	0.561
759	88.000	8.300	14.800	62	7.800	0.132	0.116	1.260	0.175	56.800	0.030	141	297	—	13.800	0.561
673	87.000	4.200	3.800	27.8	7.700	0.119	0.154	0.888	0.215	94.500	0.060	155	266	—	14.000	0.561
673	9.940	4.600	1.910	1	7.650	0.130	0.100	1.500	1.120	35.700	—	74.000	278	—	12.500	—
592	—	3.400	2.100	8	—	0.300	0.180	1.800	—	—	—	22.000	178	0.003	—	0.180
680	26.000	2.340	0.500	0	9.800	0.174	0.032	3.780	0.196	38.800	0.000	24.000	112	0.001	1.500	0.295
607	37.000	0.550	0.580	42	12.900	0.176	0.084	2.270	0.470	16.700	0.000	54.000	97.000	0.001	—	0.084
704	—	1.260	—	27.3	6.300	0.063	0.105	1.680	—	—	—	65.000	92.000	0.001	1.200	—
5.000	1.200	0.024	0.021	0	0.830	0.003	0.000	0.084	0.010	0.900	0.000	0.500	3.100	0.000	0.029	0.085
0.400	0.400	0.013	0.013	0.045	1.030	0.000	0.002	0.014	0.003	1.220	0.000	0.900	0.800	0.000	0.100	—
401	31.000	3.470	0.440	4.72	34.800	0.050	0.052	0.337	0.307	7.050	0.000	72.000	46.000	—	—	—
312	44.000	1.520	0.300	376	15.800	0.044	0.106	0.406	0.110	108	0.000	56.000	28.000	0.001	1.760	1.030
838	157	6.420	1.370	1474	17.700	0.171	0.425	0.882	0.436	262	0.000	244	100	0.002	3.420	3.380
611	141	3.120	1.440	1595	25.200	0.123	0.344	0.859	0.299	220	0.000	299	98.400	0.002	4.510	3.850
346	44.000	0.640	0.710	52.2	10.000	0.079	0.074	0.923	0.117	36.200	0.000	48.000	69.000	0.006	3.160	0.216
895	16.000	0.670	0.540	730	19.700	0.174	0.049	1.440	0.148	57.400	0.000	28.000	41.000	0.006	3.460	0.246
397	23.000	0.520	0.330	2487	28.000	0.083	0.145	0.689	0.275	25.700	0.000	32.000	62.000	0.001	2.050	5.200
602	32.000	1.830	0.870	5592	55.900	0.174	0.459	2.100	0.800	36.300	0.000	70.000	88.000	0.002	5.580	15.000
198	12.000	1.190	0.160	440	7.000	0.019	0.044	0.414	0.043	12.000	0.032	27.000	27.000	0.001	1.100	—
536	61.000	3.390	0.540	3858	13.300	0.069	0.230	2.440	0.168	—	0.000	76.000	133	0.002	6.120	—
254	14.000	0.590	0.130	76.3	21.600	0.074	0.062	0.738	0.059	11.500	0.000	8.000	29.000	0.001	2.100	0.418
529	29.000	1.450	0.380	144	36.300	0.108	0.074	1.760	0.216	7.000	0.000	63.000	46.000	0.002	1.930	0.530
4.000	3.600	0.100	0.034	21	2.000	0.010	0.010	0.200	0.016	0.750	0.000	3.000	8.000	0.000	—	—
536	28.000	1.420	0.360	137	44.600	0.114	0.076	1.640	0.270	48.400	0.000	20.000	46.000	0.001	2.900	0.535
547	50.600	1.300	0.486	490	33.100	0.259	0.216	2.590	0.130	34.100	0.000	47.100	83.800	—	—	—
308	40.000	1.500	0.900	946	5.800	0.130	0.218	1.550	0.134	34.600	0.000	44.000	92.000	0.001	4.190	—
504	32.000	0.670	0.220	1435	15.400	0.099	0.066	0.788	0.243	23.000	0.000	23.000	33.000	0.002	4.200	0.283
583	59.000	1.220	0.270	88.2	30.900	0.148	0.035	1.990	0.254	39.300	0.000	84.000	55.000	0.002	3.500	0.246
896	87.000	1.910	0.350	146	22.100	0.342	0.027	1.810	0.398	38.400	0.000	90.000	93.000	0.002	4.300	0.246
162	4.000	0.620	—	5	13.400	0.056	0.056	0.280	—	76.000	0.000	20.000	26.000	0.000	0.773	0.224
972	—	4.900	—	0	0.000	0.380	0.160	1.100	—	—	—	131	322	—	—	—
0.000	—	2.300	—	0.568	0.000	0.070	0.040	0.100	—	—	—	154	151	—	—	—
4.800	9.370	0.710	0.264	144	1.420	0.003	0.011	0.085	—	—	—	11.100	30.100	—	1.400	—
529	29.000	1.450	0.380	1505	36.300	0.108	0.074	1.760	0.216	—	0.000	63.000	46.000	0.002	1.690	0.528
539	132	3.700	0.990	647	31.600	0.042	0.248	0.634	0.187	136	0.000	195	74.000	0.003	5.080	0.047
2442	134	7.830	2.100	5.28	111	0.406	0.498	8.440	0.996	—	0.000	91.700	207	0.003	—	—
316	47.000	1.620	0.430	21.6	8.900	0.068	0.059	0.709	0.104	53.400	0.000	47.000	72.000	—	4.000	0.228
668	84.000	3.940	1.580	42.2	21.600	0.072	0.106	1.320	0.154	—	0.000	70.000	176	—	10.400	—
—		0.770		0	0.190	0.078	0.031	0.180	—	—	0.000	14.900	—	—	1.390	—
268	—	2.430	—	56.4	7.500	0.078	0.132	0.502	—	—	0.000	72.000	—	—	12.000	—
8.000	2.000	0.050	—	19.2	2.400	0.003	0.005	0.021	0.005	—	0.000	2.000	2.000	—	—	—
2442	134	7.830	2.100	647	111	0.406	0.498	8.440	0.996	—	0.000	91.700	207	0.003	—	—
1051	60.000	2.320	0.540	340	88.200	0.178	0.135	4.290	0.380	—	0.000	37.000	99.000	0.003	—	0.550
468	26.000	1.020	0.480	283	67.000	0.104	0.068	1.760	0.339	—	0.000	26.000	40.000	0.001	2.700	—
994	99.000	4.470	3.450	0	15.200	0.124	0.139	1.230	—	—	—	118	214	—	—	—
451	116	7.520	9.130	24.8	0.000	0.267	0.688	2.370	0.591	90.800	0.570	183	420	—	9.900	—
1051	60.000	2.320	0.540	340	88.200	0.178	0.135	4.290	0.380	—	0.000	37.000	99.000	0.003	—	0.550
752	82.000	0.740	3.550	43.2	—	0.389	0.152	1.090	0.340	60.700	0.000	128	264	—	6.600	—
238	13.000	0.340	0.140	5.76	1.300	0.073	0.019	0.576	0.083	13.800	0.000	5.000	22.000	—	2.690	0.029
2.000	1.000	0.050	—	0	0.900	0.006	0.003	0.021	—	0.100	0.000	5.000	5.000	0.000	—	0.000
108	18.000	1.360	—	5.7	5.200	0.032	0.025	0.248	—	30.100	0.000	37.000	21.000	—	3.970	1.140
8.000	1.000	0.210	0.100	0	0.500	0.009	0.036	0.535	0.011	2.200	0.000	1.000	10.000	0.001	0.216	0.010
—	—	0.100	0.090	0	—	—	—	—	—	1.500	0.000	—	—	0.005	0.216	0.010
2.900	1.900	0.169	0.042	2.3	0.140	0.028	0.014	0.361	0.008	1.300	0.000	3.100	8.100	—	—	0.069
185	16.000	3.810	0.260	231	17.700	0.041	0.068	0.680	—	—	0.000	35.000	23.000	—	—	—
332	25.000	4.080	0.280	0	7.800	0.071	0.061	1.780	0.356	12.500	0.000	20.000	59.000	—	3.020	—
970	48.000	1.560	1.690	93.1	24.300	0.157	0.284	2.430	0.426	19.900	0.492	292	278	—	4.410	—
501	32.000	1.270	0.460	0	8.900	0.115	0.031	3.120	0.434	12.000	0.000	13.000	65.000	—	—	—

Continued.

A Nutritive Components for Vegetables—cont'd.

Food Name	Serving Portion	WT. Gm	KCAL Kc	PROT Gm	CARB Gm	FAT Gm	CHOL Mg	SAFA Gm	MUFA Gm	PUFA Gm	SOD Mg
POTATO-SCALLOP-HOME REC	1.000 CUP	245	210	7.030	26.400	9.020	29.000	5.530	2.550	0.407	821
POTATO-SCALLOP-MIX-PREP	1.000 SERVING	28.400	26.400	0.602	3.630	1.220	—	0.748	0.344	0.055	96.800
POTATO PANCAKES-HOME REC	1.000 ITEM	76.000	495	4.630	26.400	12.600	93.000	3.420	5.350	2.540	388
PUMPKIN PIE MIX-CAN	1.000 CUP	270	282	2.930	71.300	0.340	0.000	0.176	0.043	0.019	561
RUTABAGAS-BOIL-DRAIN	1.000 CUP	170	58.000	1.880	13.200	0.320	0.000	0.042	0.040	0.142	30.000
SEAWEED-WAKAME-RAW	1.000 SERVING	28.400	12.800	0.860	2.600	0.182	0.000	0.037	0.016	0.062	248
SQUASH-ZUCCHINI-RAW-SLICED	1.000 CUP	130	19.000	1.500	3.780	0.180	0.000	0.038	0.014	0.078	3.000
SQUASH-ZUCCHINI-RAW-BOIL	1.000 CUP	180	28.000	1.140	7.080	0.100	0.000	0.018	0.008	0.038	4.000
SQUASH-ZUCCHINI-FROZ-BOIL	1.000 CUP	223	37.000	2.560	7.940	0.290	0.000	0.060	0.022	0.123	5.000
SQUASH-ZUCCHINI-ITALIA-CAN	1.000 CUP	227	65.000	2.330	15.600	0.250	0.000	0.052	0.018	0.107	850
SUCCOTASH-BOIL-DRAIN	1.000 CUP	192	222	9.730	46.800	1.530	0.000	0.284	0.298	0.732	32.000
TOMATO-RED-RAW-BOIL	1.000 CUP	240	60.000	2.680	13.500	0.650	0.000	0.091	0.096	0.262	25.000
TOMATO-STEW-COOK-HOME REC	1.000 CUP	101	59.000	1.770	10.400	2.210	0.000	0.400	0.701	0.447	374
TOMATO-RED-CAN-STEWED	1.000 CUP	255	68.000	2.370	16.500	0.360	0.000	0.051	0.054	0.148	647
ASPARAGUS-FROZ-BOIL-SPEARS	1.000 CUP	180	50.400	5.310	8.770	0.756	0.000	0.171	0.023	0.331	7.200
BEANS-LIMA-FROZ-BOIL-DRAIN	1.000 CUP	170	170	10.300	32.000	0.580	0.000	0.130	0.034	0.278	90.000
BEANS-SNAP-GREEN-RAW-BOIL	1.000 CUP	125	44.000	2.360	9.860	0.360	0.000	0.080	0.014	0.181	4.000
BEANS-GREEN-FROZ-FRENCH	1.000 CUP	135	36.000	1.840	8.260	0.180	0.000	0.041	0.007	0.093	17.000
BEANS-SNAP-GREEN-CAN-CUTS	1.000 CUP	135	27.000	1.550	6.000	0.135	0.000	0.030	0.006	0.070	339
BEANS-SNAP-WAX-RAW-BOIL	1.000 CUP	125	44.000	2.360	9.860	0.360	0.000	0.080	0.014	0.181	4.000
BEANS-SNAP-YELLOW/WAX-CAN	1.000 CUP	136	26.000	1.560	6.120	0.140	0.000	0.030	0.006	0.070	340
BEANS-MUNG-SPROUTED-BOIL	1.000 CUP	125	26.000	2.520	5.200	0.110	0.000	0.031	0.015	0.040	12.000
BEETS-CAN-SLICED-DRAIN	1.000 CUP	170	54.000	1.560	12.200	0.240	0.000	0.040	0.048	0.086	479
COWPEAS-BLACKEYE-RAW-BOIL	1.000 CUP	165	179	13.400	29.900	1.320	0.000	0.345	0.117	0.041	7.000
COWPEAS-BLACKEYE-FROZ-BOIL	1.000 CUP	170	224	14.400	40.400	1.130	0.000	0.298	0.102	0.036	9.000
BROCCOLI-RAW	1.000 CUP	88.000	24.000	2.620	4.620	0.300	0.000	0.048	0.022	0.148	24.000
BROCCOLI-RAW-BOIL-DRAIN	1.000 CUP	155	46.000	4.640	8.680	0.440	0.000	0.068	0.032	0.210	16.000
CABBAGE-WHITE MUSTARD-RAW	1.000 CUP	70.000	9.000	1.050	1.530	0.140	0.000	0.018	0.011	0.067	45.000
BROCCOLI-FROZ-BOIL-DRAIN	1.000 CUP	185	51.000	5.710	9.850	0.210	0.000	0.030	0.015	0.101	44.000
CABBAGE-COMMON-RAW-SHRED	1.000 CUP	90.000	21.600	1.090	4.830	0.162	0.000	0.021	0.012	0.078	16.200
CABBAGE-COMMON-BOIL-DRAIN	1.000 CUP	145	30.500	1.390	6.920	0.363	0.000	0.046	0.026	0.173	27.600
CABBAGE-RED-RAW-SHREDDED	1.000 CUP	70.000	19.000	0.970	4.290	0.180	0.000	0.024	0.013	0.088	7.000
CABBAGE-CELERY-RAW	1.000 CUP	76.000	12.000	0.910	2.460	0.150	0.000	0.033	0.017	0.055	7.000
CABBAGE-WHITE MUSTARD-BOIL	1.000 CUP	170	20.000	2.650	3.030	0.270	0.000	0.036	0.020	0.131	57.000
CARROT-RAW-WHOLE-SCRAPED	1.000 ITEM	72.000	31.000	0.740	7.300	0.140	0.000	0.022	0.006	0.055	25.000
CARROT-RAW-SHRED-SCRAPED	1.000 CUP	110	48.000	1.120	11.200	0.200	0.000	0.034	0.008	0.084	38.000
CARROTS-BOIL-DRAIN-SLICED	1.000 CUP	156	70.000	1.700	16.300	0.280	0.000	0.054	0.014	0.138	104
CARROTS-CAN-SLICED-DRAIN	1.000 CUP	146	34.000	0.940	8.080	0.280	0.000	0.052	0.014	0.134	352
BABY-CARROTS	1.000 SERVING	28.400	8.000	0.200	1.700	0.000	0.000	0.000	0.000	0.000	11.000
CAULIFLOWER-RAW-CHOPPED	1.000 CUP	100	24.000	1.990	4.920	0.180	0.000	0.000	0.000	0.000	15.000
CAULIFLOWER-RAW-BOIL-DRAIN	1.000 CUP	124	30.000	2.320	5.740	0.220	0.000	0.046	0.022	0.144	8.000
CAULIFLOWER-FROZ-BOIL	1.000 CUP	180	34.000	2.900	6.760	0.390	0.000	0.060	0.028	0.186	32.000
CELERY-PASCAL-RAW-STALK	1.000 ITEM	40.000	6.000	0.260	1.450	0.050	0.000	0.013	0.010	0.024	35.000
CELERY-PASCAL-RAW-DICED	1.000 CUP	120	18.000	0.800	4.360	0.140	0.000	0.038	0.028	0.072	106
COLLARDS-RAW-BOIL-DRAIN	1.000 CUP	190	27.000	2.100	5.020	0.290	0.000	—	—	—	36.000
COLLARDS-FROZEN-BOIL-DRAIN	1.000 CUP	170	61.000	5.040	12.100	0.690	0.000	—	—	—	85.000
CORN-KERNELS FROM 1 EAR	1.000 ITEM	77.000	83.000	2.560	19.300	0.980	0.000	0.152	0.288	0.464	13.000
CORN-KERNELS&COB-FROZ-BOIL	1.000 ITEM	228	118	3.920	28.100	0.920	0.000	0.144	0.272	0.438	6.000
CORN-FROZ-BOIL-KERNELS	1.000 CUP	165	134	4.940	33.700	0.120	0.000	0.018	0.034	0.056	8.000
CORN-SWEET-CREAM STYLE-CAN	1.000 CUP	256	186	4.460	46.400	1.080	0.000	0.166	0.314	0.506	730
CORN-SWEET-CAN-DRAINED	1.000 CUP	165	132	4.300	30.500	1.640	0.000	0.254	0.478	0.772	470
CUCUMBER-RAW-SLICED	1.000 CUP	104	14.000	0.560	3.020	0.140	0.000	0.034	0.004	0.054	2.000
ENDIVE-RAW-CHOPPED	1.000 CUP	50.000	8.000	0.620	1.680	0.100	0.000	0.024	0.002	0.044	12.000
LETTUCE-BUTTERHEAD-LEAVES	1.000 SLICE	15.000	2.000	0.190	0.350	0.030	0.000	0.004	0.001	0.018	1.000
LETTUCE-ICEBERG-RAW-LEAVES	1.000 SERVING	135	17.600	1.360	2.820	0.257	0.000	0.034	0.009	0.135	12.200
LETTUCE-ICEBERG-RAW-CHOP	1.000 CUP	55.000	7.150	0.556	1.150	0.105	0.000	0.014	0.003	0.055	4.950
LETTUCE-LOOSELEAF-RAW	1.000 CUP	55.000	10.000	0.720	1.960	0.160	0.000	0.022	0.006	0.090	6.000
MUSHROOMS-RAW-CHOPPED	1.000 CUP	70.000	18.000	1.460	3.260	0.300	0.000	0.040	0.004	0.120	2.000
ONIONS-MATURE-RAW-CHOPPED	1.000 CUP	160	54.000	1.880	11.700	0.420	0.000	0.070	0.060	0.164	4.000
CARROTS-FROZEN-BOIL-DRAIN	1.000 CUP	146	52.000	1.730	12.000	0.160	0.000	0.031	0.007	0.077	86.000
ONIONS-MATURE-BOIL-DRAIN	1.000 CUP	210	58.000	1.900	13.200	0.340	0.000	0.056	0.048	0.132	16.000

Mg	MAG Mg	IRON Mg	ZINC Mg	V-A RE	V-C Mg	THIA Mg	RIBO Mg	NIAC Mg	V-B6 Mg	FOL Ug	V-B12 Ug	CALC Mg	PHOS Mg	SEL Mg	FIBD Gm	V-ET mg
925	46.000	1.410	0.980	46.6	26.100	0.169	0.225	2.580	0.436	21.300	0.348	140	154	—	4.410	—
700	3.980	0.108	0.071	5.96	0.937	0.005	0.016	0.292	0.012	0.312	—'	10.200	15.900	—	0.540	—
538	24.000	1.210	0.680	26.6	0.400	0.104	0.095	1.610	0.290	21.500	0.217	21.000	78.000	—	—	—
372	43.000	2.870	0.720	2241	9.500	0.043	0.319	1.010	—	—	0.000	99.000	120	—	—	—
488	36.000	0.800	0.520	0	37.200	0.122	0.062	1.070	0.154	26.400	0.000	72.000	84.000	—	2.500	0.255
200	30.400	0.619	0.108	10.2	0.852	0.017	0.065	0.454	—	—	0.000	42.600	22.700	—	1.200	—
322	28.000	0.550	0.260	44.2	11.700	0.091	0.039	0.520	0.116	28.800	0.000	20.000	42.000	0.004	2.000	0.156
456	38.000	0.640	0.320	43.2	8.400	0.074	0.074	0.770	0.140	30.200	0.000	24.000	72.000	0.006	2.300	0.216
434	28.000	1.080	0.440	95.9	8.200	0.091	0.089	0.861	0.100	17.500	0.000	38.000	55.000	0.007	3.230	0.268
622	31.000	1.550	0.580	123	5.200	0.095	0.091	1.200	—	—	0.000	38.000	66.000	—	—	—
787	102	2.930	1.220	55.7	15.700	0.323	0.184	2.550	0.223	—	0.000	32.000	224	—	—	—
324	33.000	1.440	0.320	178	50.300	0.170	0.144	1.720	0.086	22.600	0.000	20.000	70.000	0.001	1.920	0.816
170	13.000	0.780	0.170	67.7	14.800	0.067	0.064	0.750	0.031	9.900	0.000	19.000	32.000	0.001	—	0.343
611	29.000	1.860	0.420	140	33.800	0.117	0.089	1.820	—	7.400	0.000	84.000	51.000	0.002	2.040	0.561
392	23.400	1.150	1.000	148	43.900	0.117	0.185	1.870	0.036	242	0.000	41.400	99.000	0.007	2.160	2.520
694	58.000	2.320	0.740	32.3	21.800	0.120	0.104	1.800	0.208	111	0.000	38.000	153	0.001	8.330	0.000
373	32.000	1.600	0.450	83.8	12.100	0.093	0.121	0.768	0.070	41.600	0.000	58.000	46.000	0.001	2.250	0.025
451	29.000	1.110	0.840	71.6	11.100	0.065	0.100	0.563	0.076	44.200	0.000	61.000	33.000	0.001	2.160	0.176
447	17.500	1.200	0.390	47.3	6.500	0.020	0.075	0.270	0.054	43.000	0.000	35.000	34.000	0.001	1.760	0.041
373	32.000	1.600	0.450	83.8	12.100	0.093	0.121	0.768	0.070	41.600	0.000	58.000	48.000	0.001	2.250	0.363
148	18.000	1.220	0.400	47.6	6.400	0.020	0.076	0.274	0.057	43.000	0.000	36.000	26.000	0.001	1.770	0.394
125	18.000	0.810	0.580	1.25	14.100	0.062	0.126	1.010	—	166	0.000	15.000	34.000	—	2.700	—
284	22.100	3.100	0.360	1.7	5.000	0.020	0.050	0.200	0.085	40.800	0.000	32.000	31.000	0.001	3.200	0.051
693	83.000	2.360	1.300	130	2.600	0.112	0.177	1.770	0.083	173	0.000	46.000	197	—	11.000	0.215
538	85.000	3.600	2.420	13.6	4.500	0.442	0.109	1.240	0.162	240	0.000	40.000	208	—	9.800	0.204
286	22.000	0.780	0.360	136	82.000	0.058	0.104	0.562	0.140	62.400	0.000	42.000	58.000	—	3.170	0.405
254	94.000	1.780	0.240	215	98.000	0.128	0.322	1.180	0.308	107	0.000	178	74.000	—	6.400	0.713
476	13.000	0.560	—	210	31.500	0.028	0.049	0.350	—	—	0.000	74.000	26.000	0.002	1.300	0.084
332	37.000	1.130	0.560	350	73.700	0.101	0.150	0.843	0.239	104	0.000	94.000	101	—	7.300	0.851
221	13.500	0.504	0.162	11.7	42.600	0.045	0.027	0.270	0.086	51.000	0.000	42.300	20.700	0.002	1.800	1.500
297	21.800	0.566	0.232	13.1	35.200	0.083	0.080	0.330	0.093	29.400	0.000	47.900	36.300	0.003	4.000	2.420
444	11.000	0.350	0.150	2.8	39.900	0.035	0.021	0.210	0.147	14.500	0.000	36.000	29.000	0.002	1.700	0.140
181	10.000	0.230	0.170	91.2	20.500	0.030	0.038	0.304	0.176	59.800	0.000	58.000	22.000	0.002	1.630	0.090
530	18.000	1.770	—	4.37	44.200	0.054	0.107	0.728	—	—	0.000	158	49.000	0.004	2.100	1.190
233	11.000	0.360	0.140	2025	6.700	0.070	0.042	0.668	0.106	10.100	0.000	19.000	32.000	0.002	2.030	0.317
356	16.000	0.540	0.220	3094	10.200	0.106	0.064	1.020	0.162	15.400	0.000	30.000	48.000	0.002	3.100	0.484
354	20.000	0.960	0.460	3830	3.600	0.054	0.088	0.790	0.384	21.600	0.000	48.000	48.000	0.002	5.770	0.651
262	12.000	0.940	0.380	2010	4.000	0.026	0.044	0.806	0.164	13.400	0.000	38.000	34.000	0.002	2.480	0.613
000	3.000	0.100	0.043	3249	1.600	0.007	0.011	0.131	0.021	4.200	—	6.000	6.000	0.000	—	0.128
355	14.000	0.580	0.180	2	71.500	0.076	0.057	0.633	0.231	66.100	0.000	29.000	46.000	0.001	2.670	0.030
400	14.000	0.520	0.300	1.8	68.600	0.078	0.064	0.684	0.250	63.400	0.000	34.000	44.000	0.001	2.230	0.038
250	16.000	0.740	0.240	3.6	56.400	0.066	0.096	0.558	0.158	73.800	0.000	30.000	44.000	0.001	3.240	0.054
114	5.000	0.190	0.070	5.2	2.500	0.012	0.012	0.120	0.012	3.600	0.000	14.000	10.000	0.000	0.400	0.144
340	14.000	0.580	0.200	15.6	7.600	0.036	0.036	0.360	0.036	10.600	0.000	44.000	32.000	0.000	1.200	0.432
177	21.000	0.780	1.220	349	18.600	0.032	0.082	0.448	0.080	12.400	0.000	148	19.000	0.001	2.100	—
427	52.000	1.900	0.460	1017	44.900	0.080	0.196	1.080	0.194	129	0.000	357	46.000	0.001	5.200	—
192	24.000	0.470	0.370	16.9	4.800	0.166	0.055	1.240	0.046	35.700	0.000	2.000	79.000	0.001	6.600	0.056
316	36.000	0.780	0.800	26.5	6.000	0.220	0.086	1.910	0.282	38.400	0.000	4.000	94.000	0.001	2.650	0.069
228	30.000	0.500	0.560	41.3	4.200	0.114	0.120	2.100	0.164	33.400	0.000	4.000	78.000	0.001	3.470	0.050
344	44.000	0.980	1.360	25.6	11.800	0.064	0.136	2.460	0.162	115	0.000	8.000	130	0.001	—	0.102
160	28.000	1.400	0.640	26.4	7.000	0.050	0.080	1.500	0.330	59.400	0.000	8.000	81.000	0.001	2.150	0.066
156	12.000	0.280	0.240	5.2	4.800	0.032	0.020	0.312	0.054	14.400	0.000	14.000	18.000	0.001	1.460	0.156
158	8.000	0.420	0.400	103	3.200	0.040	0.038	0.200	0.010	71.000	0.000	26.000	14.000	—	—	—
000	1.650	0.040	0.030	14.6	1.200	0.010	0.010	0.045	0.008	11.000	0.000	5.000	4.000	0.000	0.207	0.060
213	12.200	0.675	0.297	6.61	5.270	0.062	0.041	0.252	0.054	75.600	0.000	25.700	27.000	0.001	1.600	0.080
900	4.950	0.275	0.121	18.2	2.150	0.025	0.017	0.103	0.022	30.800	0.000	10.500	11.000	0.000	0.600	0.220
148	6.000	0.780	0.121	105	10.000	0.028	0.044	0.224	0.030	76.000	0.000	38.000	14.000	0.000	0.760	0.220
260	8.000	0.860	0.344	0	2.400	0.072	0.314	2.880	0.068	14.800	0.000	4.000	72.000	0.009	1.060	0.056
248	16.000	0.580	0.280	0	13.400	0.096	0.016	0.160	0.252	31.800	0.000	40.000	46.000	0.003	2.640	0.496
230	14.000	0.690	0.350	2584	4.100	0.039	0.054	0.639	0.188	15.800	0.000	41.000	39.000	0.003	5.400	0.613
318	22.000	0.420	0.380	0	12.000	0.088	0.016	0.168	0.378	26.600	0.000	58.000	48.000	0.007	1.680	0.252

Continued.

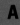

Nutritive Components for Vegetables—cont'd.

Food Name	Serving Portion	WT. Gm	KCAL Kc	PROT Gm	CARB Gm	FAT Gm	CHOL Mg	SAFA Gm	MUFA Gm	PUFA Gm	SOD Mg
ONIONS-YOUNG GREEN	1.000 ITEM	5.000	1.250	0.087	0.278	0.007	0.000	0.001	0.000	0.000	0.200
PARSLEY-RAW-CHOPPED	1.000 TBSP	4.000	1.200	0.088	0.276	0.012	0.000	0.000	0.000	0.000	1.600
PEAS-GREEN-CAN-DRAINED	1.000 CUP	170	118	7.520	21.400	0.580	0.000	0.106	0.052	0.278	372
PEAS-GREEN-FROZ-BOIL-DRAIN	1.000 CUP	160	126	8.240	22.800	0.440	0.000	0.078	0.038	0.206	140
PEPPERS-HOT-RED-DRIED	1.000 TSP	2.000	5.000	0.000	1.000	0.000	0.000	0.000	0.000	0.000	20.000
POTATO-FRENCH FRIED-RAW	1.000 ITEM	5.000	13.500	0.200	1.800	0.700	0.000	0.170	0.178	0.033	11.100
POTATO-FRENCH FRIED-FROZ	1.000 ITEM	5.000	11.100	0.173	1.700	0.438	0.000	0.208	0.178	0.033	1.500

T Mg	MAG Mg	IRON Mg	ZINC Mg	V-A RE	V-C Mg	THIA Mg	RIBO Mg	NIAC Mg	V-B6 Mg	FOL Ug	V-B12 Ug	CALC Mg	PHOS Mg	SEL Mg	FIBD Gm	V-ET mg
.800	1.000	0.095	0.022	25	2.250	0.004	0.007	0.001	—	0.685	0.000	3.000	1.650	0.000	0.083	0.006
.600	1.600	0.248	0.028	20.8	3.600	0.003	0.004	0.028	0.006	7.320	0.000	5.200	1.600	0.000	0.152	0.070
294	30.000	1.620	1.200	131	16.200	0.206	0.132	1.240	0.108	75.400	0.000	34.000	114	0.001	6.970	0.034
268	46.000	2.520	1.500	107	15.800	0.452	0.160	2.370	0.180	93.800	0.000	38.000	144	0.001	6.080	0.192
.000	3.400	0.300	0.054	130	0.000	0.000	0.020	0.200	—	—	0.000	5.000	4.000	0.000	—	—
.700	—	0.070	—	0	1.100	0.007	0.004	0.160	0.009	1.100	0.000	0.800	5.600	0.000	0.160	0.010
.900	1.100	0.067	0.021	0	0.550	0.006	0.002	0.115	0.012	0.830	0.000	0.400	4.300	0.000	0.160	0.010

APPENDIX B
CLINICAL MEASURES AND PHYSICAL EVIDENCE OF NUTRITIONAL STATUS

B

Clinical Signs and Symptoms of Various Nutrient Deficiencies

Area of Examination	Sign/Symptom	Potential Nutrient Deficiency	Area of Examination	Sign/Symptom	Potential Nutrient Deficiency
Hair	Loss	Zinc, essential fatty acids	**Skin**	Follicular hyperkeratosis	Vitamin A, essential fatty acids
	Easy pluckability	Protein, essential fatty acids		Nose-lip dryness	Niacin, pyridoxine, riboflavin
	Lackluster	Protein, zinc		Bilateral dermatitis	Niacin, zinc
	"Corkscrew" hair	Vitamin C, vitamin A	**Extremities**	Subcutaneous fat loss	kcalories
	Decreased pigmentation	Protein, copper		Muscle wastage	kcalories, protein
Eyes	Drying of conjunctiva	Vitamin A		Edema	Protein
	Corneal vascularization	Riboflavin		Osteomalacia, bone pain, rickets	Vitamin D
	Xerophthalmia	Vitamin A		Bone pain	Vitamin C
	Bitot's spots	Vitamin A	**Hematologic**	Anemia	Vitamin B-12, iron, folate, copper, vitamin E, vitamin K
GI tract	Nausea, vomiting	Pyridoxine			
	Diarrhea	Zinc, niacin			
	Mouth inflammation	Pyridoxine, riboflavin, iron		Low white cell count	Copper
	Cheilosis	Pyridoxine, iron		Low prothrombin, prolonged clotting time	Vitamin K
	Tongue inflammation	Pyridoxine, zinc, niacin, folate, vitamin B-12	**Neurologic**	Disorientation	Niacin, thiamin
	Magenta tongue	Riboflavin		Confusion	Thiamin
	Swollen, bleeding gums	Vitamin C		Nerve degeneration	Thiamin, pyridoxine, chromium
	Fissured tongue	Niacin			
	Enlarged liver	Protein		Poor coordination, feeling	Thiamin, pyridoxine, Vitamin B-12
Skin	Dry and scaling	Vitamin A, essential fatty acids, zinc	**Cardiovascular**	Congestive heart failure, enlarged heart	Thiamin
	Petechiae, ecchymoses (small hemorrhages)	Vitamin C, vitamin K		Heart degeneration	Selenium

From Ross Labortories

APPENDIX C
NUTRIENT RECOMMENDATIONS FOR CANADIANS

Summary of Examples of Recommended Nutrients Based on Energy Expressed as Daily Rates

Age	Sex	Energy kcal	Thiamin mg	Riboflavin mg	Niacin Ne[+]	n-3 PUFA[*] g	n-6 PUFA g
Months							
0–4	Both	600	0.3	0.3	4	0.5	3
5–12	Both	900	0.4	0.5	7	0.5	3
Years							
1	Both	1100	0.5	0.6	8	0.6	4
2–3	Both	1300	0.6	0.7	9	0.7	4
4–6	Both	1800	0.7	0.9	13	1.0	6
7–9	M	2200	0.9	1.1	16	1.2	7
	F	1900	0.8	1.0	14	1.0	6
10–12	M	2500	1.0	1.3	18	1.4	8
	F	2200	0.9	1.1	16	1.2	7
13–15	M	2800	1.1	1.4	20	1.5	9
	F	2200	0.9	1.1	16	1.2	7
16–18	M	3200	1.3	1.6	23	1.8	11
	F	2100	0.8	1.1	15	1.2	7
19–24	M	3000	1.2	1.5	22	1.6	10
	F	2100	0.8	1.1	15	1.2	7
25–49	M	2700	1.1	1.4	19	1.5	9
	F	1900	0.8	1.0	14	1.1	7
50–74	M	2300	0.9	1.2	16	1.3	8
	F	1800	0.8[†]	1.0[†]	14[†]	1.1[†]	7[†]
75 +	M	2000	0.8	1.0	14	1.1	7
	F[§]	1700	0.8[†]	1.0[†]	14[†]	1.1[†]	7[†]
Pregnancy (additional)							
1st Trimester		100	0.1	0.1	1	0.05	0.3
2nd Trimester		300	0.1	0.3	2	0.16	0.9
3rd Trimester		300	0.1	0.3	2	0.16	0.9
Lactation (additional)		450	0.2	0.4	3	0.25	1.5

[*]PUFA, polyunsaturated fatty acids.

[+]Niacin equivalents.

[†]Level below which intake should not fall.

[§]Assumes moderate physical activity.

From Scientific Review Committee: *Nutrition Recommendation*, Ottawa, Canada, 1990, Health and Welfare.

Summary Examples of Recommended Nutrient Intake Based on Age and Body Weight Expressed as Daily Rates

Age	Sex	Weight kg	Protein g	Vit. A RE[*]	Vit. D ug	Vit. E mg	Vit. C mg	Folate ug	Vit. B_{12} ug	Calcium mg	Phosphorus mg	Magnesium mg	Iron mg	Iodine ug	Zinc mg
Months															
0–4	Both	6.0	12[+]	400	10	3	20	25	0.3	250[†]	150	20	0.3[§]	30	2[§]
5–12	Both	9.0	12	400	10	3	20	40	0.4	400	200	32	7	40	3
Years															
1	Both	11	13	400	10	3	20	40	0.5	500	300	40	6	55	4
2–3	Both	14	16	400	5	4	20	50	0.6	550	350	50	6	65	4
4–6	Both	18	19	500	5	5	25	70	0.8	600	400	65	8	85	5
7–9	M	25	26	700	2.5	7	25	90	1.0	700	500	100	8	110	7
	F	25	26	700	2.5	6	25	90	1.0	700	500	100	8	95	7
10–12	M	34	34	800	2.5	8	25	120	1.0	900	700	130	8	125	9
	F	36	36	800	2.5	7	25	130	1.0	1100	800	135	8	110	9
13–15	M	50	49	900	2.5	9	30	175	1.0	1100	900	185	10	160	12
	F	48	46	800	2.5	7	30	170	1.0	1000	850	180	13	160	9
16–18	M	62	58	1000	2.5	10	40[‖]	220	1.0	900	1000	230	10	160	12
	F	53	47	800	2.5	7	30[‖]	190	1.0	700	850	200	12	160	9
19–24	M	71	61	1000	2.5	10	40[‖]	220	1.0	800	1000	240	9	160	12
	F	58	50	800	2.5	7	30[‖]	180	1.0	700	850	200	13	160	9
25–49	M	74	64	1000	2.5	9	40[‖]	230	1.0	800	1000	250	9	160	12
	F	59	51	800	2.5	6	30[‖]	185	1.0	700	850	200	13	160	9
50–74	M	73	63	1000	5	7	40[‖]	230	1.0	800	1000	250	9	160	12
	F	63	54	800	5	6	30[‖]	195	1.0	800	850	210	8	160	9
75 +	M	69	59	1000	5	6	40[‖]	215	1.0	800	1000	230	9	160	12
	F	64	55	800	5	5	30[‖]	200	1.0	800	850	210	8	160	9
Pregnancy (additional)															
1st Trimester			5	0	2.5	2	0	200	1.2	500	200	15	0	25	6
2nd Trimester			20	0	2.5	2	10	200	1.2	500	200	45	5	25	6
3rd Trimester			24	0	2.5	2	10	200	1.2	500	200	45	10	25	6
Lactation (additional)			20	400	2.5	3	25	100	0.2	500	200	65	0	50	6

[*]Retinol Equivalents

[+]Protein is assumed to be from breast milk and must be adjusted for infant formula.

[†]Infant formula with high phosphorus should contain 375 mg calcium.

[§]Breast milk is assumed to be the source of the mineral.

[‖]Smokers should increase vitamin C by 50%.

From Scientific Review Committee: *Nutrition Recommendations*, Ottawa, Canada, 1990, Health and Welfare.

APPENDIX D
DIETARY INTAKE ASSESSMENT

Though it may seem overwhelming at first, it is actually very easy to track the foods you eat. One tip is to record foods and beverages consumed as close as possible to the actual time of consumption.

Fill in the food record form that follows. We supply a blank copy (see the completed example in Figure 3-2). Then, to estimate the nutrient values of the foods you are eating, consult food labels and the food composition table in Appendix A or use your Mosby Diet Simple nutrition software package. If these resources do not have the serving size you need, adjust the value. If you drink $\frac{1}{2}$ cup of orange juice, for example, but a table has values for only 1 cup, halve all values before you record them. Then, consider pooling all the same food to save time; if you drink a cup of 1% milk three times throughout the day, enter your milk consumption only once as 3 cups. As you record your intake for use on the nutrient analysis form that follows consider the following tips:

- Measure and record the amounts of food eaten in portion sizes of cups, teaspoons, tablespoons, ounces, slices, or inches (or convert metric units to these units).
- Record brand names of all food products, such as "Quick Quaker Oats."
- Measure and record all those little extras, such as gravies, salad dressings, taco sauces, pickles, jelly, sugar, ketchup, and margarines.
- For beverages
  —List the type of milk, such as whole, skim, 2%, evaporated, chocolate, or reconstituted dry.
  —Indicate whether fruit juice is fresh, frozen, or canned.
  —Indicate type for other beverages, such as fruit drink, fruit-flavored drink, Kool-Aid, and hot chocolate made with water or milk.
- For fruits
  —Indicate whether fresh, frozen, dried, or canned.
  —If whole, record as number eaten and size with approximate measurements (such as 1 apple—3 inches in diameter).
  —Indicate whether processed in water, light syrup, heavy syrup, or other medium.
- For vegetables
  —Indicate fresh, frozen, canned, dried.
  —Record as portion of cup, teaspoon, or tablespoon or as pieces (such as 2 carrot sticks—4 inches long, $\frac{1}{2}$ inch thick).
  —Record preparation method.
- For cereals
  —Record cooked cereals in portions of tablespoon or cup, (a level measurement after cooking).
  —Record dry cereal in level portions of cup or tablespoons.

—If margarine, milk, sugar, fruit, or something else is added, then measure and record amount and type.

- For breads
  —Indicate whether whole wheat, rye, white, and so on.
  —Measure and record number and size of portion (biscuit—2 inches across, 1 inch thick; slice of homemade rye bread—3 inches by 4 inches, $1/4$ inch thick.
  —Sandwiches: list ALL ingredients (lettuce, mayonnaise, tomato, and so on) with amounts.

- For meats, fish, poultry, cheese
  —Give size (length, width, thickness) in inches or weight in ounces after cooking for meats, fish, and poultry (such as cooked hamburger patty—3 inches across, $1/2$ inch thick).
  —Give size (length, width, thickness) in inches or weight in ounces for cheese.
  —Record measurements only on the cooked edible part—without bone or fat that is left on the plate.
  —Describe how meat was prepared.

- For eggs
  —Record as soft or hard cooked, fried, scrambled, poached, or omelet.
  —If milk, butter, or drippings are used, specify kinds and amount.

- For desserts
  —List commercial brand or "homemade" or "bakery" under brand.
  —Purchased candies, cookies, and cakes: Specify kind and size.
  —Measure and record portion size of cakes, pies, and cookies by specifying thickness, diameter, and width or length, depending on the item.

D

Time	Minutes Spent Eating	M or S[*]	H[+]	Activity While Eating	Place of Eating	Food and Quantity	Others Present	Reason for Food Choice

[*]M or S; meal or snack
[+]Hunger (0 none; 3 maximum)

D

Now complete the nutrient analysis form as shown using your food record. A blank copy of this form also follows for your use.

Nutrient Analysis Form (Sample)

Quantity	Name	Kcalories	Protein (grams)	Carbohydrate (grams)	Fat-total (grams)	Cholesterol (milligrams)	Saturated fat (grams)	Monounsaturated fat (grams)	Polyunsaturated fat (grams)	Sodium (milligrams)	Potassium (milligrams)	Magnesium (milligrams)
1 ea.	Egg bagel-3.5 inch diam.	180	7.45	34.7	1.00	44.0	0.171	0.286	0.400	300	65.0	18.0
1 Tbs.	Jelly	49.0	0.018	12.7	0.018	–	0.005	0.005	0.005	4.00	16.0	0.720
1.5 cup	Orange juice-prep fr/frzn	165	2.52	40.2	0.210	–	0.025	0.037	0.045	3.00	711	36.0
2 ea.	Cheeseburger-McD	636	30.2	57.0	32.0	80.0	13.3	12.2	2.18	1460	314	45.8
1 ea.	Serving-French fries-McD	220	3.00	26.1	11.5	8.57	4.61	4.37	0.570	109	564	26.7
1.5 cup	Cola beverage-regular	151	–	38.5	–	–	–	–	–	15.0	4.00	3.00
4 oz.	Pork loin chop-brld-lean	261	36.2	–	11.9	112	4.09	5.35	1.43	88.2	476	34.0
1 ea.	Baked potato with skin	220	4.65	51.0	0.200	–	0.052	0.004	0.087	16.0	844	55.0
.5 cup	Peas-frozen-cooked	63.0	4.12	11.4	0.220	–	0.039	0.019	0.103	70.0	134	23.0
20 gr.	Margarine-reg/soft-80% fat	143	0.160	0.100	16.1	–	2.76	5.70	6.92	216	7.54	0.467
2 cup	Iceberg lettuce-chopped	14.6	1.13	2.34	0.212	–	0.028	0.008	0.112	10.1	177	10.1
2 oz.	French dressing	300	0.318	3.63	32.0	–	4.94	14.2	12.4	666	7.03	5.81
1 cup	2% lowfat milk	121	8.12	11.7	4.78	22.0	2.92	1.35	0.170	122	377	33.0
2 ea.	Graham crackers	60.0	1.04	10.8	1.46	–	0.400	0.600	0.400	86.0	36.0	6.00
	Totals:	2584	99.0	300	112	266	33.4	44.1	24.8	3165	3732	298
RDA or minimum requirement*		2900	58							500	2000	350
% of RDA		89	170							633	187	85

*Values from inside cover. The values listed are for a male age 19 to 24 years. Note that kcalories is just a rough estimate. It is better to base energy needs on actual energy output.

Iron (milligrams)	Zinc (milligrams)	Vitamin A (RE)	Vitamin E (milligrams)	Vitamin C (milligrams)	Thiamin (milligrams)	Riboflavin (milligrams)	Niacin (milligrams)	Vitamin B-6 (milligrams)	Folate (micrograms)	Vitamin B-12 (micrograms)	Calcium (milligrams)	Phosphorus (milligrams)	Selenium (micrograms)	Dietary Fiber (grams)
2.10	0.612	7.00	1.80	–	2.58	0.197	2.40	0.030	16.3	0.065	20.0	61.0	5.00	0.748
0.120	–	0.200	0.016	0.710	0.002	0.005	0.036	0.005	2.00	–	2.00	1.00	0.360	–
0.411	0.192	28.5	0.714	145	0.300	0.060	0.750	0.165	163	–	33.0	60.0	0.735	1.49
5.68	5.20	134	0.560	4.10	0.600	0.480	8.66	0.230	42.0	1.82	338	410	58.0	0.460
0.605	0.320	5.00	0.203	12.5	0.122	0.020	2.26	0.218	19.0	0.027	9.10	101	0.600	4.19
0.120	0.049	–	–	–	–	–	–	–	–	–	9.00	46.0	–	–
1.04	2.54	3.15	0.405	0.454	1.30	0.350	6.28	0.535	6.77	0.839	5.67	277	20.6	–
2.75	0.650	–	0.100	26.1	0.216	0.067	3.32	0.701	22.2	–	20.0	115	1.80	3.90
1.25	0.750	53.4	0.400	7.90	0.226	0.140	1.18	0.090	46.9	–	19.0	72.0	3.20	3.61
–	0.041	199	2.19	0.028	0.002	0.006	0.004	0.002	0.211	0.017	5.29	4.06	0.199	–
0.560	0.246	37.0	0.120	4.36	0.052	0.034	0.210	0.044	62.8	–	21.2	22.4	0.448	1.68
0.227	0.045	0.023	15.9		–	–	–	0.006	–	–	7.10	3.63		0.431
0.120	0.963	140	0.080	2.32	0.095	0.403	0.210	0.105	12.0	0.888	297	232	5.66	–
0.367	0.113	–		–	0.020	0.030	0.600	0.011	1.80	–	6.00	20.0	1.54	1.40
15.4	11.7	607	22.5	204	5.52	1.79	25.9	2.14	395	3.65	792	1425	98.2	17.9
10	15	1000	10	60	1.5	1.7	19	2	200	2	1200	1200	70	–
54	78	61	225	340	368	105	132	107	198	180	66	118	140	–

D

Nutrient Analysis Form (Sample)

Quantity	Name	Kcalories	Protein (grams)	Carbohydrate (grams)	Fat-total (grams)	Cholesterol (milligrams)	Saturated fat (grams)	Monounsaturated fat (grams)	Polyunsaturated fat (grams)	Sodium (milligrams)	Potassium (milligrams)	Magnesium (milligrams)
Totals:												
RDA or minimum requirement*												
% of RDA												

*Values from inside cover. The values listed are for a male age 19 to 24 years. Note that kcalories is just a rough estimate. It is better to base energy needs on actual energy output.

Iron (milligrams)	Zinc (milligrams)	Vitamin A (RE)	Vitamin E (milligrams)	Vitamin C (milligrams)	Thiamin (milligrams)	Riboflavin (milligrams)	Niacin (milligrams)	Vitamin B-6 (milligrams)	Folate (micrograms)	Vitamin B-12 (micrograms)	Calcium (milligrams)	Phosphorus (milligrams)	Selenium (micrograms)	Dietary Fiber (grams)	Vitamin E

D

For this same day you keep your food record, also keep a 24-hour record of your activities. Include sleeping, sitting, and walking, as well as the obvious forms of exercise. Calculate your kcalorie expenditure for these activities using Appendix M. Try to substitute a similar activity if your particular activity is not listed in Appendix M. Calculate the total kcalories you used for the day (Total for column 3). Here is an example of an activity record. A blank form follows for your use.

Weight (lb or kg):

| | Energy cost | | | |
Activity	Time (minutes); Convert to Hours;	Column 1 kcal/hr (from table)	Column 2 Time	Column 3 (Column 1 × Column 2)
Example for 150 lb man: Brisk Walking	0.5 hr (30 min)	299	0.5	150

Calculate total kcalories used for the day:

Weight (lb or kg):

| | Energy cost | | | |
Activity	Time (minutes); Convert to Hours;	Column 1 kcal/hr (from table)	Column 2 Time	Column 3 (Column 1 × Column 2)

Total kcalories used (from adding all of column

This Appendix is now completed. See if your professor wants you to complete more work before turning in this assignment.

APPENDIX E

U.S. Recommended Daily Allowances (U.S. RDA)

Vitamins and Minerals	Unit of Measurement	Adults and Children 4 or More Years of Age[*]	Infants	Children Under 4 Years of Age	Pregnant or Lactating Women
Protein	Grams	65[†]	25[†]	28	[‡]
Vitamin A	International Units	5000	1500	2500	8000
Vitamin D	"	400	400	400	400
Vitamin E	"	30	5.0	10	30
Vitamin C	Milligrams	60	35	40	60
Folic Acid	"	0.4	0.1	0.2	0.8
Thiamin	"	1.5	0.5	0.7	1.7
Riboflavin	"	1.7	0.6	0.8	2.0
Niacin	"	20	8.0	9.0	20
Vitamin B-6	"	2.0	0.4	0.7	2.5
Vitamin B-12	Micrograms	6.0	2.0	3.0	8.0
Biotin	Milligrams	0.3	0.05	0.15	0.3
Pantothenic Acid	"	10	3.0	5.0	10
Calcium	Grams	1.0	0.6	0.8	1.3
Phosphorus	"	1.0	0.5	0.8	1.3
Iodine	Micrograms	150	45	70	150
Iron	Milligrams	18	15	10	18
Magnesium	"	400	70	200	450
Copper	"	2.0	0.6	1.0	2.0
Zinc	"	15	5.0	8.0	15

[*]These U.S. RDA values are on most nutrition labels.

[†]If protein efficiency ratio of protein is equal to or better than that of casein. U.S. RDA is 45 g for adults, 20 g for children under 4 yrs, and 18 g for infants (see Chapter 8 and Appendix S).

[‡]Not specified because this U.S. RDA is used only in vitamin and mineral supplements for pregnant or lactating females.

E

(Proposed) Reference Daily Intakes (RDIs)[*†] (These Will Soon Replace the U.S. RDAs)

Nutrient	Unit of Measurement[*]	Adults and Children 4 or More Years of Age	Children Less Than 4 Years of Age[†]	Infants[‡]	Pregnant Women	Lactating Women
Vitamin A	Retinol equivalents[§]	875	400	375	800	1300
Vitamin C	Milligrams	60	40	33	70	95
Calcium	Milligrams	900	800	500	1200	1200
Iron	Milligrams	12	10	8.0	30	15
Vitamin D	Micrograms[‖]	6.5	10	9.0	10	10
Vitamin E	*alpha*-Tocopherol equivalents[§]	9.0	6.0	3.5	10	12
Vitamin K	Micrograms	65	15	7.5	65	65
Thiamin	Milligrams	1.2	0.7	0.4	1.5	1.6
Riboflavin	Milligrams	1.4	0.8	0.5	1.6	1.8
Niacin	Niacin equivalents[§]	16	9.0	5.5	17	20
Vitamin B-6	Milligrams	1.5	1.0	0.5	2.2	2.1
Folate	Micrograms	180	50	30	400	280
Vitamin B-12	Micrograms	2.0	0.7	0.4	2.2	2.6
Biotin	Micrograms	60	20	13	65	65
Pantothenic acid	Milligrams	5.5	3.0	2.5	5.5	5.5
Phosphorus	Milligrams	900	800	400	1200	1200
Magnesium	Milligrams	300	80	50	320	355
Zinc	Milligrams	13	10	5.0	15	19
Iodine	Micrograms	150	70	45	175	200
Selenium	Micrograms	55	20	13	65	75
Copper	Milligrams	2.0	0.9	0.6	2.5	2.5
Manganese	Milligrams	3.5	1.3	0.6	3.5	3.5
Fluoride	Milligrams	2.5	1.0	0.5	3.0	3.0
Chromium	Micrograms	120	50	33	13	130
Molybdenum	Micrograms	150	38	26	160	160
Chloride	Milligrams	3150	1000	650	3400	3400

[*]The following abbreviations are allowed: "mg" for "milligrams"; "mcg" for "micrograms"; "mcg RE" for "retinol equivalents"; "mg a-TE" for *alpha*-tocopherol equivalents"; "mg NE" for "niacin equivalents."

[†]The term "children less than 4 years of age" means persons 13 through 47 months of age.

[‡]The term "infants" means persons not more than 12 months of age.

[§]1 retinol equivalent = 1 microgram retinol or 6 micrograms *beta*-carotene; 1 *alpha*-tocopherol equivalent = 1 milligram *d-alpha*-tocopherol; 1 niacin equivalent = 1 milligram niacin or 60 milligrams of extra dietary tryptophan.

[‖]As cholecalciferol.

E

APPENDIX F
THE EXCHANGE SYSTEM

The *exchange system* is a valuable tool for quickly estimating the energy, protein, carbohydrate, and fat content of a food or meal. Using it also creates greater understanding about what one eats. Rather than memorizing the tables of composition of all foods, your work is greatly simplified by using the exchange system because it generalizes those details into a manageable framework.

The exchange system arranges food into six different categories: milk, fruit, vegetables, starch/bread, meat, and fat. These categories are designed so that after noting the proper serving size, each food within a category provides about the same amount of carbohydrate, protein, fat, and kcalories. This equality allows the exchange of foods within a category. Hence the term exchange system.

USING THE EXCHANGE SYSTEM

Using the exchange system requires knowing what foods are in each group and knowing the serving sizes for each food. We have listed the entire U.S. exchange system in this appendix. You will need to consult the exchange lists many times before you can apply the system.

Table F-1 shows the carbohydrate, protein, fat, and energy composition of each of the six exchange groups. The starch/bread group has 15 grams of carbohydrate, 3 grams of protein, and a trace of fat per exchange. The trace of fat is calculated as 1 gram of fat when the total energy contribution of an exchange is determined. The meat group is divided into three subclasses: lean, medium fat, and high fat. Each exchange has 7 grams of protein. Lean meats contain 3

TABLE F-1

The exchange lists composition (1986 edition)

Exchange List	Household Measures*	Carbohydrate (grams)	Protein (grams)	Fat (grams)	Kcalories
Starch/Bread	1 slice, ¾ cup raw, or ½ cup cooked	15	3	trace†	80
Meat	1 ounce				
Lean		—	7	3	55
Medium-Fat		—	7	5	75
High-Fat		—	7	8	100
Vegetable	½ cup cooked	5	2	—	25
Fruit	1 small piece	15	—	—	60
Milk	1 cup				
Skim		12	8	trace	90
Lowfat		12	8	5	120
Whole		12	8	8	150
Fat	1 teaspoon	—	—	5	45

The American Diabetes Association and American Dietetic Association, Exchange Lists for Meal Planning, 1986.

*Just an estimate. See exchange lists for actual amounts.

†Calculated as 1 gram for purposes of energy contribution

grams of fat per exchange, medium-fat meats have 5 grams of fat per exchange, and high-fat meats have 8 grams of fat per exchange. Meats have essentially no carbohydrate. The vegetable group contains 5 grams of carbohydrate, 2 grams of protein, and no fat per exchange. The fruit group has 15 grams of carbohydrate per exchange. Fruit has no appreciable fat or protein.

The milk group is divided into three subclasses: nonfat, lowfat, and whole. Each exchange has 12 grams of carbohydrate and 8 grams of protein. Nonfat milk has a trace of fat (calculated as 1 gram when energy content is expressed) per exchange. Lowfat milk has 5 grams of fat per exchange, and whole milk has 8 grams of fat per exchange. Finally, the fat group contains 5 grams of fat per exchange. Fats contain no appreciable amount of carbohydrate or protein.

An exchange from the starch/bread group contains 80 kcalories. Lean meats have 55 kcalories per exchange, medium-fat meats have 75 kcalories per exchange, and high-fat meats have 100 kcalories per exchange. Vegetables have 25 kcalories per exchange. Fruits have 60 kcalories per exchange. Skim milk has 90 kcalories per exchange; lowfat milk has 120 kcalories per exchange; and whole milk has 150 kcalories per exchange. Finally, fat has 45 kcalories per exchange.

TAKING A CLOSER LOOK AT THE EXCHANGE GROUPS

Before you can turn a group of exchanges into a meal plan for 1 day, you first have to see what each exchange group contains. The starch/bread group contains dry cereal, cooked cereal, rice, pasta, baked beans, corn on the cob, potatoes, bread, and tortillas. This list is not the same as that used for the Guide to Daily Food Choices. The exchange system is not concerned about the origin of the food, animal or vegetable. It is primarily concerned with the nutrient composition in terms of carbohydrate, protein, and fat of each food in a group. For example, the carbohydrate composition of potatoes resembles that of bread more than that of broccoli, although bread is not a vegetable.

The lean meat list contains round steak, lean ham, veal, chicken (without skin), fish, cottage cheese, and 95% fat-free luncheon meat. The medium-fat meat list contains T-bone steak, pork roast, lamb chops, well-drained duck and goose, salmon, mozzarella cheese, and eggs. The high-fat meat list contains prime cuts of beef (marbled), ribs, sausage, fried fish, cheddar cheese, salami, and peanut butter.

The vegetable list contains most vegetables. Some starchy vegetables were listed above in the starch/bread group. Some vegetables, such as cabbage, celery, mushrooms, lettuce, and zucchini, are free foods: their minimal energy contribution does not count in the calculations. The fruit list contains fruits and fruit juices.

The milk exchange list contains milk, plain yogurt, and buttermilk. The amount of fat in a product determines whether the serving is nonfat, lowfat, or whole.

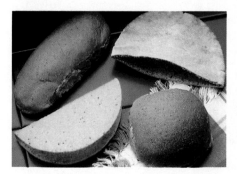 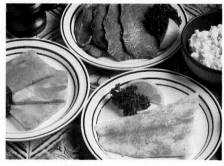

The starch/bread exchange group (left). The meat exchange group (right).

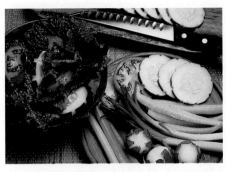
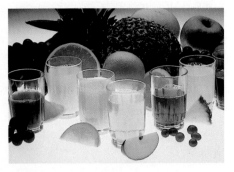

The vegetable exchange group (left). The fruit exchange group (right).

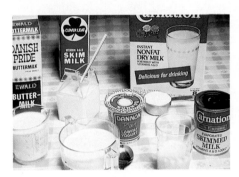
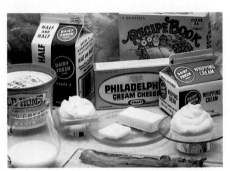

The milk exchange group (left). The fat exchange group (right).

The fat list contains margarine, mayonnaise, nuts and seeds, salad oils, olives, sour cream, and cream cheese. Bacon is considered a fat, rather than a high-fat meat.

Free foods, other than the vegetables already mentioned, include bouillon, diet soda, coffee, tea, dill pickles, and vinegar, as well as herbs and spices.

PUTTING THE EXCHANGE SYSTEM TO WORK

Let's now turn an exchange food plan into 1 day's menu. Let's say we want to consume 2000 kcalories, consisting of 55% energy from carbohydrates, 15% energy from protein, and 30% energy from fat. This can be translated into 2 lowfat milk exchanges, 3 vegetable exchanges, 5 fruit exchanges, 11 bread exchanges, 3 medium-fat meat exchanges, and 8 fat exchanges (Table F-2). Note this is only one of many possible combinations; the exchange system offers great flexibility.

Table F-3 arbitrarily separates these exchanges into breakfast, lunch, dinner, and a snack. Breakfast includes 1 lowfat milk exchange, 2 fruit exchanges, 3

TABLE F-2

Exchange patterns to get you started

Kcalories/day	1200	1600	2000	2400	2800	3200	3600
Exchange Group							
Milk (lowfat)	2	2	2	2	2	2	2
Vegetables	2	2	3	3	3	3	3
Fruit	5	4	5	8	8	10	10
Bread	4	8	11	11	15	17	20
Meat (medium fat)	2	2	3	5	5	7	8
Fat	4	7	8	9	12	12	14

These are just one set of options. More meat could be included if less milk is used, for example. The breakdown is 55% kcalories as carbohydrate, 30% kcalories as fat, 15% kcalories as protein.

TABLE F-3

Turning an exchange system plan into a menu for one day

Breakfast

1 lowfat milk exchange	1 cup 2% milk (put some on cereal)
2 fruit exchanges	1 cup orange juice
3 bread exchanges	¾ cup cold cereal, 2 pieces whole-wheat toast
2 fat exchanges	2 teaspoons margarine on toast

Lunch

4 bread exchanges	2 slices whole-wheat bread, 16 animal crackers
3 fat exchanges	2 slices bacon, 1 teaspoon mayonnaise
1 vegetable exchange	1 sliced tomato
2 fruit exchanges	1 banana (9 inches)

Dinner

3 medium-fat meat exchanges	3 ounces broiled T-bone steak
2 bread exchanges	1 large baked potato
1 fat exchange	1 teaspoon margarine
2 vegetable exchanges	1 cup broccoli
1 fruit exchange	1 kiwi fruit
1 lowfat milk exchange	1 cup 2% milk

Snack

2 bread exchanges	1 bagel
2 fat exchanges	2 tablespoons cream cheese

Prescription

	Values calculated using a computer and nutrient analysis software	
2000	kcalories	2037
55%	Carbohydrate	55%
15%	Protein	16%
30%	Fat	29%

starch/bread exchanges, and 2 fat exchanges. This total corresponds to ¾ cup cold cereal eaten with 1 cup of 2% milk, 2 slices of bread with 2 teaspoons margarine, and 1 cup of orange juice.

Lunch consists of 3 fat exchanges, 4 starch/bread exchanges, 1 vegetable exchange, and 2 fruit exchanges. This translates into 2 slices of bacon with 1 teaspoon mayonnaise, two slices of bread, and tomato. In other words, a bacon and tomato sandwich. Add to this a 9-inch banana (1 exchange = ½ banana), and 16 animal cookies.

Dinner consists of 3 medium-fat meat exchanges, 1 lowfat milk exchange, 1 fruit exchange, 2 vegetable exchanges, 1 fat exchange, and 3 starch/bread exchanges. This total corresponds to a 3-ounce broiled tenderloin steak, 1 large baked potato (1 exchange = 1 small baked potato) with 1 teaspoon of margarine, 1 cup broccoli, 1 cup of 2% milk, and 1 kiwi fruit.

Finally, we have a snack containing two starch/bread exchanges and two fat exchanges. This translates into 1 bagel with 2 tablespoons of cream cheese.

We have listed only one of many possibilities for a day's food plan. Orange juice could be exchanged for apple juice. The banana could be an apple. The tenderloin steak could be 3 ounces of chicken breast with the skin. The choices are endless.

Note that an exchange list is much easier to plan if you use individual foods as we have. However, the exchange system tables (Appendix G) list some combination foods to help you. Using combination foods, such as pizza or lasagna, just makes it more difficult to calculate the number of exchanges in a serving. For instance, lasagna has meat exchanges, vegetable exchanges, and starch/bread exchanges. With experience, you will be able to tackle such complex foods. For now, using individual foods makes learning the exchange system much easier.

To recap, Table F-3 lists the original prescription for carbohydrate, protein, fat, and energy intake. The actual percentages of carbohydrate, protein, fat, and kcalories in the diet have also been calculated using a nutrient software package and a computer. Note that the exchange system values closely match the computer analysis shown in the Table. The exchange system is a very useful tool for diet planning. If used correctly, there is no easier way to plan a precise menu pattern. Table F-1 gives you a head start in planning diets. Use this table and the following form to plan a day's diet for tomorrow. Then follow the diet you develop. Practicing this system makes it much easier to understand.

FORM F-1

Record the Exchange System pattern you have chosen in the left hand column. Then distribute the exchanges throughout the day, noting the food to be used and the serving size.

1800 Kcal/day

Exchange List	Total Exchanges to be Consumed Daily	Exchanges Consumed at Each Meal		
		Breakfast	Lunch	Dinner
Milk	2	1 c. 2% milk 1 c 1		1 c 2% milk 1
Vegetable	3		1 cup celery + carrots 1	1 c. cooked broccoli/cauliflower 2
Fruit	4	1 c. orange juice 2	1 apple 1	1/2 banana 1
Bread	10	1 c. shredded wheat cereal 2	2 slices whole wheat bread 3/4 q. pretzels 3	2 rolls 1 c. mashed potato 3 graham crackers 5
Meat	3		1 1/2 q. luncheon meat 1	2 q. baked chicken 2
Fat	7		2 teas. mayo 1	2 teas. butter 4 T. gravy 6

APPENDIX G
EXCHANGE SYSTEM LISTS

Milk exchange list

Skim milk (12 grams carbohydrate, 8 grams protein, 0 grams fat, 90 kcalories)

1 cup	skim or nonfat milk (1/2% and 1%)
1/3 cup	powdered (nonfat dry, before adding liquid)
1/2 cup	canned, evaporated skim milk
1 cup	buttermilk made from skim milk
1 cup	yogurt made from skim milk (plain, unflavored)

Lowfat milk (12 grams carbohydrate, 8 grams protein, 5 grams fat, 120 kcalories)

1 cup	2% fat fortified milk
1 cup	plain nonfat yogurt (added milk solids)

Whole milk (12 grams carbohydrate, 8 grams protein, 8 grams fat, 150 kcalories)

1 cup	whole milk
1/2 cup	buttermilk made from whole milk
1 cup	custard-style yogurt made from whole milk (plain, unflavored)

Vegetable exchange list

(5 grams carbohydrate, 2 grams protein, 0 grams fat, 25 kcalories)
1 exchange equals:
  1/2 cup cooked vegetables or vegetable juice
  1 cup raw vegetables

artichoke (1/2 medium)	cauliflower	sauerkraut
asparagus	celery	spinach cooked
beans (green, wax, Italian)	eggplant	squash, summer, zucchini
bean sprouts	green pepper	string beans (green, yellow)
beets	greens	tomato
broccoli	mushrooms, cooked	tomato juice
brussels sprouts	onions	turnips
cabbage, cooked	pea pods	vegetable juice
carrots	rhubarb	zucchini

Fruit exchange list

(15 grams carbohydrate, 0 grams protein, 0 grams fat, 60 kcalories)
1 fruit exchange equals:

1	apple (2 inches in diameter)
4 rings	dried apple
1/2 cup	apple juice
1/2 cup	applesauce (unsweetened)
4	apricots, fresh
1/2 cup	apricots, canned
7 halves	apricots, dried
1/2	banana, 9 inches

Fruit exchange list—cont'd.

3/4 cup	blackberries
3/4 cup	blueberries
1 cup	raspberries
1 1/4 cup	strawberries
1/3 melon	cantaloupe (5 inches in diameter)
12	cherries (large, raw)
1/2 cup	cherries, canned
1/2 cup	cider
1/3 cup	cranberry juice
2 1/2 medium	dates
2	figs, fresh (2 inches in diameter)
1 1/2	figs, dried
1/2	grapefruit
1/2 cup	grapefruit juice
15	grapes
1/3 cup	grape juice
1/8 melon	honeydew melon (7 inches in diameter; cubes = 1 cup)
1	kiwi (large)
3/4 cup	mandarin oranges
1/2 small	mango
1 small	nectarine (1 1/2 inches in diameter)
1 small	orange (2 1/2 inches in diameter)
1/2 cup	orange juice
1 medium or 3/4 cup	peach, fresh (2 3/4 inches in diameter)
1/2 cup or 2 halves	peach, canned
1 small or 1/2 large	pear, fresh
1/2 cup or 2 halves	pear, canned
3/4 cup	pineapple, raw
1/3 cup	pineapple, canned
1/2 cup	pineapple juice
2	plums (2 inches in diameter)
3	prunes, dried
1/3 cup	prune juice
2 tablespoons	raisins
2	tangerine (2 1/2 inches in diameter)
1 1/4 cups	watermelon (cubes)

Starch/bread exchange list

(15 grams carbohydrate, 3 grams protein, 0 grams fat, 80 kcalories)

1 starch/bread exchange equals:

Bread

1 slice	white (including French and Italian)
1 slice	whole wheat
1 slice	rye or pumpernickel
1 slice	raisin (unfrosted)
2 (2/3 ounces)	bread sticks (crisp, 4 inches long, 1/2 inch wide)
1/2 (1 ounce)	bagel, small
1/2	English muffin
1 (small)	plain roll
1/2 (1 ounce)	frankfurter bun
1/2 (1 ounce)	hamburger bun
3 tablespoons	dried bread crumbs
1	tortilla (6 inches in diameter)
1/2	pita (6 inches in diameter)

Cereal/Grains/Pasta

1/2 cup	bran flakes
3/4 cup	other ready-to-eat unsweetened cereal
1 1/2 cups	puffed cereal (unfrosted)
1/2 cup	cereal (cooked)
1/3 cup	rice or barley (cooked)

G

Cereals/Grains/Pasta—cont'd

3 tablespoons	grapenuts
1/2 cup	shredded wheat
3 tablespoons	wheat germ
1/2 cup	pasta (cooked spaghetti, noodles, macaroni)
2 1/2 tablespoons	cornmeal (dry)
2 1/2 tablespoons	flour (dry)

Crackers/Snacks

3	graham (2 1/2 inch square)
3/4 ounce	matzoh (4 inches × 6 inches)
24	oyster
4	rye crisp (2 inches × 3 1/2 inches)
6	saltines
8	animal
5 slices	melba toast
3 cups	popcorn (popped with no added fat)
3/4 ounce	pretzels

Dried Beans/Peas/Lentils

1/3 cup	dried beans, such as kidney, white, split, blackeye (cooked)
1/3 cup	lentils (cooked)
1/4 cup	baked beans

Starchy Vegetables

1/2 cup	corn
1	corn on the cob (6 inches)
1/2 cup	lima beans
1/2 cup	peas, green (canned or frozen)
1 small	potato, white (3 ounces baked)
1/2 cup	potato, mashed
1 cup	winter squash, acorn or butternut
1/3 cup	yam or sweet potato

Starch Group (With Fat)

1 starch/bread exchange
1 fat exchange

1	biscuit (2 1/2 inches across)
1/2 cup	chow mein noodles
1 (2 ounce)	corn bread (2-inch cube)
6	cracker, round butter type
10 (1 1/2 ounce)	french fries (2 inches to 3 1/2 inches)
1	muffin, plain, small
2	pancake (4 inches in diameter)
1/4 cup	stuffing, bread (prepared)
2	taco shell (6 inches across)
1	waffle (4 1/2 inches square)
4-6 (1 ounce)	whole-wheat crackers (such as Triscuits)

Meat exchange list

Lean (0 grams carbohydrate, 7 grams protein, 3 grams fat, 55 kcalories)

Beef	1 ounce	baby beef (lean) chipped beef, chuck, flank steak, tenderloin, plate ribs, round (bottom, top), all cuts rump, spare ribs, tripe
Pork	1 ounce	leg (whole rump, center shank), ham (center slices), USDA good or choice grades such as round, sirloin, flank, and tenderloin
	1 1/2 ounce	95% fat-free luncheon meat
Veal	1 ounce	leg, loin, rib, shank, shoulder, chops, roasts, all cuts except cutlets (ground or cubed)

Poultry	1 ounce	chicken, turkey, cornish hen (without skin)
	3 (1/2 cup)	egg whites, egg substitutes
Fish	2 ounces	fresh or frozen, any type canned salmon, tuna (in water), mackerel, crab, or lobster
	1 ounce	clams, oysters, scallops, shrimp
	3 ounces	sardines, drained
Cheeses	1 ounce	cottage, farmer's, or pot (lowfat), grated parmesan
Dried peas and beans	1/2 ounce	cooked

Medium fat (0 grams carbohydrate, 7 grams protein, 5 grams fat, 75 kcalories)

Beef	1 ounce	all ground beef, roast (rib, chuck, rump), steak (cubed, porterhouse, T-bone), meat loaf
Lamb	1 ounce	leg, rib, sirloin, loin (roast and chops), shank, shoulder
Pork	1 ounce	loin (all cuts tenderloin), chops, roast, Boston butt, cutlets
Poultry	1 ounce	capon, duck (domestic), goose, ground turkey, chicken with skin
Veal	1 ounce	cutlets
Organ meats	1 ounce	all types
Fish	1/4 cup	tuna (canned in oil); salmon (canned)
Cheeses	1/4 cup or 1 ounce	cottage (creamed), mozzarella (made with skim milk), ricotta, Neufchatel
Egg	1	egg
Other	4 ounces	tofu

High fat (0 grams carbohydrate, 7 grams protein, 8 grams fat, 100 kcalories)

Beef	1 ounce	brisket, corned beef (commercial), chuck (ground commercial), roasts (rib), steaks (club and rib); most USDA prime cuts of beef
Lamb	1 ounce	patties (ground lamb)
Pork	1 ounce	spare ribs, loin (back ribs), pork (ground), country-style ham, deviled ham, pork sausage
Cheeses	1 ounce	all regular cheeses (American, blue, brick, Camembert, cheddar, Gouda, Limburger, Muenster, Swiss, Monterey), all processed cheeses
Cold cuts	1 ounce	bologna, salami, pimento loaf
Frankfurter	1 ounce	(turkey or chicken)
Peanut butter	1 tablespoon	
Sausage	1 ounce	(Polish, Italian)

G

Fat exchange list

(0 grams carbohydrate, 0 grams protein, 5 grams fat, 45 kcalories)

1/8 medium	avocado	**Nuts,** 6	almonds, whole, dry roasted
1 strip	bacon, crisp	2 large	pecans, whole
1 teaspoon	butter, margarine	20 small or	peanuts, Spanish, whole
2 tablespoons	cream, light	10 large	
2 tablespoons	cream, sour	10	peanuts, Virginia, whole
1 tablespoon	cream, heavy	2 whole	walnuts
1 tablespoon	cream cheese	1 tablespoon	cashews, dry roasted
Dressing		1 tablespoon	seeds (pine, sunflower)
1 tablespoon	all varieties	2 teaspoons	pumpkin seeds
2 teaspoons	mayonnaise type	1 tablespoon	other
1 tablespoon	reduced calorie	**Oil**	
2 tablespoons	reduced calorie	1 teaspoon	corn, cottonseed, safflower, soy,
	(mayonnaise type)	**Olives**	sunflower, olive, peanut, canola
1 tablespoon	gravy, meat	10 small or 5 large	

Free Foods

A free food is any food or drink that contains less than 20 kcalories per serving. You can eat as much as you want of those items that have no serving size specified. You may eat two or three servings per day of those items that have a specific serving size. Be sure to spread them out through the day.

Drinks:
Bouillon or broth without fat
Bouillon, low-sodium
Carbonated drinks, sugar-free
Carbonated water
Club soda
Cocoa powder, unsweetened (1 tablespoon)
Coffee/Tea
Drink mixes, sugar-free
Tonic water, sugar-free
Nonnstick pan spray

Fruit:
Cranberries, unsweetened (1/2 cup)
Rhubarb, unsweetened (1/2 cup)
Vegetables:
(raw, 1 cup)
Cabbage
Celery
Chinese cabbage
Cucumber
Green onion
Hot peppers
Mushrooms
Radishes
Zucchini

Salad greens:
Endive
Escarole
Lettuce
Romaine
Spinach
Sweet substitutes:
Candy, hard, sugar-free
Gelatin, sugar-free
Gum, sugar-free
Jam/Jelly, sugar-free (2 teaspoons)
Pancake syrup, sugar-free (1-2 tablespoons)

Sugar substitutes (saccharin, aspartame)
Whipped topping (2 tablespoons)
Condiments:
Catsup (1 tablespoon)
Horseradish
Mustard
Pickles, dill, unsweetened
Salad dressing, low-calorie (2 tablespoons)
Taco sauce (3 tablespoons)
Vinegar

Seasonings:
Basil (fresh)
Celery seeds
Cinnamon
Chili powder
Chives
Curry
Dill

Flavoring extracts (vanilla, almond, walnut, peppermint, butter, lemon, etc.)
Garlic
Garlic powder
Herbs
Hot pepper sauce
Lemon

Lemon juice
Lemon pepper
Lime
Lime juice
Mint
Onion powder
Oregano
Paprika
Pepper

Pimento
Spices
Soy sauce
Soy sauce, low-sodium (lite)
Wine, used in cooking (1/4 cup)
Worcestershire sauce

APPENDIX H
THE CELL–PRIMARY SITE FOR METABOLISM

The cell is the basic unit of body structure, and it is where most metabolic reactions occur (Figure H-1). The cell is surrounded by a semipermeable membrane that controls the passage of nutrients and other substances in and out of it. Within the cell is fluid called the cytosol. Within the cytosol are small bodies called organelles that perform specific metabolic functions. The names and activities of the various cell parts are given below:

Nucleus: This spherical structure is bound by its own double membrane. Within the nucleus are chromosomes, which are long threads of DNA that contain hereditary information for directing cell protein synthesis and cell division. Although most cell types have only one nucleus, muscle cells contain many nuclei.

Mitochondria: These have their own outer membrane, as well as an inner membrane that is highly folded. The mitochondria are the major sites of energy production in the cell. Muscle cells contain many mitochondria.

Endoplasmic reticulum: This network of internal membranes serves as a communication network within the cell. Small granules called ribosomes are attached to parts of the outside of the endoplasmic reticulum, which is known as the rough endoplasmic reticulum. Ribosomes are the site for pro-

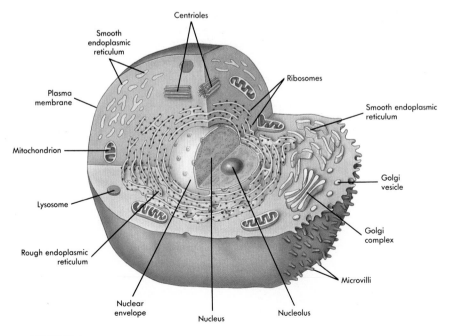

FIGURE H-1

An animal cell. Almost all human cells contain these various organelles.

tein synthesis. Fat is synthesized in other areas of the endoplasmic reticulum where there are no ribosomes, namely, the smooth endoplasmic reticulum. In muscles, this organelle (called sarcoplasmic reticulum) plays a key role in muscle contraction.

Golgi complex: This consists of stacks of flattened structures that both package proteins for export from the cell and help form other cell organelles.

Lysosomes: These small bodies contain digestive enzymes that break down worn out cell parts and other cell debris. When a lysosome fuses with a particle that is to be digested, the digestive activity begins.

Storage forms of energy: These occur in the cell as glycogen granules and lipid droplets.

H

APPENDIX I

NATIONAL CHOLESTEROL EDUCATION PROGRAM FOR ADULTS–DIETARY ADVICE

GOAL: Total blood cholesterol <200 mg/dl[*]

      LDL cholesterol <160 mg/dl or <130 mg/dl with 2 or more risk factors

If total blood cholesterol is >200 mg/dl and an individual has two or more of the following risk factors:

- Family history of coronary heart disease
- Smokes cigarettes
- Diabetes mellitus
- Obesity
- Hypertension
- Low-HDL cholesterol
- Male

Test for LDL cholesterol

If LDL cholesterol > 130 mg/dl:

- Reduce saturated fat intake to 10% of total kcalories
- Reduce total fat intake to 30% of total kcalories
- Reduce cholesterol intake to 300 mg/day

For 6 months

If unsuccessful (that is, LDL cholesterol >130 mg/dl)

- Reduce saturated fat intake to 7% of total kcalories
- Reduce cholesterol intake to 200 mg/day

For 6 months

---

[*]mg/dl represents milligrams per 100 milliliters of serum.

APPENDIX J
IMPORTANT CHEMICAL STRUCTURES IN NUTRITION

Amino Acids

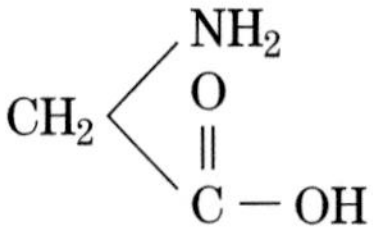

CH₂ ⟨ NH₂ / O ∥ C — OH

Glycine

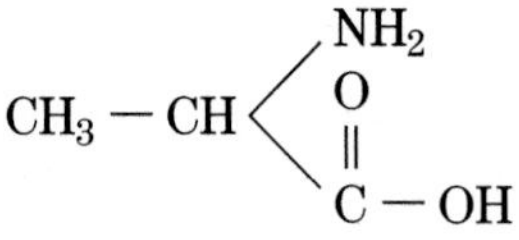

CH₃ — CH ⟨ NH₂ / O ∥ C — OH

Alanine

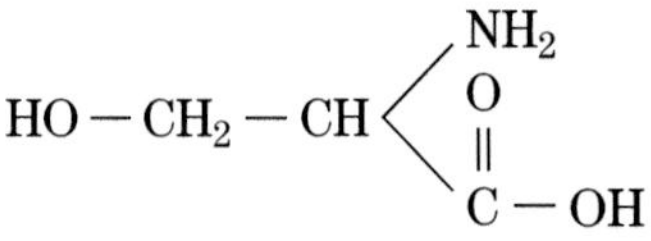

HO — CH₂ — CH ⟨ NH₂ / O ∥ C — OH

Serine

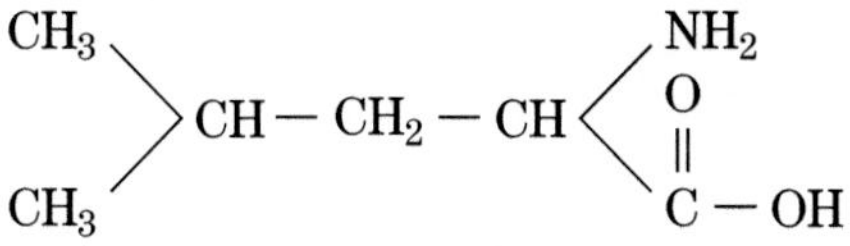

CH₃ ⟩ CH — CH₂ — CH ⟨ NH₂ / O ∥ C — OH
CH₃

**Leucine
(essential)**

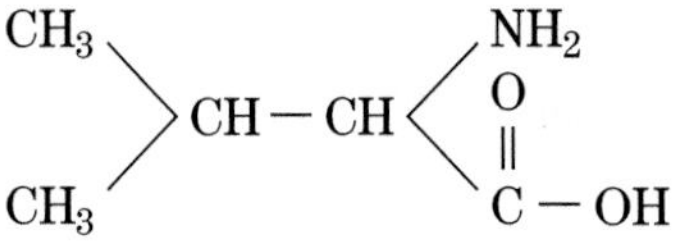

CH₃ ⟩ CH — CH ⟨ NH₂ / O ∥ C — OH
CH₃

**Valine
(essential)**

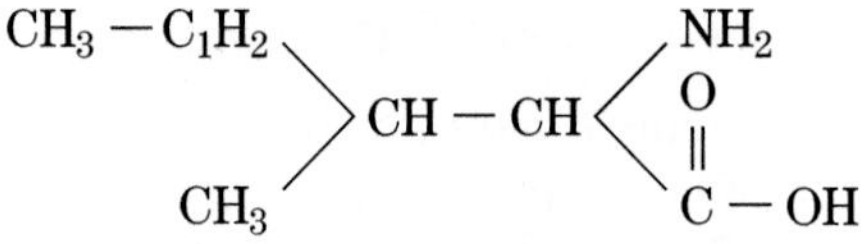

CH₃ — C₁H₂ ⟩ CH — CH ⟨ NH₂ / O ∥ C — OH
CH₃

**Isoleucine
(essential)**

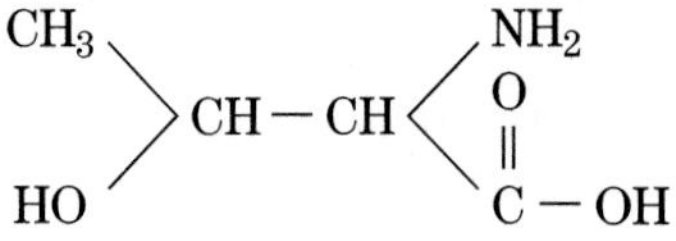

CH₃ ⟩ CH — CH ⟨ NH₂ / O ∥ C — OH
HO

**Threonine
(essential)**

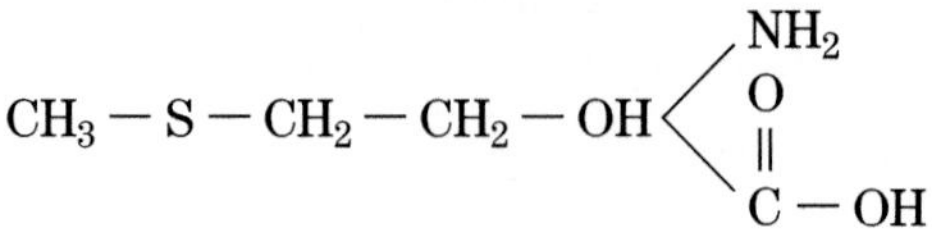

CH₃ — S — CH₂ — CH₂ — OH ⟨ NH₂ / O ∥ C — OH

**Methionine
(essential)**

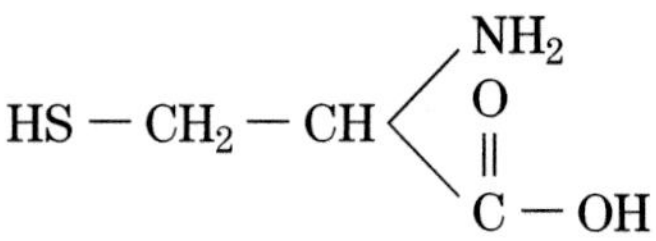

HS — CH₂ — CH ⟨ NH₂ / O ∥ C — OH

Cysteine

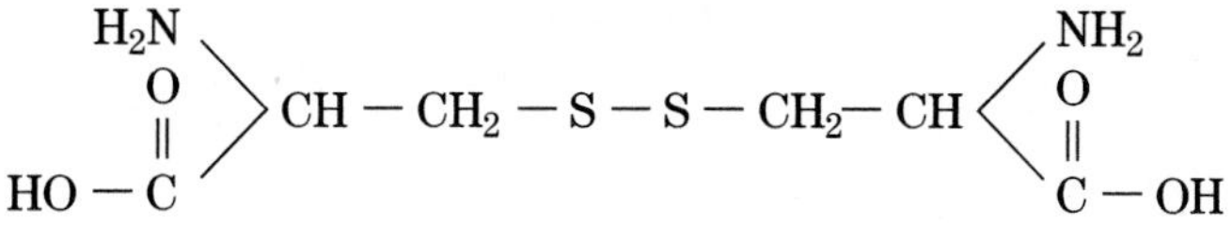

Cystine

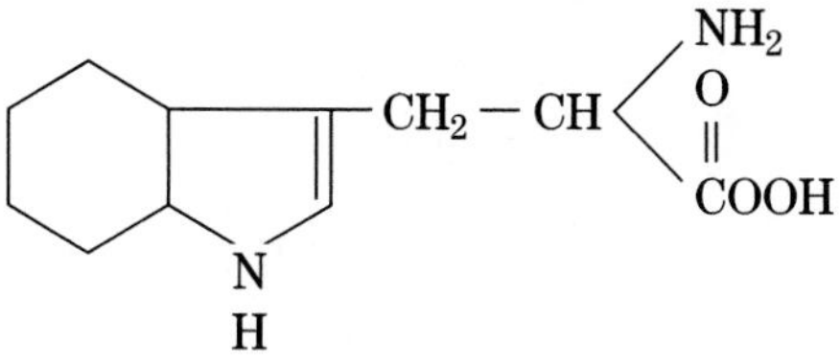

Tryptophan
(essential)

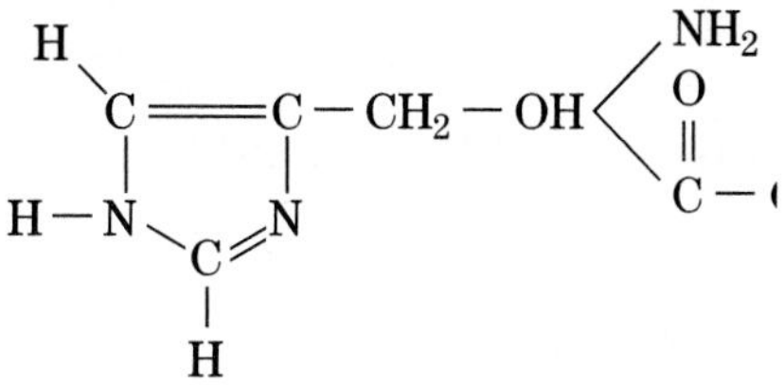

Histidine
(essential)

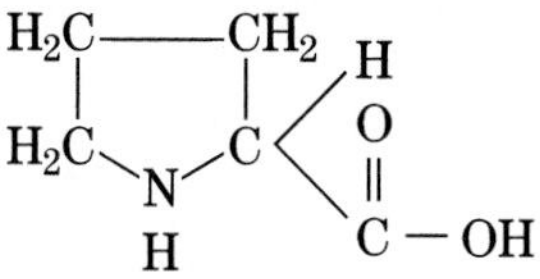

Proline

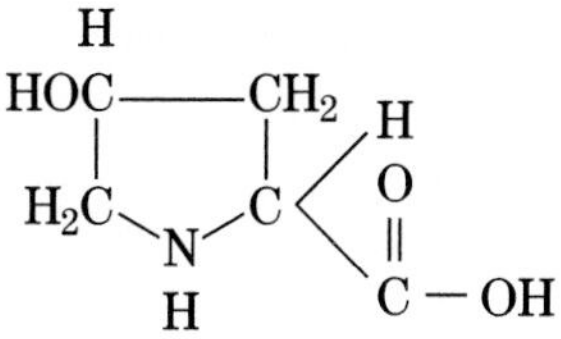

Hydroxyproline

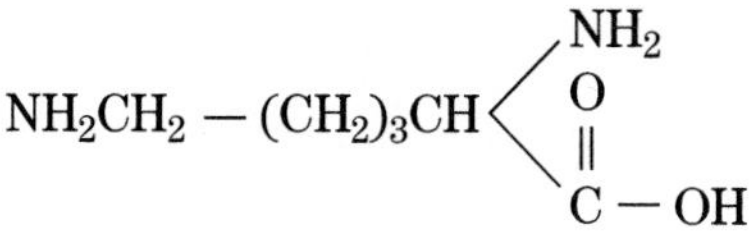

Lysine
(essential)

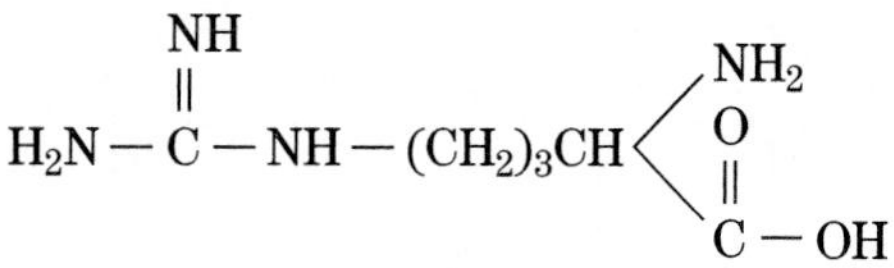

Arginine
(essential)

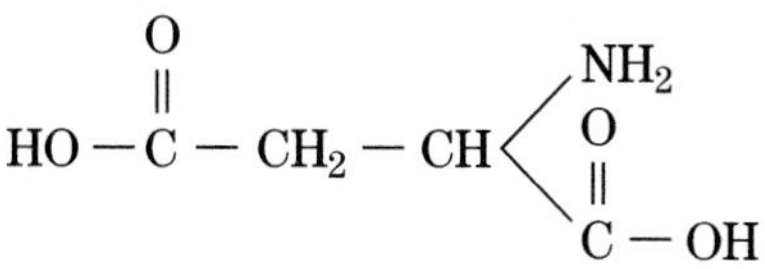

Aspartic Acid

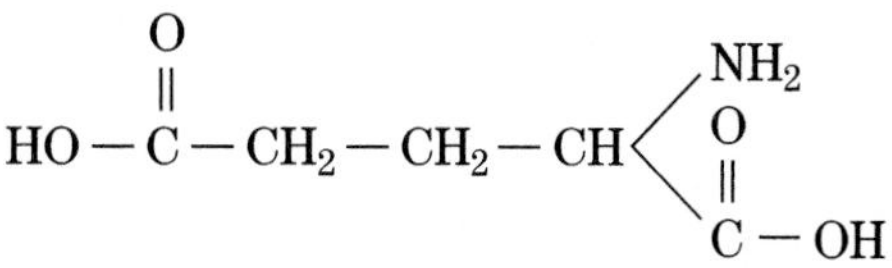

Glutamic acid

With benzene ring

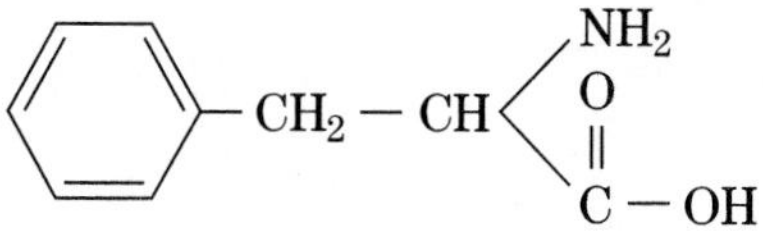

Phenylalanine
(essential)

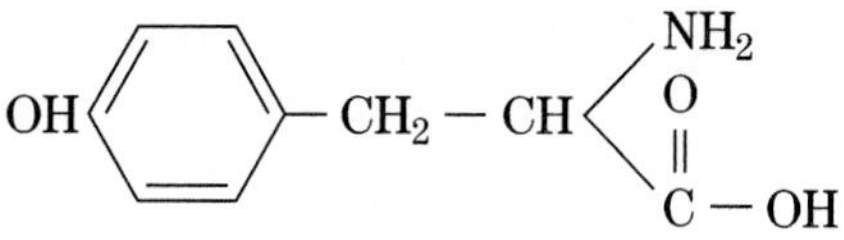

Tyrosine

Ketones

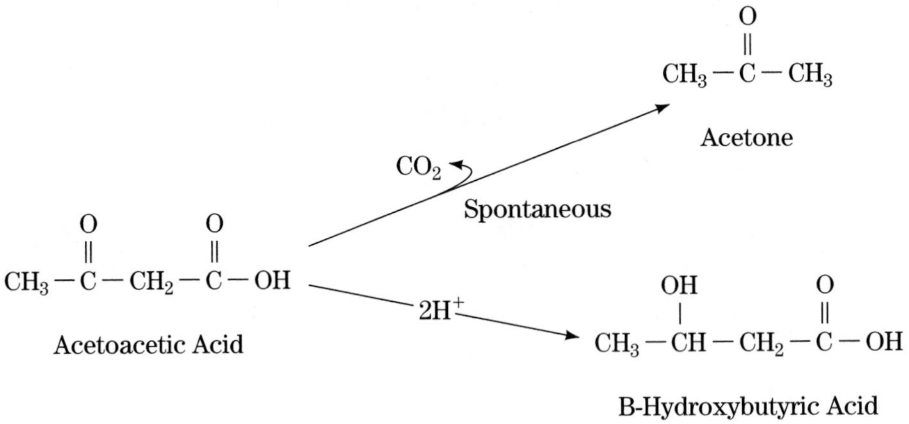

Acetoacetic Acid

Spontaneous

CO_2

Acetone

$2H^+$

B-Hydroxybutyric Acid

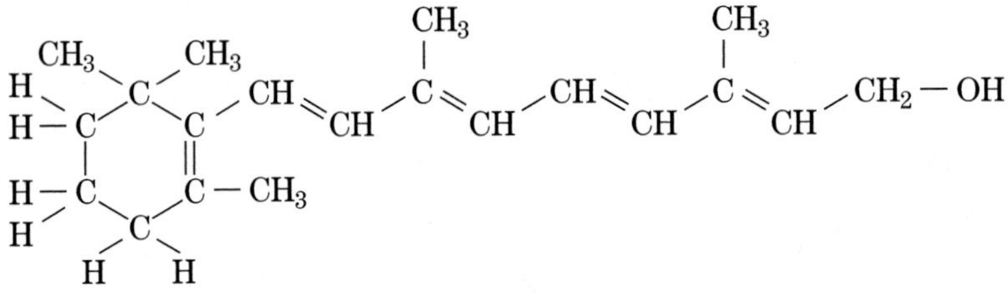

Vitamin A: retinol

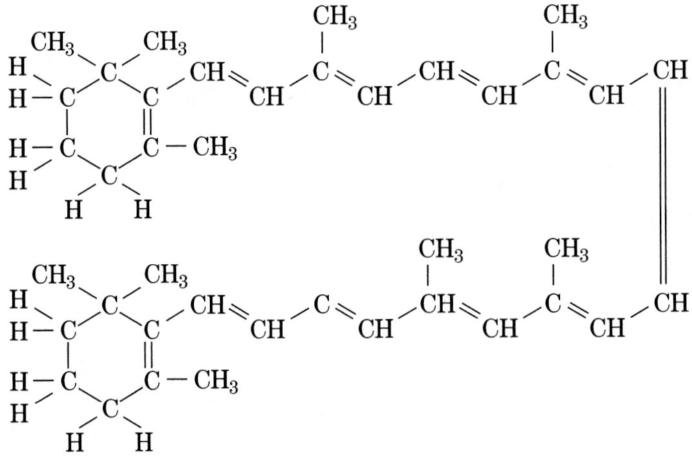

Beta-carotene

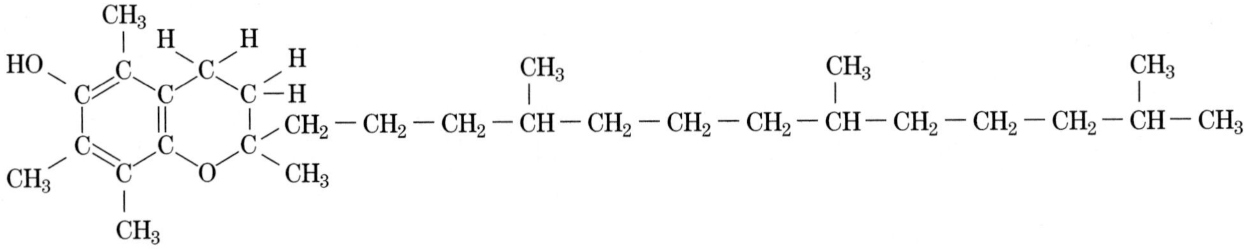

Vitamin E

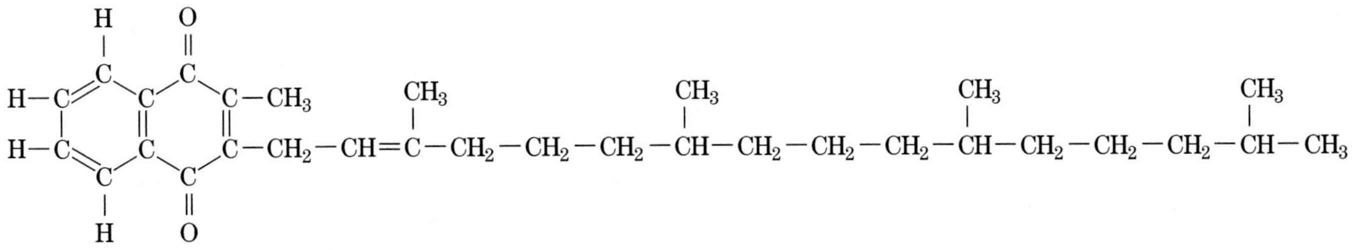

Vitamin K

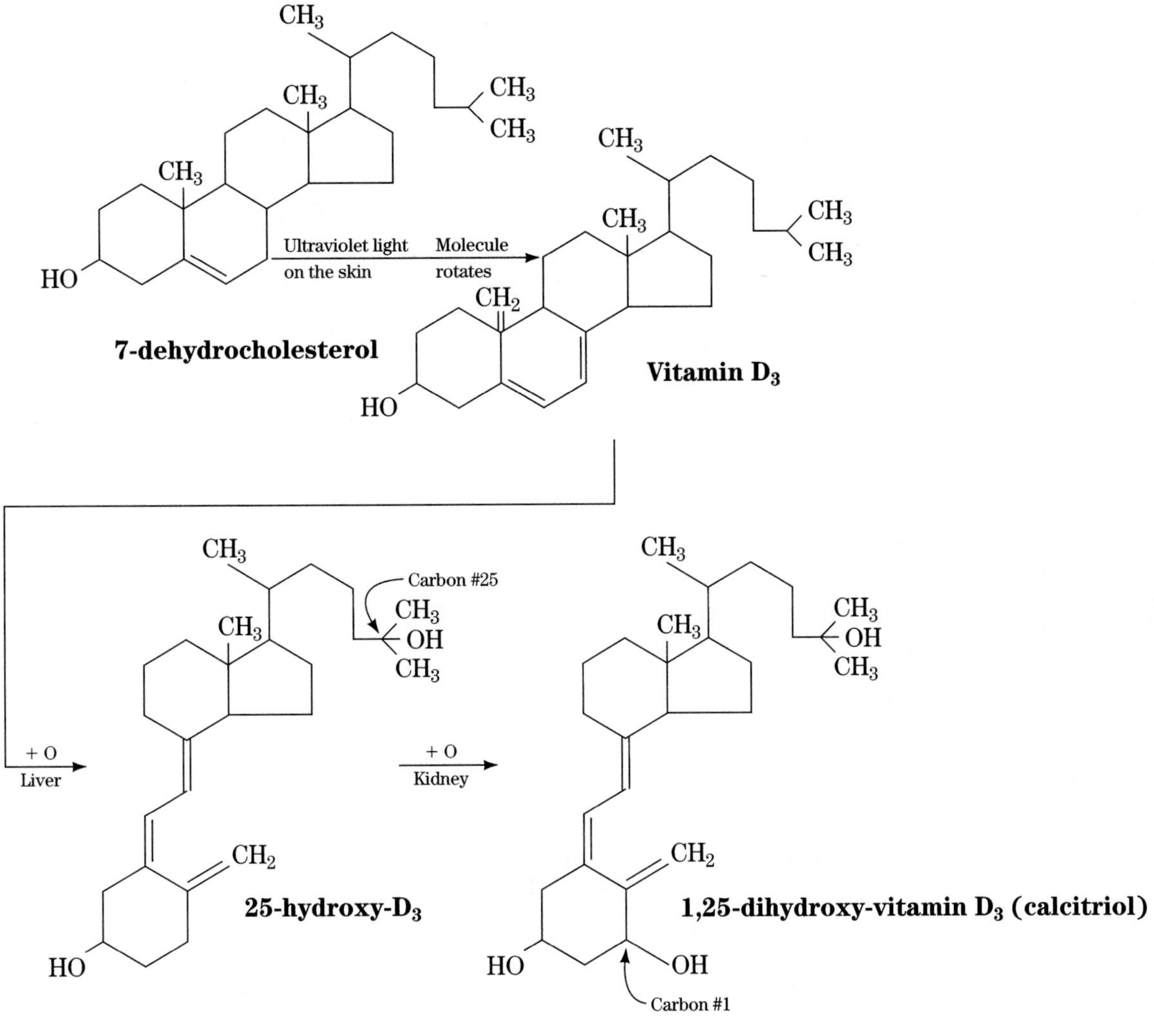

7-dehydrocholesterol → Ultraviolet light on the skin → Molecule rotates → **Vitamin D₃**

25-hydroxy-D₃

1,25-dihydroxy-vitamin D₃ (calcitriol)

Active vitamin D (calcitriol) and its precursors, beginning with 7-dehydrocholesterol

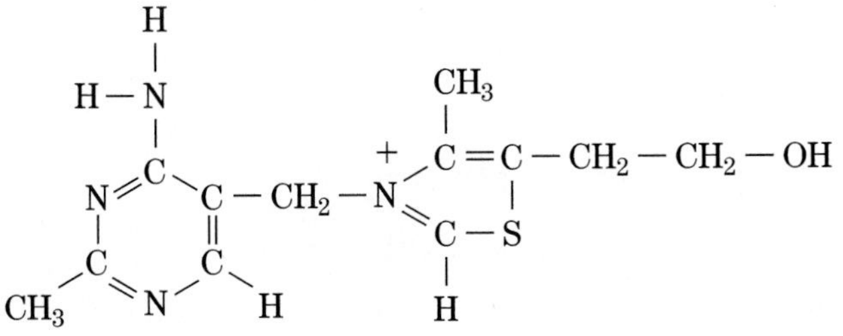

Thiamin

J

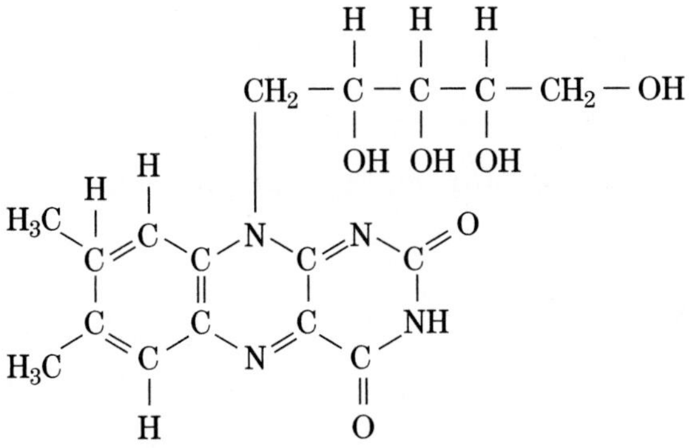

Riboflavin

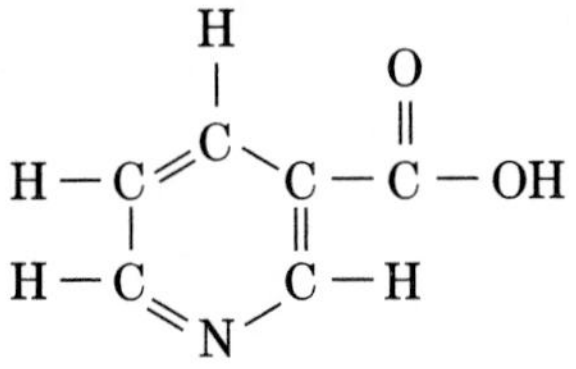

Nicotinic acid

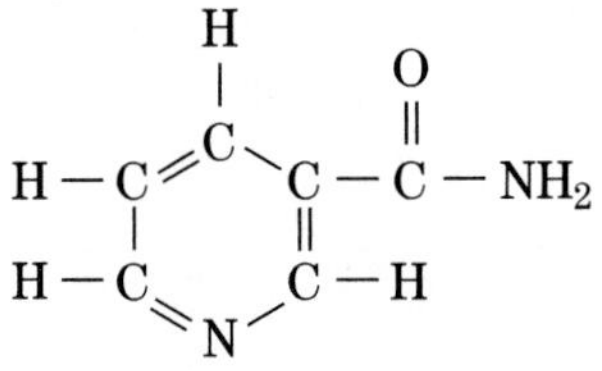

Nicotinamide

Niacin (nicotinic acid and nicotinamide).

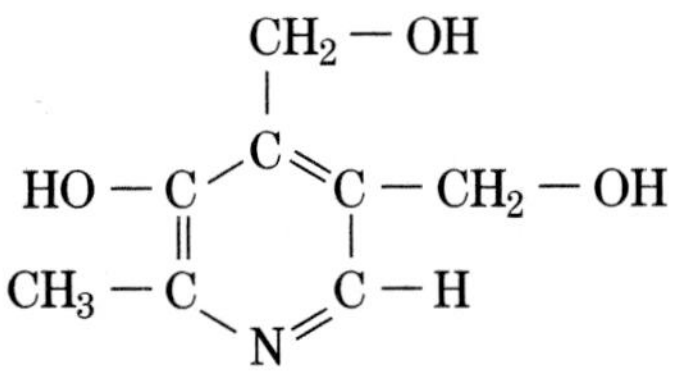

Pyridoxine

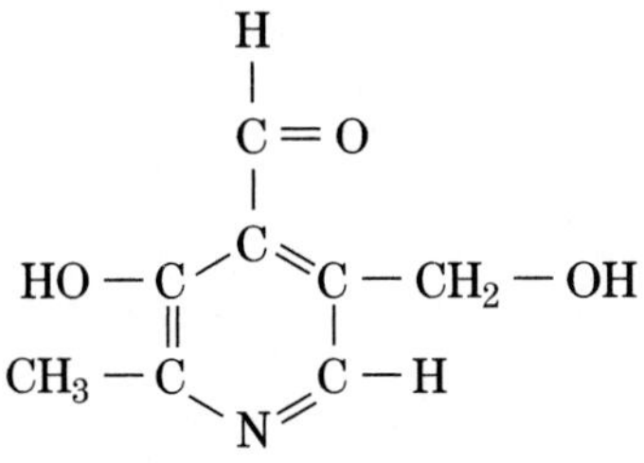

Pyridoxal

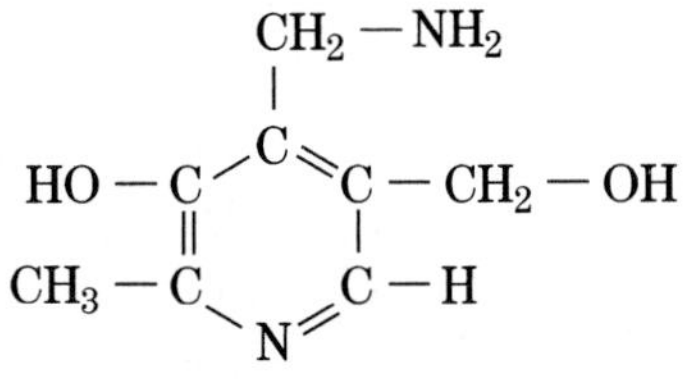

Pyridoxamine

Vitamin B-6 (a general name for three compounds—pyridoxine, pyridoxal, and pyridoxamine).

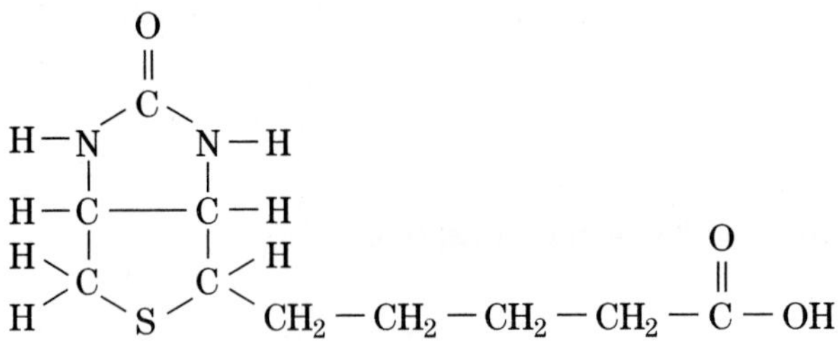

Biotin

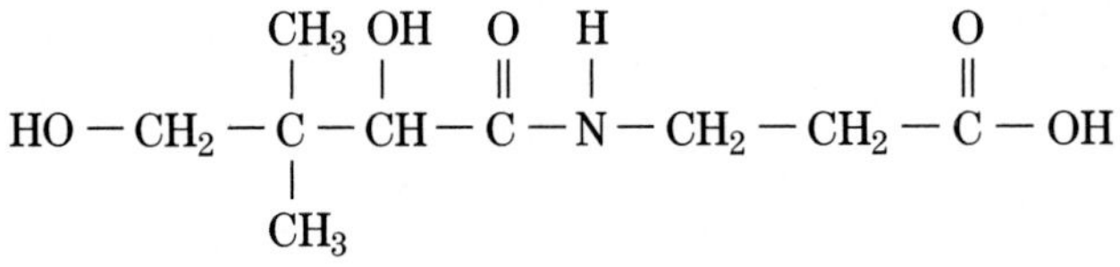

Pantothenic acid

Folate (folacin or folic acid)

Vitamin B$_{12}$ (cyanocobalamin). The arrows in this diagram indicate that the spare electrons on the nitrogens attract them to the cobalt atom.

Vitamin C

Vitamin C (ascorbic acid).

Determination of Frame Size

Method 1

Height is recorded without shoes.

Wrist circumference is measured just beyond the bony (styloid) process at the wrist joint on the right arm using a tape measure.

The following formula is used:

$$r = \frac{\text{height (cm)}}{\text{wrist circumference (cm)}}$$

Frame size can be determined as follows:

Males	Females
r > 10.4 small	r > 11.0 small
r = 9.6-10.4 medium	r = 10.1-11.0 medium
r < 9.6 large	r < 10.1 large

From Grant JP: *Handbook of total parenteral nutrition*, Philadelphia, 1980, WB Saunders.

Method 2

The patient's right arm is extended forward perpendicular to the body, with the arm bent so the angle at the elbow forms 90 degrees with the fingers pointing up and the palm turned away from the body. The greatest breadth across the elbow joint is measured with a sliding caliper along the axis of the upper arm, on the two prominent bones on either side of the elbow. This is recorded as the elbow breadth. The following tables give the elbow breadth measurements for medium-framed men and women of various heights. Measurements lower than those listed indicate a small frame size; higher measurements indicate a large frame size.

Men		Women	
Height in 1″ Heels	**Elbow Breadth**	**Height in 1″ Heels**	**Elbow Breadth**
5′2″-5′3″	$2\frac{1}{2}$-$2\frac{7}{8}$	4′10″-4′11″	$2\frac{1}{4}$-$2\frac{1}{2}$
5′4″-5′7″	$2\frac{5}{8}$-$2\frac{7}{8}$	5′0″-5′3″	$2\frac{1}{4}$-$2\frac{1}{2}$
5′8″-5′11″	$2\frac{3}{4}$-3	5′4″-5′7″	$2\frac{3}{8}$-$2\frac{5}{8}$
6′0″-6′3″	$2\frac{3}{4}$-$3\frac{1}{8}$	5′8″-5′11″	$2\frac{3}{8}$-$2\frac{5}{8}$
6′4″ and over	$2\frac{7}{8}$-$3\frac{1}{4}$	6′0″ and over	$2\frac{1}{2}$-$2\frac{3}{4}$

From Metropolitan Life Insurance Co, 1983.

APPENDIX L
CAFFEINE CONTENT OF FOODS

Beverages

*Carbonated Beverages**

cherry coke, Coca-Cola—*12 fl oz (370 g)*	46
cherry cola Slice—*12 fl oz (360 g)*	48
cherry RC—*12 fl oz (360 g)*	36
Coca-Cola—*12 fl oz (370 g)*	46
Coca-Cola Classic—*12 fl oz (369 g)*	46
cola—*12 fl oz (370 g)*	37
cola, RC—*12 fl oz (360 g)*	36
Mello Yello—*12 fl oz (372 g)*	52
Mr. Pibb—*12 fl oz (369 g)*	40
Mountain Dew—*12 fl oz (360 g)*	54
pepper type soda—*12 fl oz (368 g)*	37
Pepsi Cola—*12 fl oz (360 g)*	38

*Carbonated Beverages, Low Calorie**

diet cherry coke, Coca-Cola—*12 fl oz (354 g)*	46*
diet cherry cola Slice—*12 fl oz (360 g)*	48
diet coke, Coca-Cola—*12 fl oz (354 g)*	46
diet cola, aspartame sweetened—*12 fl oz (355 g)*	50
diet Pepsi—*12 fl oz (360 g)*	36
diet RC—*12 fl oz (360 g)*	48
Pepsi Light—*12 fl oz (360 g)*	36
Tab—*12 fl oz (354 g)*	46

Coffee

brewed—*6 fl oz (177 g)*	103
inst powder—*1 t (1.8 g)*	57
decaffeinated—*1 rd t (1.8 g)*	2
w/chicory—*1 t (1.8 g)*	37
prep from inst powder—*6 fl oz water & 1 t powder (179 g)*	57
amaretto, General Foods—*6 fl oz water & 11.5 g powder (189 g)*	60
amaretto, sugar-free, General Foods—*6 fl oz water & 7.7 g powder (185 g)*	60
decaffeinated—*6 fl oz water & 1 t powder (179 g)*	2
francais, General Foods—*6 fl oz water & 11.5 g powder (189 g)*	53
francais, sugar-free, General Foods—*6 fl oz water & 7.7 g powder (185 g)*	59
irish creme, General Foods—*6 fl oz water & 12.8 g powder (190 g)*	53
irish creme, sugar-free, General Foods—*6 fl oz water & 7.1 g powder (185 g)*	48

Beverages—cont'd

irish mocha mint, General Foods—*6 fl oz water & 11.5 g powder (189 g)*	27
irish mocha mint, sugar-free, General Foods—*6 fl oz water & 6.4 g powder (189 g)*	25
orange cappuccino, General Foods—*6 fl oz water & 14 g powder (191 g)*	73
orange cappuccino, sugar-free, General Foods—*6 fl oz water & 6.7 g powder (184 g)*	71
suisse mocha, General Foods—*6 fl oz water & 11.5 g powder (189 g)*	41
suisse mocha, sugar-free, General Foods—*6 fl oz water & 6.4 g powder (184 g)*	40
vienna, General Foods—*6 fl oz water & 14 g powder (191 g)*	56
vienna, sugar-free, General Foods—*6 fl oz water & 6.7 g powder (184 g)*	55
w/ chicory—*6 fl oz water & 1 t powder (179 g)*	38

Tea, Hot/Iced

brewed 3 min—*6 fl oz water (178 g)*	36
inst powder—*1 t (0.7 g)*	31
w/ lemon flavor—*1 rd t (1.4 g)*	25
w/ sugar & lemon flavor—*3 t (23 g)*	29
w/ sodium saccharin & lemon flavor—*2 t (1.6 g)*	36
prep from inst powder	
1 t powder in 8 fl oz water (237 g)	31
Crystal Light—*8 fl oz (238 g)*	11
w/lemon flavor—*1 t powder in 8 fl oz water (238 g)*	26
w/ sugar & lemon flavor—*3 t powder in 8 fl oz water (259 g)*	29
w/ sodium saccharin & lemon flavor—*2 t powder in 8 fl oz water (238 g)*	36

Candy

chocolate (choc)	
german sweet, Bakers—*1 oz square (28 g)*	8
semi-sweet, Bakers—*1 oz square (28 g)*	13
choc chips	
Bakers—*¼ cup (43 g)*	12
german sweet, Bakers—*¼ cup (43 g)*	15
semi-sweet, Bakers—*¼ cup (43 g)*	14
milk choc, Cadbury—*1 oz (28 g)*	15

*Caffeine-free carbonated beverages and most non-cola carbonated beverages contain no caffeine.

From Pennington JAT: *Bowes and Church's food values of portions commonly consumed*, ed 15, Philadelphia, 1989, JB Lippincott.

Continued.

Desserts

Frozen Desserts

pudding pops, Jell-O

choc—*1 pop (47 g)*	2
choc caramel swirl—*1 pop (47 g)*	1
choc fudge—*1 pop (47 g)*	3
choc van swirl—*1 pop (47 g)*	1
choc w/ choc chips—*1 pop (48 g)*	3
choc w/ choc coating—*1 pop (49 g)*	3
double choc swirl—*1 pop (47 g)*	2
milk choc—*1 pop (47 g)*	2
van w/ choc chips—*1 pop (48 g)*	1
van w/ choc coating—*1 pop (49 g)*	1

Pies

choc mousse, from mix, Jell-O—*⅛ pie (95 g)*	6

Puddings, from inst mix

choc

Jell-O—*½ cup (150 g)*	5
sugar-free, D-Zerta—*½ cup (130 g)*	4
sugar-free, Jell-O—*½ cup (133 g)*	4

choc fudge

Jell-O—*½ cup (150 g)*	8
sugar-free, Jell-O—*½ cup (135 g)*	9
choc fudge mousse, Jell-O—*½ cup (86 g)*	12
choc mousse, Jell-O—*½ cup (86 g)*	9

Desserts—cont'd

choc tapioca, Jell-O—*½ cup (147 g)*	8
milk choc, Jell-O—*½ cup (150 g)*	5

Milk Beverages

choc flavor mix in whole milk—*2-3 t powder in 8 fl oz milk (266 g)*	8
choc malted milk flavor powder	
in whole milk—*3 t powder in 8 fl oz milk (265 g)*	8
w/ added nutrients in whole milk—*4-5 t powder in 8 fl oz milk (265 g)*	5
choc syrup in whole milk—*2 T syrup in 8 fl oz milk (282 g)*	6
cocoa/hot chocolate, prep w/ water from mix—*¾ t powder in 6 fl oz water (206 g)*	4

Milk Beverage Mixes

choc flavor mix, powder—*2-3 t (22 g)*	8
choc malted milk flavor mix, powder—*¾ oz (3 t) (21 g)*	8
choc malted milk flavor mix w/ added nutrients, powder—*¾ oz (4-5 t) (21 g)*	6
choc syrup—*2 T (1 fl oz) (38 g)*	5
cocoa mix powder—*1 oz pkt (3-4 t) (28 g)*	5

Miscellaneous

baking choc, unsweetened, Bakers—*1 oz (28 g)*	25

APPENDIX M
ENERGY COST OF VARIOUS ACTIVITIES

| Activity | Body Weight | | |
	120 Pounds (54 Kilograms) Kcal/Hour	150 Pounds (68 Kilograms) Kcal/Hour	180 Pounds (82 Kilograms) Kcal/Hour
Aerobics—heavy	435	544	653
Aerobics—light	163	204	244
Aerobics—medium	272	340	408
Back-packing	489	612	734
Badminton	277	346	416
Ballroom dancing	166	208	249
Basketball—vigorous	544	680	816
Bicycling (5.5 MPH)	163	204	244
Billiards	108	136	163
Bowling	212	265	318
Calisthenics—heavy	435	544	653
Calisthenics—light	217	272	326
Canoeing (2.5 MPH)	179	224	269
Carpentry—general	272	340	408
Circuit training	604	755	906
Cleaning (F)	202	253	303
Cleaning (M)	189	236	284
Climbing (100 FT/HR)	391	489	587
Cooking (F)	146	183	220
Cooking (M)	156	195	235
Cycling (13 MPH)	527	659	791
Disco dancing	326	408	489
Ditch digging—hand	315	394	473
Dressing/showering	85	106	128
Driving	93	117	140
Eating (sitting)	75	93	112
Fencing	239	299	359
Food shopping (F)	202	253	303
Food shopping (M)	189	236	284
Football—touch	380	476	571
Gardening	174	217	261
Gardening—digging	411	514	617
Gardening—raking	176	220	264
Golf	195	244	293
Horseback riding—trotting	277	346	416
Housework—cleaning	217	272	326
Ice skating (10 MPH)	315	394	473
Jazzercize—heavy	435	544	653
Jazzercize—light	163	204	244
Jazzercize—medium	272	340	408
Jogging—medium	489	612	734
Jogging—slow	380	476	571

Continued.

Activity	Body Weight		
	120 Pounds (54 Kilograms) Kcal/Hour	150 Pounds (68 Kilograms) Kcal/Hour	180 Pounds (82 Kilograms) Kcal/Hour
Judo	636	795	955
Lawn mowing (hand)	212	265	318
Lawn mowing (power)	195	244	293
Lying—at ease	71	89	107
Piano playing	130	163	195
Racquetball—social	435	544	653
Roller skating	277	346	416
Rowboating (2.5 MPH)	239	299	359
Running or jogging (10 MPH)	718	897	1077
Scull rowing (race)	669	836	1004
Sewing—hand	104	130	156
Shuffleboard/skeet	163	204	244
Sitting quietly	68	85	102
Skiing (10 MPH)	478	598	718
Sleeping	64	80	97
Square dancing	277	346	416
Squash or handball	478	598	718
Swimming (.25 MPH)	239	299	359
Table tennis	282	353	424
Tennis	331	414	497
Volleyball	277	346	416
Walking (2.5 MPH)	163	204	244
Walking (3.75 MPH)	239	299	359
Water skiing	380	476	571
Weight lifting—heavy	489	612	734
Weight lifting—light	217	272	326
Window cleaning (F)	192	240	288
Window cleaning (M)	189	236	284
Wood chopping/sawing	315	394	473
Writing (sitting)	94	118	142

M

APPENDIX N

AN EXAMPLE OF PRENATAL VITAMIN/MINERAL SUPPLEMENTS AND PRENATAL WEIGHT GAIN CHART

NATALINS® Rx

Ingredients Vitamins	Natalins Rx Units
Vitamin A, IU	4000
Vitamin D, IU	400
Vitamin E, IU	15
Vitamin C, mg	80
Folic Acid, mg	1
Thiamin (B-1), mg	1.5
Riboflavin (B-2), mg	1.6
Niacin, mg	17
Vitamin B-6, mg	4
Vitamin B-12, mcg	2.5
Biotin, mg	0.003
Pantothenic Acid, mg	7
Minerals	
Calcium, mg	200
Iron, mg	60
Magnesium, mg	100
Copper, mg	3
Zinc, mg	25

Indications and usage

Natalins Rx tablets help asssure an adequate intake of the vitamins and minerals listed above. Folic acid helps prevent the development of megaloblastic anemia during pregnancy.

Contraindications

Supplemental vitamins and minerals should not be prescribed for patients with hemochromatosis or Wilson's disease.

Warning

Keep Natalins Rx tablets out of the reach of children.

Precautions

General

Pernicious anemia should be excluded before using this product since folic acid may mask the symptoms of pernicious anemia. The calcium content should be considered before prescribing for patients with kidney stones. Do not exceed the recommended dose.

Adverse Reactions

No adverse reactions or undesirable side effects have been attributed to the use of Natalins Rx tablets.

Dosage and Administration

One tablet daily, or as prescribed.

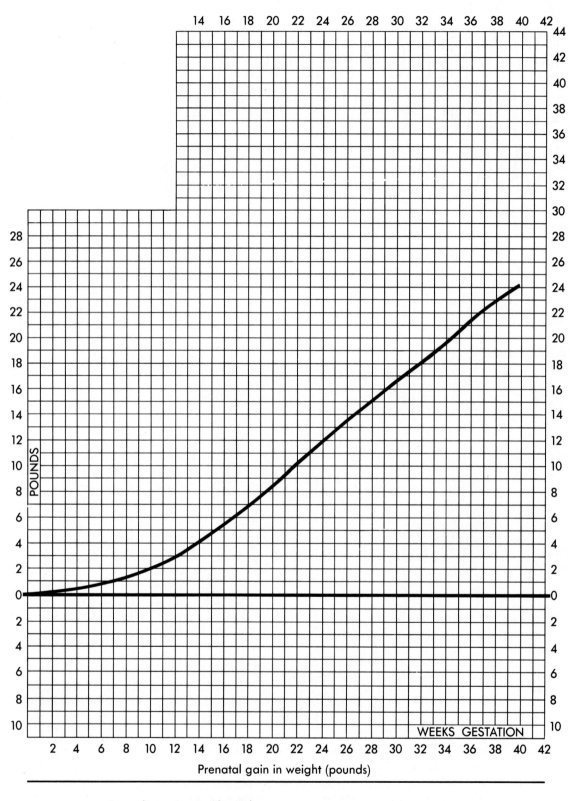

POUNDS

WEEKS GESTATION

Prenatal gain in weight (pounds)

Immediate pregravid weight: _____

Height in inches without shoes (plus one inch): _____

Standard weight: _____

(Record weight *with* shoes) _____

APPENDIX O
INFANT AND CHILD GROWTH CHARTS

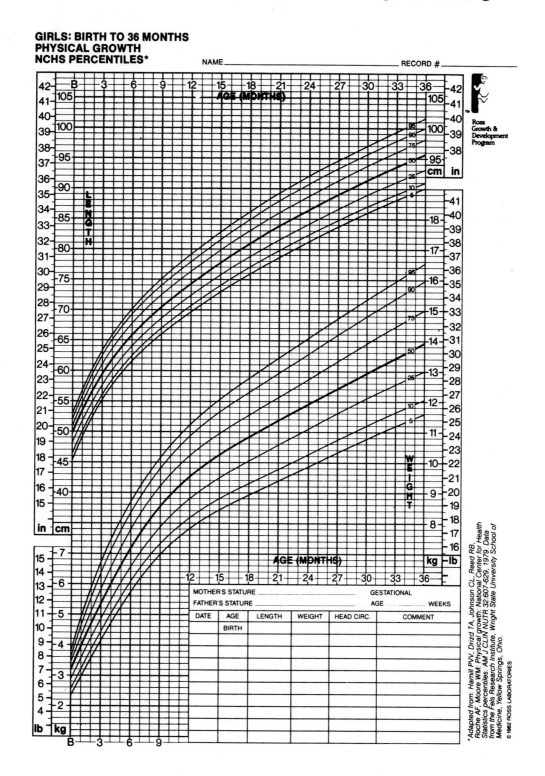

GIRLS: BIRTH TO 36 MONTHS
PHYSICAL GROWTH
NCHS PERCENTILES*

NAME _____ RECORD # _____

*Adapted from: Hamill PVV, Drizd TA, Johnson CL, Reed RB, Roche AF, Moore WM: Physical growth: National Center for Health Statistics percentiles. AM J CLIN NUTR 32:607-629, 1979. Data from the Fels Research Institute, Wright State University School of Medicine, Yellow Springs, Ohio.
© 1982 ROSS LABORATORIES

BOYS: BIRTH TO 36 MONTHS
PHYSICAL GROWTH
NCHS PERCENTILES*

NAME _____   RECORD # _____

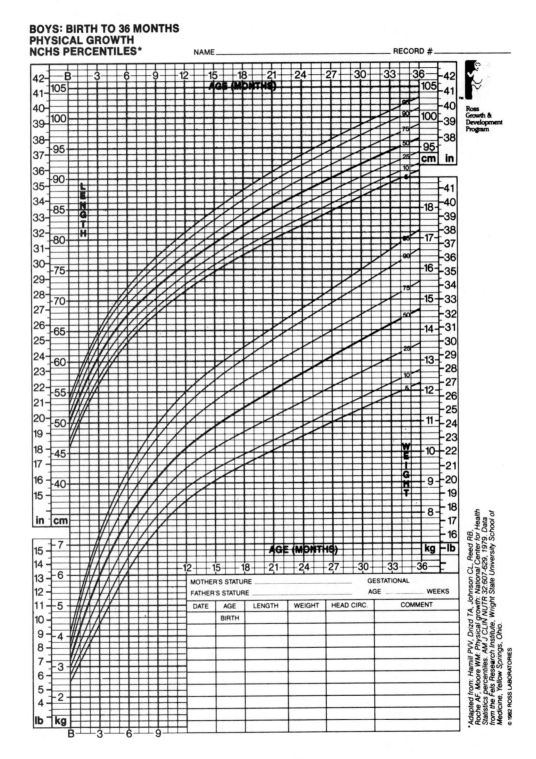

MOTHER'S STATURE _____   GESTATIONAL
FATHER'S STATURE _____   AGE _____ WEEKS

DATE	AGE	LENGTH	WEIGHT	HEAD CIRC.	COMMENT
	BIRTH				

*Adapted from: Hamill PVV, Drizd TA, Johnson CL, Reed RB, Roche AF, Moore WM. Physical growth: National Center for Health Statistics percentiles. AM J CLIN NUTR 32:607-629, 1979. Data from the Fels Research Institute, Wright State University School of Medicine, Yellow Springs, Ohio.

© 1982 ROSS LABORATORIES

Ross
Growth &
Development
Program

GIRLS: BIRTH TO 36 MONTHS
PHYSICAL GROWTH
NCHS PERCENTILES*

NAME _____ RECORD # _____

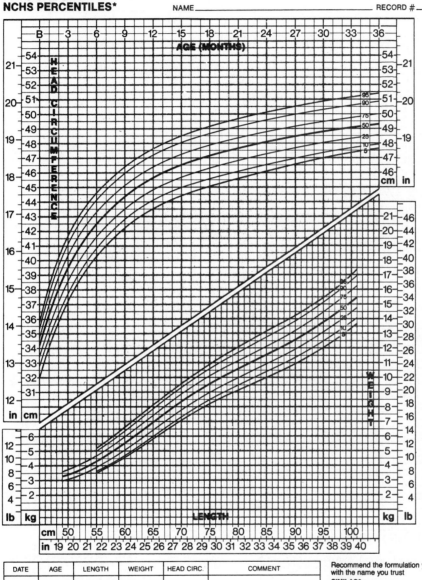

*Adapted from: Hamill PVV, Drizd TA, Johnson CL, Reed RB, Roche AF, Moore WM. Physical growth: National Center for Health Statistics percentiles. AM J CLIN NUTR 32:607-629, 1979. Data from the Fels Research Institute, Wright State University School of Medicine, Yellow Springs, Ohio.
© 1982 ROSS LABORATORIES

DATE	AGE	LENGTH	WEIGHT	HEAD CIRC.	COMMENT

Recommend the formulation you prefer
with the name you trust

SIMILAC®
SIMILAC® WITH IRON
SIMILAC® WITH WHEY
Infant Formulas

The ISOMIL® System of
Soy Protein Formulas

ADVANCE®
Nutritional Beverage

ROSS LABORATORIES
COLUMBUS, OHIO 43216
Division of Abbott Laboratories, USA

G106/JUNE 1983   LITHO IN USA

BOYS: BIRTH TO 36 MONTHS
PHYSICAL GROWTH
NCHS PERCENTILES*

NAME _____ RECORD # _____

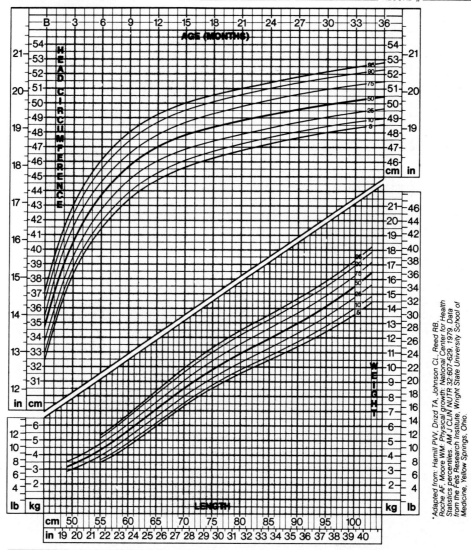

*Adapted from: Hamill PVV, Drizd TA, Johnson CL, Reed RB, Roche AF, Moore WM: Physical growth: National Center for Health Statistics percentiles. AM J CLIN NUTR 32:607-629, 1979. Data from the Fels Research Institute, Wright State University School of Medicine, Yellow Springs, Ohio.

© 1982 ROSS LABORATORIES

DATE	AGE	LENGTH	WEIGHT	HEAD CIRC.	COMMENT

Recommend the formulation you prefer
with the name you trust

SIMILAC®
SIMILAC® WITH IRON
SIMILAC® WITH WHEY
Infant Formulas

The **ISOMIL®** System of
Soy Protein Formulas

ADVANCE®
Nutritional Beverage

ROSS LABORATORIES
COLUMBUS, OHIO 43216
Division of Abbott Laboratories, USA

G105/JUNE 1983   LITHO IN USA

**BOYS: PREPUBESCENT
PHYSICAL GROWTH
NCHS PERCENTILES***

NAME _____ RECORD # _____

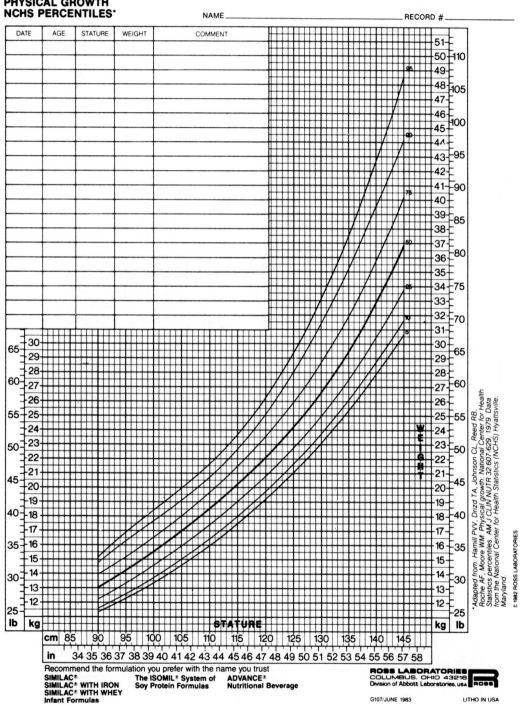

*Adapted from: Hamill PVV, Drizd TA, Johnson CL, Reed RB, Roche AF, Moore WM. Physical growth: National Center for Health Statistics percentiles. AM J CLIN NUTR 32:607-629, 1979. Data from the National Center for Health Statistics (NCHS) Hyattsville, Maryland.

© 1982 ROSS LABORATORIES

Recommend the formulation you prefer with the name you trust

SIMILAC®
SIMILAC® WITH IRON
SIMILAC® WITH WHEY
Infant Formulas

The ISOMIL® System of
Soy Protein Formulas

ADVANCE®
Nutritional Beverage

ROSS LABORATORIES
COLUMBUS, OHIO 43216
Division of Abbott Laboratories, USA

G107/JUNE 1983   LITHO IN USA

O

**GIRLS: PREPUBESCENT
PHYSICAL GROWTH
NCHS PERCENTILES***

NAME _____ RECORD # _____

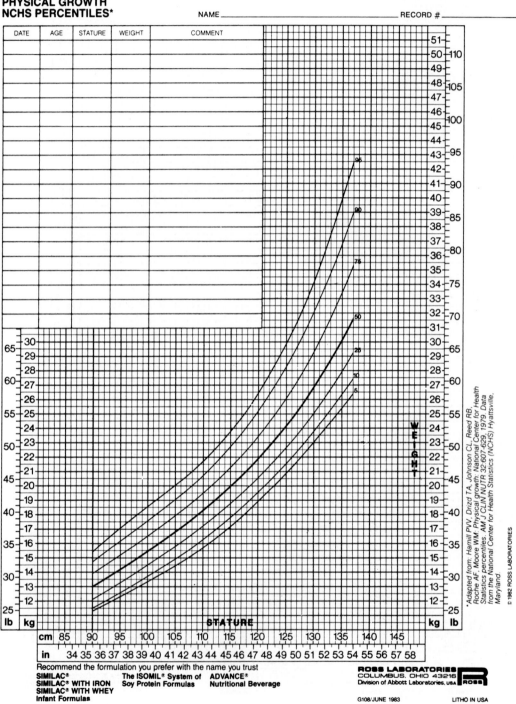

*Adapted from: Hamill PVV, Drizd TA, Johnson CL, Reed RB, Roche AF, Moore WM. Physical growth: National Center for Health Statistics percentiles. AM J CLIN NUTR 32:607-629, 1979. Data from the National Center for Health Statistics (NCHS) Hyattsville, Maryland.

© 1982 ROSS LABORATORIES

Recommend the formulation you prefer with the name you trust
SIMILAC®
SIMILAC® WITH IRON   The ISOMIL® System of   **ADVANCE®**
SIMILAC® WITH WHEY   Soy Protein Formulas   **Nutritional Beverage**
Infant Formulas

ROSS LABORATORIES
COLUMBUS, OHIO 43216
Division of Abbott Laboratories, USA

G108/JUNE 1983   LITHO IN USA

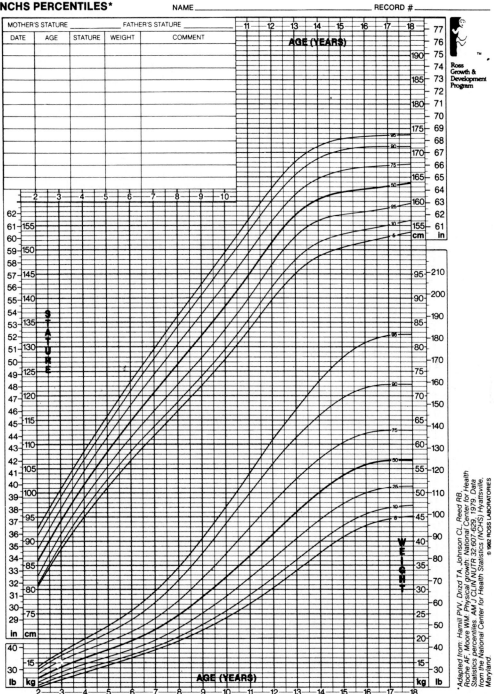

GIRLS: 2 TO 18 YEARS
PHYSICAL GROWTH
NCHS PERCENTILES*

NAME _____ RECORD # _____

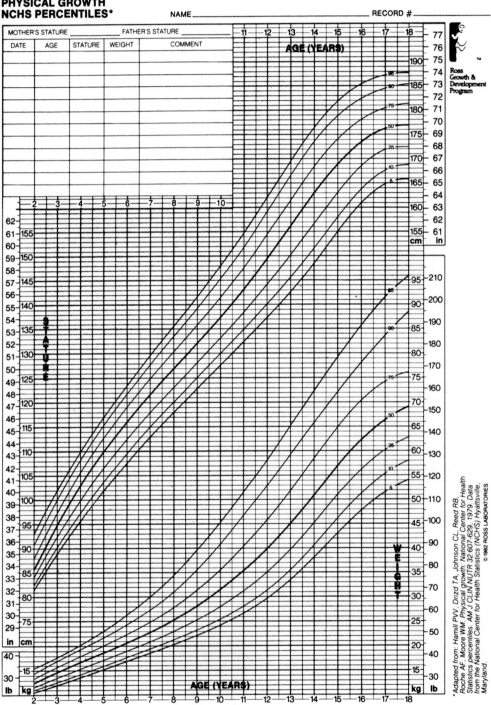

BOYS: 2 TO 18 YEARS
PHYSICAL GROWTH
NCHS PERCENTILES*

NAME _____ RECORD # _____

*Adapted from: Hamill PVV, Drizd TA, Johnson CL, Reed RB, Roche AF, Moore WM: Physical growth: National Center for Health Statistics percentiles. AM J CLIN NUTR 32:607-629, 1979. Data from the National Center for Health Statistics (NCHS) Hyattsville, Maryland.

© 1982 ROSS LABORATORIES

Ross
Growth &
Development
Program

APPENDIX P
SAFE FOOD STORAGE

Safe Food Storage and Handling Chart
—Refrigerator Storage—

The suggested time aims at maintaining good eating quality and minimizing loss of nutritive value.
Suggested maximum times for storing food in refrigerator at 34° F to 40° F

Food	Time	Special Handling
Canning food after opening		
Baby food	2-3 days	*Store covered. Don't feed baby from jar; saliva may liquefy food.*
Fish, seafood, and poultry	1 day	
Fruit	1 week	*Store all canned foods tightly covered. It is not necessary to remove food from can.*
Meats, gravy, broths	2 days	
Pickles, olives	1 month	
Sauce, tomato based	5 days	
Vegetables	3 days	
Cured and smoked meats		
Bacon, corned beef	5-7 days	*Keep wrapped. Store in coldest part of refrigerator or in a meat keeper. Times are for opened packages of sliced meats. Unopened vacuum packs keep about two weeks.*
Bologna loaves	4-6 days	
Dried beef	10-12 days	
Dry and semidry sausage (salami, etc.)	2-3 weeks	
Frankfurters, liver sausage	4-5 days	
Hams (whole, halves)	1 week	
Hams, canned (unopened)	6 months	
Luncheon meat	3 days	
Sausage, fresh or smoked	2-3 days	
Dairy products		
Butter, margarine	1-2 weeks	*Keep tightly wrapped or covered.*
Buttermilk, sour cream, or yogurt	5-14 days	
Cheese		
cottage, ricotta	5 days	*Keep all cheese tightly packaged in moisture-resistant wrap. If outside of hard cheese gets moldy, just cut away mold— it won't affect flavor.*
cream, Neufchatel	2 weeks	
hard and wax-coated cheeses		
large pieces (unopened)	3-6 months	
(opened)	3-4 weeks	
(sliced)	2 weeks	
process (opened)	3-4 weeks	*Unopened process cheese need not be refrigerated*
Cream—light, heavy, half-and-half	3 days	*Keep tightly covered. Don't return unused cream to original container. This would spread any bacteria present in leftover cream.*
Dips—sour cream, etc.		
commercial	2 weeks	
homemade	2 days	
Eggs: in shell	3 weeks	
whites	3 days	*Store in covered container.*
yolks	3 days	*Cover yolks with water; cover container.*
Milk		
evaporated (opened)	4-5 days	

Continued.

Safe Food Storage and Handling Chart
—Refrigerator Storage—cont'd.

Food	Time	Special Handling
Dairy products—cont'd		
pasturized, reliquefied nonfat dry, skimmed	3-4 days	*Keep containers tightly closed. Do not return unused milk to original container.*
sweetened condensed	4-5 days	*Remove entire lid of can to make pouring easier. Keep covered.*
Fruits and vegetables—fresh		
Fruits		
apples, melons, citrus fruits	1 week	*Do not wash fruit before storing—moisture encourages spoilage. Store in crisper or moisture-resistant bags or wrap. Wrap uncut cantaloupe, honeydew, etc., to prevent odor spreading to other foods.*
berries, cherries	1-2 days	
other fruit	3-5 days	
citrus juices, bottled, frozen, canned	6 days	
Vegetables		
beets, carrots, radishes	2 weeks	*Remove leafy tops; keep in crisper.*
mushrooms	1-2 days	*Do not wash before storing.*
shredded salad greens	1-2 days	*Keep in moisture-resistant wrap or bags.*
peas (in the pod), corn in husks	3-5 days	*Keep in crisper or moisture-resistant wrap or bags.*
other vegetables	3-5 days	*Keep in crisper or moisture-resistant wrap or bags.*
Meat, fish, and poultry—fresh uncooked		
Meats—beef, lamb, pork, and veal—chops	3-4 days	
ground meat, stew meat	1-2 days	
roasts	5-6 days	
steaks	3-5 days	
variety of meats (liver, heart, etc.)	1-2 days	
Fish and shellfish		*Store loosely wrapped. Keep in coldest part of refrigerator or in meat keeper.*
fresh cleaned fish		*Cook only live shellfish.*
including steaks and fillets	1 day	
clams, crab, lobster in shell	2 days	
seafood including shucked clams, oysters,		
scallops, shrimp	1 day	
Poultry		*Store loosely wrapped. Keep fresh poultry in coldest part of refrigerator or in meat keeper.*
ready-to-cook chicken, duck or turkey	2 days	
Other foods		
Coffee, regular	2 weeks	
Honey, jams, jellies		*Refrigeration not needed but storage life is lengthened if refrigerated.*
Nuts	2 weeks	*Refrigerate nuts after opening.*
Refrigerated biscuits, rolls, pastries, cookie dough	date on label	*Products keep better if stored in back of refrigerator where it is colder.*
Salad dressings (opened)	3 months	*Keep covered.*
Wines, table	2-3 days	*Keep tightly closed.*
cooking	2-3 months	*Keep tightly closed.*

P

Safe Food Storage and Handling Chart
—Freezer Storage—

Suggested maximum times for storing foods in freezer at 0° F.
Longer than recommended storage is not dangerous, but flavors and textures begin to deteriorate.

Food	Time	Special Handling
Dairy products		
Butter, margarine	9 months	*Store in airtight freezer containers or wrapped in freezer wrap.*
Cheese		
cream cheese	1 month	*Thaw in refrigerator.*
hard cheeses	3 months	*Thaw in refrigerator.*
Roquefort, blue, process	3 months	*Thaw in refrigerator.*
Cream—light, heavy, half-and-half	2 months	*Heavy cream may not whip after thawing. Use for cooking. Thaw in refrigerator.*
Cream, whipped	1 month	
Eggs: whites	1 year	*Store in covered container. Freeze in amounts for favorite recipes.*
yolks	1 year	
Ice cream, ice milk, sherbet	1 month	*Cover surface with plastic wrap or foil after each use to keep from drying.*
Milk	3 months	*Freezing affects flavor and appearance. Use in cooking and baking. Thaw in refrigerator.*
Fruits and vegetables		
Fruits		
berries, cherries, peaches, pears, pineapple, etc.	1 year	
citrus fruit and juice, frozen at home	1 year	
Vegetables		
home frozen	10 months	*Cabbage, celery, salad greens, tomatoes do not freeze successfully.*
purchased frozen	8 months	
Meat, fish, and poultry		
Meats—home frozen		
bacon, frankfurters, ham slices, luncheon meats	1 month	*If meat is purchased fresh on trays and in plastic wrap, check for holes. If none, freeze in this wrap for up to 1 month. For longer storage, over-wrap with foil, plastic wrap or freezer wrap.*
ground beef, lamb and veal	4 months	
ground pork	3 months	
ham, whole	2 months	
roasts		
beef	1 year	
lamb, veal	9 months	
pork	6 months	
sausage, dry, smoked	1 month	*Keep meat purchased frozen in original package.*
sausage, fresh	2 months	*Thaw and cook according to label instructions.*
steaks		
beef	1 year	
lamb, veal	9 months	
pork	6 months	
Fish		
fillets and steaks from "lean" fish—cod, flounder, haddock, sole	6 months	*To home-freeze fish, wrap in foil, plastic wrap or freezer wrap. Make packages as airtight as possible. Freeze in coldest part of freezer.*
"fatty" fish—bluefish, mackerel, perch, salmon	3 months	
breaded fish	3 months	
clams, lobster, scallops	3 months	*Keep fish purchased frozen in original wrapping.*
cooked fish or seafood	3 months	
king crab	10 months	*Thaw and cook according to label directions.*
oysters	4 months	
shrimp, unbreaded	1 year	
shrimp, breaded	4 months	

P

Continued.

Safe Food Storage and Handling Chart
—Freezer Storage—cont'd.

Food	Time	Special Handling
Meat, fish, and poultry—cont'd		
Poultry		
chicken, whole or cut-up	1 year	*Cook all thawed poultry within 1 day.*
chicken livers	3 months	
cooked poultry	3 months	
duck, turkey	6 months	
Miscellaneous		
Baked goods		
breads, baked	3 months	*Package foods tightly in foil, plastic wrap, freezer wrap or watertight freezer containers.*
breads, unbaked	2 months	
cakes		
cheesecake	3 months	
chocolate	4 months	
fruitcake	1 year	
spongecake	2 months	
yellow or pound	6 months	
pies		
cream, custard	8 months	
fruit	8 months	
Main dishes		
meat, fish and poultry pies and casseroles	3 months	*For casseroles, allow head room for expansion. Freeze in coldest part of freezer.*
TV dinners	6 months	
Nuts	3 months	

Safe Food Storage and Handling Chart
—Pantry Shelf Storage—

Suggested maximum times for sorting foods in coldest cabinets		
Food	**Time**	**Special Handling**
Canned and dried food		
Canned pineapple, tomato or sauerkraut	8 months	*Put in airtight container.*
Fruits, canned	1 year	
dried	6 months	
Gravies	1 year	*Refrigerate after opening.*
Meat, fish, poultry	1 year	
Pickles, olives	1 year	
Soups, canned, dried	1 year	
Vegetablels, canned, dried	1 year	
Herbs, spices, and condiments		
Catsup (opened)	1 month	
Herbs and spices		
whole spices, herbs	1 year	
ground spices, herbs	6 months	
Tabasco, Worcestershire	2 year+	
Mixes and packaged foods		
Cakes, prepared	1-2 days	*If butter-cream, whipped-cream or custard frostings, fillings, refrigerate.*
Cake mixes	1 year	
Casserole mixes	18 months	
Cookies, homemade	1 week	*Put in airtight container.*
packaged	4 months	*Keep box tightly closed.*
Crackers	3 months	*Keep box tightly closed.*
Frosting, in cans or mixes	8 months	

Continued.

Safe Food Storage and Handling Chart
—Pantry Shelf Storage—cont'd.

Food	Time	Special Handling
Mixes and packaged foods—cont'd		
Hot roll mix	18 months	*If opened, put in airtight container.*
Pancake mix	6 months	*Put in airtight container.*
Piecrust mix	8 months	
Pie and pastries	2-3 days	*Refrigerate whipped cream, custard, chiffon fillings.*
Potatoes, instant	18 months	
Toaster pop-ups	3 months	
Staples		
Baking powder	18 months	
Boullion cubes	1 year	
Bread crumbs, dried	6 months	
Cereals, ready-to-eat	4 months	
ready to cook	6 months	
Chocolate, premelted	1 year	
semi sweet	2 years	
unsweetened	18 months	
Coffee, cans (unopened)	1 months	*Refrigerate after opening.*
Coffee, instant (opened)	2 weeks	*Keep lid tightly closed.*
(unopened)	6 months	
Coffee lighteners (dry) (opened)	6 months	
Condensed and evaporated milk	1 year	*Refrigerate after opening.*
Flour (all types)	1 year	*Put in airtight container.*
Gelatin (all types)	18 months	
Honey, jams, syrups	1 year	
Nonfat dry milk	6 months	*Put in airtight container.*
Pasta	2 years+	*Keep tightly closed.*
Pudding mixes	1 year	
Rice, white	2 years+	*Keep tightly closed.*
Rice mixes	6 months	
Salad dressing (all types)	3 months	*Refrigerate after opening.*
Salad oil	1-3 months	
Shortening, solid	8 months	
Sugar, brown	4 months	*Put in airtight container.*
confectioners	4 months	*Put in airtight container.*
granulated, molasses	2 years+	*Keep tightly covered.*
Tea, bags	18 months	*Put in airtight container.*
instant	3 years	*Keep tightly covered.*
loose	2 years	*Put in airtight container.*
Miscellaneous		
Coconut	1 year	*Refrigerate after opening.*
Metered-calorie products, instant breakfasts	6 months	
Nuts	9 months	*Refrigerate after opening.*
Onions, potatoes, sweet potatoes	2 weeks	*For longer storage, keep below 50° F, but not refrigerated. Keep dry, out of sun.*
Parmesan cheese	2 months	
Peanut butter (opened)	2 months	
(unopened)	9 months	
Soft drinks	3 months	
Whipped topping mix	1 year	

P

COMMON FOOD ADDITIVES

This list identifies the functions of some of the more than 2800 additives allowed in the U.S. food supply.

Additive	Function	Additive	Function
A		**D**	
Acetic acid	pH control‡	Dehydrated beets	color
Acetone peroxide	mat-bleach-condit§	Dextrose	sweetener
Apidic acid	pH control‡	Diglycerides	emulsifier
Ammonium alginate	stabil-thick-tex*	Diocytl sodium sulfosuccinate	emulsifier
Annatto extract	color	Disodium guanylate	flavor enhancer
Arabinogalactan	stabil-thick-tex*	Disodium inosinate	flavor enhancer
Ascorbic acid	nutrient	Dried algae meal	color
	preservative		
	antioxidant	**E**	
Azodicarbonamide	mat-bleach-condit§	EDTA (ethylenediamine-tetraacetric acid)	antioxidant
B			
Benzoic acid	preservative	**F**	
Benzoyl peroxide	mat-bleach-condit§	FD&C Colors:	
Beta-apo-8′ carotenal	color	Blue No. 1	color
Beta carotene	nutrient	Red No. 3	color
	color	Red No. 40	color
BHA (butylated hydroxyani-sole)	antioxidant	Yellow No. 5	color
		Fructose	sweetener
BHT (butylated hydroxytolu-ene)	antioxidant		
		G	
Butylparaben	preservative	Gelatin	stabil-thick-tex*
		Glucose	sweetener
C		Glycerine	humectant
Calcium alginate	stabil-thick-tex*	Glycerol monostearate	humectant
Calcium bromate	mat-bleach-condit§	Grape skin extract	color
Calcium lactate	preservative	Guar gum	stabil-thick-tex*
Calcium phosphate	leavening†	Gum arabic	stabil-thick-tex*
Calcium silicate	anticaking‖	Gum ghatti	stabil-thick-tex*
Calcium sorbate	preservative		
Canthaxanthin	color	**H**	
Caramel	color	Heptylparaben	preservative
Carob bean gum	stabil-thick-tex*	Hydrogen peroxide	mat-bleach-condit§
Carrageenan	emulsifier	Hydrolyzed vegetable protein	flavor enhancer
	stabil-thick-tex*		
Carrot oil	color	**I**	
Cellulose	stabil-thick-tex*	Invert sugar	sweetener
Citric acid	preservative	Iodine	nutrient
	antioxidant	Iron	nutrient
	pH control‡	Iron-ammonium citrate	anticaking‖
Citrus Red No. 2	color	Iron oxide	color
Cochineal extract	color		
Corn endosperm	color	**K**	
Corn syrup	sweetener	Karaya gum	stabil-thick-tex*

Additive	Function	Additive	Function
L		Sodium benzoate	preservative
Lactic acid	pH control[‡]	Sodium bicarbonate	leavening[†]
	preservative	Sodium calcium alginate	stabil-thick-tex[*]
Larch gum	stabil-thick-tex[*]	Sodium citrate	pH control[‡]
Lecithin	emulsifier	Sodium diacetate	preservative
Locust bean gum	stabil-thick-tex[*]	Sodium erythorbate	preservative
		Sodium nitrate	preservative
M		Sodium propionate	preservative
Mannitol	sweetener	Sodium sorbate	preservative
	anticaking[‖]	Sodium stearyl fumarate	mat-bleach-condit[§]
	stabil-thick-tex[*]	Sorbic acid	preservative
Methylparaben	preservative	Sorbitan monostearate	emulsifier
Modified food starch	stabil-thick-tex[*]	Sorbitol	humectant
Monoglycerides	emulsifier		sweetener
MSG (monosidium glutamate)	flavor enhancer	Spices	flavor
		Sucrose (table sugar)	sweetener
N			
Niacinamide	nutrient	**T**	
		Tagetes (Aztec Marigold)	color
P		Tartaric acid	pH control[‡]
Paprika (and oleoresin)	flavor	TBHQ (tertiary butyl hydro-	antioxidant
	color	quinone)	
Pectin	stabil-thick-tex[*]	Thiamine	nutrient
Phosphates	pH control[‡]	Titanium dioxide	color
Phosphoric acid	pH control[‡]	Toasted, partially defatted	color
Polysorbates	emulsifiers	cooked cottonseed flour	
Potassium alginate	stabil-thick-tex[*]	Tocopherols (vitamin E)	nutrient
Potassium bromate	mat-bleach-condit[§]		antioxidant
Potassium iodide	nutrient	Tragacanth gum	stabil-thick-tex[*]
Potassium propionate	preservative	Turmeric (oleoresin)	flavor
Potassium sorbate	preservative		color
Propionic acid	preservative		
Propyl gallate	antioxidant	**U**	
Propylene glycol	stabil-thick-tex[*]	Ultramarine blue	color
	humectant		
Propylparaben	preservative	**V**	
		Vanilla, vanillin	flavor
R		Vitamin A	nutrient
Riboflavin	nutrient	Vitamin C (ascorbic acid)	nutrient
	color		preservative
			antioxidant
S		Vitamin D (D-2, D-3)	nutrient
Saccharin	sweetener	Vitamin E (tocopherols)	nutrient
Saffron	color		
Silicon dioxide	anticaking[‖]	**Y**	
Sodium acetate	pH control[‡]	Yeast-malt sprout extract	flavor enhancer
Sodium alginate	stabil-thick-tex[*]	Yellow prussiate of soda	anticaking[‖]
Sodium aluminum sulfate	leavening[†]		

Key to abbreviations: [*]stabil-thick-tex = stabilizers-thickeners-texturizers; [†]leavening = leavening agents; [‡]pH control = pH control agents; [§]mat-bleach-condit = maturing and bleaching agents, dough conditioners; [‖]anticaking = anticaking agents.

From Lehmann P: More than you ever thought you would know about food additivs, *FDA Consumer reprint*, Health and Human Services Publication No. (FDA) 79-2115, 1979.

APPENDIX R
SOURCES OF NUTRITION INFORMATION

Consider the following reliable sources of food and nutrition infomation:

Journals that Regularly Cover Nutrition Topics:

American Family Physician*
American Journal of Clinical Nutrition
American Journal of Epidemiology
American Journal of Medicine
American Journal of Nursing
American Journal of Obstetrics and
   Gynecology
American Journal of Physiology
American Journal of Public Health
American Scientist
Anals of Internal Medicine
Annual Reviews of Medicine
Annual Reviews of Nutrition
Archives of Disease in Childhood
Archives of Internal Medicine
British Journal of Nutrition
British Medical Journal
Cancer
Cancer Research
Circulation
Diabetes
Diabetes Care
Disease-a-Month
Ecology of Food and Nutrition
FASEB Journal
FDA Consumer*
Food Chemical Toxicology
Food Engineering
Geriatrics
Gastroenterology
Gut
Human Nutrition: Applied Nutrition
Human Nutrition: Clinical Nutrition

Journal of The American Dietetic
   Association*
Journal of The American Geriatric
   Society
Journal of The American Medical
   Association
Journal of Applied Physiology
Journal of Canadian Dietetic Association*
Journal of Clinical Investigation
Journal of Food Service
Journal of Food Technology
Journal of The National Cancer Institute
Journal of Nutrition
Journal of Nutritional Education*
Journal of Nutrition for the Elderly
Journal of Nutrition Research
Journal of Pediatrics
Lancet
Mayo Clinic Proceedings
Medicine and Science in Sports and
   Exercise
Nature
New England Journal of Medicine
Nutrition
Nutrition Reviews
Nutrition Today*
Pediatrics
The Physician and Sports Medicine
Postgraduate Medicine*
Proceedings of the Nutrition Society
Science
Science News*
Scientific American*

The majority of these journals will be available in college or university libraries, or in a specialty library on campus, much as one designated for health services or home economics. Have a reference librarian help you locate these sources. The asterisked (*) journals are ones we feel you will find especially interesting and useful because the number of nutrition articles presented each month or the less technical nature of the presentation.

Magazines for the Nonmedical Person that Cover Nutritional Topics:

American Health
Better Homes and Gardens
Consumer Reports

Good housekeeping
Parents
Self

Textbooks for Advanced Study of Nutrition Topics:

Food and Nutrition Board: *Recommended dietary allowances*, ed 10, Washington, DC, 1989, National Academy of Sciences.

Linder MC: *Nutritional biochemistry and metabolism with clinical applications*, New York, 1985, Elsevier Science Publishing.

Murray RK and others: *Harpers biochemistry*, ed 21, Norwalk, Conn, 1988, Appleton & Lange.

Pike RI, Brown ML: *Nutrition: an integrated approach*, ed 3, New York, 1984, John Wiley & Sons.

Present knowledge in nutrition, ed 6, 1990, The Nutrition Foundation.

Schils ME, Young ER: *Modern nutrition in health and disease*, ed 7, Philadelphia, 1988, Lea & Febiger.

Newsletters that Cover Nutrition Issues on a Regular Basis:

Contemporary Nutrition
General Mills, Inc.
Production Manager
P.O. Box 1112, Department 65
Minneapolis, MN 55440
(inexpensive)

CNI Nutrition Week
Community Nutrition Institute
2001 S. St. NW
Washington, D.C. 20009

Dairy Council Digest
National Dairy Council
6300 River Rd.
Rosemont, IL 60018
(inexpensive)

Dietetic Currents
Ross Laboratories
Director of Professional Services
625 Cleveland Ave.
Columbus, OH 43216
(free)

Environmental Nutrition
52 Riverside Dr.
New York, NY 10024

Food and Nutrition News
National Livestock and Meat Board
444 Michigan Ave.
Chicago, IL 60610
(free)

Harvard Medical School Health Letter
Department of Continuing Education
25 Shattuck St.
Boston, MA 02115

Healthline
830 Menlo Ave. #100
Menlo Park, CA 94025

National Council Against Health Fraud
    Newsletter (NCAHF)
P.O. Box 1276
Loma Linda, CA 92354

Nutrition & the M.D.
P.O. Box 2160
Van Nuys, CA 91404

Nutrition Forum
George Stickley Co.
210 Washington Square
Philadelphia, PA 19106

Nutrition Research Newsletter
P.O. Box 700
Pallisades, NY 10964

Tufts University Diet & Nutrition Letter
P.O. Box 10948
Des Moines, IA 50940

Professional Organizations with a Commitment to Nutrition Issues:

American Academy of Pediatrics
P.O. Box 1034
Evanston, IL 60204

American Cancer Society
777 Third Ave.
New York, NY 10017

American Dental Association
211 E. Chicago Ave.
Chicago, IL 60611

American Diabetes Association
2 Park Ave.
New York, NY 10016

American Dietetic Association
216 W. Jackson Blvd.
Suite 800
Chicago, IL 60606

American Geriatrics Society
770 Lexington Ave.
Suite 400
New York, NY 10021

American Heart Association
7320 Greenville Ave.
Dallas, TX 75231

R

American Home Economics Association
2010 Massachusetts Ave. N.W.
Washington, DC 20036

American Institute of Nutrition
9650 Rockville Pike
Bethesda, MD 20014

American Medical Association
Nutrition Information Section
535 N. Dearborn St.
Chicago, IL 60610

American Public Health Association
1015 Fifteenth St. N.W.
Washington, DC 20005

American Society for Clinical Nutrition
9650 Rockville Pike
Bethesda, MD 20014

The Canadian Diabetes Association
123 Edward St.
Suite 601
Toronto, Ontario M5G 1E2 Canada

The Canadian Dietetic Association
480 University Ave.
Suite 601
Toronto, Ontario M5G 1V2 Canada

The Canadian Society
   for Nutritional Sciences
Department of Foods and Nutrition
University of Manitoba
Winnipeg, Manitoba, Canada R3T 2N2

Food and Nutrition Board
National Research Council
National Academy of Sciences
2101 Constitution Ave. N.W.
Washington, DC 20418

Institute of Food Technologies
221 N. LaSalle St.
Chicago, IL 60601

National Council on the Aging
1828 L St. N.W.
Washington, DC 20036

National Institute of Nutrition
1335 Carling Ave.
Suite 210
Ottawa, Ontario, Canada K1Z 0L2

Nutrition Foundation, Inc.
1126 Sixteenth St. N.W.
Suite 111
Washington, D.C. 20036

Nutrition Today Society
428 E. Preston St.
Baltimore, MD 21202

Society for Nutrition Education
1736 Franklin St.
Oakland, CA 94612

Professional or Lay Organizations Concerned with Nutrition Issues:

Bread for the World
802 Rhode Island Ave. N.E.
Washington, DC 20018

Center for Science in the Public Interest
   (CSPI)
1755 S. Street N.W.
Washington, DC 20009

Children's Foundation
1420 New York Ave. N.W.
Suite 800
Washington, D.C. 20005

California Council Against Health Fraud,
   Inc.
P.O. Box 1276
Loma Linda, CA 92354

Food Research and Action Center (FRAC)
2011 I Street N.W.
Washington, D.C. 20006

Institute for
   Food and Development
   Policy
1885 Mission St.
San Francisco, CA 94103

La Leche League International, Inc.
9616 Minneapolis Ave.
Franklin Park, IL 60131

March of Dimes Birth Defects Foundation
(National Headquarters)
1275 Mamaroneck Ave.
White Plains, NY 10605

Overeaters Anonymous (OA)
2190 190th St.
Torrance, CA 90504

Oxfam America
115 Broadway
Boston, MA 02116

Local Resources for Advice on Nutrition Issues:

Cooperative extension agents in county extension offices
Dietitians (Contact the state or local Dietetics Association.)
Nutrition faculty affiliated with departments of food and nutrition, home economics, and
   dietetics
Nutritionists (RDs) in city, county, or state agencies

Government Agencies that are Concerned with Nutrition Issues or that Distribute Nutrition Information:

United States
Department of Agriculture (USDA)
Extension Services
3 South Building
Room 6007
Washington, DC 20250

The Consumer Information Center
Department 609K
Pueblo, CO 81009

Food and Drug Administration (FDA)
5600 Fishers Lane
Rockville, MD 20852

National Agricultural Library
10301 Baltimore Blvd.
Room 304
Beltsville, MD 20705

Food and Nutrition Information and
    Education Resources Center
National Library of Congress
Beltsville, MD 20705

Human Nutrition Research Division
Agricultural Research Center
Beltsville, MD 20705

Office of Cancer Communications
National Cancer Institute
Building 31
Room 10A18
90 Rockville Pike
Bethesda, MD 20205

National Center for Health Statistics
3700 East-West
Hyattsville, MD 20782

U.S. Government Printing Office
The Superintendent of Documents
Washington, DC 20402

Canada
Nutrition Programs
446 Jeanne Mance Building
Tunney's Pasture
Ottawa, Ontario K1A 1B4

Nutrition Services
P.O. Box 488
Halifax, Nova Scotia B3J 3R8

Nutrition Services
P.O. Box 6000
Fredericton, New Brunswick E3B 5H1

Department of Community Health
1075 Ste-Foy Rd.
Seventh Floor
Quebec, Quebec G1S 2M1

Public Health Resource Service
15 Overlea Blvd.
Fifth Floor
Toronto, Ontario M4H 1A9

Home Economics Directorate
880 Portage Ave.
Second Floor
Winnipeg, Manitoba R3G 0P1

United Nations
Food and Agriculture Organization (FAO)
North American Regional Office
1325 C St. S.W.
Washington, D.C. 20025
Via della Terma di Caracella
0100 Rome, Italy

World Health Organization (WHO)
1211 Geneva 27
Switzerland

Trade Organizations and Companies that Distribute Nutrition Information:

American Egg Board
1460 Renaissance St.
Park Ridge, IL 60068

American Institute of Banking
P.O. Box 1148
Manhattan, KS 66502

American Meat Institute
P.O. Box 3556
Washington, D.C. 20007

Best Foods
Consumer Service Department
Division of CPC International
International Plaza
Englewood Cliffs, NJ 07632

Borden Farm Products
Bordon Co.
Consumer Affairs
180 E. Broad St.
Columbus, OH 43215

Campbell Soup Co.
Food Service Products Division
375 Memorial Ave.
Camden, NJ 08101

Del Monte Teaching Aids
P.O. Box 9075
Clinton, IA 52736

Fleischman's Margarines
Standard Brands, Inc.
625 Madison Ave.
New York, NY 10022

Trade Organizations and Companies that Distribute Nutrition Information:

General Foods Consumer Center
250 North St.
White Plains, NY 10625

General Mills
P.O. Box 113
Minneapolis, MN 55440

Gerber Products Co.
445 State St.
Fremont, MI 49412

H.J. Heinz
Consumer Relations
P.O. Box 57
Pittsburgh, PA 15230

Hunt-Wesson Foods
Education Services
1654 W Valencia Dr.
Fullerton, CA 92634

Kellogg Co.
Department of Home Economics Services
Battle Creek, MI 49016

Mead Johnson Nutritionals
2404 Pennsylvania Ave.
Evansville, IN 47721

National Dairy Council
6300 N. River Rd.
Rosemont, IL 60018-4233

Oscar Mayer Co.
Consumer Service
P.O. Box 1409
Madison, WI 53701

Pillsbury Co
1177 Pillsbury Building
608 Second Ave. S.
Minneapolis, MN 55402

The Potato Board
1385 S. Colorado Blvd.
Suite 512
Denver, CO 80222

Rice Council
P.O. Box 22802
Houston, TX 77027

Ross Laboratories
Director of Professional Services
625 Cleveland Ave.
Columbus, OH 43216

Sunkist Growers Consumer Service
Division BB, P.O. Box 7888
Valley Annex
Van Nuys, CA 91409

Vitamin Nutrition Information Service
  (VNIS)
Hoffmann-LaRoche
340 Kingsland Ave.
Nutley, NJ 07110

United Fresh Fruit and Vegetables
  Association
727 N Washington St.
Alexandria, VA 22314

APPENDIX S
EVALUATION OF PROTEIN QUALITY

Are all proteins equally effective at supporting growth and maintenance? There are ways to measure how efficiently a particular protein is used. The methods we discuss here provide a means to evaluate and compare protein quality in our diet.

BIOLOGICAL VALUE

The **biological value (BV) of a protein** is a measure of how efficiently it can be turned into body tissues after it is absorbed. The efficiency depends on how closely a protein's amino acid pattern reflects the pattern of human tissue. The better the match, the more completely a food protein turns into body protein.

An easier way to measure protein absorption and retention of the amino acids in proteins is to measure nitrogen absorption and retention. Recall that nitrogen is present in all amino acids.

$$\text{Biological Value (BV)} = \frac{\text{Nitrogen retained}}{\text{Nitrogen absorbed}}$$

If the amino acid pattern in a food protein varies greatly from that of human tissue, many amino acids in the food will not be used as body protein. Their nitrogen groups are removed and excreted in the urine as urea. The carbon skeletons that remain are transformed into either glucose or fat burned for energy needs (see Figure 8-1).

Egg white protein has the highest biological value of any single protein source (Table S-1). In other words, most of the amino acids can be used to make body tissue. Milk and meat proteins also have high biological values. This makes sense because humans and other animals show similar amino acid compositions. On the other hand, plant amino acid patterns differ greatly from those of humans. For example, corn has only a moderate biological value: it will support body maintenance but not growth. Peanuts by themselves also have a poor biological value.

NET PROTEIN UTILIZATION

The biological value of a food can be adjusted to account for its digestibility. This adjusted value is called net protein utilization (NPU). Most proteins are almost entirely digested and absorbed. Typical plant sources of protein show only about a 10% lower value than animal sources. Overall, the biological value and the NPU for most individual proteins are quite similar (Table S-1).

PROTEIN EFFICIENCY RATIO

The **protein efficiency ratio (PER)** provides a less technical means for measuring a food's protein quality. FDA uses this method to set standards for food labeling. The PER compares the amount of weight gained by a growing rat after 10 or more days of eating a set amount of protein to the total protein intake over the period of time in the experiment.

S

The PER value of a food reflects its biological value.

TABLE S-1

Protein quality values of selected foods

Food	Chemical (Amino Acid) Score	BV*	NPU†	PER‡
Egg	100	100	94	3.92
Cow's milk	95	93	82	3.09
Fish	71	76	—	3.55
Beef	69	74	67	2.30
Unpolished rice	67	86	59	—
Peanuts	65	55	55	1.65
Oats	57	65	—	2.19
Polished rice	57	64	57	2.18
Whole wheat	53	65	49	1.53
Corn	49	72	36	—
Soybeans	47	73	61	2.32
Sesame seeds	42	62	53	1.77
Peas	37	64	55	1.57

NOTE: A high or low value for one measure is usually reflected in a similar value for the other measures of protein quality.

*Biological value.

†Net protein utilization.

‡Protein efficiency ratio.

$$\text{Biological Value (BV)} = \frac{\text{Nitrogen retained}}{\text{Nitrogen absorbed}}$$

CHEMICAL SCORE OF PROTEINS

A food's protein quality can be estimated by its amino acid composition. This is reflected by its **chemical score**. To calculate the chemical score, we find the amounts of each essential amino acid provided by a gram of protein in the food. Now we divide each amount by an *ideal* amount of that essential amino acid for a gram of food protein. The *ideal* protein pattern is based on the minimal amount (in milligrams) of each essential amino acid that is needed for a gram of the food protein to provide a complete protein balance.

$$\text{Biological Value (BV)} = \frac{\text{Nitrogen retained}}{\text{Nitrogen absorbed}}$$

The lowest amino acid ratio calculated for any essential amino acid is the chemical score.

To calculate a chemical score for a food, assume the *ideal* lysine level in a diet is 55 milligrams per gram of total protein. Let's assume the food is most deficient in lysine, with a concentration of 24 milligrams per gram of total protein. The chemical score for the food would be:

$$\frac{24}{55} \times 100 = 44$$

The chemical score formula resembles the concept of biological value since both are based on meeting the body's need for the right balance of essential amino acids. The main advantage of using the chemical score method is convenience; the instruments needed to measure a food's value are readily available, and neither animal nor human subjects are needed.

Given a variety of foods in a meal, the various amino acids usually combine to yield complete protein. This gives a good overall amino acid balance, hence a high chemical score for the meal. This is a key factor to consider when planning diets for young children; their diets must contain a high quality protein intake.

GLOSSARY

The Following Medical Terms and Combining Forms Are Used Frequently in the Study of Nutrition.

Term	Meaning
a-	without, from
acyl	a carbon chain
aden-, adeno-	gland
-algia	pain
aliment	food
-amine	containing nitrogen
andr-, andro-	man or male
ap-, apo-	detached
arteri-, arterio-	artery
arthr-, arthro	joint
-ase	enzyme
-blast	immature form, embryonic
brady-	slow
buli-	ox
cancr-, carcino-	malignant tumor
cardi-, cardio-	heart
centi-	divided into 100 parts
chol-, chole-, cholo-	bile, gall
cholecyst-	gallbladder
chondr-, chondrio-, chondro-	cartilage
chrom-, chromo-	color, colored
-clast	something that breaks
col-, coli-, colo-	colon
cyan-, cyano-	blue
cyt-, cyto-	cell
derm-, dermato-	skin
dextr-, dextro-	right, on or toward the right
duoden-, duodeno-	duodenum
dys-	difficult, painful
ect-, ecto-	without, outside, external
-ectomy	excision of
-ein	a protein
em-	blood
-emia	in blood
encephal-, encephalo-	brain
end-, endo-, ent-, ento-	within
enter-, entero-	intestine
erythr-, erythro-	red
esophag-, esophago-	esophagus
eu-	well, easy, good
gastr-, gastri-, gastro-	stomach
gen-	to become or produce
gloss-, glosso-	tongue
gluco-, glyc-, glyco-	sugar
gyn-, gyne-, gyneco-	woman or female (especially female reproductive organs)
hem-, hemat-	blood

Continued.

Term	Meaning
hepat-, hepato-	liver
hex-, hexa-	six
hist-, histo-	tissue
homeo-, homoeo, homoio	sameness, similarity
hydr-, hydro-	water
hyp-, hypo-	under, beneath, deficient
hyper-	excessive, above, beyond
hyster-, hystero-	uterus
idio-	one's own, peculiar to; separate, distinct
ile-, ileo-	ileum
inter-	between, among
intra-	within, during, between layers of
-itis	inflammation of
jejun-, jejuno-	jejunum
kilo-	1000 times;
lact-, lacti-, lacto-	milk
leuc-, leuk-	white, colorless
lev-, levo-	left
lip-, lipo-	fat, lipid
lith-, litho-	stone
lymph-, lympho-	waterlike
-lysis	destruction
mal-	bad, badly
malac-, malaco-	soft, a condition of abnormal softness
mega-, megalo-	large, great
meta-	after, later; change, exchange
metallo-	containing metal
micro-	divided into 1 million parts
milli-	divided into 1000 parts
mono-	one
morph-, morpho-	form, shape
my-, myo-	muscle
myel-, myelo-	marrow; spinal cord
nas-, naso-	nose, nasal
necr-, necro-	dead
nephr-, nephro-	kidney
neur-, neuro-	nerve
-oid	formed like
olig-, oligo-	few, scant
-ol	alcohol
-oma	tumor
ophthalm-, ophthalmo	eye, eyeball
-orex	mouth
-orexis	desire, appetite
ost-, oste-, osteo-	bone
-ose	sugar, carbohydrate
-osis	action, process, result, usually discussed
ot-	ear
ovari-, ovario-	ovary
ovi, ovo-	eggs
pan-	all
pancreat-, pancreato-	pancreas
para-	beside
parieto-	wall of a cavity
path-, patho-	disease
ped-	child; foot
-penia	without, lack of
-phobia	fear of
-plasm	formative, formed; cell or tissue substance
pneum-, pneumo-, pneumono-	lung
-poiesis	production
poly-	many, much
post-	after

Term	Meaning
pre-	before
prot-, proto-	first
pseud-, pseudo-	false
pulmo-, pulmon-, pulmono-	lung
pyel-, pyelo-	pelvis
pyr-	fever, fire
rect-, recto-	rectum
reni-, reno-	kidney
rhin-, rhino-	nose
-rrhagia	rupture; excessive fluid discharge
-rrhea	flow, discharge
sate	to fill
scler-, sclero-	hard, hardness
-scopy	viewing
seb-, sebi, sebo-	hard fat; sebum, sebaceous glands
semi-	half
-soma, somat-, somato-	body
-stasia, -stasis	slowing or stopping of
stenosis	narrowing of
stomat-, stomato-	mouth, stoma
-stomy	surgical opening
sub-	under, below
super	over, above
tachy-	swift, fast
thi-, thio-	containing sulfur
thromb-, thrombo-	blood clot
tox-, toxi-, toxo-	poison
trache-, tracheo-	trachea
-trophy	growth or mutation
ure-, urea-, ureo-	urine
uter-, utero-	uterus
vas-, vaso-	blood vessel
ven-, veni-, veno-	vein
vita-	life
xer-, sero-	dry

GLOSSARY TERMS

absorptive cells (ab-sorp-tiv) A class of cells that line the villi (finger projections in the small intestine) and participate in nutrient absorption.

acesulfame-K (ay-see-sul-fame) An artificial sweetener that yields no energy to the body; it is 200 times sweeter than sucrose.

achlorhydria (ay-clor-high-dre-ah) A state of reduced acid production by the stomach, primarily resulting from loss of the acid-producing cells in the stomach, a condition associated with aging.

acquired immunodeficiency syndrome (AIDS) A disease characterized by poor function of one class of white blood cells (called helper T lymphocytes). The resulting poor immune function leaves the person quite susceptible to infection, which can in turn result in rapidly failing health and death.

active absorption Absorption using a carrier and expending energy. In this way the absorptive cell can absorb nutrients, such as glucose, against a high concentration in the absorptive cells.

ad libitum (ad-lib-eh-tum) At one's desire or pleasure.

adenosine triphosphate (ATP) (ah-den-o-sin try-fos-fate) The main energy currency for cells. ATP energy is used to promote ion pumping, enzyme activity, and muscular contraction.

adipose (fat) cells (add-ih-pos) A grouping of fat-storing cells.

adipsin (ah-dip-sin) A protein that appears to be made by fat cells and that acts as a communication link between these cells and the brain.

adult-onset obesity Obesity that develops in adulthood; characteristically, the individual has a normal number of adipose cells, but each cell is enlarged because of fat storage. Also called non-insulin dependent diabetes mellitus, or type II diabetes.

aerobic (air-row-bic) Requiring oxygen.

alcohol (al-co-hall) Ethyl alcohol or ethanol. An energy-yielding substance found in beer, wine, and distilled spirits.

aldosterone (al-dos-ter-own) A powerful hormone produced by the adrenal glands that acts on the kidneys to cause sodium reabsorption and, in turn, water conservation.

alimentary canal (al-ih-men-tah-ree) Another name for the gastrointestinal (GI) tract.

alkaline (basic) pH (al-kah-line) A pH greater than 7. Baking soda in water yields an alkaline pH.

allergy (al-er-jee) An immune response that occurs when immune bodies (antibodies) react with a foreign substance (antigen).

alpha-linolenic acid (al-fah lin-oh-len-ik) A fatty acid with 18 carbon atoms and three double bonds; omega-3.

alveoli (al-ve-o-lye) The small air sacs of the lungs.

amino acid (ah-mee-noh) The building block for proteins; amino acids have a carbon in the center with a nitrogen and other atoms attached.

amniotic fluid (am-nee-ott-ik) The fluid that surrounds and protects the fetus in the uterus.

amylase (am-uh-lace) Starch-digesting enzymes from the salivary glands or pancreas.

amylopectin (am-ih-low-pek-tin) A branched-chain polysaccharide made of glucose units.

amylose (am-uh-los) A straight-chain digestible polysaccharide made of glucose units.

anabolism (an-ah-bol-iz-um) The process of building compounds.

anaerobic (an-ah-row-bic) Not requiring oxygen.

anaphylactic shock (an-ah-fih-lak-tic) A severe allergic response that results in greatly lowered blood pressure as well as respiratory and gastrointestinal distress.

androgen (an-dro-jen) A general term for hormones that stimulate development in male sex organs; testosterone is an example.

anemia (a-knee-me-a) Poor oxygen-carrying ability of the blood, caused by a reduction in the number of healthy red blood cells.

anergy (an-er-jee) Lack of an immune response to foreign compounds entering the body.

animal model A disease in animals that duplicates human disease and thus can be used to further understand human diseases.

anorexia nervosa (an-oh-rex-ee-uh ner-voh-sah) An eating disorder involving a psychological loss of appetite and self-starvation, resulting in part from a distorted body image and various social pressures associated with puberty.

anthropometry (an-throw-pom-eh-tree) The measurement of weight, lengths, circumferences, and thicknesses of the body.

antibody (an-tih-bod-ee) Blood proteins that inactivate foreign proteins found in the body, thus preventing infection.

anticarcinogens (an-tie-car-sin-o-gins) Compounds that potentially inhibit the development of cancer.

antidiuretic hormone (ADH) (an-tie-dye-your-ret-ik) A hormone secreted by the pituitary gland that acts on the kidneys to decrease water excretion.

antioxidant (an-tie-ox-ih-dant) A compound that can donate electrons to electron-seeking (oxidizing) compounds.

apolipoproteins (ape-oh-lip-oh-pro-teens) Proteins embedded in the outer shell of lipoproteins.

appetite (ap-peh-tight) The psychological drive to find and eat food, often in the absence of hunger.

arachidonic acid (air-ah-kih-don-ik) A fatty acid with 20 carbon atoms and four double bonds; omega-6.

areola (ah-ree-oh-lah) The circular dark area of skin at the center of the breast.

arithmetic ratio A group of numbers in which the difference between each number is the same.

arthritis (arth-rite-us) Inflammation at a point where bones join; the disease has many possible causes.

aseptic processing (ah-sep-tik) A method by which food and its container are sterilized simultaneously; this process allows manufacturers to produce boxes of milk that can be stored at room temperature. Variations of this process are also known as ultra-high-temperature (UHT) packaging.

aspartame (ah-spar-tame) An alternate sweetener made of two amino acids (part of proteins) and methanol; it is 200 times sweeter than sucrose (table sugar).

atherosclerosis (ath-er-oh-scleh-roh-sis) A buildup of fatty material (plaque) in the arteries, including those surrounding the heart.

atom The smallest combining unit of an element.

autodigestion (auto-dye-jes-chun) Literally, self-digestion. The stomach limits autodigestion by covering itself with a thick layer of mucous and by producing enzymes and acid only when needed for digestion of food.

autoimmune (auto-im-mune) Immune reactions against normal body cells; self against self.

avidin (av-ih-din) A protein found in raw egg whites that can bind biotin and inhibit its absorption. Cooking destroys avidin.

baryophobia (bear-ee-oh-fo-bee-ah) A poor rate of growth in children associated with parents underfeeding them in an attempt to prevent obesity and heart disease.

basal metabolism (bay-sal) The minimum energy the body requires to support itself when resting and awake. It amounts to roughly 1 kilocalorie per minute, or about 1400 kilocalories per day.

behavior contract A written agreement that lists intended changes in behavior, plans for reinforcement, and witnesses to monitor progress.

behavior chains Activities linked in a person's lifestyle, such as snacking while watching television.

beriberi (bear-ee-bear-ee) A thiamin-deficiency disorder characterized by muscle weakness, loss of appetite, nerve degeneration, and sometimes edema.

BHA and **BHT** Butylated hydroxyanisole and butylated hydroxytoluene; two common synthetic antioxidants that are added to foods.

bile A substance made in the liver and stored in the gallbladder; it is released into the small intestine to aid fat absorption.

bioavailability The degree to which an ingested nutrient is absorbed and so is available to the body.

biochemical changes Nutritional deficiency symptoms observed in the blood or urine, such as low levels of nutrient by-products or low enzyme activities. These indicate reduced biochemical functioning in the body.

bioelectrical impedance (im-pee-dance) A method of estimating total body fat by measuring the impedance (resistance) of a low-energy electrical current by the body.

biological value of a protein The body's ability to retain protein absorbed from a food.

biotechnology The use of advanced scientific techniques to alter and, ideally, improve characteristics of animals.

blood doping A technique by which an athlete's red blood cell count is increased. Blood is taken from the athlete, and the red blood cells are concentrated and then later reintroduced into the athlete.

body mass index Weight (in kilograms) divided by height squared (in meters); a value of 30 or higher indicates obesity.

bomb calorimeter (kal-oh-rim-eh-ter) An instrument used to determine the kilocalorie content of a food.

bond A sharing of electrons, charges, or attractions used to link two atoms.

brown adipose tissue (add-ih-pos) A specialized form of fat storage that produces large amounts of heat by metabolizing energy-yielding nutrients without synthesizing much usable energy for the body. Much of the energy released simply forms heat.

buffer A compound that can cause a solution to resist changes in acid-base balance.

bulimia (boo-leem-ee-uh) An eating disorder in which large quantities of food are eaten at one time (binging) and then purged from the body by vomiting, use of laxatives, or other means.

beta-carotene (beta-care-oh-teen) An orange pigment found in many fruits and vegetables, such as peaches and carrots. The body can use beta-carotene to make vitamin A.

calcitriol (kal-sih-try-ol) The active hormone form of vitamin D. A cholesterol-like substance is part of its structure.

cancer (can-sir) A condition characterized by uncontrolled growth of body cells.

carbohydrate loading The process of consuming a very high carbohydrate diet for 6 days before an athletic event to try to increase muscle glycogen stores.

carbohydrates (kar-bow-high-drates) Compounds containing carbon, hydrogen, and oxygen atoms; known as sugars and starches.

carcinogens (car-sin-oh-gins) Compounds that have the potential to cause cancer.

cardiac output The amount of blood pumped by the heart.

cardiovascular Pertaining to the heart and blood vessels.

cariogenic (care-ee-oh-jen-ik) A substance, often rich in carbohydrates, that promotes dental caries (e.g., caramels and raisins).

carnitine (car-nih-teen) A compound used to shuttle fatty acids into the cell mitochondria, allowing the fatty acids to be burned for energy.

carotenoids (care-ah-ten-oids) Pigment substances in plants that often can form vitamin A. Beta-carotene is the most active form.

casein (kay-seen) A protein found in milk that form curds; it tends to be difficult for infants to digest.

cash crops Crops grown by a country specifically for export rather than to feed the country's citizens (e.g., coffee, tea, cocoa, and bananas).

catabolic (cat-ah-bol-ik) Breaking down compounds.

catalyst (cat-uhl-ist) A compound that speeds reaction rates but is not altered by the reaction.

cell membrane An outer barrier found in animal cells. It is composed mostly of fats and proteins and surrounds each body cell.

cell A minute structure; the living basis of all plant and animal organization. Cells can both take up compounds from their environment and excrete compounds into it.

cellulose (sell-you-los) A straight-chain polysaccharide of glucose molecules that is undigestible; part of insoluble fiber.

Celsius A centigrade measure of temperature; to convert Fahrenheit temperatures to Celsius, use this formula: (degrees Fahrenheit − 32 ÷ 1.8.

centimeter A measure of length in the metric system; 100 centimeters equal 1 meter.

cerebrovascular accident (CVA) (se-ree-bro-vas-cue-lar) Death of part of the brain tissue as a result of a blood clot.

chain breaking Breaking the link between two or more behaviors that encourage overeating, such as snacking while watching television.

chemical score A ratio comparing the essential amino acid content of the protein in a food with the essential amino acid content in an ideal protein; the lowest ratio for an essential amino acid becomes the chemical score.

chemical reaction An interaction between two chemicals that changes both participants.

cholecystokinin (CCK) (koh-lee-sis-toe-ky-nin) A hormone that stimulates the release of enzymes from the pancreas and bile from the gallbladder.

cholesterol (koh-les-te-rol) A waxy fat, made only by animals, that is found in all body cells. Its structure contains multiple chemical rings.

chronic (kron-ik) Long standing, developing over time; slow to develop or resolve. When referring to disease, this indicates that the disease progress slows and tends to remain once developed, as with heart disease.

chylomicrons (kye-lo-my-kron) Dietary fats that are surrounded by a shell of cholesterol, phospholipids, and protein. Chylomicrons are made in the intestine after fat absorption and travel through the lymphatic system to the bloodstream.

chyme (kime) A mixture of stomach secretions and partly digested food.

cirrhosis (sir-roh-sis) A loss of functioning liver cells, which are replaced by nonfunctioning connective tissue. Any substance that poisons liver cells, such as alcohol, can lead to cirrhosis.

clinical symptom Generally, a change in health status noted by the individual (e.g., stomach pain) or during a physical examination.

Clostridium botulinum (claw-strid-ee-um bot-you-ly-num) A bacterium that can cause a fatal type of food poisoning.

coenzyme (koh-en-zime) The active form of many vitamins; Coenzyme forms aid enzyme function.

cognitive restructuring Changing one's frame of mind regarding eating; for example, instead of using a difficult day as an excuse to overeat, substituting other pleasures for rewards, such as a relaxing walk with a friend.

colic (call-ik) Periodic crying in a healthy infant, apparently as a result of gas buildup.

collagen (call-a-gin) The major protein form found in connective tissue, cartilage, and bone. Vitamin C aids in its synthesis.

colon (ko-lon) Another name for the large intestine.

colostrum (ko-lahs-trum) The first milk secreted during late pregnancy and the first few days after birth. This thick fluid is rich in immune factors and protein.

complementarity of proteins The ability of two food protein sources to make up for each other's insufficient contribution of specific amino acids, such that together they yield a high-quality protein diet.

complete proteins Proteins that contain ample amounts of all nine essential amino acids.

constipation A condition of infrequent bowel movements.

contingency management Forming a plan of action for responding to an environment in which overeating is likely, such as when snacks are within easy reach at a party.

control group In an experiment, the group whose habits are not altered.

cortical bone (kort-ih-kal) Dense, compact bone that comprises the outer surface and shaft of a bone.

covalent bond (ko-vay-lent) A union of two atoms formed by the sharing of electrons.

cretenism (kreet-in-ism) The stunting of body growth and mental development that results from inadequate maternal intake of iodine during pregnancy.

crude fiber The remains of dietary fiber after acid and alkaline treatment; this consists primarily of cellulose and lignins.

cystic fibrosis (sis-tik figh-bro-sis) A disease that, among other effects, often leads to overproduction of mucus, which can invade the pancreas and decrease the production of enzymes. The subsequent lack of lipase enzyme contributes to severe malabsorption of fat.

daily food guide A dietary planning tool that recommends food choices from milk and milk products; meat, fish, poultry, and beans; vegetables and fruits; and breads and cereals.

deamination (dee-am-ih-na-shun) The removal of an amino group from an amino acid.

Delaney clause A clause in the 1958 Food Additives Amendment of the Pure Food and Drug Act; it forbids the intentional (direct) addition of a compound to foods introduced after that date that has been shown to cause cancer in animals or humans.

dementia (de-men-shah) A general loss or decrease in mental function.

denature (dee-nay-ture) Alteration of a protein's three-dimensional structure, usually as a result of treatment by heat, acid or alkaline solutions, or agitation.

dental caries (kare-ees) Sites of erosion on the tooth surface. Caries are caused by the acid produced when bacteria on the tooth's surface metabolize sugar.

deoxyribonucleic acid (DNA) The site of hereditary information in cells; DNA directs the synthesis of cell proteins.

dermatitis (derm-a-tite-us) Inflammation of the skin.

diabetes mellitus (dye-uh-beet-eez mell-uh-tus) A disease characterized by high blood sugar levels that result from poor action by the hormone insulin.

diastolic blood pressure (dye-ah-stol-ik) The pressure in the bloodstream when the heart is between beats.

dietary fiber Substances in food (essentially all from plants) that are not digested by the processes in the stomach and small intestine.

dietary goals Specific goals for nutrient intake set in 1977 by a committee of the U.S. Senate.

dietary guidelines General goals for nutrient intake and diet composition set by the U.S. Department of Agriculture and the Department of Health and Human Services.

digestibility (dye-jes-tih-bil-it-ee) The porportion of food substances eaten that can be broken down in the intestinal tract and absorbed into the bloodstream.

digestion (dye-jes-tjun) The process by which food is broken down into forms that can be absorbed by the GI tract.

diphosphoglycerate (dye-foss-foe-gliss-er-ate) A compound used in the red blood cells that is involved in the release of oxygen from hemoglobin.

direct calorimetry (cal-oh-rim-eh-tree) A method of determining energy use by the body by measuring heat that emanates from the body.

disaccharides (dye-sack-uh-rides) A class of sugars formed by linking two monosaccharides.

diuretic (dye-your-et-ik) A substance that increases the flow of urine.

diverticula (dye-ver-tik-you-luh) Pouches that protrude through the wall of the large intestine. Diverticulosis is the condition of having many diverticula in the colon.

diverticulitis (dye-ver-tik-you-lite-us) An inflammation of the diverticula caused by acids produced by bacterial metabolism inside the diverticula.

double-blind study An experiment in which the subjects and researchers are unaware of the study assignment (placebo vs experimental) until it is completed.

ecosystem A "community" in nature that includes plants and animals and the environment associated with them.

ectomorph (ek-toh-morf) A body type associated with very long, thin bones and very long, thin fingers.

edema (uh-dee-muh) The buildup of excess fluid in extracellular spaces.

eicosanoids (eye-koh-san-oyds) Hormonelike compounds synthesized from polyunsaturated fatty acids; this class of compounds includes prostaglandins, thromboxanes, and leukotrienes.

eicosapenteanoic acid (EPA) (eye-koh-sah-pen-tah-no-ik) An omega-3 fatty acid with 20 carbon atoms and five double bonds; present in fish oils.

electrolytes (ih-lek-tro-lites) Compounds that break down into ions in water and thus can conduct an electrical current.

elimination diet A restrictive diet that systematically tests foods that may cause an allergic response by first eliminating suspected foods and then adding them back one at a time.

embryo (em-bree-oh) The developing human life form during the second to eighth week after conception.

emulsifier (ee-mull-sih-fye-er) A substance that can suspend fat in tiny droplets within a watery fluid.

endomorph (en-doh-morf) A body type characterized by short, stubby bones, a short trunk, and very short fingers.

endorphins (en-dor-fins) Natural body tranquilizers that may be involved in the feeding response, as well as in pain reduction.

enriched A term generally meaning that the vitamins thiamin, niacin, and riboflavin and the mineral iron have been added to a grain product to improve nutritional quality.

enzyme (en-zime) A compound that speeds the rate of a chemical process but is not altered by the process. Almost all enzymes are proteins.

epidemiology (ep-uh-dee-me-oll-uh-gee) The study of how disease rates vary between different population groups, such as the rate of stomach cancer in Japan compared with that in Germany.

epinephrine (ep-ih-nef-rin) A hormone also known as adrenaline; it is released by the adrenal gland (located near the kidneys) and various nerve endings in the body. Epinephrine increases glycogen breakdown in the liver, among other functions.

epithelial cells (ep-ih-thee-lee-ul) The surface cells that line the outside of the body and all external passages within it.

equilibrium (ee-kwih-lib-ree-um) In nutritional terms, a state in which nutrient intake equals nutrient losses; this allows the body to maintain a stable condition.

ergogenic (ur-go-jen-ic) Work producing.

essential Having no obvious, external cause.

essential amino acids The amino acids that cannot be synthesized by humans in sufficient amounts and therefore must be included in the diet; there are nine essential amino acids.

essential fatty acids Fatty acids that must be present in the diet to maintain health; these are linoleic acid and alpha-linolenic acid.

esterification (e-ster-ih-fih-kay-shun) The process of attaching fatty acids to a glycerol molecule. Removing a fatty acid is called deesterification; reattaching a fatty acid is called reesterification.

Estimated Safe and Adequate Daily Dietary Intake (ESADDI) Nutrient intake recommendations, made by the National Academy of Sciences' Food and Nutrition Board, that give a range for intake of some nutrients because not enough information is available to set a recommended daily allowance (RDA).

exchange system A grouping of foods in six lists. When the serving size for any food in a list is consumed, all foods within the list yield a similar amount of carbohydrate, fat, protein, and energy.

experiment A test conducted to examine the validity of a hypothesis.

failure to thrive Inadequate gains in height and weight in infancy, often resulting from inadequate food intake.

famine A time of massive starvation, often associated with crop failures, war, and political strife.

fasting hypoglycemia (high-po-gligh-see-me-uh) Low blood sugar that follows a day or so of fasting.

fatty acid Acids found in fat; they are composed of carbon atoms linked to hydrogen atoms, with an acidic chemical group at one end.

fat-soluble vitamin Vitamins that dissolve in substances such as ether or benzene. These vitamins include A, D, E, and K.

feeding center A group of cells in the hypothalamus that cause hunger when stimulated. These cells are also known as the lateral feeding centers.

ferritin (ferr-ih-tin) A protein compound that serves as the storage form of iron in the blood and tissues.

fetal alcohol syndrome (FAS) A group of physical and mental abnormalities in an infant caused by the mother's consumption of alcohol during pregnancy.

fetus (feet-us) A developing infant inside its mother from 8 weeks to birth.

fluoroapatite (fleur-oh-app-uh-tite) Tooth crystals containing fluoride ions that are relatively acid resistant.

food diary A written record of sequential food intake for a period of time. Details associated with the food intake are often recorded as well.

food intolerance An adverse reaction to food that does not involve the immune system.

food sensitivity A mild reaction to a substance in food that might be noticed as slight itching or redness of the skin.

fore milk The first breast milk delivered in the nursing session.

fortified A term generally meaning that vitamins, minerals, or both have been added to a food product in excess of what was originally found in the product.

fraternal twins Infants that develop from two separate ova and sperm and therefore have separate genetic identities, although they develop simultaneously in the mother.

fructose (frook-tose) A monosaccharide with six carbons found in fruits and honey.

galactose (gah-lak-tose) A six-carbon monosaccharide; an isomer of glucose.

galactosemia (gah-lak-toh-see-mee-ah) A disease characterized by the buildup of the monosaccharide galactose in the bloodstream, resulting from the liver's inability to metabolize galactose. If present at birth and left untreated, galactosemia results in severe growth and mental retardation.

gastrin (gas-trin) A hormone that stimulates the secretion of enzymes and acids in the stomach.

gastrointestinal (GI) tract (gas-troh-in-tes-tin-al) The main sites in the body used in digestion and absorption of nutrients. It consists of the mouth, esophagus, stomach, small intestine, large intestine, rectum, and anus.

gastroplasty (gas-troh-plas-tee) Surgery performed on the stomach to limit its volume to approximately 50 milliliters, about the size of a shot glass.

generally recognized as safe (GRAS) A group of food additives that in 1958 were considered safe; thus manufacturers have been allowed to use them when needed in food products.

genes The hereditary material on chromosomes that makes up DNA. Genes provide the blueprints for the production of cell proteins.

genetic engineering Alteration of genetic material in plants or animals with the intent of improving growth, disease resistance, or other characteristics.

geometric ratio A group of numbers in which the division of each number by the one to the left of it yields the same number.

gestation (jes-tay-shun) The time of fetal growth from conception to birth; a period of about 40 weeks after a woman's last normal menstrual period.

gestational diabetes (jes-tay-shun-al) A high blood glucose level that develops during pregnancy but returns to normal after birth. One cause is production of hormones by the placenta that antagonize the action of the hormone insulin.

glucagon (gloo-kuh-gon) A hormone made by the pancreas that stimulates the liver to break down glycogen into glucose; this raises the blood glucose level. Glucagon also performs other functions.

gluconeogenesis (gloo-ko-nee-oh-jen-uh-sis) The production of new glucose molecules by metabolic pathways in the cell. Amino acids usually are the source of the carbon atoms for these new glucose molecules.

glucose (gloo-kos) A six-carbon carbohydrate found in blood; in table sugar it is linked to another sugar called fructose.

glucose polymer A carbohydrate source used in some sports drinks that consists of grouping of a few glucose molecules.

glycerol (gliss-er-ol) A three-carbon alcohol used to form triglycerides.

glycogen (gligh-ko-jen) A carbohydrate made up of several units of glucose containing a highly branched structure; sometimes known as animal starch. Glycogen is the storage form of glucose, which is synthesized in the liver and muscles.

glycolysis (gligh-coll-ih-sis) The pathway that results in the breakdown of glucose into two three-carbon molecules.

goiter (goy-ter) An enlargement of the thyroid gland (located in the neck area) often caused by a lack of iodide in the diet.

goitrogens (goy-troh-jens) Substances in food that interfere with the absorption and use of iodine; they therefore may cause goiter if consumed in large amounts.

gram A measure of weight in the metric system; 28 grams equal 1 ounce, and 1 kilogram equals 2.2 pounds.

green revolution A period in the 1960s when much emphasis was placed on improving strains and cultivation practices of cereal grains such as rice, wheat, and corn.

growth hormone A pituitary hormone that produces body growth and the release of fat from storage, among other effects.

gums A group of soluble fibers containing chains of galactose, glucuronic acid, and other monosaccharides; gums characteristically are found in matter exuded from plant stems.

hazard The chances that injury will result from use of a substance.

heart attack A rapid fall in heart function caused by reduced blood flow through the heart's blood vessels. Often part of the heart dies in the process.

heart disease A disease characterized by the deposition of fatty material in the blood vessels in the heart. The fatty materials reduce blood flow through the blood vessels supplying the heart.

heartburn A pain emanating from the esophagus as a result of stomach acid backing up into the esophagus and irritating the tissue in that organ.

hematocrit (hee-mat-oh-krit) The percentage of blood that is made up of red blood cells.

heme iron (heem) Iron provided from animal tissues as hemoglobin and myoglobin. Approximately 50% of the iron in meat is heme iron; it is readily absorbed.

hemicellulose (hem-ih-sell-you-los) A group of insoluble fibers containing the monosaccharides xylose, galactose, and glucose, as well as other monosaccharides linked in an indigestible fashion.

hemochromatosis (heem-oh-krom-ah-tos-sis) A disorder of iron metabolism characterized by increased iron absorption and deposition in the liver tissue; this eventually poisons the liver cells.

hemoglobin (heem-oh-glow-bin) The iron-containing protein in red blood cells that carries oxygen to the cells and carbon dioxide away from the cells. Hemoglobin also gives blood its red color.

hemolysis (hee-mol-ih-sis) Destruction of red blood cells. The red blood cell membrane breaks down, allowing cell contents to leak into the fluid portion of the blood.

hemorrhoids (hem-or-oyds) Swollen veins of the rectum and anus; they often protrude into the anus.

hemosiderin (heem-oh-sid-er-in) An insoluble iron-protein compound found in the liver. Hemosiderin stores increase as the amount of iron in the liver exceeds the storage capacity of ferritin.

herbicide (erb-ih-side) A compound that reduces the growth and reproduction of plants.

high-fructose corn syrup A corn syrup that is 40% to 90% fructose.

high density lipoprotein (HDL) (lip-oh-pro-teen) A lipoprotein synthesized by the liver and small intestine that picks up cholesterol from dying cells and other sources and transfers it to the other lipoprotein in the bloodstream. A low HDL level increases the risk for heart disease.

hind milk (hynd) The milk secreted at the end of a nursing session; it is higher in fat than fore milk.

hormone (hore-moan) A compound secreted into the bloodstream that acts to control the function of distant cells.

hospice Hospital care that emphasizes comfort and dignity in death.

hunger The physiological drive to find and eat food.

hydrogenation (high-draw-je-nay-shun) The addition of hydrogen atoms to the double bonds of polyunsaturated and monounsaturated fatty acids to reduce the extent of unsaturation; this process turns liquid vegetable oils into solid fats.

hydrophilic (high-dro-fill-ik) Attracts water (literally means "water loving").

hydrophobic (high-dro-fo-bik) Repels water (literally means "water fearing").

hydroxyapatite (high-drox-ee-app-uh-tite) A compound composed of calcium and phosphate that is deposited into the bone protein matrix to give bone strength and rigidity.

hyperactivity A poorly defined term generally used to label inattention, irritability, and excessively active behavior in children.

hyperglycemia (high-per-gligh-see-me-uh) A high blood glucose level; that is, above 140 milligrams per 100 milliliters of blood.

hypertension (high-per-ten-shun) A condition also known as high blood pressure in which blood pressure remains persistently elevated, especially when the heart is between beats.

hypoglycemia (high-po-gligh-see-mee-uh) A low blood glucose level; that is, below 40 to 50 milligrams per 100 milliliters of blood.

hypothalamus (high-po-thall-uh-mus) A grouping of cells at the base of the brain. These cells participate in many body functions, such as regulating hunger.

hypothesis (high-poth-eh-sis) An "educated guess" by a scientist to explain a phenomenon.

identical twins Two infants that develop from a single ovum and sperm and consequently have the same genetic makeup.

in utero (in you-ter-oh) "in the uterus"; that is, during pregnancy.

incidental food additives Additives introduced into food products indirectly from environmental contamination of ingredients or during the manufacturing process.

indirect calorimetry (kal-oh-rim-eh-tree) A method of estimating energy use by the body by measuring oxygen uptake and then using formulas to convert that gas usage into kilocalorie use.

infectious disease (in-fek-shus) Any disease caused by invasion of the body by microorganisms, such as bacteria, fungi, or viruses.

infrastructure The basic framework of a system or organization. For society, this includes roads, bridges, telephones, and other basic technologies.

inorganic (in-ore-gan-ik) Free of carbon linked to hydrogen in the chemical structure.

insensible Not consciously noted by the individual.

insoluble fibers (in-sol-you-bul) Fibers that mostly do not dissolve in water and are not digested by bacteria in the large intestine. These include cellulose, some hemicellulose, and lignins.

insulin (in-suh-lin) A hormone produced by the beta cells of the pancreas. Insulin increases the synthesis of glycogen in the liver and the movement of glucose from the bloodstream into muscle and adipose cells, among other processes.

insulin-dependent diabetes mellitus A form of diabetes prone to ketosis; it requires insulin therapy.

intentional food additives Additives knowingly (directly) incorporated into food products by manufacturers.

intermediate density lipoprotein (IDL) (lih-poh-pro-teen) The product formed after a very low density lipoprotein (VLDL) has had most of its triglyceride removed.

international unit (IU) A crude measure of vitamin activity, often based on the growth rate of animals. Today these units have been replaced by more precise milligram and microgram quantities.

intracellular fluid Fluid contained within a cell.

intravenous (in-trah-veen-us) Introduced directly into the bloodstream.

intrinsic factor A proteinlike compound produced by the stomach that enhances absorption of vitamin B12.

ion an atom with an unequal number of electrons and protons. If the number of electrons exceeds the number of protons, the ion is negative. If the number of protons exceeds the number of electrons, the ion is positive.

irradiation (ir-ray-dee-ay-shun) A process whereby radiation energy is applied to foods, creating compounds within the food that destroy cell membranes, break down DNA, link proteins, limit enzyme activity, and alter a variety of other proteins and cell functions that can lead to food spoilage.

isomer (eye-so-mer) Different chemical structures for compounds that share the same chemical formula.

kcalories or kilocalories (kay-kal-oh-ree) A measure of the energy content in foods. A kilocalorie is the heat needed to raise 1000 grams (1 liter) of water 1° Celsius. This is the same as raising about 4 cups of water 2° Fahrenheit.

ketone (kee-tone) Incomplete breakdown products of fat containing three or four carbons.

ketone bodies Products of acetyl-CoA (fat) metabolism containing three to four carbon atoms: acetoacetic acid, beta-hydroxybutyric acid, and acetone. These contain a ketone group, hence the name.

ketosis (kee-toe-sis) The condition of having high levels of ketones in the bloodstream.

kidney nephrons (nef-rons) A unit of kidney cells that filter wastes out of the bloodstream.

kilogram A measure of weight in the metric system; 1 kilogram equals 1000 grams.

kjoule (kay-jool) A measure of work in which 1 kjoule equals the work needed to move 1 kilogram a distance of 1 meter with the force of 1 newton; 1 kilocalorie equals 4.8 kjoules.

kwashiorkor (kwash-ee-or-core) A disease occurring primarily in young children when disease and infections add to high demands for growth; edema, moderate weight deficit, and weakness are common symptoms. If the child consumes insufficient kilocalories and protein, kwashiorkor may result.

lactation (lak-ta-shun) The period after childbirth during which milk is produced in the woman's breasts.

lactic acid (lak-tik) A three-carbon acid formed during anaerobic cell metabolism; a partial breakdown of glucose; also called lactate.

lactovegetarian (lak-toe ve-jah-tear-ree-an) A semivegetarian food plan in which milk products are consumed as well as vegetable products.

lacto-ovo-vegetarian A semivegetarian food plan in which a person consumes plant products, dairy products, and eggs.

Lactobacillus bifidus factor (lak-toe-bah-sil-us biff-id-us) A protective factor secreted in colostrum that encourages growth of beneficial bacteria in the intestine of an infant.

lactose (lak-tose) A sugar made up of glucose linked to another sugar, called galactose.

lactose intolerance Lactose is reduced as lactase production declines. Symptoms include gas and bloating after consuming dairy products.

lanugo (lah-new-go) The downlike hair that appears after much body fat is lost as a result of semistarvation. The hair stands erect and traps air, which acts as insulation to the body, replacing that usually supplied by body fat.

larva (lar-vah) An early developmental stage in the life history of some microorganisms, such as parasites.

laxative A medication or other substance that stimulates evacuation of the intestinal tract.

lean body mass The part of the body that is free of all but essential body fat. About 2% of body fat is essential; the rest represents storage and so is not part of lean body mass. Lean body mass includes muscle, bone, organs, connective tissue, skin, and other body parts.

lecithin (less-uh-thin) A phospholipid containing two fatty acids, a phosphate group, and a choline molecule.

let-down reflex A reflex stimulated by infant suckling that causes the release (ejection) of milk from milk ducts in the mother's breasts.

life expectancy The average length of life for a given group of people.

life span The potential oldest age to which a person can survive.

lignin (lig-nin) A group of insoluble fibers made up of a multiringed alcohol (noncarbohydrate) structure.

limiting amino acid The essential amino acid in the lowest concentration in a food in proportion to body needs.

linoleic acid (lin-oh-lay-ik) A fatty acid with 18 carbon atoms and two double bonds; omega-6.

lipase (lye-pase) Fat-digesting enzymes; lipase produced by the pancreas to act in the small intestine is the most important form used in digestion.

lipectomy (lip-eck-toe-mee) Surgical removal of body fat; also known as liposuction.

lipids (lip-ids) Compounds containing carbon, hydrogen, oxygen, and sometimes other atoms. Lipids dissolve in ether or benzene and are commonly known as fats and oils.

lipogenic (lye-poh-jen-ik) Means "creating lipid." The liver is the major lipogenic organ in the body.

lipoprotein (lye-poh-pro-teen) A compound found in the bloodstream containing a core of lipids with a shell of protein, phospholipid, and cholesterol.

lipoprotein lipase (lye-poh-pro-teen lye-pase) An enzyme attached to the outside of the cells that line the bloodstream; it breaks down triglycerides into free fatty acids and glycerol.

liter (lee-ter) A measure of volume in the metric system; 1 liter equals 1.06 quarts.

lobules (lob-you-els) Sacklike structures in the breast that store milk.

long-chain fatty acids Fatty acids that contain more than 12 carbon atoms.

low birth weight (LBW) Infant weight at birth of less than 5.5 pounds (2.5 kilograms), usually because of premature birth; these infants have a higher risk of health problems.

low density lipoprotein (LDL) The product of the intermediate density lipoprotein (IDL) containing primarily cholesterol; an elevated level of LDL is strongly linked to heart disease.

low input sustainable agriculture (LISA) A form of farming that attempts to limit use of purchased materials such as manufactured fertilizers and pesticides. Use of manure and crop rotation are typical substitutes.

lower body obesity The type of obesity, called gynoid, in which fat is stored primarily in the buttocks and thigh area.

lymphatic system (lim-fat-ick) The system of vessels that can accept large particles, such as products of fat absorption, and eventually pass them into the bloodstream.

macrobiotics (mack-row-by-ah-tiks) A food plan that emphasizes vegetable foods over animal foods, often with heavy use of brown rice.

macrocyte (mac-row-site) A greatly enlarged mature red blood cell; these cells have a short life spans.

major mineral A mineral vital to health that is required in the diet in amounts greater than 100 milligrams per day.

malnutrition Failing health that results from a long-standing dietary intake that fails to meet or greatly exceeds nutritional needs.

maltose (mawl-tose) Glucose linked to glucose.

marasmus (mah-ras-mus) A disease caused essentially by starvation; the person does not consume sufficient protein and kilocalories and thus has the equivalent of severe protein-energy malnutrition. The individual will be severely underweight and have little or no fat stores, little muscle mass, and poor strength.

marginal Noticeable but not severe.

mass movement A peristaltic wave that simultaneously coordinates contraction over a large area of the colon. These contractions move material from one portion of the colon to another and from the colon into the rectum.

meconium (meh-koh-nee-um) The first stool passed by an infant after birth. It has a thick, mucuslike consistency.

medium-chain fatty acids Fatty acids that contain six to 10 carbon atoms.

megadose (meg-ah-dose) Intake of a nutrient in amounts greater than 10 times the desired 1989 RDA listed values.

megaloblast (meg-ah-low-blast) A large, immature red blood cell that results from the particular cell's inability to divide when it normally should.

menarche (men-ar-kee) The onset of menses in women, which occurs usually between 10 and 13 years of age.

menopause (men-oh-paws) The cessation of menses in women, which usually begins at about 50 years of age.

mesomorph (mez-oh-morf) A body type associated with average bone size, trunk size, and finger length.

metabolism (meh-tab-oh-liz-um) Chemical reactions that occur in the body, enabling cells to release energy from foods, convert one substance into another, and prepare end products for excretion.

meter (meet-er) A measure of length in the metric system; 1 meter equals 39.4 inches.

micelle (my-sell) A droplet of fat surrounded by a shell of water. Emulsifiers are used to produce micelles.

microgram A measure of weight in the metric system; 1 million micrograms equal 1 gram.

milligram A measure of weight in the metric system; 1000 milligrams equal 1 gram.

minerals Chemical elements used in the body to promote chemical processes and form body structures.

Minimum Requirements for Health (MRH) Nutrient intake recommendations for sodium, potassium, and chloride, as set by the National Academy of Sciences' Food and Nutrition Board.

miscarriage Loss of pregnancy that occurs before 28 weeks of gestation; also called spontaneous abortion.

molecule (mol-e-kewl) A group of like or unlike atoms that are chemically linked; it is similar to a compound, which is a group of different types of atoms bonded together in definite proportion.

monoglycerides (mon-oh-glis-er-ides) A breakdown product of a triglyceride, consisting of one fatty acid bonded to the carbohydrate glycerol.

monosaccharide (mon-oh-sack-uh-ride) A single sugar, such as glucose, that is not broken down further during digestion.

monounsaturated fatty acid A fatty acid containing one carbon-carbon double bond.

mortality Synonymous with death; rate of death.

mottle (mot-tal) Discoloration or marking of the surface of teeth caused by a high fluoride content.

mucilage (mew-sih-laj) A group of soluble fibers consisting of chains of galactose, mannose, and other monosaccharides; characteristically found in seaweed.

mucus (mew-cuss) A thick fluid, secreted by glands throughout the body, that contains a compound that is both carbohydrate and protein in nature. Mucus acts as a lubricant and a means of protection for cells.

mycotoxins (my-ko-tok-sins) A group of toxic compounds produced by molds, such as aflatoxin B-1, found on moldy grains.

myocardial infarction (my-oh-card-ee-ahl in-fark-shun) Death of part of the heart muscle.

myoglobin (my-oh-glow-bin) An iron-containing compound that transports oxygen and carbon dioxide in muscle tissue.

neurotransmitter A compound made by a nerve cell that allows communication between it and other cells.

nitrate (nye-trate) A nitrogen-containing compound used to cure meats. It gives meat a pink color and confers some resistance to bacterial growth.

no observable effect level (NOEL) The highest dose of an additive that produces no deleterious health effect in animals.

nonheme iron Iron provided from plant sources and animal tissues other than in the form of hemoglobin and myoglobin. Nonheme iron is less efficiently absorbed than heme iron.

nonessential amino acids Amino acids that can be synthesized by the body in sufficient amounts; there are 11 nonessential amino acids in the diet.

noninsulin-dependent diabetes mellitus A form of diabetes in which ketosis is not common, and insulin therapy may be used but is not often required.

nonpolar A compound with no charges.

nucleus (new-klee-us) The core of an atom; it consists of protons and neutrons.

nutrient density The ratio formed by dividing a food's contribution to the need for a nutrient by its contribution to kilocalorie needs. When the contribution to nutrient need exceeds that of kilocalorie needs, the food has a favorable nutrient density.

nutrients Chemical substances in food that nourish the body by providing energy, building materials, and factors to regulate needed chemical reactions in the body. The body either can't make these substances or can't make them fast enough for its needs.

nutrition The Council on Food and Nutrition of the American Medical Association defines nutrition as "the science of food, the nutrients and the substances therein, their action, interaction, and balance in relation to health and disease, and the process by which the organism (i.e., body) ingests, digests, absorbs, transports, utilizes, and excretes food substances."

nutrition labels A label format that must be included on foods under certain circumstances, such as when nutrients are added to foods or when a nutritional claim is made for the food. The nutrition label must follow specific guidelines set by the FDA.

nutritional status The nutritional health of a person as determined by anthropometric measures (height, weight, circumferences, and so on), biochemical measures of nutrients or their by-products in blood and urine, a clinical (physical) examination, and a dietary analysis; these elements can be remembered by the mnemonic ABCD.

nutritionist A person who advises about nutrition or works in the field of food and nutrition. In many states in the United States a person does not need formal training to use this title; some states reserve this title for registered dietitians.

obesity (oh-bees-ih-tee) A condition characterized by excess body fat, usually defined as body weight 20% above the desirable level.

oligosaccharides (ol-ih-go-sak-ah-rides) Carbohydrates that contain 3 to 10 monosaccharide units.

omega-6 fatty acid A fatty acid with its first carbon-carbon double bonds starting at the sixth carbon atom from the -CH3 end.

omega-3 fatty acid A fatty acid with its first carbon-carbon double bond starting at the third carbon atom from the CH3 end.

omnivore (ahm-nih-voor) A person who consumes foods from both plants and animals.

opportunistic infections Infections primarily seen in undernourished or otherwise weakened people.

organ A group of tissues designed to perform a specific function (e.g., the heart). An organ contains muscle tissue, nerve tissue, and so on.

organic (ore-gan-ik) Contains carbon atoms linked to hydrogen in the chemical structure.

organism (ore-gan-ih-zim) A living thing. The human body is an organism consisting of many organs that act in a coordinated manner to support life.

osmosis (oz-mos-is) The passage of solutions across a semipermeable membrane.

osmotic pressure The pressure needed to prevent particles in a solution from drawing liquid across a semipermeable membrane.

osteomalacia (os-tee-oh-mal-ay-shuh) The adult form of rickets, osteomalacia is a weakening of the bones as a result of poor calcium content. The condition is caused by a reduction in the activity of the vitamin D hormone.

osteopenia (os-tee-oh-pee-nee-ah) Decreased bone mass stemming from cancer, hyperthyroidism, or other causes.

osteoporosis (os-tee-oh-po-roh-sis) A bone disease that develops primarily after menopause in women and is characterized by a decrease in bone density.

ostomy (oss-toh-mee) A surgically created short circuit in intestinal flow in which the end point usually opens from the abdominal cavity rather than the anus, as with a colostomy.

outpatient A person treated by medical personnel outside the hospital setting; for example, in a clinic or a physician's office.

overnutrition A state in which nutritional intake exceeds the body's needs.

oxidize (ox-ih-dize) To lose an electron or gain an oxygen atom.

oxidizing compound (ox-ih-dy-zing) A compound capable of capturing an electron from another compound (or supplying oxygen to another compound). The word "oxidize" literally means to lose or gain an electron.

palatable (pal-it-ah-bull) Pleasing to the taste.

passive absorption Absorption that requires permeability of the substance through the wall of the small intestine, as well as a concentration higher in the small intestine than in the absorptive cells.

pasteurize (pas-tur-eyes) The process of heating food products to kill pathogenic microorganisms. Under one method, milk is heated at 161° F for about 20 seconds.

pathway A metabolic progression of individual steps from starting materials to ending products.

pectin (peck-tin) A group of soluble fibers containing chains of galacturonic acid and other monosaccharides; characteristically found between plant cell walls.

peer-reviewed journal A journal that publishes research only after two or three scientists (essentially peers) who were not part of the study agree that it was well conducted and that the results are fairly represented.

pellagra (peh-lahg-rah) A disease resulting from lack of the vitamin niacin in the diet; it is characterized by inflammation of the skin, diarrhea and, eventually, mental incapacity.

pepsin (pep-sin) A protein-digesting enzyme produced by the stomach.

peptide bond A bond formed to link amino acids in a protein.

peptides (pep-tydes) A few amino acids bonded together (often two to four).

percent A part of the total when the total consists of 100 parts.

peristalsis (pear-ih-stall-sis) A coordinated muscular contraction that is used to propel food down the GI tract.

pernicious anemia (per-nish-us ah-nee-mee-ah) The anemia that results from a lack of vitamin B-12 absorption; it is "pernicious" because of the associated nerve degeneration that eventually can result in paralysis.

pesticide (pest-i-side) A general term signifying that an agent can destroy bacteria, fungi, insects, rodents, or other pests.

pH A measure of the hydrogen ion concentration in a solution.

phenylketonuria (PKU) (fee-null-kee-tone-your-ee-ah) A disease in which the liver cannot readily metab-

olize the amino acid phenylalanine. Toxic by-products of phenylalanine build up in the body, leading to mental retardation.

phenylpropanolamine (fee-null-pro-pan-awl-ah-meen) An over-the-counter decongestant that has a mild appetite-reducing effect.

phosphocreatine (PCr) A high-energy compound that can be used to reform adenosine triphosphate (ATP) from adenosine diphosphate (ADP).

photosynthesis (foto-sin-tha-sis) The process by which plants use energy from the sun to produce energy-yielding compounds, such as glucose.

physiological anemia The normal increase in blood volume that occurs during pregnancy and dilutes the concentration of red blood cells, resulting in anemia; also called hemodilution.

phytobezoars (fy-tow-bee-zors) A pellet of fiber characteristically found in the stomach.

pica (pie-kah) The practice of eating nonfood items such as dirt, laundry starch, or clay.

placebo (plah-see-bo) A fake medicine used to disguise the roles of participants in an experiment.

placenta (plah-sen-tah) An organ formed only during pregnancy that secretes hormones and makes possible the transfer of oxygen and nutrients from the mother's blood to the fetus and the removal of fetal wastes.

plaque (plack) A cholesterol-rich substance deposited in the blood vessels; it contains various white blood cells, cholesterol and other lipids, and eventually calcium.

polar A compound with distinct positive and negative charges, which act like poles on a magnet.

polysaccharides (paw-lee-sack-uh-rides) Carbohydrates that contain up to 3000 or more glucose units; also known as complex carbohydrates.

polyunsaturated fatty acid A fatty acid containing two or more carbon-carbon double bonds.

portal vein (poor-tall vane) A large vein leading to the liver. Capillary blood vessels from the intestinal drain into this vein.

positive balance A state in which nutrient intake exceeds losses, resulting in a net gain of the nutrient in the body (e.g., when tissue protein is gained during growth). The opposite of this state is negative balance, in which losses exceed intake, as with starvation.

pregnancy-induced hypertension A serious disorder, also called toxemia, that can involve high blood pressure, kidney failure, convulsion, and even death of the mother and the fetus. Although the exact cause is not known, good nutrition and prenatal care can prevent or limit the severity of this disorder. Mild cases are known as preeclampsia; more severe cases are called eclampsia.

premature An infant born before 38 weeks of gestation.

premenstrual syndrome (PMS) A disorder found in some women in the days surrounding menstrual periods that is characterized by depression, headache, bloating, and mood swings.

preservatives Compounds that extend the shelf life of food by inhibiting microbial growth or by minimizing the destructive effect of oxygen and metals.

progestins (pro-jes-tins) Hormones, including progesterone, that are necessary for maintaining pregnancy and lactation.

prognosis (prog-no-sis) A forecast of a disease's course.

prolactin (pro-lack-tin) A hormone secreted by the mother that stimulates the synthesis of milk.

protein efficiency ratio A measure of protein quality in a food, as determined by the protein's ability to support the growth of a young rat.

protein-energy malnutrition (PEM) A condition that results when a person regularly consumes insufficient amounts of kilocalories and protein. The deficiency eventually results in body wasting and an increased susceptibility to infections.

proteins (pro-teens) Compounds made up of amino acids. Proteins contain carbon, hydrogen, oxygen, nitrogen, and sometimes sulfur atoms in a specific configuration. They contain the form of nitrogen most easily used by the human body.

prothrombin (pro-throm-bin) A blood protein needed for blood clotting that requires vitamin K for its synthesis.

proton (pro-ton) The part of an atom that is positively charged.

psyllium (sil-ee-um) A mostly soluble type of dietary fiber found in the seeds of the plantain plant.

quack (kwak) A person who pretends to have certain medical skills or knowledge.

R protein A protein produced by the salivary glands that enhances absorption of vitamin B-12.

radiation (ray-dee-ay-shun) Literally, that which is transmitted from a center in all directions. Various forms of radiation energy include x-rays, ultraviolet rays from the sun, and microwaves.

rancid (ran-sid) Having a disagreeable odor or taste, usually as a result of the breakdown of fat.

reactive hypoglycemia (high-po-gligh-see-mee-uh) Low blood sugar that follows a meal high in simple sugars, with corresponding symptoms of irritability, headache, nervousness, sweating, and confusion.

receptive framework The process by which a person opens and responds to learning more about a problem; it usually involves seeking more information about the issue from books and people.

receptor pathway for cholesterol uptake A process by which LDL molecules (cholesterol containing) are bound by cell receptors, with the incorporation of the LDL molecule into the cell.

Recommended Dietary Allowances (RDA) Recommended nutrient intakes that meet the needs of essentially all people of similar age and gender. These amounts are established by the Food and Nutrition Board of the National Academy of Sciences.

Recommended Nutrient Intakes (RNI) The Canadian version of the RDA.

Reference Daily Intakes (RDI) Standards of expressing nutrient content on nutrition labels. RDI figures are based on average 1989 RDA values set for a nutrient that span a particular age range, such as children over 4 years through adults. RDI will replace U.S. RDA by November, 1992.

Registered Dietitian (RD) (dye-eh-tish-shun) A person who has completed a baccalaureate degree program approved by the American Dietetic Association, has participated in a supervised professional practice program, and has passed a registration examination.

reinforcement A reaction by others in response to a person's behavior. Positive reinforcement entails encouragement; negative reinforcement entails criticism or penalty.

requirement The amount of a nutrient required by one person to maintain health; this varies from individual to individual. We do not know our individual requirements for each nutrient.

reserve capacity The extent to which an organ can preserve essentially normal function despite decreasing cell number or cell activity.

resting metabolic rate Essentially the same as the basal metabolic rate, but the individual need not meet the strict conditions for determining a basal metabolic rate. The terms often are used interchangeably.

retinoids (ret-ih-noyds) Chemical forms of preformed vitamin A; one source is animal foods.

reverse transport of cholesterol The process by which cholesterol is picked up by HDL molecules and transferred to other lipoprotein that can dispose of it.

rhodopsin (row-dop-sin) A protein involved in vision; it is made in the eye and incorporates a protein called opsin and a form of vitamin A. It is especially important to night vision.

rickets (rick-its) A deficiency disease characterized by softening of the bones because of poor calcium content. It arises from lack of vitamin D activity in the body.

risk factor A characteristic or behavior that contributes to the chances of developing an illness.

runner's anemia A condition found in athletes that involves a decrease in the blood's ability to carry oxygen; this may be caused by iron loss through perspiration, destruction of red blood cells from the impact of exercise, or increased blood volume.

saccharin (sack-ah-rin) An alternate sweetener that yields no energy to the body; it is 500 times sweeter than sucrose.

safety The relative certainty that a substance won't cause injury.

saliva (sah-ligh-vah) A watery fluid produced by the salivary glands in the mouth; it contains lubricants, enzymes, and other substances.

salt Generally refers to a mixture of sodium and chloride in a 40:60 ratio.

satiety (suh-tie-uh-tee) A state in which there is no longer a desire to eat.

satiety center A group of cells in the hypothalamus that, when stimulated, causes satiety. These cells are also known as the ventromedial satiety center.

saturated fat (sat-your-ate-ed) A fat containing no carbon-carbon double bonds in its structure.

saturated fatty acid A fatty acid with no carbon-carbon double bonds.

scavenger pathway for cholesterol uptake A process by which LDL molecules (cholesterol containing) are taken up by scavenger cells embedded in the blood vessels.

scurvy (sker-vee) The deficiency disease that results after a few weeks of consuming a diet that lacks vitamin C.

sebum (see-bum) A secretion of the sebaceous glands consisting of fats, waxes, and other substances.

secrete (se-kreet) To produce and then release a substance from a cell in the body.

secretin (see-kreh-tin) A hormone that causes bicarbonate ion release from the pancreas and slow stomach emptying.

self-monitoring A process of tracking foods eaten and conditions affecting eating; these are usually recorded in a diary, along with the location, time, and state of mind. This is a tool to help a person understand more about his or her eating habits.

semiessential amino acids Amino acids that, when consumed, spare the need to use an essential amino acid for their synthesis.

senile Related to old age.

sequesterants (see-kwes-ter-ants) Compounds that bind free metal ions. In so doing, they reduce the ions' ability to cause rancidity in compounds containing fat.

serotonin (ser-oh-tone-in) A neurotransmitter synthesized from the amino acid tryptophan that appears both to decrease the desire to eat carbohydrates and to induce sleep.

set point A term referring to the close regulation of body weight. It is not known what cells control the set point nor how it actually functions in weight regulation. There is no doubt, however, that there are mechanisms that help regulate weight.

short-chain fatty acids Fatty acids that contain fewer than six carbon atoms.

sickle cell disease An anemia that results from a malformation of the red blood cell protein hemoglobin, a condition caused by an incorrect amino acid composition in the hemoglobin protein chains. The disease can lead to anemia and episodes of severe bone and joint pain, abdominal pain, headache, convulsions, paralysis, and even death.

slough (sluf) To shed or cast off.

small for gestational age (SGA) (jes-tay-shun-al) Infants born after normal gestation length (38 weeks) but weighing less than 2500 grams (about 5.5 pounds).

sodium bicarbonate An alkaline substance made basically of sodium and carbon dioxide ($NaHCO_3$).

soluble fibers (sol-you-bull) Fibers that either dissolve or swell when in water or are metabolized by bacteria in the large intestine. Soluble fibers include pectins, gums, mucilages, and some hemicellulose.

solvent A substance in which other substances dissolve.

sphincter (sfink-ter) A circular, muscular valve that controls the flow of food in the GI tract.

Standard of Identity A means by which a manufacturer can avoid disclosing ingredients on a food label. If a food is produced according to a specific recipe on file with the FDA, the label need not carry a list of its ingredients. In such cases the manufacturer is using its Standard of Identity.

starch A carbohydrate made up of several units of glucose attached in a form that the body can digest; also a part of complex carbohydrates.

steroids (stare-oydes) A group of hormones and related compounds that are derivatives of cholesterol.

stimulus control Altering the environment to minimize the stimuli for eating; for example, removing foods from sight and storing them in kitchen cabinets.

stroke The loss of body function that results from a blood clot in the brain, which in turn causes the death of brain tissue.

subjects Participants in an experiment.

sucrose (sue-kros) Fructose linked to glucose.

symptom A change in health status noted by the person with the problem, such as a stomach pain.

synapse (sin-apps) Spaces between nerve cells. One nerve stimulates other nearby cells, including other nerve cells, by releasing chemicals that cross the synapse. These chemicals are what excites neighboring cells.

systolic blood pressure (sis-tol-ik) The pressure in the bloodstream associated with the pumping of blood from the heart.

tetany (tet-ah-nee) A body condition marked by sharp contraction of muscles and failure to relax afterward; usually caused by abnormal calcium metabolism.

theory An explanation for a phenomenon that has numerous lines of evidence to support it.

thermic effect of food The increase in metabolism occurring during the digestion, absorption, and metabolism of energy-yielding nutrients. This effect represents 5% to 10% of kilocalories consumed.

"thrifty" metabolism A metabolism that characteristically conserves more kilocalories than normal, such that the risk of weight gain and obesity is enhanced.

tissue A group of cells designed to perform a specific function; muscle tissue is an example.

tocopherols (tuh-koff-er-alls) The chemical name for some forms of vitamin E.

toxic (tok-sick) Poisonous; caused by a poison.

toxicity (tok-sis-ih-tee) The capacity of a substance to produce injury at some level of intake.

toxicology (tok-si-call-oh-gee) The scientific study of harmful substances.

trabecular bone (trah-beck-you-lar) The spongy, inner matrix of bone, found primarily in the spine, pelvis, and ends of bones.

trace mineral A mineral vital to health that is required in the diet in amounts less than 100 milligrams per day.

transamination (trans-am-ih-nat-shun) The transfer of an amino group from an amino acid to a carbon skeleton to form a new amino acid.

triglyceride (try-gliss-uh-ride) The major form of lipid in food. It is composed of three fatty acids bonded to the carbohydrate glycerol.

trimester One of the three 13- to 14-week periods that make up a normal pregnancy.

trypsin (trip-sin) A protein-digesting enzyme secreted by the pancreas to act in the small intestine.

U.S. Recommended Daily Allowances (U.S. RDA) Nutrient standards established by the FDA for use on nutrition labels. Generally the four existing versions use the highest nutrient recommendation in the appropriate age and gender category from the 1968 publication of the RDA. The version that includes children over 4 years of age and adults is most commonly seen on nutrition labels.

ulcer (ul-sir) Erosion of the tissue lining in either the stomach or the upper small intestine; usually referred to as a peptic ulcer.

undernutrition Failing health that results from a long-standing dietary intake that does not meet nutritional needs.

unsaturated fat (un-sat-your-ate-ed) A fatty acid containing one or more carbon-carbon double bonds in its structure.

urea (yur-ee-ah) A nitrogen-containing waste product found in urine. Most nitrogen excreted from the body leaves in this form.

vegan (veh-gan) A person who consumes no animal products.

vegetarian (veh-jih-tair-ee-un) A person who avoids eating animal products to a varying degree, ranging from eating no animal foods to simply not eating foods from four-footed animals.

very low density lipoprotein (VLDL) The lipoprotein that initially leaves the liver; it carries both the cholesterol and lipid newly synthesized by the liver.

very low calorie diet (VLCD) Also known as a protein-sparing modified fast (PSMF), this diet allows the consumption of 400 to 700 kilocalories per day in liquid form. Of this about 30 grams or so are carbohydrate; the rest is protein.

villi (vil-eye) Fingerlike protrusions into the small intestine that participate in digestion and absorption of food.

visual cycle A chemical process in the eye that contributes to vision. Forms of vitamin A are used in the process.

vitamins (vye-ta-mens) Carbon-containing compounds needed in very small amounts in the diet to help promote and regulate chemical reactions and processes in the body.

water-soluble vitamin Vitamins that dissolve in water; these include the B vitamins and vitamin C.

whey (way) Proteins, such as lactalbumin, found in great amounts in human milk. These are easy to digest.

whole grains Grains containing the entire seed of the plant, including the bran, germ, and endosperm (starchy interior).

xerophthalmia (zer-op-thal-mee-uh) Literally, "dry eye." A cause of blindness that results from a vitamin A deficiency. The specific cause is a lack of mucus production by the eye, a condition that leaves the eye more vulnerable to surface dirt and bacterial infections.

yo-yo dieting The practice of losing weight and then regaining it, only to lose it and regain it again. This practice in animals (and probably humans) can make it more difficult to succeed in future attempts to lose weight.

Answers to How Much Have I Learned

CHAPTER 1

1. **True.** Water is the medium in which most of the body's substances are dissolved: a lean human body is about 60% water.
2. **False.** Minerals cannot be further broken down by biochemical reactions in the body.
3. **False.** Kcalories (kilocalories) are 1000-calorie units. Although most people talk about energy units as calories, what they really mean is kcalories.
4. **True.** One gram of protein yields 4 kcalories, 1 gram of carbohydrate 4 kcalories, 1 gram of fat 9 kcalories, and 1 gram of alcohol 7 kcalories.
5. **True.** Although vitamins, like carbohydrates, fats, and proteins, contain carbon atoms, vitamins yield no energy directly to the body.
6. **True.** When nutrient intake does not meet nutrient needs, nutrient stores are used. However, once these stores are depleted, serious health problems can result.
7. **False.** Some minerals, such as calcium, are required in larger amounts than vitamins.
8. **False.** Organic describes substances in which carbon atoms are bonded to hydrogen atoms.
9. **False.** A hypothesis only leads to a theory after the hypothesis is verified numerous times in later experiments.
10. **True.** If you don't eat enough iron, you can become pale and your heart rate can increase. If severely deficient, your body's temperature control mechanism will change and you may feel cold.
11. **True.** If you overeat continually, you are likely to gain weight. This overnutrition may have long-term consequences, such as causing high blood pressure or a form of diabetes mellitus.
12. **False.** People should get their nutrients from foods rather than from supplements.

Vitamins A and D and minerals such as iron and selenium can even be harmful if taken in large amounts for long periods of time.
13. **True.** Alcoholic beverages are the third leading contributor to energy intakes in the United States.
14. **True.** Recent studies have shown that although people are concerned about their nutritional health, they often resist changing their diets.
15. **True.** No food is totally worthless. Diets, however, that don't provide enough needed nutrients can be described as *junk diets*.

CHAPTER 2

1. **False.** No scientific data show that sodium intakes for the typical North American produce hypertension in people who have normal blood pressures.
2. **True.** Manufacturers decide serving sizes. Since these can vary from product to product, it is important to note the exact serving size when comparing nutrition labels.
3. **False.** The term *sodium free* means that the product contains less than 5 milligrams of sodium per serving.
4. **False.** Moderation in sugar intake poses no health risk if good dental hygiene is practiced.
5. **False.** Vegetables, fruits, and grains should form the bulk of a diet. Meat is important, but not that much is needed for health.
6. **False.** RDA is the abbreviation for recommended *dietary* allowances.
7. **False.** No nutrient is required daily. You can maintain health for about 4 days on a diet without water and about 10 days on a diet without the vitamin thiamin.
8. **True.** While nutrient recommendations are often similar, groups of scientists from different countries may disagree with each other; for instance, compare standards for the

United States to those of Canada.
9. **False.** The RDA is a recommendation for group needs. It is not designed to provide personal nutrient requirements.
10. **False.** Active people usually need closer to 2200 to 2800 kcalories or more to meet energy needs.
11. **False.** Just meeting losses is not sufficient because children need to gain new protein tissue. Children should regularly eat more protein than they lose (positive protein balance).
12. **True.** With the exchange system we don't have to memorize what nutrients are found in all foods: it is a powerful tool for quickly and conveniently estimating the energy, protein, carbohydrate, and fat content of a food or meal.
13. **True.** Nutrient density is an important tool, especially for people on a low-kcalorie diet. It represents how many nutrients a food has compared to its kcalorie content.
14. **False.** By practicing good nutrition—following the rules of variety, balance, and moderation—a reasonably healthy person can obtain all necessary vitamins from foods.
15. **True.** All foods are low in one or more of the nutrients that we need. Milk is low in iron; eggs are low in calcium.

CHAPTER 3

1. **False.** It is commonly believed that people who cannot change their behaviors are weak willed. This destructive misconception perpetuates unsuccessful attempts to change. Instead, changing one's environment is a key to behavior change.
2. **True.** For some people, food preferences vary with emotional state. For example, eating chocolate may reduce stress for some people, while pizza may be considered solely a party food.
3. **False.** Commitment to a goal is the best predictor of

success. Realistic goal setting includes scrutiny of commitment.

4. **False.** Occasional backsliding is expected when undertaking behavioral change. This is not a reason to abandon a goal.

5. **True.** Food is more than nourishment for most people. By identifying the roles food plays in a person's life and finding appropriate substitutes for food, food habits are more easily changed.

6. **False.** Body types are partially genetically determined. Striving for an unrealistic, unattainable body type deprives a person of the success deserved for maximizing personal potential.

7. **True.** Monitoring progress from a beginning baseline yields tangible reinforcement and encouragement to a dieter.

8. **False.** Positive reinforcement helps instill self-confidence, maintain enthusiasm, and foster the self-worth that facilitates behavior change.

9. **False.** Some dieters find evenings the hardest. They restrict themselves during the day so that, by late evening, hunger and feelings of deprivation encourage overeating.

10. **False.** Diet changes need not be so restrictive. Long-term change results from practical, feasible routines that can be continued throughout life—not from starvation.

11. **True.** Even the most finicky eaters, with the guidance of nutrition experts, can have healthier diets consisting of foods they enjoy.

12. **False.** It is wiser to avoid tempting situations when initiating behavior change. Once a person is comfortable with new behaviors, it will be easier to confront and cope with problem situations.

13. **False.** Separating final behavior goals into smaller steps that are more easily and quickly achieved can give a person the confidence and motivation needed to reach the ultimate goal. It is also a key to understand that behav-iors require daily decisions, not magic pills or a once-in-a-lifetime change.

14. **True.** Even friends and relatives do not always understand a person's choices or motivations. A strong commitment to change and honesty with friends can enable one to continue a plan, even if support from others is lacking.

15. **False.** Rewarding oneself in constructive ways along each step of the plan can motivate a person to continue following the plan. Every step made toward the final goal is worth recognition.

CHAPTER 4

1. **True.** Studies show no significant differences in health risk from pesticide levels in organic and conventionally grown foods.

2. **False.** Enriched white rice has had a few nutrients replaced, but not the lost fiber.

3. **False.** Raw milk sometimes contains microorganisms that cause disease. Pasteurization usually kills these germs.

4. **False.** Exercise mostly increases the need for calories, carbohydrates, and water. Vitamin and mineral needs change very little.

5. **False.** Foods often contain natural toxins. For example, raw turnips contain substances that cause an enlargement of the thyroid gland (goiter).

6. **False.** Most physicians feel that nutrient supplements are not needed in treating most diseases.

7. **True.** Studies by the American Council on Science and Health have shown that both storekeepers and clerks frequently prescribe vitamins.

8. **False.** Federal laws require that health products be truthfully labeled. Additional verbal claims by anyone should be carefully scrutinized.

9. **True.** An extensive study by the Mayo Clinic showed that high doses of vitamin C have no value in treating colon cancer.

10. **True.** Most victims of quackery share their misinformation with others.

11. **False.** It is easy to be fooled by scientific jargon that may sound plausible but is not correct.

12. **False.** No scientific evidence supports the use of macrobiotic diets to treat anemia.

13. **False.** Whether self-prescribed or directed by others, herbal therapy can be toxic and should be first discussed with a physician.

14. **False.** Pharmacists rarely discourage people from buying what they sell.

15. **True.** Distributors are first encouraged to use the products themselves and then to persuade friends, relatives, and neighbors to become distributors.

CHAPTER 5

1. **True.** However, for many foods some digestion actually begins during cooking when protein structures soften, starch granules swell, and tough vegetable fibers are softened.

2. **True.** A special portal vein connects the intestinal tract to the liver. Many nutrients can enter the bloodstream only after passing through the liver.

3. **True.** A living person's small intestine is approximately 10 feet long; at autopsy it is approximately 23 feet because the muscles that hold it in a tensed condition relax.

4. **True.** Acid produced by the stomach would easily erode the stomach wall if mucus was not present to protect the stomach.

5. **True.** The term colon also refers to the large intestine.

6. **False.** The digestive enzymes work efficiently no matter what combination of foods is eaten.

7. **True.** Stomach enzymes require acid conditions for maximum activity, whereas the small intestine is slightly alkaline.

8. **True.** Hormones and nerves contribute to the coordination of digestive processes.

9. **True.** For about 70% of people worldwide, the ability to digest the milk carbohydrate, lactose, declines in adulthood.

10. **False.** Unless diarrhea

results, typical daily stress does not affect digestion nor absorption of food.

11. *False.* A better recommendation to try first is not to lie down after the meal and eat less next time.

12. *True.* The sugar glucose is absorbed from the small intestine into the bloodstream against a high concentration. Glucose from the bloodstream bathes cells of the intestine, so energy must be expended if more glucose in the intestinal tract is to enter the intestinal cells. Conversely, fat concentration in the intestinal cells is low, allowing fat to be passively absorbed into them.

13. *True.* The peristaltic waves that propel food down the intestinal tract require a coordination of both muscles that run lengthwise down the intestinal tract and circular muscles that surround the intestinal tract.

14. *True.* Many undigested foods that enter the large intestine are nutrient sources for bacteria there. The bacteria then make a variety of products, including gas.

15. *False.* About 95% of nutrient absorption takes place in the small intestine.

CHAPTER 6

1. *True.* Glucose combined with fructose forms sucrose, or table sugar.

2. *True.* Few carbohydrates are present in animals foods.

3. *True.* Simple sugars can be metabolized to acids by bacteria on the teeth. This acid can form dental caries (cavities).

4. *True.* Carbohydrates are important energy-supplying nutrients.

5. *False.* Crude fiber may not reflect the true amount of dietary fiber because it represents only what remains after a harsh chemical treatment—a much harsher treatment than intestinal enzymes can possibly subject fibers to. Because of this, values for crude fiber and dietary fiber for a food are not necessarily equivalent.

6. *False.* Although there is no RDA for carbohydrates, 50 to 100 grams per day is consid-

ered minimum intake.

7. *False.* The body uses dietary fiber to increase stool mass, which eases elimination.

8. *True.* One cup (8 ounces) of milk yields 12 grams of carbohydrate, which is one fourth of our minimum carbohydrate need.

9. *True.* When eaten in excess of energy needs, carbohydrates are stored as glycogen and fat.

10. *False.* Honey, like table sugar, is a simple carbohydrate.

11. *True.* About 125 pounds of simple sugars are produced each year for each American. Many nutritionists believe that this is too much. A diet including less than 50 pounds per year allows for other more healthful foods in the diet.

12. *True.* Honey may contain spores of the bacterium, *Clostridium botulinum*, which can grow in an infant's stomach and even lead to death because infant stomachs have yet to develop the strong acidic environment that adult stomachs have. Acid reduces the bacterium's growth.

13. *False.* Diabetes mellitus is a disorder of high blood glucose levels.

14. *True.* Starvation conditions promote the breakdown of proteins into amino acids in order to supply the carbon atoms needed to make needed glucose.

15. *True.* This was observed by Dr. Denis Burkitt, who attributes this phenomenon to the high dietary fiber intakes of Africans as compared with North Americans.

CHAPTER 7

1. *False.* Saturated fats are solid at room temperature.

2. *True.* Carbohydrate yields 4 kcalories per gram and fat yields 9 kcalories per gram.

3. *True.* But don't be misled by advertisers who state certain products are "cholesterol-free." The product may still contain saturated fat, which is a greater determinant of your blood cholesterol level.

4. *True.* Animal fats are rich in

saturated fat.

5. *True.* Triglyceride is the primary form of lipid in both foods and the body.

6. *False.* Fat is absolutely necessary for life because it supplies essential fatty acids used to make vital body compounds.

7. *True.* In some cases this process makes food production easier; hydrogenation prevents the oils in peanut butter from separating during storage.

8. *True.* Most fruits contain only a trace amount of fat.

9. *True.* Vitamin E helps protect against the breakdown of the double bonds in fatty acids.

10. *True.* Because vitamins A, E, D, and K are fat soluble, their absorption is enhanced by dietary fat.

11. *False.* Everyone age 20 years or more should monitor and track his or her blood cholesterol levels. (Some experts recommend that anyone over 2 years old who has a family history of premature heart disease should do the same.) Elevated blood cholesterol is a risk factor for heart disease. Early action to reduce an elevated LDL-cholesterol level is the best plan.

12. *True.* Butter, however, contains more saturated fats than tub margarine.

13. *False.* Studies of humans have shown that high doses of fish oil can raise LDL-cholesterol levels in some people and disrupt blood glucose regulation in people with diabetes mellitus.

14. *False.* Nondairy creamers often contain coconut oil, which is very high in saturated fat.

15. *False.* The best way to use diet to lower an elevated blood cholesterol level is to eat less saturated fat. Eating more soluble fiber is also quite helpful.

CHAPTER 8

1. *False.* Most of us eat such a varied assortment of food that if we consume enough kcalories it would be difficult not to have a complete protein diet that contains enough of all

nine essential amino acids.

2. **True.** Protein is particularly important for building new tissue during periods of rapid growth.

3. **True.** Only a few enzymes are composed of other compounds.

4. **False.** Even a minor change that alters the original structure can affect the protein's ultimate structure. This, in turn, could critically affect its ability to function.

5. **True.** Biological value represents the body's ability to retain the protein absorbed.

6. **True.** Milk proteins provide one of the highest possible biological values from foods. An egg white has the very best biological value, slightly better than milk.

7. **False.** People require more protein per weight when they are growing.

8. **False.** All of us, including athletes, can meet our protein needs with basic foods. Rarely is an intake greater than twice the RDA necessary.

9. **True.** For this reason trimming meats of fat and broiling them are good ideas.

10. **True.** Although lack of energy can be caused by other things, it is a symptom of severe protein-energy malnutrition.

11. **False.** Gelatin is an incomplete protein; it lacks the amino acid tryptophan. Therefore it is a poor source for supporting any protein synthesis in the body.

12. **True.** Starvation in infancy leads to marasmus, which means to waste away.

13. **False.** Plant proteins contain much dietary fiber and magnesium; in comparison, animal proteins supply the most absorbable form of iron and almost all of our vitamin B-12 intake.

14. **True.** It is over 80% protein.

15. **True.** These contain mostly carbohydrate and water.

CHAPTER 9

1. **False.** No vitamin missing from a diet for a week leads to deficiency symptoms in an initially healthy person. Earliest signs of deficiency appear with a thiamin-free diet after about 10 days. The first symptoms of a vitamin C deficiency are seen after about 20 to 40 days.

2. **True.** Mineral oil is not absorbed by the intestine. During its passage, mineral oil can dissolve fat-soluble vitamins and pull them into the colon for eventual elimination.

3. **True.** When in the active form, vitamin D, through a variety of mechanisms, can improve calcium absorption from the small intestine.

4. **True.** Vitamin A enhances night vision by participating in the formation of a compound used in the visual cycle.

5. **True.** Sunlight striking the skin converts a modified form of cholesterol into vitamin D. This is then slowly transferred from the skin into the bloodstream.

6. **True.** Vitamin K gives calcium-binding properties to proteins needed to clot blood.

7. **False.** Although vitamin B-6 does affect levels of some neurotransmitters such as serotonin, it has not been shown to have any consistent effect on premenstrual syndrome. In addition, women who take high doses of vitamin B-6 to treat PMS risk toxic effects.

8. **False.** Thiamin needs are more closely tied to carbohydrate intake because the metabolism of carbohydrate to energy requires thiamin. The more carbohydrate consumed, the more thiamin is required.

9. **True.** Milk is the best source of riboflavin in the American diet.

10. **True.** The amino acid tryptophan is converted into niacin in the body. Niacin needs then are met by consuming both niacin-containing foods and protein in the diet.

11. **True.** A niacin deficiency causes severe dermatitis and skin redness, especially where the sun strikes, as well as diarrhea and dementia.

12. **True.** Good sources of folate include green leafy vegetables and sprouts, organ meats, and orange juice.

13. **True.** Vitamin B-12 is not found in plants unless its presence is related to contamination from soil organisms, stray bacteria, or yeast.

14. **True.** Vitamin C keeps iron in a form that is absorbable.

15. **False.** High doses of vitamin C may moderately reduce the symptoms and duration of a cold; no medication can prevent colds.

CHAPTER 10

1. **False.** The terms major and trace are not designations of nutritional importance. They are classifications referring only to the amount needed for daily functioning.

2. **True.** For example, the vitamin thiamin requires magnesium to function efficiently.

3. **False.** Animal foods are often the best mineral sources, since animals concentrate the minerals they consume from plants. The exception is magnesium, which is plentiful in green plants.

4. **True.** Water evaporation from the skin requires heat energy. So when perspiration evaporates, heat energy is taken from the skin, leaving you feeling cooler.

5. **True.** About one half of the sodium consumed by Americans is supplied by processed foods. Sodium is prevalent in foods such as frozen dinners, canned soups, and convenience entrees.

6. **False.** The effectiveness of dietary calcium in entirely preventing osteoporosis has been disproven, but adequate dietary amounts can slow some bone loss in old age.

7. **False.** It is estimated that only 10% to 15% of the population has hypertension caused by excess sodium intake. These people can benefit from restricting sodium. No data establish the need for consuming a low-sodium diet if blood pressure is normal.

8. **True.** The small amounts needed by the body make trace mineral deficiencies difficult to detect in humans. Laboratory techniques are not even available to adequately measure some trace elements in tissues, and there are gaps

in our knowledge about metabolism and storage of many minerals. This hampers interpretation of laboratory results.

9. **True.** Trace minerals that have the same charge and are chemically similar often compete with each other during absorption and metabolism. This must be considered when setting the RDA for a trace mineral and when using mineral supplements.

10. **True.** Women in their child-bearing years have a greater need for iron because of their greater iron loss during menstruation.

11. **False.** The body has no efficient mechanism for eliminating excess iron. Excess iron intake can be very damaging. In response, the body carefully regulates iron absorption in an attempt to prevent excess absorption.

12. **True.** A main function of zinc is promoting growth and development. A zinc deficiency can cause poor growth in children, whereas a zinc supplement can help increase appetite and the rate of weight gain in children recovering from semistarvation.

13. **True.** In an iodide deficiency the thyroid gland expands to try to trap more iodine from the bloodstream. An enlarged gland leads to a goiter.

14. **True.** Iron metabolism depends on copper. Copper aids in the formation of the iron protein, hemoglobin.

15. **True.** Fluoride prevents dental caries in two ways. It inhibits the growth of bacteria on teeth, and it helps produce teeth that are resistant to acid.

CHAPTER 11

1. **True.** Regulation of body weight has been compared with the regulation of blood pressure. Both appear to be set to some extent, with blood pressure even more so.

2. **False.** The RDA represents an average energy need for a person performing light activity. The range given may or may not accurately estimate a person's energy needs.

3. **True.** To keep a resting body alive, there is need to maintain heart rate, respiration, body temperature, and other functions. The energy used represents basal metabolism.

4. **True.** Your body weight may be greater than a desirable figure, as predicted from the Metropolitan Life Insurance Table, but excess weight yields a health risk only if it is caused by excess body fat. Extra muscle mass poses no risk.

5. **False.** Women tend to store fat in the hip and thigh areas, whereas men tend to store fat in the abdominal area.

6. **True.** Health problems usually begin when a person exceeds desirable weight by more than 20%; the greater the difference, the greater the health risk.

7. **True.** Muscle tissue uses energy at a high rate and thus has a great influence on the basal metabolism.

8. **False.** There is little evidence that adult obesity in men is related to childhood obesity; however, there is a strong relationship between childhood and adult obesity in women.

9. **False.** Probably less than 10% of cases of obesity in America are caused by problems in thyroid or other hormone levels in the bloodstream.

10. **True.** A diet with fewer than 1200 kcalories is likely to cause hunger and fatigue. Furthermore, there is a high probability that this type of diet is a fad diet.

11. **False.** Many people regain the weight they lost within 1 year.

12. **True.** It is impractical to lose fat tissue rapidly because of the high-kcalorie deficit required.

13. **True.** Behavior modification is likely to reduce the tendency to relapse into bad habits and regain lost weight.

14. **True.** High-carbohydrate foods contain by and large fewer kcalories than high-fat foods.

15. **False.** FDA is concerned only when products are suspected of causing serious harm. There is no regulation of claims made by fad diets.

CHAPTER 12

1. **False.** A cell must first convert the energy stored in carbohydrate to ATP energy.

2. **False.** Carbohydrates and fats both provide energy for the body.

3. **False.** Only initial stages do not require oxygen to work. Ultimate burning to carbon dioxide and water does require oxygen input.

4. **True.** Complete burning of all body fuels yields carbon dioxide as one of the by-products.

5. **False.** No evidence supports this assertion.

6. **False.** Rapid weight loss, such as seen in wrestlers, can weaken the body. Long-term weight loss can reduce muscle mass and make it hard to keep glycogen stores adequate.

7. **False.** Given high kcalorie intakes of athletes, protein needs are easily met from typical food choices. No supplements are needed.

8. **True.** This is the key recommendation for carbohydrate-loading strategies.

9. **True.** The carbohydrate present can reduce glycogen use and the electrolytes can help maintain blood volume.

10. **True.** Caffeine can enhance fat use by muscles, which may improve athletic performance in some endurance events.

11. **False.** The target heart rate range to promote aerobic conditioning is 60% to 85% of maximal heart rate.

12. **False.** Warm-up exercises are important for everyone who exercises.

13. **False.** Thirst is not a good indication for fluid replacement needs. A much better guide is weight loss: 2 cups ($\frac{1}{2}$ liter) of water should eventually be consumed for every pound ($\frac{1}{2}$ kilogram) lost while exercising.

14. **False.** Loading up on carbohydrate will not be beneficial for short sprint type of exercise; it benefits exercise lasting longer than 1.5 to 2 hours.

15. **True.** Anabolic steroids are

illegal substances. They are also unsafe.

CHAPTER 13

1. **True.** Some cultures use certain foods as ceremonial foods. In the United States waffles are a breakfast food, while in England they are dessert.
2. **True.** About 5% of young women suffer from an eating disorder.
3. **False.** They have an intense fear of gaining weight.
4. **True.** This is referred to as purging.
5. **True.** People with anorexia nervosa tend to be extremely competitive.
6. **True.** People with anorexia nervosa see themselves as fat, even when they are thin.
7. **True.** But they don't like to admit it.
8. **False.** Bulimics are extremely secretive.
9. **True.** This attitude is reflected in advertisements.
10. **True.** Most people with eating disorders see themselves as inadequate.
11. **True.** People with eating disorders are often obsessively neat and highly aware of imperfections.
12. **True.** The damaging effects of late stages of these conditions increase the risk of permanent injury.
13. **True.** Bingeing and purging characterize bulimia.
14. **False.** Treatment should emphasize choice as opposed to restriction.
15. **True.** This should be suspected in children who exhibit poor growth rates.

CHAPTER 14

1. **True.** Infants weighing less than 5.5 pounds (2.5 kilograms) at birth are considered to have low birth weight. The risk of sickness and death in the early months of life is much greater for these infants.
2. **False.** During the first trimester (13 weeks), when organs and body parts are forming, the potential for birth defects is greatest.
3. **True.** The quality of the mother's diet and the amount of weight she gains during pregnancy are more important than genetic background in determining birth weight.
4. **True.** During pregnancy, an average increase of 300 kcalories per day is needed. Kcalorie demands are greatest during the second and third trimesters.
5. **True.** This range of weight gain normally allows optimal fetal development and birth weight.
6. **True.** Gaining excessive weight from eating too many kcalories is a problem for many pregnant women.
7. **False.** Eating a healthful diet requires learning wise food choices.
8. **True.** Many mineral needs, but particularly those for iron, calcium and zinc, are increased. Iron requirements usually necessitate taking supplements in addition to changing the diet.
9. **True.** Symptoms of high blood pressure may occur during pregnancy and then disappear after birth. This happens more frequently in women who have a poor nutrient intake, especially calcium.
10. **True.** Immune factors passed from mother to infant via breast milk reduce the number of respiratory and intestinal infections.
11. **True.** Almost all women are capable of breast-feeding; breast size and even having to feed twins pose no major barriers.
12. **True.** Many substances ingested by the mother, including medicines, are secreted into the milk.
13. **True.** The placenta is a specialized organ of pregnancy that both secretes hormones and allows for the transfer of oxygen, nutrients, and wastes between mother and fetus.
14. **True.** Good nutrition and health habits should begin early, ideally before pregnancy begins.
15. **False.** Cow's milk is too difficult for an infant to digest and fully metabolize until approximately 6 to 12 months of age.

CHAPTER 15

1. **True.** Although all nutrients and an adequate kcalorie intake are needed for growth, protein is particularly important for reaching one's genetic potential.
2. **True.** Infancy is a period of very rapid growth.
3. **False.** Brain growth rate is maximal at birth and continues through 2 to 4 years of age.
4. **False.** No evidence strongly links infant obesity to obesity in childhood or adulthood.
5. **False.** Infant energy needs are higher per pound.
6. **False.** Infants need relatively high-fat diets to support brain growth and supply enough energy for other growth with a small volume of food.
7. **False.** Infants are not usually developmentally or nutritionally ready for solid food until 4 to 6 months of age.
8. **True.** It is not necessary to add salt, sugar, or spices to infant foods.
9. **True.** However, little besides patience and understanding helps deal with colic. In extreme cases, a formula containing predigested protein may be helpful.
10. **True.** Cow's milk should not be fed to a child until about 6 months of age at the earliest, and preferably not until 12 months of age.
11. **True.** Cow's milk is low in iron, and the protein is more difficult to digest than that in human milk. This may cause intestinal irritation that contributes to iron losses.
12. **False.** What is eaten is most important—not when.
13. **True.** Anemia and obesity are the nutritional problems clinicians need to focus on.
14. **False.** Parents should control what food is available, but let children decide the amount to eat. With good foods available, children can reliably decide on serving size.
15. **True.** Allergic reactions can be limited by avoiding offending food.

CHAPTER 16

1. **False.** The average length of time Americans live has increased during the last century, but not the age of the oldest people.

2. **True.** Exercise can slow muscle loss, and weight lifting can even rebuild lost muscle mass.

3. **True.** Drug-nutrient interactions can be a problem at any age, but because the elderly generally take more and different combinations of drugs over a long period, nutritional status is more likely to be affected.

4. **True.** In addition, because the elderly population is rapidly growing, society will need to continue dealing with this concern.

5. **False.** Good nutrition can delay some symptoms of aging, but no diet can magically prevent aging; aging probably begins at conception.

6. **False.** The senses of smell and taste tend to decrease with age. Adding seasonings can enhance food appeal.

7. **True.** The sense of thirst may diminish with age, but not the need for fluids.

8. **True.** Stomach secretions that promote absorption of vitamin B-12 decrease with age.

9. **True.** Increasing fiber and fluid intakes can help reduce constipation.

10. **True.** Excessive intake of vitamin A supplements results in many toxicity problems. These are only a few examples (see Chapter 9).

11. **True.** Be aware of these nutrients if you are involved in the health care of elderly people or have the chance to advise elderly relatives.

12. **True.** Exercise is an important part of body maintenance.

13. **False.** This age-group varies more in physical ability than any other.

14. **True.** This dose of alcohol is high enough to cause cirrhosis in most people; even lower doses cause cirrhosis in some people, especially in women.

15. **False.** Taking zinc in RDA levels is a key practice to maintain health of the immune system, but doses about 20 times greater than RDA actually diminish immune system function.

CHAPTER 17

1. **True.** We do not realize food poisoning is so common because the symptoms mimic other disorders, such as stomach or intestinal flu.

2. **False.** Foods having the potential to cause food poisoning often show no signs of it in taste, smell, or appearance.

3. **False.** Imported foods, such as soft cheeses from Mexico, have been implicated in food-poisoning incidents. While foods are inspected when they enter the U.S. from foreign countries, there is not adequate funding to inspect all foods carefully.

4. **False.** Chemical structure—not origin—is the key to evaluating chemicals: whether a chemical is made in a laboratory or found in nature has nothing to do with its potential effects on humans. Some naturally occurring toxins in foods, such as solanine in green potatoes, are much more toxic than synthetic food additives.

5. **True.** When the pulp of an apple is exposed to oxygen, a "browning" reaction occurs. Antioxidants, such as vitamin C, can prevent this browning.

6. **True.** The growth of bacteria and fungi in foods requires sufficient free water, that is, water not bound by other food compounds. If the water content of a food is reduced considerably, the lack of free water curtails growth of bacteria and fungi.

7. **False.** Only a few of the many bacteria, fungi, viruses, and other earthly microbes are known to cause food poisoning.

8. **True.** And for this reason, foods generally should be kept cold (below 40°F or 4°C) or hot (above 140°F or 60°C).

9. **True.** The symptoms of food poisoning are abdominal bloating, gas, diarrhea, vomiting, and headache, all of which are also symptoms of stomach or intestinal flu.

10. **False.** One food-poisoning incident provides no immunity against future attacks.

11. **True.** *Salmonella* bacteria are commonly associated with chickens, especially raw chicken carcasses. Raw chicken should be handled very carefully so that juices do not contaminate other foods, thereby spreading *Salmonella* bacteria to other foods.

12. **True.** The bacterium that produces the very deadly botulism food poisoning is present in all soil.

13. **True.** *Clostridium botulinum* grows only in the absence of air. Thus it may be found in improperly canned foods and in thick foods where air is excluded from the center. Chili is an example.

14. **True.** Many viruses and parasites that may live in raw fish are destroyed by cooking. Consuming raw fish poses a significant health risk for hepatitis, parasite infections, and other health problems.

15. **False.** Aside from the alcohol present in high amounts (which over time can lead to cirrhosis of the liver), alcoholic beverages contain urethanes, which the FDA is now studying carefully to determine their risk to health. Some wines contain sulfites, which may pose a health risk for sensitive individuals.

CHAPTER 18

1. **True.** Hunger is a physiological state and can be described as an uneasiness, discomfort, weakness, or pain caused by lack of food.

2. **True.** And this poverty can be caused by unemployment, homelessness, illiteracy, poor health, and other factors.

3. **False.** Diabetes mellitus is more common when food supplies are abundant.

4. **True.** Undernutrition is also the primary cause of many nutrient deficiency diseases, such as scurvy, pellagra, anemia, and many others.

5. **True.** No other social indicator shows a wider gap between the developing and industrialized world.

6. **True.** The growing fetus needs a diet rich in vitamins, protein, and minerals.

7. **True.** Failure of children to grow is a common result of undernutrition.

8. **False.** Marginal iron deficiencies affect hundreds of millions of people worldwide.

9. **False.** Full recovery may never happen, and if it does, it is likely to take months to years.

10. **False.** The United States is in twenty-second place.

11. **True.** This is partly because the cost of housing has substantially increased, and partly because federal support for subsidized housing was cut during the 1980s.

12. **False.** Some economists estimate that world food production will continue to increase more than world population in the near future, allowing the food/population ratio to increase through the year 2000.

13. **True.** There are many reasons for this. Among them is an economic imperative to have large families. Experts believe couples will choose to have fewer children once the couple experiences an increased livelihood.

14. **True.** Most of these urban poor live in overcrowded, self-made shelter with inadequate public utilities.

15. **True.** WHO estimates that more than 1 billion people are without a safe and adequate water supply.

Credits

Front matter p. xi, Dick Luria, FPG International; p. xii, David York, The Stock Shop; p. xiii, S. Feld, H. Armstrong Roberts; p. xiv, Superstock FourByFive; p. xv, Grant Faint, The Image Bank; p. xvi, B. March, FPG International.

Chapter 1 p. 5, Bod Daemmrich, Stock Boston; p. 9, H. Abernathy, H. Armstrong Roberts; p. 13, James Schnepf, Woodfin Camp and Associates; p. 15, Wolff Communications; p. 17, Linsley Photographics; p. 19, Reprinted by permission of Universal Press Syndicate; p. 23, Mike Clemmer, Picture Group; p. 24, Daniel MacDonald, The Stock Shop; p. 25, Wolff Communications; p. 26, Tom Ebenhoh, Photographic Resources.

Chapter 2 p. 37, Superstock FourByFive; p. 39, Wolff Communications; p. 49, Courtesy of the National Cancer Institute; p. 53, International Diabetes Center, Minneapolis, MN; p. 61, Reprinted by permission of NEA, Inc.; p. 62, Wolff Communications; p. 63, Chick Harrity, U.S. News and World Report.

Chapter 3 p. 65, Wolff Communications; p. 67, Andree Abecassis, The Stock Market; p. 72, John H. Anderson, Photographic Resources; p. 80 (top), Wolff Communications; p. 80 (bottom), Reprinted with special permission of King Features Syndicate, Inc.; p. 81, Kevin Fleming, Annapolis, MD; p. 86, Ellis Herwig, The Picture Cube; p. 92 (left), Tom McCarthy, The Stock Market; p. 92 (right), Mauritius, The Stock Shop.

Chapter 4 p. 95, Marilynne Herbert; p. 99, Superstock FourByFive; p. 102, Wolff Communications; p. 107, From Hechtlinger, Adelaide: The Great Patent Medicine Era, Grosset & Dunlap, Inc., 1970; p. 111, Wolff Communications; p. 118, Reprinted with special permission of North America Syndicate, Inc.

Chapter 5 p. 123, Cecil Fox, Photo Researchers; p. 126, Science Photo Library, Photo Researchers; p. 128 (top left), H. Armstrong Roberts; p. 128 (middle right), Ed Reschke; p. 135, Superstock FourByFive; p. 136, Reprinted by permission of NEA, Inc.; p. 146, Wolff Communications; p. 148, International Diabetes Center, Minneapolis, MN.

Chapter 6 p. 151, Roy Morsch, The Stock Market; p. 154, Wolff Communications; p. 157, Roy Morsch, The Stock Market; p. 161, Carolyn Delevitt, The Stock Shop; p. 163, Linsley Photographics; p. 167, Reprinted by permission of Universal Press Syndicate; p. 169, Reprinted with special permission of North America Syndicate; p. 171, Raul R. Aguirre, The Stock Shop.

Chapter 7 p. 183, Howard Sochurek, Medichrome; p. 188, Bob Daemmrich, Stock Boston; p. 191, Wolff Communications; p. 194, Wolff Communications; p. 198, C.P. George, H. Armstrong Roberts; p. 201, National Cancer Institute, Bethesda, MD; p. 205, Reprinted by permission of Chronicle Features; p. 206, NutraSweet, Monsanto Corp.; p. 215, Reprinted by permission of NEA, Inc.; p. 216, Benda/Zefa, H. Armstrong Roberts.

Chapter 8 p. 219, Lennart Nilsson (c) Boehringer Ingleheim International GmbH; p. 224, Superstock FourByFive; p. 226, Wolff Communications; p. 232, Superstock FourByFive; p. 234, Superstock FourByFive; p. 237, FPG International; p. 242, Reprinted by permission of Universal Press Syndicate; p. 245, Reprinted by permission of NEA, Inc.

Chapter 9 p. 247, J. Trefethen, FPG International; p. 250, Reprinted by permission of United Features Syndicate; p. 257, Garry Gay, The Image Bank; p. 258, Wally McNarmee, Woodfin Camp and Associates; p. 260, George Obrenski, The Image Bank; p. 263, Al Assid, The Stock Market; p. 269, Joe Devenney, The Image Bank; p. 278, Anne Heimann, The Stock Market.

Chapter 10 p. 291, Peter Steiner, The Stock Market; p. 297, Marc Romanelli, The Image Bank; p. 299, Plessner International, The Stock Shop; p. 303, Michael A. Keller, The Stock Market; p. 303, Reprinted with special permission of King Features Syndicate, Inc.; p. 305, from Healthline, Menlo Park, CA; p. 311, Janeart Ltd., The Image Bank; p. 321, from McLaren, Donald S.: A Colour Atlas of Nutritional Disorders, ed. 1, Wolfe Medical Publications, Ltd., 1981; p. 222, John Kelly, The Image Bank.

Chapter 11 p. 337, SUMO, The Image Bank; p. 341 (top), Reprinted with special permission of King Features Syndicate, Inc.; p. 341 (middle), Reprinted with special permission of King Features Syndicate, Inc.; p. 341 (bottom), Reprinted by permission of NEA, Inc.; p. 345, Medical Graphics Corporation, St. Paul, MN; p. 340, Linsley Photographics, from Payne, W. and Hahn, D., Understanding Your Health, ed. 2, Times Mirror/Mosby College Publishing; p. 353, Robert Jones, Jr.; p. 355, Karen Kasmauski, San Diego County; p. 373, Reprinted by permission of Universal Press Syndicate.

Chapter 12 p. 375, David Stoecklein, The Stock Market; p. 378, Reprinted by permission of NEA, Inc.; p. 379, Lou Jones, The Image Bank; p. 383, Reprinted by permission: Tribune Media Services; p. 384, John Kelly, The Image Bank; p. 391, FPG International.

Chapter 13 p. 401, Cathy Lander-Goldberg, Lander Photographics; p. 406, Paul Buddle, H. Armstrong Roberts; p. 407, Wolff Communications; p. 411, Cathy Lander-Goldberg, Lander Photographics; p. 412, Reprinted by permission of Universal Press Syndicate; p. 413, Wolff Communications; p. 422, A) Culver Pictures, Inc., B) Kobal Collection, Superstock International Inc., C) Caron/Gamma Liason, D) 1991, Sports Illustrated; p. 423 (top), Wolff Communications; p. 423 (bottom), Reprinted by permission of Universal Press Syndicate.

Chapter 14 p. 427, Lennart Nilsson, Dell Publishing Co.; p. 430, Wolff Communications; p. 431, Reprinted by permission of Universal Press Syndicate; p. 432, Wolff Communications; p. 434, The Stock Market; p. 435, Reprinted by permission of Universal Press Syndicate; p. 446, William Hubbell, Woodfin Camp and Associates; p. 454, from Streissguth, A., and others: Science 109:353, 1980 Copyright, American Association for the Advancement of Science.

Chapter 15 p. 461, Pedro Coll, The Stock Market; p. 467, Edward Lettau, FPG International; p. 471, Banus March, FPG International; p. 474 (bottom), Gerd Ludwig, Woodfin Camp and Associates; p. 479, H. Armstrong Roberts; p. 480, David Hundley, The Stock Market; p. 481, Grant Faint, The Image Bank; p. 484, Mike Clemmer, Picture Group; p. 488, Paul Solomon, Woodfin Camp and Associates.

Chapter 16 p. 497, Larry Dale Gordon, The Image Bank; p. 500, Reprinted by permission of Universal Press Syndicate; p. 503, Reprinted by permission of NEA, Inc.; p. 511, John Lawlor, The Stock Market; p. 517, Lynn Johnson, Black Star; p. 519, Ron Chapple, FPG International; p. 520, Miro Vintoniv, The Picture Cube.

Chapter 17 p. 533, FPG International, p. 539, George Contorakes, The Stock Market; p. 542, Roy Morsch, The Stock Market; p. 543, Stacey Pick, Stock Boston; p. 544, Reprinted by permission of Universal Press Syndicate; p. 546, Leslie Taha, San Mateo, CA; p. 549 (top), Karen Kasmauski, Woodfin Camp and Associates; p. 549 (bottom), Reprinted by permission of Universal Press Syndicate; p. 551, Zanetti, The Stock Market; p. 561, Superstock FourByFive.

Chapter 18 p. 571, Joe Sohm/Chromosohm, The Stock Market; p. 581, Frans Lanting, Minden Pictures; p. 585, Suzanne L. Murphy, FPG International; p. 589, Reprinted by permission of Universal Press Syndicate; p. 595, Jay Freis, The Image Bank.

Index

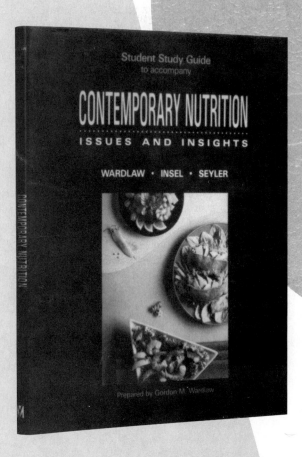

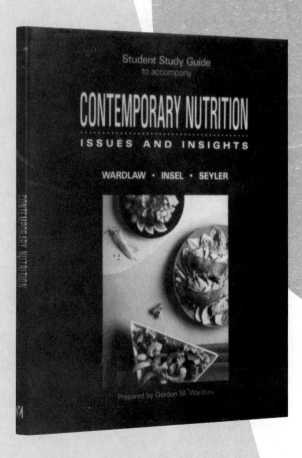